AF323792

Minimally Invasive Bariatric Surgery

Minimally Invasive Bariatric Surgery

Edited by

Philip R. Schauer, MD
Professor of Surgery, Lerner College of Medicine, Director, Advanced Laparoscopic and Bariatric Surgery, Bariatric and Metabolic Institute, The Cleveland Clinic, Cleveland, Ohio, USA

Bruce D. Schirmer, MD
Stephen H. Watts Professor of Surgery, Department of Surgery, Health Sciences Center, University of Virginia Health System, Charlottesville, Virginia, USA

Stacy A. Brethauer, MD
Staff Surgeon, Advanced Laparoscopic and Bariatric Surgery, Department of Surgery, The Cleveland Clinic Foundation, Cleveland, Ohio, USA

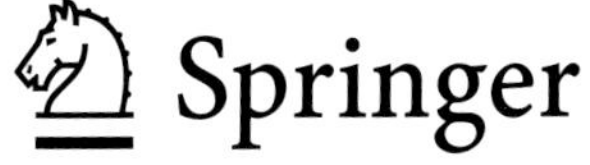 Springer

Philip R. Schauer, MD
Professor of Surgery
Lerner College of Medicine
Director
Advanced Laparoscopic and
   Bariatric Surgery
Bariatric and Metabolic Institute
The Cleveland Clinic Foundation
Cleveland, OH 44195
USA

Bruce D. Schirmer, MD
Stephen H. Watts Professor of Surgery
Department of Surgery
Health Sciences Center
University of Virginia Health System
Charlottesville, VA 22908
USA

Stacy A. Brethauer, MD
Staff Surgeon
Advanced Laparoscopic and Bariatric Surgery
Department of General Surgery
The Cleveland Clinic Foundation
Cleveland, OH
USA

The following figures are reprinted with the permission of The Cleveland Clinic Foundation: Figures 3-1 through 3-10, 19.1-1 through 19.1-3, 20.1-2, 20.1-3, 20.1-5 through 20.1-9, 21.1-1 through 21.1-9, 21.4-1 through 21.4-14, 21.8-3A and B, 21.8-5A and B, 21.86A and B, 22.1-1 through 22.1-9, and 22.2-2 through 22.2-9.

Library of Congress Control Number: 2006938046

ISBN: 978-0-387-68058-3   e-ISBN: 978-0-387-68062-0

Printed on acid-free paper.

To my endearing wife Patsy and our jewels:
Daniel, Aaron, Teresa, and Isabella.
PRS

To my wife, Geri, who sacrificed her time with
me to allow its creation.
And to my two daughters, Kate Lynn and Liza,
the joys of my life.
Finally, I wish to thank the many patients who have
placed their trust and faith in me to help them with the
medical issues of their being overweight.
BDS

To my wife, Pam, for her incredible support and
encouragement, and to our beautiful children,
Katie, Anna, and Jacob.
SAB

Preface

Over the last decade, bariatric surgeons have witnessed more dramatic advances in the field of bariatric surgery than in the previous 50 years of this relatively young discipline. These changes have certainly been fueled by the great obesity epidemic beginning in the 1970s, which created the demand for effective treatment of severe obesity and its comorbidities. The gradual development and standardization of safer, more effective, and durable operations, such as Roux-en Y gastric bypass (RYGB), biliopancreatic diversion, duodenal switch, and adjustable gastric banding account for the first wave of advances over the last decade. More recently, the advent of minimally invasive surgery in the mid-1990s accounts for the second wave of major advances.

Fifteen years ago, fewer than 15,000 bariatric procedures (mostly vertical banded gastroplasty) were performed each year in the United States, and all were performed with a laparotomy requiring nearly a week of hospitalization and six weeks of convalescence. Mortality rates exceeding 2% and major morbidity exceeding 25% was the norm. It later became apparent that the laparotomy itself accounted for much of the morbidity of bariatric surgery. It contributed to major impairment in postoperative cardiopulmonary function, which led to atelectasis, pneumonia, respiratory failure, heart failure, and lengthy stays in the intensive care unit for a significant subset of patients. Furthermore, wound complications, including infections, seromas, hernias, and dehisences were the norm rather than the exception. Hernias were so common (20–25%) that they were often considered the second stage of a bariatric procedure.

Today, more than 200,000 bariatric procedures are performed each year in the United States and almost twice that figure worldwide. Nearly all gastric banding procedures, an estimated 75% of RYGB procedures, and even some BPD procedures are performed laparoscopically, indicating that the laparoscopic approach has been widely adopted in bariatric surgery. The dramatic reduction in postoperative pain, hospital stays of only 1 to 3 days, recovery time of 2 to 3 weeks, incidence of intensive care utilization to less than 5%, along with a great reduction in cardiopulmonary complications and wound complications can be attributed to the laparoscopic approach. Operative mortality of less than 1% is now common and perhaps also attributable to laparoscopic surgery. Indeed, bariatric surgery has become safer and more desirable because of laparoscopic surgery.

This textbook, *Minimally Invasive Bariatric Surgery*, is intended to provide the reader with a comprehensive overview of the current status of bariatric surgery, emphasizing the now dominant role of laparoscopic techniques. It is our intention to address issues of interest to not only seasoned and novice bariatric surgeons, but all healthcare providers who participate in the care of the bariatric patient. Specifically, we expect surgical residents, fellows, allied health, and bariatric physicians to benefit from this book. At the onset of this book, we invited contributing authors whom we considered the most authoritative, coming up with a "Who's Who" list of bariatric surgeons. The reader will note among the authors a high degree of clinical expertise and international diversity, as well as diversity of thought. We have even included a chapter on the role of open bariatric surgery to balance the enthusiasm of the editors for minimally invasive surgery. Furthermore, we are thankful for our good fortune in recruiting authors who have been in the forefront in developing and teaching specific procedures. Although not intended to be an atlas of bariatric surgery, this text does provide detailed illustrations and descriptions of all the common procedures with technical pearls from the surgeons who introduced them to the world.

The benefits of laparoscopic surgery, however, must be balanced with the significant training challenges posed by laparoscopic bariatric surgery. Special emphasis on learning curves and training requirements are found throughout this text. A chapter on training and credentialing is included to update the reader on current guidelines.

To further enlighten the reader, we also have included chapters on special issues and controversial subjects, including laparoscopic instruments and visualization, bariatric equipment for the ward and clinic, medical treatment of obesity, hand-assisted surgery, hernia management, diabetes surgery, perioperative care, pregnancy and gynecologic issues, and plastic surgery after weight loss. Chapter 24, "Risk-Benefit Analysis of Laparoscopic Bariatric Procedures," is particularly useful in that it compares head-to-head the risks and benefits of all the major operations. Finally, we do incorporate chapters that focus on new and futuristic operations, such as sleeve gastrectomy, gastric pacing, and endoluminal/natural orifice surgery—perhaps the next wave of minimally invasive surgery.

In the wake of the laparoscopic revolution of the 1990s, minimally invasive approaches to nearly every abdominal procedure and many thoracic procedures have been devised. However, in reality, only a few common procedures are now performed with a laparoscopic approach as the standard (i.e., >50%). Laparoscopic cholecystectomy, Nissen fundoplication, and bariatric procedures represent the major triumphs thus far of the laparoscopic revolution. Perhaps, bariatric operations represent the best application of minimally invasive procedures because avoidance of an extensive laparotomy in the high-risk bariatric population provides the greatest relative benefit. We hope that you encounter as much enjoyment reading *Minimally Invasive Bariatric Surgery* as we have had writing it! Now, on to the next revolution in bariatric surgery!

Philip R. Schauer, MD
Bruce D. Schirmer, MD
Stacy A. Brethauer, MD

Acknowledgments

The editors would like to acknowledge and thank Margaret Burns, our developmental editor, for her persistence and expertise in completing this book; Tomasz Rogula, MD, PhD, for his many contributions to the content and organization of the text; Joseph Pangrace, CMI, and the medical illustration department at The Cleveland Clinic for creating many of the superbly detailed illustrations included in the book; and our editors at Springer, Paula Callaghan, Laura Gillan, and Beth Campbell, for their guidance and support during the completion of this project.

Philip R. Schauer, MD
Bruce D. Schirmer, MD
Stacy A. Brethauer, MD

Contents

Contributors

Jeffrey W. Allen, MD
Associate Professor, Department of Surgery and the Center for Advanced Surgical Technologies, University of Louisville, Louisville, KY, USA

Iselin Austrheim-Smith, BS
Senior Research Associate, Department of Internal Medicine, University of California at Davis Medical Center, Sacramento, CA, USA

F. Merritt Ayad, PhD
Assistant Clinical Professor, Department of Psychiatry, Louisiana State University School of Medicine, New Orleans, LA, USA

Gianluca Bonanomi, MD
Assistant Professor, Department of Surgery, University of Pittsburgh Medical Center, Pittsburgh, PA, USA

Franklin A. Bontempo, MD
Associate Professor, Department of Medicine, Magee-Women's Hospital, University of Pittsburgh Medical Center, Pittsburgh, PA, USA

Keith Boone, MD, FACS
Associate Clinical Professor, Department of Surgery, University of California at San Francisco, Fresno Medical Program, Fresno, CA, USA

Enzo Bortolozzi, MD
Attending, Department of Surgery, Regional Hospital, Vicenza, Italy

Stacy A. Brethauer, MD
Staff Surgeon, Advanced Laparoscopic and Bariatric Surgery, Department of General Surgery, The Cleveland Clinic Foundation, Cleveland, OH, USA

Luca Busetto, MD
Faculty, Obesity Center, University of Padova, Padova, Italy

J.K. Champion, MD, FACS
Clinical Professor, Department of Surgery, Mercer University School of Medicine, Director of Bariatric Surgery, Department of Surgery, Emory-Dunwoody Medical Center, Atlanta, GA, USA

Bipan Chand, MD
Director of Surgical Endoscopy, Department of Bariatric and Metabolic Institute, The Cleveland Clinic Foundation, Cleveland, OH, USA

Ricardo Cohen, MD
Co-Director, Center for the Surgical Treatment of Morbid Obesity, Hospital Sao Paulo, Sao Paulo, Brazil

Maurizio De Luca, MD
General and Oncological Surgeon, Department of General Surgery, San Bortolo Regional Hospital, Vicenza, Italy

Eric J. DeMaria, MD, FACS
Chief of Endoscopy and Vice Chairman of Network General Surgery, Department of Surgery, Duke University Medical Center, Durham, NC, USA

John B. Dixon, MBBS, PhD, FRACGP
Faculty, Department of Surgery, Monash University, Alfred Hospital, Melbourne, Victoria, Australia

Liza Eden Giammaria, MD, MPH
Fellow, Department of Surgery, Beth Israel Deaconess Medical Center, Boston, MA, USA

Daniel Edmundowicz, MD, MS, FACC
Associate Professor, Director of Preventive Cardiology and Outpatient Services, Department of Cardiology, University of Pittsburgh Medical Center, Pittsburgh, PA, USA

George M. Eid, MD
Assistant Professor, Department of Surgery, Magee-Women's Hospital, University of Pittsburgh Medical Center, Pittsburgh, PA, USA

Franco Favretti, MD
Attending, Department of Surgery, Regional Hospital, Vicenza, Italy

George A. Fielding, MD
Associate Professor, Department of Surgery, New York University Program for Surgical Weight Loss, New York, NY, USA

Michel Gagner, MD, FRCS, FACS
Professor and Chief, Laparoscopic and Bariatric Surgery, Department of Surgery, Weill Medical College of Cornell University, New York-Presbyterian Hospital, New York, NY, USA

Scott F. Gallagher, MD
Research Fellow, Department of Surgery, University of South Florida Health Sciences Center, Tampa, FL, USA

Victor F. Garcia, MD
Professor, Department of Pediatric Surgery, Cincinnati Children's Hospital Medical Center, Cincinnati, OH, USA

Rachel J. Givelber, MD, FCCP, D, ABSM
Assistant Professor, Department of Pulmonary, Allergy and Critical Care Medicine/Sleep Medicine Center, University of Pittsburgh, Pittsburgh, PA, USA

Carolina Gomes Goncalves, MD
Clinical Fellow, Department of General Surgery, The Cleveland Clinic Foundation, Cleveland, OH, USA

Rodrigo Gonzalez, MD
Fellow, Advanced Laparoscopic Gastrointestinal and Bariatric Surgery, Department of Surgery, University of South Tampa College of Medicine, Tampa, FL, USA

William Gourash, MSN
CRNP, Department of Minimally Invasive Bariatric and General Surgery, Magee-Women's Hospital, Pittsburgh, PA, USA

Giselle Hamad, MD
Assistant Professor, Medical Director of Minimally Invasive General Surgery and Bariatrics, Department of Surgery, Magee-Women's Hospital, University of Pittsburgh Medical Center, Pittsburgh, PA, USA

Kelvin Higa, MD, FACS
Assistant Clinical Professor, Department of Surgery, University of California at San Francisco, Fresno Medical Program, Fresno, CA, USA

Dennis Hong, MD, MSc, FRCSC
Surgeon, Department of Surgery, Good Samaritan Hospital, Portland, OR, USA

Dennis Hurwitz, MD
Clinical Professor of Surgery (Plastic), Department of Surgery, University of Pittsburgh Medical School, Pittsburgh, PA, USA

Sayeed Ikramuddin, MD, FACS
Associate Professor, Co-Director, Center for Minimally Invasive Surgery, Department of Surgery, University of Minnesota, Minneapolis, MN, USA

Thomas H. Inge, MD, PhD
Assistant Professor, Department of Pediatric Surgery, Cincinnati Children's Hospital Medical Center, Cincinnati, OH, USA

Mohammad K. Jamal, MD
Assistant Professor, Department of Surgery, University of Iowa Carver College of Medicine, Iowa City, IA, USA

Jay C. Jan, MD
Bariatric Surgeon, Department of Surgery, Good Samaritan Hospital, Portland, OR, USA

Daniel B. Jones, MD, MS, FACS
Associate Professor, Department of Surgery, Harvard Medical School; Director, Bariatric Program; Chief, Section of Minimally Invasive Surgery, Beth Israel Deaconess Medical Center, Boston, MA, USA

Kenneth B. Jones, Jr., MD, FACS
Medical Director, Bariatric Surgery Center, Department of Surgery, Christus Schumpert Medical Center, Shreveport, LA, USA

Timothy D. Kane, MD
Assistant Professor, Department of Surgery, Division of Pediatric General and Thoracic Surgery, Children's Hospital of Pittsburgh, Pittsburgh, PA, USA

Sangeeta Kashyap, MD
Associate Staff, Department of Endocrinology, Diabetes and Metabolism, The Cleveland Clinic Foundation, Cleveland, OH, USA

Julie Kim, MD
Assistant Professor, Department of Surgery, Tufts University School of Medicine, Tufts–New England Medical Center, Boston, MA, USA

Tommaso Maccari, MD
Attending, Department of Endoscopic and Gastrointestinal Medicine, Hospital Sant Antonio, Padova, Italy

Alessandro Magon, MD
Attending, Department of Surgery, Regional Hospital, Vicenza, Italy

Vicki March, MD
Clinical Instructor, Department of Medicine, University of Pittsburgh School of Medicine, Pittsburgh, PA, USA

Louis F. Martin, MD
Professor, Department of Surgery, Louisiana State University School of Medicine, New Orleans, LA, USA

Samer G. Mattar, MD
Medical Director, Clarian Bariatric Center, Indianapolis, IN, USA

Ronald Matteotti, MD
Research Fellow, Department of Surgery, Weill Medical College of Cornell University, New York-Presbyterian Hospital, New York, NY, USA

Kathleen M. McCauley, JD
Partner, Department of Medical Litigation, Goodman, Allen, and Filetti, Glen Allen, VA, USA

Carol A. McCloskey, MD
Assistant Professor, Department of Surgery, University of Pittsburgh Medical Center, Magee-Women's Hospital, Pittsburgh, PA, USA

W. Scott Melvin, MD
Professor, Division of General and Gastrointestinal Surgery, Department of Surgery, Ohio State University Hospital, Columbus, OH, USA

Dean J. Mikami, MD
Assistant Professor, Division of General and Gastrointestinal Surgery, Department of Surgery, Ohio State University Hospital, Columbus, OH, USA

Edward C. Mun, MD, FACS
Assistant Professor, Department of Surgery; Director, Bariatric Surgery, Harvard Medical School, Beth Deaconess Medical Center, Boston, MA, USA

Michel M. Murr, MD, FACS
Director of Bariatric Surgery, Tampa General Hospital, Tampa, FL, USA

Ninh T. Nguyen, MD
Chief, Division of Gastrointestinal Surgery, Department of Surgery, University of California, Orange, CA, USA

Paul E. O'Brien, MD, FRACS
Chairman, Department of Surgery, Monash University, Alfred Hospital, Melbourne, Victoria, Australia

Ariel Ortiz Lagardere, MD, FACS
Professor, Department of Surgery, UABC School of Medicine, University of Baja California, Tijuana, Mexico

Emma J. Patterson, MD, FACS, FRCSC
Medical Director, Bariatric Surgery Program, Department of Surgery, Legacy Health System, Portland, OR, USA

Kim M. Pierce, MD
Clinical Instructor, Department of Medicine, University of Pittsburgh Medical Center, Magee-Women's Hospital, Pittsburgh, PA, USA

Ramesh C. Ramanathan, MD, FRCS
Assistant Professor, Department of General Surgery, University of Pittsburgh, Magee-Women's Hospital, Pittsburgh, PA, USA

Christine J. Ren, MD
Assistant Professor, Department of Surgery, New York University School of Medicine, New York, NY, USA

Tomasz Rogula, MD
Staff Surgeon, Bariatric and Metabolic Institute, Department of General Surgery, Cleveland Clinic, Cleveland, OH, USA

James C. Rosser, Jr., MD
Chief, Minimally Invasive Bariatric Surgery, Beth Israel; Director, Advanced Medical Technology Institute, Beth Israel, New York, NY, USA

Vivian M. Sanchez, MD
Instructor, Harvard Medical School, Section of Minimally Invasive Surgery, Beth Israel Deaconess Medical Center, Boston, MA, USA

Mark H. Sanders, MD, FCCP, D, ABSM
Professor, Departments of Medicine and Anesthesiology, Division of Pulmonary, Allergy and Critical Care Medicine/Sleep Medicine Center, University of Pittsburgh, Pittsburgh, PA, USA

Michael G. Sarr, MD, FACS
Masson Professor of Surgery, Department of Surgery, Mayo Clinic College of Medicine, Rochester, MN, USA

Philip R. Schauer, MD
Professor of Surgery, Lerner College of Medicine; Director, Advanced Laparoscopic and Bariatric Surgery, Bariatric and Metabolic Institute, The Cleveland Clinic Foundation, Cleveland, OH, USA

Bruce R. Schirmer, MD
Stephen H. Watts Professor of Surgery, Department of Surgery, Health Sciences Center, University of Virginia Health System, Charlottesville, VA, USA

Crystal T. Schlösser, MD, FACS
Attending Surgeon, Department of Surgery, Abbott Northwestern Hospital/Minneapolis Bariatric Surgeons, Minneapolis, MN, USA

Benjamin E. Schneider
Instructor, Department of Surgery, Beth Israel Deaconess Medical Center, Harvard Medical School, Boston, MA, USA

Gianni Segato, MD
Attending, Department of Surgery, Regional Hospital, Vicenza, Italy

Saraswathy Shekar, MB, BS, FFARCS(I)
Clinical Assistant Professor, Department of Anesthesiology, University of Pittsburgh Medical Center Presbyterian Hospital, Pittsburgh, PA, USA

Vadim Sherman, MD, FRCS(C)
Fellow, Department of General Surgery, The Cleveland Clinic Foundation, Cleveland, OH, USA

Scott Shikora, MD
Professor, Department of Surgery, Tufts University School of Medicine, Tufts–New England Medical Center, Boston, MA, USA

Mark Stephens, MB, BS, FRACP
Attending, Chesterville Day Hospital, Melbourne, Victoria, Australia

Harvey Sugerman, MD
Emeritus Professor of Surgery, Department of Surgery, Virginia Commonwealth University, Richmond, VA, USA

Michael Tarnoff, MD
Assistant Professor, Department of Surgery, Tufts–New England Medical Center, Boston, MA, USA

Paul A. Thodiyil, MD
Fellow, Department of Surgery, The Cleveland Clinic Foundation, Cleveland, OH, USA

Michael Williams, MD
Chief, Department of Surgery, Emory-Dunwoody Medical Center, Atlanta, GA, USA

Alan Wittgrove, MD, FACS
Medical Director, Wittgrove Bariatric Center, Scripps Memorial Hospital, La Jolla, CA, USA

Bruce M. Wolfe, MD
Professor, Department of Surgery, Division of General Surgery, Oregon Health and Science University, Portland, OR, USA

Panduranga Yenumula, MD
Assistant Professor, Department of Surgery, Michigan State University, Lansing, MI, USA

1
Pathophysiology of Obesity Comorbidity: The Effects of Chronically Increased Intraabdominal Pressure

Harvey J. Sugerman

Severe obesity is associated with multiple comorbidities that reduce the life expectancy and markedly impair the quality of life. Morbidly obese patients can suffer from central (android) obesity or peripheral (gynoid) obesity or a combination of the two. Gynoid obesity is associated with degenerative joint disease and venous stasis in the lower extremities. Android obesity is associated with the highest risk of mortality related to problems due to the metabolic syndrome or syndrome X, as well as increased intraabdominal pressure (IAP). The metabolic syndrome is associated with insulin resistance, hyperglycemia, and type 2 diabetes mellitus (DM), which in turn are associated with nonalcoholic liver disease (NALD), polycystic ovary syndrome, and systemic hypertension (1–7). Increased IAP is probably responsible in part or totally for obesity hypoventilation, venous stasis disease, pseudotumor cerebri, gastroesophageal reflux disease, stress urinary incontinence, and systemic hypertension. Central obesity is also associated with increased neck circumference and sleep apnea.

A previous clinical study of patients with obesity hypoventilation syndrome noted extremely high cardiac filling (pulmonary artery and pulmonary capillary wedge) pressures, as high as or higher than in patients with congestive heart failure (CHF), but most of these patients were not in heart failure. It was initially hypothesized that this could have been secondary to hypoxemic pulmonary artery vasoconstriction; however, the pressures remained elevated following gastric surgery for obesity despite post-operative mechanical ventilation and correction of both hypoxemia and hypercarbia. This pressure returned to normal within 6 to 9 months after surgically induced weight loss (8). High lumbar cerebrospinal fluid (CSF) pressures were noted in obese women with pseudotumor cerebri (also known as idiopathic intracranial hypertension). Resolution of headache and marked decreases in CSF pressures were noted when restudied 34 ± 8 months following gastric bypass (GBP) surgery (Fig. 1-1) (9). The cause(s) of these phenomena remained unexplained until women with stress overflow urinary incontinence, in whom resolution of the problem occurred within months following GBP surgery, underwent measurement of urinary bladder pressures (UBPs) in the gynecologic urodynamic laboratory before and 1 year following obesity surgery (10). These women were noted to have extremely high UBPs that normalized following surgically induced weight loss. Their pressures were as high as, or even higher than, UBPs noted in critically ill patients with an acute abdominal compartment syndrome where treatment is urgent surgical decompression (11,12). It was hypothesized that severely obese patients with central obesity have a chronic abdominal compartment syndrome with high UBPs, as an estimate of an increased intraabdominal pressure (IAP), and this would be related to a number of obesity comorbidity problems.

Animal Studies

Several studies have been performed to evaluate the effects of acutely elevated IAP in a porcine model, using either an infusion of isosmotic polyethylene glycol normally used for bowel cleansing (Go-Lytely®) or an intraabdominal balloon, on the cardiovascular, pulmonary, and central nervous systems. Polyethylene glycol was chosen, as it is not osmotically active, and it neither should be absorbed into the central circulation in significant amounts nor cause significant decreases in intravascular volume. Urinary bladder pressures correlated well ($r = 0.98$, $p < .0001$) with directly measured IAP in this model. Acutely elevated IAP produced hemodynamic changes characterized by decreased cardiac output, increased filling pressures, and increased systemic vascular resistance (Fig. 1-2). Pulmonary effects were hypoxia, hypercarbia, increased inspiratory pressure, and elevated pleural pressure (13). These changes are consistent with the pulmonary pathology characteristic of obesity hypoventilation syndrome. As IAP increased, pleural

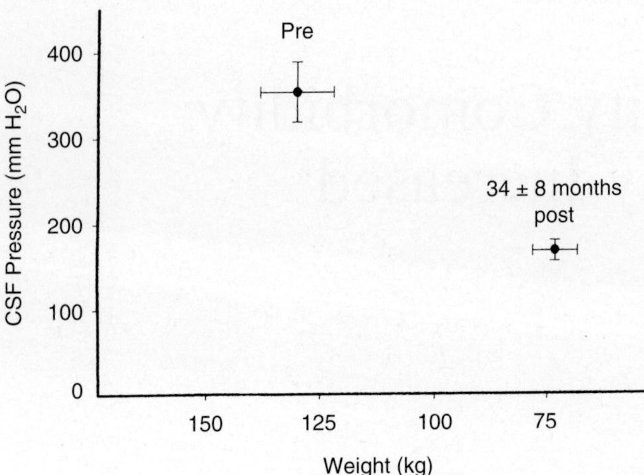

FIGURE 1-1. Elevated cerebrospinal fluid (CSF) pressure prior to, and significant ($p < .001$) decrease 34 ± 8 months following, gastric surgery for severe obesity associated with pseudotumor cerebri. [Sugerman et al. (9), with permission.]

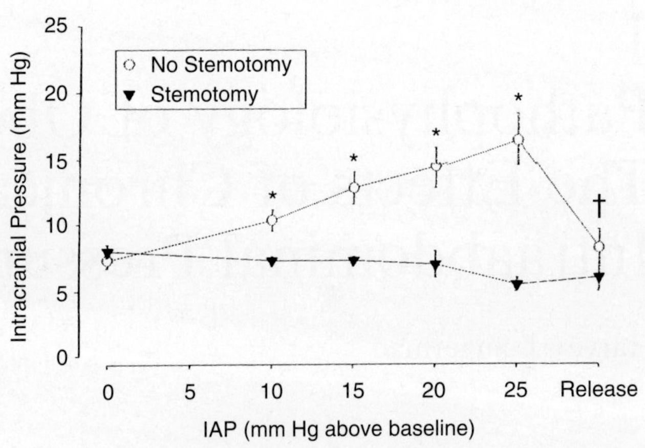

FIGURE 1-3. Progressive increase in directly measured intracranial pressure with increasing intraabdominal pressure associated with the intraabdominal instillation of iso-osmotic polyethylene glycol in an acute porcine model and prevention of this increase in animals that had undergone a median sternotomy and pleuropericardiotomy. [Bloomfield et al. (14), with permission.]

pressure, central venous pressure, and intracranial pressure also increased (Fig. 1-3). When pleural pressure was prevented from rising by midline sternotomy and incision of the pleura and pericardium, the effects of rising IAP on the cardiovascular, pulmonary, and central nervous systems were all negated, except for the decrease in cardiac output (14). Acute elevation of IAP caused increases in both plasma renin activity (PRA) and aldosterone levels (Figs. 1-4 and 1-5) (15).

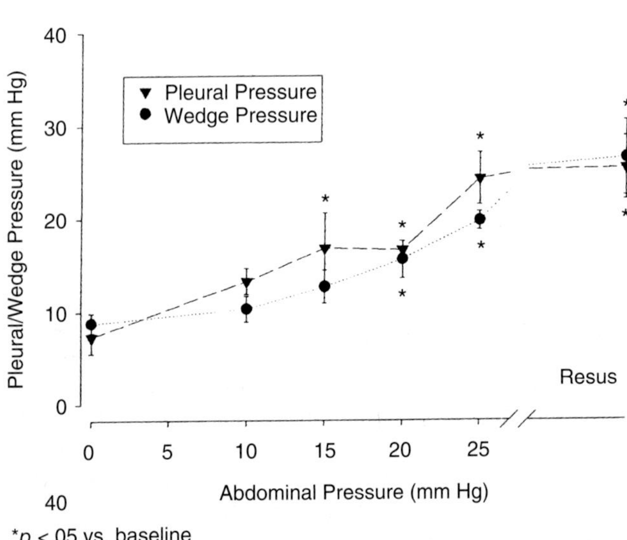

*$p < .05$ vs. baseline

FIGURE 1-2. Progressive increase in pleural pressure and pulmonary artery wedge (occlusion) pressure with increasing intraabdominal pressure associated with the intraabdominal instillation of iso-osmotic polyethylene glycol in an acute porcine model. Resus, resuscitation. [Ridings et al. (13), with permission.]

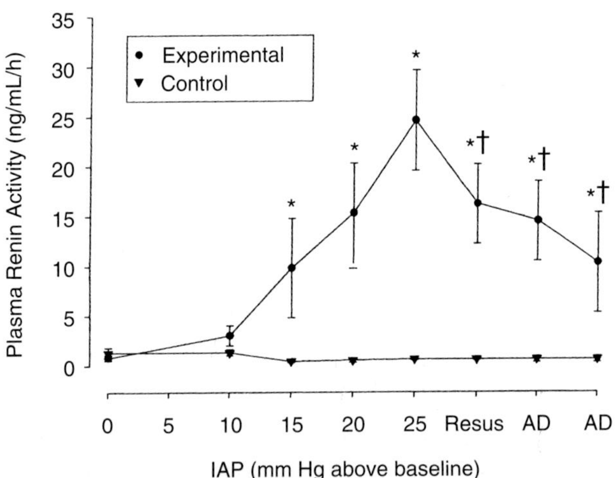

FIGURE 1-4. Progressive increase in plasma renin activity with increasing intraabdominal pressure (IAP) associated with the intraabdominal instillation of iso-osmotic polyethylene glycol in an acute porcine model as compared to control animals that did not have their IAP increased; effect of volume expansion (resuscitation) and 30 and 60 minutes after abdominal decompression (AD). *$p < .05$ versus baseline and control animals; †$p < .05$ versus pre-resuscitation value. [Bloomfield et al. (15), with permission.]

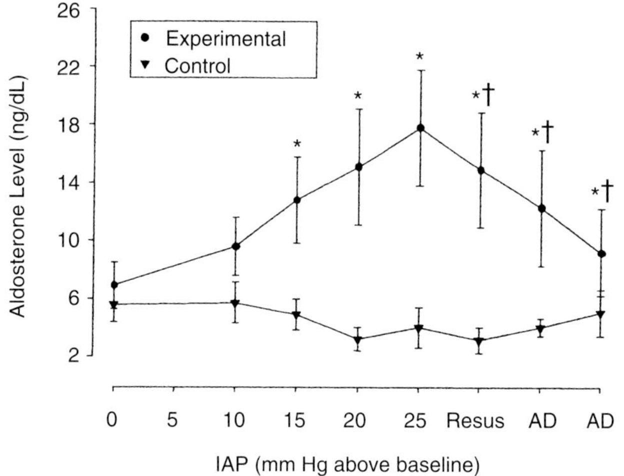

FIGURE 1-5. Progressive increase in serum aldosterone levels with increasing intraabdominal pressure (IAP) associated with the intra-abdominal instillation of iso-osmotic polyethylene glycol in an acute porcine model as compared to control animals that did not have their IAP increased; effect of volume expansion (resuscitation) and 30 and 60 minutes after abdominal decompression (AD). $*p < .05$ versus baseline and control animals; $†p < .05$ versus pre-resuscitation value. [Bloomfield et al. (15), with permission.]

Clinical Studies

During the course of this research it was noted that conditions known to increase IAP such as pregnancy, laparoscopic pneumoperitoneum, and ascites are associated with pathologic consequences also encountered in the morbidly obese, such as gastroesophageal reflux, abdominal herniation, stress overflow urinary incontinence, and lower limb venous stasis (16–20). Thus, the comorbidities that are presumed to be secondary to increased IAP in

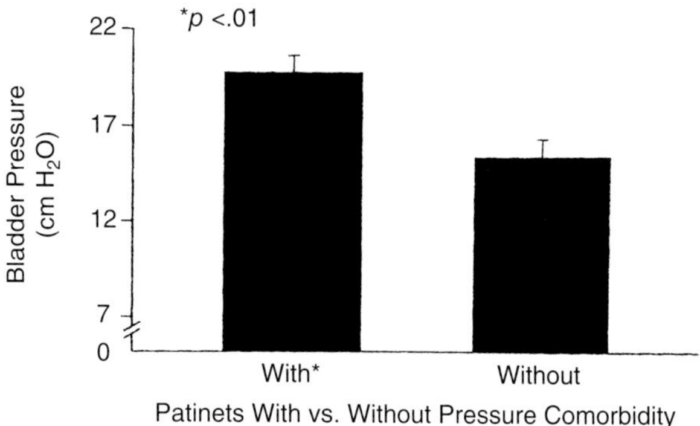

FIGURE 1-7. Increased urinary bladder pressure in the 67 patients with intraabdominal pressure-related morbidity and in 17 patients without IAP-related morbidity. [Sugerman et al. (21), with permission.]

obese patients include CHF, hypoventilation, venous stasis ulcers, gastroesophageal reflux disease (GERD), urinary stress incontinence, incisional hernia, pseudotumor cerebri, proteinuria, and systemic hypertension.

In a study of 84 patients with severe obesity prior to GBP surgery and five nonobese patients prior to colectomy for ulcerative colitis, it was found that obese patients had a significantly higher UBP (18 ± 0.7 vs. 7 ± 1.6 cm H_2O, $p < .001$) which correlated with the sagittal abdominal diameter (SAD, $r = 0.67, p > .001$, Fig. 1-6) and was greater ($p > .05$) in patients with (compared to those without) morbidity presumed due to increased IAP (Fig. 1-7) (21). The waist/hip ratio (WHR) correlated with UBP in men ($r = 0.6, p > .05$) but not in women ($r = -0.3$), supporting the concept that the SAD is a better reflection of central obesity than the WHR. In 15 patients studied before and 1 year after GBP, there were significant ($p > .001$) decreases in weight (140 ± 8 to 87 ± 6 kg), body mass index (BMI) (52 ± 3 to 33 ± 2 kg/m^2), SAD (32 ± 1 to 20 ± 2 cm, Fig. 1-8),

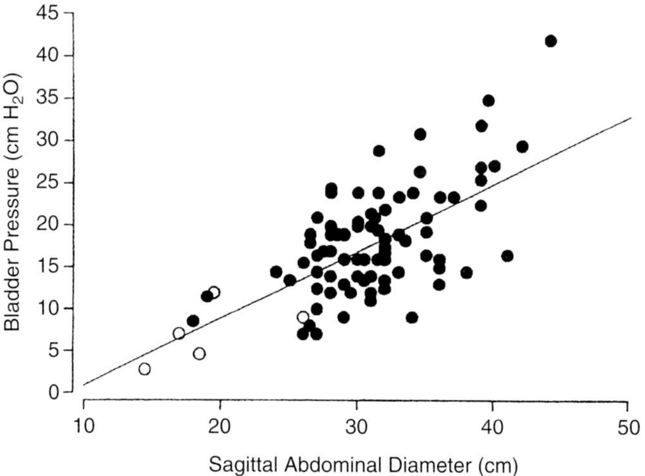

FIGURE 1-6. Correlation between urinary bladder pressure and sagittal abdominal diameter in 84 morbidly obese patients (•) and five control nonobese patients (o) with ulcerative colitis, $r = 0.67$, $p < .0001$). [Sugerman et al. (21), with permission.]

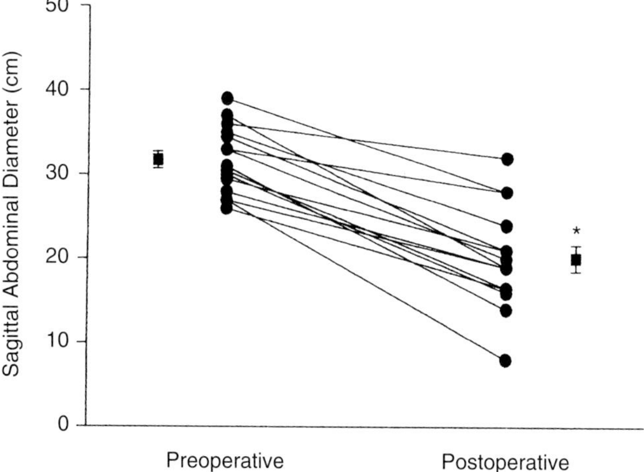

FIGURE 1-8. Sagittal abdominal diameter before and 1 year after surgically induced weight loss. • = individual patient, ■ = mean ± standard error of the mean. $*p < .0001$. [Sugerman et al. (11), with permission.]

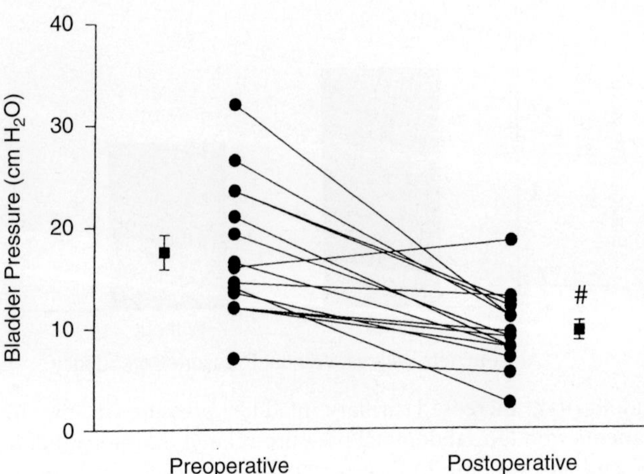

FIGURE 1-9. Urinary bladder pressure before and 1 year after surgically induced weight loss. • = individual patient, ■ = mean ± standard error of the mean. *$p < .0001$. [Sugerman et al. (11), with permission.]

UBP (17 ± 2 to 10 ± 1 cm H_2O, Fig. 1-9), and obesity comorbidity with the loss of $69\% \pm 4\%$ of excess weight (11).

Discussion

The relationship of central obesity to the constellation of health problems known collectively as the metabolic syndrome appears well established (3,7). However, this has been presumed to be due to increased visceral fat metabolism. Increased UBP and its relationship to increased IAP has been used in postoperative patients as an indication for emergent reexploration and abdominal decompression for an acute abdominal compartment syndrome to correct oliguria and increased peak inspiratory pressures with mechanical ventilation (12,22). The decision to perform emergency abdominal decompression is usually taken when the UBP is ≥25 cm H_2O. In the study of obese patients prior to GBP surgery, 11 patients had UBPs ≥25, four ≥30, and one ≥40 cm H_2O. It became apparent after our previous study where we found very high UBPs in severely obese women with stress overflow urinary incontinence (10) that centrally obese patients may have a chronic abdominal compartment syndrome. We have also found a significantly higher ($p < .001$) risk of incisional hernia following surgery for obesity (20%) than after colectomy in mostly nonobese patients with ulcerative colitis (4%) where two thirds of the colitis patients were taking prednisone and had a much larger incision (19). Four of the seven incisional hernias in the colitis group occurred in patients with a BMI ≥30. Presumably, this increased risk of incisional hernia was due to an increased IAP in the obese patients.

Urinary bladder pressures were significantly higher in patients with comorbid factors mechanistically associated with elevated IAP than in patients with obesity-related problems that are not considered to be secondary to an increased IAP. The abdominal pressure–related morbidity factors chosen have been documented in pregnancy and cirrhotics with ascites, as well as obese patients, and included hypoventilation, venous stasis disease, GERD, urinary incontinence, pseudotumor cerebri, and incisional hernia. In another report we have found that obese women with pseudotumor cerebri have increased SAD, thoracic pressures as measured transesophageally, and cardiac filling pressures (23). In addition, hypertension was considered to be probably related to IAP, through one or more of the following mechanisms: (1) increased renal venous pressure, (2) direct renal compression (24), and (3) an increased intrathoracic pressure leading to a decreased venous return and decreased cardiac output. Each of these may lead to activation of the renin-angiotensin-aldosterone system, leading to sodium and water retention and vasoconstriction. The increased renal venous pressure could lead to a glomerulopathy with proteinuria. It is currently hypothesized that the hypertension seen in the morbidly obese is secondary to insulin-induced sodium reabsorption. However, systemic hypertension in the morbidly obese may not be associated with hyperinsulinemia, and these patients have been noted to have a decreased renal blood flow (RBF), glomerular filtration rate (GFR), and proteinuria (25).

Although the UBPs were measured supine in anesthetized, paralyzed patients and these pressures could be altered by the upright position, we believe the data to be clinically relevant. First, in the stress incontinence study the pressures rose even further when the patient assumed a sitting or standing position (10). Second, these pressures likely would be even higher in the absence of muscle paralysis. Third, most individuals spend 6 to 8 hours sleeping in a supine or lateral decubitus position. Many severely obese patients, especially those with sleep apnea and hypoventilation, have found that they must sleep in the sitting position, presumably to lower the effect of the increased IAP on their thoracic cavity. It is also for this reason that patients with pseudotumor cerebri have more severe headaches in the morning upon awakening.

Although an increased WHR is a recognized measurement of central obesity and metabolic complications, we found a poor correlation between the WHR and UBPs in women but a good correlation in men. This is probably the result of the diluting effect of peripheral obesity, commonly present in women, on the estimate of central obesity. The greater problem of central obesity in men was reinforced by the finding of a greater SAD and UBP in men compared to women despite an equal BMI (11). Unlike the WHR, the SAD provided good positive correlations with UBP in both men and women, corroborating the computed tomography (CT) scan data reported by Kvist et al. (26,27) that the SAD is a better reflection of central obesity than the WHR.

In the study of UBP in patients following GBP surgery, significant weight loss was associated with a marked reduction in both pressure-related and non–pressure-related comorbidity, except for incisional hernias and the need for cholecystectomy. Much of the improvement in comorbidity was based on subjective reports by patients rather than on objective data such as sleep apnea (respiratory disturbance) index from sleep polysomnography or acid reflux episodes from 24-hour pH monitoring. This improvement may have been exaggerated by the patients' sense of euphoria over their significant weight loss and their desire to please the investigative team. To obtain objective follow-up data would be expensive and difficult in the current managed-care environment in the United States. Several studies have documented improvement following surgically induced weight loss in conditions such as urinary incontinence (10), respiratory insufficiency including sleep apnea and hypoventilation (8,28), type 2 diabetes (29), GERD (30), pseudotumor cerebri (9), hyperlipidemia (31), female sexual hormone dysfunction (32), hypertension (31,33), and cardiac dysfunction (8).

These possible pathophysiologic consequences of increased IAP (hypertension, peripheral edema, proteinuria, increased CSF pressures, increased cardiac filling pressures, and increased hepatic venous pressures) suggest that the chronic abdominal compartment syndrome could be responsible for toxemia of pregnancy. This hypothesis is supported by the increased association of preeclampsia in primiparas (where the abdomen has never been stretched before), twin pregnancies, morbid obesity where an increased IAP is predictable, and its correction with parturition. We are in the process of developing an externally applied device that reduces IAP, and we plan to use this device to treat severely obese patients with systemic hypertension, venous stasis disease, GERD, obesity hypoventilation, and pseudotumor cerebri. Results of these studies should provide further data to evaluate the proposed hypothesis that increased IAP is responsible for these comorbidities. Furthermore, this device may prove to be therapeutic in women with preeclampsia/eclampsia, obviating the need to urgently deliver a very premature infant with its attendant morbidity and mortality.

References

1. Eckel RH, Grundy SM, Zimmet PZ. The metabolic syndrome. Lancet 2005;365(9468):1415–1428.
2. Grundy SM, Brewer HB Jr, Cleeman JI, et al. Definition of metabolic syndrome: Report of the National Heart, Lung, and Blood Institute/American Heart Association conference on scientific issues related to definition. Circulation 2004;109(3):433–438.
3. Third Report of the National Cholesterol Education Program (NCEP) Expert Panel on Detection, Evaluation, and Treatment of High Blood Cholesterol in Adults (Adult Treatment Panel III) final report. Circulation 2002;106(25): 3143–3421.
4. Ong JP, Elariny H, Collantes R, et al. Predictors of nonalcoholic steatohepatitis and advanced fibrosis in morbidly obese patients. Obes Surg 2005;15(3):310–315.
5. Mattar SG, Velcu LM, Rabinovitz M, et al. Surgically-induced weight loss significantly improves nonalcoholic fatty liver disease and the metabolic syndrome. Ann Surg 2005;242(4):610–617; discussion 618–620.
6. Escobar-Morreale HF, Botella-Carretero JI, Alvarez-Blasco F, et al. The polycystic ovary syndrome associated with morbid obesity may resolve after weight loss induced by bariatric surgery. J Clin Endocrinol Metab 2005; 90(12):6364–6369.
7. Johnson D, Prud'homme D, Despres JP, et al. Relation of abdominal obesity to hyperinsulinemia and high blood pressure in men. Int J Obes Relat Metab Disord 1992; 16(11):881–890.
8. Sugerman HJ, Baron PL, Fairman RP, et al. Hemodynamic dysfunction in obesity hypoventilation syndrome and the effects of treatment with surgically induced weight loss. Ann Surg 1988;207(5):604–613.
9. Sugerman HJ, Felton WL 3rd, Salvant JB Jr, et al. Effects of surgically induced weight loss on idiopathic intracranial hypertension in morbid obesity. Neurology 1995;45(9): 1655–1659.
10. Bump RC, Sugerman HJ, Fantl JA, McClish DK. Obesity and lower urinary tract function in women: effect of surgically induced weight loss. Am J Obstet Gynecol 1992;167(2):392–397; discussion 397–399.
11. Sugerman H, Windsor A, Bessos M, et al. Effects of surgically induced weight loss on urinary bladder pressure, sagittal abdominal diameter and obesity co-morbidity. Int J Obes Relat Metab Disord 1998;22(3):230–235.
12. Ertel W, Oberholzer A, Platz A, et al. Incidence and clinical pattern of the abdominal compartment syndrome after "damage-control" laparotomy in 311 patients with severe abdominal and/or pelvic trauma. Crit Care Med 2000; 28(6):1747–1753.
13. Ridings PC, Bloomfield GL, Blocher CR, Sugerman HJ. Cardiopulmonary effects of raised intra-abdominal pressure before and after intravascular volume expansion. J Trauma 1995;39(6):1071–1075.
14. Bloomfield GL, Ridings PC, Blocher CR, et al. A proposed relationship between increased intra-abdominal, intra-thoracic, and intracranial pressure. Crit Care Med 1997; 25(3):496–503.
15. Bloomfield GL, Blocher CR, Fakhry IF, et al. Elevated intra-abdominal pressure increases plasma renin activity and aldosterone levels. J Trauma 1997;42(6):997–1004; discussion 1004–1005.
16. Dent J, Dodds WJ, Hogan WJ, Toouli J. Factors that influence induction of gastroesophageal reflux in normal human subjects. Dig Dis Sci 1988;33(3):270–275.
17. Fantl JA. Genuine stress incontinence: pathophysiology and rationale for its medical management. Obstet Gynecol Clin North Am 1989;16(4):827–840.

18. Nagler R, Spiro HM. Heartburn in late pregnancy. Manometric studies of esophageal motor function. J Clin Invest 1961;40:954–970.
19. Sugerman HJ, Kellum JM Jr, Reines HD, et al. Greater risk of incisional hernia with morbidly obese than steroid-dependent patients and low recurrence with prefascial polypropylene mesh. Am J Surg 1996;171(1):80–84.
20. Skudder PA, Farrington DT. Venous conditions associated with pregnancy. Semin Dermatol 1993;12(2):72–77.
21. Sugerman H, Windsor A, Bessos M, Wolfe L. Intra-abdominal pressure, sagittal abdominal diameter and obesity comorbidity. J Intern Med 1997;241(1):71–79.
22. Kron IL, Harman PK, Nolan SP. The measurement of intra-abdominal pressure as a criterion for abdominal re-exploration. Ann Surg 1984;199(1):28–30.
23. Sugerman HJ, DeMaria EJ, Felton WL 3rd, et al. Increased intra-abdominal pressure and cardiac filling pressures in obesity-associated pseudotumor cerebri. Neurology 1997;49(2):507–511.
24. Harman PK, Kron IL, McLachlan HD, et al. Elevated intra-abdominal pressure and renal function. Ann Surg 1982;196(5):594–597.
25. Scaglione R, Ganguzza A, Corrao S, et al. Central obesity and hypertension: pathophysiologic role of renal haemodynamics and function. Int J Obes Relat Metab Disord 1995;19(6):403–409.
26. Kvist H, Chowdhury B, Grangard U, et al. Total and visceral adipose-tissue volumes derived from measurements with computed tomography in adult men and women: predictive equations. Am J Clin Nutr 1988;48(6):1351–1361.
27. Kvist H, Chowdhury B, Sjostrom L, et al. Adipose tissue volume determination in males by computed tomography and 40K. Int J Obes 1988;12(3):249–266.
28. Sugerman HJ, Fairman RP, Sood RK, et al. Long-term effects of gastric surgery for treating respiratory insufficiency of obesity. Am J Clin Nutr 1992;55(2 suppl):597S–601S.
29. Pories WJ, MacDonald KG Jr, Morgan EJ, et al. Surgical treatment of obesity and its effect on diabetes: 10–y follow-up. Am J Clin Nutr 1992;55(2 suppl):582S–585S.
30. Deitel M, Khanna RK, Hagen J, Ilves R. Vertical banded gastroplasty as an antireflux procedure. Am J Surg 1988;155(3):512–516.
31. Gleysteen JJ, Barboriak JJ, Sasse EA. Sustained coronary-risk-factor reduction after gastric bypass for morbid obesity. Am J Clin Nutr 1990;51(5):774–778.
32. Deitel M, To TB, Stone E, et al. Sex hormonal changes accompanying loss of massive excess weight. Gastroenterol Clin North Am 1987;16(3):511–515.
33. Foley EF, Benotti PN, Borlase BC, et al. Impact of gastric restrictive surgery on hypertension in the morbidly obese. Am J Surg 1992;163(3):294–297.

2
The Medical Management of Obesity

Vicki March and Kim Pierce

Although health practitioners traditionally have not been trained in the medical management of obesity, they attain expertise in the treatment of its comorbidities—those conditions associated with, exacerbated by, or even caused by obesity, such as coronary artery disease, hypertension, type 2 diabetes, obstructive sleep apnea, degenerative joint disease, cancers (endometrium, colon, renal cell, breast, and prostate), gout, nonalcoholic steatohepatitis (NASH), polycystic ovary (PCO) syndrome, and other gynecologic conditions (Table 2-1).

Even though the numbers of individuals classified as overweight and obese have reached epidemic proportions in the United States, affecting the majority of Americans (1), and rapidly approaching tobacco use as the leading preventable cause of death in this country (2,3), there remain numerous obstacles to the discussion of obesity in the clinical setting. First, most medical professionals have not had the training necessary to address the subject adequately. In addition, many overweight individuals who have failed diets do not return for follow-up visits. Furthermore, a clinician knowledgeable about weight management might not be allotted sufficient time during the office visit. To compound these difficulties, insurance companies often deny claims when obesity is listed as the primary diagnosis. Unfortunately, out-of-pocket costs of comprehensive medical weight management programs may be prohibitive. This chapter presents an overview of the nonsurgical management of obesity in adults. Although the increase in pediatric and adolescent obesity and its concomitant conditions is alarming (4), the management of obesity in this population is beyond the scope of this chapter, and only brief mention will be made.

The Approach to the Obese Patient

Spectrum of Treatment

The spectrum of obesity treatment has been broad and overlapping, and consists of a variety of dietary maneuvers, nutritional education, exercise, cognitive-behavioral therapy, pharmacotherapy, group support, self-help, and surgery. The measurement of the body mass index (BMI) has become a useful tool in determining the type(s) of treatment. The BMI, which is defined as the weight in kilograms divided by the square of the height in meters, allows identification of the overweight or obese patient as follows: normal, BMI = 18.5 to 24.9; overweight, BMI = 25 to 29.9; class I obesity, BMI = 30 to 34.9; class II obesity, BMI = 35 to 39.9; class III obesity, BMI = 40 or greater (Table 2-2). In considering modes of treatment, it is important for the clinician to be aware that as the BMI increases, so do all-cause morbidity and mortality (5,6). Thus, weight loss interventions become more aggressive as the BMI increases. The more extreme recommendations stem not only from the higher morbidity and mortality associated with higher BMIs but also from the heightened difficulty patients experience in achieving substantial and durable weight loss. Although bariatric surgery is reserved for patients with BMIs greater than 35 with comorbidities or greater than 40 without comorbidities, many persons who are surgical candidates have BMIs that far exceed these numbers. The operative risk in these heaviest individuals is so great (7,8) that some surgeons attempt to lower patients' BMIs prior to surgery.

It has been demonstrated repeatedly that most people who lose weight gain it back, and gain even more (9,10). The comprehensive weight-loss models, which incorporate dietary adjustments, exercise, behavioral modification, and group support, have been the most successful in maintaining weight loss (9,10). People who receive ongoing follow-up after losing weight have the least regain of weight (9,10).

The Office Visit

The History

When evaluating an overweight or obese patient in the setting of either a general or bariatric practice, the

TABLE 2-1. Obesity-related comorbidities

Cardiovascular	Genitourinary
Coronary artery disease	Preeclampsia
Congestive heart failure	Polycystic ovarian syndrome
Hypertension	Infertility
Diastolic dysfunction	Amenorrhea
Cor pulmonale	Dysfunctional uterine bleeding
Peripheral vascular disease peripheral edema	Menorrhagia
Lymphedema	Urinary incontinence
Pulmonary	Testicular atrophy
Obstructive sleep apnea	Nephrologic
Cor pulmonale	Chronic renal insufficiency
Asthma	Primary nephrotic syndrome proteinuria
Peripheral edema	Dermatologic
Lymphedema	Venous stasis
Insomnia	Cellulitis
Endocrinologic	Tinea corporis
Dyslipidemia	Alopecia
Diabetes mellitus types 1 and 2	Hirsutism
Gestational diabetes mellitus	Hidradenitis suppurativa
Insulin resistance	Acanthosis nigricans
Metabolic syndrome	Telangiectasia
Polycystic ovarian syndrome	Striae
Gynecomastia	Neoplastic
Testicular atrophy	Breast
Hematologic	Colon
Pulmonary embolism	Endometrial
Venous thrombosis hypercoagulable state	Prostate
Endothelial dysfunction	Renal cell
Gastroenterologic	Psychological
Nonalcoholic steatohepatitis	Depression
Cholelithiasis	Anxiety
Reflux	Personality disorder
Hiatal hernia	Bulimia
Esophageal dysmotility	Anorexia
Constipation	Eating disorders
Irritable bowel syndrome	Body dysmorphic syndrome
Musculoskeletal	Insomnia
Degenerative joint disease	Neurologic
Gout	Cerebrovascular accident
Lumbago	Pseudotumor cerebri
Fibromyalgia	Meralgia paresthetica

clinician should obtain information pertinent to the patient's weight, including an assessment of the patient's knowledge about diet and exercise, previous weight loss attempts, and exercise patterns. Intake questionnaires that request details about diet, exercise, psychosocial factors, and stress can be used as starting points in the interview. The clinician should identify medications that cause weight gain, and assess obesity-related comorbidities, underlying genetic or hormonal disorders, and the presence of psychiatric conditions, with particular attention to eating disorders—anorexia nervosa, binge-eating disorder, and bulimia. Because there is not yet a clear evidence-based algorithm for the care of the obese patient, treatment must be planned individually.

The Physical Examination

At the initial visit, the patient's height should be measured, and at the initial and all subsequent visits, the weight should be obtained and the BMI calculated or obtained from a chart. In patients younger than 20 years of age, once the BMI is obtained, the percentage BMI must then be determined from an age-specific and gender-specific growth chart. An individual in greater than the 85th percentile is considered "at risk for overweight" or "overweight," and an individual in greater than the 95th percentile is considered "overweight" or "obese." The terminology varies because of the concern about social stigma attached to the word *obesity* in the pediatric population (11).

In adult patients with a BMI less than 35, a waist circumference measurement can be an adjunct in predicting a patient's cardiovascular risk factors. This measurement has largely supplanted the waist/hip ratio (WHR) measurement because it is easier to obtain and yields the same information. A circumference greater than 35 inches in a female and 40 inches in a male indicates the presence of the metabolic syndrome, which is characterized by

TABLE 2-2. Body mass index

BMI	Normal						Overweight					Obese										Extreme Obesity															
	19	20	21	22	23	24	25	26	27	28	29	30	31	32	33	34	35	36	37	38	39	40	41	42	43	44	45	46	47	48	49	50	51	52	53	54
Height (Inches)																		Body Weight (pounds)																			
58	91	96	100	105	110	115	119	124	129	134	138	143	148	153	158	162	167	172	177	181	186	191	196	201	205	210	215	220	224	229	234	239	244	248	253	258
59	94	99	104	109	114	119	124	128	133	138	143	148	153	158	163	168	173	178	183	188	193	198	203	208	212	217	222	227	232	237	242	247	252	257	262	267
60	97	102	107	112	118	123	128	133	138	143	148	153	158	163	168	174	179	184	189	194	199	204	209	215	220	225	230	235	240	245	250	255	261	266	271	276
61	100	106	111	116	122	127	132	137	143	148	153	158	164	169	174	180	185	190	195	201	206	211	217	222	227	232	238	243	248	254	259	264	269	275	280	285
62	104	109	115	120	126	131	136	142	147	153	158	164	169	175	180	186	191	196	202	207	213	218	224	229	235	240	246	251	256	262	267	273	278	284	289	295
63	107	113	118	124	130	135	141	146	152	158	163	169	175	180	186	191	197	203	208	214	220	225	231	237	242	248	254	259	265	270	278	282	287	293	299	304
64	110	116	122	128	134	140	145	151	157	163	169	174	180	186	192	197	204	209	215	221	227	232	238	244	250	256	262	267	273	279	285	291	296	302	308	314
65	114	120	126	132	138	144	150	156	162	168	174	180	186	192	198	204	210	216	222	228	234	240	246	252	258	264	270	276	282	288	294	300	306	312	318	324
66	118	124	130	136	142	148	155	161	167	173	179	186	192	198	204	210	216	223	229	235	241	247	253	260	266	272	278	284	291	297	303	309	315	322	328	334
67	121	127	134	140	146	153	159	166	172	178	185	191	198	204	211	217	223	230	236	242	249	255	261	268	274	280	287	293	299	306	312	319	325	331	338	344
68	125	131	138	144	151	158	164	171	177	184	190	197	203	210	216	223	230	236	243	249	256	262	269	276	282	289	295	302	308	315	322	328	335	341	348	354
69	128	135	142	149	155	162	169	176	182	189	196	203	209	216	223	230	236	243	250	257	263	270	277	284	291	297	304	311	318	324	331	338	345	351	358	365
70	132	139	146	153	160	167	174	181	188	195	202	209	216	222	229	236	243	250	257	264	271	278	285	292	299	306	313	320	327	334	341	348	355	362	369	376
71	136	143	150	157	165	172	179	186	193	200	208	215	222	229	236	243	250	257	265	272	279	286	293	301	308	315	322	329	338	343	351	358	365	372	379	386
72	140	147	154	162	169	177	184	191	199	206	213	221	228	235	242	250	258	265	272	279	287	294	302	309	316	324	331	338	346	353	361	368	375	383	390	397
73	144	151	159	166	174	182	189	197	204	212	219	227	235	242	250	257	265	272	280	288	295	302	310	318	325	333	340	348	355	363	371	378	386	393	401	408
74	148	155	163	171	179	186	194	202	210	218	225	233	241	249	256	264	272	280	287	295	303	311	319	326	334	342	350	358	365	373	381	389	396	404	412	420
75	152	160	168	176	184	192	200	208	216	224	232	240	248	256	264	272	279	287	295	303	311	319	327	335	343	351	359	367	375	383	391	399	407	415	423	431
76	156	164	172	180	189	197	205	213	221	230	238	246	254	263	271	279	287	295	304	312	320	328	336	344	353	361	369	377	385	394	402	410	418	426	435	443

Source: http://www.nhlbi.nih.gov/guidelines/obesity/bmi_tbl2.htm.

hypertension, abdominal obesity, insulin resistance, low high-density lipoprotein (HDL) cholesterol, and high triglycerides, and is linked to an increased risk of cardiovascular events (12).

Some practitioners find body fat analysis a useful gauge in quantifying the fitness of the overweight individual; however, measurements may not be consistent. At this time, a body fat analysis is not recommended in the routine care of the overweight or obese person. Blood pressure and pulse should be measured at each visit. The physical exam often reveals underlying and often under-diagnosed medical diseases. Pertinent physical findings in a bariatric examination include neck circumference to assess for the risk of obstructive sleep apnea (greater than 16 inches in women and 17 inches in men confers increased risk) and acanthosis nigricans (AN). Polycystic ovary syndrome and Cushing's syndrome have many similarities on physical examination. A PCO patient, by definition female, is likely to present with hirsutism, oligomenorrhea or infertility, and acne. Striae, buffalo hump, muscle wasting, and moon-like facies are more specific to a syndrome of hypercortisolism. Hypothyroidism may be suspected with a history of rapid weight gain and findings on physical examination of goiter, lateral eyebrow thinning, and skin changes.

The Laboratory Evaluation

Pertinent initial tests include a fasting lipid profile, fasting blood glucose, and renal, liver, and thyroid function tests. If fasting blood glucose is greater than 100 mg/dL (the most recent criterion for impaired fasting blood glucose), the test should be repeated and a glucose tolerance test considered. Hemoglobin A_{1c}, fasting insulin, and C-peptide levels can be used to guide treatment in both the metabolic syndrome and type 2 diabetes. If diabetes is present, a urine microalbumin level and hemoglobin A_{1c} should be ordered. An electrocardiogram should be included and may uncover weight-related abnormalities, such as left ventricular hypertrophy, right ventricular strain, ischemia, or arrhythmias.

Treatment Modalities

General Considerations

Individuals in whom weight loss is contraindicated include women who are either pregnant or lactating, persons with unstable psychiatric illnesses, and those with other medical conditions, such as immunologic diseases or malignancies, which could be exacerbated with caloric restriction. Others who have gained less than 20 pounds during adulthood, and are without comorbidities and have BMIs between 25 and 25.9, can be encouraged simply to avoid weight gain and can be educated about how to do so, perhaps merely by increasing exercise.

The initial objective for most weight-loss candidates is a reduction of 10% of baseline weight. In addition to having a beneficial effect on health, this degree of weight loss is usually achievable in about 6 months (13). Once this 10% target is attained, the clinician and patient can decide if further weight loss is necessary.

Diet

Loss of weight requires an energy deficit, which can be achieved both through adjustment of diet and activity. A unit of energy is 1 kilocalorie (kcal), which is the quantity of energy required to raise 1 kg of water by 1°C. For weight maintenance, most humans require anywhere between 1500 and 2500 kcal (heretofore called the colloquial "calories"). To lose 1 pound in 1 week, it is necessary to create a calorie deficit of 3500 calories, or 500 fewer calories a day, for 7 consecutive days. Dietary approaches to weight loss include total fasting, very low calorie diets (VLCDs), low-calorie diets (LCDs), balanced deficit diets, and fad diets. Near- or total-fasting diets have been used for rapid weight reduction, with daily caloric intake of less than 400 calories. These "starvation diets" should rarely be recommended, because of serious consequences including lean body mass loss, fluid and electrolyte abnormalities, decrease in resting metabolic rate, cardiac arrhythmias, and nutrient deficiencies (14). A VLCD is a diet with caloric intake between 400 and 800 calories a day, a significant reduction in calories. It is reserved for individuals with BMIs greater than 30, or BMIs greater than 27 in patients with comorbidities, and who have failed to lose weight with more conventional diets. Another term often used to describe this diet is *protein-sparing modified fast* (PSMF). A VLCD is indicated for persons in whom a rapid, substantial weight loss would ameliorate life-threatening conditions related to the obesity (14). For example, VLCDs have been used in bariatric surgery candidates in whom a preoperative reduction in weight might reduce significantly the operative risk (15).

The VLCDs are often commercially produced meal substitutes (such as shakes, hot beverages, nutrition bars, soups) that incorporate essential nutrients including the recommended daily allowance of vitamins, and are formulated as complete dietary replacements. Another approach to VLCDs is utilizing over-the-counter meal substitutes (beverages or nutrition bars are most common) for two meals a day, with the third meal composed of high-quality lean protein and vegetables. As an alternative to meal substitution, a careful diet plan using real food can be devised with the assistance of a dietitian, who can suggest weekly menu plans and grocery lists, as well as vitamin and mineral supplements. In the latter two instances, the protein intake should be from 1 to 1.5 g of protein per kilogram of ideal body weight per day, and multivitamins must be prescribed to prevent deficiencies. Patients must be monitored closely with clinician visits and laboratory evaluations. Potential complications of VLCDs are symptomatic cholelithiasis, cardiac arrhythmias, and exacerbation of underlying medical conditions. Common side effects include orthostatic hypotension, constipation, dry skin and brittle nails, hair loss, and menstrual irregularities.

The LCDs, which average 1 to 2 pounds a week of weight loss, are recommended to many overweight and obese individuals (6). They are diets ranging from 800 to 1500 calories a day. It remains unclear which type of LCD works best or is the most healthful. The more traditional LCD is a lower fat regimen, and includes lean protein, complex carbohydrates, and less than 30% fat. The Adult Treatment Panel II (ATP II; the second report of the Expert Panel on the Detection, Evaluation and Treatment of High Blood Cholesterol in Adults) has suggested a "step I" LCD (energy deficit of 500 to 1000 calories a day) with the following composition: total fat, 30% or less of total calories; protein, about 15% of total calories; and carbohydrates, 55% or more of total calories (15). Additional recommendations include a fiber intake of 20 to 30 g per day, a calcium intake of 1000 to 1500 mg per day, and a sodium intake of no more than 2400 mg per day. Included is the recommendation to consume five to nine servings of fruits and vegetables per day, because these higher-densities, lower-calorie foods are satisfying and therefore may encourage adherence. In addition to being helpful with weight loss, diets high in fruits, vegetables, and fiber have been shown to reduce the incidence of certain cancers and type 2 diabetes. Currently, only 1% of U.S. children are meeting all of the nutritional recommended daily allowance (RDA) guidelines, and only 30% are meeting the fruit and vegetable guidelines (16,17). In a study of children and parents, there was an improvement in percentage of subjects overweight at the end of the study in families whose only instruction was to eat more fruits and vegetables (18).

On some LCDs, individuals are instructed to eliminate certain foods, such as sweets. More recently, however, those on LCDs have been encouraged to include all foods, but practice portion control. Underestimation of serving sizes often sabotages attempts at weight loss. Although a serving size of fish, poultry, or beef is only 3 oz—the size of a deck of cards—restaurant portions are often several times larger. Therefore, education about portion sizes may decrease daily caloric intake by hundreds of calories. By practicing gauging by sight portions of various foods and by weighing or measuring foods when eating at home, patients learn how to judge appropriate serving sizes when eating out. These balanced deficit diets are modified versions of LCDs, with less restrictive daily caloric intakes.

Although the medical community has raised objections to low-carbohydrate diets, several recent studies suggest that both weight loss and maintenance are at least as, if not more, effective than the more conventional LCD described above, although a consensus has not yet been reached concerning recommendations of such diets (19–22). The regimens do not require calorie counting, but instead propose unrestricted quantities of protein, an "induction" phase in which only minimal quantities of carbohydrate (20 g/day, or 80 calories) are permitted, and some limitations on fat intake.

Health professionals should advise against "fad" diets, which may be dangerous, such as those that incorporate "cleansing" programs such as coffee enemas, or only one or two types of food, exemplified by the cabbage soup diet or the grapefruit diet. These diets not only may lead to nutritional deficiencies, dehydration, and electrolyte abnormalities, but also are so unpalatable that their use is usually short-lived and followed by rebound weight gain.

Exercise

The benefits of exercise in any weight loss regimen cannot be overemphasized. The greatest health advantages result when people exercise for 60 minutes, most days of the week (4 to 7 days), and there is evidence that lesser amounts are also beneficial. Moderate, consistent exercise without calorie deficit does not seem to result in weight loss, but has been shown to be a crucial factor in weight maintenance. During the weight-loss phase, increasing activity has been shown to enhance health by improving cardiovascular fitness and lipid metabolism, improving bone density, preventing or delaying the onset of type 2 diabetes mellitus, increasing lean body mass and strength, controlling depression and anxiety, promoting a sense of well-being, increasing resistance to infection, improving energy level and quality of sleep, and reducing symptoms of degenerative joint disease (DJD) (23–25).

Having patients complete activity questionnaires can help the clinician establish safe, realistic exercise goals and determine a patient's exercise preferences. The role of the clinician is to assess the patient's physical capabilities, reinforce the benefits of exercise, and help the patient ease into a medically safe exercise program.

Abnormalities in cardiac and pulmonary function may limit the patient's tolerance to exercise. Other impediments to exercise include hypertension, venous stasis disease, and degenerative joint disease as well as additional comorbidities of obesity. In this group of patients, recommending a rigorous exercise plan would be inappropriate and medically unsafe. A full assessment including pulmonary and cardiac evaluations is recommended for this population. An exercise stress test should be considered in asymptomatic individuals with diabetes mellitus or other cardiovascular risk factors (26).

Behavioral and Cognitive Strategies

Through a variety of techniques, based on the theory that behaviors are learned, and that thoughts leading to behaviors can be changed, overweight and obese individuals can be taught to recognize their less healthful behavior patterns with respect to eating and exercise and substitute more healthful ones that will eventually lead to weight loss, maintenance of lost weight, and improved health. Behavioral and cognitive therapies are goal oriented, and are often employed in combination in either group or individual settings. Even commercial weight loss programs use these approaches, incorporating a variety of strategies, including patient education, patient support, and problem solving. The ultimate challenge is to make these changes in thought and behavior durable. There is evidence that a variety of behavioral therapies as adjuncts to both weight loss and weight maintenance are effective, but that long-term efficacy depends on consistent, professional reinforcement of the new habits even after weight loss and throughout maintenance (6,27).

The first step to modifying behavior is the desire to change. Therefore, the clinician must first assess the patient's stage of readiness. This is especially true in a primary care setting, where patients' priorities are varied. The stages of readiness are precontemplation, when a person is not even thinking about change yet; contemplation, when a person has begun to think about change but is not yet prepared to act; preparation, when a person begins to get ready to act; action, when a person has begun to take the action necessary to make the change; and maintenance of the altered behavior. The action stage is often triggered by a defining moment, during which the patient experiences an epiphany that leads to a change in behavior.

A positive patient–clinician relationship can help enhance weight loss endeavors, especially if the patient has suffered the emotional consequences of discrimination or ostracism. Obese persons may feel alienated, which may lead to low self-esteem, shame, and reluctance to seek help. The relationship with the patient may be improved if the clinician employs the following tools: empathic communication; formation of a patient–clinician partnership; understanding one's own and the patient's cultural biases, values, and health beliefs regarding weight and nutrition; and promotion of respect, support, and acceptance of these patients. Patient education and behavior modification can be provided by a variety of health professionals such as primary clinicians, behavioral therapists, dietitians, and exercise physiologists.

Weight maintenance frequently is even more challenging than weight loss. There is substantial evidence that in the majority of individuals who actually reach or approach a goal weight, the lifestyle changes are often abandoned, supervision is discontinued, and weight regain occurs (6,27,28) usually to or even above previous levels. Many people do not know how to maintain lower weights, and believe they can revert to their old ways without regaining. Even after bariatric surgery, there can be weight regain because despite eating restrictions imposed by the altered anatomy, patients may learn to circumvent these limitations.

Evidence supports the continued role of health professionals after weight loss is accomplished (6). Although by the time weight is lost, individuals usually are cognizant of healthful diet and activity styles, it is not knowledge alone that predicts successful weight maintenance. The same evaluation and strategies described above should be sustained and reinforced, ideally with medical oversight. Long-term success is more likely in individuals who tend to eat an average of 1580 calories a day (24% fat, 19% protein, and 56% carbohydrates); eat five times a day, eat breakfast, eat out no more than three times a week, weigh themselves at least once a week, and continue an exercise regimen. Other predictors of success include continued self-monitoring, and continued contact with a health professional. Those who regain lost weight tend to participate in restrictive or inconsistent dietary patterns, have negative coping styles, experience unusual life stresses, and continue emotion-driven binge-eating patterns (29–32).

Pharmaceutical Interventions

Due to our growing understanding of the pathophysiology and pathogenesis of obesity, and the use of molecular biology to study energy balance, more than 150 new drugs are in developmental stages, with more than 44 now in human clinical trials at the time of this writing (33). As the extremely complex hormonal regulation of appetite and weight in normal-weight and obese individuals becomes understood, new pharmaceutical agents can be more precisely targeted along these regulatory pathways.

Medications are not recommended for use in isolation, but rather as adjuncts to diet, exercise, and behavioral modification. Patients who are optimal candidates for pharmacologic intervention have BMIs of 30 or greater, or BMIs of 27 or greater with comorbidities (6). Some experts recommend that medications be used only after a failure to lose a significant amount of weight after 6 months of nonpharmacologic therapies (6). In randomized, placebo-controlled trials, there have been reports of weight loss significantly greater with weight-loss medication when combined with lifestyle changes than with placebo, although differences are modest (6).

Efficacy is predicted by short-term outcome. Pharmacologic intervention is most likely to be successful (10% or more of body weight reduction after 12 months) if a patient loses 2 kg or more in the first month of use, or if the weight falls to 5% or more below baseline after 3 months of use (6,34). A satisfactory ultimate response to medication is considered a 10% loss; an excellent response is 15% or greater. Weight loss medication does not cure obesity; a rebound in weight is predictable when the medication is stopped, and, even if continued, the medication may lose some effectiveness.

Only a few of the medications have been approved for long-term use by the Food and Drug Administration (FDA); however, many bariatric specialists prescribe them off-label for long-term use and find them both effective and safe. Some specialists report excellent results and few adverse effects when the medications are used intermittently during both the weight loss and maintenance phases (33–37). However, neither long-term nor intermittent uses of most medications prescribed for weight loss are supported by clinical evidence.

In the past, drugs used for weight loss have been found to be unsafe and to pose clinical risk. Medications taken off the market include fenfluramine, which in the combination of phentermine/fenfluramine (phen-fen) was associated with a risk of valvular heart disease and pulmonary hypertension (38,39); dexfenfluramine (an isomer of fenfluramine), which was also associated with a higher risk of valvular disease and pulmonary hypertension (9,40); and phenylpropanolamine, an over-the-counter decongestant that was associated with an increased incidence of hemorrhagic stroke in women who used it (41). For a variety of reasons, multiple other medications are no longer used. These include thyroid hormone, dinitrophenol, dexamphetamine, amphetamine, digitalis, rainbow pills, human chorionic gonadotropin, dexfenfluramine, aminorex, and chlorphentermine.

Currently, pharmaceutical options include the pure sympathomimetic agents, which include the prototype, phentermine, as well as diethylpropion, phendimetrazine, benzphetamine, and ephedrine. All are noradrenergic, potentiating the release of norepinephrine, which binds to hypothalamic β-adrenergic receptors and, to a lesser extent, the release of dopamine. These medications all cause anorexia (a reduction in appetite) through an as yet unclear mechanism. Both phentermine and diethylpropion, which are the only ones approved by the FDA for the short-term treatment of obesity (up to 12 weeks), are schedule intravenous (IV) drugs and considered by the FDA to have addictive potential, although this potential seems to be quite low (33). Phentermine, the most frequently prescribed agent of its class, was shown to be efficacious in a 36-week, placebo-controlled trial. Caution must be exercised when a clinician chooses to prescribe any of these medications off-label, or differently from those uses approved by the FDA. A careful tracking mechanism should be in place, and each patient should sign an off-label consent form (9,33).

Sibutramine, a weight-loss medication which is FDA-approved for long-term use (9), is a serotonin and norepinephrine reuptake inhibitor that acts as an appetite suppressant and, in rodents, seems to have a thermogenic effect (not yet established in humans). Multiple other clinical trials have demonstrated efficacy of this medication. The major adverse reaction of sibutramine is an increase in diastolic blood pressure, even in the presence of significant weight loss, and even with the improvement of other parameters, such as low-density lipoprotein (LDL) and total cholesterol and hemoglobin A_{1c} (42,43).

Another class of agent that is FDA-approved for long-term use is exemplified by orlistat, which is in the nutrient-partitioning category. As a pancreatic lipase inhibitor, it alters fat metabolism by preventing hydrolysis of ingested fat to fatty acids and glycerol, thereby reducing the absorption of ingested fat by 33% (44). Since fat-soluble vitamins may be poorly absorbed with this medication, multiple vitamin supplementations are recommended. The efficacy has been established in placebo-controlled studies (45). A further benefit of orlistat is an improvement in serum lipid levels, which cannot be explained by weight loss alone (46). Major adverse reactions include fecal soiling, oiliness, and incontinence. The fact that the adverse effects increase as ingested fat increases may itself deter individuals from consuming fat-laden, calorie-dense foods. Orlistat, among other medications, is now being evaluated for use in overweight adolescents (9).

In patients with metabolic syndrome, PCO, insulin resistance, and type 2 diabetes, metformin is an optimal medication, because unlike other oral hypoglycemic agents, it not only does not cause weight gain, but also may result in some weight loss. It also improves insulin sensitivity as well as the lipid profile, and may delay the onset of overt diabetes mellitus.

Drugs with Potential that Are on the Horizon

Several new and promising agents that are not yet approved by the FDA are endogenously produced peptides. The discovery of leptin, a hormone secreted by adipocytes, caused initial excitement among researchers and in the press because the absence of it seemed to cause obesity in mice and the administration of it in these mice caused weight loss. However, when it was found that leptin levels are increased in obese humans, and that they suffer from leptin resistance, the excitement waned. Very large doses of leptin do seem to overcome this resistance (47). Glucagon-like peptide (a fragment of the hormone glucagon) may reduce food intake in humans (48). Although there is conflicting data on the weight loss actions of peptide YY, which is produced in the human gut, the substance has been shown to decrease appetite and food intake in both normal-weight and obese human subjects; caloric intake was reduced by as much as 30% in these subjects via suppression of serum levels of ghrelin, an appetite-stimulating hormone (49).

A medication called Axokine, which is a recombinant human modified variant of ciliary neurotrophic factor (CNTF), was associated with unintentional weight loss in some patients taking it for amyotrophic lateral sclerosis. This finding triggered a randomized clinical trial of obese subjects, in which Axokine produced dose-related weight losses (50). In another trial, many patients developed antibodies to this agent, which was then ineffective; however, it remained effective in those without the antibody response (50).

Rimonabant (SR141716), which is a cannabinoid receptor-1 antagonist, antagonizes cannabinoid hyperphagia in mice both by reducing food intake transiently and then by sustaining weight loss when food intake normalized, suggesting an increase in metabolic rate (51).

Research involving herbal supplements, such as green tea, guar gum, and hydroxycitric acid, has not yet ascertained that they result in significant weight loss. Ephedra, because of its serious adverse effects, was ultimately banned by the FDA (52).

Conclusion

In the United States, the incidence of overweight and obesity now affects the majority of the population. As obesity surpasses smoking as the major cause of mortality in the U.S., it becomes the epidemic of the new millennium. Despite extensive coverage in the media and the burgeoning of weight loss products and programs, the disturbing trend is not reversing. And although the numbers of bariatric practitioners are increasing, there is still a vast shortage of effective medical weight loss programs and medical professionals trained in bariatrics. Eradication of this new scourge will require a commitment as well as action from the community at large, the medical profession, insurance companies, academic institutions, school boards, corporations, politicians, and families.

References

1. Hedley AA, Ogden CL, Johnson CL, Carroll MD, Curtin LR, Flegal KM. Prevalence of overweight and obesity among US children, adolescents, and adults, 1999–2002. JAMA 2004;291:2847–2850.
2. Mokdad A, Marks J, Stroup D, Gerberding J. Actual causes of death in the Unites States, 2000. JAMA 2004;291:1238–1245.
3. Fontaine KR, Redden DT, Wang C, Westfall AO, Allison DB. Years of life lost due to obesity. JAMA 2003;289:187–193.
4. Dietz WH. Overweight in childhood and adolescence. N Engl J Med 2004;350:855–857.
5. Overweight, obesity, and health risk. National Task Force on the Prevention and Treatment of Obesity. Arch Intern Med 2000;160:898–904.
6. Lenfant C. Clinical Guidelines on the Identification, Evaluation, and Treatment of Overweight and Obesity in Adults: The Evidence Report. Bethesda: National Institutes of Health, 1998.
7. Savel RH, Gropper MA, Macura JM, Lazzaro RS. Management of the Critically Ill Obese Patient. www.uptodate.com, 2004.
8. Brolin RE. Gastric bypass. Surg Clin North Am 2001;81:1077–1095.
9. Yanovski SZ, Yanovski JA. Obesity. N Engl J Med 2002;346:591–602.
10. Methods for voluntary weight loss and control. NIH Technology Assessment Conference Panel. Consensus Development Conference, 30 March to 1 April 1992. Ann Intern Med 1993;119:764–770.
11. Roldan EO. Childhood and Adolescent Obesity—Treatment of the Obese Patient. American Board of Bariatric Medicine Review Course, Scottsdale, Arizona, May 5, 2004.
12. Grundy SM, Brewer HB Jr, Cleeman JI, Smith SC Jr, Lenfant C. Definition of metabolic syndrome: Report of the National Heart, Lung, and Blood Institute/American Heart Association conference on scientific issues related to definition. Circulation 2004;109:433–438.
13. Blackburn G. Effect of degree of weight loss on health benefits. Obes Res 1995;3(suppl 2):211s–216s.
14. National Task Force on the Prevention and Treatment of Obesity NIH. Very low-calorie diets. JAMA 1993;270:967–974.
15. National Cholesterol Education Program. Second Report of the Expert Panel on Detection, Evaluation, and Treatment of High Blood Cholesterol in Adults (Adult Treatment Panel II). Circulation 1994;89:1333–1445.
16. Munoz KA, Krebs-Smith SM, Ballard-Barbash R, Cleveland LE. Food intakes of US children and adolescents compared with recommendations. Pediatrics 1997;100:323–329.
17. Food and Nutrition Intakes by Children 1994–1996, 1998. U.S. Department of Agriculture, Agricultural Research Service, 1999:Table Set 17.
18. Epstein LH, Gordy CC, Raynor HA, Beddome M, Kilanowski CK, Paluch R. Increasing fruit and vegetable intake and decreasing fat and sugar intake in families at risk for childhood obesity. Obes Res 2001;9:171–178.
19. Daniels SR. Abnormal weight gain and weight management: are carbohydrates the enemy? J Pediatr 2003;142:225–227.
20. Brehm BJ, Seeley RJ, Daniels SR, D'Alessio DA. A randomized trial comparing a very low carbohydrate diet and a calorie-restricted low fat diet on body weight and cardiovascular risk factors in healthy women. J Clin Endocrinol Metab 2003;88:1617–1623.
21. Samaha FF, Iqbal N, Seshadri P, et al. A low-carbohydrate as compared with a low-fat diet in severe obesity. N Engl J Med 2003;348:2074–2081.
22. Foster GD, Wyatt HR, Hill JO, et al. A randomized trial of a low-carbohydrate diet for obesity. N Engl J Med 2003;348:2082–2090.

23. Slentz CA, Duscha BD, Johnson JL, et al. Effects of the amount of exercise on body weight, body composition, and measures of central obesity: STRRIDE—a randomized controlled study. Arch Intern Med 2004;164:31–39.

24. Ross R, Dagnone D, Jones PJ, et al. Reduction in obesity and related comorbid conditions after diet-induced weight loss or exercise-induced weight loss in men. A randomized, controlled trial. Ann Intern Med 2000;133:92–103.

25. Jakicic JM, Marcus BH, Gallagher KI, Napolitano M, Lang W. Effect of exercise duration and intensity on weight loss in overweight, sedentary women: a randomized trial. JAMA 2003;290:1323–1330.

26. Gibbons RJ, Balady GJ, Bricker JT, et al. ACC/AHA 2002 guideline update for exercise testing: summary article. A report of the American College of Cardiology/American Heart Association Task Force on Practice Guidelines (Committee to Update the 1997 Exercise Testing Guidelines). J Am Coll Cardiol 2002;40:1531–1540.

27. Wadden TA, Foster GD. Behavioral treatment of obesity. Med Clin North Am 2000;84:441–461, vii.

28. Methods for Voluntary Weight Loss and Control. Proceedings of NIH Technology Assessment Conference. Bethesda, Maryland, 30 March–1 April 1992. Ann Intern Med 1993; 119:641–770.

29. Fletcher AM. Thin for Life. Boston, Houghton Mifflin, 1994.

30. Klem ML, Wing RR, McGuire MT, Seagle HM, Hill JO. A descriptive study of individuals successful at long-term maintenance of substantial weight loss. Am J Clin Nutr 1997;66:239–246.

31. Shick SM, Wing RR, Klem ML, McGuire MT, Hill JO, Seagle H. Persons successful at long-term weight loss and maintenance continue to consume a low calorie, low fat diet. J Am Dietetic Assoc 1998;98:408–413.

32. McGuire MT, Wing RR, Klem ML, Seagle HM, Hill JO. Long-term maintenance of weight loss: do people who lose weight through various weight loss methods use different behaviors to maintain their weight? Int J Obes 1998;22:572–577.

33. Hendricks EJ. Pharmacotherapy—Treatment of the Obese Patient, 2004 American Board of Bariatric Medicine Review Course, Scottsdale, Arizona, 2004.

34. Obesity National Task Force on the Prevention and Treatment of Obesity. Long-term pharmacotherapy in the management of obesity. JAMA 1996;276:1907–1915.

35. Munro JF, MacCuish AC, Wilson EM, Duncan LJ. Comparison of continuous and intermittent anorectic therapy in obesity. Br Med J 1968;1:352.

36. Stallone DD. Long-term use of appetite suppressant medications: rationale and recommendations. Drug Dev Res 1992;26:1–20.

37. Stafford RS, Radley DC. National trends in antiobesity medication use. Arch Intern Med 2003;163:1046–1050.

38. Jick H, Vasilakis C, Weinrauch LA, Meier CR, Jick SS, Derby LE. A population-based study of appetite-suppressant drugs and the risk of cardiac-valve regurgitation. N Engl J Med 1998;339:719–724.

39. Khan MA, Herzog CA, St Peter JV, et al. The prevalence of cardiac valvular insufficiency assessed by transthoracic echocardiography in obese patients treated with appetite-suppressant drugs. N Engl J Med 1998;339:713–718.

40. Weissman NJ, Tighe JF Jr, Gottdiener JS, Gwynne JT. An assessment of heart-valve abnormalities in obese patients taking dexfenfluramine, sustained-release dexfenfluramine, or placebo. Sustained-Release Dexfenfluramine Study Group. N Engl J Med 1998;339:725–732.

41. Kernan WN, Viscolli CM, Brass LM, et al. Phenylpropanolamine and the risk of hemorrhagic stroke. N Engl J Med 2000;343:1826.

42. Bray GA, Blackburn GL, Ferguson JM, et al. Sibutramine produces dose-related weight loss. Obes Res 1999;7:189–198.

43. Fujioka K, Seaton TB, Rowe E, et al. Weight loss with sibutramine improves glycaemic control and other metabolic parameters in obese patients with type 2 diabetes mellitus. Diabetes Obes Metab 2000;2:175–187.

44. Guerciolini R. Mode of action of orlistat. Int J Obes Relat Metab Disord 1997;21(suppl 3):S12–23.

45. Heck AM, Yanovski JA, Calis KA. Orlistat, a new lipase inhibitor for the management of obesity. Pharmacotherapy 2000;20:270–279.

46. Tonstad S, Pometta D, Erkelens DW, et al. The effect of the gastrointestinal lipase inhibitor, orlistat, on serum lipids and lipoproteins in patients with primary hyperlipidaemia. Eur J Clin Pharmacol 1994;46:405–410.

47. Hukshorn CJ, Saris WH, Westerterp-Plantenga MS, Farid AR, Smith FJ, Campfield LA. Weekly subcutaneous pegylated recombinant native human leptin (PEG-OB) administration in obese men. J Clin Endocrinol Metab 2000;85:4003–4009.

48. Flint A, Raben A, Astrup A, Holst JJ. Glucagon-like peptide 1 promotes satiety and suppresses energy intake in humans. J Clin Invest 1998;101:515–520.

49. Batterham RL, Cohen MA, Ellis SM, et al. Inhibition of food intake in obese subjects by peptide YY3–36. N Engl J Med 2003;349:941–948.

50. Ettinger MP, Littlejohn TW, Schwartz SL, et al. Recombinant variant of ciliary neurotrophic factor for weight loss in obese adults: a randomized, dose-ranging study. JAMA 2003;289:1826–1832.

51. Cota D, Marsicano G, Tschop M, et al. The endogenous cannabinoid system affects energy balance via central orexigenic drive and peripheral lipogenesis. J Clin Invest 2003; 112:423–431.

52. Bent S, Tiedt TN, Odden MC, Shlipak MG. The relative safety of ephedra compared with other herbal products. Ann Intern Med 2003;138:468–471.

3
Evolution of Bariatric Minimally Invasive Surgery

Iselin Austrheim-Smith, Stacy A. Brethauer, Tomasz Rogula, and Bruce M. Wolfe

The present state of minimally invasive bariatric surgery is the result of separate but parallel progress in the fields of bariatric surgery and minimally invasive surgery, with the ultimate combination of the two. Thus, minimally invasive surgery evolved from its early beginnings to the performance of advanced laparoscopic procedures, prior to the establishment and acceptance of the techniques for minimally invasive bariatric surgery. Similarly, bariatric surgery evolved substantially such that the establishment of bariatric surgical procedures using minimally invasive techniques was initially a matter of adapting accepted bariatric surgical procedures to the minimally invasive methodology.

History

The recognition that morbid obesity is a life-threatening disease that produces multiple comorbidities, which is well established at the present time, evolved slowly. Prior to the development of modern medicine, it was considered a sign of affluence and prestige to be overweight, if not morbidly obese. Early attempts to control obesity in the modern era of medicine and surgery were dominated by jaw wiring (1). While conceptually understandable, jaw wiring proved unsuccessful because it still allowed patients to consume high-calorie liquids. In addition, the teeth could not withstand permanent wiring of the jaws so it would have to be reversed at some point. Other associated issues included difficulty in maintaining oral hygiene, dental infection, danger of vomiting, difficulty with upper respiratory infection, local pain, loosening of wires, and high rate of weight regain (1). Thus, one of the most critical concepts of bariatric surgery was recognized: the requirement for a permanent procedure with permanent protection or action against recurrent obesity.

Induction of Malabsorption

The modern era of bariatric surgery began in the 1950s with the concept that limiting the length of the small intestine by surgical induction of short bowel syndrome and secondary malabsorption would represent an optimal approach to accomplishment and maintenance of major weight loss in patients with morbid obesity (2,3). Jejunocolic bypass was initially performed (Fig. 3-1), but it uniformly caused excessive malabsorption and related complications such as uncontrollable diarrhea, dehydration, electrolyte imbalance, and liver dysfunction. The jejunocolic surgery was abandoned and the operations ultimately revised to a jejunoileal bypass (Fig. 3-2). This new procedure achieved widespread popularity in the late 1960s and early 1970s despite a lack of scientific study of its mechanisms of action and relatively high complication rates (4). Although long-term weight loss was variable, 65% of patients maintained a mean loss of ≥50% of excess weight (4). Jejunoileal bypass laid the foundation for malabsorptive procedures and helped shape bariatric surgery (5).

Actual Mechanisms of Action

Malabsorption was created by a surgically induced short gut syndrome, so it was originally thought that diarrhea was the cause of weight loss. However, due to rectal complications and intense anal irritation, it was determined that the actual cause of weight loss was the diminished caloric intake in an attempt to alleviate the diarrhea (6). This idea was confirmed with careful metabolic balance studies done in the mid-1970s, in which the reduced intake accounted for the majority of the weight loss in patients with intestinal bypasses (7,8). This diminished intake was due not only to diarrhea but also to a change in eating habits representing a learned behavior (6). The patients soon learned that if they were to control their diarrhea sufficiently to be able to function in society, they could consume only minimal fat and minimal nutrients prior to venturing out of their homes. In addition, a major reduction of total intake, particularly fat intake, was required to avoid excessive loss of electrolytes and also reported. Other nutrient deficiencies developed over a longer interval of time, including vitamin deficiency with secondary neuropathies and bone demineralization and protein malnutrition. Additional complications of the intestinal bypass, which seemed to be partially due to bacterial activity in the bypassed intestine, included hepatic decomposition and arthritis. Alterations of luminal calcium, fatty acid, and oxalate absorption led to paradoxical hyperabsorption of ingested oxalate and secondary nephrolithiasis or chronic renal failure (6). Scopinaro et al. (9) performed studies that showed that most of the undesirable side effects of the jejunoileal bypass were caused by toxins from bacterial overgrowth in the unused excluded bowel. As adaptation to the short gut syndrome progressed, the capacity to digest and absorb carbohydrate remarkably increased. Patients would thus experience cessation of weight loss and variable regain of weight, in some cases back to the original weight, despite continued malabsorption of certain nutrients, hepatic decomposition, arthritis, and nephrolithiasis (6). This failed experience with a purely malabsorptive procedure must not be forgotten when devising new bariatric surgical procedures.

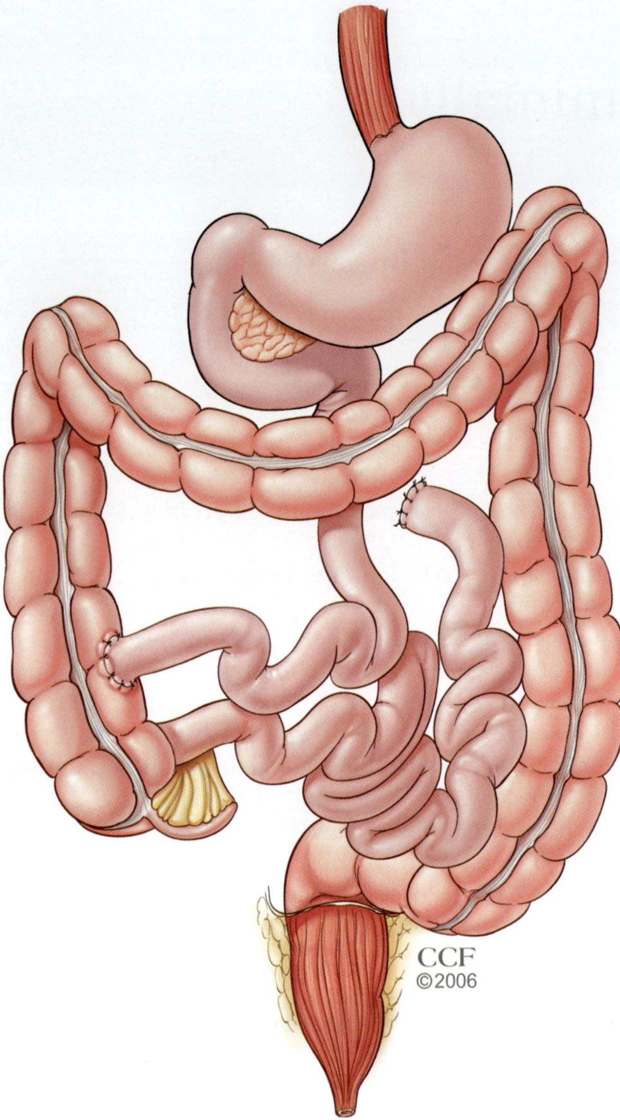

FIGURE 3-1. Jejunocolic bypass. (Courtesy of the Cleveland Clinic Foundation.)

minerals, with resultant life-threatening hypokalemia, hypocalcemia, and other deficiencies. The role of neuroendocrine signals resulting from the presence of luminal nutrients in the distal gut remains incompletely studied, but it serves as a promising mechanism for stimulating diminished intake.

Complications

While frequent diarrhea and flatulence were major social problems for the patients, it was in fact the incidence of unacceptable complications that forced a purely malabsorptive approach to bariatric surgery to be abandoned. Specifically, loss of potassium, calcium, and magnesium were a constant threat and frequently led to rehospitalization. Deaths due to losses of these electrolytes were

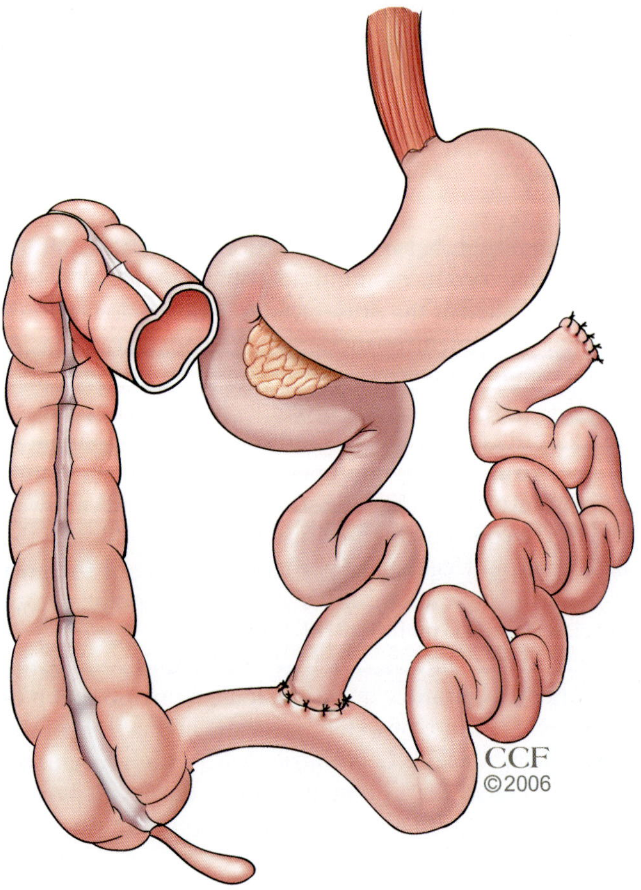

FIGURE 3-2. Jejunoileal bypass. (Courtesy of the Cleveland Clinic Foundation.)

Gastric Restriction

In response to the popularity and widespread application of intestinal bypass for morbid obesity and the associated complication and mortality rates, in 1966 Mason and Ito (10) at the University of Iowa set out to devise an entirely different conceptual approach to bariatric surgery, resulting in gastric restriction. They had observed that women who had undergone partial gastrectomy for peptic ulcer disease had difficulty gaining weight and therefore remained underweight. The initial procedure that they performed involved the creation of a small 100- to 150-mL gastric pouch with a Billroth II–type loop gastrojejunostomy (Fig. 3-3). In the late 1970s, conversion of the Billroth II gastrectomy into a Roux-en-Y anastomosis became a very common procedure in an effort to combat bile reflux esophagitis and gastritis (11). In 1979, Mason began performing the gastric bypass, creating a smaller gastric pouch, gastric transection, and the use of a jejunal Roux-en-Y limb of various lengths.

Gastroplasty

Early in their experience, Mason and others became concerned about the immediate postoperative complications

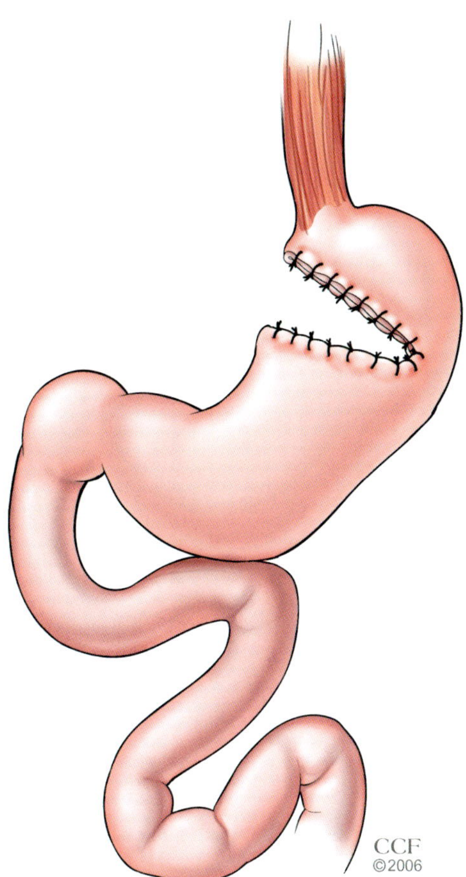

FIGURE 3-4. Gastroplasty with horizontal partial transection. (Courtesy of the Cleveland Clinic Foundation.)

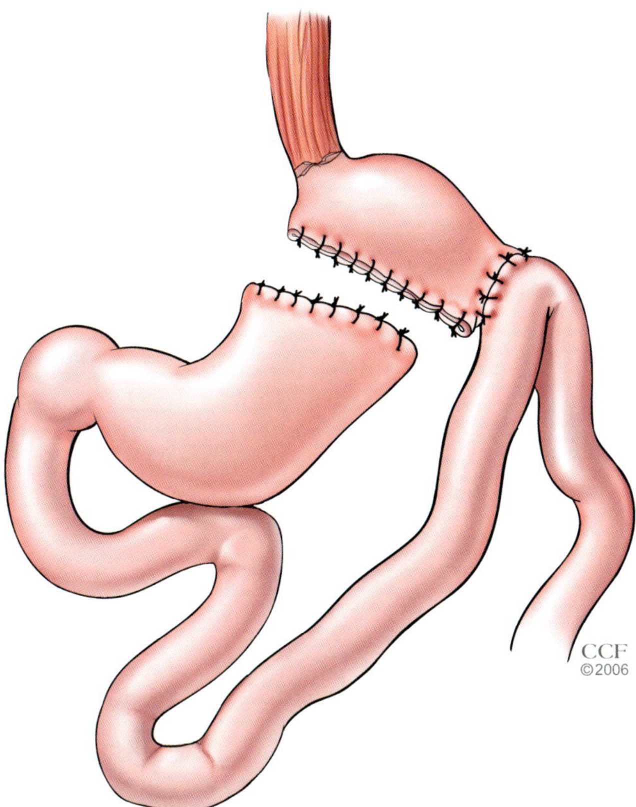

FIGURE 3-3. Gastric bypass with loop gastrojejunostomy as performed by Mason and Ito (10). (Courtesy of the Cleveland Clinic Foundation.)

that followed the early gastric bypass procedures. Therefore, efforts were made to establish gastric restrictive procedures based on various types of gastroplasty. Various relatively simple procedures were devised in which stomach partitioning was done (Fig. 3-4) (12,13). In the late 1970s, gastric restrictive operations became the choice of most bariatric surgeons because they were relatively safe and proved to be generally effective, at least in the short term (11).

Introduced in 1971, gastroplasty was developed with the idea of controlling energy intake by creating a small upper stomach to limit food and liquid intake and small outlet to limit the rate of passage of food and liquid into the intestine (6). Gastroplasty does have advantages over gastric bypass, such as the ease of performing the operation and its associated safety. In contrast, the gastroplasty does require more careful control over food choices as it lacks the malabsorptive component of the gastric bypass (6). Dilation of the pouch and stoma, between the gastric partition and body of the stomach, was thought to be the reason for the rapid failure of these procedures. As a result of inadequate weight loss, revisions of the gastroplasty were common. In response, Mason and others developed the vertical banded gastroplasty (Fig. 3-5), a

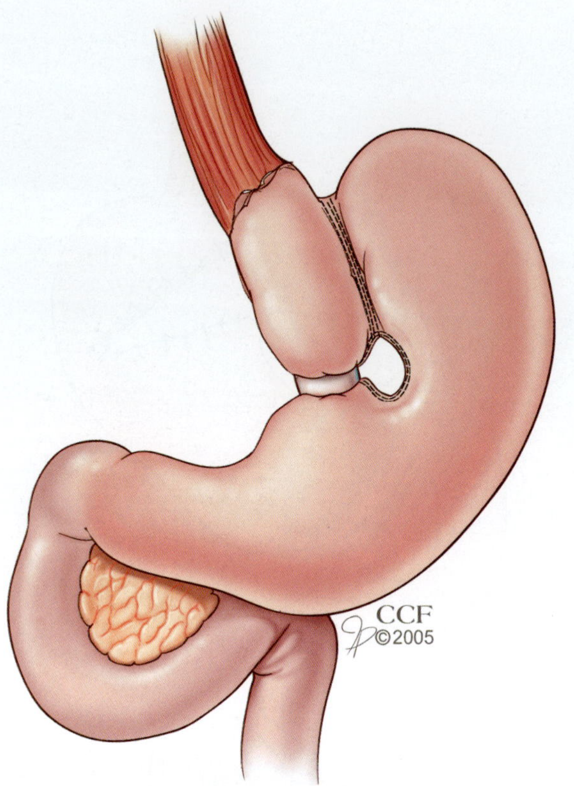

FIGURE 3-5. Vertical banded gastroplasty. (Courtesy of the Cleveland Clinic Foundation.)

Combined Malabsorptive and Restrictive Procedures

The next generation of malabsorptive procedures was mainly dominated by two procedures: the biliopancreatic diversion and the duodenal switch. Scopinaro et al. (9) developed the biliopancreatic diversion, drawing on the concept that the combination of gastric restriction and malabsorptive components to a bariatric surgical procedure would lead to superior weight loss compared to the gastric bypass. They hypothesized that the unacceptable complications of intestinal bypass could be prevented by avoiding the stagnant lumen of the intestinal bypass and maintaining the forward flow of bile and pancreatic juice in the bypassed limb. Scopinaro et al. (16) began working with dogs to develop a malabsorptive procedure that would correct morbid obesity without the undesirable side effects of the jejunoileal bypass. Based on these experimental studies, the biliopancreatic diversion (BPD) was developed to consist of a partial gastrectomy and distal mixing of ingested nutrients with bile and pan-

partitioning of the stomach with reinforcement by either a ring of prosthetic mesh or Silastic ring of the stoma between the partition and body of the stomach.

Vertical Banded Gastroplasty

Vertical banded gastroplasty (VBG) came to be the predominant bariatric procedure in the United States in the mid- to late 1980s. Unsatisfactory long-term weight loss in the VBG patients led to several randomized trials comparing gastric bypass to VBG (14,15). These studies uniformly showed superior weight loss following gastric bypass compared to VBG and led to the transition to Roux-en-Y gastric bypass as the predominant bariatric surgical procedure in the mid-1990s.

Gastric Banding

Gastric banding was first performed during the early 1980s by Wilkinson and Peloso, Kolle and Molina, and Oria (Fig. 3-6) (5). The original procedure used a fixed band to create a narrow gastric outlet. This procedure currently involves the placement of an inflatable silicone band around the upper stomach, which, connected to a subcutaneous port, allow for adjustments to the band (Fig. 3-7).

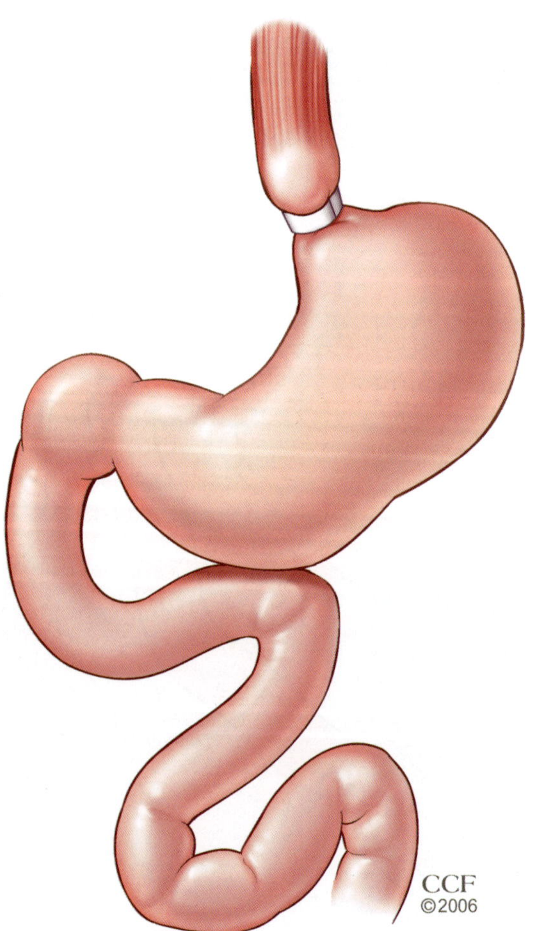

FIGURE 3-6. Nonadjustable gastric banding. (Courtesy of the Cleveland Clinic Foundation.)

creatic juice. This delayed digestion and absorption of nutrients added a malabsorptive component to the restriction of the partial gastrectomy (Fig. 3-8).

The BPD was modified by Marceau et al. (17) and Hess and Hess (18) to include a duodenal switch (DS) in which the partial gastrectomy preserved the pylorus by creating an anastomosis of the long Roux-en-Y limb to the postpyloric duodenum (Fig. 3-9) (17,18).

Further research is required to determine the mechanisms of action by which any of these bariatric procedures produce and maintain weight loss. Restrictive procedures physically limit the amount that can be ingested at one time but also stimulate learned behavior changes by negative feedback of an unpleasant experience if the small gastric pouch is overdistended or vomiting occurs. Dumping symptoms and diarrhea also stimulate learned behaviors. Malabsorption of macronutrients can contribute to weight loss by stimulating neuroendocrine signals to appetite and satiety centers of the central nervous system (CNS).

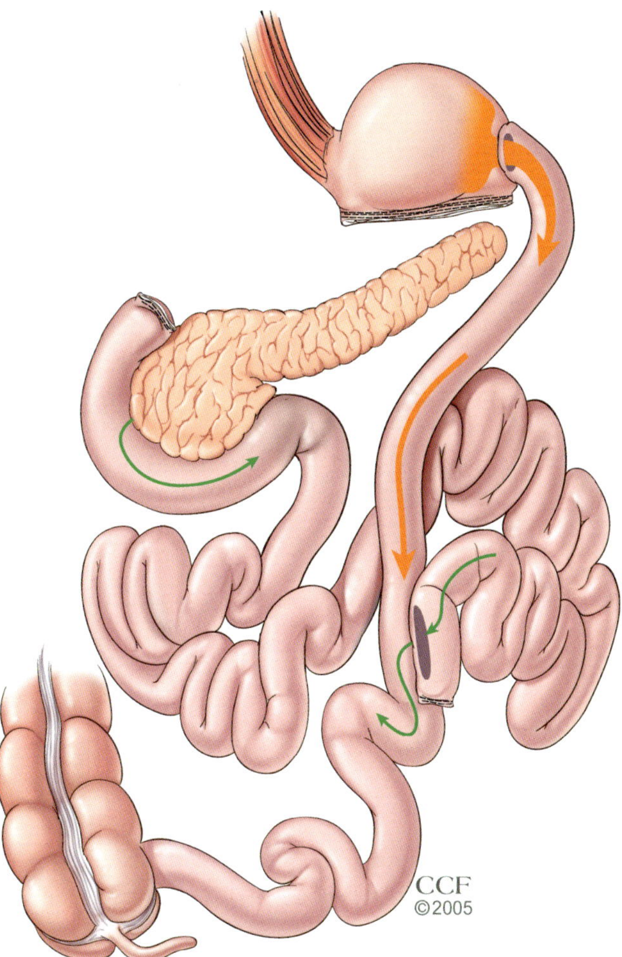

Figure 3-8. Biliopancreatic diversion. (Courtesy of the Cleveland Clinic Foundation.)

Minimally Invasive Bariatric Surgery

Minimally invasive techniques emerged in bariatric surgery in the early 1990s, and the first operations performed laparoscopically were gastric restriction procedures. Initial reports consisted of placement of a fixed, Silastic gastric band in 1993 (19) followed by laparoscopic placement of an adjustable gastric band (20). Results of these procedures were comparable to those of the open technique, but adjustments in technique were necessary to minimize complications related to improper band placement or slippage. Considerable experience with laparoscopic adjustable gastric banding (LAGB) has accrued since these early reports, and the current method utilizes the pars flaccida technique to minimize the incidence of gastric prolapse through the band (21). The LAGB was approved for use in the United States in 2001 and is growing in popularity due to less technical difficulty compared to gastric bypass and low morbidity and mortality rates.

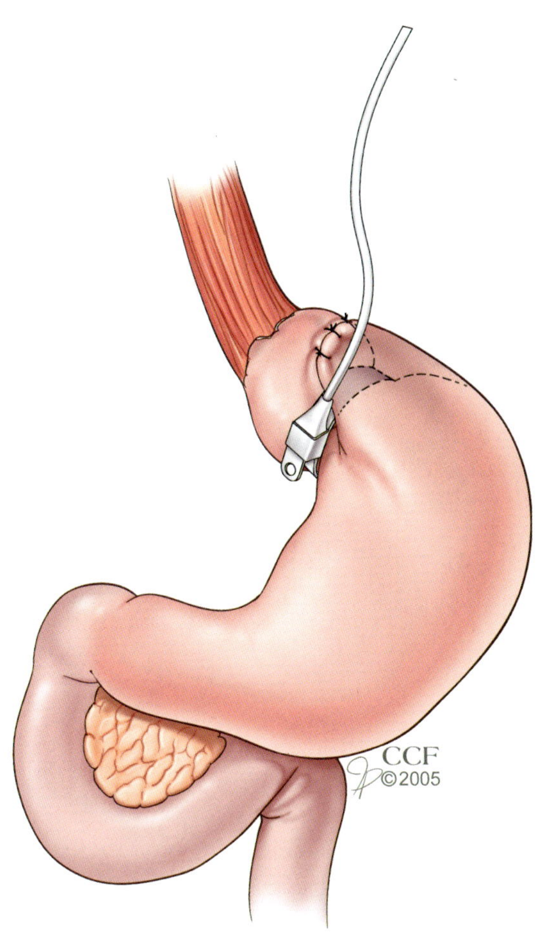

Figure 3-7. Laparoscopic adjustable gastric banding. (Courtesy of the Cleveland Clinic Foundation.)

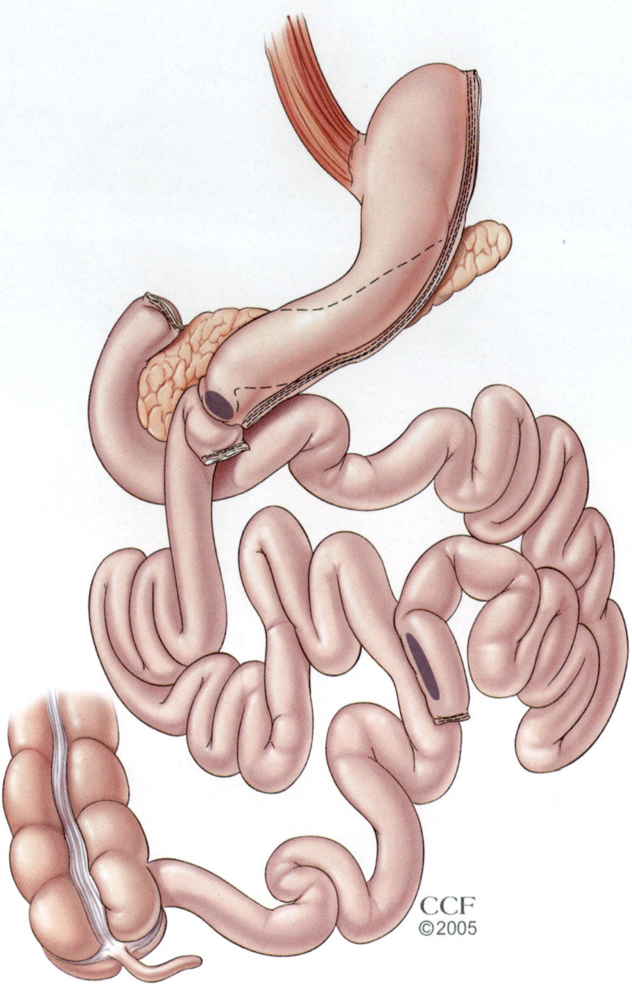

FIGURE 3-9. Duodenal switch. (Courtesy of the Cleveland Clinic Foundation.)

Over the last four decades, there have been many different bypass procedures attempted, but the Roux-en-Y gastric bypass has prevailed as the most effective and durable of these. Given the advantages of laparoscopy with other general surgery procedures, it was a logical step to attempt gastric bypass using a minimally invasive approach. The feasibility of the laparoscopic gastric bypass was demonstrated by Wittgrove et al. (22) in 1994. Small series in the late 1990s followed this initial study and reported weight loss and comorbidity resolution similar to those of the open approach (23,24). Since that time there have been several large studies demonstrating the safety and efficacy of laparoscopic Roux-en-Y gastric bypass (RYGB) (25–29) and three randomized controlled trials comparing laparoscopic RYGB to open RYGB (30–32). Some authors have advocated the use of hand-assisted laparoscopic gastric bypass to overcome the steep learning curve with this procedure (33–35). Although techniques for specific parts of the operation differ among studies, the laparoscopic RYGB replicates

the open procedure from an anatomical standpoint (Fig. 3-10). The type of gastrojejunal anastomosis performed varies, but primarily includes three common techniques. The originally described method of transoral placement of the anvil for a circular stapled anastomosis is still used by Wittgrove with a low complication rate. Other techniques (hand-sewn or linear stapler) have been developed, but this has been less of an evolution than a matter of surgeon preference and experience.

The first laparoscopic BPD/DS was performed by Gagner in 1999. There are currently seven series (with 467 patients total) demonstrating the feasibility of laparoscopic BPD or DS (36). These procedures are technically difficult and are performed by only a few surgeons who have extensive experience with the open procedure. The largest series by Rabkin et al. (37) (345 patients) used a hand-assisted technique. Laparoscopic BPD/DS

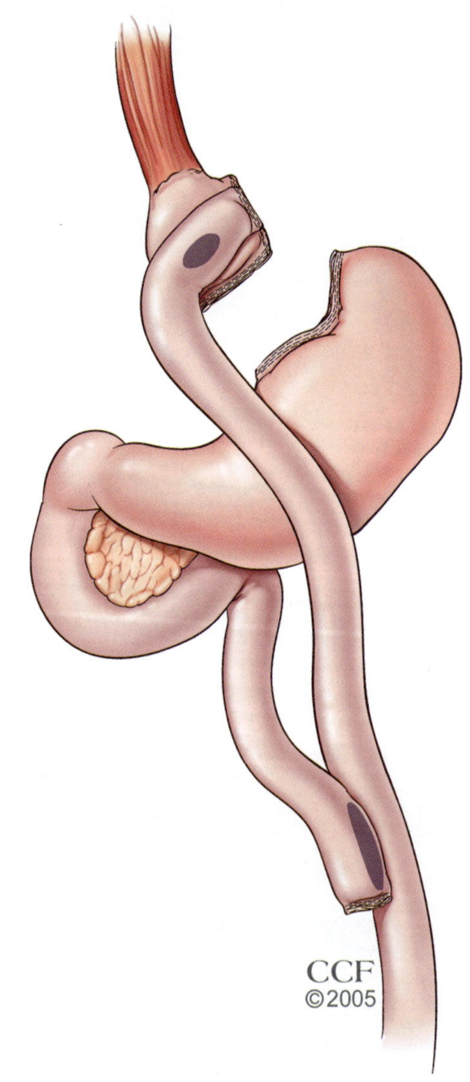

FIGURE 3-10. Roux-en-Y gastric bypass. (Courtesy of the Cleveland Clinic Foundation.)

has a higher complication rate compared to gastric bypass or banding and a mortality rate as high as 5% (36). More experience is needed with this procedure before adequate comparisons can be made to other laparoscopic bariatric procedures.

Other minimally invasive bariatric procedures have been developed as well. Laparoscopic placement of gastric pacing leads has been evaluated in the United States and Europe. This procedure has resulted in approximately 20% excess weight loss at 2 years with better results in carefully selected patients (38). Endoscopic intragastric balloon placement can be used as a primary weight loss procedure in conjunction with dietary modifications (39) but has also been used effectively to produce short-term weight loss prior to bariatric or other procedures (40).

In the next decade, there will be many new developments in bariatric surgery. The evolution of minimally invasive weight loss surgery is still in its early stages and there are many opportunities to improve on existing procedures and develop new ones. As new technologies emerge, endoluminal and transgastric procedures will be tested to achieve weight loss with reduced morbidity.

References

1. Rodgers S, Burnet R, Goss A, et al. Jaw wiring in treatment of obesity. Lancet 1977;1:1221–1222.
2. Kremen AJ, Linner JH, Nelson CH. An experimental evaluation of the nutritional importance of proximal and distal small intestine. Ann Surg 1954;140:439–448.
3. Rucker RD Jr, Chan EK, Horstmann J, Chute EP, Varco RL, Buchwald H. Searching for the best weight reduction operation. Surgery 1984;96:624–631.
4. Deitel M. Overview of operations for morbid obesity. World J Surg 1998;22:913–918.
5. Buchwald H. Overview of bariatric surgery. J Am Coll Surg 2002;194(3):367–375.
6. Mason EE. Surgical Treatment of Obesity. Philadelphia, London, Toronto: WB Saunders, 1981.
7. Bray GA, Barry RE, Benfield JR, Castelnuovo-Tedesco P, Rodin J. Intestinal bypass surgery for obesity decreases food intake and taste preferences. Am J Clin Nutr 1976; 29:779–783.
8. Condon SC, Janes NJ, Wise L, Alpers DH. Role of caloric intake in the weight loss after jejunoileal bypass for obesity. Gastroenterology 1978;74:34–37.
9. Scopinaro N, Gianetta E, Civalleri D, Bonalumi U, Bachi V. Bilio-pancreatic bypass for obesity: II. Initial experience in man. Br J Surg 1979;66:618–620.
10. Mason EE, Ito C. Gastric bypass in obesity. Surg Clin North Am 1967;47(6):1345–1351.
11. Deitel M. Surgery for the Morbidly Obese Patient. Philadelphia: Lea & Febiger, 1989.
12. Gomez CA. Gastroplasty in the surgical treatment of morbid obesity. Am J Clin Nutr 1980;33(2 suppl):406–415.
13. Pace WG, Martin EW Jr, Tetirick T, Fabri PJ, Carey LC. Gastric partitioning for morbid obesity. Ann Surg 1979;190: 392–400.
14. Sugerman HJ, Londrey GL, Kellum JM, et al. Weight loss with vertical banded gastroplasty and Roux-Y gastric bypass for morbid obesity with selective versus random assignment. Am J Surg 1989;157:93–102.
15. Hall JC, Watts JM, O'Brien PE, et al. Gastric surgery for morbid obesity. The Adelaide Study. Ann Surg 1990;211: 419–427.
16. Scopinaro N, Gianetta E, Civalleri D, Bonalumi U, Bachi V. Bilio-pancreatic bypass for obesity: I. An experimental study in dogs. Br J Surg 1979;66(9):613–617.
17. Marceau P, Hould FS, Potvin M, Lebel S, Biron S, Biliopancreatic diversion (duodenal switch procedure). Eur J Gastroenterol Hepatol 1999;11(2):99–103.
18. Hess DS, Hess DW. Biliopancreatic diversion with a duodenal switch. Obes Surg 1998;8:267–282.
19. Catona A, Gossenberg M, La Manna A, Mussini G. Laparoscopic gastric banding: preliminary series. Obes Surg 1993; 3(2):207–209.
20. Catona A, La Manna L, La Manna A, Sampiero C. Swedish adjustable gastric banding: a preliminary experience. Obes Surg 1997;7(3):203–205; discussion 206.
21. O'Brien PE, Dixon JB, Laurie C, Anderson M. A prospective randomized trial of placement of the laparoscopic adjustable gastric band: comparison of the perigastric and pars flaccida pathways. Obes Surg 2005;15(6):820–826.
22. Wittgrove AC, Clark GW, Tremblay LJ. Laparoscopic gastric bypass, Roux-en-Y: preliminary report of five cases. Obes Surg 1994;4(4):353–357.
23. Wittgrove AC, Clark GW. Laparoscopic gastric bypass, Roux-en-Y: experience of 27 cases, with 3–18 months follow-up. Obes Surg 1996;6(1):54–57.
24. Wittgrove AC, Clark GW, Schubert KR. Laparoscopic gastric bypass, Roux-en-Y: technique and results in 75 patients with 3–30 months follow-up. Obes Surg 1996;6(6):500–504.
25. DeMaria EJ, Sugerman HJ, Kellum JM, et al. Results of 281 consecutive total laparoscopic Roux-en-Y gastric bypasses to treat morbid obesity. Ann Surg 2002;235(5):640–645; discussion 645–647.
26. Higa KD, Ho T, Boone KB. Laparoscopic Roux-en-Y gastric bypass: technique and 3-year follow-up. J Laparoendosc Adv Surg Tech A 2001;11(6):377–382.
27. Papasavas PK, Hayetian FD, Caushaj PF, et al. Outcome analysis of laparoscopic Roux-en-Y gastric bypass for morbid obesity. The first 116 cases. Surg Endosc 2002; 16(12):1653–1657.
28. Schauer PR, Ikramuddin S, Gourash W, et al. Outcomes after laparoscopic Roux-en-Y gastric bypass for morbid obesity. Ann Surg 2000;232(4):515–529.
29. Wittgrove AC, Clark GW. Laparoscopic gastric bypass, Roux-en-Y—500 patients: technique and results, with 3–60 month follow-up. Obes Surg 2000;10(3):233–239.
30. Lujan JA, Frutos MD, Hernandez Q, et al. Laparoscopic versus open gastric bypass in the treatment of morbid obesity: a randomized prospective study. Ann Surg 2004; 239(4):433–437.
31. Nguyen NT, Goldman C, Rosenquist CJ, et al. Laparoscopic versus open gastric bypass: a randomized study of out-

comes, quality of life, and costs. Ann Surg 2001;234(3): 279–289; discussion 289–291.

32. Westling A, Gustavsson S. Laparoscopic vs open Roux-en-Y gastric bypass: a prospective, randomized trial. Obes Surg 2001;11(3):284–292.

33. Rodriguez DI, Jackson JD Jr, Delcambre JB, et al. Hand-assisted laparoscopic (HAL) gastric partition with roux-en-Y intestinal bypass. Surg Technol Int 2004;12:87–102.

34. Gould JC, Needleman BJ, Ellison EC, et al. Evolution of minimally invasive bariatric surgery. Surgery 2002;132(4): 565–571; discussion 571–572.

35. Sundbom M, Gustavsson S. Hand-assisted laparoscopic Roux-en-Y gastric bypass: aspects of surgical technique and early results. Obes Surg 2000;10(5):420–427.

36. Gagner M, Matteotti R. Laparoscopic biliopancreatic diversion with duodenal switch. Surg Clin North Am 2005; 85(1):141–149, x–xi.

37. Rabkin RA, Rabkin JM, Metcalf B, et al. Laparoscopic technique for performing duodenal switch with gastric reduction. Obes Surg 2003;13(2):263–268.

38. Shikora SA. "What are the Yanks doing?" the U.S. experience with implantable gastric stimulation (IGS) for the treatment of obesity—update on the ongoing clinical trials. Obes Surg 2004;14(suppl 1):S40–48.

39. Hodson RM, Zacharoulis D, Goutzamani E, et al. Management of obesity with the new intragastric balloon. Obes Surg 2001;11(3):327–329.

40. Doldi SB, Micheletto G, Di Prisco F, et al. Intragastric balloon in obese patients. Obes Surg 2000;10(6):578–581.

4
Essential Characteristics of the Successful Bariatric Surgeon: Skills, Knowledge, Advocacy

James C. Rosser, Jr. and Liza Eden Giammaria

The age-adjusted prevalence of overweight and obesity in the United States of adults of ages 20 to 74 reveals the tremendous challenge that faces modern society. According to the National Health and Nutrition Examination Study II (NHANES II) from 1976 to 1980, 47% of the above age group were overweight [body mass index (BMI) ≥25] and 15% were obese (BMI ≥30). The NHANES III (1988–94) found that 56% were overweight and 23% were obese. The NHANES IV (1999–2000) found that 64% were overweight and 31% were obese. More recent data do not offer any encouragement that this trend will be reversed in the near future (1).

The prevalence is high in many ethnic minorities, especially women who are African American, Mexican American, Native American, Pacific Islanders, Puerto Ricans, and Cuban Americans. Compounding this alarming trend is the fact that these minority groups are growing in number in the United States. Therefore, this health care issue must be addressed as quickly as possible. In addition, this is not just a problem in the United States. The prevalence of obesity continues to increase in many countries around the world; it is the price that is paid for social evolution and development. Nutrition and fitness countermeasures must be part of a long-range plan to achieve an ultimate solution. Unfortunately, these initiatives will not show results for some time to come. For those already stricken, this disease is aggressively resistant to dietary and exercise intervention, and these patients need help now.

All of this translates into a tremendous number of patients eligible for a lifesaving weight loss surgical procedure. Fourteen million people in the United States have a BMI of 36 to 39, but only those who have obesity-related comorbidities are currently candidates for surgical therapy. Even with this restriction this represents a large number of individuals. Furthermore, eight million people have a BMI of 40 or above (1). Clearly a large segment of the U.S. population is eligible for weight loss surgery now. With several high-profile celebrities publicly disclosing that they chose a surgical option for the treatment of their obesity, the stigma associated with this treatment has eased. Subsequently, weight-loss surgery is rapidly gaining popularity and generating skyrocketing consumer demand. From 2000 to 2001, the number of cases increased from 55,000 to 77,000. In 2002 a total of 116,000 procedures were done, with 15,000 of these being laparoscopic adjustable band procedures. The number of procedures for 2004 was 140,000, with perhaps 25,000 being bands. Current data suggest that this trend has continued with over 200,000 procedures performed in 2006.

The number of surgeons qualified to perform this procedure safely is in no way increasing as fast as demand. In the year 2000 there were approximately 500 general surgeons who included bariatrics as a major component of their practice. This increased to 696 in 2001, 865 in 2002, 1143 in 2003, and over 1500 in 2004. Many have theorized that high-volume centers could expand capacity and cover the demand. But this is not a likely scenario because the average high-volume center can increase capacity by only 33% each year. In addition, there is a trend for these procedures to be done with the laparoscopic approach. As reported by Schauer et al. (2), the learning curve associated with this procedure is probably the steepest of any minimally invasive operation to date. This increase in the required skill level further hinders efforts to train more surgeons in this procedure. Increased liability and decreased reimbursements are additional factors that combine to produce a situation in which there is going to be a shortage of qualified surgeons that perform these procedures safely. This crisis has arisen in part because many insurance companies do not provide coverage for this treatment option.

All these factors place tremendous pressure on medical schools and teaching hospitals to train surgeons in this type of surgery, because traditional educational paradigms are not designed to efficiently generate the number of providers that are needed. Surgeons must possess a superior surgical skill set and cognitive foundation to provide the total care requirements for these patients and to perform these procedures in a minimally invasive fashion. Also, aspiring bariatric surgeons must be motivated by more than just the prospect of expanding their practice and benefiting financially. They must serve as advocates for patients who are outcasts in our social hierarchy, a group that not only is laden with the burden of excess adipose tissue but also is discriminated against in society and in employment (3). New approaches must be found for helping the nutritionally challenged.

Skill

The skills necessary to competently and safely perform laparoscopic weight reduction procedures include accurate targeting, two-dimensional (2D) depth perception compensation, bimanual dexterity, and two-hand choreography. These skills must not be present in just a rudimentary fashion but rather must be present at a superior and advanced level. Furthermore, surgeons must not depend solely on technology to achieve operative efficiency and patient safety. They must be capable of protecting the patient and successfully completing a procedure even in the face of equipment malfunction. This requires the surgeon to be able to suture intracorporeally under endoscopic guidance, which is the most difficult task to perform in the laparoscopic environment. But it is absolutely essential if the patient is to be afforded the same safety net in the minimally invasive environment that is provided with open surgery.

The acquisition and mastery of the suturing skill set traditionally was thought to require intensive and prolonged training. In the demanding environment of minimally invasive weight loss surgery, suturing is a necessity and not an accessory skill set. A number of skill development programs have been established to teach the skills required in the minimally invasive environment. One such program is the McGill Inanimate System for Training and Evaluation of Laparoscopic Skills (MISTE) developed by Gerald Fried and colleagues at McGill University. A derivative of this system has been used as the basis for the Fundamentals of Laparoscopic Surgery (FLS) program developed by the Society of American Gastrointestinal and Endoscopic Surgeons (SAGES) and is now embraced by the American College of Surgeons, and the Society of Laparoscopic Surgery. These excellent programs concentrate on basic skills but are not focused exclusively on intracorporeal suturing.

The Rosser Top Gun Laparoscopic Skills and Suturing Program is a competitive interactive curriculum that has been validated as an effective and efficient method to transfer laparoscopic skills and suturing capability to this type of surgery. Details on this program have been reported in the literature (4). This is a very structured program with the student/instructor ratio recommended to be 4:1. Level I can be conducted in 1.5 days. It is built around the premise that validated preparatory drills can establish skills that can assist in the execution of a validated intracorporeal suturing algorithm. There also is an emphasis on nondominant hand skill development. A CD-ROM is available that covers the curriculum and provides detailed instruction in the suturing process. Another noteworthy feature is the availability of a large database that provides objective evidence of one's skill capability as compared to one's peers. The program's validated remote education platform with online follow-up facilitates further skill development (5). The program incorporates progressively increasing degrees of difficulty, from level I (basic skills and suturing course), to level II (master's course), to level III (anastomosis course).

In the early development of the program, the time required to perform the tasks was the only quantifiable parameter used. Top Gun and other inanimate trainer-based programs were appropriately criticized for this shortcoming because time is not the only performance-defining variable. But these programs did not assess the surgeon's accuracy in any other way (6). Furthermore, programs such as Top Gun are limited by the need for an increased instructor/student ratio to maintain dynamic quality control of performance without errors (4). With no quantifiable assessment of accuracy, traditional computer training programs are unable to address variables such as the surgeon's economy of motion. The requirement of multiple proctors to ensure proper technique also increases cost, and it discourages self-study for participants whose schedules are already full (7).

The inadequacies of the computer training programs, including their low reliability and dependence on virtual reality systems, have necessitated the creation of hybrid devices that use laparoscopic instrumentation and videoscopic display. These systems provide visual realism and tactile feedback, thus improving the computer training programs for surgeons (8). Hybrid devices also integrate measures designed to address the major flaws in computer training systems, namely their inability to address the surgeon's accuracy and economy of motion.

The Rosser Inanimate Proctor (RIP) is designed to provide the user with experience in complex instrument manipulation as well as in the execution of a procedural protocol that promotes efficient acquisition of surgical skill and suturing in the endoscopic environment. It has been an integral part of Rosser's Top Gun program since 2001. The device tests an individual's skills using tasks that have been validated for both construct and content validity (4,9). This means that the scores have been proven to correlate with the level of surgical experience, and that the tests measure psychomotor skills and not just anatomic knowledge. The device limits the performance of tasks to a small designated area. This forces the participant to execute the tasks exhibiting economy of motion with error recognition, as the errors are automatically recorded. The device also has a light and buzzer that activate whenever errors are committed. This device represents potential stand-alone instructional capability that could greatly reduce the personnel infrastructure necessary to execute the program. A database similar to the original program has been established. The introduction of this device has clearly upgraded Top Gun, and other platforms are moving in this direction as well.

In summary, it must be stressed that the establishment, maintenance, and maturation of skill in the minimally invasive environment is the foundation for developing competence in laparoscopic weight-loss surgery and other advanced laparoscopic procedures. Acquisition of such skills is essential to minimize complications early in one's experience, especially since the learning curve for weight-loss procedures is considered to include the first 100 procedures that one performs (2). This is the steepest of any minimally invasive procedures. No matter what skill program is used, the neophyte as well as the experienced weight-loss surgeon should be prepared to make the sacrifices needed to develop these necessary skill sets.

Knowledge

The cognitive knowledge base that is needed to participate in the surgical care of nutritionally challenged patients has been frequently underestimated. For some casual observers it would seem that bariatric surgery is just an extension of basic gastrointestinal surgery, and there is no appreciable change in approach to the execution of weight-loss procedures or postprocedural care considerations. But nothing could be further from the truth if one aspires to be a successful bariatric surgeon. The chronicled history of over 50 years of bariatric procedure development must become part of the surgeon's immediate recall, and the scientific evolution of weight-loss procedures must be taken into consideration when evaluating newly introduced surgery options. Skill is not the only training issue of substance. Good surgical judgment is a requirement for good operative outcome. It is important to know not only how to do something, but also what to do and when to do it. Constant situational awareness with attention to detail and to every aspect of the technique of weight-loss surgery places another extraordinary demand on the surgeon. This is especially true with the gastric bypass procedure performed under laparoscopic guidance. One must become a student of the intricate details and their sequence of occurrence.

Knowledge about the mechanism of action, the efficacy of the procedure, and the validation of long-term results of all types of weight-loss surgery must be mastered. The type of procedure chosen will dictate adjustments in long-term treatment. This is imperative in treating not only patients presenting for first-time procedures but also patients who have had previous procedures and experienced complications or require revisional surgery. The surgeon must be knowledgeable about the procedure's complications and how to treat them, such as anastomotic leaks and postoperative plantar compression syndrome secondary to prolonged extreme reverse Trendelenburg positioning without adequate padding of the feet.

Knowledge of the literature must not stop with procedural or perioperative care issues; the surgeon must understand the pathophysiology of comorbidities. Also, a competent grasp of this information is important if the surgeon is to properly educate the patient and nonsurgical colleagues. The surgeon must correct the many misperceptions that patients and nonsurgical colleagues have regarding weight-loss surgery.

It is very difficult to achieve through traditional educational resources the full scope of the skill and knowledge required for a successful bariatric surgeon. Residency programs will not produce enough competent surgeons in this exploding field for quite some time. Patient demand and the sheer numbers associated with the obesity epidemic have overwhelmed our traditional surgical training system. Compounding this issue is that, similar to the development of laparoscopic cholecystectomy, a concentrated effort in weight-loss surgery did not start in the medical schools, and they have been slow to respond to the changing clinical landscape. In spite of these issues, we cannot repeat the educational errors of the past by attempting to meet patient demand by training surgeons in brief courses with limited lab animal surgical experience.

One-year fellowships have historically provided focused and extended clinical opportunities for specialized areas of study. A surgeon can take a year of specialized study that includes both cognitive and surgical skill development in weight-loss procedures. It is a valid, traditional methodology, and these programs are increasingly being funded. But this approach is hampered by the fact that the number of programs is still and will always be limited, and it does not address the immediate need of training general surgeons in the performance of weight-loss procedures. It also does not provide an opportunity for experienced bariatric surgeons who would like to convert to the minimally invasive approach. It would be financially catastrophic for most surgeons to take a year off from their practices.

Therefore, other options must be considered. The effort must subscribe to traditional training values but be flexible enough to address the constraints placed on the practicing surgeon. In view of these requirements, the mini-fellowship system offers the most feasible option. Orthopedic surgery responded in a similar fashion with the rapid expansion of technique approaches (i.e., hand, shoulder, athletic reconstruction mini-fellowships). The mini-fellowship system that is currently in place for bariatric surgery has limitations that must be addressed. It must expand the clinical exposure it provides from experts, and it must provide a more structured curriculum with quantifiable assessment of the participant's skills and clinical decision making.

The proposed system consists of two components that work in concert with each other: the *core competency* phase and the *clinical competency* phase. Each phase takes 3 weeks, but the core competency program may take longer than that for surgeons with time constraints who are attending part-time. The core competency phase is a highly structured cognitive and skill development program that establishes and enhances one's execution of procedures in the minimally invasive environment. This program closely monitors student progress with objective parameters. It consists of formal lectures, review of pertinent materials, research assignments, laboratory exercises, and practical experience, with observation of procedures both on site and via video conferencing. Further clinical exposure is provided by structured videotapes of the techniques of leading surgeons that are reviewed and analyzed by other surgeons in the field.

The curriculum has the flexibility to address customized procedures. For instance, the clinical portion of the core competency program may be modified to address selected areas of interest, such as weight-loss surgery, colon surgery, foregut surgery, etc. This program is limited to a small number of surgeons so that close supervision and individual attention can be given to every participant. Detailed performance assessments are made on every student to provide feedback as well as documentation for future credentialing. The documentation system is based on that used for the aviation qualification system. Qualification to fly a certain type of aircraft is dependent on two primary factors, cognitive and experience, based on the number of hours spent in the flight simulator as well as in the actual aircraft. Experience is measured by the number of hours involved in directed activity. Instructor observation is also a very important part of aviation training. For instance, to become fully qualified as a single-engine noncommercial pilot, along with educational requirements, one has to have about 40 hours of documented experience. To progress to a more advanced aircraft, a certain number of hours on a less sophisticated aircraft must be achieved.

This aviation training has been adapted to surgeon training by the proposed mini-fellowship program. Table 4-1 lists the number of hours spent on each component of the core competency mini-fellowship, totaling over 300 structured educational hours. Rosser initiated such a program in 1997 and since that time six courses have been taught. A total of 38 fellows have been trained. Over that same time period, only six fellows have graduated from the traditional 1-year program. This educational program has the potential to generate a greater number of graduates, and to become a more attainable option for many surgeons. One must question whether or not this type of program produces a well-trained surgeon. But considering the lack of structure, the restricted clinical exposure, and the lack of performance assessment in most current 1-year programs, this approach offers assets that could offset the program's limited time duration. Another feature of this program is that the participants are trained to be trainers and are exposed to the most up-to-date knowledge and skill transfer techniques. This "train the trainer" approach enables each mini-fellowship graduate not only to perform procedures but also to teach others.

Once the core competence program is completed, the surgeon can go on to a 6-week clinical competence mini-fellowship. Schauer at the University of Pittsburgh, and more recently at the Cleveland Clinic, instituted such a program, which provides hands-on surgery experience. However, the programs raise the issues of licensing and lawsuits. Schauer has addressed these issues, and his program was established in accordance with local and state medical governing rules and regulations. In addition, this clinical mini-fellowship trains surgeons in certain emerging surgical procedures while minimizing the learning curve. More of these programs will be developed in the future, but the number of programs will be limited by local and state rules and regulations. Probably not all states will allow this innovative approach to be followed. Consequently, a similar option using centers in other countries could be a feasible alternative. They can offer a less complicated medicolegal climate, excellent teaching, and exotic clinical material. But one must be cautious in embarking on this course, because if participants enter the program without the core competency component, the benefit of the clinical exposure will be suboptimal. The successful completion of the core competency mini-fellowship establishes skill and cognitive

TABLE 4-1. Hourly activity of an average participant in the core competency preceptorship

	Components of core competency	Total hours
	Hours completed in basic, advanced, and master's level skill and suturing development	94.0
9	Animal labs	61.0
23	Clinical lectures	29.5
11	Cases on-site	29.0
18	CD-ROM and video cases	24.0
	Instruction in advanced technology	21.25
11	Video conferences observed in advanced minimally invasive procedures	19.5
	Course instructor	15.0
	Multimedia and special practice development	5.5
5	Special procedural deconstruction format	4.5
		303.25

milestones that help to ensure the maximum benefit of the clinical mini-fellowship.

After completing the mini-fellowship the surgeon is ready to offer these cutting-edge clinical services to patients. But at first the surgeon should be mentored by an experienced surgeon if possible, who can intervene in the procedure if necessary. In view of the concern for patient safety, guidelines have been suggested as to when the surgeon can perform advanced procedures. Mentoring and proctoring are now strong components of the credentialing process. For example, the American Society for Bariatric Surgery (ASBS) has published "Guidelines for Granting Privileges in Bariatric Surgery" that includes a strong proctoring and mentoring component, because more needs to be done to prepare surgeons to execute new procedures, and nontraditional methodologies need to be evaluated to help accomplish the desired goals.

Unfortunately, there is only a very limited mentor pool. How do we expand the availability of the mentor pool? Telemedicine offers a potential solution. It involves the use of telecommunications for the delivery of health care with the provider being located at a remote site. Telementoring represents an advanced telemedical application that can provide real-time guidance and instruction to a surgeon in a remote location utilizing audio, video, and other telecommunications technologies. Telementoring addresses the safety issue by facilitating an extended clinical education opportunity (ECEO) no matter where the patient and the operating surgeon are located.

However, the promise of telementoring cannot be fulfilled unless a structured methodology is followed and effective outcomes are quantifiably assessed. Rosser has suggested such a methodology. The components of this algorithm include (1) preprocedural assessment and enhancement of surgical skills, (2) establishment of a standardized approach to the procedure, (3) use of practical information, (4) use of a telementoring simulation laboratory, and (5) use of telemedical applications. This system facilitates expanding the use of telementoring services, and the safety net for patients can be broadened (10).

Advocacy

Even with the adoption of all of the aforementioned programs and strategies, another element must be added to ensure the successful surgical treatment of the nutritionally challenged patient. Developing excellent surgical skills is not enough; surgeons also must become advocates for the morbidly obese. Many surgeons would prefer to be just technicians, but surgery is only the first step to a lasting cure. Surgeons must address the society's ignorance about obesity. The struggle for the nutritionally challenged is lifelong and must be aggressively addressed each day. Other members of the weight-loss surgery team may be better qualified to address these issues, but the surgeon can provide intellectual leadership.

Being a bariatric advocate begins with the realization that the disease entity presents unique treatment challenges. The patients have special structural requirements. For example, chairs with arms should not be placed in the nutritionally challenged patients' reception area. Large and extra large paper gowns should be provided for the physical examination. Bathrooms need to have commodes that are of the pedestal type and not suspended from the wall. Suspended commodes can snap off the wall when the patient sits down. Air conditioning should be set low enough so that obese patients will not sweat profusely. The staff members must be sensitive when interacting with patients who are candidates for weight-loss surgery. They should not refer to patients as being obese or fat. They should show respect and consideration for the mobility constraints of these patients, and should allow the patients to move slowly. They also must realize that many patients are extremely sensitive about their weight. Thus the scales should be placed in a secluded area, and all examinations should be conducted in private rooms. Staff members should be discreet in their conversations with patients and with other staff. Comments that are overheard can be taken out of context, and the patients could feel intimidated into withholding important information that could be critical to their successful recovery.

Advocacy also entails addressing the fact that nutritionally challenged patients are also discriminated against by others, who believe that obesity is not a disease but rather the manifestation of the most blatant form of self-destructive behavior. But obesity *is* a disease and the most reliable cure for morbid obesity is surgery, as the National Institutes of Health (NIH) and the medical and surgical communities have stated (11). In spite of this, many believe that obese individuals just lack willpower and thus are not deserving of the attention and intervention traditionally afforded other medical conditions. Substance abusers are treated more respectfully than the morbidly obese. Size discrimination is the last bastion of institutionalized bigotry. In our society the nutritionally challenged are inhumanely subjected to jokes, stereotyping, and profiling. In television and the movies, obesity is used as the foundation of comic satire. The obese experience job discrimination, the lack of public facility access, verbal insensitivity, social rejection, and isolation. These patients are systematically denied the appropriate medical care for this recognized disease entity because of health insurance restrictions. With patients facing this difficult road to proper care, it is imperative that bariatric surgeons be their allies and advocates.

References

1. Weighing the options: criteria for evaluating weight-management programs (1995). In: Thomas PR ed. Washington, DC: National Academy Press, 1995.
2. Schauer P, Ikramuddin S, Hamad G, Gourash W. The learning curve for laparoscopic Roux-en-Y gastric bypass is 100 cases. Surg Endosc 2003;17:212–215.
3. Melcher J, Bostwick GJ Jr. The obese client: myths, facts, assessment and intervention. Health Soc Work 1998;23(3): 195–202.
4. Rosser JC, Rosser LE, Savalgi RS. Skills acquisition and assessment for laparoscopic surgery. Arch Surg 1997;132: 200–204.
5. Rosser JC, Rosser LE, Savalgi RS. Objective evaluation of a laparoscopic surgical skill program for residents and senior surgeons. Arch Surg 1998;133(6):657–661.
6. Smith CD, Farrell TM, McNatt SS, Metreveli RE. Assessing laparoscopic manipulative skills. Am J Surg 2001;181:547–550.
7. Bridges M, Diamond DL. The financial impact of teaching surgical residents in the operating room. Am J Surg 1999; 177:28–32.
8. Hamilton EC, Scott DJ, Fleming JB, et al. Comparison of video trainer and virtual reality training systems on acquisition of laparoscopic skills. Surg Endosc 2002;16:406–411.
9. Pearson AM, Gallagher AG, Rosser JC, Satava RM. Evaluation of structured and quantitative training methods for teaching intracorporeal knot tying. Surg Endosc 2002;16: 130–137.
10. Rosser JC, Gabriel NH, Herman B, Murayama M. Telementoring and Teleproctoring. World J Surg 2001;11:1438–1448.
11. Livingston E, Fink A. Quality of life cost and future of bariatric surgery. Arch Surg 2003;138:383–388.

5
Bariatric Surgery Program Essentials

Tomasz Rogula, Samer G. Mattar, Paul A. Thodiyil, and Philip R. Schauer

Obesity has grown to epidemic proportions in our society (1). This frightening trend is being highlighted by the news media and by periodic calls for action from government officials (2). Family practitioners and general surgeons are coming under increasing market pressures to provide medical or surgical solutions for patients who seek significant and durable weight loss. Morbidly obese patients have multiple diagnoses, and surgeons who embark on this specialty quickly realize that the safest and most effective approach to managing these patients is through a comprehensive multidiscipline program.

This chapter presents a multidisciplinary approach to the bariatric surgery patient. We describe the components of a successful, comprehensive bariatric program including the essential staff, the ancillary personnel, the material infrastructure, and educational and patient support strategies.

Patient Selection Criteria for Bariatric Surgery

Some patients who consider themselves overweight may request a bariatric operation, but specific criteria must be met for bariatric surgery. Patients must be aware that these operations are not primarily aesthetic, but are performed to prevent the pathologic consequences of morbid obesity. A thorough preoperative evaluation will discover previously undiagnosed comorbidities in many patients, and these conditions must be optimally managed prior to surgery.

Patients with a BMI of ≥40, or ≥35 with comorbidity, are generally eligible for bariatric surgery. Attempted weight loss in the past by supervised diet regimens, exercise, or medications is required. Patients should be highly motivated to comply with the postoperative dietary and exercise regimens and follow-up schedule. The NIH consensus recommendations discussed bariatric surgery for patients 18 to 60 years old. In our experience, however, bariatric surgery may be equally safe and effective in older adults. Despite some controversies, many authors agree that carefully selected adolescent patients with morbid obesity should be considered for bariatric surgery.

Generally, patients who are unable to undergo general anesthesia because of cardiac, pulmonary, or hepatic disease, and those who are unwilling or unable to comply with postoperative lifestyle changes, diet, micronutrient supplementation, or follow-up, are considered unsuitable candidates.

Close patient follow-up and a multidisciplinary approach are necessary for the success of a bariatric surgery program. Patients referred long distances to a large bariatric center are difficult to follow long term and are often unable to regularly participate in support groups where they had their surgery performed (6). Every effort should be made to contact these patients at regular intervals after surgery.

Patients are most commonly referred for bariatric surgery by their primary care physicians (PCPs). These physicians need to understand the risks and benefits of modern bariatric procedures. They also need to be familiar with the mandatory changes in lifestyle and eating habits that patients must adopt after surgery. This can only be achieved with periodic "outreach" lectures and seminars delivered to PCPs by bariatric surgeons and physicians who are experts in the field. These educational opportunities allow PCPs to meet specialist surgeons and physicians, thereby fostering strong collaborative relationships and referral sources. The end result is a generalized awareness by the PCPs of the problems posed to patients as a result of morbid obesity, the medical and surgical solutions available for treatment, and the requirements for a durable and sustained positive outcome. Clearly, better informed PCPs, in turn, help foster patient cooperation and compliance with recommended postoperative guidelines (7).

Components of a Bariatric Program

Professional Bariatric Surgery Team

Active collaboration with multiple patient care disciplines including nutrition, anesthesiology, cardiology, pulmonary medicine, orthopedic surgery, endocrinology, psychiatry, and rehabilitation medicine is essential. A dietitian can help patients adjust to postoperative dietary guidelines and food choices. Patients participate in a program of behavioral adjustment, exercise rehabilitation therapy, and a patient support group under the direction of qualified personnel (8).

The treatment of morbid obesity should begin with simple lifestyle changes in diet. Initially, the patient's PCP usually addresses the diagnosis of morbid obesity and associated comorbidities. Exercise regimens and medications may be recommended as the initial therapeutic strategies.

A multidisciplinary approach to the evaluation of the potential surgical candidate is critical. Apart from dietary consultation, patients may require evaluation by a psychiatrist, psychologist, cardiologist, pulmonary specialist, or endocrinologist, depending on their comorbidities. Ideally, these specialists should have an interest in bariatric patients and should consider themselves part of the bariatric team.

Dietary Evaluation

Bariatric surgeons often consider themselves metabolic surgeons, in recognition of the fact that weight-loss surgery significantly alters metabolism. An extreme form of this is severe protein-calorie malnutrition that can follow certain malabsorptive operations. The goal of any bariatric procedure is to achieve a negative energy balance without compromising protein and micronutrient absorption.

Different types of procedures (restrictive, malabsorptive, or a combination) achieve this balance between weight loss and malnutrition to different degrees. Regardless of the procedure being performed, though, thorough preoperative nutrition education and postoperative nutrition follow-up are mandatory. A well-known effect of bariatric operations is a reduction of appetite, at least for the first 5 to 6 months after surgery. Patients and family members should be made aware of this side effect, and caregivers should ensure that the postoperative patient is achieving adequate protein intake and hydration. Dumping syndrome in patients undergoing bypass procedures can result in an aversion to sweets. Patients must be made aware of this phenomenon, understand its causes, and, more importantly, learn to avoid precipitating factors.

Patients' dietary regimens must meet their daily requirements of proteins. Nutrition counselors are trained to deliver advice on the proper identification of protein sources and the preparation of meals to render them more palatable. They will also advise patients on proper chewing and swallowing techniques and give tips regarding solid and liquid intake. Patients are required to know the hazards of insufficient fluid intake and are counseled to drink fluids throughout the day, pausing before meals. The daily administration of vitamins and supplements is critical for postoperative bariatric surgery patients, and it is incumbent on surgeons to reinforce compliance with vitamin supplementation. Surgeons have been held liable for complications of vitamin deficiencies, particularly neurologic manifestations that may result from inadequate intake. Easy access to nutrition counselors and periodic laboratory assessment of nutrition parameters may reduce the occurrence of the preventable complications.

Nutrition counselors should also assess a patient's ability to comply with the required dietary modifications imposed by bariatric surgery. Patients should be motivated to accept and reliably follow dietary guidelines. They must also understand the potential repercussions of nonadherence. In addition to providing dietary advice to patients, the nutritionist on the bariatric team provides invaluable information to the bariatric surgeon regarding potential problems with patient compliance.

Psychological Evaluation

Some bariatric programs do not include psychologists as members of the bariatric team and simply refer patients elsewhere for psychological evaluation. This is not ideal, as psychological support of the morbidly obese patient is essential. These patients are often diagnosed with depression, anxiety, or other stress-related conditions. There are often problems with body image and low self-esteem. In addition to offering invaluable support, psychologists assess the patient's mental status and counsel the patient regarding the lifelong changes required after bariatric surgery. Several instruments for psychological assessment of morbidly obese patients in the preoperative and postoperative periods have been developed and validated, and are in wide use. The Moorehead-Ardelt questionnaire is an example of such a tool (9).

Education of patients should be emphasized in every bariatric program. For example, knowledge of the "rules of eating" and the "rules of vomiting" are essential for good outcomes following gastric restrictive surgery (10). Patient knowledge, psychosocial adaptation, and motivation may play crucial roles in achieving desirable outcomes. Discrepancies between a patient's ideal weight goals and a reasonable weight loss goal after surgery need to be addressed. Limited data currently exist to guide patient selection for bariatric surgery (or to match a specific patient type with a specific procedure), and well-designed studies are needed to provide more precise guidance with respect to psychological factors (10).

Postoperative nausea, depression, and even remorse are relatively common for several months following surgery. Both the patient and the surgeon must be aware of these symptoms, and the physician should delineate the physical issues from the psychological. Thorough preoperative screening and careful patient selection does not identify or eliminate all potential problems. Psychological intervention is sometimes useful in achieving overall patient stability and emotional well-being. This underscores the important role of the psychologist throughout the patient's entire treatment experience (11).

Expert Consultants

Medical conditions frequently associated with morbid obesity include cardiovascular, pulmonary, endocrine, metabolic, hematological, and many other diseases (see Chapter 2). The availability of consultants and experts in these fields is critical. Consultants should be appropriately trained and be familiar with the specific pathophysiologic consequences of morbidly obese patients. In general, their role is to determine with a certain degree of confidence the eligibility of candidates to withstand the rigors of major surgery and the required physical demands during the postoperative period. The primary aim of preoperative consultations is to adequately prepare patients for general anesthesia, particularly with regard to cardiac and pulmonary function. Additionally, patients with sleep apnea should have special preoperative training by an experienced consultant. Patients with life-threatening myocardial ischemia should be revascularized prior to weight-loss surgery. These experts need to be readily available in the immediate postoperative period and in the long-term care of these patients.

Extensive evaluation prior to weight-loss surgery is mandatory in every case. Thorough history taking and clinical examinations will guide clinicians to diagnose previously unrecognized diseases. Appropriate diagnostic algorithms should be used to investigate all comorbidities for which the patient is at risk.

Anesthesiology for Bariatric Surgery

Anesthesiologists who are charged with managing bariatric patients undergoing major surgery should be experienced in diagnosing and treating immediate or imminent life-threatening conditions, such as a difficult airway, hypoventilation syndrome, sleep apnea, congestive heart failure, renal insufficiency, and venous thromboembolism. Anesthesiologists who manage bariatric patients undergoing laparoscopic operations must be cognizant of the pulmonary and hemodynamic changes that occur upon establishing and maintaining prolonged pneumoperitoneum. There should be more than one experienced anesthesiology staff member available at all times for these cases. Morbidly obese patients have little cardiopulmonary reserve and deteriorate rapidly when an airway or cardiac event occurs. Because establishing an emergency airway can be extremely difficult in these patients even for an experienced anesthesiologist, the surgeon should be present during intubation, extubation, and transfer to the recovery room in the event that a surgical airway is needed.

Hypertension, left ventricular hypertrophy, myocardial ischemia, and atherosclerosis are more common in morbidly obese patients than in the normal-weight population. Perioperative myocardial infarction is a major concern in these patients. Preoperative assessment of cardiovascular system must be thorough and should establish the patient's cardiac risk for a bariatric procedure.

Laboratory tests should include hemoglobin and platelet count, glucose, blood urea, and electrolytes. An electrocardiogram and chest x-ray should be performed, and patients with a history of myocardial ischemia should undergo invasive cardiac testing.

A primary concern of anesthesia in morbidly obese patients is the difficult airway that is typical of this population. This is compounded by impaired pulmonary function. Obese patients have decreased expiratory reserve volume (ERV), inspiratory capacity, vital capacity, and functional reserve capacity (FRC). Additionally, drug pharmacokinetics differ in morbidly obese patients. Changes in volume of distribution include smaller than normal fraction of total body water, greater adipose tissue content, altered protein binding, and increased blood volume. Possible changes in renal and hepatic function also have to be taken into consideration when administrating drugs to obese patients.

The perioperative risk is also increased due to potential postoperative respiratory and thromboembolic complications. A thoracic epidural can be used as an intra- and postoperative adjunct for pain control, particularly for patients undergoing open procedures. A carefully planned and executed anesthetic plan can reduce operative risk to an acceptable level in the majority of patients (12).

Preoperative Workshops and Support Groups

Support groups are an important part of the bariatric program. In these small group settings, patients can freely discuss successes and problems with other patients and bariatric staff members. This is frequently one of the most valuable sources of information and reinforcement for bariatric surgery patients. Family members may play an important role in such settings, and an informal setting should be maintained for these meetings to promote participation. Effective group activities include the preoperative workshops or seminars and a regularly scheduled postoperative support group.

During preoperative educational workshops patients obtain information from bariatric clinic staff and from other patients. This is a mutually beneficial exercise between prospective patients and bariatric program health providers. Additionally, patients become acquainted with the program, the personnel, and the path they will follow during their preoperative and postoperative course. The risks and benefits of procedures can be introduced and the importance of compliance with supplementation and with exercise can be emphasized. This is also an opportunity for the staff and the surgeon to observe patients' interactions and become acquainted with the patients. The program for these workshops should be organized and the material concisely presented with audio-visual aids and printed material. Following the presentations, a question-and-answer period with the surgeon will prompt a variety of pertinent discussions.

Support groups are mainly offered to patients who underwent bariatric surgery and are in the recovery phase. However, we also invite prospective patients to join support groups. This allows them to discuss the dramatic changes they will undergo with patients who are actively losing weight. These workshops primarily address the medical, nutritional, psychological, and social issues that postoperative patients may experience. Tips and advice are frequently delivered by more experienced patients. Invited speakers may offer additional experience or perspectives. The role of the bariatric program staff at these meetings should be to facilitate the discussions and to ensure that false information is not disseminated.

Postoperative workshops can provide the following: (1) support for patient compliance and praise for success; (2) instruction about life after surgery, including nutrition, psychological aspects, and exercise and dieting techniques; (3) recognition of new kinds of self-nurturing; (4) a forum in which patients share their experiences; (5) a friendly, safe atmosphere for family members and significant others so that they may also understand and recognize the issues they face as their loved one loses weight; and (6) an atmosphere of true caring and concern for the long-term well-being of the patients (Table 5-1) (13).

TABLE 5-1. Goals of preoperative patient education

Encourage patient's compliance and offer praise for success
Prepare patient for life after surgery, including nutrition, exercise, and dieting
Identify patient's problems
Identify and help patient develop new kinds of self-nurturing
Encourage patient's participation in a forum or group where others understand the challenges and difficulties associated with change (positive or negative change)
Create a friendly, safe atmosphere where patients can bring spouses, parents, and significant others; emphasize that spouses must also recognize their own issues related to the dramatic changes occurring with their loved one
Provide an opportunity for surgical candidates to learn from postoperative patients in a supportive atmosphere

Requirements for Hospitals

A bariatric surgery program can be established only with the full support and commitment of the health care institution in which it will function. This often requires a major paradigm shift for hospitals that have not previously committed to caring for these patients. Acceptance of the bariatric program must occur at every level within the institution. Often, the first goal is to convince the administration and consultants that morbid obesity is a life-threatening disease that can be treated with bariatric surgery. Once this philosophy is accepted by the hospital administration and the staff members who will care for these patients, then planning the necessary infrastructure can begin. Next, a task force or team led by the bariatric surgeon should evaluate the available resources and decide what is needed to provide hospital access, comfort, and safety to the bariatric patient population.

Morbidly obese patients must feel welcome within the hospital. Appropriately sized furniture in the waiting rooms and examination rooms is required. Specific equipment including weight scales, blood pressure cuffs, and patient transport gurneys, and wheelchairs should be appropriately sized. The inpatient rooms should be specially designed for bariatric patients to provide maximum safety and comfort. Chapter 6 provides a detailed description of bariatric office and hospital equipment.

Bariatric Surgery Database

An electronic database is an essential part of any bariatric program, and it is a valuable resource for both clinical and research purposes. Patients can be easily followed for many years, and specific information can be rapidly accessed. The success of a bariatric program should be measured according to defined outcomes such as weight loss, morbidity and mortality, and the percentage of patients receiving long-term follow-up, and this can easily be achieved with a variety of database programs. A well-designed database allows quick analysis of patient outcomes and can identify areas that need improvement. Some bariatric programs use commercially available software and others have software developed to specifically meet the clinical and research needs of the program.

Bariatric Surgery Program Web Site

Creating a Web site for the bariatric surgery program provides an opportunity for patients to quickly learn about the strengths of the program, the personnel, and the institution. It can also provide a vast amount of information to patients through frequently asked questions, links to other Web sites, and other informational presentations. It also provides the surgeon an opportunity to state the mission of the bariatric surgery program, the pre- and postoperative pathways, and the procedures offered.

The Web site can also provide initial access to the bariatric clinic. Patients can complete screening questionnaires online and, if they are appropriate candidates, can be invited to an educational workshop through this same site. Some bariatric programs offer Internet-based chat rooms and forums where patients can talk to each other, contact the surgery program personnel, or request prescription refills. This method of communication is frequently more efficient and practical than conventional telephone messages.

Future Developments

The number of bariatric surgeries performed in the United States will increase dramatically over the next few years. Bariatric surgery is likely to become one of the mainstays of general surgery training and practice, and the shift from open to laparoscopic surgery is attracting increasing numbers of surgeons to the field.

Despite these changes, there is an increasing need for the implementation of weight reduction health policies and the development of comprehensive bariatric programs that include medical and surgical care. There are vast research opportunities in bariatric surgeries as well, and these will focus on the mechanisms of weight loss, glucose metabolism, the durability of the procedures, and the optimal procedure for patients based on their BMI, comorbidities, psychological profile, and eating habits (14).

Public health policy needs to further address this epidemic before it becomes a critical public health and financial crisis. These efforts should include awareness and assistance programs to facilitate access to bariatric surgery, given that only about 1% of eligible patients are currently being referred for weight-loss surgery. These policies also need to address the socioeconomic and ethnic disparities in the morbidly obese population. Individual health care systems and centers performing bariatric surgery also need to address the access and financial limitations faced by many patients who qualify for bariatric surgery (15).

Conclusion

As the worldwide epidemic of obesity continues its exponential growth, the demand on surgeons to safely and effectively treat patients with this disease will also grow.

Because morbid obesity is a disease that affects nearly every system in the body, it can only be managed by a diverse group of skilled practitioners who are dedicated to the treatment of this life-threatening condition. To adequately treat these patients, a comprehensive program must be in place that can fully evaluate prospective patients and prepare them mentally and physically for surgery and the permanent lifestyle changes they will need to adopt. Such a comprehensive program requires a multidisciplinary team approach, a strong fundamental infrastructure, and total institutional commitment.

References

1. Mokdad AH, et al. Prevalence of obesity, diabetes, and obesity-related health risk factors, 2001. JAMA 2003; 289(1):76–79.
2. International Food Information Council Foundation, Trends in Obesity-Related Media Coverage, November 2003: http://www.ific.org/research/obesitytrends.cfm
3. Livingston EH. Obesity and its surgical management. Am J Surg 2002;184(2):103–113.
4. Gastrointestinal surgery for severe obesity: National Institutes of Health Consensus Development Conference Statement. Am J Clin Nutr 1992;55(2 suppl):615S–619S.
5. Kuczmarski RJ, et al. Increasing prevalence of overweight among US adults. The National Health and Nutrition Examination Surveys, 1960 to 1991. JAMA 1994;272(3): 205–211.
6. Shikora SA, Abrahamian GA, Gaines CE. Can a bariatric surgery program succeed without close patient proximity? The experience in a military medical center. Obes Surg 1994;4(3):238–243.
7. Choban PS, et al. Bariatric surgery for morbid obesity: why, who, when, how, where, and then what? Cleve Clin J Med 2002;69(11):897–903.
8. Walen ML, Rodgers P, Scott JS. The multi-disciplinary team. Obes Surg 2001;11(1):98.
9. DiGregorio JM, Moorehead MK. The psychology of bariatric surgery. Obes Surg 1994;4(4):361–369.
10. Kral JG. Selection of patients for anti-obesity surgery. Int J Obes Relat Metab Disord 2001;25(suppl 1):S107–S112.
11. Higa KD, et al. Narcotic withdrawal syndrome following gastric bypass—a difficult diagnosis. Obes Surg 2001;11(5): 631–634.
12. Munsch Y, Sagnard P. [The anesthetist's point of view in the surgical treatment of morbid obesity.] Ann Chir 1997;51(2): 183–188.
13. Algazi LP. Transactions in a support group meeting: a case study. Obes Surg 2000;10(2):186–191.
14. Buchwald H. Overview of bariatric surgery. J Am Coll Surg 2002;194(3):367–375.
15. Livingston EH, Ko CY. Socioeconomic characteristics of the population eligible for obesity surgery. Surgery 2004; 135(3):288–296.

6
Essential Bariatric Equipment: Making Your Facility More Accommodating to Bariatric Surgical Patients

William Gourash, Tomasz Rogula, and Philip R. Schauer

Persons with morbid and super-morbid obesity have special ergonomic needs that are often not met by conventional hospital equipment and furniture. Hospitals with programs specifically addressing the surgical and medical needs of this population have an obligation to provide for their patients' comfort and safety throughout their entire hospital stay. Anticipating the needs of the bariatric patient requires some experience, and meeting those needs requires some familiarity with what is available. Further, the reader is encouraged to consider this to be an ongoing endeavor of prioritizing both essential and nonessential expenditures and of evaluating the results of these decisions.

This chapter addresses these questions: What is bariatric equipment? Why does our facility or program need bariatric equipment? How can our facility or program become more accommodating to bariatric surgery patients with bariatric equipment? What are the essential equipment items that we should consider?

Definition

What is bariatric equipment? Broadly speaking, it is all of the technology utilized to administer health care to the morbidly obese population. Technology is the knowledge and application of principles involved in the production of objects for the accomplishment of specific ends (1).

In this chapter we further restrict our discussion to the equipment used in caring for patients undergoing bariatric surgical procedures, although much of the information is broadly applicable to caring for obese patients in any health care setting. Equipment can be categorized with respect to its function: diagnostic or therapeutic. Equipment may have a specific role in the bariatric surgical process: preoperative, operative, and postoperative. This chapter focuses on the preoperative and postoperative needs. Operative equipment and instruments are covered in Chapter 10.

Rationale

Florence Nightingale recognized that healing took place in a "therapeutic patient environment" and by "putting the patient in the best condition for nature to act upon him" (2). The increasing prevalence of obese and morbidly obese persons essentially mandates that health care facilities of all levels work toward making their facilities safe and effective for the specific needs resulting from large patient size and its accompanying comorbid conditions (3). The combination of large size and often-limited mobility must also be accommodated. Safety is the most compelling reason for making health care facilities more accommodating to the needs of the morbidly obese patient (4,5). Better therapeutic and diagnostic outcomes can also be achieved with advanced planning and accommodation (3,6). Modifications that safely enhance mobility have the additional benefit of preventing morbidity (7). Safety for the health care staff is based on the need to prevent musculoskeletal injuries significantly associated with moving and physically caring for the morbidly obese patient. Many of these accidents and injuries are related to the use of conventional but inadequate equipment, especially for transferring and transporting patients (8–10).

Decreasing morbidity, especially that related to immobility, will enhance patient outcomes. Complications related to immobility include respiratory insufficiency, atelectasis, pneumonia, deep vein thrombosis, pulmonary embolism, decubitus ulcers, hygiene-related skin problems, and falls (4,5). Improved equipment can also decrease lengths of stay, accidents involving obese family members, and the nursing time spent improvising for the needs of the obese because of the lack of bariatric equipment or because of inadequate space (11).

Diagnostic testing may also be hampered by inadequate equipment. Failure to perform routinely ordered tests because of patient size puts the bariatric patient at risk. Problems may be encountered in the simple measurement of blood pressure or weight without appropriate bariatric tools. Obtaining accurate results from upper gastrointestinal tract series, computed tomography scans, polysomnograms, and cardiac stress tests requires meeting the specific needs presented by the patient's size, weight, and limited mobility.

Efficiency of care is related to the availability of bariatric equipment. Prolonged waiting time for transport may be caused by the unavailability of staff or equipment, and wastes not only time but also energy and money. Enhanced satisfaction of the patient, families, and staff is clearly related to readily available and properly sized equipment. A patient who is cared for safely, efficiently, appropriately, and in a timely manner will see the facility and the caregivers as being prepared and competent. The caregivers will be better able to focus on the patient's clinical and personal needs without the distraction or even resentment caused by an increased risk of injury (7,9–12). Rehabilitation may be possible only with specialized equipment, including walkers or parallel bars, that provides the extra space and durability needed.

Investigation and Planning

In our experience the approach that has worked best to coordinate the implementation in bariatric equipment was the development of a bariatric task force (BTF). This can be a problem-oriented group that is established on a temporary basis, but optimally the task force would function as a permanent committee that reviews the needs and concerns of bariatric patients. Equipment and physical plant issues in particular require ongoing attention (evaluation, updating, new construction, etc.). Prior to establishing the BTF, a presentation to senior staff and department administrators by a knowledgeable individual or group can provide an introduction to bariatric patients, equipment, surgical procedures, and surgical results for the hospital that can go a long way toward building goodwill and support for a BTF. The BTF should have a broad representation from all departments, including administration, parking, environmental services, transport, purchasing, nursing (intensive care units, intermediate care units, medical-surgical floors, clinics, administration, home care, bariatric coordinators, case managers, enterostomal therapy, outpatient surgery units, postanesthesia care units, operating room, and emergency room), nutrition, social work, physical therapy, radiology, cardiology, and pulmonology, as well as surgeons and midlevel practitioners.

The BTF should first undertake an assessment of facility's assets and limitations with respect to the physical layout and available conventional and bariatric patient care equipment (3,4). Questions to ask are the following: How has the facility been managing thus far with morbidly obese patients? Which practitioners have had an interest in these patients (e.g., nurses, enterostomal therapist, physical therapist, pulmonologist)? What are the weight and width limitations of the currently available equipment and furniture, including chairs in waiting rooms and hospital beds? Who are the vendors of the bariatric equipment already in use? What are the present policies for the utilization of bariatric equipment? What distances must patients travel from the clinic and the acute care areas to the diagnostic testing areas? The committee also should systematically review each step of the patient's hospital stay.

A second area of investigation should focus on what bariatric equipment is available for purchase. There are a number of reputable sources of information on products and vendors, one of the most useful being the bariatric equipment catalog available from the American Society for Bariatric Surgery (ASBS). Vendors typically have Web sites with listings of a wide range of bariatric products with links (e.g., www.sizewiserentals.net).

A third area of investigation should focus on the characteristics of the patients expected to make up the service population, in view of the hospital's prior experience with morbidly obese patients. The bariatric surgeons should be questioned with respect to their expectations for maximum and median weight and body mass index (BMI). In our practice, the first 500 patients had a weight range from 190 to 473 pounds (86 to 215 kg) with BMIs from 35 to 69. Thus contingency plans for patients weighing greater than 500 pounds (227 kg) and patients with BMIs greater than 70 were needed, recognizing that there would be a relatively small number of these patients.

One of the goals of these investigations is to prioritize purchases and other adaptations in the environment. The BTF should also develop criteria for the utilization of the new equipment. For example, in our institution we did not have a dedicated bariatric surgical floor, and there were hospital beds in the facility of a variety of vintages and models. The standard hospital beds had a variety of weight limits [350 to 500 pounds (159 to 227 kg)] and widths [34 to 36 inches (86 to 91 cm)]. The lowest of these weight limits had to become the maximum permitted for the use of a standard hospital bed. Similarly, the mattresses on the beds also had weight ratings of 325 to 400 pounds (147 to 182 kg). This led to the protocol that all patients with a weight over 325 pounds (147 kg) or a BMI greater than 55 (to capture the width parameter) would require a bariatric bed (13). Criteria-based protocols help to utilize the hospital resources most effectively and allow for preplanning as the patient population changes (6).

Essential Bariatric Equipment

Utilization of bariatric equipment does not ensure proper health care but can greatly improve the quality and safety of care (7). Both patients and caregivers should receive specific instructions for using specialized bariatric equipment properly in order to fully benefit from the advantages that this equipment offers.

This review of bariatric furniture and equipment that should be considered is based on the available literature and the authors' experience in caring for 4000 bariatric surgical patients (3,5,6,8,13–18). The discussion follows the surgical patient through the entire hospital stay, which is divided clinically into the preoperative, operative, and postoperative periods. Since the operative period is discussed in detail in Chapter 10, this chapter reviews the equipment needs of the preoperative and postoperative morbidly obese patient. Table 6-1 lists the bariatric equipment along with contact information for some of the vendors.

TABLE 6-1. Bariatric equipment information

Patient transfer (most commonly used size: 34-inch; use 39-inch for very large patients)		
Hovermatt	Web site: www.hovermatt.com	1-800-471-2776
AirPal	Web site: www.airpal.com	1-800-633-4725
Reliant 600 Patient Lift, Invacare Corporation	Web site: www.invacare.com	1-800-333-6900
Beds (bed and mattress weight capacity 1000 lb, 39-inch mattresses)		
Wheelchairs		
(size: 26-, 28-, and 30-inch widths, seat depths 22 inches, 750-lb weight capacity)		
Commode chairs		
(width 30 inches, weight capacity 750 lb, seat depth 23 inches)		
Invacare Corporation	Web site: www.invacare.com	1-800-333-6900
KCI (BariKare)	Web site: www.kci1.com	1-888-275-4524
Shower chair (width 30 inches, weight capacity 750 lb, seat depth 23 inches)		
Hill-Rom	Web Site: www.hill-rom.com	1-800-433-6245
KCI	Web site: www.kci1.com	1-888-275-4524
SIZEWise Rentals	Web site: www.sizewise.net	1-800-814-9389
Invacare Corporation	Web site: www.invacare.com	1-800-333-6900
Scales		
(weight capacity 600–880 lb)		
Scale-Tronix	Web site: www.scale-tronix.com	1-800-873-2001
Tanita Corp. of America	Web site: www.tanita.com	1-800-TANITA8
Health O Meter	Web site: www.sunbeam.com	(Division of Sunbeam)
Furniture		
Nemschoff	Web site: www.nemschoff.com	1-800-203-8916
Chair: 260-0815 OB15		
Sauder Manufacturing	Web site: www.saudermanufacturing.com	1-800-537-1530
Chair: Special Edition Series 30 and 40-inch widths		
Folding Chair–Lifetime Inc.	Web site: www.lifetime.com	1-800-225-3865
Examination tables		
Midmark	Web site: www.midmark.com	1-800-MIDMARK
United Metal Fabricators	Web site: www.umf-exam.com	1-800-638-5322
Hausmann Inc.	Web site: www.hausmann.com	1-888-428-7626
Stretchers		
Stryker Medical Inc.	Web site: www.med.stryker.com	1-800-STRYKER
Hill-Rom Services Inc.	Web site: www.hill-rom.com	1-800-433-6245
Gendron Inc.	Web site: www.gendronic.com	1-800-537-2521
Recent blood pressure technology		
Vasotrac	Web site: www.vasotrac.com	
Medwave Inc.	Web site: www.medwave.com	1-800-894-7601
Gowns/pants		
Size 10XL, and 3XL		
Superior Pad Outfitters	Web site: www.superiorpad.com	1-888-855-7970

Preoperative

Some patients will not be able to come to the facility by independent means and will require an ambulance. The team should collect information on the ambulance services in the surrounding area and how they are equipped for the transportation of morbidly obese patients. A number of modifications can be made to ambulance equipment and to transportation protocols to ensure that the service provided is a safe, efficient, comfortable, and dignified experience (12).

Transportation Equipment: Wheelchairs and Stretchers

Transportation equipment, especially wheelchairs and stretchers, are needed. In the past, many facilities invested in oversized wheelchairs, as this was one of the first areas where it was recognized that one size does not fit all. Initially, manufacturers simply took the standard wheelchair design and made it wider to accommodate the larger patients' needs. However, a good bariatric wheelchair is specifically engineered for the extra weight as well as size of the morbidly obese patient. It should come in a number

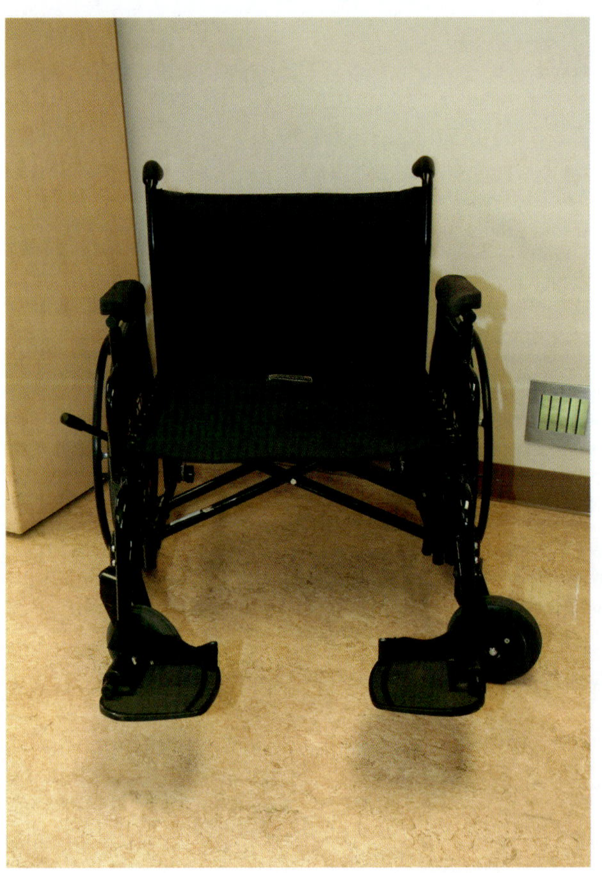

FIGURE 6-1. Bariatric wheelchair. (Courtesy of Invacare Corp., Elyria, OH, and Bariatric and Metabolic Institute, Cleveland Clinic Foundation, Cleveland, OH.)

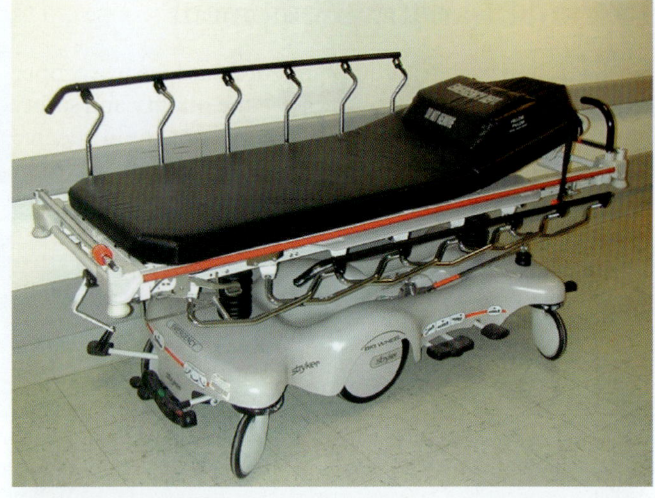

A

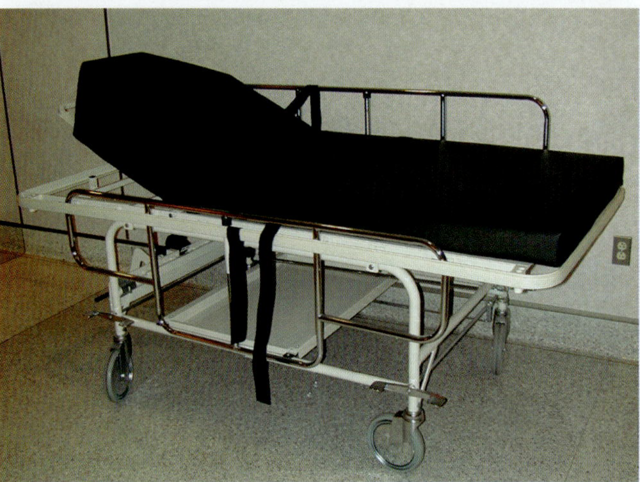

B

FIGURE 6-2. (A) Standard gurney. (B) Bariatric gurney. (Courtesy of Stryker, Kalazoo, MI.)

of widths [24 to 30 inches (60 to 76 cm)] and have a weight capacity of at least 750 pounds (340 kg) (Fig. 6-1).

Similarly, stretchers were not designed for the morbidly obese patient, and increasing weight limit modifications have been incorporated over the years. A good stretcher for the bariatric patients will have the appropriate weight rating in addition to adjustability of the head section and overall height. A crucial factor is the stretcher width. Space is a limiting factor in the successful passage through elevators, hallways, and doorways, but the width of the stretcher affects patient comfort and the potential for pressure morbidity. Many facilities use stretchers such as the Stryker M series (Kalamazoo, MI) with a weight limit of 500 to 700 pounds (227 to 317 kg), a height range of 20.75 to 34.5 inches (53 to 87 cm), a patient surface width of 26 to 30 inches (66 to 76 cm), (with a side-rails-up width of 33.5 to 37 inches (85 to 94 cm) (Fig. 6-2A). These are adequate for the majority of patients provided that they are not to be used for

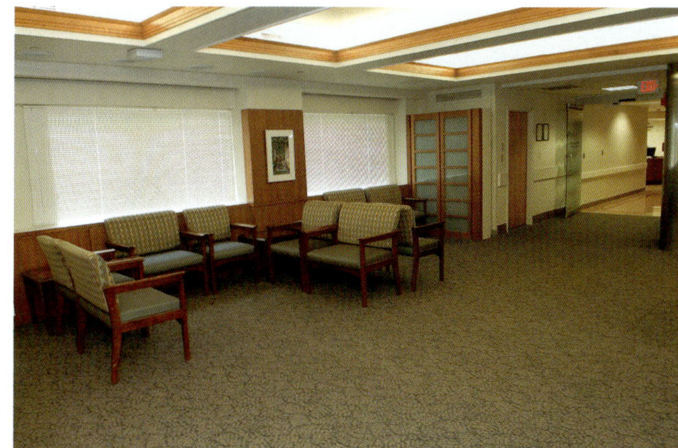

A

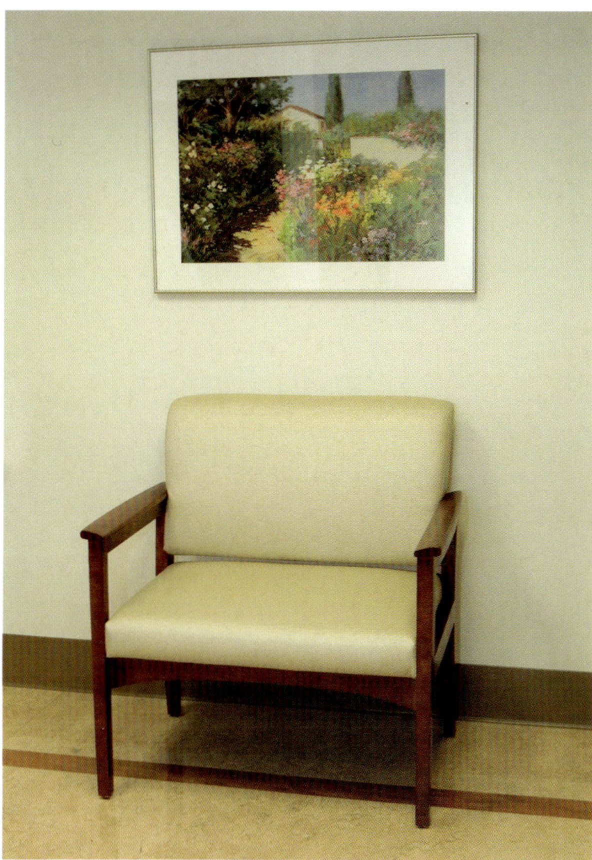

B

FIGURE 6-3. (A) Bariatric waiting room. (B) Bariatric chair in vital signs area. (A,B: Courtesy of Bariatric and Metabolic Institute, Cleveland Clinic Foundation, Cleveland, OH; B: Courtesy of Sauder Manufacturing, Archbold, OH.)

testing and emergency treatment areas, should be tested in advance.

Chairs

One of the common concerns of morbidly obese patients is that they will break furniture, especially chairs, or get stuck in a chair, causing them extreme embarrassment or even injury. Typically the chairs in medical office waiting rooms are not weight rated specifically or are rated up to only 300 pounds (136 kg). Their widths are usually from 20 to 24 inches (50 to 60 cm) and often have width-limiting arms. A bariatric chair should have a width of 28 to 44 inches (72 and 112 cm) and a weight rating of 600 to 750 pounds (272 to 341 kg) (Fig. 6-3). Another important factor is the height of the chair. Some morbidly obese persons are also of short stature. Adjustability of the chair height is a feature offered on some models. These chairs can be used in waiting rooms, patient rooms, recovery rooms, and hallways.

For group information sessions or support groups that patients attend, a portable and relatively inexpensive folding chair is suitable. These chairs have weight capacities up to 500 pounds (227 kg), are without arms, and offer flexibility in seating arrangements for discussions (Fig. 6-4).

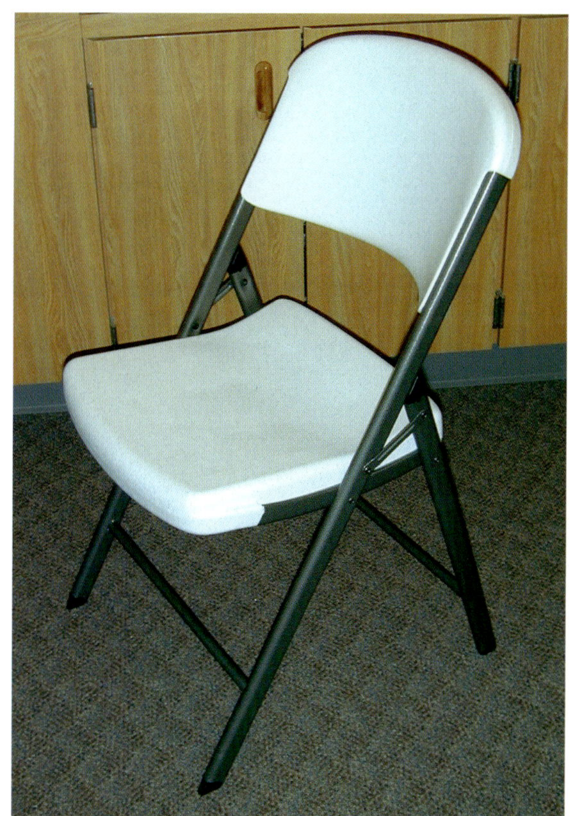

FIGURE 6-4. Folding chair with weight limit of 500 pounds. (Courtesy of Lifetime Products, Inc., Clearfield, UT.)

extended periods due to pressure ulcer concerns. All facilities should have the availability of a bariatric stretcher for those instances where these limitations are exceeded. A bariatric stretcher has a weight limit of 1000 pounds (454 kg) and a patient surface width of 39 inches (99 cm) (Fig. 6-2B). These dimensions make it more difficult to negotiate in tight halls, elevators, and rooms, and the patient's route to critical areas, including diagnostic

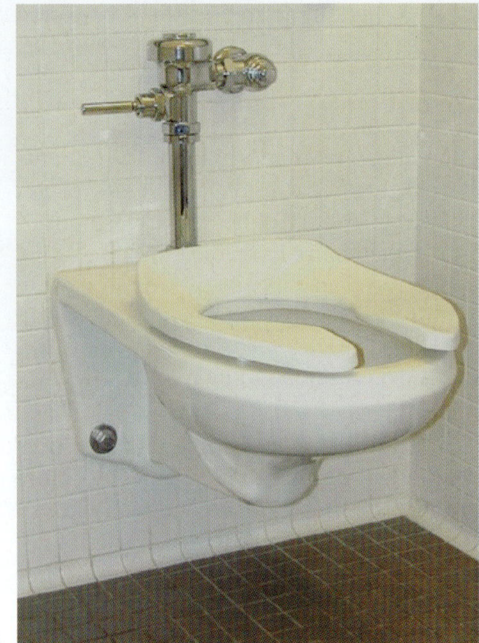
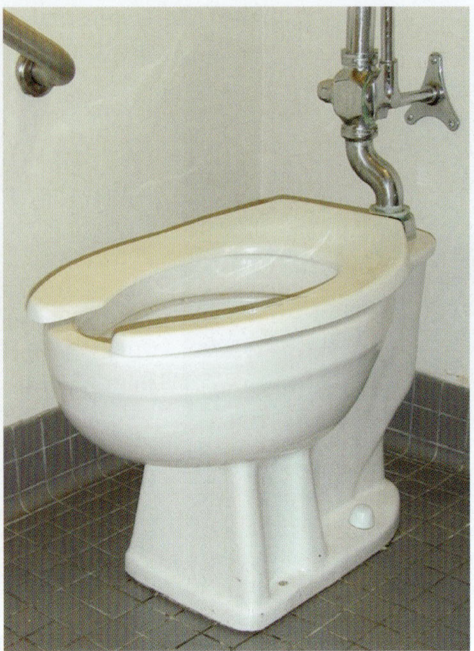
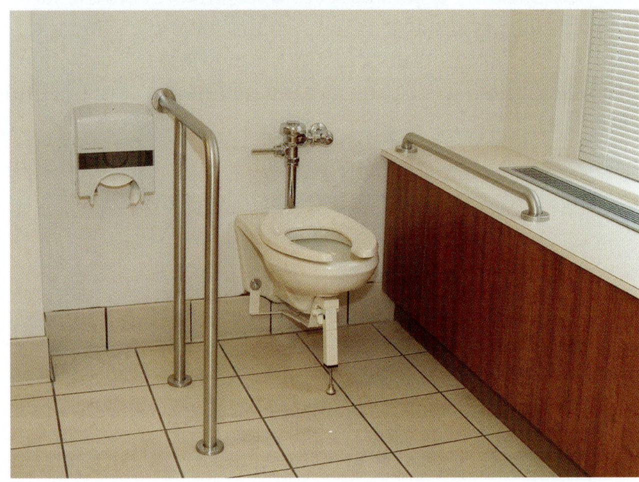

FIGURE 6-5. (A) Wall-mounted commode. (B) Pedestal commode. (C) Hand rails and adequate space around the commode. (Courtesy of Bariatric and Metabolic Institute, Cleveland Clinic Foundation, Cleveland, OH).

Commodes

Another important item to address is the commode. The standard wall-mounted model (Fig. 6-5A) is not safe, as it can snap off the wall when an obese person sits on it. Additional structural support can be added under the standard wall-mounted commode to provide sufficient weight-bearing capacity, but pedestal commodes, which are floor mounted, are preferable. Beginning April 2000 the American National Standards Institute (ANSI) standard for pedestal commodes was increased to 500 pounds (227 kg) (Fig. 6-5B). In addition, the commode should have adequate surrounding space to accommodate the morbidly obese patient (Fig. 6-5C).

Scales and Height-Measuring Devices

Easy and accurate measurement of weight and height in bariatric patients is essential to calculate the BMI and to track clinical changes associated with fluid management. A number of manufacturers have responded to this challenge with an array of products. Our team has used two scales, the Scale-Tronix model 5002 (White Plains, NY) (Fig. 6-6A) and model 6702W (Fig. 6-6B). The important features of a scale are accuracy, stability, an ample standing platform, a weight limit of at least 750 pounds (340 kg), portability, attachable height gauge, and wheelchair accessibility. These models have weight limits of 880 pounds (400 kg). Many products come with a height

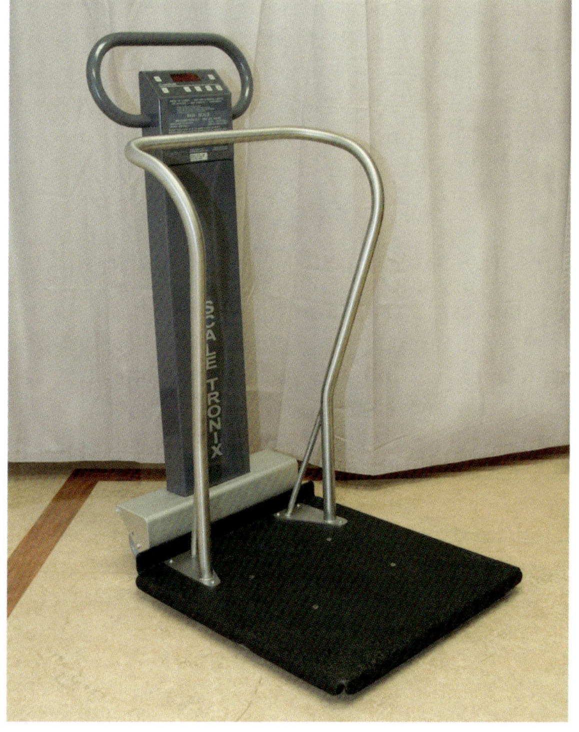

A

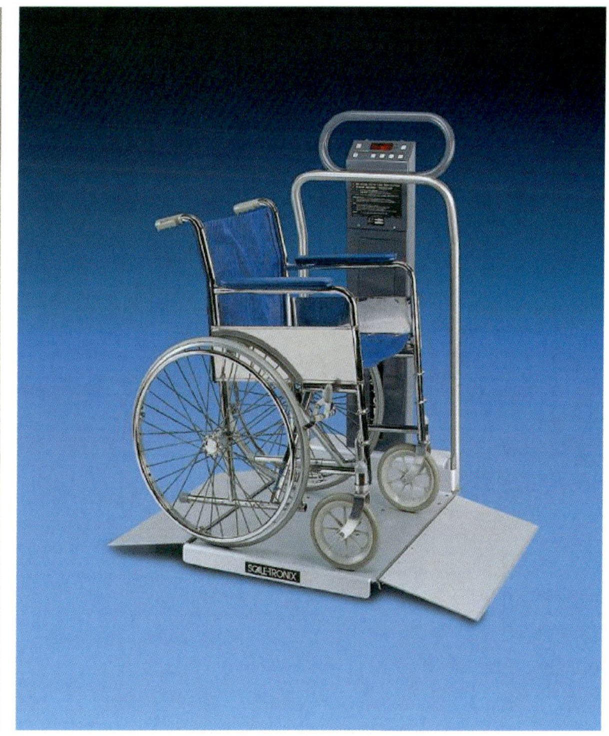

B

FIGURE 6-6. (A) Movable bariatric scale with weight limit of 880 pounds. (Courtesy of Bariatric and Metabolic Institute, Cleveland Clinic Foundation, Cleveland, OH). (B) Wheelchair-accessible bariatric scale. (Courtesy of Scale-Tronix, White Plains, NY.)

measure attached. Generally one scale will not meet the demands of both portability and wheelchair accessibility.

Blood Pressure Monitoring (Standard Cuffs and New Technology)

It is commonly understood that a large cuff is required to get an accurate measurement in morbidly obese patients.

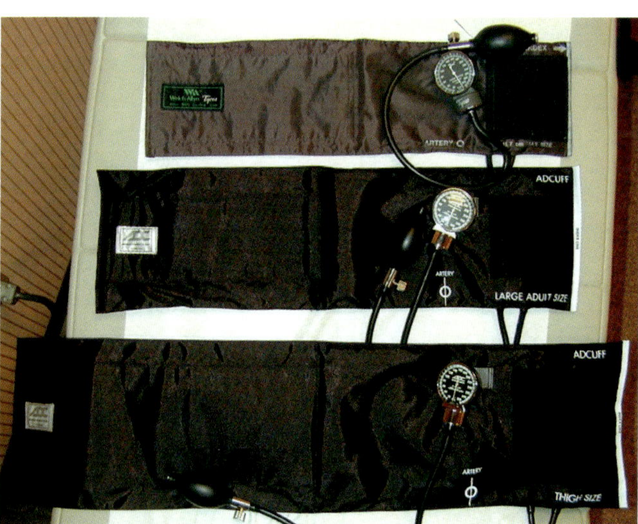

FIGURE 6-7. Multiple sizes of blood pressure cuffs. (Top, Welch Allyn, Skaneateles Falls, NY; middle and bottom, American Diagnostic Corporation, Hauppauge, NY.)

This requires specialized equipment. The large adult size or the thigh size cuffs must be readily available in clinics (Fig. 6-7). Even with the appropriate-sized cuff, simultaneous comparisons with an arterial line measurement show significant discrepancies. Overall, the technology of noninvasive blood pressure evaluation (sphygmomanometry) has changed little over the last 100 years. More recently, however, approaches that measure the waves and pulsations from the radial artery have become available and may well have an increasing utilization in the morbidly obese patient (19). An example is the Vasotrac (Medwave Inc., Arden Hills, MN). These devices are relatively easy to apply, noninvasive, comfortable, and accurate (Fig. 6-8).

Examination Tables

Morbidly obese persons may have difficulty climbing up on the examination table, and they may destabilize the table by using the attached step. Standard examination tables are often at a fixed height of 33 inches (84 cm) with a 7-inch (18 cm) step. In finding a table appropriate for obese patients, both the table's height and stability must be taken into account. The needs of a majority of obese patients are met by tables like the Ritter Barrier-Free™ (Midmark Corp., Versailles, OH) model 223, which has powered height adjustments from 18 to 37 inches (45.7 to 94 cm), a weight limit of 400 pounds (181.4 kg), and a width of 28 inches (72 cm) (Fig. 6-9). However, the power

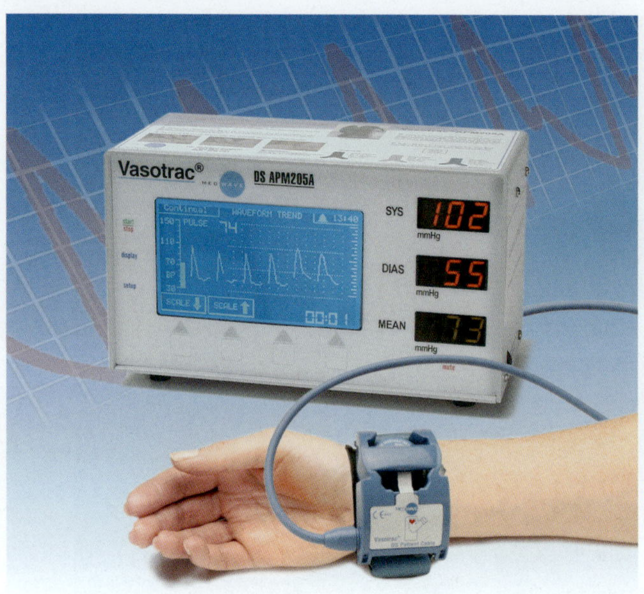

FIGURE 6-8. Vasotrac noninvasive radial artery blood pressure monitor. (Courtesy of Medwave, Inc., Arden Hills, MN.)

overall imaging power. Currently, we use the General Electric Discovery ST 16, which has a weight rating of 450 pounds (204 kg), a gantry diameter of 70 cm, and a circumference of 220 cm (86.5 inches). The newer GE Lightspeed VCT volume CT scanner has the same limits but improved imaging power technology.

Cardiac Risk Stratification Equipment

Cardiac risk stratification in high-risk morbidly obese patients in preparation for bariatric surgery has many limitations. The most frequently used single photon emission computed tomography (SPECT) myocardioperfusion study has weight limitations of about 300 pounds (137 kg) due to the camera. The planar scans can be performed in patients up to 400 pounds but the risk of false positives increases at the higher weights. Dobutamine stress echocardiogram studies can be performed on

lift function serves only up to 400 pounds (181.4 kg). For super-obese patients, a bariatric examination table such as the Ritter Model 244 is helpful, as it has a 850-pound (385-kg) weight limit, a powered height range of 18 to 34 inches (45.7 to 86.4 cm), a width of 32 inch (81.3 cm), and a powered back rest that rises to 65 degrees.

Upper Gastrointestinal and Computed Tomography Scans

Preoperative and postoperative upper gastrointestinal studies and abdominal computed tomography (CT) scans are frequently required to assess comorbid conditions, variant anatomy, and complications such as leak of the anastomosis (20). Even in the best of circumstances, the quality of these studies may be inferior in an obese patient, but it is important that the patient's size be accommodated by the diagnostic facilities and equipment (21).

Fluoroscopy equipment has limitations in the image quality and weight limits regarding articulation of the table. Full articulation of most tables has a weight limit of 300 pounds (137 kg). The footboards on the tables have weight limits of 300 to 350 pounds (137 to 159 kg) depending on the model. Larger patients' studies are often obtained in the standing position (on the floor) with a sacrifice of optimal image control.

The limitations with abdominal CT scanning in the bariatric patient relate to the weight limitations of the power table, the diameter of the entry port, and the

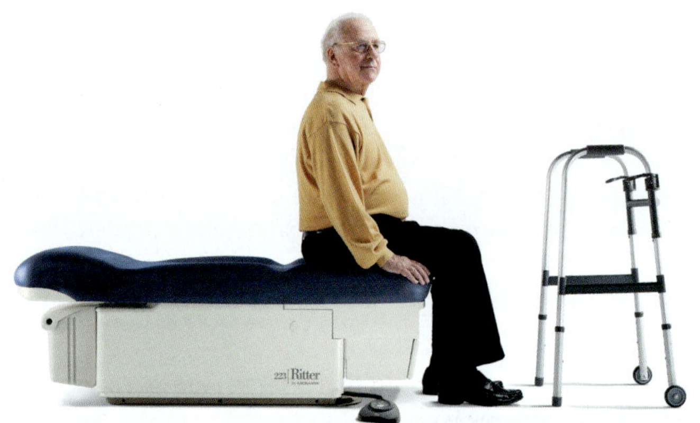

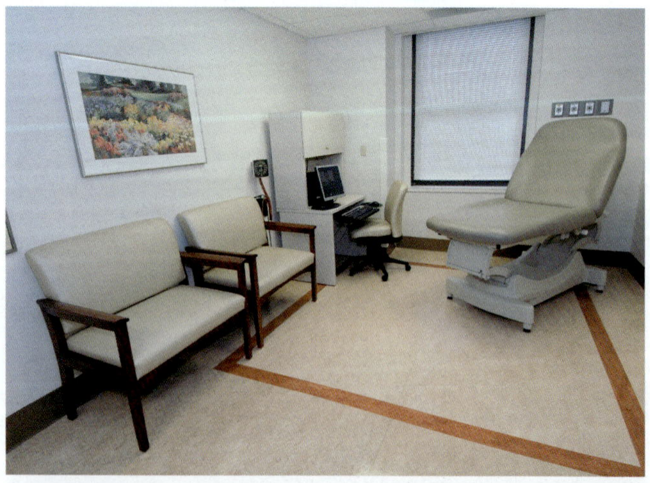

FIGURE 6-9. (A) Standard examination table (Courtesy of Midmark Corp, Versailees, OH.) (B) Bariatric examination room and table. (Courtesy of Bariatric and Metabolic Institute, Cleveland Clinic Foundation, Cleveland, OH.)

morbidly obese patients, but anatomic and operator variability decreases the accuracy and reliability. Cardiac catheterization, the gold standard in risk stratification, is difficult to perform technically due to vascular access problems and has weight limitations of 350 pounds (159 kg) due to the table. A limited catheterization without table articulation or on an alternative stretcher can be performed as an alternative. These equipment weight and performance limitations leave cardiac risk stratification in obese patients in a less than optimal state especially at weights greater than 400 pounds (182 kg), which can be altogether prohibitive for some studies.

Postoperative

Beds and Mattresses

In the operating room it is helpful to transfer the patient to the bed using a transfer device (see Chapter 10). Standard hospital beds have weight ratings of 350 to 500 pounds (159 to 227 kg). It is important to check with the manufacturer for the weight rating for each model and vintage. Most recent models have weight ratings of up to 500 pounds (227 kg), which would serve the majority of patients. The standard mattress on the bed also will have a weight rating, often 300 to 500 pounds (136 to 227 kg). They also are available in a number of different types of surfaces. It is appropriate to routinely use a pressure reduction mattress, recognizing the high risk for developing pressure ulcerations (7,22).

The width of the patient and bed must be considered. Standard hospital beds are typically from 34 to 36 inches (86 to 91 cm), often with the critical care beds tending to be the narrowest. Manufacturers recommend that a patient be fitted for the need for a bariatric bed by having the patient measured lying flat. This is not often practical prior to surgery. We and others have adopted utilization of the BMI to take into account the width of the patient (23). Our criteria-based protocol calls for a bariatric bed and wheelchair for those patients weighing 325 pounds (150 kg) or more or with a BMI of 55 or greater.

Special bariatric beds offer a number of options requiring choices at the time of purchase or rental. There are two types of entry: side entry (as with standard beds) (Fig. 6-10A), and bottom entry (Fig. 6-10B). Some beds easily allow both types. The side entry bed looks more like the standard hospital bed and may have less stigma for the majority of bariatric surgical patients who are for the most part easily ambulatory. The bottom entry beds can often be converted into a chair position to facilitate ambulation and possibly lead to fewer staff injuries related to patient ambulation. Other features to take into consideration are the type of side rail adjustment, the

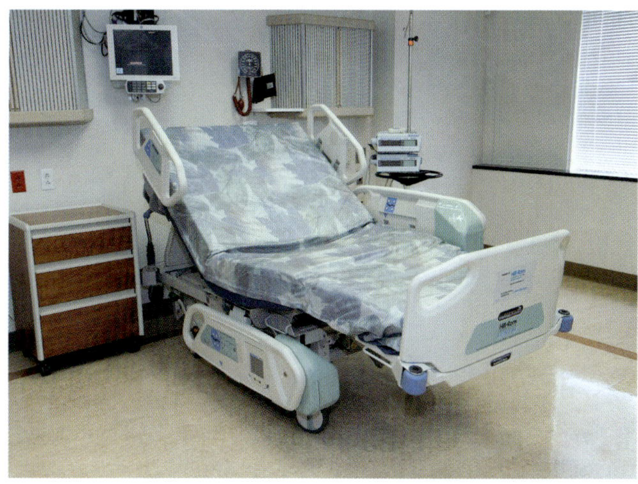

A

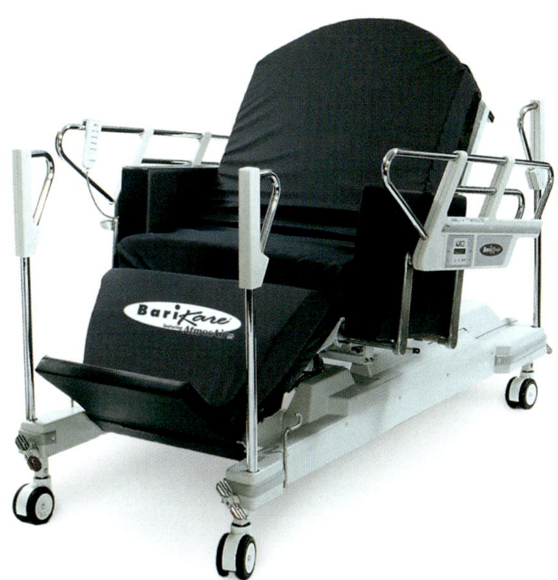

B

FIGURE 6-10. (A) Side entry bariatric bed. (Courtesy of Hill-Rom. © 2006 Hill-Rom Services, Inc. Reprinted with permission. All rights reserved; and Bariatric and Metabolic Institute, Cleveland Clinic Foundation, Cleveland, OH). (B) Bottom entry bariatric bed (Courtesy of BariKare, KCI, San Antonio, TX.)

wheels and locks, the height adjustment parameters, the ability to attach over-bed trapezes, built-in scales, and the complexity and ease of use of the hand controls. Another important consideration is that the bed should be able to be placed in at least 45 degree of reverse Trendelenburg position easily, as this is the optimum position for pulmonary function, given that many of the patients have ventilatory comorbid conditions (obstructive sleep apnea, obesity hypoventilation syndrome, and restrictive lung disease) and may in some cases require tracheotomy and ventilatory support (24).

Hospital Patient Room Layout, Equipment, and Fixtures

The layout of the hospital room is the basic building block of a bariatric nursing unit and most influential in the administering of nursing care postoperatively. A dedicated unit with a dedicated staff is most preferable but at present is not the norm. The driving force in the design and layout is the large patient size and weight, requiring many pieces of oversized and extremely durable equipment (already noted) and providing safety in the staff's negotiating around the patient.

In an effort to establish industry standards, Hill-Rom Services, Inc. formed the Bariatric Room Design Advisory Board (BRDAB), which made a number of recommendations with respect to room space, target maximum weight tolerance for room equipment and fixtures, and the equipment a patient room should have (11). The board recommended 5 feet (152 cm) of space around a bed to allow for the passage of oversized equipment (Fig. 6-11A), which thus necessitates an overall room size of at least 13 feet (4 m) in width and 15 ft (4.6 m) in depth from the corridor. The opening for this space should be ideally 60 inches (152 cm) with an unequally divided leaf-swinging door, one leaf being 42 inches (107 cm). The BRDAB set a target maximum of 1000 pounds (454 kg) as a recommendation for room equipment and fixture weight tolerance. In many cases this would not be possible at present. The board recommended that other room equipment for consideration would be a bedside chair (specification as noted in an earlier section) and a lift. Lifts are essential to have available due to the high number of staff and patient injuries associated with patient lifting and transfer (25). The board suggested that a mobile portable lift is most appropriate due to its flexibility in accommodating the patient in any part of the

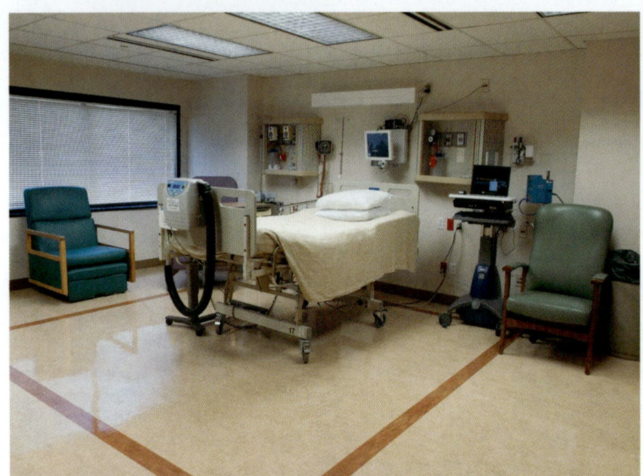

A

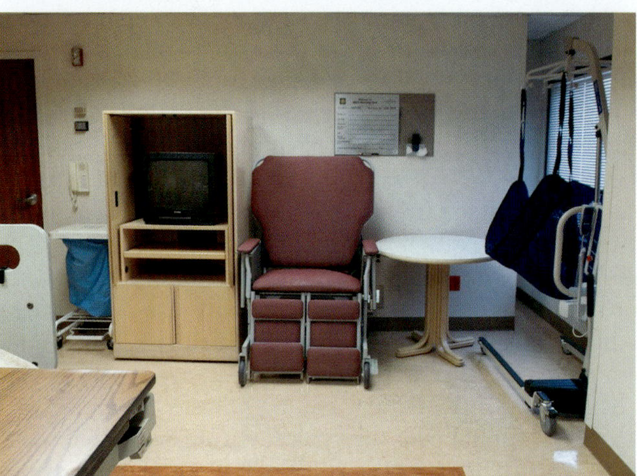

B

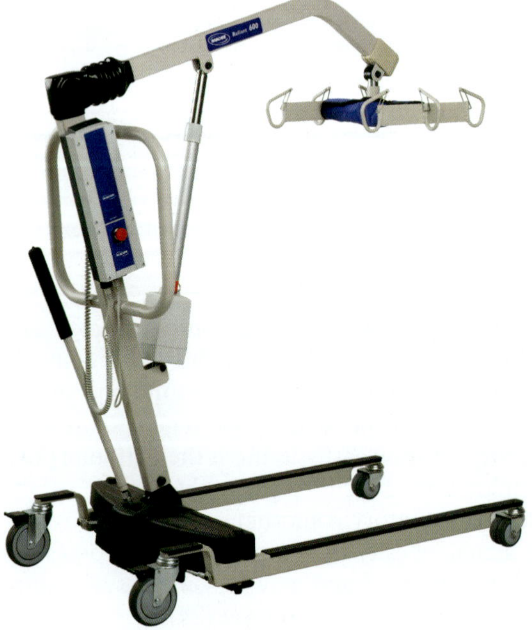

C

FIGURE 6-11. (A) Bariatric inpatient room with adequate space around bed. (Courtesy of Bariatric and Metabolic Institute, Cleveland Clinic Foundation, Cleveland, OH.) (B) Bariatric recliner chair in inpatient room and patient lift (right). (Courtesy of Bariatric and Metabolic Institute, Cleveland Clinic Foundation, Cleveland, OH.) (C) Patient lift with electric motor and 600-lb weight capacity. (Courtesy of Invacare Corp., Elyria, OH.)

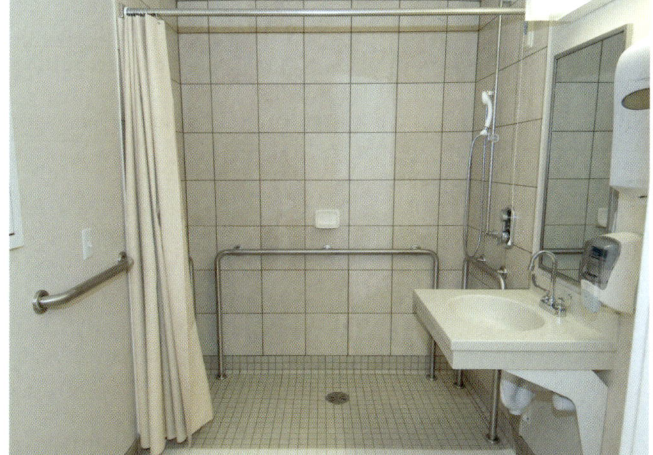

A

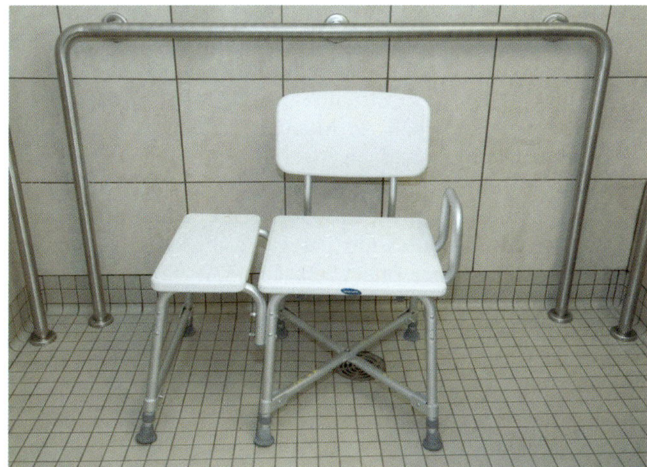

B

FIGURE 6-12. (A) Large shower room with unobstructed access to shower. (Courtesy of Bariatric and Metabolic Institute, Cleveland Clinic Foundation, Cleveland, OH). (B) Shower chair (Courtesy of Sizewise Rentals, www.sizewise.net.)

room (Fig. 6-11B). One example of a mobile lift is the Invacare Reliant 600 (Elyria, OH) that features an electric motor and a lift of up to 660 pounds (300 kg) (Fig. 6-11C).

Hygiene Items: Toilets, Showers, Gowns/Pants

Personal hygiene can be difficult for the bariatric surgical patient due to space limitations, limited mobility, and the need for a durable environment. Toileting requires a bathroom with an opening of 60 inches (152 cm) in width, to accommodate the width of the widest wheelchair. Commodes require hand rails to enable the patient to self assist. For those patients with minimal mobility but able to bear weight and to transfer, a bedside commode is an excellent option preferable to the use of a bedpan. It especially allows for increased safety, comfort, and dig-

nity. It should have a width of at least 30 inches (76 cm) and a weight capacity of at least 750 pounds (341 kg).

The BRDAB recommends that a shower space be at least 45 square feet (4.17 square meters), large enough to accommodate the assistance of two caregivers and wheelchair access. Each patient room may not have enough space available, so a reasonable option for showering is a communal shower, which we have at our facility, and the feedback from patients has been excellent. The BRDAB also recommends waterproof walls and floor, with a drainage sloping floor without curbs for easy entry and exit (Fig. 6-12A). A portable shower chair/bench, either a commode chair combination model or a stand-alone, is a necessity (Fig. 6-12B).

The availability of appropriate fitting hospital clothing is essential to patient safety, hygiene, and dignity. Since the morbidly obese are also not all the same size or shape, a few sizes of gowns (3X to 10X) and pants (X to 4X) should be readily available. The gowns should accommodate peripheral intravenous lines.

Many severely obese patients have chronic osteoarthritis affecting their backs, hips, and knees. Postoperatively and upon discharge from the hospital, these patients may temporarily require walkers to avoid falls during their recovery from surgery. The walker model should be one that is designed specifically for the bariatric patient. These walkers have a wide base and an adjustable height, and can support up to 700 pounds of weight (Fig. 6-13). A wheel kit can be added to provide additional assistance with ambulation.

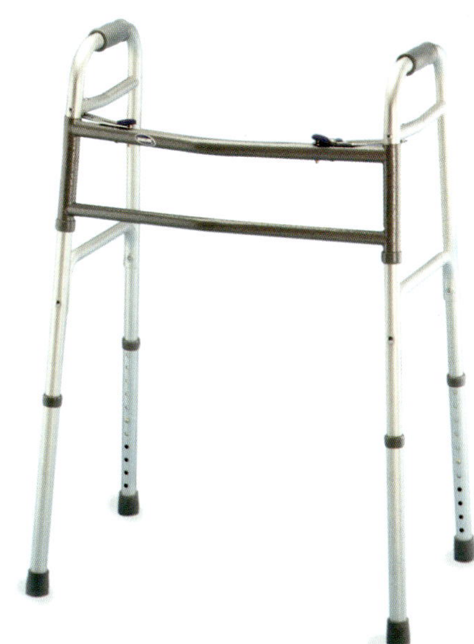

FIGURE 6-13. A walker designed for bariatric patients has a deep and wide frame, adjustable height, and can support up to 700 pounds. A wheel kit can be added if needed. (Courtesy of Invacare Corp., Elyria, OH.)

Periodic Reevaluation

It is important to reevaluate patient anthrometric data, the equipment utilization numbers, comorbidity related to immobilization, accidents or falls involving patients, staff injuries, and overall surgical outcome data. Bariatric surgical programs including surgeons, staff, patient characteristics, and facilities will mature over time and require further evaluation of equipment needs and use criteria.

Conclusion

Bariatric equipment includes all of the technology used to administer health care to the morbidly obese patient. This equipment is essential in providing quality bariatric surgical care by providing for safety, reducing morbidity, and enhancing mobility, thereby promoting the best possible outcomes. Further, adequately sized accommodations and equipment allow for accurate diagnostic testing and reduce stress and wasted time. These benefits promote the dignity of the patients, improving the satisfaction of patients, families, and staff. To achieve this, a facility must investigate its own resources, limitations, and patient base, based on its current management of morbidly obese patients, and survey the bariatric equipment market. A bariatric task force is a good organizational structure to coordinate this activity. Ultimately, criteria-based protocols will be developed to guide the appropriate utilization of bariatric equipment resources. These will need to be revised intermittently as the program matures and technology advances. The process requires ongoing communication among clinicians, administrators, and equipment manufacturers in the further refinement and development of additional technology to better care for the morbidly obese patient (3,6).

Acknowledgments. William Gourash would like to thank Judy Myers and the staff on 5300 of Magee Women's Hospital of the University of Pittsburgh Health System for their innovation and excellent nursing care; Susan Gallagher for her years of numerous contributions to care of the morbidly obese; and Laura Smolenak, RN, for sharing her insight into the morbidly obese; Amy Haller for sharing her knowledge of bariatric equipment; and his family, especially his wife, Linda M. Gourash, for their patience and editing.

References

1. Gallagher S. Ethics: the human element of advanced technology. Ostomy Wound Management 2003;49(4):24–28.
2. Nightingale F. Notes on Nursing: What It Is and What It Is Not. New York: Dover, 1860.
3. Foli MB, Collier MS, MacDonald KG, Pories WF. Availability and adequacy of diagnostic and therapeutic equipment for the morbidly obese patient in an acute care setting. Obes Surg 1993;3:153–156.
4. Barr J, Cunneen J. Understanding the bariatric client and providing a safe hospital environment. Clin Nurse Specialist 2001;15(5):219–223.
5. Sarr MG, Gelty CL, Hilmer DM, et al. Technical and practical considerations involved in operations on patients weighing more than 270 kg. Arch Surg 1995;130(1):102–105.
6. Gallagher SM, Arzouman J, Lacovara J, et al. Criteria-based protocols and the obese patient: planning care for a high-risk population. J Ostomy Wound Manag 2004;50(5):32–44.
7. Gallagher SM. Restructuring the therapeutic environment to promote care and safety for the obese patient. J Wound Ostomy Continence Nurs 1999;26(6):292–297.
8. Nguyen NT, Moore C, Stevens M, Chalifoux S, Mavandadi S, Wilson SE. The practice of bariatric surgery at academic medical centers. J Gastrointest Surg 2004;8(7):856–860.
9. Retsas A, Pinikahana J. Manual handling activities and injuries among nurses: an Australian hospital study. J Adv Nurs 2003;31(4):875–883.
10. Gallagher S. Caring for the overweight patient in the acute care setting: Addressing caregiver injury. J Healthcare Safety, Compliance Infect 2000;4(8):379–382.
11. Harrell JW, Miller B. Big challenge. Designing for the needs of bariatric patients. Health Facil Manag 2004;17(3):34–38.
12. Weiss J, Perham D, Forrest J. Build you own bariatric unit: Southwest ambulance creates a better way to transport obese patients. J EMS 2003;28(12):36–45.
13. Gourash W. Bariatric equipment: making your facility more accommodating for the morbidly obese. Presented at the University of Pittsburgh School of Medicine and the Minimally Invasive Surgery Center of the University of Pittsburgh Medical Center, February 2001.
14. Hilmer D. Technical considerations of bariatric surgery in the Super obese. Surg Technol 1994;26(7):8–13.
15. AORN Bariatric Surgery Guideline. AORN J 2004;79(5):1026–1052.
16. Recommendations for facilities performing bariatric surgery. Bull Am Coll Surg 2000;85:20–23.
17. Martin LF, Burney M, Faitor-Stampley V, Wheeler T, Raum WJ. Preparing a hospital for bariatric patients. In: Martin LF, ed. Obesity Surgery. New York: McGraw-Hill, 2003:161–172.
18. Martinez-Owens T, Lindstrom W. Special needs of the bariatric surgical office. In: Martin LF, ed. Obesity Surgery. New York: McGraw-Hill, 2003:111–132.
19. Helmut H, Mandadi G, Eagon C, Pulley D, Kurz A. Intraoperative blood pressure measurement on the wrist is more accurate than on the upper arm in morbidly obese patients. Abstract presented at the American Society of Anesthesia 2004 annual meeting.
20. Blachar A, Federle MP, Pealer K, Ikramuddin D, Schauer PR. Gastrointestinal complication of laparoscopic Roux-en-Y gastric bypass surgery: clinical and imaging findings. Radiology 2002;23(3):625–632.

21. Uppot PN. How obesity hinders image quality and diagnosis in radiology. Bariatrics Today 2005;1:31–33.

22. Brown SJ. Bed surfaces and pressure sore prevention: an abridged report. Orthop Nurs 2001;20(4):30–40.

23. Fruto LV, Malancy K, Forbis J, Cochran J. Development of decision guidelines for specialty bed/mattress selection for obese patients. Ostomy Wound Manag 1997;43(3): 66.

24. Burns SM, Egloff MB, Ryan B, Carpenter R, Burns JE. Effect of body position on spontaneous respiratory rate and tidal volume in patients with obesity, abdominal distention and ascites. Am J Crit Care 1994;3(2):102–106.

25. Evanoff B, Wolf L, Aton E, Canos J, Collins J. Reduction in injury rates in nursing personnel through introduction of mechanical lifts in the workplace. Am J Ind Med 2003; 44:451–457.

7
Bariatric Surgery Training

Stacy A. Brethauer and Philip R. Schauer

The number of bariatric procedures performed worldwide has increased dramatically over the last decade (1). Factors contributing to this increase include (1) the rising prevalence of obesity in industrialized countries; (2) increasing awareness of the societal costs of this epidemic; (3) the introduction of minimally invasive approaches to bariatric surgery; and (4) a growing body of literature supporting the safety, effectiveness, and durability of bariatric surgery. The United States has the highest prevalence of adult and childhood obesity in the world (2), and the increasing number of bariatric surgeries performed over the last decade is a reflection of this troubling epidemic (Table 7-1).

The introduction of laparoscopic bariatric procedures in the late 1990s has been a major contributor to the rising popularity of this specialty. This approach has attracted surgeons interested in advanced laparoscopy and patients who demand less invasive procedures. This rapid increase in bariatric procedures has also highlighted the need for specialized training and credentialing procedures for bariatric surgeons. The Society of American Gastrointestinal and Endoscopic Surgeons (SAGES) and the American Society for Bariatric Surgery (ASBS) have jointly put forth guidelines suggesting specific credentialing procedures to perform bariatric surgery (3). Additionally, the ASBS has developed guidelines for fellowship training in bariatric surgery that ensure an academically sound and clinically diverse experience for trainees (4). In the past, surgeons were self-taught or underwent a brief period of proctoring prior to practicing bariatric surgery. This approach has largely been replaced by formal training during residency or fellowships. This chapter reviews the options currently available to complete adequate training in bariatric surgery, credentialing procedures, fellowship training guidelines, and future directions for training in bariatric surgery.

The Learning Curve

Surgical training entails various learning curves, principally for the acquisition of technical skills and for patient management. Both of these areas are relevant to bariatric surgery and must be addressed to achieve competency in this discipline. The concept of a learning curve applied to a specific procedure emerged in the late 1980s as surgeons with experience in open cholecystectomies had higher complication rates in their early laparoscopic experience. Each new laparoscopic procedure introduced since then has been accompanied by a body of literature describing its specific learning curve (5–8). This learning curve typically represents the number of cases required to achieve complication rates similar to those seen in the open approach.

While laparoscopic adjustable gastric banding is less technically demanding than bypass procedures, several procedure-specific complications can occur early in a surgeon's experience. In O'Brien and Dixon's (9) series of 1120 Lap Bands (Inamed Health, Santa Barbara, CA), complications were more common during their early experience. Gastric prolapse through the band occurred in 125 (25%) of the first 500 patients but occurred in only 28 (4.7%) of the last 600 patients. Erosion of the band into the stomach occurred in 34 patients (3%); all occurred in the first 500 patients. The Italian collaborative study group for the Lap Band demonstrated that, among 1863 patients, gastric pouch dilation occurred in 5% of patients overall (10). Two thirds of these complications occurred during the center's first 50 cases and the incidence of gastric pouch dilation decreased as surgeons gained experience with the procedure.

Laparoscopic gastric bypass is an advanced laparoscopic procedure that has a relatively steep learning curve. This procedure requires advanced laparoscopic skills including intracorporeal suturing, creating anasto-

TABLE 7-1. Estimated number of bariatric procedures performed in the United States

Year	Bariatric procedures per year
1992–1996	15,000–20,000
1997–1999	20,000–30,000
2000	38,000
2001	48,000
2002	63,000
2003	104,000
2004	140,000

Data from the American Society for Bariatric Surgery.

moses in different quadrants of the abdomen, difficult exposure techniques, gastrointestinal stapling, and two-hand dissection techniques. The intraabdominal anatomy of the morbidly obese patient (large stores of visceral fat, hepatomegaly, adhesions from previous surgery) adds to the challenge of performing this operation. With respect to the learning curve for laparoscopic gastric bypass, one report found that wound infections, anastomotic leaks, operative times, and technical complications decreased significantly after 100 cases (11). Oliak et al. (12) found that operative time and complications decrease significantly after the first 75 cases, and others have also demonstrated decreased complication rates with increasing experience (13).

Skill Acquisition

The number of cases required to gain proficiency in advanced laparoscopic or bariatric procedures are rarely acquired during surgical residency (Table 7-2) (14,15). In 2004, the average number of bariatric procedures (open and laparoscopic) completed during the chief residency year was 5.8, and while this is up from an average of 2.8 in 2000, it is still far fewer than the recommended number to achieve a minimal level of competency (35 cases) (16) or overcome the learning curves (75 to 100 cases) for

these procedures. In addition to experience in the operating room, practicing advanced laparoscopic procedures with animal models can significantly augment the training experience for surgeons at all levels (17). Laparoscopic training devices can also be used to objectively evaluate surgical skills, overcome deficiencies, and monitor progress (18,19).

Procedure-specific training can be obtained during short courses or weekend workshops that provide didactic training and hands-on training with an animal model (20). These courses are often attended by surgeons who have advanced laparoscopic skills but want to learn bariatric procedures. Additionally, open bariatric surgeons seeking initial exposure to the laparoscopic approach can benefit from these short workshops. However, these short courses typically do not provide adequate training to perform the procedures independently.

The mini-fellowship concept involves a focused, short-term training experience in bariatric surgery and may be the best option for a practicing surgeon who wants to start a bariatric practice. The mini-fellowship is a 6- to 12-week experience designed for a surgeon who has advanced laparoscopic skills but needs to gain experience with bariatric procedures. The goal is to acquire the experience necessary to meet bariatric surgery privileging requirements as outlined in the ASBS (21). The trainee must acquire a license in the state in which they will be training and obtain hospital privileges. The mini-fellowship exposes the trainee to all aspects of bariatric surgery including preoperative evaluation, open and laparoscopic procedures, routine and complicated postoperative management, and long-term postoperative care. The didactic component of the mini-fellowship includes textbook reviews, journal clubs, and participation in clinical conferences. Additionally, the trainee gains exposure to the program's organizational structure, personnel requirements, equipment and hospital requirements, and administrative issues unique to bariatric surgery.

TABLE 7-2. Bariatric and advanced laparoscopic cases completed during general surgery residency in the United States

Procedure	1999–2000	2000–2001	2001–2002	2002–2003	2003–2004
Bariatric*					
Average number performed by all residents	5.0	6.7	9.5	11.2	12.1
Total cases reported	4,960	6,871	9,560	11,027	12,354
Laparoscopic Nissen					
Average number performed by all residents	5.4	6.2	5.9	5.9	5.1
Total cases reported	5,341	6,334	5,944	5,740	5,230
Laparoscopic colectomy					
Average number performed by all residents	1.9	2.3	3.1	3.9	4.6
Total cases reported	1,815	2,366	3,186	3,850	4,689

* Open and laparoscopic.
Data from Residency Review Committee for General Surgery National Report, www.acgme.org.

Patient Management

The second learning curve associated with bariatric surgery involves the overall management of the morbidly obese patient. This includes understanding the pathophysiology of obesity, the indications for bariatric surgery, recognition and treatment of complications specific to bariatric surgery, and the long-term management of patients postoperatively. This experience can rarely be acquired during residency training because of the relatively low volume of bariatric surgery patients. Training in a high-volume bariatric surgery environment such as a formal fellowship program is the optimal way to gain exposure to these aspects of bariatric surgery and to learn these patient management skills.

American Society for Bariatric Surgery Suggested Guidelines for Granting Privileges in Bariatric Surgery

The first ASBS guidelines were published in 2000 (3). It is important to note that neither SAGES nor ASBS is a credentialing organization. Individual hospitals or health systems are responsible for granting clinical privileges. Most credentialing committees, though, have adopted the credentialing guidelines proposed by specialty boards or specialty societies.

The current guidelines are a modification of the original guidelines enacted by the ASBS and are divided into five categories (21), as discussed in the following subsections.

Global Credentialing Requirements

The global credentialing requirements are as follows:

1. The applicant should have credentials at an accredited facility to perform gastrointestinal and biliary surgery.

2. The applicant should document that he or she is working within an integrated program for the care of the morbidly obese patient that provides ancillary services such as specialized nursing care, dietary instruction, counseling, and support groups.

3. The applicant should document that there is a program in place to prevent, monitor. and manage short-term and long-term complications.

4. The applicant should document that there is a system in place to provide and encourage follow-up for all patients.

Follow-up visits should be directly supervised either by the bariatric surgeon of record or by other health care professionals who are appropriately trained in perioperative management of bariatric patients and are part of an integrated program. While applicants cannot guarantee patient compliance with follow-up recommendations, they should demonstrate evidence of adequate patient education regarding the importance of follow-up as well as adequate access to follow-up.

Experience Required to Train Applicants

The ASBS recommends that an experienced bariatric surgeon willing to serve as trainer for applicants should meet the global credentialing requirements and have experience with at least 200 bariatric procedures in the appropriate category of procedure in which the applicant is seeking privileges prior to training the applicant. The new guidelines also define operative experience broadly to include not only procedure performance but also global care of the bariatric patient, encompassing preoperative and postoperative management.

Open Bariatric Surgery Privileges Involving Stapling or Division of the Gastrointestinal Tract

The surgeon should meet the global credentialing requirements and document an operative experience of 15 open bariatric procedures (or subtotal gastric resection with reconstruction) with satisfactory outcomes during either general surgery residency or postresidency training supervised by an experienced bariatric surgeon. Surgeons who primarily perform laparoscopic bariatric surgery may obtain open bariatric surgery privileges after documentation of 50 laparoscopic cases and at least 10 open cases supervised by an experienced bariatric surgeon.

Laparoscopic Bariatric Surgical Privileges for Procedures Involving Stapling or Division of the Gastrointestinal Tract

The surgeon must meet the global credentialing requirements and (1) have privileges to perform open bariatric surgery at the accredited facility, (2) have privileges to perform advanced laparoscopic surgery at the accredited facility, and (3) document 50 cases with satisfactory outcomes during either general surgery residency or postresidency training under the supervision of an experienced bariatric surgeon.

Bariatric Surgery Privileges for Procedures that Do Not Involve Stapling or Division of the Gastrointestinal Tract

The surgeon must meet the global credentialing requirements and (1) have privileges to perform advanced laparoscopic surgery at the accredited facility, and (2) document 10 cases with satisfactory outcomes during either general surgery residency or postresidency training under supervision of an experienced bariatric surgeon.

American Society for Bariatric Surgery Guidelines for Comprehensive Fellowship Training in Bariatric Surgery

The ASBS has proposed a formal curriculum to standardize fellowship training in bariatric surgery (Table 7-3). This curriculum provides a foundation of cognitive, clinical, and technical experience for general surgeons who plan to make bariatric surgery part of their practice after fellowship. The establishment of the Minimally Invasive Surgery Fellowship Council has formalized the application and selection process for surgeons interested in advanced laparoscopic and gastrointestinal surgery

(22). Bariatric surgery comprises a major part of many of the fellowships offered by the fellowship council, and the guidelines offered by the ASBS provide a standardized framework for these training programs.

Ultimately, an examination based on a curriculum of bariatric surgery fundamentals may become part of a formal certification process for bariatric surgery. In the meantime, efforts should be made on the part of fellows and program directors to work toward this type of formal education for future bariatric surgeons. This type of self-governance and quality control within the bariatric community will lend credibility to the field and offer reassurance to patients, payers, and referring physicians.

Continued Assessment of Outcomes

The ASBS recommends that the local facility should review the surgeon's outcome data within 6 months of initiation of a new program and after the surgeon's first

TABLE 7-3. ASBS Guidelines for comprehensive fellowship training in bariatric surgery (4)

Cognitive
- Fellows and at least one faculty member attend periodic teaching sessions
- Format can include textbook review, journal club, peer-review conferences, or teaching rounds
- The topics to be covered include:
  1. Epidemiology of obesity
  2. History of bariatric surgery
  3. Physiology and interactive mechanisms in morbid obesity
  4. Preoperative evaluation of the bariatric patient including comorbidities
  5. Psychology of the morbidly obese patient
  6. Essentials of a bariatric program
  7. Postoperative management of the bariatric patient
  8. Laparoscopic versus open access in the bariatric patient
  9. Restrictive operations
  10. Gastric bypass
  11. Malabsorptive procedures
  12. Revisional weight loss surgery
  13. Managing postoperative complications
  14. Nutritional deficiencies related to bariatric surgery
  15. Obesity in childhood and in the elderly
  16. Outcomes of bariatric surgery
- Attendance at quarterly morbidity and mortality conference focusing on bariatric cases and perioperative care issues
- Attendance at regular multidisciplinary conferences with nonsurgical specialists who treat obesity (nutrition, psychology, endocrinology, etc.)
- Attend at least one bariatric surgery support group during fellowship
- Complete at least one research project during fellowship

Clinical and technical
- Gain exposure to more than one type of weight loss operation
- Participate in at least 100 bariatric operations including:
  - Minimum of 50 procedures involving stapling/anastomosis of the gastrointestinal tract
  - At least 10 purely restrictive operations
  - At least 5 open procedures
- Primary surgeon in majority (>51%) of cases (perform key components of the operation)
- Participate in perioperative care including:
  - 50 preoperative evaluations
  - 100 postoperative inpatient encounters
  - 100 postoperative outpatient encounters
- Performance evaluation with program director every 6 months during fellowship
- Maintain current log of cases and complications

50 procedures (performed independently) as well as at regular intervals thereafter to confirm patient safety. In addition, the surgeon should continue to meet global credentialing requirements for bariatric surgery at the time of reappointment.

Conclusion

Bariatric surgery is a discipline that requires not only specialized surgical skills but also specific expertise in managing the morbidly obese patient. Laparoscopic bariatric operations are generally complex and require advanced skills such as intracorporeal suturing, stapling, and exposure techniques. Furthermore, bariatric patients are often complex, high-risk surgical candidates secondary to their underlying, and often severe, comorbidities. Therefore, to build a successful program and achieve desirable outcomes, surgeons must master the technical skills required for the operations as well as the knowledge and clinical skills to manage these complex patients.

Comprehensive, structured, and supervised training is the key to achieving desirable outcomes in bariatric surgery. The era of the weekend training course as the sole source of procedure training is over. It has been replaced with formal, supervised training in the form of a formal fellowship or mini-fellowship experience. As the obesity epidemic grows and the number of bariatric procedures continues to rise, these training programs will play a vital role in producing surgeons capable of successfully managing this complex disease.

References

1. Buchwald H, Williams SE. Bariatric surgery worldwide 2003. Obes Surg 2004;14(9):1157–1164.
2. Ogden CL, Carroll MD, Curtin LR, et al. Prevalence of overweight and obesity in the United States, 1999–2004. JAMA 2006;295(13):1549–1555.
3. American Society for Bariatric Surgery. Society of American Gastrointestinal Endoscopic Surgeons. Guidelines for laparoscopic and open surgical treatment of morbid obesity. Obes Surg 2000;10:378–379.
4. American Society for Bariatric Surgery. Core curriculum for ASBS fellowship training. http://www.asbs.org/html/about/asbsguidelines.html.
5. Deziel DJ, Millikan KW, Economou SG, et al. Complications of laparoscopic cholecystectomy: a national survey of 4,292 hospitals and an analysis of 77,604 cases. Am J Surg 1993;165(1):9–14.
6. Liem MS, van Steensel CJ, Boelhouwer RU, et al. The learning curve for totally extraperitoneal laparoscopic inguinal hernia repair. Am J Surg 1996;171(2):281–285.
7. Poulin EC, Mamazza J. Laparoscopic splenectomy: lessons from the learning curve. Can J Surg 1998;41(1):28–36.
8. Wishner JD, Baker JW Jr, Hoffman GC, et al. Laparoscopic-assisted colectomy. The learning curve. Surg Endosc 1995;9(11):1179–1183.
9. O'Brien PE, Dixon JB. Weight loss and early and late complications the international experience. Am J Surg 2002;184:42S–45S.
10. Angrisani L, Furbetta F, Doldi SB, et al. Lap Band adjustable gastric banding system: the Italian experience with 1863 patients operated on 6 years. Surg Endosc 2003;17:409–402.
11. Schauer P, Ikramuddin S, Hamad G, Gourash W. The learning curve for laparoscopic Roux-en-Y gastric bypass is 100 cases. Surg Endosc 2003;17(2):212–215.
12. Oliak D, Ballantyne GH, Weber P, et al. Laparoscopic Roux-en-Y gastric bypass: defining the learning curve. Surg Endosc 2003;17(3):405–408.
13. Wittgrove AC, Clark GW. Laparoscopic gastric bypass, Roux-en-Y—500 patients: technique and results, with 3–60 month follow-up. Obes Surg 2000;10(3):233–239.
14. Cottam DR, Mattar SG, Lord JL, Schauer PR. Training and credentialing for the performance of laparoscopic bariatric surgery. Soc Laparosc Surg Rep 2003;2:15–21.
15. Park A, Witzke D, Donnelly M. Ongoing deficits in resident training for minimally invasive surgery. J Gastrointest Surg 2002;6(3):501–507; discussion 507–509.
16. Dent TL. Training and privileging for new procedures. Surg Clin North Am 1996;76(3):615–621.
17. Wolfe BM, Szabo Z, Moran ME, et al. Training for minimally invasive surgery. Need for surgical skills. Surg Endosc 1993;7(2):93–95.
18. Rosser JC, Rosser LE, Savalgi RS. Skill acquisition and assessment for laparoscopic surgery. Arch Surg 1997;132(2):200–204.
19. Rosser JC Jr, Rosser LE, Savalgi RS. Objective evaluation of a laparoscopic surgical skill program for residents and senior surgeons. Arch Surg 1998;133(6):657–661.
20. Lord JL, Cottam DR, Dallal RM, et al. The impact of laparoscopic bariatric workshops on the practice patterns of surgeons. Surg Endosc 2006;20(6):929–933.
21. American Society for Bariatric Surgery's guidelines for granting privileges in bariatric surgery. Surg Obes Relat Dis 2006;2(1):65–67.
22. Swanstrom LL, Park A, Arregui M, et al. Bringing order to the chaos: developing a matching process for minimally invasive and gastrointestinal postgraduate fellowships. Ann Surg 2006;243(4):431–435.

8
Patient Selection, Preoperative Assessment, and Preparation

Michael Tarnoff, Julie Kim, and Scott Shikora

The overall safety of bariatric surgery has steadily improved as technology and experience with these procedures have evolved. Mortality and complication rates have fallen dramatically as a result of improvements in surgical technique (including minimally invasive strategies), better patient monitoring and anesthetic management, and increased recognition of the unique perioperative needs of the severely obese surgical patient. Outcome results have also improved with a better understanding of the importance of preoperative screening and patient preparation.

Bariatric surgery is the marriage of a complicated group of operative procedures with a complex patient population. There are numerous issues in the preparation and management of these patients. Perioperative complications have the potential to be devastating, and weight loss failure can be damaging not only to the health of an individual patient, but also to the practice of bariatric surgery. From preoperative selection to the intraoperative and early postoperative management, understanding the unique requirements of this patient population is vital for minimizing the risk of complications and maximizing the potential for durable weight loss and improved health.

Obese patients present numerous clinical challenges. The obesity-associated comorbid conditions predictably raise the risks of perioperative morbidity and mortality (Table 8-1). Many of these conditions are underdiagnosed in this population. Unrecognized sleep apnea can have dramatic and potentially fatal consequences in the immediate postoperative period. Hypertension, asthma, and diabetes commonly occur and, if untreated, may complicate perioperative care. Altered body habitus yields undefined modifications of immune function, rendering patients unusually susceptible to perioperative complications. Derangements in body composition complicate the dosing of medications and anesthetics. Radiographic studies are often unattainable or of poor quality. In general, every aspect of even typical perioperative care becomes challenging when treating these patients. Given the complexity of the perioperative management, anything less than long-term success should not be tolerated. Additionally, nonmedical factors must not be ignored. Even with appropriate perioperative management, performing surgery on a patient who is behaviorally or medically unsuitable for surgery may lead to a poor outcome. As a result, a thorough understanding of proper patient selection for surgical candidacy, appropriate preoperative evaluation, and preparation are vital to a successful practice in obesity surgery. This chapter reviews the highlights of these issues.

Patient Selection

While bariatric surgery is currently the only modality that offers durable weight loss, it is appropriate for only a small subset of patients. Standards for patient selection have been established. In 1991, the National Institutes of Health (NIH) consensus statement defined the minimal criteria for patient selection (1,2). This document proclaimed that surgery should be considered only for those patients who have a body mass index (BMI) of ≥40 without comorbidity, or 35 to 39 if they also suffer from obesity-related comorbidities. Candidates for surgery should have failed attempts to achieve sustainable weight loss with nonoperative strategies (1,2). Given the risks of weight loss surgery, surgeons must assure themselves that patients seek these interventions only after sufficient attempts at all other strategies have been made.

The NIH statement also mandates that bariatric surgery be performed in the context of a multidisciplinary program. Patients need be exposed to many nonsurgical clinicians such as bariatric internists, psychologists or other behavioral therapists, and dietitians. This mandate serves to ensure that patients address the environmental and psychosocial aspects of morbid obesity, as these factors likely play a role in long-term efficacy after surgery.

TABLE 8-1. Obesity-associated medical conditions

Cardiovascular
  Cardiomyopathy
  Cerebrovascular disease
  Coronary artery disease
  Dyslipidemia
  Hypertension
  Sudden death
Endocrine
  Amenorrhea
  Diabetes mellitus
  Hirsutism
  Infertility
Hepatobiliary/gastrointestinal
  Hepatic steatosis
  Gallstones
  Gastroesophageal reflux
  Steatohepatitis
Miscellaneous
  Chronic fatigue
  Malignancies
  Pseudotumor cerebri
  Urinary stress incontinence
Musculoskeletal/skin
  Accident proneness
  Chronic back pain
  Degenerative joint disease
  Diaphoresis
  Hernia
  Immobility
  Infections
  Intertriginous dermatitis
Psychological
  Depression
  Low self-esteem
  Poor quality of life
  Poor relationships
  Suicide
Pulmonary/respiratory
  Dyspnea
  Obesity hypoventilation
  Obstructive sleep apnea
  Asthma
Venous disease
  Deep vein thrombosis
  Lower limb edema
  Pulmonary embolus
  Venous stasis
  Venous stasis ulcers

Currently there are no universally accepted guidelines for the age limitations for surgery. The NIH guidelines recommended surgery only for patients older than 18 years but did not suggest a maximum age. Bariatric surgery at the extremes of age raises several important questions. For children and adolescents, one must question whether there is sufficient maturity to make the life-altering decision to undergo obesity surgery. Further, success after any of these procedures is likely dependent on long-term behavioral modification. It is unclear whether such young patients can commit to altering their lifestyle. With childhood obesity now recognized as a growing epidemic, surgical intervention for children or adolescents is now routinely offered. To date, only small numbers of children have undergone these procedures, and good long-term results have been reported (3).

For the elderly, questions of increased risk, inability to modify lifestyle, and life expectancy have all been raised and are as yet unanswered. However, better perioperative patient management as well as advancements in minimally invasive techniques have enabled many surgeons to offer surgery to older patients (4). Currently, many bariatric programs accept patients who are in their sixth decade of life, assuming that they are otherwise appropriate candidates. In our practice, we have safely operated on patients who were in their seventh decade of life and have found that there were no significant differences in morbidity, mortality, weight loss, or long-term outcome for our older patients when compared with our younger patients.

Patient Evaluation and Preoperative Preparation

Even for patients who meet the NIH standards, surgeons are not obligated to operate on all such patients who present to their office. Patients can be denied surgery for behavioral, medical, surgical, or other reasons. However, unlike the NIH guidelines, the contraindications to surgery are not codified or standardized. It is vitally important to be able to screen out patients unlikely to succeed before proceeding with surgery. Those patients considered to be good operative candidates need to be carefully and thoroughly prepared. Unlike other surgeries, bariatric surgery requires patients to make long-term dietary and behavioral changes. A comprehensive evaluation and preparation process should be undertaken. In our program, this includes the intervention of a multidisciplinary group of clinicians. This team includes behavioral health specialists, dietitians, internists, surgeons, and physicians' assistants. Each of these clinicians provides important input into patient selection, management, and follow-up. Success following bariatric surgery, in our opinion, is more likely to occur when patients are subjected to this multidisciplinary approach.

A thorough psychological evaluation is performed by a psychiatrist, psychologist, or other trained behavioral therapist. This evaluation should focus on weight history, social situation, life stresses, and dietary history to identify problem areas that may negatively impact on results. Patients must not display evidence of eating disorders such as severe bulimia that may preclude compliance with the postoperative dietary restrictions. In addition, they must show evidence of stress and dietary control, supportive relationships, and a stable living environment

TABLE 8-2. Behavioral exclusions for surgery

Absolute
  Significant psychiatric disorder or major depression
  Severe mental retardation
  Self-destructive lifestyle
  Active bulimia
  Drug or alcohol abuse
  Inability to comprehend the necessary behavioral changes for
    surgery
  Inability to integrate basic lifestyle adjustments preoperatively
Relative
  Patients who are abusive to staff members
  Patients who miss several office appointments
  Patients who are overly pushy about an operative date or want to
    forgo or abbreviate the preoperative process
  Patients who actively abuse tobacco
  Patients who gain weight during the preoperative process
  Patients who are untruthful or withhold information
  Patients who have already failed a bariatric procedure

(5). Immediately after surgery and beyond, behavioral support in the form of individual counseling sessions or support groups is very beneficial to help patients with the dramatic changes in lifestyle, eating, and body image. This has been shown to improve results (6).

Behavioral screening for surgical candidacy is important for long-term success (Table 8-2). Patients with significant psychiatric disorders or mental retardation should rarely be considered for surgery. In addition, a strong history of substance abuse or self-destructive behavior may also preclude patients from consideration. Other behavioral attributes that may not represent absolute contraindications for surgery, but should, at the very least, raise red flags, include abusive behavior to staff members, missed appointments, short temper, impatience with the speed of the process, or pleading to abbreviate the process. In addition, in our program, we view smoking, significant alcohol consumption, or weight gain during the evaluation and preparation process as symbolic of noncompliance and will not offer surgery to patients who demonstrate these traits. It should be understood that these decisions are subject to individual practice patterns, as little, if any, data exist to guide therapy in these situations. Finally, patients who have failed a previous bariatric procedure (particularly if the anatomy is intact by x-ray) should be approached cautiously.

Since many morbidly obese patients suffer from a wide range of medical conditions, they are at increased risk of perioperative complications (5). Therefore, a thorough history is taken and a physical examination is performed to affirm known comorbidities and to uncover conditions such as sleep apnea or diabetes, which are often underdiagnosed. Screening laboratory testing in our program include a complete blood count, liver function testing, hemoglobin A_{1c}, iron, total iron binding capacity, vitamin B_{12}, folate, vitamin D and calcium, thyroid screening, and serum lipids. Since rapid weight loss has been associated with the development of gallstone disease, gallbladder ultrasonography is performed on all patients undergoing surgery. Those identified to have cholelithiasis can undergo concomitant cholecystectomy. Alternatively, Ursodiol can be prescribed following surgery to reduce the risk of gallstone formation (7). The role of routine cholecystectomy in the context of bariatric surgery has been debated. Most authors agree that patients with symptomatic cholelithiasis should undergo concomitant cholecystectomy. Despite this, there is little consensus on the most appropriate management of patients with asymptomatic gallstone.

Obesity-associated medical conditions are commonly seen in severely obese patients and are often the reason for seeking surgical weight loss. However, some medical conditions might preclude patients from surgery (Table 8-3). These include diseases that are considered end-stage or life threatening and are not expected to improve with weight loss, such as terminal cancer. Additionally, patients in extremely poor health in whom the operative risks would be prohibitive or those considered to have a very poor quality of life that would not be expected to improve with weight loss, probably should not undergo surgery.

There are far fewer surgical reasons to exclude patients from surgery than medical or behavioral reasons. However, it is important to review the reports from all of the patient's prior abdominal surgeries. Some of this information can be obtained from a thorough history and physical examination, but it should be supplemented by obtaining the operative reports and radiographic studies. Previous gastrointestinal surgery may alter the operative options. For instance, patients who have had major or several lower abdominal procedures or small bowel resections may be better served by gastric banding or vertical banded gastroplasty than by gastric bypass. Patients who have had a Nissen fundoplication or have failed after gastric banding might be technically difficult to convert to a gastric bypass, and therefore a duodenal switch procedure might be considered. Also, multiple previous abdominal surgeries, other gastric procedures, abdominal radiation, or liver transplantation may be considered relative contraindications for bariatric surgery.

TABLE 8-3. Medical exclusions for surgery

Severe comorbid diseases that would create unacceptably high
  operative risk
Incurable diseases (cancer, AIDS, cirrhosis)
Unstable diseases (congestive heart failure, unstable angina, thyroid
  disease)
Gastrointestinal diseases (Crohn's, dysmotilities)
Overall poor quality of life that would not be expected to improve
  with weight loss

Dietary counseling should be initiated preoperatively and continued following surgery in order to teach and then reinforce the skills for making appropriate food choices (5). Persistent, maladaptive eating behaviors and dietary indiscretion are common problems in both the preoperative and postoperative setting. After surgery, dietary indiscretion can lead to persistent vomiting, pain, and even weight loss failure. Thoughtful evaluation and counseling provided by these allied health professionals serves as an invaluable asset to patients and surgeons alike.

Some surgeons routinely test for *Helicobacter pylori* infection, which occurs in morbidly obese patients with similar frequency to that seen in the general population (8). Despite this, upper gastrointestinal (GI) tract pathology following gastric bypass surgery is unusual. Since after gastric bypass there is anatomic exclusion of the antrum from the environment, *H. pylori* is unlikely to be of any consequence in the postoperative setting. We employ selective evaluation of the upper GI tract in patients with a strong history of peptic ulcer disease, gastritis, or malignancy, and reconsider offering gastric bypass to the occasional patient who may need long-term upper GI tract surveillance.

Specialty consults such as cardiology, pulmonary, and endocrinology are obtained when appropriate. All newly diagnosed conditions should be treated and the patient medically optimized before proceeding with surgery. Additional testing such as sleep studies and echocardiography are employed when appropriate.

Preoperative weight loss may also be beneficial for reducing perioperative complications. To date, there are no randomized prospective trials that evaluate the role of preoperative weight loss. Despite this, we routinely ask super-obese patients to lose approximately 10% of their total body weight before surgery. This is usually successfully achieved with the guidance of our clinicians. In our experience, such weight loss accomplishes two important goals. First, a 10% total weight loss leads to significant reductions in the volume of visceral fat (9). The liver becomes less fatty and easier to retract. The omentum and small bowel mesentery gain mobility. This greatly reduces the technical demands of the procedure and may reduce the operative complications. In a recent retrospective analysis, we demonstrated that preoperative weight loss improved perioperative safety and efficacy in performing laparoscopic gastric bypass in the super-obese whose BMI was greater than 60. Second, we believe that from a behavioral standpoint, patients who comply with a preoperative weight-loss regimen are more likely to have long-term success with weight-loss surgery. Such patients demonstrate their ability to modify their behavior and eating patterns and typically become more motivated to achieve the long-term goals they set. On the contrary, patients who fail to comply with preoperative weight loss are perhaps less likely to achieve long-term, durable success. At present, these issues are debatable and future scientific evaluation is warranted.

During the preoperative preparatory process, patient education is one of the most important components. Extensive teaching, counseling, and supervised dietary instructions are provided. A description of the surgery including the risks and benefits is provided to ensure that patients have a thorough understanding of the potential operative complications as well as the anatomic changes that they are consenting to have done. A good understanding of these operative changes of gastric capacity and function, dietary restrictions, and potential long-term nutritional concerns is critical to a good outcome.

Intraoperative Management

At the time of surgery, a number of factors must be considered. Attention must be given to proper patient positioning on the operating room table, adequate intravenous management (peripheral vs. central), safe airway management (standard intubation vs. awake fiberoptic), and balanced anesthesia. Most bariatric surgeons use some form of thromboprophylaxis and often more than one modality (10). These include unfractionated heparin, low-molecular-weight heparins, pneumatic compression sleeves, etc. Patient positioning on the table may also affect the risk of thrombosis, as some surgeons prefer the lithotomy position to the supine, but the latter is much more popular.

Intravenous antibiotics are routinely administered before creation of the incision (11,12). This reduces the likelihood of a wound infection. In open surgery, the risk of wound infection is stated to be as high as 10%. This is dramatically reduced in the laparoscopic experience (13). Given the increased body weight, the customary dose of a single gram of a first-generation cephalosporin may not be adequate. Forse et al. (12) found that administering 2 g was more effective. However, with the great heterogeneity of this population for both weight and body composition, there is probably no single recommendation that will be sufficient for all of these patients.

We advocate at least two large-bore (18 gauge or greater) peripheral IVs and do not routinely use central access or arterial line monitoring. While this scheme works in the vast majority of patients, any patient presenting with additional high-risk factors (e.g., coronary artery disease, severe pulmonary dysfunction, and so forth) should probably be monitored more closely with use of these more invasive methods.

Although it may seem intuitive, it is still important to mention that the instruments and operating room equipment must be adequate for extremely obese patients. For open surgery, this includes adequate room lighting and retractors large enough for the deep abdominal cavity. For laparoscopic surgery, standard-length instruments and trocars usually suffice, though long ultrasonic dissectors, suction/irrigators, telescopes, and blunt graspers are helpful.

Postoperative Management

Postoperative management must focus on both standard postoperative issues as well as those that are more pertinent to the obese patient. At the completion of surgery, the patient should be transferred to the appropriate ward for recovery and convalescence. We routinely send patients to the recovery room for a period of at least 5 hours, after which time the vast majority are cleared to go to a regular surgical ward. Exceptions to this rule include patients with sleep apnea who typically require continuous oxygen monitoring, as well as any patient whose status is questionable. These individuals require monitored care until they stabilize. We routinely begin patients with sleep apnea on continuous positive airway pressure (CPAP) on the evening of postoperative day 1. Studies support the notion that earlier use of CPAP is safe and appropriate (14). Additionally, there is no scientific evidence to validate the concept that CPAP jeopardizes the integrity of fresh gastrointestinal anastomoses. Pulmonary toilet and gas exchange must be carefully monitored. Abdominal surgery and the subsequent pain from the incision(s) lead to respiratory splinting. Incentive spirometry, keeping the head of the bed elevated, and early ambulation all reduce the likelihood of atelectasis and pneumonia.

No consensus exists in the literature as to whether obesity is an independent risk factor for thromboembolic events (10). However, despite the lack of compelling data, most bariatric surgeons would agree that extremely obese patients are at high risk. Factors that increase risk in this patient population include hypercoagulable states (15), abdominal surgery, impaired ambulation, postoperative bed rest, and preexisting vascular insufficiency. A recent survey of American Society for Bariatric Surgery (ASBS) members by Wu and Barba (10) found an incidence of 2.63% for deep vein thrombosis (DVT) and 0.95% for pulmonary embolism (PE). In this survey, 95% of respondent surgeons used some form of prophylaxis. Similar results were seen in a study by Eriksson and colleagues (16). They reported a 2.3% incidence of clinical DVT for gastric procedures for weight loss despite prophylaxis.

Unfortunately, thromboembolic risk is not alleviated by laparoscopic surgery. These minimally invasive procedures are touted to decrease postoperative immobilization, increase ambulation, and attenuate the acute-phase response of abdominal surgery. However, these benefits may be offset by additional risk factors such as the effects of pneumoperitoneum on venous return and prolongation of the operative time. Therefore, it would be reasonable to provide thromboprophylaxis to all patients undergoing bariatric surgery.

There is also no consensus among bariatric surgeons as to what constitutes the best method of thromboprophylaxis. Prophylaxis can include many different modalities used singly or in combinations. Simple devices that enhance venous return, reduce venous stasis, and stimulate fibrinolysis include elastic stockings and intermittent pneumatic compression sleeves. Early ambulation is also beneficial in reducing the risk of thrombosis. This is greatly facilitated by the use of specialized mechanical beds that can flex up to a sitting position and allow easy access onto and off.

Unfractionated heparin given subcutaneously has long been effective for decreasing the incidence of DVTs but carries the risks of thrombocytopenia and hemorrhage (17). Low-molecular-weight heparins are currently popular because they have better bioavailability and a longer elimination than standard heparin (18). Studies that have compared the two have generally found similar success at preventing DVTs with a slightly higher bleeding incidence for standard heparin (18,19). Unfortunately, the low-molecular-weight heparins are more costly, and the appropriate dosing for the extremely obese is not known. For high-risk patients and those who have a contraindication to anticoagulation, a vena caval filter placed preoperatively, may be necessary. In our program, we use intermittent compression sleeves on the lower extremities and twice daily or three times daily subcutaneous injections of unfractionated heparin. High-risk patients receive vena caval filters or may be prescribed low-molecular-weight heparin for a period of time after discharge from the hospital.

Once a DVT or PE has been diagnosed, it is important to quickly institute treatment. Traditional treatment includes full anticoagulation with intravenous heparin. Once the international normalized ratio (INR) becomes therapeutic, patients are converted over to oral warfarin. Recent studies, however, have suggested that low-molecular-weight heparin administered subcutaneously was equally effective as intravenous standard heparin (20).

Pain control is vitally important for early ambulation and pulmonary toilet. This can be accomplished with patient-controlled analgesia (PCA) using narcotics or intravenous nonsteroidal antiinflammatory drugs such as ketorolac. Preemptive and multimodal strategies have also been shown to be effective (21). Care must be taken to titrate narcotics for maximal comfort without compromising respiration. Epidural analgesia is also effective but may be difficult to initiate in the obese and not necessary for laparoscopic procedures. Our current practice for patients undergoing laparoscopic bariatric surgery is to use morphine PCA until postoperative day 2, at which point most patients tolerate oral narcotics. Intravenous ketorolac is used liberally in most cases. The vast majority of these patients report cessation of narcotics by postoperative day 5.

As with operative fluid management, postoperative fluid administration must be titrated to provide sufficient fluids yet avoid overload. If necessary, central venous catheterization might be necessary in the setting of poor peripheral access or when central venous pressures are necessary to determine fluid status. It is quite common for morbidly obese patients to be oliguric in the perioperative period. The oliguric state generally resolves by the morning of postoperative day 1 and, in the absence of other symptoms, is of little consequence. In contrast, persistent oliguria or anuria can represent a potential problem such as intraabdominal sepsis and should prompt a diagnostic workup.

The resumption of oral intake occurs rather early after most bariatric procedures. We routinely begin patients on one ounce of water every hour on postoperative day 1. On postoperative day 2, we progress patients to ad lib noncaloric clear liquids including sugar-free gelatin, broth, and juice. A high-protein, low-fat, vitamin- and mineral-supplemented liquid diet is started on day 3 and serves as the mainstay of the post–bariatric surgery diet for the subsequent 2 weeks. Soft solid foods are begun by week 2 and patients are then slowly advanced to a more regular, sugar-free, low-fat diet by 1 month. Most patients are discharged from the hospital by the second or third day after surgery after they demonstrate the ability to successfully tolerate nutritious liquid diet. Persistent vomiting during this time frame is a rare event, and although usually secondary to dietary indiscretion, should prompt diagnostic evaluation to exclude mechanical obstruction.

Conclusion

Bariatric surgery represents the union of complex surgical procedures with a population of high-risk patients. Good results occur when appropriately selected patients are properly prepared and then well cared for after surgery. While over 14 million American adults would qualify for surgery if based solely on their adiposity, many would ultimately be poor candidates for surgery. These determinations would include those patients whose underlying health and past surgical history would cause unacceptably high operative risk, as well as those patients who would have acceptable operative risk but whose behavioral makeup would lead to poor postoperative outcomes. It is therefore essential for the bariatric surgeon to carefully assess each prospective surgical candidate from medical, surgical, and behavioral perspectives, and then comprehensively prepare those patients. In addition, during and after surgery, these patients require a high degree of attention and surveillance. Understanding the unique requirements of this patient population and providing the appropriate attention to details is vital for minimizing the risk of complications and maximizing the potential for a good start on the long road to weight loss and improved health.

References

1. Gastrointestinal surgery for severe obesity. National Institutes of Health Consensus Development Conference Statement. Am J Clin Nutr 1992;55:615s–619s.
2. Mason EE. Vertical banded gastroplasty for obesity. Arch Surg 1982;117:701–706.
3. Strauss RS, Bradley LJ, Brolin RE. Gastric bypass surgery in adolescents with morbid obesity. J Pediatr 2001;138:499–504.
4. MacGregor AMC, Rand CS. Gastric surgery in morbid obesity. Outcome in patients aged 55 and older. Arch Surg 1993;128:1153–1157.
5. Kim JJ, Tarnoff ME, Shikora SA. Surgical treatment for extreme obesity: evolution of a rapidly changing field. Nutr Clin Pract 2003;15:13–22.
6. Nicolai A, Ippoliti C, Petrelli MD. Laparoscopic adjustable gastric banding: essential role of psychological support. Obes Surg 2003;12:857–863.
7. Sugerman HJ, Brewer WH, Shiffman ML, et al. A multicenter, placebo-controlled, randomized, double-blind, prospective trial of prophylactic ursodiol for the prevention of gallstone formation following gastric-bypass-induced rapid weight loss. Am J Surg 1995;169:91–97.
8. Renshaw AA, Rabaza JR, Gonzalez AM, et al. Helicobacter pylori infection in patients undergoing gastric bypass surgery for morbid obesity. Obes Surg 2001;11:281–283.
9. Despres JP. Dyslipidaemia and obesity. Baillieres Clin Endocrinol Metab 1994;8:629–660.
10. Wu EC, Barba CA. Current practices in the prophylaxis of venous thromboembolism in bariatric surgery. Obes Surg 2000;10:7–14.
11. Pories WJ, van Rij AM, Burlingtham BT, et al. Prophylactic cefazolin in gastric bypass surgery. Surgery 1981;90: 426–432.
12. Forse RA, Karam B, MacLean LD, et al. Antibiotic prophylaxis for surgery in morbidly obese patients. Surgery 1989;106:750–757.
13. Schauer PR, Ikramuddin S, Gourash WF, et al. Outcomes after laparoscopic roux-en-y gastric bypass for morbid obesity. Ann Surg 2000;232:515–529.
14. Huerta S, De Shields S, Shpiner R, et al. Safety and efficacy of postoperative continuous positive airway pressure to prevent pulmonary complications after Roux-en-Y gastric bypass. J Gastrointest Surg 2002;6:354–358.
15. Batist G, Bothe A, Bern M, et al. Low antithrombin III in morbidity obesity: returns to normal with weight reduction. J Parenter Enteral Nutr 1983;7:447–449.
16. Eriksson S, Backman L, Ljungstrom K-G. The incidence of clinical postoperative thrombosis after gastric surgery for obesity during 16 years. Obes Surg 1997;7:332–335.

17. Collins R, Scrimgeour A, Yusuf S, et al. Reduction of fatal pulmonary embolism and venous thrombosis by perioperative administration of subcutaneous heparin. N Engl J Med 1988;318:1162–1173.
18. Kakkar VV, Cohen AT, Edmonson RA, et al. Low molecular weight versus standard heparin for prevention of venous thromboembolism after major abdominal surgery. Lancet 1993;341:259–265.
19. Nurmohamed MT, Rosendaal F-R, Buller R, et al. The efficacy and safety of low-molecular heparin versus standard heparin in general and orthopedic surgery: a meta-analysis. Lancet 1992;340:152–156.
20. Lensing AW, Prins MH, Davidson BL, et al. Treatment of deep vein thrombosis with low-molecular weight heparins: a meta-analysis. Arch Intern Med 1995;155:601–607.
21. Shumann R, Shikora S, Weiss JM, et al. A comparison of multimodal perioperative analgesia to epidural pain management after gastric bypass surgery. Anesth Analg 2003;96:469–472.

9
The Evolving Role of the Psychologist

F. Merritt Ayad and Louis F. Martin

In the past decade the widespread expansion of the American waistline has driven the increased demand for bariatric surgery. Although obesity surgery has been extant for over 30 years, recent improvements in surgical techniques and the dramatic rise in public awareness have accelerated the pace of both its development and utilization. The changing role of the psychologist in the university-based weight management center has been part of this evolution. The major sources of the change in the psychologist's role are the following: problems with patient adherence to medical and surgical treatments, developments in the areas of health psychology and behavioral medicine, psychology billing code expansion by the American Medical Association's Current Procedural Terminology (CPT) Editorial Panel, recommendations from published guidelines for bariatric surgery practice and research, clinical implications of obesity surgery outcome research, and the recent developments in our understanding of the change process.

This chapter addresses how these changes have affected the practice of psychology in the specialized area of obesity surgery and discusses the need for psychological services during each phase of obesity surgery treatment. The assessment, preparation for surgery, and postoperative adjustment phases each requires its own combination of psychological services. These combinations are rarely the same for any two patients.

We do not have enough research on postoperative follow-up after obesity surgery, especially long-term follow-up. Patients who do not return for scheduled follow-up, the varying amounts of follow-up provided among surgeons, and the time and expense of longitudinal research all contribute to this problem. There has been more media coverage of successful bariatric surgery cases compared to the not so successful ones. To help the greatest number of people, we must learn more about the patients who never reach a healthy weight, as well as those who never build enough lean muscle, or who regain excess weight anywhere from months to years to decades

after surgery. Surgeons who are not part of a comprehensive weight management clinic are less likely to have a multidisciplinary format for follow-up care that includes a selection of behavioral modification protocols. Even among university-based weight management centers, there is a great deal of variability in the amount of follow-up assessment and treatment offered, as well as the composition of the team that provides it. Anecdotal information suggests that up to 50% of patients who undergo gastric bypass do not maintain their greatest weight loss 5 to 10 years later. It is speculated that patient nonadherence to dietary and activity recommendations and the lack of adequate medical or psychological follow-up are related to this phenomenon. Of the 50% who do well, some received behavioral modification from the clinic that did the surgery, some became involved with groups and information services on the Internet, and others have formed their own groups and support systems within their communities. With gastric banding surgeries, the behavior modification component may be even more essential because patients are able to tolerate a wider variety of foods compared to gastric bypass patients. It is estimated that up to 40% of gastric bands are eventually removed due to nonadherence, complication development, lack of psychological intervention, or any combination of these.

In our clinic we have had patients with no previous psychiatric disorder develop severe depression, or become addicted to pain medication (or alcohol) after bariatric surgery. We have referred depressed patients for aggressive pharmacotherapy and psychotherapy both pre- and postoperatively who later committed suicide despite our best efforts. We have had patients refuse to follow the postsurgical dietary and exercise requirements who prior to surgery appeared to be cooperative with and invested in the program. To our amazement, some particularly rebellious patients have attended our ongoing support group in order to boast of their newfound ability to eat foods that were in clear violation of the dietary protocol they had agreed to follow. Others refused to eat after surgery, became malnourished, lost lean muscle mass and hair, and later returned for follow-up only after friends and relatives expressed grave concerns about them. Some patients developed a formal eating disorder after surgery, while others had eating problems for which there was no agreed upon nomenclature or treatment protocol. For years we were perplexed by some of these occurrences. However, the recent work in the areas of treatment adherence, motivation, stages of change, and treatment matching have improved our understanding and have provided us with models for better integration of theory with practice. This chapter reviews only selected aspects of these developments, as a comprehensive effort could fill several texts. While obesity surgery psychology is not a formal subspecialty at the present time, it may become one some day.

How Should a Psychologist Be Used in a Bariatric Practice?

In the early developmental stages of obesity surgery, the clinical psychologist was primarily utilized to determine whether a given patient demonstrated sufficient psychological stability to safely undergo obesity surgery. Patients were "cleared" for surgery or deemed unsuitable. Some psychologists provided individual or group treatment for unstable patients to help them become stable enough for surgery. Currently, however, there are a growing number of psychologists who provide many additional services for the university-based weight management center. Developments in areas of health promotion, disease prevention, and behavioral medicine have expanded the possible roles. These services may include coordinating care with other mental health professionals; encouraging patient participation in support and psychoeducational groups; working with spouses and other family members to enhance the surgery patient's cooperation; helping all staff members to promote adherence; preventing relapse of unhealthy behavior by supporting patient efforts to develop coping skills; and reevaluating patients over time to monitor the impact of interventions and to modify them when necessary. Ideally, a psychologist should be an integral member of the multidisciplinary team. The psychologist needs to be acquainted with each phase of the treatment process, and have a deep appreciation for the range of clinical courses that flow from surgical obesity interventions. It is essential for the psychologist to be familiar with the follow-up protocols provided by the surgery clinic and with the frequency and nature of the postoperative psychosocial complications that have been identified by clinic staff.

Reich et al. (1) studied the differences between psychologists who delivered behavioral health services on-site (e.g., at a primary care clinic) versus the solo practice office. The on-site psychologists made consultation easier for physicians and relieved them of having to spend additional time and effort on patients with problematic psychological conditions. The on-site psychologist often spared patients the time and effort involved in finding an outside psychologist and arranging the initial appointment. Inclusion of a psychologist in routine practice was believed to lessen the stigma many patients associated with assessment for psychological and behavioral aspects of illness. On-site psychologists benefited greatly from this relationship in that they received up to four times the annual new referrals compared to solo practitioners doing similar kinds of work (1).

Having a psychologist as a member of the treatment team also improves the quality of psychological assessments and treatment recommendations. In their investigation of clinical versus actuarial judgment, Dawes et al. (2) found that many clinical decisions are made repeatedly without the possibility of self-correction because clinicians never received feedback about outcomes. Meehl (3) concluded that the ability of a psychologist to make clinical predictions is dependent on the degree of structure of the data set, the manner in which the clinician combines data to reach a judgment, the number of times the clinician has confronted the task before, the degree to which the clinician received feedback and cross-replicated the predictive algorithms, and whether the task matched the clinician's experience. In this vein, Weston and Weinberger (4) stated that "a clinician whose goal is valid prognostication would do well to rely on a standard set of items, make judgments at an appropriate level of inference that capitalizes on skills likely to have developed through clinical training and experience, make multiple such judgments that can then be aggregated, and avoid prognosticating outside his or her area of expertise" (p. 599). They also cautioned that statistical prediction can be premature when judges lack information or adequate knowledge of the relevant variables and their relative contributions.

Psychologists who are asked to consult from independent offices are usually cut off from feedback that could improve their recommendation and intervention strategies with successive cases. Also, they do not have the chance to follow nearly as many patients longitudinally as psychologists who interact daily with a bariatric treatment team. The unfortunate reality is that many weight management programs do not have the budget or patient volumes to hire a full-time psychologist. A reasonable compromise under these circumstances is to have the psychologist to whom the clinic regularly refers patients for psychological assessment also run the support groups for pre- and postsurgery patients, as well as provide as much of the individual and family intervention as is feasible. This allows the psychologist to receive the ongoing feedback on assessments necessary to improve the assessment battery, modify recommendations as new patient data emerges over time, and gain a better understanding of the natural history of obesity surgery.

The role of the psychologist in the arena of health care is changing. It is no longer adequate to rely solely on a psychotherapy model where mental illness and behavior disturbances are diagnosed and treated. In 2001, the American Psychological Association modified its mission statement to read as follows: "to advance psychology as a science and profession and as a means of promoting health and welfare." Today, many psychologists function as health care providers who focus on the factors that interfere with physical functioning and recovery, ways of improving health and maintaining wellness, and methods that encourage collaboration within a multidisciplinary treatment team (5). There is also a rapidly growing movement within psychology called "positive psychology" (6). Positive psychology has been embraced by clinicians who have broken free from the mold of viewing clients primarily as patients with mental illnesses who need treatment. From the lens of positive psychology, clients are also viewed as individuals who seek performance enhancement, skill development, or support of their inherent need to find balance and maintain a healthy lifestyle. This approach is a good fit for the many obesity surgery candidates who do not have a diagnosable psychiatric disorder.

New Billing Codes

For years, a major problem for psychologists working in primary and specialty care medical clinics was reimbursement. Insurers would not pay for many of the services that health psychologists had been trained to provide, especially if the patient did not meet criteria for a major psychiatric disorder. Psychologists had to have their fees "bundled" with other assessment and treatment packages of the clinic (usually at significantly reduced rates), or provide psychological services for only those patients who were affluent enough to pay for them out of pocket. However, in 2001, psychologists succeeded in gaining new CPT codes for health assessment and intervention services that may be covered by third-party insurers. The codes added services for improvement of patient adherence, symptom management, promotion of healthy behaviors, treatment of health-related risk taking behaviors, and assistance with overall adjustment to physical illness. Here is a brief summary of these codes:

- 96150—initial assessment of psychological, behavioral, and social factors affecting the patient's health
- 96151—reassessment to determine need for further treatment
- 96152—intervention provided to an individual to modify psychological, behavioral, and social factors affecting health
- 96153—intervention provided to a group (e.g., social support group; smoking cessation group)
- 96154—intervention provided to a family with the patient present
- 96154—intervention service provided to family without the patient present

The Assessment Phase

With regard to the assessment phase in the bariatric surgery clinic, the role of the psychologist should not simply be one of assessing whether the patient is psychiatrically stable enough to have surgery in the near future. There are many reasons for going beyond a one-shot psychological screening. Some patients deny or minimize important symptom domains that rely on self-report, and the truth about their behavior can only be learned through development of a trusting relationship over time. Others have recurrent psychiatric conditions that are characterized by exacerbations and remissions. The assessment phase is a recursive one. It is likely to be woven in and out of the other phases since reassessment is often used to serve as a feedback mechanism that determines whether treatments are working. Assessments of conditions that significantly impair the mental aspects of perception, reasoning, mood, memory, judgment, and impulse control are necessary, as problems in these domains can definitely interfere with postoperative treatment adherence and ultimate health. However, it is becoming evident that an initial evaluation of these domains is not sufficient for optimum treatment planning and clinical management. The psychologist must repeatedly assess subtler factors that interfere with the commitment necessary to achieve postoperative success, and the degrees to which patients acknowledge their contribution to ill health. This type of evaluation may involve analysis of ongoing interpersonal factors that interact with problematic eating patterns, motivation for change, willingness to expend the time and energy needed for adequate planning for surgery, and the capacity to adhere to the many postoperative protocols and essential follow-up care. Patients with significant impediments to any of these areas will need intervention and reassessment before they can be cleared for surgery. Sometimes the first choice of intervention does not work, due to either nonadherence or a mismatch between the treatment and the client. Various combinations of cognitive, behavioral, psychodynamic, educational, motivational, and interpersonal interventions may be needed preoperatively. Some patients without significant preoperative problems will need to be reevaluated postoperatively when complications develop that are related to psychosocial adjustment problems, eating disorders, or psychiatric disorders.

Wadden and Foster (7) and Wadden and Phelan (8) have published obesity assessment models that rely on clinical interviews, self-report scales, and self-monitoring reports over time. Crowther and Sherwood (9) have published guidelines for the assessment of eating disorders, and emphasize that assessment should occur throughout treatment to guide and evaluate it. Along these lines, we have come to believe that it is important to move beyond the idea that it is sufficient for a surgeon to send an obesity surgery candidate for an interview and an MMPI (Minnesota Multiphasic Personality Inventory) with any licensed psychologist and thus meet the obligation for preoperative psychological assessment. Morbid obesity is usually the result of a complex set of disorders, and understanding them requires experience with many cases and extensive knowledge in order for a psychologist to competently make important judgments that affect surgical treatment.

Familiarity with the psychological factors involved in problems with sleep, pain, stress, injury, disability, addiction, eating disorders, and other compulsive behaviors is critical because these disturbances may contribute to weight gain. Also some understanding of the various comorbid conditions (e.g., hypothyroidism, diabetes, hypertension, and cardiovascular disease) as well as good general clinical skills with a broad range of psychiatric disorders is necessary. The MMPI is a test that most surgeons remember from either college or medical school. It is known to be well researched and to have proven utility in the areas of mental health, forensics, and pain management. However, it has not been particularly successful in predicting bariatric surgery outcomes. Stunkard and Wadden (10) reviewed studies that attempted to create subtypes of psychological functioning in severely obese subjects. They found that the MMPI had a great deal of variability in the makeup and number of subtypes formed using its symptom, personality, and validity subscales. They concluded that the findings clearly demonstrated the heterogeneity of severe obesity, but failed to define useful empirically derived subgroups. In another study, Wadden and Stunkard (11) reviewed research that compared the MMPIs of severely obese patients with those of patients presenting for other medical or surgical procedures and found that the severely obese were not more disturbed. The authors concluded,

These findings do not mean, as McReynolds reported, that obese persons are free of psychological problems. Some overweight adults, adolescents, and children have severe depression and anxiety and require professional attention. Moreover, there is reason to believe that many overweight persons experience adverse psychological effects that are not measured by standard personality and psychopathology inventories. Such effects are likely to involve weight-specific problems. (p. 1064)

The MMPI-2 requires about 2 hours for the average patient to complete its 567 items, and the language of the instrument can be problematic for clients with low intellectual or educational levels. Although some clinicians are satisfied with the pairing of the MMPI-2 and the Millon Behavioral Health Inventory in the assessment of obesity surgery patients, concerns arise when several other scales are also routinely used in an assessment battery. If patients are going to be given many instruments to complete, inclusion of long omnibus screening tools are likely to lead to fatigue, anger, or misleading data in some instances.

The bulk of recently published studies on the psychological assessment of obesity surgery candidates use batteries of shorter scales for the assessment of health-related quality of life, subjective ratings of physical limitation(s), depression, anxiety, body image, dietary restraint and disinhibition, binge eating, bulimia, emotional eating, and social support, to name a few. The advantage of brief scales is that after trials of interventions for targeted symptoms (or syndromes), a given scale can be easily readministered to assess treatment effectiveness (multiple times if necessary). There is still no consensus on which assessment tools are best for assessing obesity surgery candidates. Assessment methods found to be most useful in state-of-the-art research protocols may not always be practical in daily clinical practice where more compromises have to be made. There may be cultural and demographic factors that would make a given scale useful in one community but not in another. A structured interview might better assess a certain disorder with one subgroup while a scale might be preferable for the same disorder with a different subgroup. Because of the heterogeneity of the morbidly obese population, some clinicians may use a standard battery composed of relatively short scales, and then follow up with more comprehensive measures in situations where there are clinical signs or processes requiring further investigation (e.g., intellectual impairment, psychosis). In addition to assessment for psychiatric disorders that may interfere with the understanding and capacity to implement the pre- and postoperative requirements for success, it makes clinical sense for the psychologist to assess those areas known to be related to relapse and nonadherence.

The theory and practice of relapse prevention developed for substance abusers can be profitably applied to obesity surgery patients who have histories of compulsive eating or unmanageable food cravings. Witkiewitz and Marlatt (12) have reconceptualized relapse within a "dynamic" model that facilitates integration of the multiple influences that trigger and operate within a high-risk situation. They listed the following psychosocial areas known to contribute to relapse: low self-efficacy, negative outcome expectancies, craving, motivational problems, negative affect states, poor coping or self-regulation, and dysfunctional interpersonal determinants. The authors emphasized the importance of situational dynamics related to a person's unique self-organizing processes. Self-organization was defined as the interaction of background factors (e.g., years of substance abuse, family history, social support, and comorbid psychopathology), physiologic states, cognitive processes, and coping skills. The authors stated, "The reconceptualized dynamic model of relapse allows for several configurations of distal and proximal relapse risk factors. Distal risks are defined as stable predispositions that increase an individual's vulnerability to lapse, whereas proximal risks are immediate precipitants that actualize the statistical probability of a lapse" (p. 229). For example, a proximal risk could be an argument with one's boss, whereas a distal one could be long-standing conflict with authority figures related to unresolved issues with a primary caregiver from childhood. Contextual factors such as walking by a bakery, for example, may mediate between other risk factors and a poor food choice.

This new model of relapse does not presume that certain factors are more influential than others, but attempts to identify meaningful interactions among them that are then used to guide clinical decisions. Application of this model requires assessment of both the "tonic" processes that contribute to chronic vulnerability for relapse, and the "phasic" ones related to situational cognitive, affective, and physical states, as well as the coping skills utilized. Obviously, multiple assessments over time are needed for the identification of the processes contributing to the lapses and relapses for a given individual. Perri (13) has been a major contributor in the effort to integrate relapse prevention models with obesity treatment. He stated, "In general, the longer obese clients remain in contact with treatment providers, the longer they adhere to necessary behaviors." His research has found that in order to prevent relapse, "clients may need the assistance of a health care professional at the time they are experiencing the initial slip or lapse."

Also with regard to assessment, there is a great deal to be gained from review of the proceedings from international and national expert panels on the treatment of obesity. While psychologists are a long way from having formal standards of practice, many useful guidelines have emerged from these panels. In 1997, the World Health Organization (WHO) held a summit in Geneva entitled, "Obesity: Preventing and Managing the Global Epidemic" (14). The WHO report of these meetings was published in 1998, and emphasized the view that an effective weight management strategy depends on "a comprehensive analysis of the individual's degree of obesity, his or her associated risks, co-existing illnesses, social and personal situation, and a history of those problems and precipitating factors which lead to weight gain" (p. 210). This document addressed the inconsistencies in the literature that compared obese and nonobese people on standard psychological tests, and recommended the work of Friedman and Brownell (15) as a guide for improving our understanding of the clinically relevant differences among healthy, obese, morbidly obese, and super-obese patients. These authors addressed the shortcomings of first-generation research in this area. They proposed a second generation of research that would identify factors that are likely to place obese people at risk for psychological problems and suffering.

Currently, there is no standard system for classifying levels of psychological risk for obesity surgery candidates, and there is no widely accepted system for grouping patients into subtypes from a psychological perspective. Friedman and Brownell (15) proposed a third generation of studies that will use the risk factors derived from second-generation studies and their association with psychological characteristics and look for causal links and cause-and-effect models. It is likely that psychologists will play an important role in the development of a set of sturdy, empirically derived psychosocial risk factors for poor surgical outcomes, and also the enabling factors for good ones.

Special Considerations in the Assessment of Depression

The most common psychiatric disorder associated with obesity is depression. The etiology of depression is heterogeneous. People may develop depression after a host of medical problems. The list is very long, but ones that typically co-occur with obesity are sleep disorders, chronic pain, hypothyroidism, injury with disability, surgery with protracted physical limitation, diabetes, cardiovascular disease, cancer, pulmonary disease, and other disorders producing significant discomfort, distress, or loss of function. In these cases, psychologists may choose to use the *Diagnostic and Statistical Manual of Mental Disorders*, fourth edition, text revision (DSM-IV-TR) (16), and refer to the category of "depression secondary to a general medical condition" rather than to the category of "major depressive disorder."

Decreased self-care is often seen in severely depressed patients. This means that depression can make it more difficult to treat the medical conditions that contributed to its development. Further complicating matters is that the decreased self-care, poor concentration, and self-injurious behaviors attributable to the depressive syndrome may lead to the development of new medical problems. It is also important to recognize that depression can be secondary to a variety of primary psychiatric disorders such as panic disorder, posttraumatic stress disorder, schizophrenia, etc. Adequate treatment of the primary disorder is often required before secondary depression will remit fully. Also worthy of consideration are the genetically determined forms of depression, which in the worst cases develop without the usual triggers of loss, insult, injury, illness, trauma, or frustrated needs. Most commonly, there is an interaction between genetic and environmental factors. However, the more episodes an individual has, the less they tend to be related to the magnitude of the external stressors.

Many of our obese patients have their own unique combination of biological, psychological, and social variables that contribute to the development of depression. To be effective, treatment must often address both the symptoms and the known causes of the patient's depression. It is important to recognize that even after adequate treatment, the mood disorder may recur, especially if postoperative complications develop or if the patient's expectations with regard to what surgery will "fix" are not met 1 year or longer after surgery. The course of recurrent depression is variable. According to the DSM-IV-TR (16),

"Some evidence suggests that the periods of remission generally last longer early in the course of the disorder. The number of prior episodes predicts the likelihood of developing subsequent Major Depression Disorder. At least 60% of individuals with Major Depressive Disorder, Single Episode, can be expected to have a second episode. Individuals who have had two episodes have a 70% chance of having a third, and individuals who have had three episodes have a 90% chance of having a fourth." (p. 372)

Recent data on the natural history of depression also suggest that the risk of repeated episodes of depression over a 10- to 15-year period exceeds 85% (17). Also, Judd (18) found that individuals with major depressive disorder will have on average four episodes of approximately 20 weeks' duration each, as well as other symptoms of depression during periods of partial remission. The implications for the assessment of depression in obesity patients are obvious. One cannot rely on a one-time assessment and be assured that a currently asymptomatic patient with a history of major depression will not develop a major depressive episode before or after surgery. Therefore, ongoing monitoring of patients and repeat assessments are much preferred over the single cross-sectional evaluation that attempts to predict future disturbance based on one sampling of data.

It is also important to remember that certain forms of substance abuse are known to contribute to characteristic forms depression (e.g., alcohol-induced mood disorder; cocaine-induced mood disorder) and that a subgroup of obese patients abuse alcohol or drugs in addition to food. Obviously, the psychologist must facilitate the treatment of substance abuse and have it well under control before any serious planning for surgery may occur.

Many investigators have addressed the fact that depression may develop de novo in certain individuals who become obese, due to the discrimination and prejudice they experience in school, in the job market, at the workplace, in the dating scene, on airplanes or other crowded spaces, or simply when out in public. Also, an individual may become depressed due to the helplessness caused by the physical limitations and discomfort associated with obesity or from its comorbid conditions. Patients who were depressed before becoming obese probably have a phenomenology somewhat different from those who became depressed after obesity developed. The low energy associated with both obesity and depression can increase avoidance of exercise. The subgroup of depressed patients who have constant somatic complaints (pre- or postoperatively) in lieu of experiencing sadness can drive a weight management center to distraction until the patient's mood disorder is treated. Both depression and obesity are known to contribute to impairment in social and occupational areas of functioning, and together may exponentially increase the level of stress for the morbidly obese patient. Feelings of helplessness may be increased when the obese patient becomes depressed, and may interfere with the patient's ability to follow the pre- or postoperative protocols.

Weight gain may also be a symptom of depression. Significant weight loss or weight gain is one among many criteria for major depressive disorder. With regard to the latter, the DSM-IV-TR states that there must be increased appetite nearly every day for at least a 2-week period or a change of more than 5% body weight in a month, and the patient may crave specific foods such as sweets or carbohydrates (16). The hypothesis that certain depressed individuals crave and ingest foods that elevate serotonin (or other neurotransmitter systems) in order to self-medicate has been proposed by researchers in the areas of nutrition, eating disorders, and holistic medicine. Other investigators have found that gorging on food elevates the body's endogenous opioids in some people, and that these individuals may achieve a desired state of numbness and escape from whatever is felt to be intolerable. These eating phenomena may not be what Hippocrates meant when he said, "Let food be your medicine and medicine be your food."

The psychological factors that contribute to depression could fill many books, but some of the typical ones found in the histories of obese patients are related to experiences of neglect, abuse (physical, emotional, or sexual), or other traumatic experiences that lead to some form of biopsychosocial dysregulation. The loss of important others through death, divorce, or other forms of termination are common causes of depression. Likewise, the loss of another's love, trust, or respect may contribute to depression. Also, the loss of anything highly valued (e.g., employment, possessions, skills, status, faith, or power) can be depressogenic. Pessimism, feelings of helplessness or hopelessness, excessive guilt, and other negative cognitions are common factors in the development and maintenance of depression. Interpersonal factors such as infidelity, spousal addiction, feeling controlled by a family member, receiving excessive criticism, or noninvolvement of significant others are common contributing factors in both depression and overeating. In other patients, the inability to establish intimate relationships may contribute to depression.

Skill or coping deficits in various life domains may contribute to excessive frustration and depression in some patients. The literature on coping and addictive behavior suggests that there are three general categories of coping: *problem-focused coping,* in which the person does something to change the situation; *emotion-focused coping,* in which the person deals mainly with the emotional reaction to the stressor; and *avoidant coping,* in which the person turns attention away from the stressful situation (19). Tennen et al. (19) found that emotion-focused and avoidant coping best predicted alcohol consumption levels. Obese patients say that they eat for comfort, or to get rid of bad feelings, or as a distraction from circumstances that cause distress.

In their relapse prevention efforts with obese patients, Perri et al. (20) found that when problem-solving interventions were added to standard behavioral treatments for obesity, the outcomes were better. In essence, Perri and colleagues had better obesity treatment outcomes when they improved problem-focused coping in their patients.

Assessment of Emotional Eating

Since the 1950s there has been consistent support for the fact that some people overeat in response to stress, emotional tension, intolerable emotional pain, conflict, or frustrating life circumstances (21). Hamburger (21) classified emotional eating into four patterns: nonspecific emotional eating, in which any negative emotion can trigger it; eating to compensate for intolerable life situations; eating to ward off symptoms of an underlying psychiatric disorder (e.g., depression); and insatiable craving or addiction to food. These categories were not mutually exclusive. Bruch (22) referred to "active phases of obesity," in which emotional eating and weight gain are prominent, and stable phases of obesity, in which weight is stable and there is less emotional eating. The phasic nature of emotional eating can pose challenges for clinicians attempting to assess it and treat it. Also, emotional eating may be done secretly, making it difficult for family members or significant others to help clinicians reliably assess it. This phenomenon has been referred to as "stress eating."

Many of the painful life situations discussed previously may contribute to depression, emotional eating, obesity, or all three in a given individual. Some people emotionally eat only when overwhelmed by multiple stressors (e.g., financial, relationship, and health problems). Others emotionally eat in response to a single stressor or a specific type of distress. Rand (23) found that 79% of the obese subjects compared to 9% of the normal-weight subjects gained 10 pounds or more during periods of major life stress such as marriage, divorce, job change, or death of a family member. The magnitude of the stressor needed to trigger emotional eating varies from person to person, as does the subjective degree of distress associated with that trigger. In their review of how obese patients who seek treatment differ from those who don't, Fitzgibbon et al. (24) stated that the former "reported elevated levels of distress and increased emotional eating in response to negative emotional reactions."

Polivy and Herman's (25) review of the binge-eating disorder literature found that stress and negative mood were the most frequently cited precipitants of binge eating. Also, negative emotional states have shown a strong relationship with relapse in patients with various types of substance abuse disorders. In Marlatt's (26) original study of relapse precipitants, "negative affect" was the unambiguous predictor of lapses following treatment. Leon and Chamberlain (27–29) studied subjects who lost weight after treatment and classified them as either "maintainers" or "regainers." The regainers had difficulties with a wide range of emotional states, whereas maintainers had difficulty mainly with loneliness and boredom. In his review of emotional eating, Ganley (30) cited studies that described patients who ate to avoid social encounters, ward off sexual feelings, or deal with many forms of interpersonal and family dysfunction. He concluded, "Although social determinants have rarely been the focus of investigation, these studies suggest that obesity and emotional eating may be deeply embedded in relationship attitudes, roles, interactions, and the regulation of emotion" (p. 353).

Rodin et al. (31) reviewed laboratory experiments showing that when obese subjects restrained their eating, this restraint was overridden by emotional arousal or anxiety. Studies showing that some overweight individuals had greater reactivity to pain, stress, and other types of emotional arousal compared to normal-weight subjects were also reviewed. It is important to recognize that patients who do not meet DSM-IV-TR criteria for a psychiatric disorder may have a clinically significant degree of emotional eating nonetheless. Thus, while these areas overlap somewhat, one cannot assume that emotional eating has been ruled out simply by a low depression or anxiety index. Some patients are not consciously aware of their emotions or cannot accurately label them, which makes the assessment of anxiety, depression, and emotional eating difficult. It also important to keep in mind that some obesity surgery candidates minimize their degree of depression or anxiety because they fear that admission of psychiatric symptoms may slow down their progress toward their goal of surgery. Others simply do not want the double stigma of being both obese and mentally ill. Therefore, it makes sense for psychologists to evaluate for presence of emotional eating pre- and postoperatively, and then help emotional eaters develop better coping mechanisms. Arnow et al. (32) have developed an emotional eating scale with established reliability and validity. It is a one-page measure that the average patient can complete in less than 5 minutes, making it ideal for serial assessment.

Assessment of Eating Disorders

There are significant challenges to the accurate assessment of eating disorders in obese patients. There is a great deal of shame associated with these behaviors, and patients often deny or minimize them. There is disagreement in the field about how best to assess the eating disorders commonly associated with obesity. Scales, structured interviews, semistructured interviews, and unstructured interviews have all been used in both research and clinical practice.

A recent development in public health and substance abuse treatment is the "harm reduction" model (33,34). This model accepts that human beings are going to use food, alcohol, and drugs for pleasure, fun, stress reduction, or coping with frustrated needs or overwhelming experiences. While abstinence may be a viable goal for some people, it is not for others. In harm reduction treatment, clients learn about the continuum of use, abuse, and addiction. Responsible use is that which has a low risk of causing harm to self or others. Practitioners of harm reduction have found that many, if not most, patients reveal accurate information about their substance use only when the clinician has proven to be trustworthy, nonjudgmental, and noncontrolling over time. This pattern clearly obtains in a subgroup of obese patients with coexisting eating disorders. We have had patients finally reveal the truth about their preoperative eating behavior a year or more after undergoing bariatric surgery.

The WHO document reviewed some of the eating disorders associated with obesity, such as binge eating, night eating syndrome, and nocturnal sleep-related disorder.

Binge Eating

Up to 30% of the obese patients seeking medical help binge eat large quantities of food with a subjective feeling of loss of control. Binge eating is associated with more severe mood problems, and a greater incidence of comorbid psychopathology. Binge eaters are more likely to drop out of behavior modification programs for weight loss than non–binge eating obese patients. Edelman (35) found that in addition to the frustration attendant to being on diets, binge eaters may also overeat in response to fatigue, feeling sorry for oneself, loneliness, family discord, or occupational frustration. Studies are inconsistent with regard to the degree of risk that preoperative binge eating has for development for postoperative disordered eating. However, it makes clinical sense to treat binge eating preoperatively. Fairburn and Wilson (36) have developed the most widely accepted cognitive-behavioral treatment for binge eating. Also, some binge eaters have shown reduction in disordered eating behavior after pharmacologic intervention with medications such as fluoxetine, sibutramine, and topiramate (37); phentermine (38); fluvoxamine (39); d-fenfluramine (40); and desipramine (41).

Night Eating Syndrome

This disorder was initially described by Stunkard et al. (42) and was characterized by the triad of morning anorexia, evening hyperphagia, and insomnia. Often night eating syndrome (NES) included depression with an unusual circadian pattern (i.e., minimal morning depression that progressed throughout the day and night). Patients eat 25% to 50% of their daily calorie intake *after* the evening meal. Many of these patients get out of bed at night to eat after having difficulty sleeping. It is hypothesized that this disorder may be more common in obese patients who have sleep apnea. Stunkard's research found NES to occur in about 1.5% of the general population and in 8.9% of obese adults. Rand et al. (43) found that 27% of obese patients seeking surgical intervention reported night eating syndrome. Contrasted to binge eating, which tends to occur in a shorter, more discrete amount of time and is often characterized by rapid eating, night eating can go on for many hours and usually into the next morning. Birketvedt et al. (44) believe that NES may be related to a malfunctioning stress response and are investigating the neuroendocrine pathophysiology of the hypothalamic-pituitary-adrenal (HPA) axis. They reported that, worldwide, 50% of night eaters are obese and 50% are not. Recent classification efforts have recommended that a patient must demonstrate night eating for a period of 3 months in order to receive the diagnosis.

Nocturnal Sleep-Related Disorder

This disorder has also been referred to as "sleep eating." It occurs when patients are somewhere between wakefulness and sleep. They may appear sound asleep to others when eating. They may eat strange combinations of foods and have little or no memory of eating. Although first described in 1955, this disorder had not attracted much scientific interest until recently. Some investigators conceptualize nocturnal sleep-related disorder (NSRD) as a sleep disorder, and view the ingestion of foods that elevate brain serotonin levels as the effort to medicate the sleep disturbance.

Grazing

This disorder of eating behavior was not addressed in the WHO document. Saunders (45) has described grazing as a high-risk behavior that most frequently occurs in postoperative bariatric surgery patients with previous histories of binge eating disorder (or a subsyndromal variant of it). Most patients who have obesity surgery are unable to consume what the DSM-IV-TR research criteria require for a diagnosis of binge eating disorder, that is, "an amount of food that is definitely larger than most people would eat in a similar period of time under similar circumstances." However, grazing retains some of the other DSM-IV-TR criteria: a sense of lack of control, eating until feeling uncomfortably full, and eating when not hungry. Saunders feels that whether grazing is referred to as subthreshold, a partial syndrome, or atypical, it has a significant negative impact on the daily functioning of bariatric surgery patients. It may impede the progress of the bariatric surgery both in terms of healthy phase-appropriate food selection and optimum weight loss. It may also contribute to a premature plateau or weight regain over time. Saunders found that of the 64 patients she followed longitudinally, 60% reported binge eating or grazing preoperatively. Of this high-risk group, 80% reported feelings of loss of control over eating. The preoperative binge eaters reported a shift to grazing at an average of 6 months after surgery, while the preoperative grazers also experienced a return of the behavior at 6 months, but it worsened between months 12 and 18. Some of her subjects reported a desire to "test the limits" of what they could eat without gaining weight, while others were actively seeking the "comfort of the too full feeling they had experienced before surgery." Importantly, some of these patients induced vomiting to avoid gaining weight.

Saunders identified psychological factors associated with grazing that are similar to those described in the binge-eating literature: creation of good/bad food dichotomies and labeling the self as bad when eating foods from that category, feelings of deprivation triggering out of control eating, and patients' belief that they were about to fail at yet another attempt at weight loss. Saunders noted that when patients believed that they would no longer have food cravings after surgery, they became distressed when craving arose. Also, those who had dysphoria trigger binge eating preoperatively were likely to have other feelings of disappointment postoperatively that triggered grazing behavior three to five times per week. Saunders found that problems with spouses, family members, and friends often became intertwined with dysfunctional eating, as well as body image and identity problems. She recommended a modified form of cognitive-behavioral therapy for postoperative grazers.

The Preparation for Surgery Phase

Any of the conditions discovered in the assessment phase known to increase surgical risk, decrease the likelihood of adherence to postoperative protocols, or cause the patient excessive distress should be treated in the preparation for surgery phase. In some cases, clearance for surgery is contingent on a specified amount of symptom reduction (e.g., a Beck Depression Index score below 20). In 1996, the American Obesity Association (AOA) and Shape Up America published *Guidelines for Treatment of Adult Obesity*. The information was compiled by a committee of obesity experts chosen by Surgeon General C. Everett Koop. A patient-oriented version was prepared in 1998 (46). This document stated that patients with symptoms of bulimia nervosa or unstable mental illness such as schizophrenia or bipolar disorder should not have any form of weight-loss treatment until their symptoms remit and until the patient has been stable for a sufficient period of time. Obese patients who binge and purge are at risk of overeating or returning to self-induced vomiting after surgery. They should be referred to a therapist specializing in eating disorders and be symptom free for a minimum of 6 months before undergoing obesity surgery.

Schizophrenia was an exclusion criterion during the evolution of bariatric surgery. However, research in recent years has shown that some individuals with schizophrenia may do well postoperatively, especially if they have good social and family support (47). Clinicians need to ensure that the patient with severe mental illness is clinically stable for a significant period of time before surgery (e.g., 6 months to a year), that a strong and informed support system is in place to monitor and assist with the postoperative protocols, and that planning has been made for ensuring long-term psychotropic medication adherence. Some of the newer antipsychotic agents are much more effective than older drugs for selected patients. However, a major problem with some of these medicines is that they cause significant weight gain. Clinicians need to consider these factors when they select drugs for maintenance therapy as opposed to acute stabilization treatments.

The AOA/Shape Up America document also recommended treatment for depression, anxiety, and high levels of stress before and during weight reduction treatment. The committee acknowledged the research that found excessive stress to be associated with increased body weight pre- and postoperatively. It was noted that weight loss may exacerbate depression in some individuals. Psychological reevaluation every 3 to 6 months was suggested. The contributors strongly recommended an evaluation specifically aimed at assessing readiness for weight loss. This evaluation should include the assessment of motivation, readiness to make a long-term commitment, and the timing of interventions. Patients in the midst of a divorce, serious financial difficulty, or an abusive marriage should postpone surgery until they have improved their situation. Patients who are about to relocate to a new geographical area or make a career change, for example, may need to delay obesity surgery until they have adjusted to such major life developments. Psychologists may be needed to assist surgery candidates with any life situation that could significantly interfere with the effort, time, and resources required to follow a graduated dietary protocol for a year, engage in regular exercise, or to faithfully return to the program for follow-up visits.

The WHO report stressed the importance of family involvement, and reviewed literature that has shown that the body weight and attitudes of a patient's spouse can have a major impact on the amount of weight lost and successful maintenance (14). Obese patients with normal-weight partners tend to lose more than those with obese partners. Success is greater when a spouse also makes an effort to lose weight with the patient. Dropout rates are reduced when the patient's spouse is included in the weight control program. In light of these findings, it makes sense to include spouses and significant life partners in the preoperative support groups and in some cases additional couples therapy. Likewise, inclusion of both patient and partner in postoperative groups or counseling may be helpful.

The use of certain substances or the cessation of others may contribute to weight gain. Alcohol consumption may disinhibit dietary restraint and lead to overeating, and cannabis use is known to stimulate appetite. Stimulant cessation may lead to weight gain. The WHO document addressed weight gain associated with smoking cessation, especially in people who smoke more than 15 cigarettes per day. Smoking cessation, according to the WHO, should be a higher priority than weight loss in obese patients who smoke, as there is strong research indicating that smoking has a greater negative impact on morbidity and mortality. Alcohol consumption was also addressed in the report. Alcohol is associated with increased risk of excess body fat development, and a number of obese patients drink. Oxidation of ingested alcohol is given priority over other macronutrients. When alcohol consumption meets the body's energy needs, it allows more of the energy from food to be stored. The psychologist may be consulted for the management of smoking, drug, and alcohol use at the weight management center.

In 2000, the National Institutes of Health (NIH), in conjunction with the National Heart, Lung, and Blood Institute and the North American Association for the Study of Obesity, published *The Practical Guide: Identification, Evaluation, and Treatment of Overweight and Obesity In Adults,* which was revised in 2002 (48). It made the following suggestions for overcoming barriers to treatment adherence: A nonjudgmental and nonblaming attitude on the part of clinicians is critical. Building a partnership with the patient and working with the patient to set achievable goals is important. When a patient does not select an area that appears in need of change, then inquiry and discussion about the costs and benefits of that area tend to work better than ordering the patient to do it. Once patients decide that they are committed to changing an area, it is important to assess their degree of confidence in their ability to achieve it (i.e., self-efficacy). Effective goals are specific, attainable, and forgiving in that they do not require perfect achievement. Examining the circumstances connected with unmet goals can facilitate developing new and more effective strategies.

The *Practical Guide* conceptualized weight loss as a "journey" and not a "destination," and suggested teaching patients to view lapses as "inevitable opportunities to learn how to be more successful." An important goal-setting strategy suggested by the *Practical Guide* is the following:

Before beginning treatment, results of the physical examination and laboratory tests should be shared with the patient. Emphasis should be placed on any new findings, particularly those associated with obesity that would be expected to improve with weight loss. The patient should focus on improvements in these health parameters, rather than focus on achieving an ideal body weight or a similarly large weight loss that may or may not be attainable. . . . By focusing patients on medical rather than cosmetic benefits of weight loss, you may better help them to attain their goals. (p. 40)

Adherence

Over two decades ago, surveys emerged indicating that one of the most common sources of treatment failure in medicine was patient noncompliance. Within the last decade this phenomenon has not changed much, but the language we use and the way we understand it has evolved. Webster defined "compliance" as conformity, yielding to the wishes of another, or submitting to the desire, demand, proposal, or coercion of another. "Adherence" is defined as sticking to, giving support, and maintaining loyalty or fidelity. The old "M. Deity" portrayal of the medical doctor who tells patients what to do in the manner of an imperious parent, and who does not discuss treatment options or costs with patients, is no longer tenable. Patients today are armed with rapid access to vast amounts of information via the Internet, and have developed skills at obtaining second opinions and medical comparison shopping. Many will no longer tolerate a paternalistic relationship with their physician. "Doctor's Orders" are passé.

In the past, patients labeled as noncompliant were often viewed as having negative character traits. The current term, *adherence,* is more neutral and describes the extent to which a patient follows through with previously agreed-upon actions. It implies cooperation rather than submission. Adherence may refer to keeping appointments, taking prescriptions, attending support groups, or completing other tasks between appointments. Current research on nonadherence shows that certain physician, treatment team, and institutional variables contribute to the problem of nonadherence and caution against blaming the patient alone for poor treatment outcome.

Dunbar-Jacob and Mortimer-Stephens (49) reviewed the literature dealing with adherence in chronic disease, and found that as many as 60% of persons with chronic disorders are poorly adherent to treatment. This group found that the costs of nonadherence are greater than $100 billion per year, and up to 40% of hospital readmissions are related to this phenomenon. The most common reason for missed medication was forgetting. The second most common was "symptom management," that is, when symptoms increase the patient increases the dose, or when symptoms decrease the patient takes less of it. The third most common reason for a missed medication dose was schedule disruption (e.g., travel, dining out, work demands, and other interruptions). Dunbar-Jacob's group also looked at physician variables in the treatment of diabetes, hypertension, and heart disease. Patients with good adherence often had doctors who reported more job satisfaction, had busier clinics in terms of visits per week, and more often provided patients with definite future appointments than the doctors whose patients showed poor adherence.

Zweben and Zuckoff (50) reviewed the adherence literature and found the following reasons for low adherence: low acceptance of the problem; having reservations about the nature, extent, and severity of the problem; and lacking the sense of safety necessary to give up what is familiar for an uncertain future. In reviewing the literature on failure to adhere to plans that patients had developed, Polivy and Herman (51) identified four primary types of overestimation: (1) the amount of change possible; (2) the speed of change; (3) the ease of change; and (4) the reward of change (e.g., "If I lose weight, I will meet the man of my dreams, get a great job, and live happily ever after"). They concluded, "Expectations often exceed what is feasible and lead people to reject more modest achievable goals. The best is the enemy of the good" (p. 679). Engle and Arkowitz (52) have observed that some patients view medication adherence, going to the doctor, or even reading literature about their illness as unpleasant reminders of their "weakened state of health." To avoid this dysphoria, patients turn a blind eye to their treatment. Engle and Arkowitz have produced an excellent new text on the reasons that patients do not change, together with strategies for overcoming barriers to health care adherence.

Heidenreich (53) found that poor adherence was related to cost and complexity of the medical regimen, patient variables, and provider variables. He also described some of the dangers of nonadherence. Using antihypertensive medications as an example, when patients do not take their prescribed dosages and do not effectively communicate this to their physician, the dose may be erroneously increased. When this process goes through several cycles, a medical emergency may result should the patient begin taking the medication at the last prescribed dose.

Wing et al. (54) concluded that adherence mediated the relationship between depression and health outcomes. Her group reviewed the literature that found depression to be associated with poor outcome in a variety of medical conditions, and that as many as 60% of depressed patients did not adhere to a 9-month antidepressant regimen. In reviewing the literature on renal disease, angina, cancer, and arthritis, Wing's group found that depressed patients were three times as likely to be nonadherent when compared to nondepressed ones. After myocardial infarction, depressed patients reported lower adherence to exercise, low-fat diet, stress reduction, and use of prescription medication. Wing et al. listed the following as possible explanations for the lower adherence rates found in depressed medical patients when compared to nondepressed ones: depressed patients report greater feelings of hopelessness and may not expect treatment to be effective; some are socially isolated, and good social support is related to adherence; cognitive impairment in depressed patients may affect their ability to remember to take medication or other recommendations given by the physician; and finally, depressed patients may not have the energy to carry out treatment recommendations. Wing's group has found that by increasing a patient's activity level, a depressive episode may be prevented. They have found that some patients who maintained their activity level did not have a recurrence of depression even when weight was regained. The authors concluded that interventions that contribute to a feeling of empowerment improve adherence.

Nemeroff (55) reviewed antidepressant adherence and found that as many as 44% of patients discontinue antidepressant treatment within the first 3 months. The main causes of poor adherence with antidepressants were poor doctor–patient relationships, lack of patient education, and unpleasant adverse side effects. Gianetti (56) described the following basics of good physician communication skills: elicit the patient's perspective, assess how much the patient wants to be involved in decision making, assess the patient's perception of the disease and its treatment, address patient concerns, offer options and explanations, periodically check for understanding, and encourage the patient to express concerns about the regimen. He identified patient beliefs about antidepressants that contribute to poor adherence: "the medication is addictive"; "medication is a 'crutch' "; "I will not be able to tolerate the side effects"; "I will never be able to stop the medication"; "if I don't feel better immediately, the medication is not working"; "medicine cannot solve my problems"; and "medication will make me tired all the time." In addition to these, we have observed other beliefs: "I am not myself on the medication"; "the medication makes me a zombie"; and "I lose my vitality and 'edge' when on the medication." Legitimate complaints of side effects such as sexual dysfunction, decreased libido, sleep difficulties, weight gain, and others should be distinguished from faulty beliefs and addressed appropriately.

Vergouwen et al. (57) investigated the differing impact on antidepressant nonadherence that educational versus collaborative care interventions had. Patient education programs included discussion of side effects, reviewing the information leaflet with the patient during the initial visit, and mailing personalized information directly to patients. Collaborative care programs were systematic approaches to the improvement of patient education with the active involvement of other health care providers such as mental health professionals, nurses, and care extenders. The interventions were multimodal in that they affected the patient, physician, and the system of care. These interventions increased the following: patient education, length and frequency of visits, surveillance of adherence, education and training of clinicians, and the use of feedback and recommendations made by care extenders. The collaborative care model was found to contribute to better adherence to the pharmacologic treatment of depression.

Gianetti (56) developed the following counseling model for psychologists to improve antidepressant adherence: (1) establish a therapeutic alliance with the patient; (2) destigmatize the illness; (3) encourage the positive health beliefs associated with the treatment of depression; (4) emphasize that the benefits outweigh the costs of taking medication; (5) dispel irrational beliefs regarding the disease state and medication treatment; (6) use behavioral interventions to tailor the regimen to the lifestyle of the patient and collaborate with the prescribing doctor to reduce the impact of side effects (e.g., change of medication type, timing of the dose, or use of long-acting or "extended-release" medications); and (7) use collaborative agreements among treating health care professionals (e.g., pharmacist, physician, and psychotherapist) to continually monitor and evaluate adherence.

The Postoperative Adjustment Phase

The studies investigating the relationship between psychosocial factors and surgical outcome have been inconsistent. Because of this, research has been unable to inform clinical practice to an optimal degree. The factors investigated have varied from study to study. Also, different scales have been used to assess the same variable across studies. Future investigative efforts will need better coordination among research sites. Despite these problems, useful trends have emerged in the literature and are addressed in this section.

In the medical domain, many studies have placed the outcome premium on weight loss. This can be misleading. For example, a patient who loses more weight than another may not be healthier if the former did not comply with recommended dietary and activity guidelines. Across studies, the mean length of time that elapsed from the date of surgery to the last weight measurement has varied a great deal. Since most patients lose weight during the first 6 months after surgery (whether they adhere to the protocols or not), subjects are much more homogeneous (with respect to weight loss) at this point in time. They are less so 5 years postoperatively. Brownell and Wadden (58) pointed out that group averages of weight loss may lead to incorrect inferences about individuals, and that intraindividual variability (e.g., cycles of loss, regain, loss) may be missed. The percentage of subjects who have maintained weight loss at 2 years may constitute a different subset of the sample than those who maintained their weight loss at 5 years. The authors cautioned that attributing change to a single intervention is often misleading because of the many concurrent treatments and lifestyle change efforts that most patients are involved in. Also, the more precise goal of surgery is to reduce fat while preserving lean body mass (59). Some patients have too little muscle preoperatively, and actually need to gain a significant amount of muscle in order to become healthy. The holy trinity of adequate protein, water, and activity levels is essential for optimal muscle development. The psychologist may need to be consulted when patients do not adequately adhere to the dietary, vitamin, and exercise protocols.

In 1991, The National Institutes of Health published a "Consensus Statement on Gastrointestinal Surgery for Severe Obesity" (60). This document stressed the importance of *lifelong* medical follow-up after obesity surgery, yet some surgeons and too many patients choose to neglect this aspect of this risky but effective set of surgical procedures. Patients are expected to go for laboratory measurements and examinations at 1 or 2 weeks postoperatively, again at 4 weeks, then between 2 and 5 months, again between 6 and 12 months, and then once a year for life unless there are complications that require more frequent visits. Follow-up may reveal psychological factors related to problems with pain management, wound care, Gastrostomy-tube care (when applicable), diet, supplement use, and activity level. Also during follow-up various clinicians may discover problems with social adjustment, work, sexual functioning, substance abuse, marital and family functioning, etc., where involvement of the psychologist will be important. The consensus statement concluded,

Quality-of-life considerations in patients undergoing surgical treatment for obesity must be considered, as there must be reorientation and adjustment to the side effect of a changing body image. Euphoria can be seen in patients during the early postoperative period. Some patients, however, may experience significant late postoperative depression. Some patients have depressive symptoms that are not improved by surgically induced weight loss. (p. 9)

The consensus statement further recommended that

Evaluation of the psychosocial changes that occur during weight reduction is needed. Standardized, reliable, and valid questionnaires and structured interviews should be developed to evaluate patients' expectations about changes and the psychosocial changes they actually experience during weight loss and maintenance. (p. 12)

The AOA/Shape Up American group summarized the behavioral research on lifestyle change strategies and recommended the following: self-monitoring of eating and activity through diaries; stress management through the use of strategies to cope with stressful events (e.g., meditation and relaxation techniques) or to reduce them (e.g., problem-solving skill training); stimulus control, whereby patients identify cues in their environment that are associated with under exercising and unhealthy eating and counter them (e.g., substitute healthy responses for unhealthy ones); reinforcement of helpful lifestyle changes with use of rewards, contingency management, and social support from friends or family; cognitive restructuring, which focuses on modification of self-defeating thoughts and feelings, helps patients change faulty attitudes and beliefs, and confronts unrealistic goals and body image distortions; social influence procedures, such as learning to elicit support from others, and identifying saboteurs with the aim of converting them into supporters; and relapse prevention, which is the identification of high-risk situations and development and implementation of plans to avoid or minimize risk. The group also stressed the importance of helping patients learn to forgive themselves for lapses, and to view them as opportunities for learning.

Marcus and Elkins (61) found that patients who attended postoperative support groups had better obesity surgery outcomes than those who did not. The NIH *Practical Guide* (48) suggested that failure to achieve weight loss after treatment requires assessment of the following areas: energy intake of food and alcohol (using both recall and daily logs); energy expenditure (using a physical activity diary); attendance records for behavior modification sessions; recent negative life events; family and societal pressures; and evidence of detrimental psychiatric problems (e.g., depression, eating disorder). This guide's review of the prediction literature concluded that most behavioral predictors have been unable to strongly and consistently predict obesity treatment outcome. However, "self-efficacy" (i.e., patients' confidence that they can succeed) has been a modest but consistent predictor of success.

Motivation for Change

In August 2004, the National Institutes of Health Obesity Task Force released its *Strategic Plan for NIH Obesity Research*" (62). The document stated, "There is no single cause of all human obesity . . . thus, no single prevention or treatment strategy is likely to work for everyone." The plan encouraged work that leads to a better understanding of the mechanisms for changing behavior and maintaining that change, and specifically mentioned the importance of studying motivational strategies that promote weight loss and maintenance. With regard to bariatric surgery, Bond et al. (63) emphasized that "theory-driven change interventions designed to promote appropriate new health behaviors and strengthen resiliency against temptation to engage in old behaviors should be implemented before and after surgery" (p. 851). Bond's group recommended the use of the transtheoretical model of behavior change commonly referred to as the "stages of change" (SOC) model. Prochaska et al. (64,65) developed the SOC model by integrating accepted empirically supported treatments with research on the self-change process. Brownell and Wadden (58) stated that the SOC model "is potentially helpful in the obesity field because it may help explain the large variation in response to treatment and may permit interventions to be targeted to individuals" (p. 512). The SOC model has been used in the successful lowering of smoking, alcohol consumption, substance use, overeating, and unhealthy food choices. This model has been effectively applied to both the initiation of healthy behavior and the modification or cessation of unhealthy behavior (66).

The SOC model is based on the study of people who made important life changes (e.g., smoking cessation, decreased alcohol consumption, or weight loss) on their own. The investigators found that while individuals had a range of tools they used to successfully change, effective changers tended to use different tools at different stages of the change process. Five well-defined stages of change were enunciated. Success requires passage through each stage, but not necessarily linearly. Most people progress, regress, and progress and regress again as they improve their change skills. The authors used a spiral to visually depict their model, and explained that most people spiral up and down through several cycles before achieving lasting success. Analogous to the development of musical or athletic abilities, error and failure experiences cannot be avoided in the process of developing good habits and extinguishing bad ones. Error and failure experiences are valuable forms of learning. Repetition, refinement, and creativity are all part of the change process. Another positive aspect of the SOC model is that it does not view relapses of old behavior as proof that all the patient's change efforts have failed. Rather, these events are seen as part of the natural process of change that must be addressed and managed. The implications for the treatment of chronic illness will become abundantly clear as each of these stages is described in turn.

Precontemplation

People at this stage minimize or deny having a problem. They do not intend to change their behavior. It does not matter if family, doctors, friends, or coworkers tell them that they have a problem. It is not their problem until they are ready to view it as such. Most patients who come to an obesity surgery specialty clinic realize that they are obese. However, there is a great deal of variability among patients in their experience of being obese. Some are pressured by family to get an evaluation for gastric bypass, but when they discover the risks of surgery or that there is no guarantee that it can be completed laparoscopically, they may panic and withdraw from the program. Others appear oblivious to the seriousness of their obesity. A common example is the patient with a body mass index greater than 45 and significant dyspnea who rates his health as "excellent." Some see the surgery as a magic bullet that will change them with little effort on their part. Others believe that their psyche has been immune to the state of being obese, or that their experiences and psychological makeup have not contributed to the development of their obesity. These are the patients who resist the preoperative psychological evaluation and declare, "My only problem is the weight!" Thus, while most patients who come to a bariatric surgery clinic are in the contemplation stage with regard to being too fat, they may be in the precontemplation stage with regard to the behaviors and conditions that led to their obesity.

Contemplation

These patients are tiring of how they feel. They may begin to wonder what allowed them to get so big. Or they may have recently realized the magnitude of their weight problem. For example, a woman who has worn large flowing outfits for years may see the huge backside of someone in a home video and with horror realize that *she* is this huge person. She may have spent years telling herself that she is going to change, but now feels a stronger urge to do something. People in the contemplation stage are typically ambivalent. They still want what

they want when they want it, but also desire to be healthier, more comfortable, and more attractive to others. The contemplative person has not made a firm commitment to action. Patients may stay in this stage for a long time, even years. A crisis or emergency can raise patient awareness, and may create a greater sense of necessity for change. For example, a 29-year-old morbidly obese man who is diagnosed with congestive heart failure may honestly reevaluate his lifestyle during recovery. He decides to have obesity surgery, and then does some serious planning.

Preparation

In this stage, people plan to take action in the next month. They review the ways they have tried and failed in the past. They dedicate energy to finding new ways to change or improving old ones, and develop backup plans should a given method fail. While individuals in this stage may not have completely resolved their ambivalence, their internal seesaw had tipped in the direction of change. They need to continue to convince themselves that change is in their best interest. According to the SOC model, patients who cut short the preparation stage usually fail during the action stage. Successful ones prepare carefully, have a firm plan with sufficient detail, and have learned what change processes will be necessary to make it to the action and maintenance stages.

Action

The SOC authors caution that action does not mean permanent change. However, the action stage is when the most visible modification of behavior and one's environment occurs. A person solidly in the action stage has made a major commitment of time and energy. No excuses are acceptable. Change is the priority. Because this is the time when others notice the patient's efforts most, action may be equated with change. The developers of SOC feel that this is a mistake, since the more challenging work is usually during the maintenance phase. Obesity surgery patients need to understand that surgery is only the beginning. They have a lifetime of hard work ahead of them. The once morbidly obese singer Carnie Wilson recently addressed a packed auditorium in New Orleans. Referring to her new body she said, "Gastric bypass was 25%. I had to do the other 75%. They did not do brain surgery on me. I have new mental, emotional, and physical challenges every single day."

Maintenance

This stage is reached when a person has gone 6 months without a lapse. For example, if a woman eats food that is not allowed on the postoperative diet, then it is 6 months from that point in time before she can be considered at maintenance. If a man stops exercising for a week due to work stress, then he must return to month 1 of the action phase. Maintenance is a time when gains are consolidated from all the preceding stages. Maintenance is the hardest phase. It is where most self-changers fail. The developers of SOC have found maintenance to be much more difficult to achieve than action. The goal is to avoid relapse. While patients may not be able to eat their presurgery amounts for a long time, if ever, they will be able to relapse by eating unhealthy foods, taking in too many calories from alcohol, grazing, losing muscle and gaining fat, or by falling off of their regular activity schedule.

Matching Interventions with Stage of Change

A "stepped-care" (67,68) model of treatment is a good beginning point for thinking about treatment matching. Sobell and Sobell (69) state, "The goal of a stepped model is to have the treatment of choice be (a) least intrusive, (b) least restrictive, (c) least costly, (d) likely to have a good outcome, (e) appealing to consumers." If an intervention does not work initially, then a quantitative increase of the same intervention can be made (e.g., higher dose of antidepressant), or a qualitative change to a different intervention could be tried (e.g., switch to psychotherapy). The Sobells suggested that the decision about the next step should be made on a case-by-case basis. At our weight management center it is common for us to discover moderate to severe depression during the initial evaluation. When patients express a preference for a mode of intervention (e.g., medication or psychotherapy), we suggest that they try their preferred method when feasible, and then reassess the depression after a few months. With patients who have histories of untreated abuse, trauma, or neglect, we also recommend psychotherapy because of the likelihood that the patient's enduring problems with self-regulation will not respond to medication alone. When there is suicidal ideation we may recommend medication and psychotherapy simultaneously, recognizing that the seriousness of the clinical risk overrides the cost and restriction factors. Should a patient present a high risk of suicide that cannot be safely lowered on an outpatient basis, we will require a brief psychiatric hospitalization.

Models from the treatment of patients with dual diagnoses (i.e., the combination of substance abuse and psychiatric disorders) can be usefully applied to the treatment of obese patients who have two or more interacting disorders. Smyth (70) reviewed the implications for integrated, parallel, and sequential interventions. Integrated intervention treats two or more disorders under the same roof. Parallel intervention involves the patient's concurrent participation in two or more treatment programs. Sequential intervention involves the enrollment of a patient in a second program some time after the first one has ended, a third sometime after the second has been completed, etc. The clinical situation and the composition of the weight management center staff will determine which of these models should be used in a given treatment situation.

Miller and Rollnick (71) are the developers of a set of interventions that have been happily married with the stages of change model. Their model of therapy is called motivational interviewing (MI). They believe that motivation is an interpersonal process and define their method as "a client-centered, directive method for enhancing intrinsic motivation to change by exploring and resolving ambivalence." Generally speaking, most patients who come to a weight management center for obesity surgery have acknowledged, to some degree, that their weight is a problem. However, many have not come to terms with the factors that led to their weight problem, and may not really want to. Another excellent resource for learning and teaching motivational techniques is a U.S. Department of Health and Human Services publication, *Treatment Improvement Protocol: Enhancing Motivation for Change in Substance Abuse Treatment* (72).

Precontemplation Interventions

Motivational interviewing describes four types of precontemplators: reluctant, rebellious, resigned, and rationalizing. Reluctant ones lack knowledge, and want to avoid information about their problem. They may fear change. They may not want to experience the discomfort involved in changing. According to MI, these patients need careful listening, sensitive feedback, and empathy.

Rebellious ones may be heavily invested in the problem behavior. They may have unresolved issues from adolescence and may appear hostile and resistant to change. The clinical goal, according to MI, is to provide freedom for these patients to express feelings about change, and then to subtly redirect their energy in a positive direction over time. When a clinician readily agrees that no one can force the patient to change, this nonadversarial attitude may diffuse the strength of the patient's argumentative stance. After a less conflictual climate has been developed, MI recommends providing a menu of options, with encouragement to think about the available choices. The clinician should then view small incremental changes as progress.

Resigned precontemplators lack the energy and investment for dealing with certain problems. They may feel helpless or hopeless. The goal with these patients, according to MI, is to instill hope and explore barriers to change.

The developers of MI stressed the importance of helping these patients to see that relapse is common, and that it does not have to be viewed as a failure. Helping these patients to understand that they will need to try many times before they finally succeed is very important. These patients need to view behavior change as difficult but not impossible. The authors of MI stressed that the key is to help the patient build confidence little by little, and that a clinician's belief in the patient's ability to change is a strong predictor of outcome.

Rationalizing precontemplators may appear to be know-it-alls, or may believe that their behavior is the result of someone else's problem. Motivational interviewing explains that empathy and reflective listening works best with this group. The clinician may need to have a rationalizer describe all the good things about the problem behavior so the patient sees that the clinician is not solely invested in proving them wrong. With the precontemplative group, less intervention often leads to more improvement. Sobell and Sobell (69) state, "What (i.e., content) clinicians say and how (i.e., style) they say it can have a powerful effect in motivating clients to change" (p. 218). The models of client-centered therapy (73), self psychology (74,75), and other forms of psychotherapy that view empathy as the primary agent of change work well with precontemplators. Once trust is developed, and the patient begins to move from precontemplation to contemplation, the clinician may be able to help patients identify the defense mechanisms that keep them from facing certain problems.

Contemplation Interventions

As stated earlier, the contemplation stage is characterized by ambivalence. Even though patients may want to lose weight with bariatric surgery, they may not have come to terms with the problems underlying the unhealthy eating behavior. Norcross and Prochaska (76) have explained that "action without insight" usually leads to failure. They point out that "raising awareness" and "emotional work" are the objectives of treatment at the contemplation stage. Patients at this stage need to understand the reasons they overeat, and what personal obstacles block the road to change. Patients are especially ambivalent about changing the way they eat. Food may be an obese patient's primary source of pleasure. Eating may be a response to present or past dysfunctional interpersonal experiences. Eating and drinking alcohol may be a person's most relied upon methods for stress reduction. While some problem drinkers find total abstinence easier to achieve than moderate drinking, no one can completely abstain from eating.

The SOC developers noted that chronic contemplators substitute thinking for acting. These patients fear failure, and would rather stay the way they are than fail again.

Some require absolute certainty before they are willing to change. Others wait for the "magic moment" to change. Conversely, premature action is also a risk factor for this group. The SOC developers have found that some contemplators make desperate and impulsive attempts at change to escape the pain of worrying. However, without adequate planning of the action and maintenance processes, failure is likely. After impulsive change efforts, patients may become even more convinced that they cannot change successfully. Prochaska et al. (65) have found that when pushed by others to change prematurely, contemplators may make a feeble change effort and then say, "See? I told you I couldn't do it."

The SOC model has found that techniques for change must be presented only after contemplators have learned more about their problem, have developed awareness of their ambivalence and defense mechanisms, and have confronted the fears that interfere with change. The aspects of psychodynamic, gestalt, cognitive, psychoanalytic, interpersonal, dialectical behavior, and other psychotherapies that deal with these areas are useful with contemplators, but only up to a point. After this first phase of "consciousness raising" is accomplished, the second phase involves helping patients learn more about their own habits, their medical disorders, and the eventual realities of the disease processes should they fail to address them. Next, the patient's own personal target behaviors should be defined. It is helpful to use specific data from the patient's labs and other measurements when defining target behaviors.

Cognitive-behavioral and behavioral therapies deal more with the direct measurement of behavior than psychodynamic and experiential ones, and will be utilized more and more as the patient progresses from the latter parts of contemplation through the preparation, action, and maintenance stages. The SOC stresses that patients need to collect the "right" data, and cautions that informal monitoring can be misleading. The SOC developers tell patients, "Don't assume you know your intake. Measure it." The SOC recommends "formal monitoring" to help the patient become more aware of exactly what needs to be changed, and to gain an accurate baseline that can be used later for comparison with action and maintenance data.

The SOC also describes the importance of a "functional analysis" to help patients understand some of the underlying mechanisms of their eating behavior. Patients are taught the "antecedent-behavior-consequences" approach to behavior analysis. A patient may learn that conflict with others or disappointments may trigger the urge to eat something unhealthy. Or, self-statements such as "I deserve this" or "This will make me feel better" may emerge prior to a slip. The SOC recommends having patients make a written list of self-statements that they have used to justify problem eating, and then encourages them to counter each statement. The authors also explain that the consequences of maladaptive behavior may strengthen it. For example, if a woman feels more relaxed after binge eating, then she is likely to do it again even though it concerns and disappoints her family members. The pleasure, stress reduction, or momentary feelings of freedom associated with unhealthy eating are powerful reinforcers. However, with repeated analysis, the patient's ambivalence may become a more significant source of discomfort. As the therapeutic process begins the work, SOC has found that patients will begin to ask themselves questions such as: "Can I consider myself healthy at this weight?" "Can I consider myself rational if I continue to gain weight?" "Can I feel responsible if I eat too much?" "Will my self-esteem go up if my weight goes down?" "Can I become successful if I cannot cope with stress?" "What will I lose by changing my eating and activity level?" "What time, energy, pleasures, or fantasies must I sacrifice in order to change?" (65).

A key aspect of MI involves helping patients identify their core values (e.g., being a well-balanced person; being the best parent they can be; having good character; earning career success commensurate with their talent and potential, etc.), and then helping patients examine whether their behavior is congruent with these values. Both MI and SOC advocate the use of the "decisional balance" developed by Janus and Mann (77) for moving patients from contemplation to preparation. The patient must list all the positive and negative aspects of the target behavior(s). In general, patients continue a self-destructive behavior because of some perceived benefit from doing so. Likewise, they avoid a healthy behavior change because the status quo is valued more than perceived benefits of change. Systematic weighing of the pros and cons must be done repeatedly until the pros of change outweigh the cons. Change that occurs before this is premature according to SOC theory.

Preparation Interventions

According to the SOC model, when patients reach the preparation stage they plan to take action within the next month. They may still need to convince themselves at times that action is what is best for them, but are much less ambivalent than they were in previous stages. The therapeutic goal at this stage is the development of a firm commitment to change. Prochaska et al. (65) believe that the patient needs to focus more on the future and less on the problematic past during this stage. All the necessary information about the patient's problem(s) has been gathered by this time, and now the focus is on the most suitable action plan to overcome the problem(s). The authors have found that people who shortcut the planning stage often experience ineffectual change. At the same time, SOC cautions that putting off action for too long can erode commitment, just as premature action can decrease self-efficacy.

Patients in the preparation stage need to develop a firm and detailed plan of action. They must review methods they used to attempt change in the past and decide which ones will be abandoned, timed differently, or modified. They also need to consider new methods of change and skill development. Helping patients deal with the inevitable anxieties surrounding change is part of the psychotherapeutic job. There are never guarantees that an important life change will be completely successful. The SOC addresses the importance of helping patients make small steps that increase courage. Once a date is set for surgery (or other obesity intervention), a patient may have an urge to return to the ambivalence of the contemplation phase. The clinician must help the patient combat this. The patient must fight her rationalizations that serve to delay action. The anticipated disruptions to important areas of life must be accepted as the price that must be paid for change.

The SOC research has found that telling supportive others about one's plan to change makes backing out more difficult. The authors have called this "going public." The SOC developers caution that the preparation stage is not the time to review the positive aspects of the maladaptive behavior, as this could weaken the patient's will and conviction toward change. During preparation for surgery, for example, patients need to focus on the benefits of surgical weight loss: better health; increased ability to travel, dance, and perform other activities that were previously impossible; better functioning on the job; better self-esteem; and an increased sense of personal freedom. Change must become the person's highest priority, and this requires the firm dedication of energy, time, and resources.

In their application of MI, Miller and Rollnick (71) have found that the amount of realistic detail patients' plans contain is a good indicator of how close they are to action. A plan that has been given little thought should be considered a red flag that the patient is not ready for action. When a patient has a limited range of change strategies, MI recommends giving examples that the clinician has seen others successfully use, or providing the patient with a menu of options to choose from. The patient needs to be able to remember these strategies. Also, the MI authors suggest having the patient create a list of the difficulties or obstacles that are likely to come up during the change process, and to develop a plan for combating each one.

Action Interventions

As mentioned previously, action does not mean permanent change. However, this stage requires the greatest commitment of time and energy. Because the patient gets the most recognition and approval from others during this stage, there is the likelihood that others will be less appreciative and supportive during the even more difficult work involved in maintaining change. The SOC emphasizes that some of the nonvisible changes are just as important as the visible ones for success. Among these, the authors list the following: changes in levels of awareness, changes in emotions, changes in self-image, and changes in thinking. A subgroup of morbidly obese patients view surgery as the magic cure that will improve their lives with little effort on their part. In contrast, prepared surgery candidates are aware that they eat for comfort or other emotional reasons and have been countering their urges to emotionally eat preoperatively by house cleaning, taking showers, listening to music, meditating, playing with a pet, praying, exercising, etc. After surgery, these patients are more likely to utilize those tools that have proven successful for them. At our weight management clinic we stress the importance of having a repertoire of self-soothing behaviors, including portable ones that can be accessed while driving, at one's place of employment, or even at the airport.

The SOC emphasizes that the most beneficial substitute for problem behavior is exercise. The authors explain that because a person's internal cues for eating, smoking, and drinking alcohol are experienced as physical urges, successful self-changers must learn to "transform these urges into cues for exercise." Prochaska et al. (65) state,

Omitting exercise from a self-change plan is like fighting a foe with one hand tied behind your back. You may still win, but the odds are against you. Inactive people are not only in poor condition for dealing with physical problems, they are frequently also in poor psychological condition for coping with distress that can accompany change. If you are too busy to exercise, you are simply too busy. (p. 177)

The SOC also advocates the use of a cognitive-behavioral intervention termed "counterthinking" during the action phase. It is advised that patients remove absolutes or imperatives from their internal dialogues. When patients tell themselves that they must be perfect, that everyone must like them, or that they must be very competent at everything they do, they are setting themselves up for unnecessary internal pressure. The SOC research has found that this pressure can lead to lapses from the change plan. Patients who cannot counterthink on their own may need psychotherapy. The SOC emphasizes the need for patients to separate their sense of what they "need" from what they "desire." The SOC authors explained that when frustrated "desires" are experienced as frustrated "needs," there is more distress. However, when desires are experienced in a less essential way (i.e., as merely desires) they are easier to modify.

The SOC stresses the importance of "environmental control" during the action stage. This is where patients lower the probability of unhealthy behaviors by decreasing the opportunity for them in their environment. Patients who keep junk food in the house "for the kids" are asking for trouble. We encourage the whole family to eat more healthily in our support groups. Most children will learn to love fruit if they have sufficient exposure to it. A related area is that of cues. For example, the SOC explains that if one's critical parents are a significant trigger for emotional eating, the solution is not to avoid them forever. Rather, one must learn new ways of dealing with them. Psychologists can use exposure techniques combined with relaxation training, which allows patients to decrease emotional arousal and find more adaptive responses to hypercritical others. The SOC has also found that it is empowering for patients to determine how much time they will spend with difficult relatives, and under what conditions they will leave.

Other tools recommended for the action stage by the developers of the SOC are the behavior therapy techniques of reminders, rewards, contracting, shaping, and helping relationships. Reminders involve the use of planned cues for a desired behavior. Some of our patients buy a daily planner and write in the times for their protein shakes, solid food, and water intake, as well as the time allotted for their daily exercise. Others prefer palm pilots, their personal computer, or a watch with an alarm that prompts them every 2 to 3 hours reminding them it is time to eat. Prochaska et al. (65) have found that posting signs that read "Relax" may help, as well as putting a stop sign on the refrigerator. Rewards help people improve self-esteem and reinforce a desired behavior. Punishment does not generally lead to adaptive behavior. The SOC research has found that resisting temptation does not feel rewarding to most people. Certain individuals benefit from positive self-statements such as "good job" or "way to go." Others need a more concrete form of reward like a new outfit, or a day at the beach.

Contracting is a more formal reward system. Patients write contracts with themselves. For example, "I will put five dollars into a reward fund for every inch I lose, or every 50 miles I walk." The SOC has found that written contracts are more powerful than spoken ones. Shaping, according to SOC, is a more realistic process than complete and immediate change. The authors recommend the use of a step-by-step approach with reinforcement following every step. Helping relationships are important for major life changes. The SOC believes that patients may need to educate family and friends with regard to what is experienced as helpful and what is not. The authors recommend a ratio of three compliments to one criticism. They have found that scolding, nagging, preaching, shaming, and guilt trips do not help the change process. Too few compliments for one person may be a patronizingly excessive number for another. Patients need to help their significant others to calibrate the rewards they provide. They may need to explicitly say, for example, that when they are really down they need a massage, but when they are doing well a hug will do. Patients need to determine what they find most meaningful in terms of support. At the same time, however, the requested supportive behaviors need to be realistic and practical for the supportive other(s).

If a support group is not available, then the patient needs to find one or create one. Prochaska et al. (65) stated, "Local support groups made up of people with the same problem(s) can reinforce, guide through rough spots, and remind you of the benefits of changing." At our clinic, we deal with the support issue prior to surgery whenever possible. If the patient has significant marital problems, we recommend couples therapy. If the family is dysfunctional we recommend family therapy. If the person is alone in life, we encourage them to stay in our support group and develop outside relationships with group members, or participate in Internet chat rooms for bariatric surgery patients. However, new problems with the support system (or lack thereof) may develop during the action stage that will need to be addressed.

Maintenance Interventions

If a person who overeats in response to stress develops new coping strategies prior to surgery, the risk of overeating after bariatric surgery may be lessened but not necessarily eradicated. The SOC has found that a behavior such as overeating must be replaced by a healthier lifestyle, and that the attraction of unhealthy foods will continue to be there long after the habit of eating the food was ostensibly broken. The SOC has found that most people in the maintenance phase need to remind themselves that they are still vulnerable. Overconfidence is a danger sign frequently associated with relapse, according to the SOC developers.

High-risk situations must be identified, and the patient needs to have a repertoire of interventions to deal with situations that cannot be avoided. There is much that can be learned from relapse-prevention methods developed for alcohol and drug abuse that can be profitably adapted to compulsive eating in obese patients. Perri et al. (20) have made significant progress in the extension of relapse prevention interventions to obese patient populations. Perri et al. (13,78) also developed useful techniques for the facilitation of weight-loss maintenance.

The SOC research has found that the most common threats to maintenance are social pressures, internal challenges, and "special situations." It is much harder to maintain a behavior change if family or friends overtly or covertly encourage a deviation from it. Family therapy may be indicated after surgery if patients are unable to modify the family system on their own. Internal chal-

lenges, according to SOC, usually result from defective thinking such as overconfidence or excessive self-blame. The SOC has found that appropriate blame may renew commitment to change, but too much blame demoralizes and lowers commitment. Cognitive-behavioral therapy may be needed if patients are unable to modify defective thinking on their own.

"Special situations" are those that create an unusual or intense degree of temptation. According to SOC, these are usually not anticipated and may pose serious threats to confidence, conviction, and ultimately commitment. For example, an obese middle-aged man who retired from his career and then devoted his energy to caring for his ailing mother did well after gastric bypass until his mother died unexpectedly. After that, he stopped exercising, resumed smoking, and began drinking at a bar every night. He regained much of his weight, and eventually died. The SOC authors state, "Renewing commitment is especially important when you are trying to modify regularly occurring behaviors. Maintaining weight loss is a constant issue for people with weight problems, and requires frequent boosts of commitment. . . . Redoubling commitment is a critical part of maintaining change" (p. 211). The authors also suggest that patients must continue environmental control. Obese patients must avoid people with the same unhealthy eating habits, review their personal reasons for changing, and return to the decision balance exercise when necessary. Learning how to manage "slips" is critical in order to prevent "slides." Self-help books may help a subgroup of obesity surgery patients prevent relapse. In other cases, a psychologist well versed in behavior modification and relapse prevention may be needed to help those who are unable to learn these skills on their own.

The SOC research has identified some common challenges with helping relationships during the maintenance phase. For example, people who were supportive during the action stage may be less so during the maintenance stage. Having someone to talk to during a crisis may prevent a lapse from turning into a relapse. The SOC suggests that some patients may need to revise their contract with others during the maintenance stage (e.g., give others permission to point out overconfidence, risk taking, or signs that old behavior is returning). Attendance at an obesity surgery support group can be invaluable during this stage. The SOC explains that patients may revert to a short-term perspective when a long-term one is necessary for success. The authors have found that family, friends, and therapists need to help the patient to give up the notion of a quick fix and to repeatedly help the patient to accept the fact that short-term ecstasies create long-term agonies. Finally, it is important for all participants in the patient's life to understand that the goal of obesity surgery is to improve the patient's quality of life for the rest of the person's life.

Conclusion

The role of the psychologist in the practice of obesity surgery has evolved considerably since the late 1960s. This chapter has reviewed how the role has grown from psychological screening to include treatment planning, individual and group therapy, couples and family therapy, health promotion, treatment adherence, motivational interviewing, coping skills training, relapse prevention, and treatment outcome assessment. We have also described how CPT codes are now in place that allow psychologists to receive reimbursement for these services. However, bariatric surgery remains a relatively young field, and all of us involved with it have a long way to go in terms of learning and improving both our theories and techniques. Too little published literature deals with the increasingly significant percentage of patients who do not permanently maintain their postoperative success. To better understand this problem, we need to develop consensus on a core battery of tests to be used in research and practice, recognizing that different sites will need to add various interviews, scales and measures to accommodate particular characteristics of the population(s) they serve. Once a battery is established, we will need large multisite collaborative studies to develop empirically based subtypes, with the eventual hope of developing treatment protocols that best fit each subtype. While most psychologists have intuitions about degrees of psychosocial risk for postoperative complications, we must develop empirically derived risk factors so that we can assign patients to high-, moderate-, and low-risk groups with greater confidence and consistency among sites. Also, while some excellent preliminary work has been conducted on motivation enhancing interventions and application of the stages of change model with obesity surgery patients, we need much more research and refinement in this area. Finally, the role that interpersonal stress and dysfunction plays in postoperative weight gain needs much more attention.

References

1. Reich L, Romano I, Kolbasovsky A. Primary Care partnership benefits psychologists and patients. National Psychol 2004;13(5):22.
2. Dawes R, Faust D, Meehl P. Clinical versus actuarial judgment. Science 1989;243:1668–1674.
3. Meehl PE. Clinical versus statistical prediction. Minneapolis: University of Minnesota Press, 1954.
4. Weston D, Weinberger J. When clinical description becomes statistical prediction. Am Psychol 2004;59:595–613.
5. Dittman M. CPT codes: use them or lose them. Monit Psychol 2004;October:58–59.
6. Seligman M, Csikszentmihalyi M. Positive psychology: an introduction. Am Psychol 2000;55:5–14.
7. Wadden W, Foster G. Behavioral assessment of markedly obese patients. In: Wadden TA, VanItallie TB, eds. Treatment of the Seriously Obese Patient. New York: Guilford Press, 1992:290–330.
8. Wadden T, Phelan S. Behavioral assessment of the obese patient. In: Wadden TA, Stunkard AJ, eds. Handbook of Obesity Treatment. New York: Guilford Press, 2002:186–226.
9. Crowther J, Sherwood N. Assessment. In: Garner DM, Garfinkel PI, eds. Handbook of Treatment for Eating Disorders, 2nd ed. New York: Guilford Press, 1997:34–49.
10. Stunkard A, Wadden T. Psychological aspects of severe obesity. Am J Clin Nutr 1991;55:524s–532s.
11. Wadden T, Stunkard A. Social and psychological consequences of obesity. Ann Intern Med 1985;103(6 pt 2):1062–1067.
12. Witkiewitz K, Marlatt G. Relapse prevention for alcohol and drug problems: that was Zen, this is Tao. Am Psychol 2004;59(4):224–235.
13. Perri M. Improving maintenance of weight lost in behavioral treatment of obesity. In Wadden TA, Stunkard AJ, eds. Handbook of Obesity Treatment. New York: Guilford Press, 2002:357–379.
14. Obesity: preventing and managing the global epidemic. Report of a World Health Organization Consultation on Obesity, Geneva, 1998.
15. Friedman M, Brownell K. Psychological correlates of obesity: moving to the next research generation. Psychol Bull 1995;117(1):3–20.
16. American Psychiatric Association. Diagnostic and Statistical Manual of Mental Disorders, 4th ed., text revision (DSM-IV-TR). Washington, DC: American Psychiatric Association Press, 2000.
17. Mueller T, Leon A, Keller M, et al. Recurrence after recovery from major depressive disorder during 15 years of observational follow-up. Am J Psychiatry 1999;156:1000–1006.
18. Judd L. The clinical course of unipolar major depressive disorders. Arch Gen Psychiatry 1997;54:989–991.
19. Tennen H, Affleck G, Armeli S, et al. A daily process approach to coping. Am Psychol 2000;55:626–636.
20. Perri M, McKelvy W, Renjilian D, Nezu A, Shermer R, Viegener B. Relapse prevention training and problem-solving therapy in the long-term management of obesity. J Consult Clin Psychol 2001;69:722–726.
21. Hamburger W. Emotional aspects of eating. Med Clin North Am 1951;35:483–499.
22. Bruch H. Eating Disorders. New York: Basic Books, 1973.
23. Rand C. Psychoanalytic treatment of obesity. In: Wolman BB, ed. Psychological Aspects of Obesity: A Handbook. New York: Van Nostrand Reinhold, 1982.
24. Fitzgibbon M, Stolley M, Kirschenbaum D. Obese people who seek treatment have different characteristics than those who do not seek treatment. Health Psychol 1993;12(5):342–345.
25. Polivy J, Herman C. Etiology of binge eating: psychological mechanisms. In: Fairburn CF, Wilson GT, eds. Binge Eating: Nature, Assessment and Treatment. New York: Guilford Press, 1993:173–205.

26. Marlatt G. Craving for alcohol, loss of control, and relapse: a cognitive behavioral analysis. In: Nathan PE, Loberg T, eds. New Directions in Behavioral Research and Treatment. New York: Plenum Press, 1978:271–314.

27. Leon G, Chamberlain K. Emotional arousal, eating patterns and body image as differential factors associated with varying success in maintaining weight loss. J Consult Clin Psychol 1973a;40:474–480.

28. Leon G, Chamberlain K. Comparison of daily eating habits and emotional states of overweight persons successful or unsuccessful in maintaining weight loss. J Consult Clin Psychol 1973;41:108–115.

29. Leon G. Personality, body image, and eating pattern changes in overweight persons after weight loss. J Consult Clin Psychol 1975;31:618–623.

30. Ganley R. Emotion and eating in obesity: a review of the literature. Int J Eating Disord 1989;8(3):343–361.

31. Rodin J, Schank D, Striegel-Moore R. Psychological factors in obesity. Med Clin North Am 1989;73(1):47–66.

32. Arnow B, Kenardy J, Agras S. The emotional eating scale: the development of a measure to assess coping with negative affect by eating. Int J Eating Disord 1995;18(1):79–90.

33. Des Jarlais D. Harm reduction: a framework for incorporating science into drug policy. Am J Public Health 1995;85:10–12.

34. Denning P. Practicing Harm Reduction Therapy: An Alternative Approach to Addictions. New York/London: Guilford Press, 2004.

35. Edelman B. Binge-eating in normal weight and overweight individuals. Psychol Rep 1981;49:739–746.

36. Fairburn C, Wilson G. Binge Eating: Nature, Assessment, and Treatment. New York: Guilford Press, 1993:361–404.

37. Carter W, Pindyck J. Pharmacologic treatment of binge-eating disorder. Prim Psychiatry 2003;10(10):31–36.

38. Devlin M, Goldfein J, Carino J, Wolk S. Open treatment of overweight binge eaters with phentermine and fluoxetine as an adjunct to cognitive behavioral therapy. Int J Eating Disord 2000;28:325–332.

39. Hudson J, McElroy S, Raymond N, et al. Fluvoxamine in the treatment of binge-eating disorder: a multicenter placebo-controlled, double-blind trial. Am J Psychiatry 1998;155:1756–1762.

40. Stunkard A, Berkowitz R, Tanrikut C, Reiss E, Yound L. d-Fenfluramine treatment of binge eating disorder. Am J Psychiatry 1996;153:1455–1459.

41. Agras W, Telch C, Arnow B, et al. Weight loss, cognitive-behavioral, and desipramine treatments in binge eating disorder: an additive design. Behav Ther 1994;25:225–238.

42. Stunkard A, Grace W, Wolff H. The night-eating syndrome: a pattern of food intake among certain obese patients. Am J Med 1955;19:78–86.

43. Rand C, Macgregor M, Stunkard A. The night eating syndrome in the general population and among post-operative obesity surgery patients. Int J Eating Disord 1997;22:65–69.

44. Birketvedt G, Florholmen J, Sundsfjord J, et al. Behavioral and neuroendocrine characteristics of night-eating syndrome. JAMA 1999;282:657–663.

45. Saunders R. "Grazing": high-risk behavior. Obes Surg 2004;14:98–102.

46. Shape Up America and the American Obesity Association; Koop CE, Keller GC, eds. Guidelines for the Treatment of Adult Obesity, 2nd ed. Bethesda, MD: Shape Up America, 1998.

47. Hamoui N, Kingsbury S, Anthone G, et al. Surgical treatment of morbid obesity in schizophrenic patients. Obes Surg 2004;14:349–352.

48. National Institutes of Health; National Heart, Lung, and Blood Institute, and North American Association for the Study of Obesity. The Practical Guide: Identification, Evaluation, and Treatment of Overweight and Obesity in Adults. Washington, DC: NIH, 2002.

49. Dunbar-Jacob J, Mortimer-Stephens M. Treatment adherence in chronic disease. J Clin Epidemiol 2001;54:S57–S60.

50. Zweben A, Zuckoff A. Motivational interviewing and treatment adherence. In: Miller WR, Rollnick S, eds. Motivational Interviewing: Preparing People for Change, 2nd ed. New York: Guilford Press, 2002:299–319.

51. Polivy J, Herman C. If at first you don't succeed: false hopes and change. Am Psychol 2002;57(9):677–689.

52. Engle D, Arkowitz H. Ambivalence in Psychotherapy, Facilitating Readiness to Change. New York: Guilford, 2006.

53. Heidenreich P. Patient adherence: the next frontier in quality improvement. Am J Med 2004;117:130–132.

54. Wing R, Phelan S, Tate D. The role of adherence in mediating the relationship between depression and health outcomes. J Psychosom Res 2002;52:877–881.

55. Nemeroff C. Improving antidepressant adherence. J Clin Psychiatry 2003;64(suppl 18):25–30.

56. Giannetti V. Adherence with antidepressant medication. P T Dig 2004;13:42–47.

57. Vergouwen A, Bakker A, Katon W, et al. Improving adherence to antidepressants: a systematic review of interventions. J Clin Psychiatry 2003;64:1415–1420.

58. Brownell K, Wadden T. Etiology and treatment of obesity: understanding a serious, prevalent, and refractory disorder. J Consult Clin Psychol 1992;60(4):505–517.

59. Raum W. Postoperative medical management of bariatric patients. In: Martin LF, ed. Obesity Surgery. New York: McGraw-Hill, 2004:133–159.

60. National Institutes of Health, United States Department of Health and Human Services. Gastrointestinal Surgery for Severe Obesity: Consensus Statement, NIH Consensus Development Conference, March 25–27, 1991, Vol. 9, No. 1.

61. Marcus J, Elkins G. Development of a model for a structured support group for patients following bariatric surgery. Obes Surg 2004;14:103–106.

62. National Institutes of Health United States Department of Health and Human Services. Strategic Plan for NIH Obesity Research: A Report of the NIH Obesity Research Task Force. Washington, DC: NIH, 2004.

63. Bond D, Evans R, Demaria E, et al. A conceptual application of health behavior theory in the design and implementation of a successful surgical weight loss program. Obes Surg 2004;14:849–856.

64. Prochaska J, DiClemente C, Norcross J. In search of how people change: applications to addictive behaviors. Am Psychol 1992;47:1102–1114.

65. Prochaska J, Norcross J, DiClemente C. Change for Good: A Revolutionary Six-Stage Program for Overcoming Bad Habits and Moving Your Life Positively Forward. New York: Avon, 1994.

66. Diclemente C, Velasquez M. Motivational interviewing and the stages of change. In: Miller WR, Rollnick S, eds. Motivational Interviewing. New York: Guilford Press, 2002: 201–216.

67. Foulds J, Jarvis M. Smoking cessation and prevention. In: Calverly P, Pride N, eds. Chronic Obstructive Pulmonary Disease. London: Chapman Hall, 1995:373–390.

68. Davison G. Stepped care: doing more with less? J Consult Clin Psychol 2000;68:580–585.

69. Sobell L, Sobell M. Using motivational interviewing techniques to talk with clients about their alcohol use. Cogn Behav Pract 2003;10:214–221.

70. Smyth N. Motivating persons with dual disorders: a stage approach. J Contemp Human Serv 1996;77:606–614.

71. Miller W, Rollnick S. Motivational Interviewing, 2nd ed. New York: Guilford Press, 2002.

72. Miller WR. Enhancing motivation for change in substance abuse treatment: Treatment Improvement Protocol (TIP) Series. Rockville, MD: United States Department of Health and Human Services, Substance Abuse and Mental Health Services Administration, 1999.

73. Rogers C. Client-Centered Therapy. Boston: Houghlin-Mifflin, 1951.

74. Kohut H. The Restoration of the Self. New York: International Universities Press, 1977.

75. Wolf E. Treating the Self: Elements of Clinical Self-Psychology. New York: Guilford Press, 1988.

76. Norcross J, Prochaska J. Using the stages of change. Harvard Ment Health Lett 2002;May:5–7.

77. Janus I, Mann L. Decision-Making: A Psychological Analysis of Conflict, Choice, and Commitment. New York: Free Press, 1977.

78. Perri M, McAllister D, Gange J, Jordan R, McAdoo W, Nezu A. Effects of four maintenance programs on the long-term management of obesity. J Consult Clin Psychol 1988;56: 529–534.

10
Operating Room Positioning, Equipment, and Instrumentation for Laparoscopic Bariatric Surgery

William Gourash, Ramesh C. Ramanathan, Giselle Hamad, Sayeed Ikramuddin, and Philip R. Schauer

Since 1995, the number of laparoscopic bariatric surgical procedures has dramatically increased both in the United States and in other countries. These advanced laparoscopic operations offer the advantage of more rapid recovery and dramatically reduced wound complication with established efficacy. For optimal efficiency and outcomes, laparoscopic procedures on obese patients require specialized laparoscopic equipment and instrumentation, including staplers and hand instruments, which are used with individual skill and coordinated teamwork to facilitate patient positioning, laparoscopic access, insufflation, visualization by camera, energy sources for transection and coagulation, flexible endoscopy, and voice activation and robotics, and to provide a fully integrated operating room layout.

Laparoscopic surgery is technologically intensive, and the surgeon must be thoroughly familiar with the equipment and instrumentation of laparoscopy in addition to understanding the treatment conditions (1,2).

Morbidly obese patients present multiple obstacles and specific characteristics that may require modifications to the technology normally used for laparoscopic procedures. In particular, excessive abdominal adiposity interferes with visualization and freedom of instrument movement, and frequently requires instruments of exceptional length and strength. Laparoscopic approaches in obese surgical patients require advanced skills in intracorporal stapling, suturing, and hemostasis techniques, and flexible endoscopy. Comorbid medical conditions may reduce patient tolerance of intraabdominal CO_2 and necessitate alternative means of maintaining visualization (1).

This chapter describes our use of technology for bariatric patients based on an experience with over 4000 laparoscopic Roux-en-Y gastric bypass (LRYGBP) procedures. It is assumed that the surgeon is familiar with the application of laparoscopic instruments and equipment as they apply to the general patient undergoing minimally invasive surgery (3,4). Detailed information regarding the engineering and technology behind the equipment is available from many excellent sources (5–9). It is certainly recognized that there may be alternative equipment or approaches that are equally or more suitable, and that optimal choices will change with time and the availability of newer technologies.

Patient Positioning

The main goals in the positioning of a morbidly obese patient in preparation for bariatric surgery are safe transfer to the operating room table, neutral positioning of the major joints and extremities, avoidance of pressure injuries to skin or nerves, accessibility of the operative field by surgical team, and security of the patient on the table (10,11). Due to anatomic considerations of some morbidly obese persons, attention to detail as well as some creativity may be needed to achieve these goals.

The patient is brought to the operating room by stretcher. We have found lateral transfer devices that utilize hover technology (Hovermatt, HoverTech International, Bethlehem, PA) enable the team to move the patient to the operating table and back to the transport stretcher or bed in a secure and comfortable manner. It requires at least two staff members, one on each side of the patient with minimal lifting or pulling force. This device has decreased patient and staff injuries (Fig. 10-1).

We place the patient in the supine position with legs together and arms abducted. The patient is secured at the waist with table straps. Sometimes the patient is secured also at the legs depending on body size and the operating table model. The patient's weight should be evenly distributed on the table without parts of the torso or limbs hanging over the side. Side-rail extensions can be use to augment the width of the table. Pneumatic compression devices that accommodate the super-obese patient are placed on the patient at this time. These devices counter potentially severe venous stasis resulting

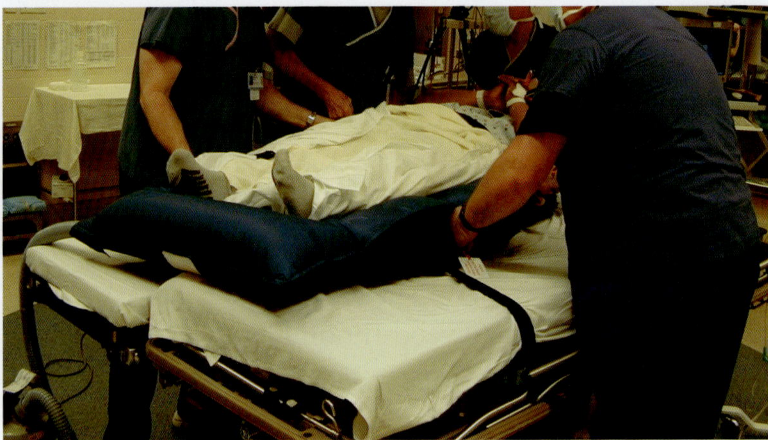

Figure 10-1. Use of lateral transfer device to move patient on and off operating table.

from the use of pneumoperitoneum and the reverse Trendelenburg position. We recommend using sequential compression devices (SCDs), which are placed prior to induction around the calves and thighs (Fig. 10-2) (12). There may be certain anatomic considerations that prevent the utilization of the thigh type and require other options such as the calf or foot models.

After the induction of general anesthesia and endotracheal intubation, a urinary catheter is inserted (often requiring two staff members, one for retraction of skin folds and one for insertion), and a Bovie grounding pad is placed usually on the anterior thigh. A footboard is placed on the table so the feet will have a secure base to rest when the patient is in the extreme reverse Trendelenburg position. To ensure that the weight is borne on the soles of the feet resting on the footboard, tape may be used on the legs to maintain a neutral and classic anatomic position.

The surgeon stands on the patient's right side along with the scrub nurse; the first assistant and the camera operator are on the patient's left side. The arms may be left out if adequate room is available or one or both may be tucked. Occasionally, when tucking an arm, a metal or plastic limb holder (sled) may be required to secure the arm at the side. This approach also serves to protect the arm.

The base of a stationary retractor-holding device may be attached to the table at this time. Care must be taken that it does not come in direct contact with the patient's skin to avoid pressure injury or electrocautery conduction.

Prior to prepping and draping the patient, a final check is made of all pressure points, especially alongside the arms, hands, head, and feet. Table attachments must be padded appropriately to avoid pressure or nerve injuries. Security of the patient on the table and neutrality of joint positioning of the extremities are also confirmed again (Fig. 10-2). Of special note, undue pressure on the gluteal area should be avoided. A rare complication of rhabdomyolysis has been reported, especially in patients with a body mass index (BMI) 60 or greater. Consequences of rhabdomyolysis include renal failure and death (13,14). Heating blankets are helpful in preventing hypothermia related to heat loss from evaporation and continuous insufflation, particularly during operations of long duration.

After prepping and draping the abdomen, setting up the equipment on the field, and assembling the operating room (OR) team, the working field will appear as depicted in Figure 10-3. Some surgeons prefer the "French" or "between the legs" positioning in which the patient's legs are abducted and the surgeon stands

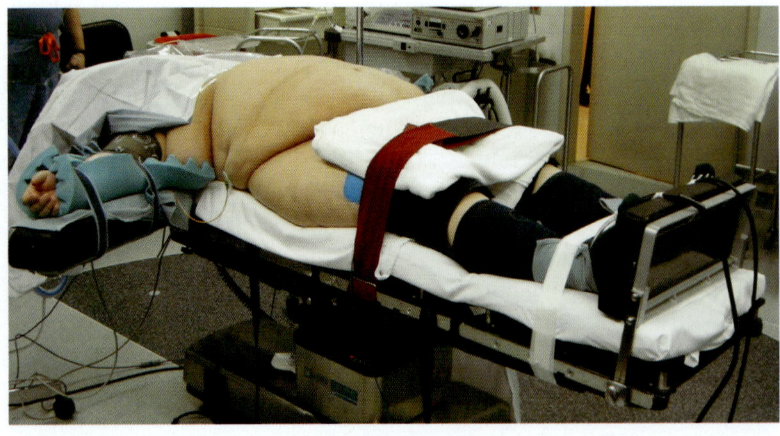

Figure 10-2. Patient positioning and application of sequential compression device. Inspect for areas of significant pressure, circulatory compromise, neutral positioning of extremities, and patient security on table prior to prepping and draping the abdomen.

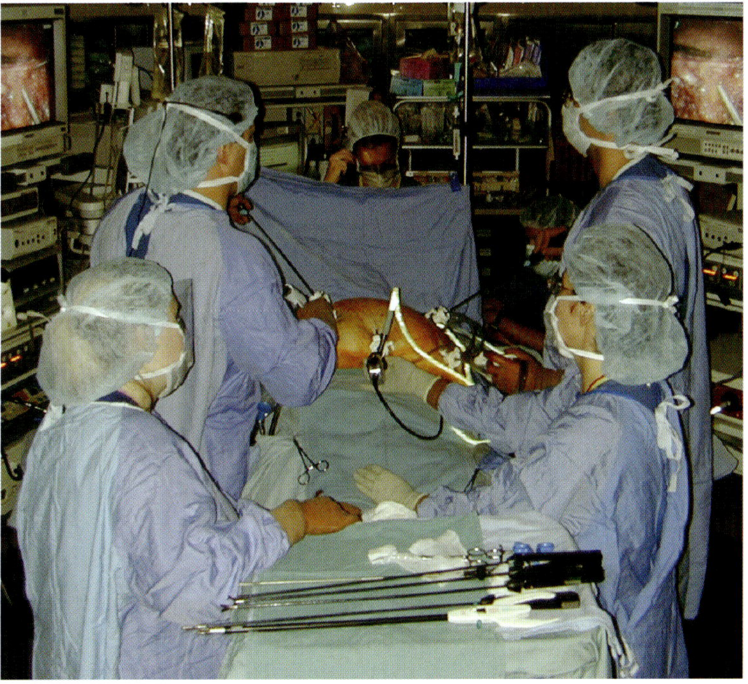

FIGURE 10-3. The operating team members in their places. The primary surgeon is to the patient's right. The first assistant is across from the primary surgeon. The second assistant and scrub nurse are at the foot of the bed.

between them with assistants and OR technicians flanking him/her. This is described in other publications. A limitation of this approach is that there may be little space between the legs due to the girth of the thighs or of the surgeon.

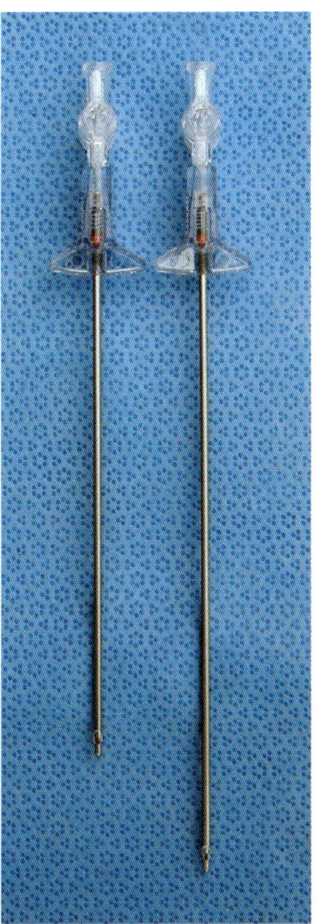

FIGURE 10-4. Standard and long Veress needles. (Copyright © 2006 United States Surgical, a division of Tyco Healthcare Group LP, with permission. All rights reserved.)

Laparoscopic Access

The Veress Needle Approach

A Veress needle can be used to establish pneumoperitoneum in the obese patient as it is technically very difficult to perform an open cut-down (Hasson) technique. A long-length Veress needle of 150 mm (Autosuture, Division of Tyco Healthcare, Mansfield, MA) (Fig. 10-4) is inserted using a subcostal incision in the left upper quadrant. The 2-mm needle has a spring-loaded blunt inner cannula that automatically extends beyond the needle point once the abdominal cavity has been entered. This blunt cannula has a side hole to permit entry of CO_2 gas into the abdominal cavity. S-shaped retractors can also be helpful for blunt dissection through the subcutaneous fat to expose the anterior fascia to facilitate Veress needle placement. Correct position of the Veress needle after it has passed through the abdominal wall can be verified by methods such as the water drop test. In obese patients, opening intraabdominal pressures may be high (up to 10 to 12 cm H_2O). We have found that placing traction using a suture at the incision site helps to stabilize the abdominal wall during the insertion of the needle and to facilitate the gas flow into the abdomen after the needle is in place.

Insertion of Trocars

In addition to being safe and reliable, trocars and cannulas for laparoscopic bariatric surgery should minimize air leaks, secure readily to the abdominal wall, allow rapid exchange of instruments of various diameters, and be of sufficient length to reach the peritoneal cavity without

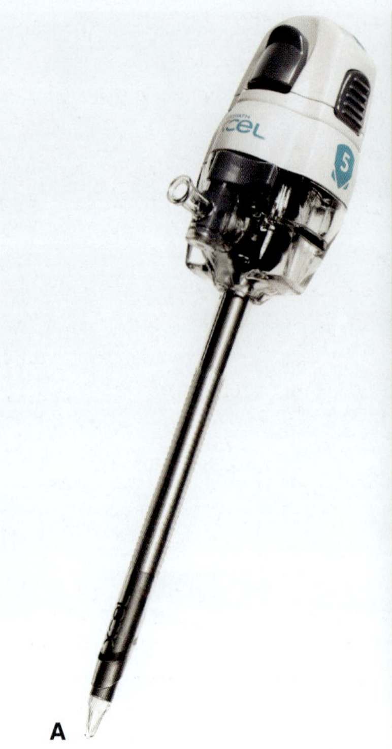

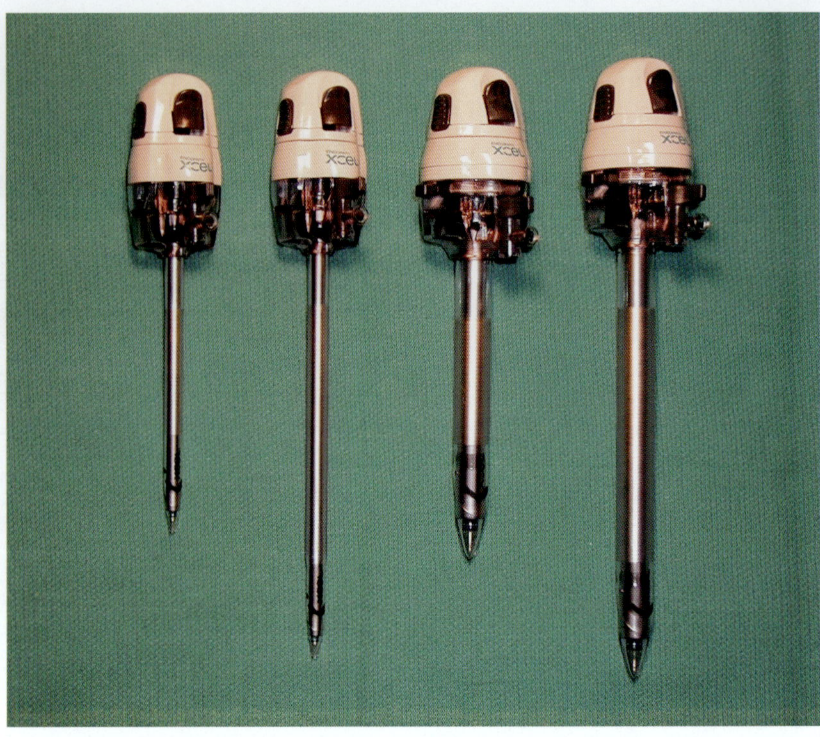

FIGURE 10-5. (A) A 5-mm optical viewing trocar can be used to obtain direct access to the peritoneal cavity without pneumoperitoneum. The distinct layers of subcutaneous fat, fascia, muscle, preperitoneal fat, and the peritoneum are identified as the trocar passes through them. (B) The 5- and 12-mm trocars (100 cm and 150 cm lengths). These clear-tipped bladeless trocars can also be used for optical entry into the peritoneal cavity. Endopath Xcel. (Courtesy of Ethicon Endo-Surgery, Inc. All rights reserved.)

causing excessive disruption of the abdominal fascia. We currently use a 5-mm optical viewing trocar (XCEL, Ethicon Endo-Surgery, Inc., Cincinnati, OH) for initial access to the peritoneal cavity (Fig. 10-5A). The 5-mm scope is placed into the trocar after the camera is white balanced. The focus is adjusted on the end of the clear trocar tip. The trocar is placed through a 5-mm incision and the fatty, fascial, and muscular layers of the abdominal wall are directly visualized as the trocar passes through them. After the tip of the trocar passes through the preperitoneal fat and the peritoneum, the camera and obturator are removed and the abdominal cavity is insufflated. Once pneumoperitoneum is established, the remaining trocars are placed under direct visualization. Trocars with 100-mm shafts are usually sufficient, but occasionally extra-long trocars (150 mm) are required for the patient with an excessively thick abdominal wall (Fig. 10-5B).

A spiral cannula sheath that screws into the fascia can be placed onto the shaft of the trocar to reduce the risk of dislodgment. We usually secure the first trocar placed in the patient's left upper quadrant to the skin with a suture for added security. After the insertion of the first trocar, a standard 25-gauge spinal needle can be helpful in locating the precise intraabdominal location for the placement of additional trocars (Fig. 10-6). Local anesthetic is injected into the preperitoneal space once the trocar site and trajectory are determined with the spinal needle.

Insufflator

In laparoscopic surgery, exposure depends on insufflation of the peritoneal cavity with CO_2 to create a pneumoperitoneum. The insufflator monitors the current intraabdominal pressure and regulates the flow of CO_2 from a pressurized reservoir. A desired intraabdominal pressure is selected and the flow of gas is automatically regulated. The front liquid-crystal display (LCD) screen on the insufflator displays the current intraabdominal pressure, the preset desired pressure, the current rate of CO_2 insufflation, the volume of gas infused, and the residual volume in the CO_2 tank. Alarms signal high intraabdominal pressures, excessive gas leak, and low gas level in the CO_2 tank. The rate of insufflation can be adjusted from 1 L/min up to 40 L/min. Our standard preset intraabdominal pressure is 15 mm Hg, but we will intermittently use higher pressure (16 to 18 mm Hg) when better exposure is needed or a lower pressure when instrument length is insufficient.

Visualization

Technology that provides the surgeon with a clear view of the operating field has been critical to the development of advanced laparoscopic procedures. Safe and efficient performance of a laparoscopic procedure is dependent on the quality of visualization. Since the surgeon is not able to touch and palpate the tissues directly, a clear crisp bright image is mandatory at all times. There are no "blind" maneuvers in laparoscopy. Components that create and maintain the image have steadily improved.

There are several conditions specific to laparoscopic bariatric surgery that make obtaining an adequate image challenging. In the morbidly obese patient, the voluminous abdominal cavity expanded by the pneumoperitoneum requires more light for visualization than that required for the nonobese patient. Viscera are often enlarged by fatty infiltration. Copious adipose tissue covering mesentery, omentum, and viscera may crowd the view and obscure the landmarks of interest. Instrumentation that will allow viewing around or over or under such tissue is necessary. Other instruments are needed to enable adequate exposure. Inadvertent contact of the laparoscope lens with adipose tissue causes soiling of the lens, resulting in a poor-quality image. Equipment that minimizes such contacts and allows quick and effective cleaning of the lens is also critical. In bariatric patients, lens fogging often results from the rapid insufflation of relatively cool CO_2 that may be increased due to small air-leaks at the trocar sites.

Laparoscope

The laparoscope uses the Hopkins rod lens system, which consists of a series of quartz rod lenses and a fiber bundle surrounding the rod lens for transmission of light (5,6). The eyepiece of the laparoscope is connected to the camera by means of a coupler adapter.

Standard laparoscopes have a length of approximately 32 cm and have diameters that range from 2 to 10 mm. Scopes are angled to various degrees, most commonly from a 0- to 45-degree orientation. Angled scopes provide more flexibility in viewing internal structures and provide access to areas that would be "blind" to 0-degree scopes. However, they require some additional skill to operate, and the angling decreases light transmission slightly.

For our bariatric procedures, we have a variety of laparoscopes available: 30 and 45 degrees with 5- and 10-mm diameters (Fig. 10-8) (Stryker Endoscopy, Kalamazoo, MI). Typically we use a 5-mm, 45-degree scope, initially at the 5-mm entrance site to visualize the other port placements. A 10-mm-diameter, 45-degree angled laparoscope is used for the balance of the procedure, as we have found that it provides the best field of

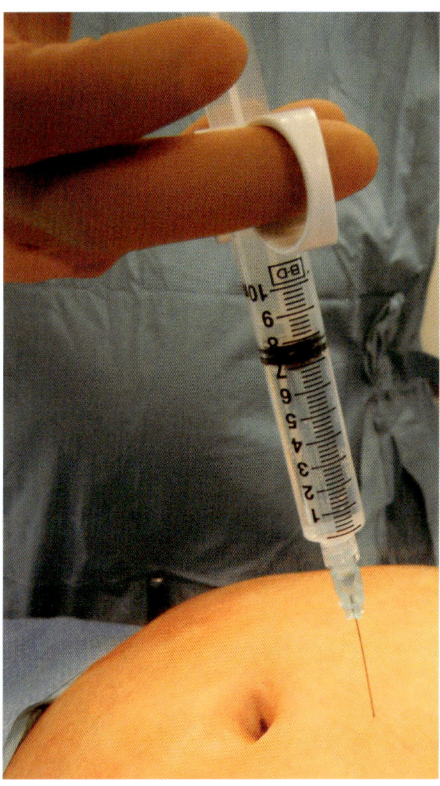

FIGURE 10-6. Spinal needle placed through abdominal wall to help with port positioning. Local anesthetic is injected into the preperitoneal space under laparoscopic visualization prior to port placement.

Gas leakage can be very troublesome during laparoscopic bariatric procedures, especially if a circular stapling technique is in use. A high-flow insufflator (40 L/min) is highly recommended to accommodate a gas leakage from small air leaks at port sites, instrument exchanges, and intraabdominal suction (Fig. 10-7). We usually use two insufflators set at high flow during gastric bypass procedures to provide added compensation for gas leakage and to prevent delay should one CO_2 canister become empty.

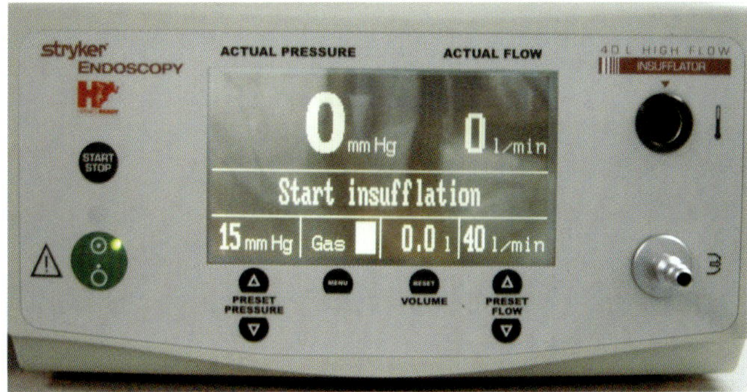

FIGURE 10-7. High-flow insufflator. (Courtesy of Stryker, Kalamazoo, MI.)

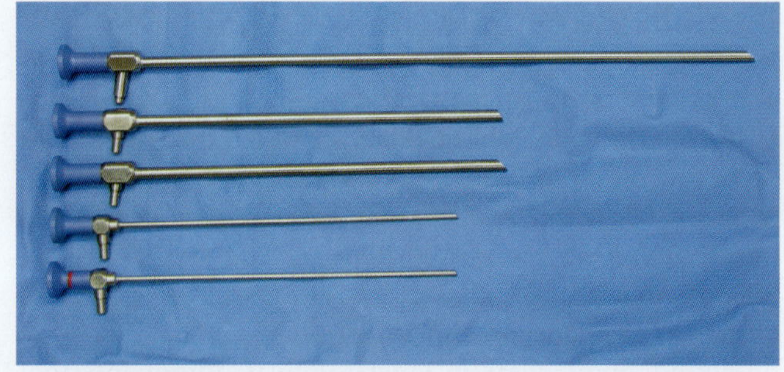

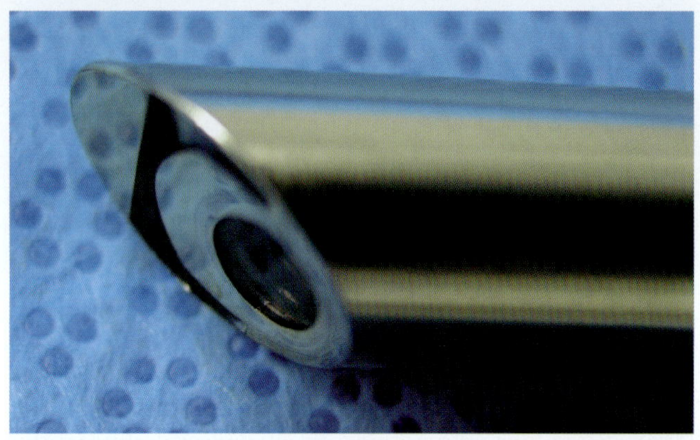

FIGURE 10-8. Standard and long length laparoscopes, 5- and 10-mm diameters (A). Angled 45 degree laparoscope (B). (Courtesy of Stryker, Kalamazoo, MI.)

view, especially in extremely obese patients. An extra long laparoscope (45 to 50 cm) is sometimes necessary and very helpful in super-obese patients. Excessive abdominal wall thickness, together with a large expanded abdominal cavity, does not allow for a close-up view of distant sites (e.g., the esophagogastric junction) using the standard-size scopes; extra-long scopes are also helpful during the use of any type of scope-holding instrument or robot that takes up functional scope length in establishing the connection.

An important scope accessory is a stainless steel scope warmer canister filled with hot sterile water for cleaning the scope and preventing lens fogging (Applied Medical, Rancho Santa Margarita, CA). We carefully attach this canister to the drapes for fast access, insulating it from the patient with a towel (Fig. 10-9). We have generally found that the antifog solutions are not helpful.

Video Camera

Miniature lightweight cameras, weighing as little as 40 g, are now in use, providing excellent resolution and color rendition, which are essential for laparoscopic bariatric surgery. The miniature camera uses a charge-coupled device (CCD) chip containing approximately 300,000 light-sensitive pixels on the chip surface measuring only about $\frac{1}{2}$-inch on the diagonal. Three-chip cameras have

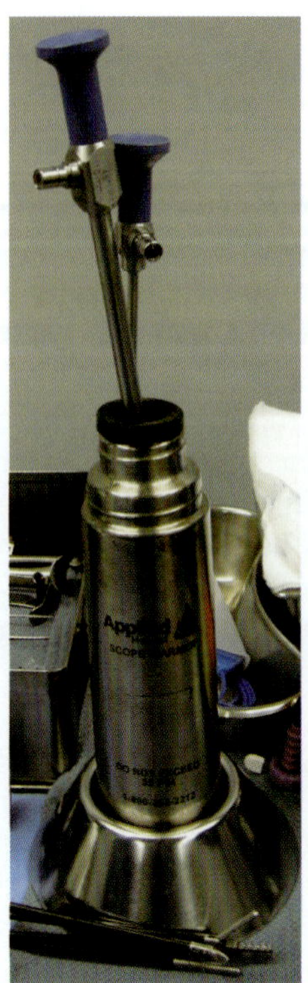

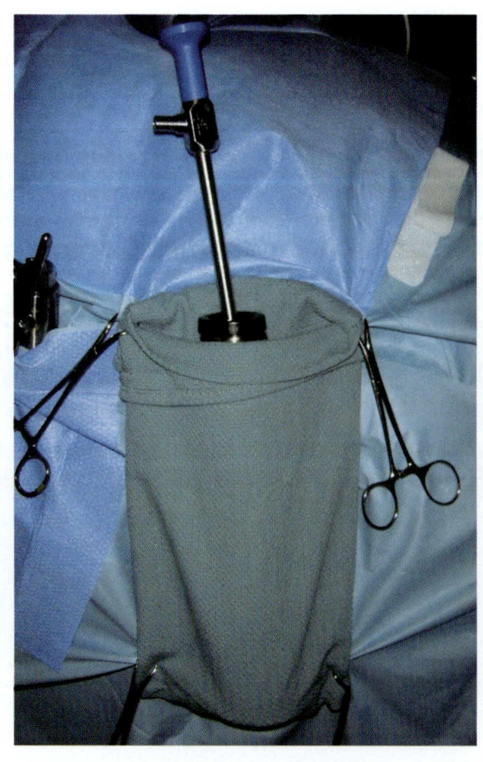

FIGURE 10-9. (A) Laparoscope warmer decreases fogging. (B) The laparoscope warmer should be attached to the surgical drapes for easy access. (Courtesy of Applied Medical, Rancho Santa Margarita, CA.)

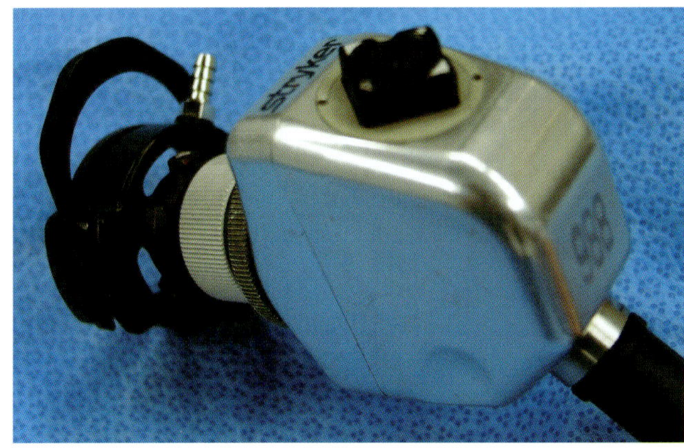

FIGURE 10-10. Three-chip video camera. (Courtesy of Stryker, Kalamazoo, MI.)

become the industry standard; each chip provides one of the three primary colors: red, green, and blue. There are a number of options for this type of equipment including the Stryker Endoscopy seventh-generation three-chip camera (model 988) (Fig. 10-10), which has a resolution of greater than 900 lines (compared to 470 to 560 lines for most single-chip cameras). This camera is extremely light sensitive (<1 Lux) and therefore effective in producing a usable image.

A C-mount endoscopic coupler permits rapid attachment of the camera to whichever lap scope is in use. The coupler also has a focusing knob. The camera head control buttons enable the user to adjust grain, digital zoom, and printer modalities. The camera is connected to the power supply and electronic control by cable. The system is further enhanced using voice activation technology from Hermes (Stryker Endoscopy) to control adjustments of white balance, gain, shutter, and digital enhancement (see Voice Activation Technology, below).

Light Source and Light Cable

Laparoscopy requires a high-intensity light source for an adequate video image of the operative field. A xenon or metal halide bulb with a life span of about 250 hours is typically used because it provides the desirable color temperature in the range of daylight (5500 K). An automatic adjustment as well as a manual override is available (to over- or underilluminate if needed). Interaction between the camera and the light source allows automatic adjustment of the illumination intensity with changes in light level at the camera CCD surface. This greatly reduces annoying glare.

The light is transmitted from the bulb to the scope through a fiber optic light cable that should be replaced if more than 15% broken fibers are noted. A full benefit of the light source depends on proper connection of the cable to the light source and the telescope. The light cables should not be autoclaved and must be sterilized in either ethylene-oxide or glutaraldehyde.

Video Monitor

The video monitor providing the laparoscopic image should be of the highest quality. We utilize monitors of both the traditional cathode ray tube (CRT) type (Sony Corporation) as well as those of the new flat-panel digital design (Stryker Endosurgery). As monitor and camera technology is trending toward higher definition digital capability, the flat-panel monitor technology will possibly replace the CRT type. The monitors are placed opposite the surgeon and the assistant on carts or towers or are suspended on booms.

Operating Tables

The operating table must provide maximum tilt and rotation and allow gravity to shift abdominal structures to allow full visualization (Fig. 10-11). For bariatric procedures, the operating table must have the capacity to support super-obese patients up to the maximum weight with which the surgeon is comfortable. Many standard general purpose OR tables have weight limits of about 227 kg (500 pounds), which are adequate for 95% or more of the cases in most bariatric practices (Fig. 10-12). It is advisable to check with the manufacturer regarding the specific weight limitations of the specific operating table model and vintage. Bariatric practices that include patients with weights greater than 227 kg require access to an operating room table that can accommodate them safely. Many general-purpose tables have been modified to accommodate the greater weight with some loss in the angle of tilt and Trendelenburg/reverse Trendelenburg in the interest of ensuring stability. This trade-off has become less necessary due to improving weight ratings and articulation in recent operating table technology. Important bed accessories include side extenders, footboards, straps, and padding to safely secure the patient to the bed and prevent injuries.

Hand Instrumentation

Grasping Instruments

Hand instruments are available with many different features and preferences. Our preference has been for

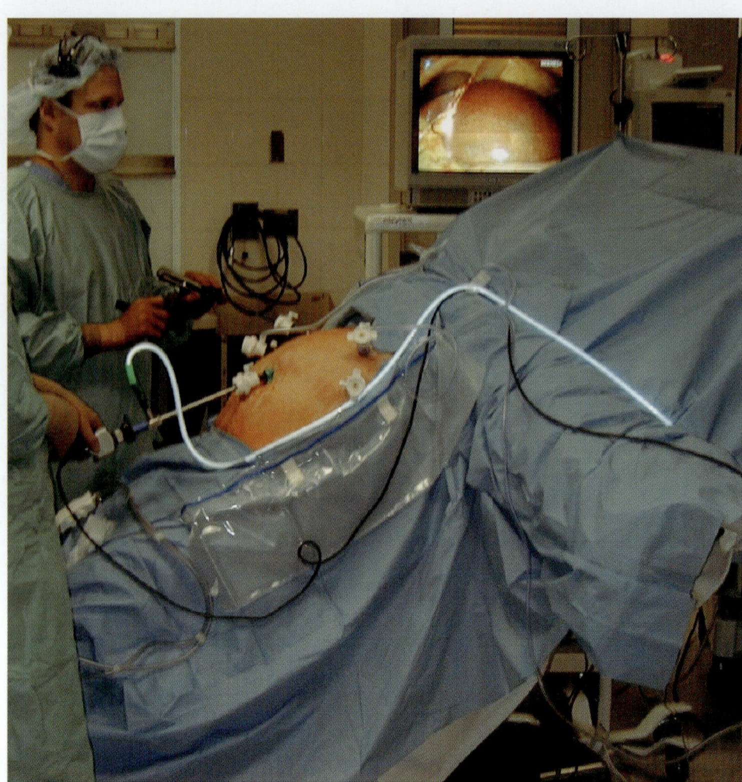

Figure 10-11. Operating table in full reverse Trendelenburg position.

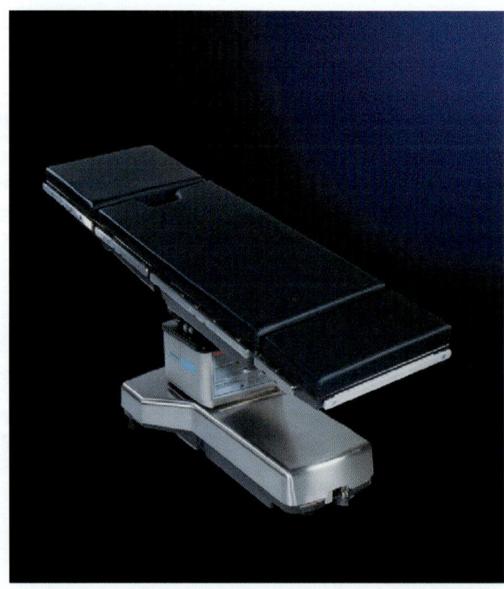

Figure 10-12. Standard Amsco(R) 3085 SP Surgical Table rated to hold a 1000-lb (454-kg) patient in normal orientation or a 500-lb (227-kg) patient in reverse orientation. (Courtesy of Steris Corp., Mentor, OH. Steris is a registered trademark of Steris Corporation. All rights reserved.)

"in-line" design (as opposed to a pistol-grip design and for instruments where ratcheted handle control can be turned on and off along with finger-controlled rotation of the shaft). For the super-obese patient, instrument length is an important factor. Many instruments are available in standard (32 cm) and extra-long lengths (45 cm) (Fig. 10-13). For laparoscopic bariatric surgery, atraumatic and traumatic grasping hand instruments are needed. An atraumatic grasper is required to manipulate bowel without causing injury. We use a 5-mm atraumatic grasper (Snowden Pencer, Tucker, GA) that features fine teeth and a broad tip design, which provide a secure grip without traumatizing tissue. The 5-mm traumatic ("crocodile") grasper (Snowden Pencer) features tissue herniation channels and long contoured jaws to provide secure grasping ability. It is excellent for holding the stomach and omentum.

Retracting Instruments and Instrument Stabilizers

Anterior and cephalad retraction of the left lobe of the liver is required to expose the gastroesophageal region. A number of devices work effectively for this purpose;

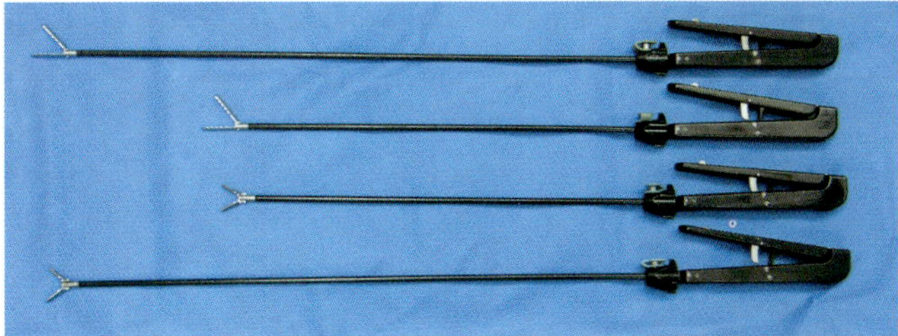

FIGURE 10-13. Hand instrumentation. Standard and long length grasper. Traumatic graspers are shown on top and atraumatic graspers for use on the small bowel are shown at the bottom. (Courtesy of Snowden Pencer, Tucker, GA.)

they must be strong enough to retract large, heavy livers without trauma to the organ tissue. The 5-mm diameter Endoflex Retractor (Snowden Pencer) is effective; it assumes a triangular configuration when tightened (Fig. 10-14). The retractor is usually held in a stationary position by means of an external holding device attached to the OR table such as the Fast Clamp System (Snowden Pencer) (Fig. 10-15). For extremely large livers, a recent modification of the Endoflex liver retractor called the Big D type is available to help stabilize and provide exposure. We have had a few occasions in the past where we have used two retractors at once.

Suction Irrigation Devices

A suction/irrigation instrument clears the surgical field of pooling blood and keeps the abdominal cavity free from smoke and vapor. The StrykerFlow 2 (Stryker Endoscopy) is a 5-mm disposable instrument with reusable probe tips that performs the function of both suction and irrigation through a single common channel. The probe tips come in a standard (32-cm) working length as well as an extra-long (45-cm) working length that is crucial for the super-obese patient (Fig. 10-16).

Suturing Instruments

Standard laparoscopic needle drivers and sutures and suturing devices such as the Endostitch™ (Autosuture,

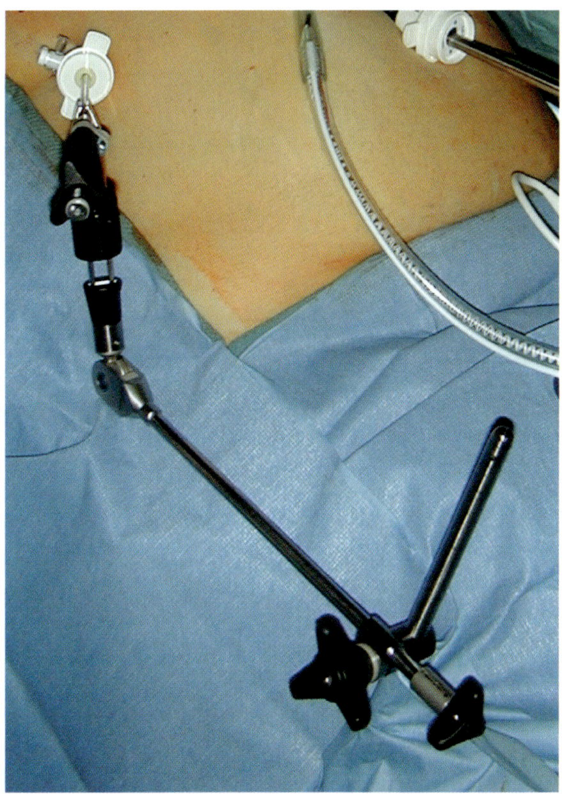

FIGURE 10-15. Table mounted instrument holding device. (Courtesy of Snowden Pencer, Tucker, GA.)

Division of Tyco Healthcare) are suitable for laparoscopic bariatric surgery. We utilize the Endostitch to facilitate endoscopic suturing. The 10-mm-diameter disposable Endostitch has a double pointed shuttle needle with the thread mounted at the center of the needle (Fig. 10-17). Double action jaws allow the needle to be passed back and forth by squeezing the handle and maneuvering the toggle switch, eliminating regrasping and repositioning the needle. The Endostitch is compatible with a variety of absorbable (e.g., Polysorb™, Autosuture, Division of Tyco Healthcare) and nonabsorbable sutures (e.g., Surgidek™, Autosuture, Division of Tyco Healthcare). The Endostitch is used during the Roux-en-Y gastric bypass (RYGBP) for approximating the bowel for the enteroenterostomy and for oversewing the gastrojejunostomy (two-layer closures).

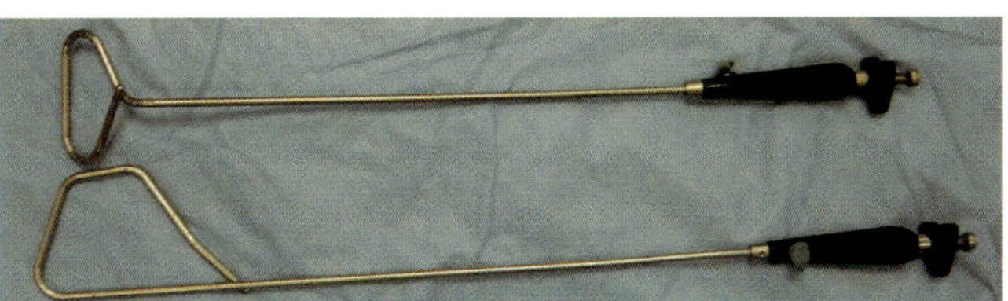

FIGURE 10-14. Flexible liver retractors, 5mm. Standard and "big D" type. (Courtesy of Snowden Pencer, Tucker, GA.)

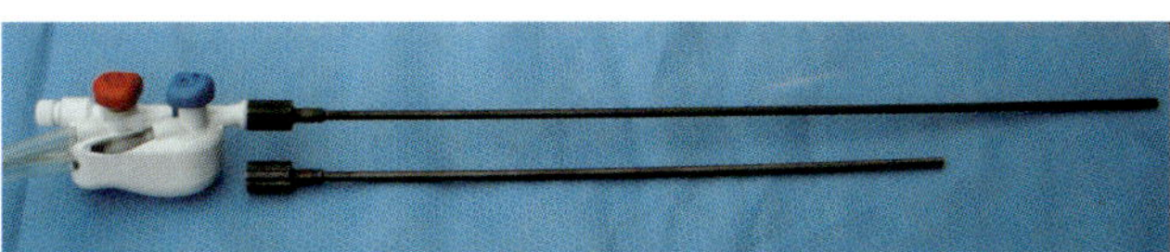

FIGURE 10-16. Suction irrigator: standard and long length tips. (Courtesy of Stryker, Kalamazoo, MI.)

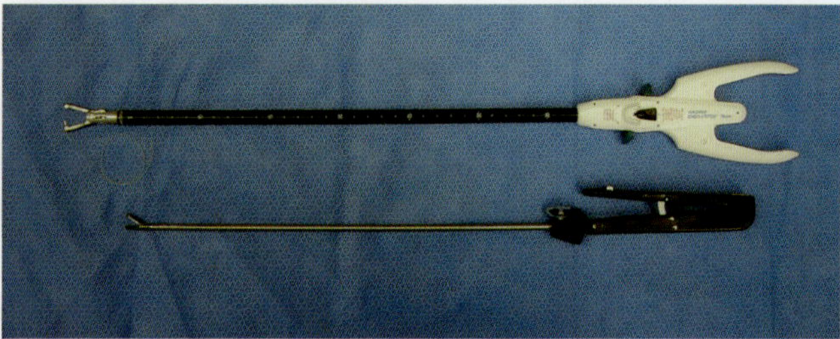

FIGURE 10-17. Endostitch and in-line laparoscopic needle driver. (Copyright © 2006 United States Surgical, a division of Tyco Healthcare Group LP, with permission. All rights reserved.)

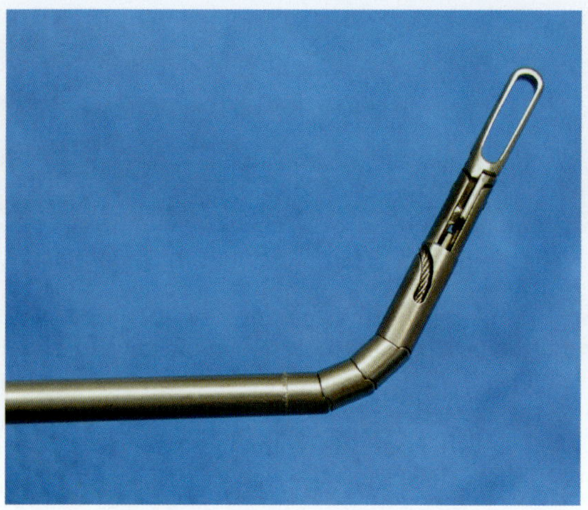

FIGURE 10-19. Fenestrated articulating grasper helps with dissection at the angle of His. (Courtesy of Snowden Pencer, Tucker, GA.)

Atraumatic Bowel Clamps

The laparoscopic bowel clamp is a 10-mm-diameter instrument that has long jaws with serrations that provide a secure atraumatic grip. It has a ratcheted handle for locking the jaws. It is available in a straight and curved jaw and is used to clamp the small bowel (Roux limb) before performing endoscopy to prevent distal insufflation of the small bowel (Fig. 10-18).

Specialized Grasping Instruments

Another grasping instrument suitable for handling bowel is the fenestrated grasper (Karl Storz Endscopy); it has broad, fenestrated jaws that provide a large surface for gently grasping and holding tissue. This instrument is used primarily for handling the small bowel and for measuring the length of the Roux limb during RYGBP. There is a mark machined into the instrument at a distance of 10 cm for the tip. We utilize this instrument for measurement of the Roux limb.

The fenestrated articulating grasper instrument (Snowden Pencer) has an articulating tip that forms a gentle curve of about 45 degrees when the handles are closed (Fig. 10-19). The instrument can be used to help in the dissection and identification of the angle of His and the development of a passage for the stapler to use as a guide. In the retrocolic retrogastric approach, this instrument is very useful in passing the Roux limb through the retrocolic and retrogastric tunnel up to the gastric pouch before performing the anastomosis.

Suture Passer for Trocar Site Closure

To prevent trocar site hernias, we close all ports of 10 mm or greater with a strong absorbable suture such as O-Polysorb. There are a number of devices available for passing sutures through the abdominal wall fascia. We use the Carter-Thomason CloseSure System (Inlet Medical Inc., Eden Prairie, MN) (Fig. 10-20A), which facilitates full-thickness closure. It is a disposable device that comes with guides (pilots) of varying diameters and in a standard and long length (CloseSure XL) to accommodate very thick abdominal walls (Fig. 10-20B). The angle projected by the guide allows for an adequate purchase of fascial tissue. This device used without the guide is valuable to ligate abdominal wall bleeders and to repair small umbilical, ventral and incisional hernias noted at the time of the laparoscopic bariatric surgery.

Lap-Band Passing Instrument

The O'Brien Lap-Band Placer (Automated Medical Products Corp., Edison, NJ) is a specialized instrument used to pass the lap band behind the stomach from the greater curve of the stomach at the angle of His to the

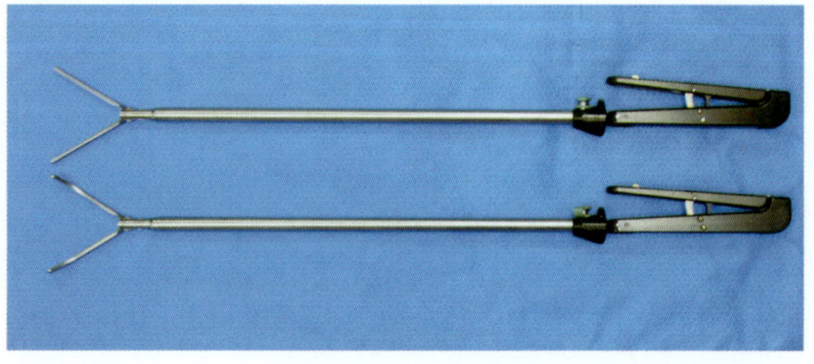

FIGURE 10-18. Atraumatic bowel clamps: straight and curved tips. (Courtesy of Snowden Pencer, Tucker, GA.)

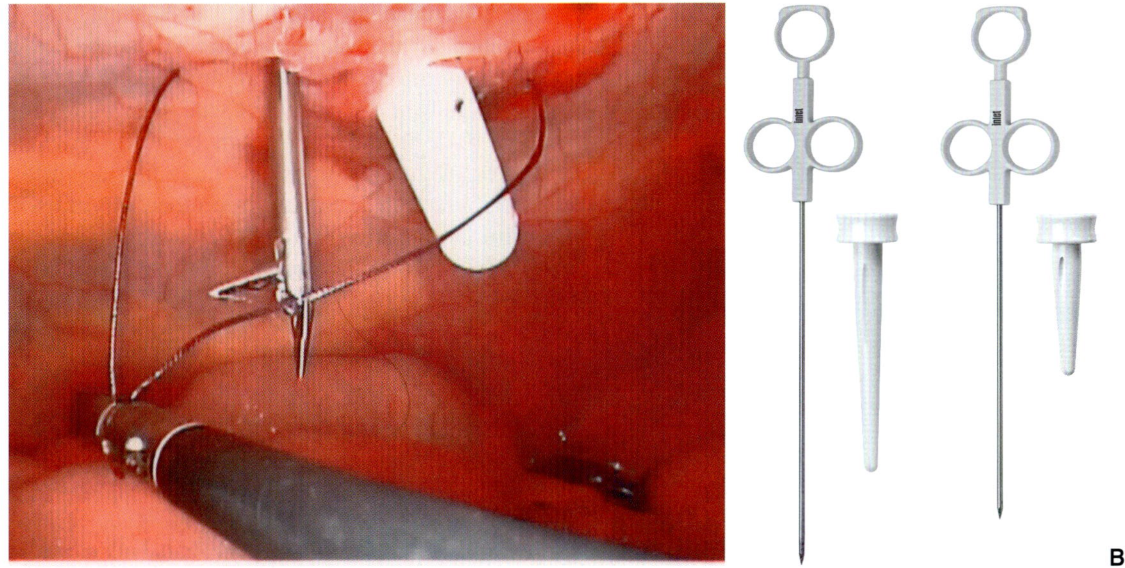

A   **B**

FIGURE 10-20. (A) Suture passer device facilitates closure of trocar sites and can be used to close small ventral hernias. (B) Standard length (right) and the Closure XL system (left) that provides added length for fascial closure in bariatric patients. (Courtesy of Inlet Medical, Eden Prairie, MN.)

lesser curve. The round tubing of the lap band is placed in the groove at the tip and is pulled behind the stomach (Fig. 10-21).

Other Hand Instruments

We use disposable endoscopic shears for cutting tissues when a laparoscopic scissor is needed. These endoscopic shears are 5 mm with a rotating shaft and a 16-mm curved blade. A reliably sharp blade is one of its major advantages.

In the event of bleeding where a clip is needed, we use the multiload disposable clip applier with titanium clips. It is available in 5- and 10-mm-diameter sizes. Compared to single clip units, the multiload units considerably increase the speed and efficiency with which hemostasis can be accomplished.

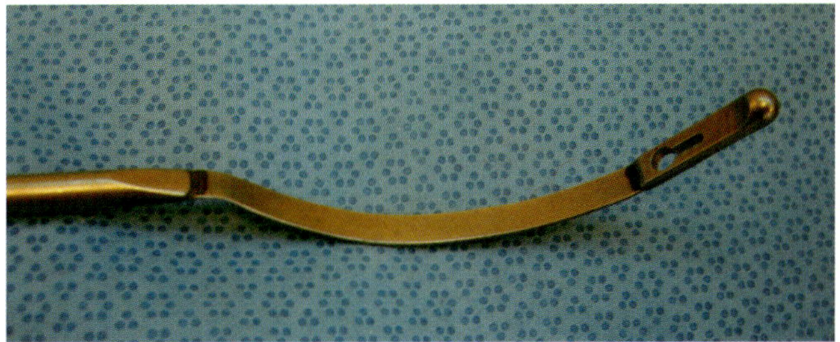

FIGURE 10-21. The O'Brien Lap-Band Placer. (Courtesy of Automated Medical Products Corp., Edison, NJ.)

Energy Sources for Transecting and Coagulation

In general laparoscopy, dividing tissues and achieving hemostasis, can be obtained with standard unipolar or bipolar electrocautery. Ultrasonic transection and coagulation may be preferable for extremely vascular tissue such as mesentery. The Ultrasonic Shears™ (Autosuture, Division of Tyco Healthcare) and the Harmonic Scalpel™ (Ethicon Endo-Surgery) are ultrasonically activated instruments that provide excellent transaction and hemostasis while eliminating the problem of electrical arc injury associated with unipolar electrocautery. The instruments have a stationary jaw and a blade that vibrates at a high frequency (55,000 Hz). The heat generated by this frequency denatures collagen and forms a coagulant that instantly seals small blood vessels. Minimal heat is generated in the tissue through friction; the lateral spread of thermal energy is 1 to 2 mm.

Ultrasonic instruments are available in 5-mm diameter and are short (15.7-cm working length) or long (38-cm working length), with finger-controlled rotating shaft (Fig. 10-22). They are activated by controls on the handle or a foot switch that adjusts the blade frequency and the speed of tissue cutting and hemostasis. These instruments produce water vapor that can obscure vision in the laparoscopic fields similar to the smoke created by intracorporeal electrocautery.

During LRYGBP, we employ ultrasonic dissection liberally, especially for dissection along the lesser and

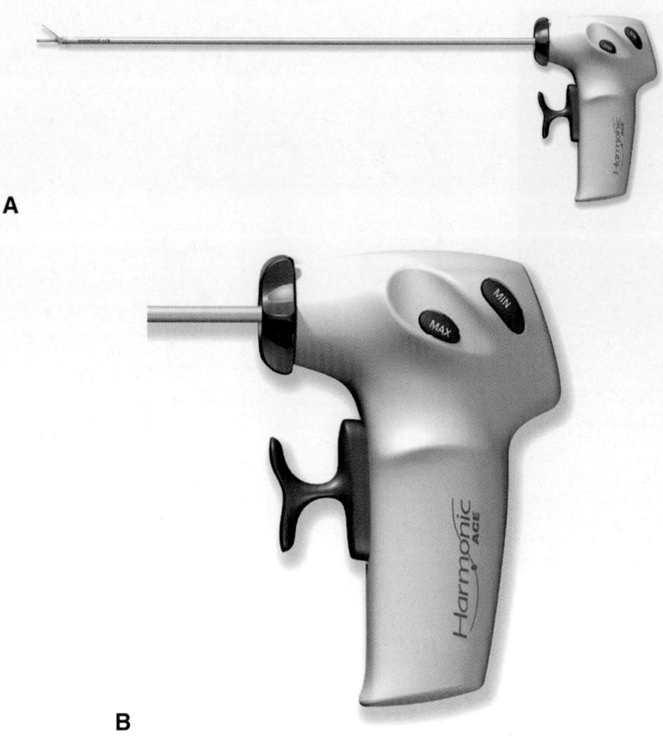

FIGURE 10-22. (A,B) Ultrasonic dissecting shears with hand controls. Harmonic ACE. (Courtesy of Ethicon Endo-Surgery, Inc. All rights reserved.)

greater curves of the stomach for gastric pouch creation, for making enterotomies in the stomach and small intestine, and for dividing the omentum.

Staplers: Linear and Circular

Linear Staplers

An endoscopic linear stapler that creates at least two (preferably three) rows of staples on each side of the transected tissue is an extremely important instrument required for many laparoscopic procedures especially laparoscopic RYGBP. It can be used to transect hollow viscera, to divide highly vascular tissue such as mesentery,

and to create an anastomosis. We use the Endopath Echelon 60 disposable stapler (Ethicon Endo-Surgery, Inc., Cincinnati, OH) that applies two triple rows of staples before dividing the tissue with an advancing knife (Fig. 10-23). The stapler can be reloaded for use with tissues of varying thickness including a white load (2.5 mm), blue load (3.5 mm), green load (4.1 mm), and a gold cartridge (3.8 mm) that is used primarily for thicker tissue compressible to 1.8 mm. The stapler fits down a 12-mm trocar. We use the blue load to create the gastric pouch and gastrojejunostomy and the white load to divided the small bowel and mesentery and to create the jejuno-jejunostomy. The green load is useful for revisional bariatric surgery or in cases where the tissue is unusually thick or indurated.

Circular Staplers

A circular endoluminal stapler can be used to create the gastrojejunal anastomosis during laparoscopic RYGB. The Endopath Circular Stapler (Ethicon Endo-Surgery, Inc.) uses two rows of circular staples with an inner circular knife to create a circular anastomosis (Fig. 10-24). The stapler (21 or 25 mm) is typically inserted through an enlarged port site in the left upper quadrant. The anvil can be placed into the pouch using transoral or transgastric techniques. Various methods of anvil insertion into the gastric pouch have been devised, including insertion through a gastrostomy or insertion through the mouth with guidance into the pouch through the esophagus using a pull wire. When using the pull-wire technique with the circular stapler, anvils can be modified to rotate the head of the anvil parallel with the shaft to facilitate transoral passage. The modification requires the removal of the spring and metal plate on the underside of the anvil, swinging the head of the anvil parallel to the shaft, and stabilizing the head of the anvil with a suture (Fig. 10-25). The pull wire is looped though the pointed end and it is ready to be pulled into place in the stomach through the esophagus. Other surgeons do not perform this modification and gently pull the intact anvil down the esophagus with a guidewire or nasogastric tube while subluxing the patient's jaw.

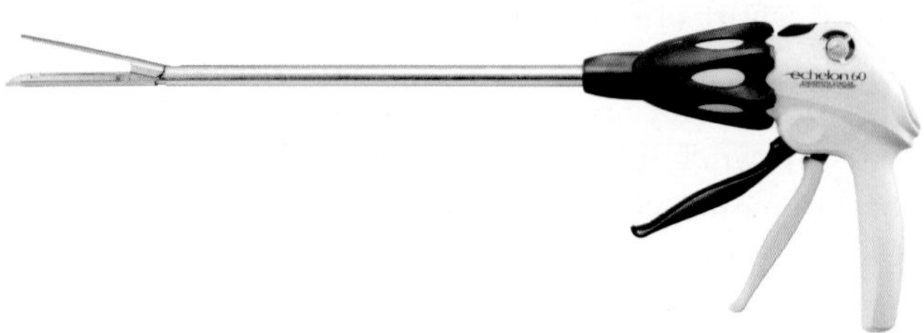

FIGURE 10-23. Laparoscopic linear cutting stapler. Echelon 60. (Courtesy of Ethicon Endo-Surgery, Inc. All rights reserved.)

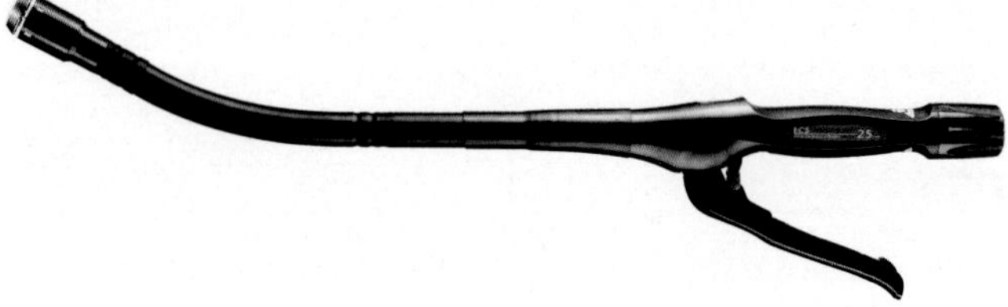

FIGURE 10-24. 25 mm circular stapler used to create a circular stapled gastrojejunostomy. ECS 25. (Courtesy of Ethicon Endo-Surgery, Inc. All rights reserved.)

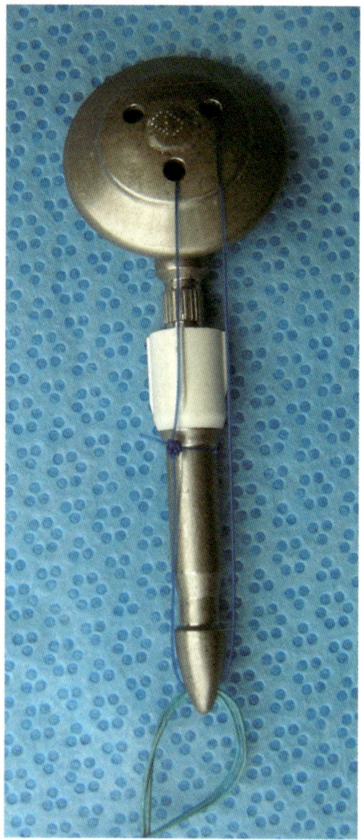

FIGURE 10-25. Some circular stapler anvils can be modified to allow the anvil head to fold parallel to the shaft. A suture can be used to maintain this configuration, which can facilitate transoral passage of the anvil. (Copyright © 2006 United States Surgical, a division of Tyco Healthcare Group LP, with permission. All rights reserved.)

Flexible Endoscopy

Flexible endoscopy serves several useful functions during the course of the LRYGBP. A two-camera system, one each for the laparoscope and endoscope, facilitates this approach. Both camera systems are fed through a digital mixer producing the two images on the same monitor as a "picture-in-picture" format allowing both the surgeon and the endoscopist to visualize both activities simultaneously.

At the completion of the LRYGBP a flexible endoscope is used to examine the gastrojejunal anastomosis. The scope is inserted beyond the anastomosis into the Roux limb prior to completing the final layer of the anastomosis. This serves to size the anastomosis (standard gastroscope is 30 French in diameter). Intraluminal insufflation of the submerged anastomosis is used to inspect for air leaks. After leak testing, the endoscope is used to examine the anastomosis for bleeding and the viability of the gastric pouch.

Endoscopy facilitates placement of the anvil into the gastric pouch during use of the circular stapler for the gastrojejunal anastomosis. Unless the transgastric tech-

nique is employed, an endoscopic snare and pull wire are needed for this technique.

Voice Activation Technology

A major innovation in operating room procedure has been the introduction of voice control technology such as Hermes (Intuitive Surgical, Sunnyvale, CA and Stryker Endoscopy). This technology provides a centralized and simplified interface for a surgeon to Hermes-compatible medical devices through voice commands. The system requires a computer control unit associated with other accessory units that are networked with multiple Hermes-ready devices. The system may include a Hermes OR control center, a Hermes port expander, a Hermes phone unit, and a ATW-R73 UHF synthesized diversity receiver (Audio-Techniques/Stryker Endoscopy) (Fig. 10-26). The surgeon wears a wireless headphone/microphone transmitter (ATW-T75 Transmitter (Audio Techniques/Stryker Endoscopy), and is able to control and operate the devices throughout the procedure. This saves time and decreases dependence on circulating nurses or technicians. A voice card is programmed for each individual surgeon. This is inserted into the control unit and allows voice recognition. Hermes allows the surgeon to voice-control the camera, light source, insufflator, video/image recorder, printer, telephone, operating table, operating room lights, and Intuitive Surgical's robotics systems such as the Automated Endoscopic System for Optimal Positioning (AESOP).

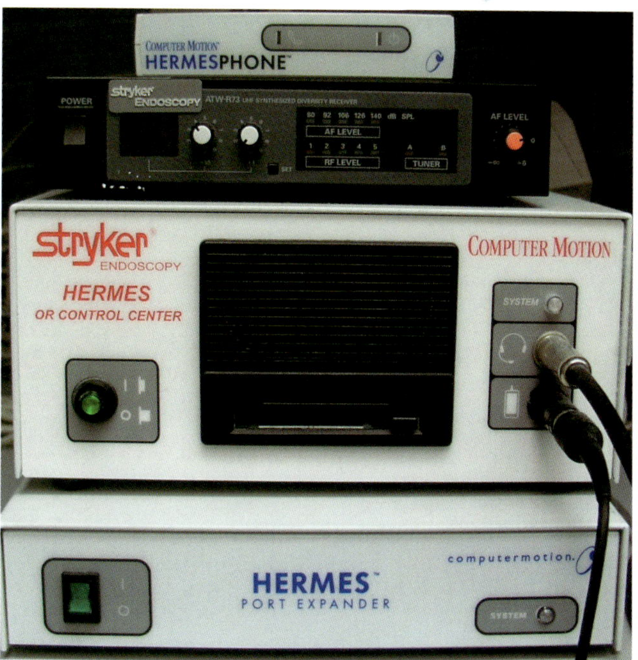

FIGURE 10-26. Voice activation unit. (Courtesy of Audio-Techniques/Stryker Endoscopy, Kalamazoo, MI.)

The Hermes system provides both visual (on the video monitor) and digitized voice feedback to the surgical team. Voice-activated control is especially appropriate to bariatric laparoscopic procedures because of the multiple adjustments and readjustments of multiple complicated medical devices during the course of the operation. Safety and quality of patient care appear to be enhanced by returning focus from the technology to the patient (15).

Operating Room Layout

The organization and layout of the operating room are as crucial to efficient surgery as the equipment used. Space for transfer of morbidly obese patients to and from the operating table must be provided, as well as space for the number of personnel needed for the transfer. Vital equipment must be in easy reach without obstructing movement of the operating staff. Many teams use mobile towers to house equipment.

Over the last 5 years, operating rooms specialized for minimally invasive procedures have made significant strides. These operating rooms employ boom technology for efficient space utilization and integrate electrical, fiber optic, computer, communication, digital, video, voice activation, and piped gas technologies. These have been called fully integrated or "intelligent" operating rooms and go by the trade names of EndoSuite, i-Suite (Stryker Endoscopy), Supersuite (Berchtold Corporation), and

OR1 (Karl Storz Endoscopy). These are clearly the wave of the present and future (Fig. 10-27). Efficient design of these operating rooms will likely improve overall operating efficiency and safety (16). The advantages in efficiency and safety appear to justify the cost, as these complex procedures become increasingly frequent in many medical centers.

Robotics

Robotic Assistance

Robotics and voice activation combine with great advantage. Examples include the AESOP, a Food and Drug Administration (FDA)-approved surgical robot (Intuitive Surgical) and the more complex Da Vinci Surgical System (Intuitive Surgical). The AESOP system is capable of holding the laparoscope and altering its position in response to the surgeon's verbal commands. A major advantage over human maneuvering of the laparoscope is that the device can store in its memory several set arm positions, allowing the surgeon quickly to return or advance to viewing positions previously found to be desirable. Other advantages over human assistants are the elimination of nonpurposeful movement, delayed movement, and inadvertent lens soiling.

Effective use of AESOP depends on acquiring skill through extensive experience. Because of the complexity of maneuvering in the upper and mid-abdomen, surgeons must allow for a learning curve. Preliminary studies have

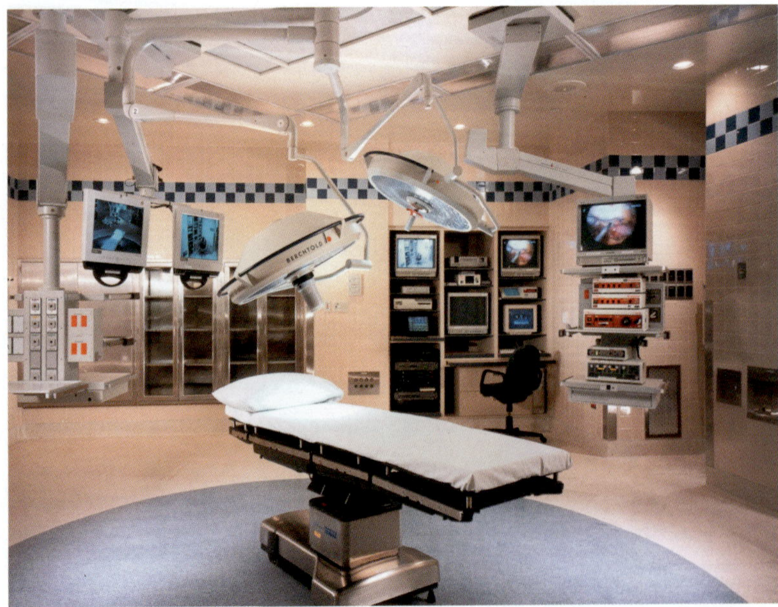

Figure 10-27. Fully integrated minimally invasive operating room. (Courtesy of Stryker/Berchtold.)

shown that the benefits of the robotic arm include improved operating room efficiency with reduction in operating time and a cost savings to the institution (17–19).

The Da Vinci Surgical System is an FDA-approved laparoscopic surgical robot that might be termed "full service." It provides much more than just a robotic arm. The system is capable of performing surgical cutting, dissecting, suturing, and tissue retraction, as well as providing visualization. It provides improved dexterity, greater surgical precision, improved minimal access, increased range of motion, and reproducibility. A number of clinical investigators have been involved with trials of this robot in laparoscopic bariatric surgery (20,21). These early studies note that laparoscopic bariatric surgery using the Da Vinci robot is safe and feasible but will require further investigation.

Conclusion

Proper use and understanding of a wide array of laparoscopic equipment and instrumentation greatly aids the team's ability to meet the technical needs of more challenging operative situations. Not all of the technology presented in this chapter is necessary to complete every bariatric procedure, but surgeons who perform laparoscopic bariatric surgery should be familiar with the wide range of instrumentation available. A listing of the disposable and reusable instrumentation needed for a typical LRYGBP case is provided (Tables 10-1 and 10-2). As current techniques are improved upon and new bariatric procedures are developed, bariatric surgeons will need to keep abreast of the latest instrumentation in order to maximize operating room efficiency and safety.

TABLE 10-1. Laparoscopic Roux-en-Y gastric bypass disposable instrumentation

GIA anastomotic method			
1	Echelon 60 Endopath stapler	12 mm, straight	(EC 60)
4–5	Disposable staple reloads	60 mm, 3.5 blue	(ECR60B)
4–5	Disposable staple reload	60 mm, 2.5 white	(ECR60W)
1–2	Disposable staple reloads (thick tissue, revision cases)	60 mm, 3.8 gold	(ECR60G)
1	Endo Stitch USS (#173016)		
3–5	Reloads of 2-0 Surgadec for the USS Endostitch	(173021)	
4–6	Reloads of 2-0 Polysorb for the USS Endostitch	(170070)	
1	Endoshears USS 5 mm (#176643) or Ethicon Endo-Surgery 5 mm	(5DCS)	
1	Clip Applier USS 10 mm large, green or Ethicon 10 mm MED/LG	(176625)	
		(ER320)	
1	Harmonic Ace Ultrasonic Scalpel, 5 mm, Ethicon	(ACE36P)	
1	150 mm USS Surgineedle Veress needle (if not using optical trocars)	(172016)	
1	Carter-Thomason CloseSure System (XL for thick abdominal wall)	(CTXL)	
Trocars			
	Four 5-mm Ethicon Endpath Xcel, bladeless 100 mm	(B5LT)	
	Two 12-mm Ethicon ENDOPATH XCEL, bladeless 100 mm	(B12LT)	
Suction irrigator			
	1 StrykeFlow 5 mm suction irrigation system		
	(utilized reusable cannula tips 32 and 45 cm)		
Circular stapler anastomotic method (requires all of the above plus the instrumentation below)			
1	Endoscopic curved intraluminal stapler		
	Ethicon Endopath ILS 21 mm	(ECS21)	
	Ethicon Endopath ILS 25 mm	(ECS25)	
Cook translumbar aortic catheter		(076828)	
1	"Pull" blue PEG wire (Microinvasive)	(6399)	
1	Endoscopic snare (Microinvasive)		
Alternatively, the anvil can be secured to the cut end of an 18-French nasogastric tube and passed transorally into the gastric pouch			

TABLE 10-2. Laparoscopic Roux-en-Y gastric bypass reusable instrumentation

Item name	Item No.	Company	No. in set
Routine set			
Crocodile grasper (traumatic) (32 cm)	90-7064	Snowden-Pencer	2
Crocodile grasper (traumatic) (45 cm)	90-7264	Snowden-Pencer	2
Diamond jaw atraumatic dissector (32 cm)	90-7041	Snowden-Pencer	3
Diamond jaw atraumatic dissector (45 cm)	90-7271	Snowden-Pencer	3
Endo-right angle	90-7031	Snowden-Pencer	1
Right angle electrode	89-7200	Snowden-Pencer	1
Tapered curved dissector	90-7033	Snowden-Pencer	1
Hasson "S" retractor narrow	88-9113	Snowden-Pencer	1 set
Hasson "S" retractor wide	88-9114	Snowden-Pencer	1 set
Monopolar cord	88-9199	Snowden-Pencer	1
Instrument tray	88-6275	Snowden-Pencer	1
Scopes			
30 degree, 10 mm	502-357-030	Stryker	1
45 degree, 10 mm	502-357-045	Stryker	1
30 degree, 5 mm	502-585-030	Stryker	1
45 degree, 5 mm	502-585-045	Stryker	1
45 degree, 10 mm extra long	502-657-045	Stryker	1
Scope warmer			
Scope warmer canister	C3001	Applied Medical	1
Base for scope warmer	C3002	Applied Medical	1
Seals for scope warmer	C3101	Applied Medical	1
Table-mounted instrument holding device			
Fast Clamp System	89-8950	Snowden Pencer	1
Liver retractors			
80-mm triangular liver			
Retractor 5 mm	89-6110	Snowden-Pencer	1
"Big D" diamond flex liver retractor	89-8216	Snowden Pencer	1
Bowel instruments			
DeBakey clamp, straight, 10 mm	90-7052	Snowden Pencer	1
DeBakey clamp, curved, 10 mm	90-7054	Snowden Pencer	1
Specials			
Diamond flex articulating			
Atraumatic grasper 40 degree	89-0509	Snowden-Pencer	1
Bougie 34-French or Olympus endoscope			
bowel grasper	33331C	Storz	1
Diamond-jaw needle holder	90-7016	Snowden Pencer	1
O'Brien Lap-Band placer		Automated Medical Products Corp.	1
StrykeProbe and tips, 5 mm (32 and 45 cm)		Stryker Endoscopy	1

Acknowledgment. We thank the Operating Room staffs at the University of Pittsburgh Medical Center–Presbyterian and Magee Women's Hospital of the University of Pittsburgh Medical System and especially Deneen Beatty, Michelle Jackson, and Brent McConnell for their assistance and support.

References

1. Ramanathan RC, Gourash W, Ikramuddin S, Schauer PR. Equipment and instrumentation for laparoscopic bariatric surgery. In: Deitel M, Cowan GSM, eds. Update: Surgical for the Morbidly Obese. Toronto: FD-Communications, 2000:277–290.

2. Carbonell AM, Joels CS, Sing RF, Heniford BT. Laparoscopic gastric bypass surgery: equipment and necessary tools. J Laparoendosc Adv Surg Tech 2003;13(4):241–245.

3. Schauer PR, Ikramuddin S, Gourash W. Laparoscopic Roux-en-Y gastric bypass: a case report at one-year follow-up. Laparoendosc Adv Surg Tech 1999;9:101–106.

4. Schauer PR, Ikramuddin S, Gourash W, Ramanathan R, Luketich JD. Outcomes of laparoscopic Roux-en-Y gastric bypass for morbid obesity. Ann Surg 2000;232(4):515–529.

5. Coller JA, Murray JJ. Equipment. In: Ballantyne GH, Leahy PL, Modlin IL, eds. Laparoscopic Surgery. Philadelphia: WB Saunders, 1994:3–14.

6. Spencer MP, Madoff RD. Imaging. In: Ballantyne GH, Leahy PL, Modlin IL, eds. Laparoscopic Surgery. Philadelphia: WB Saunders 1994:15–21.

7. Berci G, Paz-Partlow. Videoendoscopic technology. In: Toouli J, Gossot D, Hunter JG, eds. Endosurgery. New York: Churchill Livingstone, 1996:33–39.

8. Prescher T. Video imaging. In: Toouli J, Gossot D, Hunter JG, eds. Endosurgery. New York: Churchill Livingstone, 1996:41–54.

9. Melzer A. Endoscopic Instruments-conventional and intelligent. In: Toouli J, Gossot D, Hunter JG, eds. Endosurgery. New York: Churchill Livingstone, 1996:69–95.

10. AORN Bariatric Surgery Guideline. AORN J 2004;79(5): 1026–1052.

11. Schauer PR, Gourash W, Hamad G, Ikramuddin S. Operating set up and patient positioning for laparoscopic gastric bypass. SAGES Manual. New York: Springer-Verlag, 2005.

12. Nguyen NT, Cronan M, Braley S, Rivers R, Wolfe BM. Duplex ultrasound assessment of femoral venous flow during laparoscopic and open gastric bypass. Surg Endosc 2003;17:285–290.

13. Collier B, Goreja MA, Duke BE. Postoperative rhabdomyolysis with bariatric surgery. Obes Surg 2003;13(6):941–943.

14. Mognol P, Vignes S, Chosidow D, Marmuse JP. Rhabdomyolysis after laparoscopic bariatric surgery. Obes Surg 2004; 14:91–94.

15. Luketich JD, Fernando HC, Buenaventura PO, Christie NA, Grondin SC, Schauer PR. Results of a randomized trial of HERMES-assisted versus non-HERMES-assisted laparoscopic antireflux surgery. Surg Endosc 2002;16(9): 1264–1266.

16. Kenyon TAG, Urbach DR, Speer JB, et al. Dedicated minimally invasive surgery suites increase operating room efficiency. Surg Endosc 2001;15:1140–1143.

17. Kavoussi LR, Moore RG, Adams JB, et al. Comparison of robotic versus human laparoscopic camera control. J Urol 1995;154:2131–2136.

18. Omote K, Feussner H, Ungeheuer A, et al. Self-guided robotic camera control for laparoscopic surgery compared with human camera control. Am J Surg 1999;177:321–324.

19. Dunlap KD, Wanzer L. Is the robotic arm a cost effective tool? AORN J 1998;68:265–272.

20. Nguyen NT, Hinojosa MW, Finley D, Stevens M, Paya M. Application of robotics in general surgery: initial experience. Am Surg 2004;70(10):914–917.

21. Jacobsen G, Berger R, Horgan S. The role of robotic surgery in morbid obesity. J Laparoendosc Adv Surg Tech A 2003; 13(4):279–283.

11
Access to the Peritoneal Cavity

Crystal T. Schlösser and Sayeed Ikramuddin

Inherent in all minimally invasive surgery is acquiring safe, efficient, and cost-effective access to the cavity of interest. Bariatric surgery presents some challenges for achieving peritoneal access because of the patient's body habitus, limitations of the current equipment, and comorbidities. The goals of access include excellent abdominal exposure, ingress for instruments, egress of specimens, and minimization of complications.

Historical Methods

Pelviscopy introduced concepts of peritoneal access, peritoneal physiology, and the unique constraints of three-dimensional surgery using two-dimensional imaging. Initial laparoscopy methods amalgamated urologic, gynecologic, and thoracic instrumentation, and adapted the original Veress needle design of the 1930s to provide diagnostic pneumoperitoneum for operative procedures (1). Complications with this access device prompted mini-laparotomy techniques in which the abdominal cavity was entered in the traditional manner under direct visualization and placement of a large-bore cannula through which laparoscopy could proceed (2). Further refinements of both techniques have occurred, as well as the development of novel access devices engineered to reduce the axial force needed for entrance into the peritoneal cavity (rotating screw-type devices) (3).

The ideal access device is simple, fast, allows rapid pneumoperitoneum, has minimal complications (or preferably none), and is reusable for cost-effectiveness. This model device has yet to be developed, and is a goal for future research efforts.

Entry Method

Regardless of the access device chosen, certain surgical principles can maximize surgeon effectiveness and minimize complications. Careful attention to patient preparation and a supine position without tilt, rotation, or Trendelenburg positioning is crucial. Malposition can lead to errors in a surgeon's three-dimensional imagery of the patient's anatomy, causing disorientation related to the position of the great vessels, and translocate viscera to a location where injury may neither be expected nor recognized expeditiously. Physical examination of the patient should note scars and their quality as well as umbilical or other body piercings that may be associated with intraperitoneal adhesions.

Important considerations in access planning include a decision about abdominal cavity expansion. Options include standard carbon dioxide pneumoperitoneum, which causes drying and cooling of the visceral and parietal peritoneum. This is associated with increased pain (especially referred diaphragmatic pain), decreased body temperature, and morphologic changes in peritoneal mesothelial cells of uncertain significance (4,5). Alternative media such as helium have recently been reported, as has hydrodistention. Gasless options like abdominal wall lifting are also reported, but none of these options are currently appropriate in the bariatric surgery patient.

Strategies for achieving pneumoperitoneum are no insufflation, preinsufflation, and insufflation only after open access has been achieved. Management of intra-abdominal pressures must center on patient safety: One needs sufficient pressure to allow adequate exposure for safe operation, but yet low enough to avoid restriction of ventilation, hypercarbia, or impaired venous return.

Closed Methods

The Veress needle is a 2-mm blunt-tipped needle designed for induction of pneumothorax without injury to the lung (1). It has a spring-loaded tension-sensing blunt tip that retracts against resistance from fascia and peritoneum, promptly recoiling after passage through

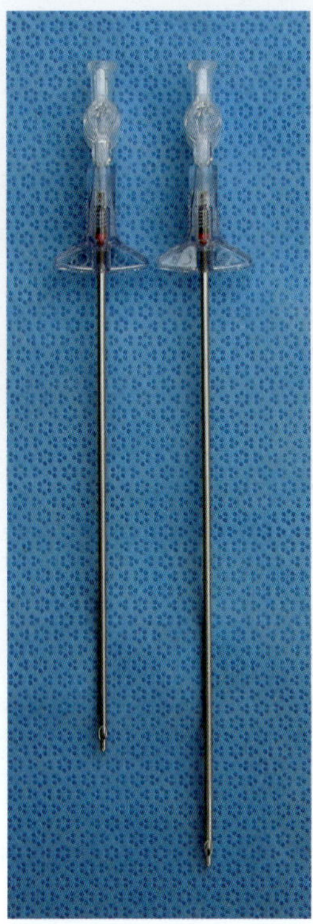

FIGURE 11-1. Standard and long Veress needles. (Copyright © 2006 United States Surgical, a division of Tyco Healthcare Group LP, with permission. All rights reserved.)

these layers. This allows the cutting needle to penetrate tissue, but yet protect viscera. Insufflation is accomplished through the needle lumen after intraperitoneal placement. It has been the access of choice for almost 40 years in many countries, especially in the field of gynecology. Long Veress needles are available for patients with thick abdominal wall such as the bariatric patient (Fig. 11-1).

A common entry site is the umbilicus, using manual countertraction against the abdominal wall to create negative intraabdominal pressure. The needle's port is open to room pressure, which has the effect of moving the abdominal wall farther from the viscera as soon as the peritoneum is breached. Unfortunately, other structures fixed against the abdominal wall or retroperitoneum may be unable to move and be injured. Alternatively, high-speed passage into the abdomen, before the blunt needle tip resets, can injure structures. Not recognizing intraperitoneal placement might encourage advancement of the needle, also potentially damaging organs.

In obese patients, umbilical exposure can be difficult, the ability to lift the abdominal wall may be impaired, and overgrowth of bacteria or yeast may exist. As a result, an alternative site of needle placement at Palmer's point (left costal margin, between the midclavicular and anterior axillary lines) is preferred. The major organ underlying this area is the omentum; access is enhanced by the tethering effect of the lower ribs and cartilage on

the rectus, its sheath, and the underlying peritoneum. Here the superior epigastric arterial plexus is usually medial and less likely to be injured than at other sites; however, care should be taken to avoid medial displacement of the needle tip as force is applied. At the umbilicus, the needle should be directed at a 45-degree angle toward the pelvis, in exactly the midline (avoid aortic bifurcation and iliac vessels). A suture can be placed through the skin to provide traction at the umbilicus. At Palmer's point, the Veress needle is inserted perpendicular to the skin (Fig. 11-2).

One should aspirate the needle to sure that blood, succus, or stool is not present. One drop of saline placed at the hub should enter the peritoneal cavity by gravity or by creation of negative intraperitoneal pressure with an abdominal lift. The onset of carbon dioxide insufflation should show a pressure of 5 to 8 mm Hg; higher pressures (>20 mm Hg) suggest preperitoneal or subcutaneous instillation of gas. No maneuver can definitively confirm intraperitoneal placement, however, and vascular or visceral injury can occur even when these tests are conducted accurately with negative results. Optical visualization via the needle has been advocated as being a safer technique, but it would seem simply to diagnose an injury sooner rather than actually prevent one (6).

Schwartz et al. (7) describe a method of dislodging and keeping the omentum off the needle tip in morbidly obese patients. They describe flow enhancement to 1 to 2

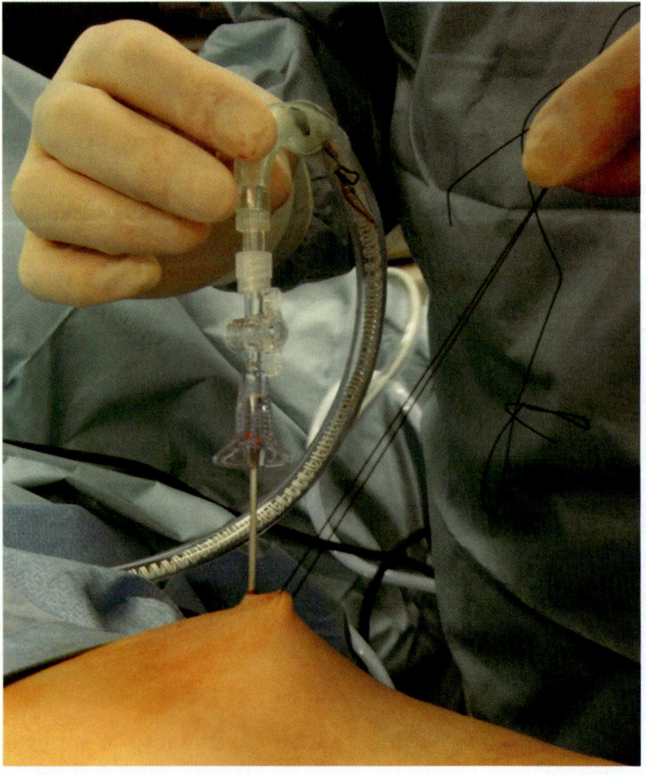

FIGURE 11-2. A traction suture can be used to lift the abdominal wall adjacent to the Veress needle.

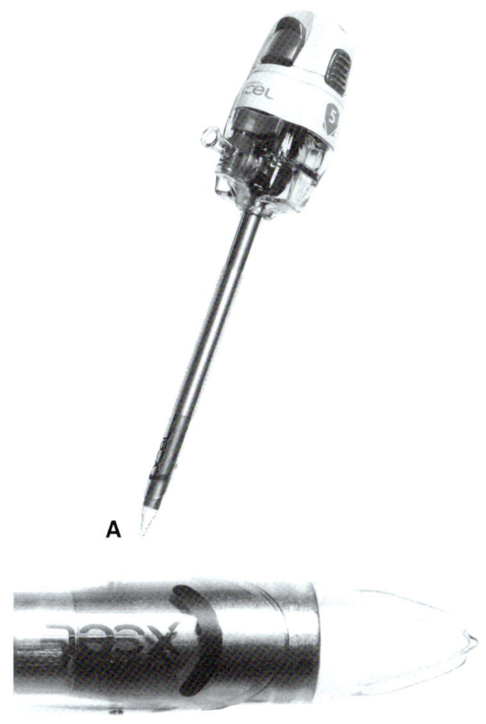

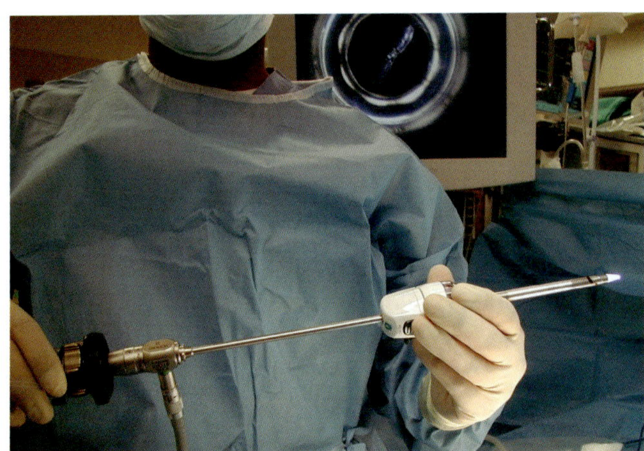

FIGURE 11-3. (A,B) Optical viewing trocar with a bladeless tip. Endopath Xcel. (Courtesy of Ethicon Endo-Surgery, Inc. All rights reserved.)

L/min by "shaking" the needle; they use short, rapid, circular motions, inscribing an ellipse with the tip. They report no mortality or vascular trauma from this technique in 600 consecutive morbidly obese patients; one seromuscular injury to the transverse colon was closed laparoscopically without sequelae.

After achieving a pressure of 15 mm Hg, primary ports are placed either at the Veress needle site or at an alternative site, taking care to maximize surgeon body mechanics to avoid excessive excursion of the trocar. Methods to minimize complications include raising the table to waist height, using the shortest ports that will achieve peritoneal entrance, avoiding reaching across the table to place ports, and positioning the surgeon's nondominant hand along the sheath to prevent excess insertion (8).

Direct trocar placement without pneumoperitoneum is performed at the umbilicus in a manner similar to Veress needle placement described above. Precise location and trajectory to the inferior sagittal midline is emphasized. The complication rate is similar to Veress needle use in most studies (0.3%), including a large meta-analysis (9–11). Another option is a fascial-dilating long conical head that provides a rectus sheath "hooking" maneuver to lift the fascia and promote negative intraabdominal pressure during puncture (45 cadavers studied). This is similar to another screw-type device recently described for use in the bariatric population (3,12).

Another direct system was designed to provide real-time visual feedback to the blind passage of an initial

trocar, with or without pneumoperitoneum. One system (Visiport, United States Surgical, Norwalk, CT) uses a bladed tip to incise layers; the other (Endopath Xcel, Ethicon Endo-Surgery, Cincinnati, OH) (Fig. 11-3) has a transparent conical bladeless terminal (Fig. 11-4). Both are designed for coaxial laparoscopic examination of the layers as they are traversed. The theory is that, with

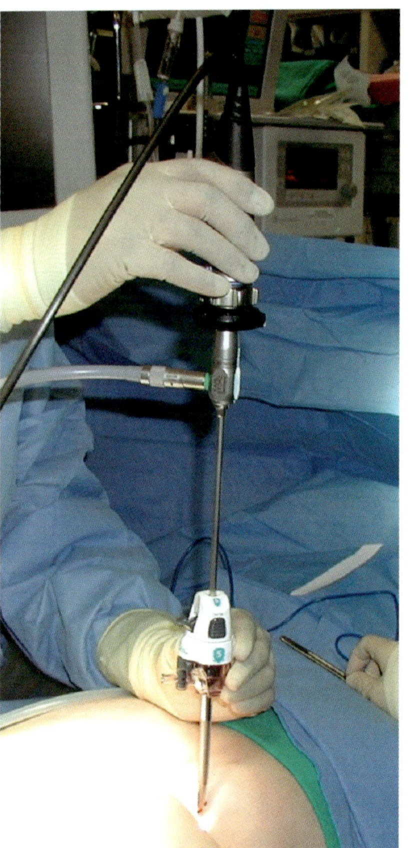

FIGURE 11-4. A 5-mm optical viewing trocar can be used to obtain access to the peritoneal cavity. (A) The camera is focused on the clear tip of the obturator. (B) The layers of the abdominal wall are directly viewed as the trocar passes through them. Endopath Xcel. (Courtesy of Ethicon Endo-Surgery, Inc. All rights reserved.)

observation, injury can be avoided. Early published experience described a low complication rate (13); however, a review of national databases shows a much higher rate, with 79 serious complications, 37 major vascular injuries, and four deaths from 1994 to 2000 (14). Meta-analysis reveals a trend toward more complications with the devices (and with Veress needles) compared to an open approach in general surgery applications (15).

Open Methods

Hasson et al. (2) described complications from Veress needle use and advocated an "open" approach with a 1- to 1.5-cm incision at the umbilicus, exposing the fascia and peritoneum under direct vision. A blunt obturator-cannula system (Fig. 11-5) is then inserted directly into the abdomen, anchored in place by fascial sutures used to close this incision later. Advantages include an extremely low (but not absent) risk of aortic injury (16), faster insufflation, and the ability to gain access in a hostile abdomen. Disadvantages include extremely difficult exposure in obese patients, perception of a higher degree of difficulty, and a slightly higher risk of bowel injury. In addition, maintenance of a leak-free seal around the port in severely obese individuals is often problematic. There is a possible selection bias in reported series, as this is used more in reoperative surgery and when access is expected to be unsuccessful with other

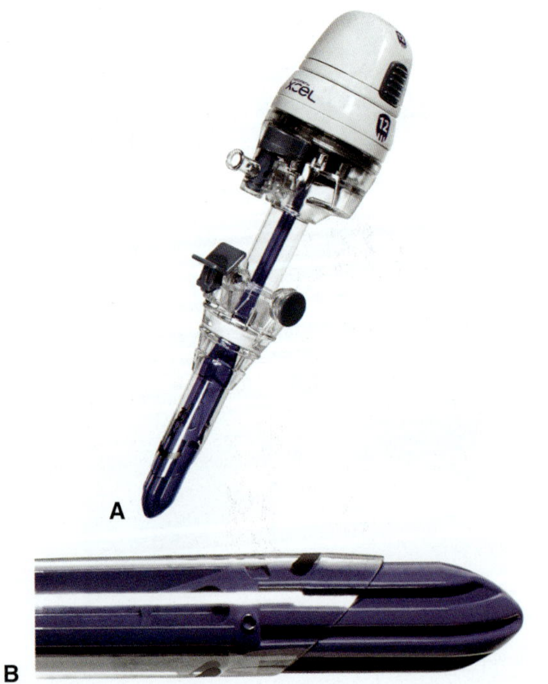

FIGURE 11-5. (A,B) Blunt trocar for use with the open technique of abdominal access. Endopath Xcel. (Courtesy of Ethicon Endo-Surgery, Inc. All rights reserved.)

techniques. The time duration of the definitive operation is equal to that with Veress access (2).

A modification of the Hasson technique is a "mini-open" transumbilical incision for placement of a 5-mm blunt cannula under direct vision. It does not use fascial anchoring sutures, is recommended for an uncomplicated abdomen, and has limited applicability to the morbidly obese population (17). Senapati et al. (18) describe a "semi-open" alteration of the Hasson technique by opening the linea alba, but passing a blunt tapered trocar through the peritoneum blindly. They described one minor liver injury in 241 patients. Balloon-tipped blunt ports are used extensively in inguinal hernia repair, and are beginning to be used for intraperitoneal procedures as well. Cost factors may limit the broader use of these devices (19).

Abdominal Evaluation

Regardless of access technique, on inserting a laparoscope, one should inspect the abdomen for inadvertent injury, with careful attention to mesentery, omentum, retroperitoneum, abdominal wall, and adjacent bowel. The abdomen should be desufflated immediately for hypotension, bradycardia, or the inability to ventilate properly. Expeditious re-inspection of the field laparoscopically (at a lower abdominal pressure) should include an assiduous search for vascular injury. If unexplained hypotension persists, conversion to laparotomy to more fully explore the retroperitoneum should be considered. A high index of suspicion is vital to avoid exsanguination from a major vessel laceration.

Secondary Access

Additional portals of entry for working and retracting instruments are needed in multiple sites. Commonly used types are pyramidal cutting tips, retractable blades, retractable "safety" shields, conical tapered tips, radial dilating cannulae, and screw devices. All should be placed perpendicular to the abdominal wall under constant direct laparoscopic vision. Trocars of different lengths can be used depending on the thickness of the abdominal wall (Fig. 11-6). In morbidly obese patients, this may not allow acceptable degrees of freedom of movement within the operative field, due to the thickness of the subcutaneous tissues. Anticipated use of the particular port and its instrumentation should be carefully considered, and ports should be angled to maximize freedom within the desired range. This requires considerable experience and is a great source of frustration in the early learning curve in bariatric surgery.

Comparison of different cannulae show mixed results. Radial dilating ports show smaller fascial and muscular

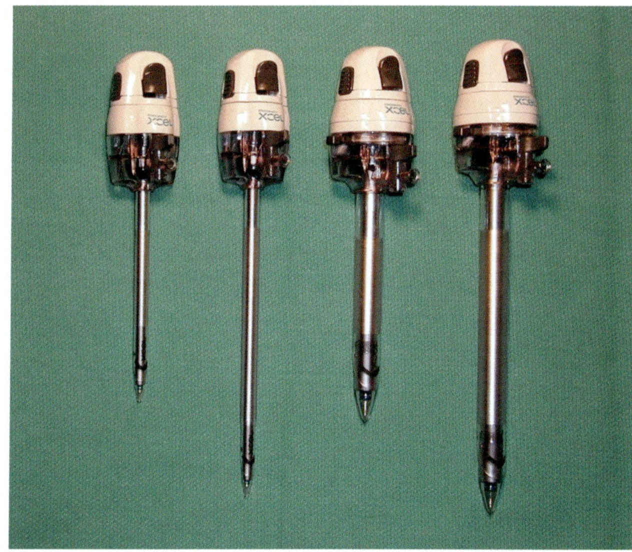

FIGURE 11-6. Trocars of different lengths and diameters should be available, particularly when operating on morbidly obese patients; 5- and 10-mm trocars 100 mm and 150 mm in length are shown. Endopath Xcel. (Courtesy of Ethicon Endo-Surgery, Inc. All rights reserved.)

defects with decreased nociception (20). It appears that the threaded screw [Endoscopic threaded imaging port (EndoTIP); Karl Storz Endoscopy America, Culver City, CA], which uses lateral spreading forces rather than axial forces, and conical ports have a lower incidence of abdominal wall vessel injury (3,21). "Safety" shields on cutting trocars have not reduced injury rates, and underreporting is common with 408 major injuries reported to the Food and Drug Administration (FDA) from 1993 to 1996, despite much lower aggregate numbers observed in the descriptive medical literature (22,23).

Complications

Mortality from access injury is estimated at 0.05%, with anesthesia complications, vascular injury, and delayed diagnosis of bowel injury as the three leading causes. Morbidity is more difficult to estimate. Historically, reports from Germany in 300,000 gynecologic patients undergoing minor procedures from 1978 to 1982 showed an overall access complication rate of 0.04% (24). Despite advances in technique, instrumentation, knowledge of the anatomy and physiology of pneumoperitoneum, and better training, rates are essentially unchanged. Catarci et al.'s (25) retrospective survey-based review of 12,919 procedures showed a 0.05% major vascular, 0.06% visceral, and 0.07% minor vascular injury incidence. Meta-analysis of prospective, randomized studies showed major complications of 0% to 2% in open access and 0% to 4% with closed access. The low fre-

quency of injuries and relatively small sample size compared to power requirements make conclusions as to safety unsubstantiated. However, there was a clear trend toward fewer visceral and vascular injuries with an open technique (15,16). Despite this, the open technique can have catastrophic major vascular injuries (26,27), and vigilance is necessary. As noted, use of open laparoscopic access in the severely obese patient is technically difficult.

Multiple mechanisms for injury are present, and immediate recognition is vital to limit patient morbidity and mortality. The most common injuries are from Veress needles or direct trocar tips used in closed entry. These injuries may not be recognized initially due to the advancement and then retraction of the device during its blind excursion. Cited causes of access injury include excessive force, inadequate skin incision, excessive laxity of the abdominal wall, inadequate pneumoperitoneum, and incomplete use of balancing motor forces that avoid unplanned advancement of the device. Learning appropriate surgeon body mechanics and knowing the patterns of injury can help reduce risk (23). Typical lesions described are aortic bifurcation, left iliac vein, and right iliac artery lacerations. These have close proximity to the umbilicus, and their retroperitoneal location can obscure the initial recognition of injury; vasoconstriction can temporarily stop bleeding, contributing to the lack of recognition of the problem. Bowel injuries frequently are small, have surrounding seromuscular spasm, and may not be suspected. Delay in the diagnosis, especially with partially contained retroperitoneal tears (visceral or vascular), can cause exsanguination, sepsis, peritonitis, abscess, enterocutaneous fistula, and death (28).

Underreporting of access-related complications is common, possibly due to the retrospective nature of many studies or variable attribution of causation of injury (assuming bowel injury is from cautery rather than access). Selection bias is likely, as experience levels are high in sites of large trials, often excluding smaller institutions and individual practitioners, thus skewing data. To address this issue, FDA device complication registries from 1993 to 1996 were reviewed, and they showed 408 access-related injuries, 87% with disposable trocars with "safety" shields; 26 deaths were reported in this series. The aorta (23%) and vena cava (15%) were most commonly injured. Concern about device malfunction was raised in 10%; however, only one of 41 allegations was verified (18).

In the bariatric population, the higher incidence of left upper quadrant primary access can shift injury attention to visceral, omental, and epigastric vessels. Visceral vessel injury is rarely identified when there is overlying mesenteric fat and peritoneum. Omental and epigastric vessel injury is usually more obvious, but again, vasoconstriction can sequester this injury until after the operation is over, leading to postoperative hemorrhage. Bowel injury from access is less common in the bariatric population, with the exception of the transverse colon (7,29).

Laceration of the epigastric vessels is rarely reported but is common anecdotally, as techniques for controlling such bleeding are numerous throughout the literature. Options include applying pressure with the inciting port or instruments placed through other ports, horizontal mattress suture, enlarging the port with direct visualization and ligation, and placement of a tamponade device (usually a Foley catheter pulled snugly against the abdominal wall) (28). The prevalence and impact of such complications is unmeasured.

Other abdominal wall complications involve nerve damage (transection with motor or sensory loss, neuropraxia, partial laceration with resultant neuroma formation) and muscular impairment (scarring causing spasm, chronic pain, laceration with local loss of function). These are poorly defined and unlikely to be quantified. Acute dehiscence is not reported in laparoscopic gastric bypass (29). Herniation does occur; however, there is difficulty in estimating the number of cases for two reasons. Asymptomatic patients are rarely diagnosed, and symptomatic patients may have vague intermittent symptoms attributed to the postoperative state. Rates from 0.02% to 1.8% have been reported, but data from 3464 cases showed a 0.47% rate (29). Richter's hernia may be more common than in open bariatric surgery, and should be considered in any patient with acute abdominal pain. Prevention of hernia should focus on reducing myofascial defect size, use of blunt trocars, closure of any port defect of 10mm or greater, and direct visualization of closure.

Miscellaneous adverse events include carbon dioxide dissection from Veress misplacement and leakage about a port, which can be extensive and spread to the mediastinum, neck, or even pericardium. Untreated, this can cause cardiovascular embarrassment directly from compressive forces, or indirectly from hypercapnia (30). Other unintended outcomes include pneumothorax, adhesion avulsion with bowel laceration or bleeding, and cardiac arrhythmias.

Conclusion

Access procedures are not standardized and the ideal device and technique has not been identified. The choice of access should be modified to match patient risk factors and surgeon experience. To identify complications promptly, one needs a high index of suspicion with any unexpected or unusual operative findings, hypotension, or other deviations from routine operations. Conversion to laparotomy should always be considered in such situations and should not be considered a failure.

References

1. Veress VJ. Eine nadel für gefahrlose Anwendung des Pneumoperitoneums. Gastroenterologia 1961;96:150–152.
2. Hasson HM, et al. Open laparoscopy: 29-year experience. Obstet Gynecol 2000;96:763–766.
3. Ternamian AM, Deitel M. Endoscopic threaded imaging port (EndoTIP) for laparoscopy: experience with different body weights. Obes Surg 1999;9:44–47.
4. Hazebroek EJ, et al. Impact of temperature and humidity of carbon dioxide pneumoperitoneum on body temperature and peritoneal morphology. J Laparoendosc Adv Surg Tech A 2002;12(5):355–364.
5. Wills VL, Hunt DR. Pain after laparoscopic cholecystectomy. Br J Surg 2000;87(3):273–284.
6. Schaller G, Kuenkel M, Manegold BC. The optical "Veress-needle"-initial puncture with a minioptic. Endosc Surg Allied Technol 1995;3(1):55–57.
7. Schwartz ML, Drew RL, Andersen JN. Induction of pneumoperitoneum in morbidly obese patients. Obes Surg 2003; 13:601–604.
8. Munro MG. Laparoscopic access: Complications, technologies, and techniques. Curr Opin Obstet Gynecol 2002;14: 365–374.
9. Jacobson MT, et al. The direct trocar technique: an alternative approach to abdominal entry for laparoscopy. JSLS 2002;6(2):169–174.
10. Merlin TL, et al. Systematic review of the safety and effectiveness of methods used to establish pneumoperitoneum in laparoscopic surgery. Br J Surg 2003;90:668–679.
11. Yerdel MA, et al. Direct trocar insertion versus Veress needle insertion in laparoscopic cholecystectomy. Am J Surg 1999;177:247–249.
12. Tansatit T, et al. Dilating missile trocar for primary port establishment: a cadaver study. J Med Assoc Thai 2002; 85(suppl 1):S320–326.
13. String A, et al. Use of the optical access trocar for safe and rapid entry in various laparoscopic procedures. Surg Endosc 2001;15(6):570–573.
14. Sharp HT, et al. Complications associated with optical access laparoscopic trocars. Obstet Gynecol 2002;99:553–555.
15. Molloy D. Laparoscopic entry: a literature review and analysis of techniques and complications of primary port entry. Aust N Z J Obstet Gynaecol 2002;42(3):246–254.
16. Hanney RM, et al. Use of the Hasson cannula producing major vascular injury at laparoscopy. Surg Endosc 1999;13: 1238–1240.
17. Carbonell AM, et al. Umbilical stalk technique for establishing pneumoperitoneum. J Laparoendosc Adv Surg Tech A 2002;12(3):203–206.
18. Senapati PSP, et al. "Semi-open" blunt primary access to the abdominal cavity during laparoscopic surgery: A new technique. J Laparoendosc Adv Surg Tech 2003;13(5):313–315.
19. Bernik TR, et al. Balloon blunt-tip trocar for laparoscopic cholecystectomy: Improvement over the traditional Hasson and Veress needle methods. J Laparoendosc Adv Surg Tech 2001;11(2):73–78.
20. Tarnay CM, Glass KB, Munro MG. Incision characteristics associated with six laparoscopic trocar-cannula systems:

a randomized, observer-blinded comparison. Obstet Gynecol 1999;94:89–93.

21. Hurd WW, Wang L, Schemmel MT. A comparison of the relative risk of vessel injury with conical versus pyramidal laparoscopic trocars in a rabbit model. Am J Obstet Gynecol 1995;173:1731–1733.

22. Campo R, Gordts S, Brosens I. Minimally invasive exploration of the female reproductive tract in infertility. Reprod Biomed Online 2002;4(suppl 3):40–45.

23. Chandler JG, Corson SL, Way LW. Three spectra of laparoscopic entry access injuries. J Am Coll Surg 2001;192(4):478–491.

24. Riedel HH, et al. German pelviscopic statistics for the years 1978–1982. Endoscopy 1986;18:219–222.

25. Catarci M, et al. Major and minor injuries during the creation of pneumoperitoneum: A multicenter study on 12919 cases. Surg Endosc 2001;15:566–569.

26. Soderstrom RM. Injuries to major blood vessels during endoscopy. J Assoc Gynecol Laparosc 1997;4:395–398.

27. Vilos GA. Litigation of laparoscopic major vessel injuries in Canada. J Am Assoc Gynecol Laparosc 2000;7:503–509.

28. Philips PA, Amaral JF. Abdominal access complications in laparoscopic surgery. J Am Coll Surg 2001;192(4):525–536.

29. Podnos YD, et al. Complications after laparoscopic gastric bypass: A review of 3464 cases. Arch Surg 2003;138:957–961.

30. Kent III RB. Subcutaneous emphysema and hypercarbia following laparoscopic cholecystectomy. Arch Surg 1991;126:1154–1156.

12
Comparison of Open Versus Laparoscopic Obesity Surgery

Ninh T. Nguyen and Bruce M. Wolfe

Background

Bariatric surgery was developed in the mid-1950s with the introduction of jejunoileal bypass, and was expanded in the 1960s with the Roux-en-Y gastric bypass (GBP) (1). Recently, there has been an increase in the demand for bariatric surgery and in turn an increase in the number of surgeons interested in learning bariatric surgery. This increase in enthusiasm and growth in the field of bariatric surgery is related, in a large part, to the development of the laparoscopic approach to bariatric surgery. Laparoscopic gastric banding was first reported in 1993 (2). In 1994, the preliminary techniques of both laparoscopic vertical banded gastroplasty and laparoscopic GBP were reported in the literature (3,4). By 2000, even a complex bariatric operation such as the biliopancreatic diversion with duodenal switch was attempted laparoscopically (5). At the current writing, essentially all commonly performed bariatric operations can be done by the laparoscopic technique.

To understand the development of laparoscopic bariatric surgery, we must understand the history of laparoscopic surgery. Laparoscopic surgery was developed in the late 1980s with the introduction of laparoscopic cholecystectomy. This single operation revolutionized and paved the way for surgeons to perform abdominal surgery using a less invasive approach. In the decade after the introduction of laparoscopy, the laparoscopic technique was applied to all areas of general surgery. By 1992, laparoscopic cholecystectomy had become the new standard for symptomatic cholelithiasis even before randomized trials demonstrated its clinical benefits (6).

Similar to the enthusiasm for laparoscopic cholecystectomy, we are beginning to see an increase in the demand for bariatric surgery with the introduction of the laparoscopic approach to bariatric surgery. The consumer views laparoscopic bariatric surgery as a minimally invasive procedure with less postoperative pain, lower morbidity, and a faster recovery. This notion of improved outcomes with laparoscopic bariatric surgery was derived from the public's perception of improved outcome after laparoscopic cholecystectomy and other laparoscopic operations such as laparoscopic solid organ removal, laparoscopic Nissen fundoplication, and laparoscopic ventral hernia repair. However, can we assume that the clinical benefits observed for these laparoscopic operations also apply to laparoscopic bariatric surgery? To answer this question, it is important to consider that laparoscopic bariatric surgery is performed in a different patient population (the morbidly obese) with more preexisting medical conditions, and the operation is often longer and technically more difficult than a routine laparoscopic cholecystectomy or Nissen fundoplication. Therefore, the debate about laparoscopic vs. open bariatric surgery is important, as the benefits observed after other laparoscopic operations do not necessarily apply to the morbidly obese. In addition, an understanding of the pros and cons of laparoscopic bariatric surgery is necessary, as many surgeons are now considering developing a laparoscopic bariatric surgery practice and many morbidly obese patients are seeking this surgical option.

Since Roux-en-Y GBP is the most commonly performed bariatric operation in the United States, this chapter discusses the differences between the laparoscopic and open approaches to GBP and the differences between laparoscopic and open bariatric surgery, reviews the important measures of outcome when comparing two different operative techniques, emphasizes the importance of a valid comparison, and reviews the differences in both the physiologic and clinical outcomes between the two techniques.

Is Laparoscopic Bariatric Surgery a Better Operation?

Is laparoscopic GBP truly a better operation than open GBP? This is an important question. Proponents for the laparoscopic approach have stated that the benefits of laparoscopic GBP should be similar to the benefits observed for other laparoscopic operations such as cholecystectomy, removal of solid organs, and Nissen fundoplication. Intuitively, the benefits of laparoscopy should apply to morbidly obese patients undergoing Roux-en-Y GBP as long as the laparoscopic operation can be performed safely and the fundamentals of the open surgery are followed. The potential benefits of laparoscopic bariatric surgery include less postoperative pain, less blood loss, shorter hospital stay, faster recovery, fewer wound complications, and better cosmesis. In addition, proponents for the laparoscopic approach have stated that laparoscopic GBP is safe when performed by surgeons who have experience in the laparoscopic technique. In contrast, opponents of the laparoscopic approach have stated that laparoscopic GBP is associated with a longer operative time and has an increased risk for complications such as anastomotic leak and bowel obstruction. Furthermore, in the hands of an experienced surgeon, open GBP can be performed through a relatively small upper abdominal incision, often in 1.5 hours, and most patients can be discharged within 3 days. Therefore, open bariatric surgery should be the gold standard operation until evidence-based clinical trials demonstrate that the benefits of laparoscopic bariatric surgery outweigh those of open bariatric surgery.

Certainly a randomized trial comparing laparoscopic vs. open bariatric surgery is the best method of evaluating a new operative treatment. The strength of a randomized trial is the random allocation of patients to treatment groups and is currently the most accepted evidence-based method for examining a new hypothesis. With a large sample size, the randomization process will by chance risk-adjust the two study groups with an end point of homogeneity between the groups. However, a randomized trial, by its design, lacks generalization, and the results can only be interpreted in the context of the stringent criteria set forth in the trial. In addition to the method of evaluation, it is equally important to determine which outcomes to measure and with what method to measure them. Some of the questions that need to be addressed include the following: (1) Is there any evidence to support the notion that laparoscopic GBP results in a reduced surgical injury compared with open GBP? (2) Is there any evidence to support the clinical advantages of laparoscopic GBP? (3) Are the benefits of the laparoscopic approach outweighed by the theoretical risk of a higher complication rate and longer operative time?

Fundamental Differences

It is important to understand the fundamental differences between the laparoscopic and open approaches to bariatric surgery to understand the possible differences in clinical outcomes between the two operations. The primary differences between the two procedures are the length of the abdominal incision (the method of access), the method of exposure, and the extent of operative trauma. Open GBP is commonly performed through an upper abdominal midline incision, whereas laparoscopic GBP is performed through five or six small abdominal access incisions. The methods of exposure during open GBP are the use of abdominal wall retractors and mechanical retraction of the abdominal viscera. In contrast, the methods of exposure during laparoscopic GBP are the use of pneumoperitoneum to create a working space and gravity for displacement of the abdominal viscera. By reducing the length of the surgical incision and eliminating the need for mechanical retraction of the abdominal wall and viscera, we believe that the operative trauma after laparoscopic GBP is reduced compared with that of open GBP. However, the use of carbon dioxide and the pressure effects of pneumoperitoneum during laparoscopic surgery can result in alteration of many intraoperative bodily functions. Carbon dioxide absorption occurs during pneumoperitoneum and can result in systemic hypercarbia, hypercapnia, and respiratory acidosis. In addition, the increased intraabdominal pressure at 15 mm Hg intraoperatively may affect body organs such as the lung, heart, and kidneys.

Important Measures of Outcome

When comparing the outcomes of a single operation performed by two different techniques, it is crucial to understand which outcome measures are important. The measures of outcome can be evaluated from the standpoint of the surgeon, the patient, or the health system. The surgeon tends to evaluate outcome using concrete evidence such as operative time, length of hospital stay, and morbidity. The health system looks at outcome globally through clinical performance measures and takes into account the length of hospitalization, quality of care, utilization of services, and cost. Most procedures are based on a per diem rate, and any laparoscopic procedure that shortens hospitalization may be scrutinized. In contrast, looking from a patient perspective, what is truly important is patients' satisfaction with their operative experience, the amount of postoperative pain/discomfort, and the time duration of functional recovery. With so many different clinical outcome measures, it is important for an investigator to use good measures of outcome and to determine how to measure these outcomes. Opinions vary regarding the most appropriate measures of outcome, but it is important to understand how these measures may be used by physicians to improve practice patterns and how it can change their decision making.

Some of the commonly used measures of outcome include operative time and length of hospital stay. A short operative time is always preferable, but as the sole outcome measure has never been shown to correlate with a better operative outcome. Similarly, the length of hospital stay can be misleading, as it represents only the period of hospitalization that is considered to be safe before discharging a patient. However, knowing what we know about the results of laparoscopic cholecystectomy, patients who underwent open vs. laparoscopic cholecystectomy can be discharged on the same postoperative day but have different views about their experience. Although discharged on the same postoperative day, one patient can be comfortable and feel well while another can be uncomfortable because of persistent postoperative pain or discomfort and difficulty in mobilization.

Other parameters for measurement of outcome include postoperative pain and convalescence. The extent of postoperative pain can be multifactorial, but an important indicator in the extent of postoperative pain is the degree of surgical injury. A minor procedure is often associated with lower postoperative pain compared with a major operation. Recovery is also a good parameter for measurement of outcome, as patients undergoing a minor operation tend to recover faster than patients undergoing a major operation. However, the method of quantifying the time and type of recovery is variable. The two most frequently used parameters for measurement of recovery are time to return to work and time to return to activities of daily living. Time for return to work is clearly a poor parameter of assessment, as this parameter is subjective based on the patient's willingness to return to work. Some patients delay returning to work even though they are physically capable of doing so. Time for return to activities of daily living is a better parameter but is still too generalized and does not specify exactly the types of activities. A more specific definition of activities of daily living should include patients' recovery based on their physical, social, and sexual functioning, and general health. Another important measure of outcome is the extent of operative injury, based on the premise that the improved outcome after laparoscopic GBP is related to the reduced surgical injury compared to open GBP.

Valid Comparison

A comparison between laparoscopic and open bariatric surgery is valid only if the laparoscopic operation is similar to that of the open operation and the surgeon has passed the learning curve of the laparoscopic approach. We must compare apples to apples. For example, initially one of the criticisms of surgeons performing laparoscopic GBP was the omission of the important step of closing the mesenteric defects. Because of this omission, late bowel obstruction was observed in the early series of laparoscopic GBP, which prompted surgeons to begin closing all mesenteric defects (7). Since laparoscopic GBP is a complex advanced laparoscopic operation, passing the learning curve of the laparoscopic approach is an equally important task to ensure a valid comparison of the two techniques. In a prospective randomized trial comparing laparoscopic vs. open GBP, Westling and Gustavsson (8) reported no significant differences between the two techniques in postoperative pain, length of hospital stay, and length of sick leave from work, based on an intention-to-treat analysis. In their trial of 51 patients (30 laparoscopic and 21 open), conversion to laparotomy occurred in seven (23%) of 30 laparoscopic operations. Their study demonstrated that laparoscopic GBP is a technically difficult operation and that any comparison of the two operations (laparoscopic vs. open) must be performed once the surgeon has passed the learning curve of the laparoscopic operation.

There is a learning curve for all new laparoscopic operations. However, the learning curve for laparoscopic GBP is steeper than most other advanced laparoscopic operations. On a relative scale measuring the degree of technical difficulty, with 1 being the easiest and 10 being the most difficult laparoscopic procedure, we consider laparoscopic GBP to be a 9. Unlike laparoscopic cholecystectomy, laparoscopic GBP requires knowledge of bowel transection and reconstruction techniques and a large number of stapling and suturing tasks.

Physiologic Basis of Improved Outcome in Laparoscopic Bariatric Surgery

The primary premise of improved outcome after laparoscopic bariatric surgery is the reduced surgical insult to the host. Surgical insult or the extent of surgical injury is related to the extent of injury to the abdominal wall (skin, fascia) and intraabdominal viscera. However, it is a difficult task to quantify the extent of surgical injury between laparoscopic and open GBP. We previously examined this question by indirect measurement of third-space fluid accumulation after laparoscopic and open GBP (9). Surgical injury often results in accumulation of edema known as third-space fluid, and the degree of third-space fluid accumulation is often proportional to the extent of surgical trauma. We indirectly measured the extent of third-space fluid accumulation by measurement of the intraabdominal pressure. The abdominal cavity is a single cavity, and the presence of any postoperative fluid accumulation such as tissue and bowel edema, bowel distention, or intraperitoneal hemorrhage can result in an elevation of intraabdominal pressure. By measuring the bladder pressure (indirect measurement of intraabdominal pressure), we reported that the intraabdominal pressure after laparoscopic GBP was significantly lower than after open GBP on postoperative days 1, 2, and 3 (9). In addition, the intraabdominal pressure returned to within baseline values by day 2 in the laparoscopic group, whereas the intraabdominal pressure continued to be elevated even on postoperative day 3 in the open group.

Another method for evaluating the severity of surgical injury is measurement of the systemic stress response. The magnitude of the systemic stress response has been shown to be proportional to the degree of operative trauma. Interleukin-6 is a nonspecific proinflammatory cytokine and its level has been shown to correlate with the severity of operative injury. We previously reported that postoperative concentrations of interleukin-6 were significantly lower after laparoscopic GBP than after open GBP (10). These findings suggest that the operative injury after laparoscopic GBP is lower than the operative injury after open GBP, substantiating the physiologic benefits of the laparoscopic approach.

Clinical Outcomes

Postoperative Pain

Postoperative pain is an important measure of outcome, as it can be measured objectively. The degree of postoperative pain after open GBP is associated with the length of the surgical incision and the extent of operative dissection and operative trauma. In our prospective randomized trial comparing laparoscopic vs. open GBP, we reported that laparoscopic GBP patients used significantly less intravenous morphine sulfate than open GBP patients on the first postoperative day (46 ± 31 mg vs. 76 ± 39 mg, respectively) (11). Despite the higher amount of self-administered morphine sulfate, open GBP patients still reported higher visual analog scale pain scores than laparoscopic GBP patients (11). After discharge, open GBP patients continued to report higher visual analog scale pain scores on postoperative day 7 compared with laparoscopic GBP patients.

Complications

Initial reports of laparoscopic GBP suggested a higher leak rate after laparoscopic GBP than after open GBP (12,13). The relatively higher leak rate after laparoscopic GBP is likely related to the learning curve of the laparoscopic procedure. For example, Wittgrove and Clark (13) reported nine anastomotic leaks (3.0%) in their first 300 laparoscopic GBP procedures and only two leaks (1.0%) in their subsequent 200 laparoscopic GBP procedures.

The reduced incidence of wound infections after laparoscopic GBP is one of the easily recognized advantages of the laparoscopic approach (14). Wound infection after open GBP is a complicated problem, since it requires the opening of a large wound and a prolonged course of wound care. Conversely, wound infection after laparoscopic GBP can be managed easily with opening of the trocar incision and a short course of local wound care.

Another clinical advantage of laparoscopic GBP is the reduced incidence of a late incisional hernia. The incidence of a postoperative incisional hernia after open GBP can be as high as 20% (15). The majority of these incisional hernias require operative intervention, which likely increases the cost associated with open GBP. By reducing the size of the surgical incision, the risk of ventral hernia after laparoscopic GBP is essentially eliminated.

Recovery

Recovery can be measured subjectively by determining the patient's time to return to activities of daily living. We previously reported that laparoscopic GBP patients had a more rapid return to activities of daily living than did open GBP patients (16). In addition, we analyzed recovery based on the patients' ability to return to physical, social, and sexual functioning and the perception of their overall health. The short form SF-36 health survey was administered preoperatively and at 1, 3, and 6 months postoperatively. The SF-36 has questions that address patients' physical and social functioning and the perception of their general health. We used the Moorehead-Ardelt Quality-of-Life (QOL) questionnaire to specifically assess the patients' sexual interest/activity. From the SF-36 survey, we learned that recovery based on physical and social functioning at 1 and 3 months postoperatively was faster after laparoscopic GBP compared with open GBP (16). In addition, the score for the perception of overall health was higher in laparoscopic GBP patients than in open GBP patients when the health survey was measured at 1 month postoperatively. From the Moorehead-Ardelt QOL questionnaire, we learned that laparoscopic GBP patients had more sexual interest or resumed sexual activity earlier than open GBP patients at 3 months postoperatively (16). Overall, the results from our trial demonstrated that laparoscopic GBP patients had a faster recovery in the context of physical, social, and sexual functioning than open GBP patients. In addition, laparoscopic GBP patients perceived themselves to be in better overall health than open GBP patients in the first month after surgery—hence a perception of faster recovery.

Conclusion

Laparoscopic GBP is a complex advanced laparoscopic operation that accomplishes the same objectives as open GBP but avoids a large upper midline abdominal incision. The primary differences between laparoscopic and open bariatric surgery are the method of access and the method of exposure. By reducing the size of the surgical incision and the operative trauma associated with operative exposure, the surgical insult is less after laparoscopic compared with open bariatric surgery. We have reported a reduction in the surgical insult after laparoscopic GBP and believe that this is the physiologic basis for the observed clinical advantages of laparoscopic GBP. The important clinical advantages of laparoscopic GBP are not the reduced length of hospitalization but the reduction in postoperative pain, lower rate of wound-related complications, and faster recovery. Given the current available data, laparoscopic bariatric surgery should be the new standard for the treatment of morbid obesity as long as the surgeon has passed the learning curve of the laparoscopic approach.

References

1. Buchwald H. Overview of bariatric surgery. J Am Coll Surg 2002;194:367–375.
2. Catona A, Gossenberg M, La Manna A, Mussini G. Laparoscopic gastric banding: preliminary series. Obes Surg 1993;3;207–209.
3. Wittgrove AC, Clark GW, Tremblay LJ. Laparoscopic gastric bypass, Roux-en-Y: preliminary report of five cases. Obes Surg 1994;4:353–357.
4. Hess DW, Hess DS. Laparoscopic vertical banded gastroplasty with complete transection of the staple-line. Obes Surg 1994;4:44–46.
5. Ren CJ, Patterson E, Gagner M. Early results of laparoscopic biliopancreatic diversion with duodenal switch: a case series of 40 consecutive patients. Obes Surg 2000;10;514–523.
6. Eubanks S, Schauer PR. Laparoscopic Surgery. In: Sabiston DC, Lyerly HK, eds. Textbook of Surgery: The Biological Basis of Modern Surgical Practice, 15th ed. Philadelphia: WB Saunders, 1997:791.
7. Nguyen NT, Ho HS, Palmer LS, Wolfe BM. A comparison study of laparoscopic versus open gastric bypass for morbid obesity. J Am Coll Surg 2000;191:149–157.
8. Westling A, Gustavsson S. Laparoscopic vs open Roux-en-Y gastric bypass: a prospective, randomized trial. Obes Surg 2001;11:284–292.
9. Nguyen NT, Lee SL, Anderson JT, et al. Evaluation of intra-abdominal pressure after open and laparoscopic gastric bypass. Obes Surg 2001;11:40–45.
10. Nguyen NT, Goldman CD, Ho HS, Gosselin RC, Singh A, Wolfe BM. Systemic stress response after laparoscopic and open gastric bypass. J Am Coll Surg 2002;194:557–567.
11. Nguyen NT, Lee SL, Goldman C, et al. Comparison of pulmonary function and postoperative pain after laparoscopic versus open gastric bypass: a randomized trial. J Am Coll Surg 2001;192:469–476.
12. Schauer PR, Ikramuddin S, Gourash W, et al. Outcomes after laparoscopic Roux-en-Y gastric bypass for morbid obesity. Ann Surg 2000;232:515–529.
13. Wittgrove AC, Clark GW. Laparoscopic gastric bypass, Roux-en-Y 500 patients: technique and results, with 3–60 month follow-up. Obes Surg 2000;10:233–239.
14. Higa KD, Boone KB, Ho T. Complications of the laparoscopic Roux-en-Y gastric bypass: 1,040 patients- what have we learned? Obes Surg 2000;10:509–513.
15. Kellum JM, DeMaria EJ, Sugerman HJ. The surgical treatment of morbid obesity. Curr Probl Surg 1998;35:791–858.
16. Nguyen NT, Goldman C, Rosenquist CJ, et al. Laparoscopic versus open gastric bypass: a randomized study of outcomes, quality of life, and costs. Ann Surg 2001;234:279–289.

13
Anesthesia for Bariatric Surgery: What a Surgeon Needs to Know

Saraswathy Shekar

With the continuing success of bariatric surgery, laparoscopic bariatric procedures are becoming the standard of care for treatment of morbid obesity. Morbid obesity surgical procedures make up 1% to 2% of anesthetic practice. This chapter reviews the factors that are relevant to the perioperative care of these patients.

Pathophysiology of Morbid Obesity

Pulmonary System

Airway

The airway is one of the most important concerns when anesthetizing this group of patients. The increased fat deposition in the cheeks and neck and the large breasts make direct laryngoscopy difficult. There is excessive palatal, pharyngeal, and supralaryngeal soft tissue, which may also contribute to difficult mask ventilation after induction of general anesthesia. Limited neck extension due to cervical fat pads also makes laryngoscopy difficult. The incidence of difficult intubation in the obese in previous studies has been reported as high as 13% to 15.5% (1–5).

Brodsky et al. (4), in their study of difficult intubation factors in the morbidly obese, determined that large neck circumference and high Mallampati score were the only predictors of potential intubation problems. Associated sleep apnea may be contributory to difficult intubation (6) and difficult mask ventilation (6–8).

Obstructive Sleep Apnea (OSA)

About 5% of patients with morbid obesity have OSA. The presence of redundant tissue narrows the pharynx at baseline, and the negative intrapharyngeal pressures caused by inspiration leads to further narrowing of the airway (8). Increased fat deposition in the pharynx results in decreased patency. This increases the likelihood that relaxation of the upper airway muscles after induction of anesthesia or after extubation will collapse the soft-walled pharynx between the uvula and epiglottis (9–11). Some reports have suggested an increased perioperative risk of OSA patients for upper-airway obstruction, oxygen desaturation, and cardiorespiratory arrest (11,12). Obstructive sleep apnea may be undiagnosed and hence it should be suspected in every obese patient presenting for surgery and anesthesia.

Pulmonary Function in Obesity

The morbidly obese patient can become hypoxemic in several ways. There is an increase in thoracic fat pads, which cause a restriction in chest wall movement. This contributes to reduced compliance of the chest cage. There is reduced pulmonary compliance, probably related to increased pulmonary blood volume secondary to the increased cardiac output (Fig. 13-1). The obese patient typically has a restrictive pattern on pulmonary function testing. All these factors contribute to hypoxemia in the morbidly obese patient, especially in the perioperative period.

Obesity Hypoventilation Syndrome

In patients with long-standing OSA, there is an alteration in the control of breathing and there are episodes of apnea without respiratory effort. These episodes are associated with a progressive desensitization of the respiratory centers to hypercapnia. These are initially nocturnal, but eventually the patient develops the obesity hypoventilation syndrome, which is characterized by obesity, hypersomnolence, hypoxia, hypercapnia, pulmonary hypertension, polycythemia, and right ventricular failure. Total pulmonary compliance is reduced by 60% in these patients (13,14), and they are at very high risk from anesthesia and surgery.

Cardiovascular System

Obesity is an independent risk factor for coronary artery disease, especially in patients younger than 50 years of

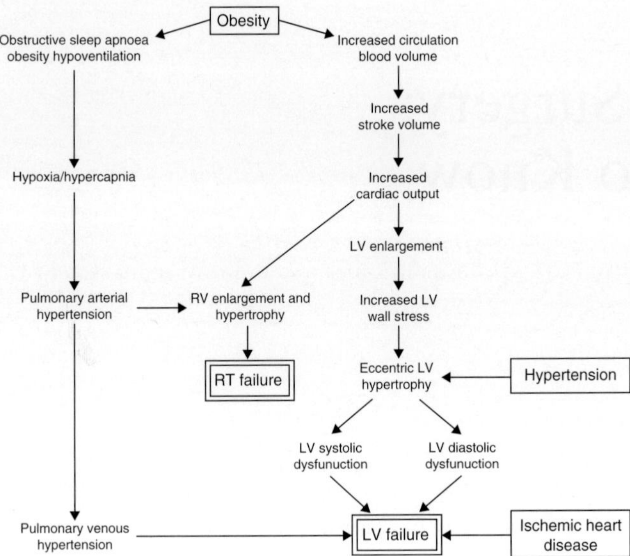

FIGURE 13-1. The etiology of obesity cardiomyopathy and its association with right-sided heart failure, systemic hypertension, and ischemic heart disease. LV, left ventricular; RV, right ventricular.

age (15). Obesity cardiomyopathy can occur in persons with severe and long-standing obesity. The cardiac output is increased as a consequence of the greater requirements of increased lean body mass, and is maintained by an increased stroke volume and high normal heart rate, and sustained by an increase in ventricular mass. Left ventricular hypertrophy and left ventricular diastolic dysfunction are also present, which are made worse by systemic hypertension or coronary artery disease (CAD) (Fig. 13-1). Right ventricular structure and function may be similarly affected by pulmonary hypertension related to chronic hypoxemia associated with OSA and obesity hypoventilation syndrome. The term *obesity cardiomyopathy* is applied when these cardiac structural and hemodynamic changes result in congestive heart failure (16).

Patients with morbid obesity also have high rates of sudden, unexpected cardiac death. The increase in left ventricular (LV) mass also implies an increase in nonmuscular tissue that plays a role in the development of electrical abnormalities, heart failure, and sudden death (17). Atrial fibrillation is more common in the obese when there is atrial dilation and left ventricular diastolic dysfunction (18).

Gastrointestinal System and Endocrine Systems

Obese patients are believed to be at risk for developing aspiration pneumonia. This has been ascribed to abnormal gastric emptying, increased intragastric volumes, and

hence an increased risk of aspiration (19), but this has been challenged (20). The risk of aspiration is also increased due to the increased incidence of hiatal hernia and raised intraabdominal pressure. It is possible that medications that increase gastric pH and reduce gastric volumes, such as proton pump inhibitors, can help reduce this complication. However, there is no evidence to support their routine use because of the infrequent incidence of aspiration and the multiplicity of factors that are associated with this complication. Indeed, the routine prescription of these drugs has not been recommended in the American Society of Anesthesiologists guidelines (21).

About 90% of morbidly obese patients show histologic abnormalities of the liver (22). One third of patients have fatty change involving more than 50% of hepatocytes. Nonalcoholic steatohepatitis (NASH) may be present with or without liver dysfunction (22). This has implications in the metabolism of inhaled and other drugs used in anesthetic practice. Preoperative liver function tests should be obtained. There is an increased incidence of type 2 diabetes mellitus, hypercholesterolemia, and hypothyroidism in this group of patients. Serum glucose control poses an additional problem in the obese diabetic patient population.

Renal System

There is increased glomerular filtration rate (by 40%) secondary to the increased cardiac output. Glomerulomegaly is common and often asymptomatic. Frequently, ensuing focal and segmental glomerulosclerosis may well be related to alterations in intraglomerular hemodynamics and may result in heavy proteinuria (23). Prolonged pneumoperitoneum during laparoscopic gastric bypass significantly reduces intraoperative urine output but does not adversely alter postoperative renal function (24).

Pharmacokinetics in Obesity

Obese people have larger absolute lean body masses (LBMs) as well as fat masses than nonobese individuals (25). Highly lipophilic substances such as barbiturates and benzodiazepines and propofol have increased volumes of distribution. There is high hepatic extraction and conjugation and hence no signs of drug accumulation when propofol was studied in morbidly obese patients (26).

Plasma cholinesterase activity increases in proportion to body weight. There is also a larger extracellular fluid compartment, and hence the absolute dosage of succinylcholine is increased. In an obese patient the dose of succinylcholine should be based on actual body mass, and not lean body mass (27). Lemmens et al. (28) recommend a dose of 1 mg/kg of succinylcholine for ideal intubating conditions (28).

There is no change in absolute clearance, volume of distribution, and elimination half-life of atracurium because of its lack of dependence on organ elimination. Vecuronium has impaired hepatic clearance and increased volume of distribution and leads to delayed recovery time. Vecuronium needs to be given per estimated lean body weight (29). Pancuronium has low lipid solubility, and the requirements may be increased in obese patients.

The two newer volatile anesthetics desflurane and sevoflurane have ideal pharmacologic properties for rapid induction and emergence from anesthesia in the morbidly obese. In a comparative study of propofol, desflurane, and isoflurane in morbidly obese patients undergoing laparoscopic gastroplasty, postoperative immediate and intermediate recoveries were more rapid after desflurane than after propofol or isoflurane anesthesia. This advantage of desflurane persists for at least 2 hours after surgery and is associated with both an improvement in patient mobility and a reduced incidence of postoperative desaturation (30).

Sevoflurane provides safe and better intraoperative control of cardiovascular homeostasis in morbidly obese patients undergoing laparoscopic gastric banding, with the advantage of a faster recovery and earlier discharge from the postanesthesia care unit (PACU) than does isoflurane (31). Sevoflurane, however, is known to release fluoride ions during metabolic degradation, and obese patients are at higher risk. Peak plasma levels of 50 μmol/L (the theoretical threshold for renal toxicity) are reached within 2 hours of sevoflurane anesthetic in obese patients without evidence of impaired renal function (32). The mechanism of enhanced biotransformation of volatile anesthetics by obese patients is not well understood. The theory that the lipid solubility of volatile anesthetics prolongs the recovery period in morbidly obese patients has been challenged (33). It is postulated that the delayed waking up from inhaled anesthetic is due to altered sensitivity of the central nervous system.

Recent studies, however, have found no clinically relevant difference in recovery in the PACU in obese patients anesthetized with desflurane or sevoflurane using the bispectral index (BIS) to monitor anesthetic depth (34,35).

Opiates have a larger volume of distribution in the obese because of their lipophilicity (25), but because of normal clearance their pharmacokinetics may be similar to those of nonobese patients. Dosing of fentanyl should be based on total body water (TBW). Dexmedetomidine is a specific α_2-adrenergic receptor agonist with antinociceptive and sedative properties that recently has been found to reduce requirements for inhaled agent, providing better control of heart rate and blood pressure and

improved postoperative analgesia. There is less ventilatory depression due to reduced narcotic use (36).

Total intravenous anesthesia techniques (TIVA) with propofol, alfentanil, or fentanyl and remifentanil can be safely used, but the incidence of postoperative nausea and vomiting is high in the remifentanil group (37). Remifentanil has similar pharmacokinetics in the lean and the obese. It is hydrolyzed by the blood and tissue esterases, resulting in rapid metabolism to inactive products. It also provides hemodynamic stability on induction and emergence (38,39).

Perioperative Management

Preoperative Evaluation

Pulmonary evaluation may include assessment for sleep apnea in the form of overnight pulse oximetry or polysomnography, especially in patients with overt history of snoring, daytime somnolence, or hypertension, or in patients whose collar size is greater than 17 inches (40). This method assesses the severity of sleep apnea and the need for continuous positive airway pressure (CPAP)/bi-level positive airway pressure (BiPAP), which needs to be instituted before surgery. This is important because the patient needs time to adjust to the equipment and optimize appropriate opening pressure with maximum comfort (8).

Preoperative lung function tests may be indicated in patients with chronic obstructive pulmonary disease, asthma, and smoking history. However, the body mass index (BMI) or preoperative lung function tests are not accurate predictors of postoperative pulmonary events. Preoperative medication history is important since some patients may have cardiac side effects including valvular disease (fenfluramine/dexfenfluramine) and pulmonary hypertension (above and mazindol).

Arterial CO_2 is a good predictor for the requirement of postoperative ventilation. Asthma, if present, should be optimized, and smoking ideally stopped 4 to 6 weeks prior to surgery. Metered dose inhalers of β_2-agonists/steroids should be continued perioperatively. Patients are usually advised to bring in their CPAP equipment for postoperative use.

Patients presenting for bariatric surgery should have a complete cardiopulmonary evaluation, including stress testing as indicated. The cardiovascular system is to be evaluated in all these patients since some of them cannot be assessed by their functional capacity [performing 4 metabolic equivalents (Mets)]. A 12-lead electrocardiogram may reveal evidence of left ventricular hypertrophy in patients with systemic hypertension and right ventricular hypertrophy in patients with sleep apnea syndrome and pulmonary hypertension. Transthoracic echocardiograms may be technically difficult, and transesophageal echocardiograms may be necessary to evaluate cardiac function in these patients. Some obese patients with symptoms of systemic and pulmonary congestion present with normal systolic function; however, diastolic function is often abnormal (41).

An echocardiogram provides valuable baseline function, and a digital subtraction echocardiogram (DSE) evaluates the development of segmental wall motion abnormalities when the heart is stressed.

The American College of Cardiology Guidelines (42) should be followed in these patients, as in other presurgical patients, bearing in mind that there are patient and equipment limitations in assessing cardiopulmonary function. For instance, cardiac catheterization can be performed only in patients weighing less than 500 pounds. Right heart catheterization may be indicated in patients with long-standing sleep apnea syndrome and obesity hypoventilation syndrome to assess the presence and severity of pulmonary hypertension. Concurrent cardiac medications, especially beta-blockers, need to be taken preoperatively and continued perioperatively. Angiotensin-converting enzyme (ACE) inhibitors may contribute to intraoperative hypotension (43).

Other preoperative considerations include airway assessment, and optimizing other medical conditions such as hypertension and diabetes. Venous access may be difficult; central venous access may be needed occasionally.

Airway assessment must be done with the patent in the seated and supine positions and should include the following (44):

1. Assessment of head and neck flexion, extension, and lateral rotation
2. Assessment of mouth opening (at least three finger-breadths), dentition and temporomandibular joint mobility
3. Assessment of thyromental distance
4. Assessment of size of tongue in relation to the oropharynx—the Mallampati classification (classes 1–4)
5. Assessment of presence of excessive pharyngeal tissue and enlarged tonsils

A past history of intubations may be helpful, but not if the patient has gained weight since then. Any patient with Mallampati class 3 or higher, in the presence of obstructive sleep apnea, is a candidate for awake intubation (awake look or fiberoptic). This is to avoid the "cannot intubate/cannot ventilate" situation, which is a possibility.

Antisialogogues may be necessary for awake intubations, especially fiberoptic intubations. Adequately topicalizing the hypopharynx is key to performing awake intubations. Anxiolysis with benzodiazepines may be used judiciously. Patients with gastroesophageal reflux disease (GERD) or hiatal hernia will benefit from H2-

receptor antagonists and nonparticulate antacid like sodium citrate. Metoclopramide may hasten gastric emptying but is ineffective in the presence of narcotics.

Intraoperative Management

The American Society of Anesthesiology (ASA) standard monitors are used, but invasive blood pressure monitoring may be necessary in patients with CAD, OSA, or pulmonary hypertension. Appropriate-size blood pressure cuffs should be used, otherwise the blood pressure will be overestimated. Central venous access may be needed in case of difficult venous access, but pulmonary artery catheters are rarely needed in laparoscopic procedures except in patients with severe cardiopulmonary disease.

The head and the neck of the patient should be placed in the so-called sniffing position, which consists of 30-degree flexion of the neck on the chest and 15-degree extension of the head at the atlanto-occipital joint necessary to bring into line the pharyngeal, oral, and laryngeal axes for a better laryngoscopic view.

An ideal way of achieving this position is by stacking blankets below the patient's shoulders and head such that the head, upper body, and shoulders are significantly elevated above the chest. The positioning should be such that an imaginary horizontal line should connect the patient's sternal notch with the external auditory meatus (45) (Fig. 13-2).

Anesthetic induction is traditionally accomplished using a rapid sequence technique. This has been ques-

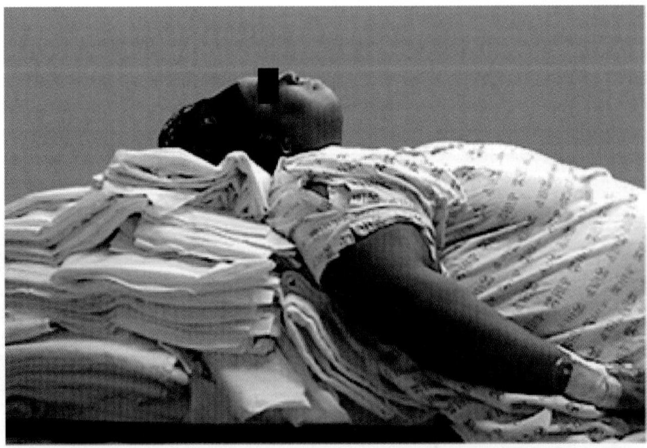

Figure 13-2. A morbidly obese patient in position for direct laryngoscopy. An imaginary horizontal line should connect the patient's sternal notch with the external auditory meatus. This is achieved by stacking blankets below the upper body, head and shoulders. (Levitan RM. Airway Cam Video Series, vol 3: Advanced Airway Imaging and Laryngoscopy Techniques. Wayne, PA: Airway Cam Technologies, 2003, with permission.)

tioned recently since the incidence of aspiration is lower than hypoxemia, and cricoid pressure (especially incorrectly applied) induced difficulties in laryngoscopy in these patients, especially in the presence of OSA (46). Establishing the adequacy of mask ventilation with cricoid pressure may be helpful in fasted nondiabetic obese patients having elective surgery.

All operating rooms catering to this group of patients should be equipped with difficult airway management devices like laryngeal mask airways (LMA) gum elastic bougies, different types of laryngoscope blades, short handles, fiberoptic scopes, and transtracheal jet ventilators. The intubating laryngeal mask airway (ILMA) or fast-track LMA have been used successfully for airway management in morbidly obese patients (47).

Anesthetic management does not differ from a standard general anesthetic for a laparoscopic procedure except in patients with severe pulmonary hypertension and significant cardiopulmonary disease. Hypoxia, hypercarbia, and acidosis may worsen pulmonary hypertension and should be avoided. Nitrous oxide is best avoided under such circumstances. Narcotics should be used judiciously in patients with OSA since they have increased risk of narcotic-induced upper airway obstruction after extubation.

Correct positioning of the tip of the endotracheal tube is essential to avoid an additional untoward endobronchial intubation or accidental extubation.

Abdominal insufflation and changes in table position (especially by voice activated table movement) lead to more frequent movements of the endotracheal tube in obese patients undergoing laparoscopic versus open gastroplasty.

Tiberiu Ezri et al. (48) compared the incidence of movements of the endotracheal tube within the trachea in morbidly obese patients undergoing laparoscopic gastroplasty with those undergoing open gastroplasty. Significant movement of the endotracheal tube was detected in laparoscopic procedures more often. This movement was associated with changes in the operating table position or abdominal gas insufflation specific to laparoscopic procedures more than in open abdominal surgery. Endobronchial intubation in these patients can result in severe hypoxemia.

It is crucial to have enough slack in the breathing circuit while harnessed onto the "tube tree" since endotracheal tubes have been inadvertently pulled out while a patient was placed in the steep reverse Trendelenburg position by the surgeon [using a voice-activated operating room (OR) table].

Intraoperative ventilation may be difficult, but larger tidal volumes do not improve oxygenation (49). Hypercapnia may be permitted during the period of pneumoperitoneum to prevent high airway pressures, which can cause barotrauma, as long as the $PaCO_2$ returns to baseline prior to emergence. The use of positive end-expiratory pressure (PEEP) may improve respiratory function more in the obese than in normal patients (50).

Clinical evaluation of volume status is difficult in the obese patient, especially when the intraabdominal pressure is increased and the urine output consequentially decreased.

Deep vein thrombosis (DVT) prophylaxis is required for all patients because these patients are hypercoagulable. Subcutaneous heparin or low-molecular-weight heparin is used. Pneumatic compression stockings in combination with the above medication are the current practice, and they need to be put on the patient prior to induction. Compression devises placed on the feet rather than the thighs or legs are easier to place and keep in place postoperatively.

These patients require specialized OR tables (weight capacity up to 1200 lb) with a footrest to support them in the steep reverse Trendelenburg position. Positioning of the patient to avoid nerve injuries is important since patients with extreme body habitus have a greater incidence of nerve injuries (51). All extremities must be cushioned and in a neutral position. It is important to remove the nasogastric tube prior to gastric stapling since there have been instances where the tube was stapled to the stomach.

Effects of Pneumoperitoneum

Morbidly obese patients have reduced lung volumes, decreased functional residual capacity (FRC), increased closing capacity (CC) leading to small airways closure, ventilation/perfusion mismatching, and an increase in the physiologic intrapulmonary shunt. These phenomena are exacerbated by supine positioning, general anesthesia, muscle relaxation, and institution of mechanical ventilation where a cephalad shift of the diaphragm and a blood shift into the chest could cause a further 50% decrease in FRC with worsening of hypoxemia (52).

Laparoscopic surgery is associated with more important intraoperative respiratory and circulatory changes than open procedures. Pneumoperitoneum induces changes in pulmonary mechanics and gas exchange. An intraabdominal insufflation pressure of 15 mm Hg is usually the safe upper limit with respect to pulmonary and hemodynamic effects. In the morbidly obese, abdominal insufflation causes moderate alterations in pulmonary mechanics, which are not accompanied by alterations in gas exchange. However, the insufflation pressures are frequently higher than 15 mmHg since the weight of an obese abdominal wall requires more pressure for elevation.

The previously mentioned factors (supine position, general anesthesia, muscle relaxation) are more important in contributing to hypoxemia in the obese; the abdominal insufflation is of minor significance.

In a study by Dumont et al. (53) of respiratory mechanics in morbidly obese patients undergoing laparoscopic gastroplasty, abdominal insufflation to 18 mm Hg caused a significant decrease in respiratory system compliance (31%), and a significant increase in peak (17%) and plateau (32%) airway pressures at constant tidal volume with a significant hypercapnia but no change in arterial oxygen saturations. Respiratory system compliance and pulmonary insufflation pressures returned to baseline values after abdominal deflation (53).

The hemodynamic response to laparoscopic surgery in the obese is characterized by an increase in cardiac output (due to increased heart rate), and neither the systolic nor diastolic blood pressure in patients without manifest cardiovascular disease is significantly affected by the introduction of pneumoperitoneum and positioning of the patient for surgery (54). This of course depends on the insufflating pressure. Intraabdominal pressures (IAPs) greater than 20 mm Hg compress the inferior vena cava, reducing venous return and decreasing cardiac output.

Postoperative Management

The pharyngeal musculature of severely obese patients, especially those with a history of sleep apnea, is sensitive to all anesthetics and narcotics, and thus recovery (i.e., maintaining airway patency) may take longer. These patients need to be extubated only when completely awake and following commands. The upright position helps improve FRC and oxygenation. A lubricated nasopharyngeal airway may be left in place prior to extubation. If in doubt, patients should be ventilated until fully awake.

Patients who are on CPAP/BiPAP may need to be placed on the machine earlier to prevent a pulmonary atelectasis and hypoxemia. Bilevel CPAP has been shown to significantly reduce pulmonary dysfunction after upper abdominal surgery in obese patients (55). General anesthesia in obese patients can generate much more atelectasis than in nonobese patients. Postoperative atelectasis remained unchanged for at least 24 hours in these patients, whereas atelectasis disappeared in the nonobese (56). Phillips and colleagues (57) reported no difference between obese and nonobese patients in the risk of pulmonary complications after laparoscopic cholecystectomy.

Patients with sleep apnea have rebound rapid eye movement (REM) sleep on the third postoperative day, which has been associated with increased prolonged apnea and myocardial events (58,59). It is thus important to observe patients with moderate to severe sleep apnea in a monitored care environment postoperatively.

The absorption of intramuscular narcotics may be unpredictable. Intravenous narcotics should be administered cautiously in patients with OSA and obesity hypoventilation syndrome. Deaths have been reported from parenteral narcotics administered to obese OSA patients (52). Postoperative analgesia is best administered by patient-controlled analgesia (PCA). Regional techniques are not routinely performed for laparoscopic bariatric procedures. Epidural anesthesia is useful in selected open bariatric procedures in providing excellent analgesia and reducing postoperative pulmonary complications.

Some of these patients develop esophageal spasm-like pains in the chest in the postoperative period, which may mimic ischemic myocardial ischemic pain. It usually responds to antacids and H2-receptor antagonists.

Conclusion

Morbidly obese patients present special risks for the anesthesiologist. All comorbid conditions should be evaluated and optimized prior to these elective procedures. This requires a team approach and adequate communication among the surgical team members and anesthesia providers. Overall, laparoscopic surgery confers definite advantages for the morbidly obese population. Awareness of and preparation for the unique needs and problems of morbidly obese patients undergoing either open or laparoscopic surgery will optimize outcomes and minimize anesthesia-related complications.

References

1. Buckley FP, Robinson NB, Simonowitz DA, et al. Anaesthesia in the morbidly obese. A comparison of anaesthetic and analgesic regimens for upper abdominal surgery. Anaesthesia (England) 1983;38(9):840–851.
2. Rose DK, Cohen MM. The airway: problems and prediction in 18,500 patients. Can J Anaesth 1994;41:372–383.
3. Wilson ME, Spiegelhalter D, Robertson JA, Lesser P. Predicting difficult intubation. Br J Anaesth 1988;22:969–973.
4. Brodsky JB, Lemmens HJM, Brock-Utne JG, Vierra M, Saidman LJ. Morbid obesity and tracheal intubation. Anesth Analg 2002;94:732–736.
5. Juvin P, Lavaut E, Dupont H, et al. Difficult tracheal intubation is more common in obese than in lean patients. Anesth Analg 2003;97(2):595–600.
6. Hiremath AS, Hillman DR, James AL, Noffsinger WJ, Platt PR, Singer SL. Relationship between difficult tracheal intubation and obstructive sleep apnea. Br J Anaesth 1998;80:606–611.
7. Barsh CI. The origin of pharyngeal obstruction during sleep. Sleep Breathing 1999;3:17–21.
8. Tung A, Rock P. Perioperative concerns in sleep apnea. Curr Opin Anesthesiol 2001;14(6):671–678.
9. Barthel SW, Strome M. Snoring, Obstructive sleep apnea, and surgery. Med Clin North Am 1999;83:85–96.

10. Strollo PJ, Rogers RM. Obstructive sleep apnea. N Engl J Med 1996;334;99–104.

11. Gentil B, Liebhart A, Fleury B. Enhancement of postoperative desaturation in heavy snorers. Anesth Analg 1995; 81:389–392.

12. Rennotte MT, Baele P, Aubert G, Rodenstein DO. Nasal continuous positive airway pressure in the perioperative management of patients with obstructive sleep apnea submitted to surgery. Chest 1995;107:367–374.

13. Sharp JT, Henry JP, Sweany SK, et al. The total work of breathing in normal and obese men. J Clin Invest 1964; 43:728.

14. Rochester DF, Enson Y. Current concepts in the pathogenesis of the obesity-hypoventilation syndrome, Am J Med 1974;57:402.

15. Hubert HB, Feinleib M, McNamara PM, Castelli WP. Obesity as an independent risk factor for cardiovascular disease: a 26-year follow-up of participants in the Framingham Heart Study. Circulation 1983;67(5):968–977.

16. Alpert MA. Obesity cardiomyopathy: pathophysiology and evolution of the clinical syndrome. Am J Med Sci 2001; 321(4):225–236.

17. Contaldo F, Pasanisi F, Finelli C, de Simone G. Obesity, heart failure and sudden death. Nutr Metab Cardiovasc Dis 2002;12(4):190–197.

18. Wang TJ, Parise H, Levy D, et al. Obesity and the risk of new-onset atrial fibrillation. JAMA 2004;292:2471–2477.

19. Vaughan RW, Bauer S, Wise L. Volume and pH of gastric juice in obese patients. Anesthesiology 1975;43(6):686–689.

20. Harter RL, Kelly WB, Kramer MG, Perez CE, Dzwonczyk RR. A comparison of the volume and pH of gastric contents of obese and lean surgical patients. Anesth Analg 1998;86:147–152.

21. American Society of Anesthesiologists Task Force on Preoperative Fasting. Practice guidelines for preoperative fasting and the use of pharmacologic agents to reduce the risk of pulmonary aspiration: application to healthy patients undergoing elective procedures. Anesthesiology 1999;90(3): 896–905.

22. Clain DJ, Lefkowitch JH. Fatty liver disease in morbid obesity. Gastroenterol Clin North Am 1987;16(2):239–252.

23. Cohen AH. Pathology of renal complications in obesity. Curr Hypertens Rep 1999;1(2):137–139.

24. Nguyen NT, Perez RV, Fleming N, Rivers R, Wolfe BM. Effect of prolonged pneumoperitoneum on intraoperative urine output during laparoscopic gastric bypass J Am Coll Surg 2002;195(4):476–483.

25. Cheymol G. Effects of obesity on pharmacokinetics. Clin Pharmacokinet 2000;39(3):215–231.

26. Servin F, Farinoti R, Harberer JP, et al. Propofol infusion for maintenance of anesthesia in morbidly obese patients receiving nitrous oxide: a clinical and pharmacokinetic study. Anesthesiology 1993;78;657–665.

27. Bentley JB. Pseudocholinesterase activity, and succinylcholine requirement. Anesthesiology 1982;57(1):48–49.

28. Lemmens HJM, Brodsky JB. The dose of succinylcholine in morbid obesity. Anesth Analg 2006;102(2):438–442.

29. Weinstein JA, Matteo RS, Ornstein E, Schwartz AE, Goldstoff M, Thal G. Pharmacodynamics of vecuronium and atracurium in the obese surgical patient. Anesth Analg 1988;67:1149–1153.

30. Juvin P, Vadam C, Malek L, et al. Postoperative recovery after desflurane, propofol, or isoflurane anesthesia among morbidly obese patients: a prospective randomized study. Anesth Analg 2000;91:714–719.

31. Torri G, Casati A, Albertin A, et al. Randomized comparison of isoflurane and sevoflurane for laparoscopic gastric banding in morbidly obese patients. J Clin Anesth 2001; 13(8):565–570.

32. Higuchi H, Satoh T, Arimura S, Kanno M, Endoh R. Serum inorganic fluoride levels in mildly obese patients during and after sevoflurane anesthesia. Anesth Analg 1993;77:1018–1021.

33. Cork RC, Vaughan RW, Bentley JB. General anesthesia for morbidly obese patients—an examination of postoperative outcomes. Anesthesiology 1981;54:310–313.

34. Arain SR, Barth CD, Shankar H, Ebert TJ. Choice of volatile anesthetic for the morbidly obese patient: sevoflurane or desflurane. J Clin Anesth 2005;17(6):413–419.

35. Luc EC, De Baerdemaeker SJ, Nadia MM, et al. Postoperative results after desflurane or sevoflurane combined with remifentanil in morbidly obese patients. Obes Surg 2006;16:728–733.

36. Feld JM, Hoffman WE, Stechert MM, Hoffman IW, Ananda RC. Fentanyl or dexmedetomidine combined with desflurane for bariatric surgery. J Clin Anesth 2006;18(1):24–28.

37. Gaszynski TM, Strzelczyk JM, Gaszynski WP. Postanesthesia recovery after infusion of propofol with remifentanil or alfentanil or fentanyl in morbidly obese patient. Obes Surg 2004;14:498–504.

38. Egan TD, Huizinga B, Gupta SK. Remifentanil pharmacokinetics in obese versus lean patients. Anesthesiology 1998;89:562–573.

39. Salihoglu Z, Demiroluk S, Demirkiran N, Kose Y. Comparison of effects of remifentanil, alfentanil and fentanyl on cardiovascular responses to tracheal intubation in morbidly obese patients. Eur J Anaesthesiol 2002;19(2):125–128.

40. Johns MW. A new method for measuring daytime sleepiness: the Epworth sleepiness scale. Sleep 1991;14(6):540–545.

41. Kaltman AJ, Goldring RM. Role of circulatory congestion in the cardiorespiratory failure of obesity. Am J Med 1976; 60:645–653.

42. Eagle KA, Berger PB, Calkins H, et al. ACC/AHA guideline update for perioperative cardiovascular evaluation for noncardiac surgery—executive summary: a report of the American College of Cardiology/American Heart Association Task Force on Practice Guidelines (Committee to Update the 1996 Guidelines on Perioperative Cardiovascular Evaluation for Noncardiac Surgery). J Am Coll Cardiol 2002;39(3):542–553.

43. McConachie I, Healy TE. ACE inhibitors and anaesthesia. Postgrad Med J 1989;65(763):273–274.

44. Adams JP, Murphy PG. Obesity in anaesthesia and intensive care. Br J Anaesth 2000;85(1):91–108.

45. Brodsky JB, Lemmens HJM, Brock-Utne JG, Saidman LJ, Levitan R. Anesthetic considerations for bariatric surgery:

proper positioning is important for laryngoscopy. Anesth Analg 2003;96:1841–1842.

46. Freid EB. The rapid sequence induction revisited: obesity and sleep apnea syndrome. Anesthesiol Clin North Am 2005;23(3):551–564.

47. Freppier J. Airway management using the intubating laryngeal mask airway for the morbidly obese patient. Anesth Analg 2003;96(5):1510–1515.

48. Ezri T, Hazin V, Warters D, Szmuk P, Weinbroum AA. The endotracheal tube moves more often in obese patients undergoing laparoscopy compared with open abdominal surgery. Anesth Analg 2003;96:278–282.

49. Bardoczky GI, Yernault JC, Houben JJ, d'Hollander AA. Large tidal volume ventilation does not improve oxygenation in morbidly obese patients during anesthesia. Anesth Analg 1995;81:385–388.

50. Pelosi P, Ravagnan I, Giurati F, et al. Positive end-expiratory pressure improves respiratory function in obese but not in normal subjects during anesthesia and paralysis. Anesthesiology 1999;91(5):1221–1231.

51. Warner MA, Warner ME, Martin JT. Ulnar neuropathy, incidence outcome and risk factors in sedated or anesthetized patients. Anesthesiology 1994;81:1332–1340.

52. Damia G, Mascheroni D, Croci M, Tarenzi L. Perioperative changes in functional residual capacity in morbidly obese patients. Br J Anaesth 1988;60: 574–578.

53. Dumont L, Mattys M, Mardirosoff C, Vervloesem N, Alle J, Massaut J. Changes in pulmonary mechanics during laparoscopic gastroplasty in morbidly obese patients. Acta Anaesthesiol Scand 1997;41(3):408–413.

54. Fried M, Krska Z, Danzig V. Does the laparoscopic approach significantly affect cardiac functions in laparoscopic surgery? Pilot study in non-obese and morbidly obese patients. Obes Surg 2001;11(3):293–296.

55. Joris J, Sottiaux T, Chiche JD, Luten I, Lamy M. Bi-level CPAP (BIPAP) reduces the postoperative restrictive pulmonary syndrome in obese patients after gastroplasty. *Br J Anaesth* 1994;**72**(suppl 1):A111.

56. Eichenberger A, Proietti S, Wicky S, et al. Morbid obesity and postoperative pulmonary atelectasis: an underestimated problem. Anesth Analg 2002;95(6):1788–1792.

57. Phillips EH, Carroll BJ, Fallas MJ, Pearlstein AR. Comparison of laparoscopic cholecystectomy in obese and non-obese patients. Am Surg 1994;60:316–321.

58. Knill RL, Moote CA, Skinner MI, Rose EA. Anesthesia with abdominal surgery leads to intensive REM Sleep during the first postoperative week. Anesthesiology 1990;73:52–61.

59. Peiser J, Ovnat A, Uwyyed K, Lavie P, Charuzi I. Cardiac arrhythmias during sleep in morbidly obese sleep-apneic patients before and after gastric bypass surgery. Clin Cardiol 1985;8(10):519–521.

14
Pneumoperitoneum in the Obese: Practical Concerns

Ninh T. Nguyen and Bruce M. Wolfe

Background

The laparoscopic approach to bariatric surgery was first reported in the early 1990s (1). With refinement of the laparoscopic approach to bariatric surgery, particularly laparoscopic gastric bypass, there has been a tremendous growth in the field of bariatric surgery. Patients view laparoscopic bariatric surgery as a less invasive approach and are more likely to seek laparoscopic surgical therapy for the treatment of morbid obesity. With an increase in the demand for bariatric surgery, there is also an increase in the number of surgeons interested in learning laparoscopic bariatric surgery. There has also been an increase in the number of institutions providing laparoscopic bariatric surgery workshops and growth in membership of the American Society for Bariatric Surgery. Therefore, it is important for surgeons performing laparoscopic bariatric surgery to understand the fundamental differences between laparoscopic and open surgery and possible intraoperative adverse consequences of pneumoperitoneum in the morbidly obese.

Fundamental Differences Between Laparoscopic Versus Open Bariatric Surgery

The benefits of laparoscopic bariatric surgery include reduced tissue trauma, less postoperative pain, and a faster postoperative recovery (2). The fundamental differences between the laparoscopic and open approaches to bariatric surgery are the method of access and method of exposure. Surgical access is generally obtained through an upper midline incision in open bariatric surgery and through five small abdominal incisions in laparoscopic bariatric surgery. Surgical exposure of the operative field includes the use of surgical retractors during open surgery and the use of carbon dioxide gas during laparo-

scopic surgery. Carbon dioxide (CO_2) gas has been used since the introduction of laparoscopic cholecystectomy in the late 1980s and has been the preferred gas medium for laparoscopy. Adverse consequences of CO_2 pneumoperitoneum include peritoneal absorption of CO_2 and hemodynamic alteration of various body organs from the increased intraabdominal pressure. Absorption of CO_2 can lead to hypercarbia and eventual systemic acidosis. The increased intraabdominal pressure at 15 mm Hg during laparoscopy has been shown to result in alteration of the vascular, renal, hepatic, and cardiorespiratory systems (3–6).

The physiologic effects of pneumoperitoneum have been thoroughly examined in the nonobese; however, few studies have examined these effects in the morbidly obese. In addition, laparoscopic gastric bypass is a complex operation and is often associated with a longer operative time than most other commonly performed laparoscopic procedures. A longer operative time during laparoscopic gastric bypass translates to a longer exposure for the patient to the adverse effects of pneumoperitoneum. Therefore, it is important for surgeons performing laparoscopic bariatric surgery to understand the physiologic effects of pneumoperitoneum in the morbidly obese.

Carbon Dioxide Absorption During Pneumoperitoneum

The use of CO_2 during pneumoperitoneum can result in systemic absorption and alteration of the acid–base balance. Absorption of CO_2 across the peritoneum is normally eliminated through the lungs because of its high aqueous solubility and diffusibility. However, if intraoperative ventilation is impaired, CO_2 absorption can result in hypercarbia, hypercapnia, and even acidosis. Intraoperative monitoring using end-tidal CO_2 ($ETCO_2$) is an important indicator of hypercarbia; however, $ETCO_2$

levels can underestimate the level of arterial partial pressure of CO_2 ($PaCO_2$). In a study of laparoscopic gastric bypass, Nguyen et al. (7) reported that $ETCO_2$ levels increased by 15% and $PaCO_2$ levels increased by 9% from baseline after abdominal insufflation; $PaCO_2$ levels remained stable during open gastric bypass but increased from 38 to 42 mm Hg during laparoscopic gastric bypass. In addition, pH levels decreased during laparoscopic gastric bypass. Therefore, appropriate changes in respiratory rate, tidal volume, and minute ventilation are necessary to prevent hypercarbia and acidosis. Dumont et al. (8) reported that minute ventilation increased by 21% in morbidly obese patients who underwent laparoscopic gastroplasty. Nguyen et al. (7) reported that respiratory rate was increased by 25% to minimize the rise of $ETCO_2$ and $PaCO_2$, and minute ventilation was increased by 21% during laparoscopic gastric bypass.

Absorption of CO_2 also increases pulmonary CO_2 excretion. By measuring the amount of pulmonary CO_2 excretion, Tan and colleagues (9) estimated that the volume of CO_2 absorbed from the peritoneal cavity ranged from 38 to 42 mL/min during laparoscopy. Nguyen et al. (7) reported that at baseline the total volume of exhaled CO_2 per min (VCO_2) ranged from 201 to 222 mL/min. During open gastric bypass (GBP), VCO_2 levels remained stable, whereas VCO_2 levels increased by 29% during laparoscopic gastric bypass. Assuming that the measured VCO_2 during open GBP is the direct product of metabolic CO_2 production, the amount of absorbed CO_2 during laparoscopic gastric bypass can be estimated by taking the difference in VCO_2 levels between the laparoscopic and open GBP groups. The estimated rate of CO_2 absorption during laparoscopic gastric bypass, therefore, ranges from 19 to 39 mL/min (7).

Increased Intraabdominal Pressure During Pneumoperitoneum

Pneumoperitoneum results in a state of acute elevation of intraabdominal pressure. Typically, the intraabdominal pressure is set at 15 mm Hg during laparoscopic gastric bypass to provide adequate visualization of the operative field. The pathophysiologic changes during pneumoperitoneum can adversely affect various body organs as the normal intraabdominal pressure of nonobese individual is 5 mm Hg or less (10). In contrast, morbidly obese patients have a chronic state of elevated intraabdominal pressure at baseline (11). The intraabdominal pressure of obese patients has been reported to be as high as 9 mm Hg (10). We believe that abdominal insufflation at 15 mm Hg is better tolerated in the morbidly obese because these patients have an intrinsically elevated intraabdominal pressure at baseline.

Hemodynamic Changes During Pneumoperitoneum

Abdominal insufflation has been shown to alter mean arterial pressure and heart rate. Dexter et al. (12) reported that heart rate and mean arterial blood pressure increased during laparoscopic cholecystectomy. Meininger et al. (13) noted an increase in heart rate, but mean arterial pressure remained stable during laparoscopic radical prostatectomy. In a comparative study of obese and nonobese individuals, Fried and colleagues (14) reported that heart rate increased after pneumoperitoneum in both nonobese and obese individuals; however, obese individuals had a more pronounced increase in the heart rate level. In morbidly obese patients who underwent Roux-en-Y GBP, Nguyen et al. (15) reported that heart rate and mean arterial pressure increased during both laparoscopic and open GBP.

Hepatic Function During Pneumoperitoneum

Transient elevation of liver enzymes has been reported after laparoscopic operations even though no adverse clinical consequences have been observed (16,17). Halevy and colleagues (16) reported transient increases in the level of hepatic transaminases (alanine aminotransferase and aspartate aminotransferase) after laparoscopic cholecystectomy, which returned to normal range by 72 hours postoperatively. One of the mechanisms for this clinical finding is the effect of increased intraabdominal pressure on portal venous flow. Knowledge of this mechanism is important particularly in the morbidly obese as these patients tend to have preexisting liver disease. For example, Gholam and colleagues (18) noted that 84% of subjects who underwent Roux-en-Y GBP had steatosis, and Spaulding et al. (19) reported that there is a high prevalence (56%) of nonalcoholic steatohepatitis in morbidly obese subjects.

Few studies have examined the effects of pneumoperitoneum on postoperative hepatic function in the obese. Nguyen et al. (20) reported a sixfold elevation of hepatic transaminase levels peaking at 24 hours after laparoscopic GBP that returned to baseline levels by the third postoperative day. The increase in hepatic transaminase levels suggests acute hepatic damage. The mechanisms for alteration of postoperative hepatic function include direct operative trauma to the liver, the use of general anesthetics, and the effects of increased intraabdominal pressure on portal venous flow. Direct operative trauma to the liver occurs as a result of electrocautery or mechanical retraction of the liver. Certain anesthetic agents, metabolized through the liver, can be hepatotoxic and result in elevation of postoperative hepatic function. Lastly, an acute increase in the intraabdominal pressure at 15 mm Hg during laparoscopy has been shown to result in reduction of portal venous flow, as the normal portal venous pressure is often less than 10 mm Hg (21). A reduction in portal venous blood flow during pneumoperitoneum may lead to hepatic hypoperfusion and acute hepatocyte injury. In a clinical study of laparoscopic cholecystectomy, Jakimowics et al. (3) reported a 53% reduction in portal blood flow with abdominal insufflation to 14 mm Hg. Although acute elevation of hepatic transaminase has been observed after laparoscopic GBP, pneumoperitoneum in the morbidly obese is considered safe in patients with normal baseline liver function. Further study is needed to evaluate the safety of pneumoperitoneum in obese patients with preexisting liver dysfunction (e.g., liver cirrhosis) undergoing laparoscopic GBP.

Intraoperative Pulmonary Mechanics During Pneumoperitoneum

The increased intraabdominal pressure at 15 mm Hg during laparoscopy can adversely affect intraoperative pulmonary mechanics. Pneumoperitoneum has been shown to decrease respiratory compliance and increase airway pressure. The mechanism for this physiologic change is the increased intraabdominal pressure with cephalad shift of the diaphragm. Respiratory compliance consists of both lung and chest wall compliance. In a randomized trial comparing pulmonary mechanics during cholecystectomy performed by an abdominal wall lift method or pneumoperitoneum, Lindgren and colleagues (22) reported higher respiratory compliance during the abdominal lift method than during pneumoperitoneum. Similar findings occurred in the morbidly obese. Nguyen et al. (7) reported that respiratory compliance decreased significantly during both laparoscopic and open GBP. However, laparoscopic GBP was associated with a greater reduction in respiratory compliance compared with open GBP (42% vs. 29%, respectively). The reduction in respiratory compliance during open GBP is presumed from the use of abdominal wall retractors. The reduction in respiratory compliance during laparoscopic GBP is presumed from the increased intraabdominal pressure and cephalad shifts of the diaphragm.

Increased intraabdominal pressure during laparoscopy also increases the airway pressure. Without ventilatory changes, peak inspiratory pressure can increase by 17% to 109% during laparoscopy (23). Galizia and colleagues (24) reported a significant increase in the peak inspiratory pressure (PIP) in patients who underwent laparoscopic cholecystectomy but no change in the PIP in patients who underwent cholecystectomy by the open or abdominal wall lifting technique. In morbidly obese patients, Nguyen et al. (7) reported no significant change in PIP during open GBP, but PIP increased by 12% during laparoscopic GBP; in response to the rise in PIP, tidal volume was decreased by 7%.

Renal Function During Pneumoperitoneum

Acute increase in the intraabdominal pressure has been shown to impair renal function. Kron and colleagues (25) reported that rapid elevation of intraabdominal pressure to greater than 25 mm Hg resulted in acute renal insufficiency and that abdominal decompression caused immediate improvement in renal function. Even at an abdominal pressure of 15 mm Hg, laparoscopy has been shown to impair renal function. A decrease in intraoperative urine output has been documented during laparoscopic operations (26,27). In a trial comparing laparoscopic adrenalectomy with gasless laparoscopic adrenalectomy, Nishio and colleagues (26) demonstrated that urine output decreased significantly with abdominal insufflation and improved upon desufflation. In a swine model, McDougall et al. (28) demonstrated that the degree of intraoperative oliguria is dependent on the level of increased intraabdominal pressure. Few studies have examined the effect of pneumoperitoneum on renal function in the obese. Nguyen et al. (29) reported that pneumoperitoneum at 15 mm Hg during laparoscopic GBP significantly reduced intraoperative urine output. In contrast, intraoperative urine output remained stable during open GBP. Urinary output during laparoscopic GBP was 31% to 64% lower than that of open GBP (29).

There are several mechanisms for diminished urine output during laparoscopic operations. First, pneumoperitoneum has a direct pressure effect on the renal parenchyma. In a swine model, Chiu et al. (5) confirmed that renal cortical perfusion decreased by 60% with abdominal insufflation to 15 mm Hg and returned to preinsufflation level after desufflation. Second, pneumoperitoneum has a direct pressure effect on the renal vasculature, resulting in decreased renal blood flow. In a swine study, Are and colleagues (30) demonstrated that renal blood flow decreased by 36% below baseline as measured by radioactive microspheres. A third mechanism for diminished urine output during laparoscopic operations is the release of antidiuretic hormone (ADH) that regulates body osmolality and an increase in serum levels of vasopressin. Antidiuretic hormone (ADH) facilitates water reabsorption in the distal tubules and concentrates the urine. Ortega et al. (31) reported higher ADH concentrations during laparoscopic cholecystectomy than during open cholecystectomy. In a study of morbidly obese subjects, Nguyen et al. (29) reported that

ADH levels increased by fourfold during laparoscopic GBP.

Despite intraoperative oliguria, pneumoperitoneum is considered clinically safe as there is no clinical evidence of perioperative renal damage. Nishio et al. (26) reported no change in serum creatinine after laparoscopic adrenalectomy when compared with gasless laparoscopic adrenalectomy. Nguyen et al. (29) also reported no significant changes in blood urea or serum creatinine levels in patients who underwent laparoscopic GBP. Additionally, creatinine clearance was reported to be in the normal range on both the first ($150 \pm 59\,\mathrm{mL/min}$) and second ($145 \pm 41\,\mathrm{mL/min}$) postoperative day in patients who underwent laparoscopic GBP (11).

Venous Stasis During Pneumoperitoneum

According to Virchow's triad, the risks for development of deep venous thrombosis (DVT) include the presence of endothelial injury, a hypercoagulable state, or venous stasis. Although the relative risks for development of DVT after laparoscopic operations compared with open operations are unknown, the effect of increased intraabdominal pressure during pneumoperitoneum on the femoral vasculature is of concern. Many investigators have reported that the increased intraabdominal pressure and reverse Trendelenburg position during laparoscopy may promote venous stasis (32,33). The increased intraabdominal pressure at $15\,\mathrm{mm\,Hg}$ commonly used during laparoscopy has a direct compressive effect on the inferior vena cava and iliac veins and decreases lower extremity venous flow. By the force of gravity and compressive effects of abdominal viscera on the iliac veins, the reverse Trendelenburg position has also been shown to decrease femoral venous flow, hence promoting venous stasis (32). In a study of laparoscopic cholecystectomy, Millard et al. (33) reported that a combination of pneumoperitoneum and 30-degree reverse Trendelenburg position decreased peak systolic velocity of the common femoral vein by 42%. Ido et al. (32) also reported that abdominal insufflation significantly reduced femoral vein velocity, and the addition of the reverse Trendelenburg position has an additive effect. Similar findings have been observed in the obese. Nguyen et al. (34) reported that the increased intraabdominal pressure and reverse Trendelenburg position are independent factors for reduction of femoral peak systolic velocity in patients who underwent laparoscopic GBP. Increased intraabdominal pressure to $15\,\mathrm{mm\,Hg}$ during laparoscopic GBP significantly reduced peak systolic velocity and increased the cross-sectional area of the femoral vein. Combining pneumoperitoneum with the reverse Trendelenburg position has an additive effect and

reduces femoral peak systolic velocity by 57% of the baseline value (34).

The use of sequential compression devices during laparoscopy has been shown to reverse the reduction in femoral peak systolic velocity (35). Sequential compression devices provide a sequential pressure gradient starting from the ankle up to the thigh. The pressure gradient accelerates blood flow, facilitates venous emptying, and therefore prevents venous stasis. Millard et al. (33) and Schwenk et al. (35) reported that the use of sequential compression devices reversed the reduction of femoral peak systolic velocity to baseline values during laparoscopic cholecystectomy. In contrast, the use of sequential compression devices in morbidly obese subjects was only partially effective in augmenting the femoral peak systolic velocity. Nguyen et al. (34) reported that the use of sequential compression devices reversed the reduction in femoral peak systolic velocity by 45%; however, the femoral peak systolic velocity was still lower than baseline by 38%. The ineffectiveness of sequential compression devices in returning femoral peak systolic velocity to baseline in morbidly obese patients is attributed to their larger calves and thighs (34). Therefore, DVT prophylaxis for morbidly obese patients undergoing laparoscopy should include a combination of sequential compression devices and antithrombotic measures.

Cardiac Function During Pneumoperitoneum

The hemodynamic effects of pneumoperitoneum on cardiac function have been extensively examined in nonobese individuals. Clinical studies evaluating the effects of CO_2 pneumoperitoneum on cardiac function have documented variable results. These studies used either intraoperative Swan-Ganz catheterization or transesophageal echocardiography for evaluation of cardiac function. Several investigators have demonstrated a reduction in cardiac output during pneumoperitoneum (36,37), whereas others have reported no change (38,39). Westerband et al. (37) reported a 30% decrease in cardiac index in patients who underwent laparoscopic cholecystectomy. Joris and colleagues (36) also demonstrated that cardiac index decreased by 20% of preoperative values immediately after insufflation, which recovered after desufflation. Conversely, Kraut et al. (38) and Dorsay et al. (39) using transesophageal echocardiography reported no change in cardiac output in patients who underwent laparoscopic cholecystectomy.

Few studies have examined the effects of pneumoperitoneum on cardiac function in the obese. In a small study of 12 patients who underwent laparoscopy, Fried et al. (14) compared cardiac function of six morbidly obese individuals with six normal body weight subjects.

Morbidly obese subjects had an increase in cardiac output after abdominal insufflation. In a larger study of morbidly obese subjects who underwent laparoscopic and open GBP, Nguyen et al. (15) noted a mild decrease in cardiac output after abdominal insufflation by 6% and a reduction in stroke volume by 8% from baseline. In contrast to the results observed in the nonobese, studies with obese subjects demonstrated minimal cardiac depression during pneumoperitoneum. We hypothesized that abdominal insufflation at 15 mm Hg is better tolerated in the morbidly obese patients due to their chronically elevated intraabdominal pressure compared with nonobese patients.

Although the primary mechanism for alteration of cardiac function is the increased intraabdominal pressure, other factors may play a role, including the reverse Trendelenburg position, hypercarbia, and hypovolemia. In an animal model, Ho and colleagues (40) attributed the cardiovascular depression to systemic acidosis. A combination of hypercarbia and acidosis can decrease myocardial contractility. However, Declan Fleming et al. (41) demonstrated that even helium insufflation reduces cardiac output, which suggested that the increased intraabdominal pressure was the primary cause for cardiac depression. In addition, hypercarbia is normally avoided in the clinical setting by increasing in the minute ventilation, and a moderate rise in the $PaCO_2$ should not contribute to cardiac depression. The reverse Trendelenburg position has been demonstrated by Joris and colleagues (36) to reduce cardiac index by 18% when compared with the supine position in healthy adults. Hypovolemia is another factor that may account for the reduction of cardiac output during pneumoperitoneum. Hypovolemia reduces the preload and hence reduces cardiac output. The increased intraabdominal pressure also decreases preload by impeding venous return. Therefore, a euvolemic preoperative volume status of the patient is very important to minimize any cardiac depression related to the initiation of abdominal insufflation.

The physiologic mechanism for reduction in cardiac output associated with increased intraabdominal pressure is believed to be the increase in systemic vascular resistance. Declan Fleming and colleagues (41) reported that systemic vascular resistance significantly increased after abdominal insufflation to 15 mm Hg and decreased with desufflation. In a trial comparing open vs. laparoscopic GBP, Nguyen et al. (15) noted that open GBP was not associated with an alteration in the systemic vascular resistance. However, laparoscopic GBP resulted in an immediate increase in the systemic vascular resistance upon insufflation and returned to baseline by 1.5 hours after initiation of pneumoperitoneum. The timing of the increase in the systemic vascular resistance correlates with the timing of the reduction in cardiac output and stroke volume. The results from these studies suggest that an increase in the systemic vascular resistance is the primary event leading to a reduction in cardiac output. In addition, cardiac depression observed after pneumoperitoneum is often transient. In a laparoscopic cholecystectomy study, Zuckerman and Heneghan (42) reported that reduction in cardiac output and index occurred immediately after abdominal insufflation but returned to baseline levels 10 to 15 minutes after abdominal insufflation. Nguyen et al. (15) reported that cardiac output levels recovered after a transient depression and increased above baseline by 2.5 hours after abdominal insufflation; at desufflation, cardiac output increased by 42.8% above baseline.

Conclusion

Laparoscopic bariatric surgery is now a common approach for the treatment of morbid obesity. It is important for surgeons performing laparoscopic bariatric surgery to understand the physiologic consequences of pneumoperitoneum in the morbidly obese and its clinical end points. During pneumoperitoneum, the two factors that can result in adverse physiologic changes are absorption of CO_2 and increased intraabdominal pressure. Absorption of CO_2 during abdominal insufflation can lead to hypercarbia and hypercapnia, and alter the acid–base balance. Making appropriate ventilatory changes is mandatory to minimize these physiologic changes. The increased intraabdominal pressure can adversely affect respiratory mechanics, femoral venous flow, and renal, cardiac, and hepatic function. The increased intraabdominal pressure reduces pulmonary compliance and increases the airway pressure. Increased intraabdominal pressure also decreases femoral vein systolic velocity and enhances venous stasis. Clinically, urine output is often low during laparoscopy, and one of the mechanisms for this finding is the reduction in renal blood flow from the increased intraabdominal pressure. The increased intraabdominal pressure can also reduce cardiac output, which is related to an increase in systemic vascular resistance. There is also an alteration of hepatic transaminases, which is possibly related to a reduction in portal venous flow during pneumoperitoneum. Despite the adverse consequence of pneumoperitoneum, laparoscopic bariatric surgery is considered safe. However, we do not advocate the laparoscopic approach for morbidly obese patients with significant preexisting renal, hepatic, cardiac, or respiratory dysfunction.

References

1. Wittgrove AC, Clark GW, Tremblay LJ. Laparoscopic gastric bypass, Roux-en-Y: preliminary report of five cases. Obes Surg 1994;4:353–357.

2. Nguyen NT, Goldman C, Rosenquist CJ, et al. Laparoscopic versus open gastric bypass: a randomized study of outcomes, quality of life, and costs. Ann Surg 2001;234:279–289.

3. Jakimowics J, Stultiens G, Smulders F. Laparoscopic insufflation of the abdomen reduces portal venous flow. Surg Endosc 1998;12:129–132.

4. Beebe DS, McNevin MP, Crain JM, et al. Evidence of venous stasis after abdominal insufflation for laparoscopic cholecystectomy. Surg Gynecol Obstet 1993;176:443-447.

5. Chiu AW, Chang LS, Birkett DH, Babayan RK. The impact of pneumoperitoneum, pneumoretroperitoneum, and gasless laparoscopy on the systemic and renal hemodynamics. J Am Coll Surg 1995;181:397–406.

6. Hirvonen EA, Poikolainen EO, Paakkonen ME, Nuutinen LS. The adverse hemodynamic effects of anesthesia, head-up tilt, and carbon dioxide pneumoperitoneum during laparoscopic cholecystectomy. Surg Endosc 2000;14:272–277.

7. Nguyen NT, Anderson J, Fleming NW, Ho HS, Jahr J, Wolfe BM. Effects of pneumoperitoneum on intraoperative respiratory mechanics and gas exchange during laparoscopic gastric bypass. Surg Endosc 2004;18:64–71.

8. Dumont L, Mattys M, Mardirosoff C, et al. Changes in pulmonary mechanics during laparoscopic gastroplasty in the morbidly obese patient. Acta Scand Anesth 1997;41: 408–413.

9. Tan PL, Lee TL, Tweed WA. Carbon dioxide absorption and gas exchange during pelvic laparoscopy. Can J Anaesth 1992;39:677–681.

10. Sanchez NC, Tenofsky PL, Dort JM, Shen LY, Helmer SD, Smith RS. What is normal intra-abdominal pressure? Am Surg 2001:67:243–248.

11. Nguyen NT, Lee SL, Anderson JT, et al. Evaluation of intra-abdominal pressure after open and laparoscopic gastric bypass. Obes Surg 2001;11:40–45.

12. Dexter SP, Vucevic M, Gibson J, McMahon MJ. Hemodynamic consequences of high- and low-pressure capnoperitoneum during laparoscopic cholecystectomy. Surg Endosc 1999;13:376–381.

13. Meininger D, Byhahn C, Bueck M, et al. Effects of prolonged pneumoperitoneum on hemodynamics and acid-base balance during totally endoscopic robot-assisted radical prostatectomies. World J Surg 2002;26:1423–1427.

14. Fried M, Krska Z, Danzig V. Does the laparoscopic approach significantly affect cardiac functions in laparoscopic surgery? Pilot study in non-obese and morbidly obese patients. Obes Surg 2001;11:293–296.

15. Nguyen NT, Ho HS, Fleming NW, et al. Cardiac function during laparoscopic vs open gastric bypass: a randomized comparison. Surg Endosc 2002;16:78–83.

16. Halevy A, Gold-Deutch R, Negri M, et al. Are elevated liver enzymes and bilirubin levels significant after laparoscopic cholecystectomy in the absence of bile duct injury? Ann Surg 1994;219:362–364.

17. Saber AA, Laraja RD, Nalbandian HI, Pablos-Mendez A, Hanna K. Changes in liver function tests after laparoscopic cholecystectomy: not so rare, not always ominous. Am Surg 2000;66:699–702.

18. Gholam PM, Kotler DP, Flancbaum LJ. Liver pathology in morbidly obese patients undergoing Roux-en-Y gastric bypass surgery. Obes Surg 2002;12:49–51.

19. Spaulding L, Trainer T, Janiec D. Prevalence of non-alcoholic steatohepatitis in morbidly obese subjects undergoing gastric bypass. Obes Surg 2003;13:347–349.

20. Nguyen NT, Braley S, Fleming NW, Lambourne L, Rivers R, Wolfe BM. Comparison of postoperative hepatic function after laparoscopic versus open gastric bypass. Am J Surg 2003;186:40–44.

21. Jakimowics J, Stultiens G, Smulders F. Laparoscopic insufflation of the abdomen reduces portal venous flow. Surg Endosc 1998;12:129–132.

22. Lindgren L. Koivusalo AM, Kellokumpu I. Conventional pneumoperitoneum compared with abdominal wall lift for laparoscopic cholecystectomy. Br J Anaesth 1995;75:567–572.

23. Sharma KC, Brandstetter RD, Brensilver JM, Jung LD. Cardiopulmonary physiology and pathophysiology as a consequence of laparoscopic surgery. Chest 1996;110: 810–815.

24. Galizia G, Prizio G, Lieto E, et al. Hemodynamic and pulmonary changes during open, carbon dioxide pneumoperitoneum and abdominal wall-lifting cholecystectomy. Surg Endosc 2001;15:477–483.

25. Kron IL, Harman PK, Nolan SP. The measurement of intra-abdominal pressure as a criterion for abdominal re-exploration. Ann Surg 1984;199:28–30.

26. Nishio S, Takeda H, Yokoyama M. Changes in urinary output during laparoscopic adrenalectomy. BJU Int 1999;83: 944–947.

27. Harman PK, Kron IL, McLachlan HD, Freedlender AE, Nolan SP. Elevated intra-abdominal pressure and renal function. Ann Surg 1982;196:594–597.

28. McDougall EM, Monk TG, Wolf JS, et al. The effect of prolonged pneumoperitoneum on renal function in an animal model. J Am Coll Surg 1996;182:317–328.

29. Nguyen NT, Perez RV, Fleming N, Rivers R, Wolfe BM. Effect of prolonged pneumoperitoneum on intraoperative urine output during laparoscopic gastric bypass. J Am Coll Surg 2002;195:476–483.

30. Are C, Kutka M, Talamini M, et al. Effect of laparoscopic antireflux surgery upon renal blood flow. Am J Surg 2002;183:419–423.

31. Ortega AE, Peters JH, Incarbone R, et al. A prospective randomized comparison of the metabolic and stress hormonal responses of laparoscopic and open cholecystectomy. J Am Coll Surg 1996;183:249–256.

32. Ido K, Suzuki T, Kimura K, et al. Lower-extremity venous stasis during laparoscopic cholecystectomy as assessed using color Doppler ultrasound. Surg Endosc 1995;9:310–313.

33. Millard JA, Hill BB, Cook PS, Fenoglio ME, Stahlgren LH. Intermittent sequential pneumatic compression in prevention of venous stasis associated with pneumoperitoneum during laparoscopic cholecystectomy. Arch Surg 1993;914-919.

34. Nguyen NT, Cronan M, Braley S, Rivers R, Wolfe BM. Duplex ultrasound assessment of femoral venous flow during laparoscopic and open gastric bypass. Surg Endosc 2001;192:469–476.

35. Schwenk W, Bohm B, Fugener A, Muller JM. Intermittent pneumatic sequential compression (ISC) of the lower

extremities prevents venous stasis during laparoscopic cholecystectomy. A prospective randomized study. Surg Endosc 1998;12:7-11.

36. Joris JL, Noirot DP, Legrand MJ, Jacquet NJ, Lamy ML. Hemodynamic changes during laparoscopic cholecystectomy. Anesth Analg 1993;76:1067–1071.

37. Westerband A, Van De Water JM, Amzallag M, et al. Cardiovascular changes during laparoscopic cholecystectomy. Surg Gynecol Obstet 1992;175:535–538.

38. Kraut EJ, Anderson JT, Safwat A, Barbosa R, Wolfe BM. Impairment of cardiac performance by laparoscopy in patients receiving positive end-expiratory pressure. Arch Surg 1999;134:76–80.

39. Dorsay DA, Greene FL, Baysinger CL. Hemodynamic changes during laparoscopic cholecystectomy monitored with transesophageal echocardiography. Surg Endosc 1995; 9:128–133.

40. Ho HS, Saunders CJ, Gunther RA, Wolfe BM. Effector of hemodynamics during laparoscopy: CO_2 absorption or intra-abdominal pressure? J Surg Res 1995;59:497–503.

41. Declan Fleming RY, Dougherty TB, Feig BW. The safety of helium for abdominal insufflation. Surg Endosc 1997;11: 230–234.

42. Zuckerman RS, Heneghan S. The duration of hemodynamic depression during laparoscopic cholecystectomy. Surg Endosc 2002;16:1233–1236.

15
Postoperative Assessment, Documentation, and Follow-Up of Bariatric Roux-en-Y Surgical Patients

Edward C. Mun, Vivian M. Sanchez, and Daniel B. Jones

Bariatric procedures are major operations often performed on high-risk patients with multiple comorbidities. Meticulous postoperative assessment and management may avoid preventable complications. Early identification and treatment of postoperative complications may be lifesaving. Documentation and long-term follow-up may prevent complications and monitor the surgical outcomes. For these reasons, the American Society of Bariatric Surgeons (ASBS) has provided strict guidelines for centers performing bariatric surgery. The three main bariatric surgery center requirements are as follows: (1) The center should have an integrated program in which the pre- and postoperative care of a bariatric patient is performed by a multidisciplinary clinical staff of surgeons, bariatric internists, nurses, psychologists, physical therapists, nutritionists, and other consultants. (2) Surgeons and bariatric centers should document the follow-up on a regular basis for 5 years in at least 50% of patients who have undergone a restrictive procedure or 75% of patients who have had a malabsorptive procedure. (3) New surgeons performing bariatric surgery must have their outcomes assessed after the first 6 months. Clinical pathway management protocols for postoperative care may further improve the quality of care while shortening the length of stay (LOS) and thereby reducing cost (1,2). This chapter discusses major postoperative assessment and management issues.

Postoperative Assessment in Hospital

Management of patients following a bariatric procedure in the intensive care unit (ICU) is rarely necessary but should be available. Patients with severe cardiopulmonary dysfunction such as valvular heart disease, significant coronary artery disease, and heart failure may require postoperative use of electrocardiogram and Swan-Ganz hemodynamic monitoring. Patients with severe obstructive and restrictive pulmonary diseases may benefit from prolonged postoperative intubation. Most patients, however, can be safely extubated in the operating room and managed in the recovery room where patients' vital signs, oxygen saturation, and urine output are closely monitored for respiratory and hemodynamic stability prior to transfer to the ward.

If any signs of acute bleeding or respiratory failure are noted during the immediate postoperative period, no time is wasted for reexploration or reintubation. Blood pressure, heart rate, urine output, and skin capillary refill are monitored closely for signs of hypovolemia. If drains and tubes (e.g., gastrostomy) are placed, their output is closely monitored for amount and nature (bloody vs. serous). Serial hematocrit is obtained if the amount of blood loss is uncertain. Coagulation studies are performed in patients with active bleeding, and appropriate factors are replaced to facilitate the control of the bleeding. Oxygen saturation, respiratory rate, peripheral cyanosis, and the work of breathing are also monitored closely to check the adequacy of spontaneous breathing. Blood gas level should be obtained if suspicion of hypoxemia or hypercarbia exists. Because many morbidly obese patients have baseline hypoxia and hypercarbia, documentation of these numbers preoperatively in high-risk patients may help determine the degree of postoperative respiratory insufficiency.

Patients with obstructive sleep apnea (OSA) are placed on either a nasal continuous positive airway pressure (CPAP) or bi-level PAP machine immediately postoperatively; this has been shown to reduce the need for tracheostomy (3). Patients with suspected severe OSA may benefit from a preoperative sleep study, and must be fitted with appropriate apparatus before the procedure so the custom-fitted mask is available for the postoperative care period. Postoperative use of CPAP does not lead to an increased incidence of leaks despite the positive pressure (4). Patients with significant asthmatic history should be given well-timed bronchodilator treatments intra- and postoperatively to reduce pulmonary complications.

Frequent auscultation of lung fields should start in the recovery room.

Pain control by morphine or other narcotics in the form of patient-controlled analgesia (PCA) may be initiated in the recovery room. PCA appears to be safe and superior to intramuscular (IM) injection in achieving analgesic and sedative effects in post–bariatric surgery patients (5). Ketorolac, when included in the cocktail of anesthetics in patients undergoing bariatric procedures, may help reduce the incidence of nausea and vomiting, and facilitates quick awakening from anesthesia (6). Unless specific contraindications exist, ketorolac (Toradol) may be used as an adjunct to PCA to lower postoperative pain.

Many surgeons are removing the nasogastric tube (NGT) early or avoiding it altogether. In postlaparotomy patients the NGT is associated with discomfort (7), atelectasis, pneumonia (8,9), and increased gastroesophageal reflux (10). In one study, routine postoperative NGT decompression in Roux-en-Y gastric bypass (RYGBP) patients specifically did not demonstrate benefits in preventing postoperative complications (11). Placement of the NGT in response to postoperative ileus is usually avoided in gastric bypass patients because it carries a significant risk of perforation due to the altered anatomy and may even fail to adequately decompress the gastrointestinal tract due to the Roux-en-Y anatomy.

Once transferred out of the ICU or recovery room, most patients are monitored on the ward for 2 to 3 days prior to discharge. Several serious postoperative complications can occur during this period, and attention is paid to identifying the signs of these complications as early as possible.

Pulmonary embolus remains one of the leading causes of mortality following gastric bypass (12), and thus all patients are urged to ambulate as early as possible on the evening of surgery. Although no consensus for perioperative prophylaxis exists, many bariatric surgeons employ both pneumatic compression devices (pneumoboots) as well as subcutaneous heparin (13). Low-molecular-weight heparin may be more effective than unfractionated heparin, but at higher doses more bleeding complications may occur. Although venous stasis during laparoscopic gastric bypass is greater than during an open procedure because of greater degrees of reverse Trendelenburg positioning as well as increased pneumoperitoneum (14), the incidence of pulmonary embolus is similar in both approaches (12,15–17). No evidence-based literature exists to suggest an optimal deep vein thrombosis (DVT)/pulmonary embolism (PE) prophylaxis.

Patients with low oxygen saturation, shortness of breath, pleuritic chest pain, labored breathing, leg swelling, and pain should be evaluated for PE and DVT. Computed tomographic (CT) angiography, pulmonary angiography, or lower extremity duplex scan can be obtained to make the diagnosis. Lung scan is less specific. Some patients, however, may not be able to undergo these diagnostic studies due to their size. If PE or DVT is confirmed by a study or the level of clinical suspicion is high, the patient is immediately anticoagulated with heparin and then Coumadin. In rare patients in whom anticoagulation is contraindicated, a mechanical filter may be placed in the inferior vena cava to lower the risk of continued clot embolization. In patients identified as high risk for PE due to a history of previous thromboembolic disease, venous stasis disease, or inability to ambulate (e.g., wheelchair-bound), heparin may be prescribed for an extended period even after discharge from the hospital.

During workup of PE, leaks may go unrecognized and the diagnosis delayed. Gastric bypass requires multiple areas of visceral transection and anastomosis, and thus gastrointestinal leak can occur from a failure at any of these suture or staple lines. Subsequent peritonitis accounts for much of the mortality and morbidity of the procedure. The incidence of leak in more recent laparoscopic series ranges from 0% to 5.1% and is comparable to that of the open series (15–21). While the signs and symptoms of a leak are quite nonspecific in sedated postoperative patients in pain, an index of suspicion for a leak should be maintained during the early postoperative period. The most sensitive signs are tachycardia and respiratory compromise. Unexplained tachycardia especially greater than 120 beats per minute, respiratory distress, fever, severe pain/tenderness, low urine output, and hypotension are associated with gastrointestinal leak, which should be suspected early if these signs are present (22). Radiographic studies utilizing contrast materials such as upper gastrointestinal (UGI) series or CT may help making the diagnosis (22–25). A negative study must not deter a surgeon from reexploring if the level of suspicion for a leak is high.

Management of a leak if a patient is hemodynamically unstable or septic includes prompt operative (open or laparoscopic) washout of peritoneal contamination, broad drainage of the affected area, identification and repair of the visceral defect, broad-spectrum antibiotics, and possibly creation of gastrostomy for drainage and feeding. In patients with minimal symptoms and no hemodynamic instability, a contained leak may be managed with percutaneous drainage, antibiotic therapy, and total parenteral nutrition (TPN) and/or a feeding gastrostomy. Similarly, a closed suction drain such as a Jackson-Pratt (JP), placed at the time of the initial operation, may control a small leak and thus may avoid another procedure in selected cases.

Acute gastric distention is a rare but potentially devastating complication. The gastric remnant is a blind pouch and may become distended if paralytic ileus or distal mechanical obstruction exists postoperatively. Iatrogenic injury to vagal fibers along the lesser curvature may result in impaired emptying of the bypassed stomach. Progressive distention may ultimately lead to rupture of the gastric remnant, spillage of massive gastric contents, and subsequent severe peritonitis from contamination with acid, bile, pancreatic enzymes, and bacteria. Its toxic contents combined with the large size of inoculums make this complication much more serious than the leakage occurring at the gastrojejunostomy. Upper abdominal fullness, distention, tympany, and hiccups should be taken seriously during the early postoperative period, and should promptly be assessed with a kidney, ureters, and bladder (KUB) x-ray or a CT scan looking for a large gastric bubble. Although gastrostomy is not performed routinely by most surgeons at the initial gastric bypass operation, drainage of the gastric remnant can prevent the rare but sometimes fatal complication, and should be considered in elderly, advanced diabetics, and after revisional surgeries where the integrity of the vagus nerve function is in doubt and gastric emptying may be slowed.

Bleeding from surgical sites, anastomoses, or staple lines can occur intraluminally, and may present with hematemesis, melena, and hematochezia with or without hemodynamic instability. Most anastomotic bleeding stops spontaneously, but may require correction of coagulopathy if present or transfusion of blood products. There have been anecdotal reports that upper endoscopy with injection of sclerosing agents has been successful in controlling acute anastomotic bleeding. We routinely use a histamine blocker for 4 weeks postoperatively; however, it is unclear whether that may lower the incidence of anastomotic ulcer (26). Intraperitoneal bleeding may be more difficult to detect and should be suspected if a patient becomes pale, tachycardic, hypotensive, or has bloody JP drainage. In general, slow postoperative bleeding may resolve with transfusion; however, ongoing hemorrhage or hemodynamic instability should prompt immediate reexploration.

Wound infection is more common in open than in laparoscopic gastric bypass in a randomized study (10.5% vs. 1.3%) (19). As these procedures are clean but contaminated with gastric and intestinal flora, infection may arise from direct inoculation of bacteria during surgery and may manifest during the early postoperative period. Most open-surgery patients develop a sizable subcutaneous seroma, which may get secondarily infected if skin closure is not maintained adequately. Although wound infection following laparoscopic bariatric procedures is uncommon (19,21), removal of gastrointestinal tissues through a port site may lead to contamination. Thus, all incisions should be carefully inspected for the presence of signs of wound infection such as erythema, tenderness, fluctuance, and purulent drainage. Patients should be instructed to look for these signs upon discharge.

Incentive spirometry and ambulation are excellent prophylaxis and treatment for atelectasis. All patients are encouraged to ambulate the same day of surgery with assistance. If there is a persistent low-grade temperature despite aggressive chest physical therapy, particularly with productive cough, pneumonia must be ruled out with chest x-ray and sputum culture.

Uncomplicated patients are advanced in diet stages (Table 15-1) during the early postoperative period. Bariatric programs differ in their approaches to advancing the diet, but, in general, patients begin with liquids and gradually progress to solids. Frequent sips of water are emphasized to avoid dehydration. Patients are maintained on high-protein, low-fat liquid diet for the first 3

TABLE 15-1. Postoperative gastric bypass diet

Stage	Diet	Examples	Location	Timing	Amount
I	Sips	Water	In hospital	POD 1	30 cc/hr
II	Clear liquids	Broth, diet Snapple, Crystal Light, decaffeinated tea	In hospital	POD 2	90 cc serving (30 cc/hr)
III	Full liquids, high protein	Carnation Instant Breakfast (no sugar), low-fat milk, yogurt, diet custard, soup with low-fat milk, popsicle	In hospital/home	POD 2 and at home for 3 weeks	3–5 servings/day calories: 600–800 protein: 60–80 g/day fluid: 3 L/day
IV	Pureed solids, high protein, low sugar	Continue protein shakes, ground beef, fish, egg whites, tofu	Home	POD 21–27 and then for 4 weeks	4–6 servings/day
V	Modified fat and fiber, low sugar, high quality protein	Same as stage IV, chicken, turkey, cheese, pork, yogurt	Home	POD 60	4–6 servings/day

POD, postoperative day.

weeks. Liquid diet can provide adequate hydration, daily protein, and caloric requirements. Solid foods are introduced gradually in stages to avoid early impaction of inadequately chewed food leading to retching and vomiting. Because the micropouch is unable to provide adequate mechanical grinding action of the intact stomach, initially solids must be either pureed or chewed properly for the passage through the narrow stoma. Medications should be crushed or switched to liquid forms if available. Preoperative instruction as well as postoperative counseling by the nutrition service is important to avoid frequent nausea and vomiting.

Most of the preoperative medications should be restarted as early as possible. If available, liquid forms are preferred during the early postoperative periods. The psychological well-being of the patient should be monitored closely during this stressful period, and preoperative antidepressants are usually resumed to avoid depression. Type 2 diabetes improves rapidly following Roux-en-Y gastric bypass, almost independent of the weight loss. Patients' serum glucose is carefully monitored with frequent finger-stick checks. Oral hypoglycemic agents and long-acting insulin are usually discontinued postoperatively to prevent episodes of hypoglycemia. Most patients can be managed with sliding scale short-acting regular insulin. Total daily insulin requirements are recorded during the early hospitalization to estimate the outpatient daily dose upon discharge. Hypertension also improves quite rapidly postoperatively. Many patients are discharged on a fewer number of antihypertensive agents or more frequently on reduced doses of these medications. In general, diuretics should not be abruptly discontinued as patients may retain fluid.

Postoperative Follow-Up

Early

If no major immediate postoperative complications are noted, the patients can be discharged when adequate oral hydration and control of postoperative pain can be achieved. Instructions are reviewed carefully with the patients and the arrangements are made for follow-up visits with the surgeon, dietitian, psychologist, and primary care physician. Patients should be evaluated in an outpatient clinic at regular intervals during the first year of the procedure.

Adequate self-hydration is of utmost importance during the early follow-up period. Strategies to ensure proper delivery of adequate amounts of fluid and nutrition during this period should be reviewed with the patient in detail. Patients should be evaluated carefully in the clinic by paying a close attention to vital signs, peripheral perfusion, orthostasis, and so on. They are also

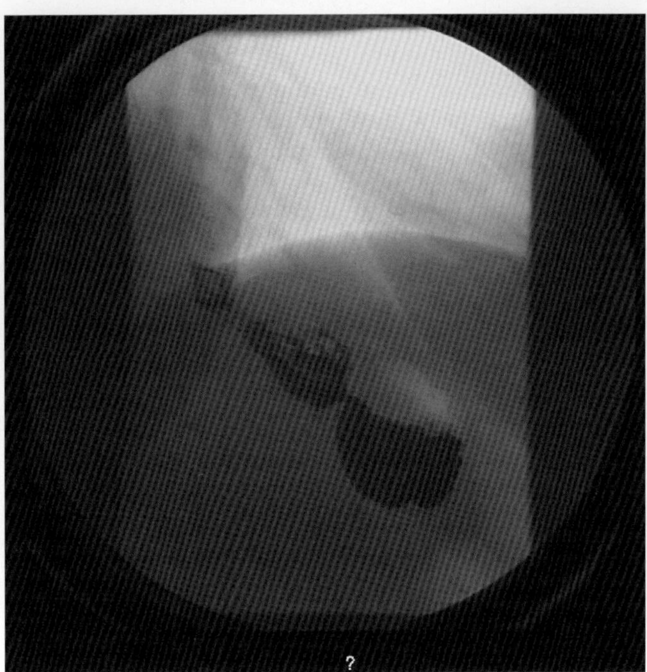

FIGURE 15-1. Upper gastrointestinal series demonstrating a gastrojejunal stricture.

questioned about urinary frequency and amount. If dehydration is suspected, electrolytes and urinary ketones are checked to confirm the diagnosis. Dehydration, if identified, should be aggressively treated with intravenous fluids.

Although dietary management following bariatric surgery is widely variable, most patients will advance in a gradual fashion from liquid to solid diet. Dysphagia to solids, especially if progressive, should raise the suspicion of anastomotic stenosis, and should be evaluated with UGI or an upper endoscopy (Fig. 15-1). Confirmed gastrojejunal stenosis should be treated promptly with endoscopic balloon dilation to avoid development of food aversion and protein calorie malnutrition (27).

Incisions are checked for infection, seroma, or an early hernia development. Incisional hernia is more common in open surgery patients and will require a repair eventually. Repair of incisional hernias may fail if the patients are still significantly obese. If possible, a formal repair is deferred until a significant weight loss occurs (>1 year).

All medications are reviewed and adjusted if necessary. A blood pressure measuring device can be purchased for postoperative home-use by the patients. The insulin dose must be frequently adjusted by the primary care physician to prevent hypoglycemia. It is important that the patients are kept in a close communication with their endocrinologist, cardiologist, or internist upon discharge, as their medications need to be adjusted frequently.

Late

Patients who recover from the early postoperative period are then followed long-term from surgical, medical, nutritional and psychosocial aspects. Late surgical complications include a potential development of gallstone-related diseases, anastomotic ulcers (Fig. 15-2), incisional hernias, and small bowel obstruction from adhesions, internal hernia, and volvulus.

Rapid weight loss is associated with formation of gallstones and 36% of post–gastric bypass patients may develop gallstones if not prophylaxed (28). Patients who retain gallbladder after weight loss surgeries are routinely prophylaxed with a 6-month course of Ursodiol, as this has been shown to be effective in reducing the incidence of gallstone formation (29–31). Patients presenting with postprandial abdominal pain, nausea, and vomiting should be ruled out for gallstones with ultrasound. Because the duodenum is bypassed, an endoscopic retrograde cholangiopancreatography (ERCP) may not be technically feasible in patients suspected of choledocholithiasis, cholangitis, or gallstone pancreatitis, although successful ERCP has been reported in post–gastric bypass patients by experienced endoscopists. Placement of gastrostomy tube at the time of gastric bypass with a radiopaque marker may facilitate a future endoscopic surveillance and possible therapy of the gastric remnant and duodenum. Diagnostic options include hepatic 2,6-dimethyliminodiacetic acid (HIDA) scan, percutaneous transhepatic cholangiography (PTC), or magnetic resonance cholangiopancreatography (MRCP). Therapeutic maneuvers for patients with gallstones in the common bile duct include PTC drainage with stone retrieval, and more definitively, open or laparoscopic cholecystectomy with common bile duct exploration.

Patients with chronic unremitting abdominal pain, particularly associated with eating, should be tested for occult blood in the stool, as an anastomotic ulcer may be the cause of their pain. Strong suspicion of an anastomotic ulcer should precipitate the performance of a diagnostic upper endoscopy. Chronic nonsteroidal antiinflammatory medication use, *Helicobacter pylori* infection, and nonabsorbable suture materials may be associated with ulcer disease in gastric bypass patients. Diagnosis is made using flexible upper endoscopy. Patients with anastomotic ulcers are treated with proton pump inhibitors and eradication of *H. pylori* infection if indicated. A follow-up esophagogastroduodenoscopy (EGD) should be performed to monitor the progress. Indications for surgery include active or recurrent bleeding not responding to medical treatment, perforation leading to peritonitis, chronic pain with nonhealing ulcer on EGD, or gastrogastric fistula as a result of the ulcer.

Symptoms of abdominal pain, nausea, vomiting, and distention should also lead to a careful workup to rule out mechanical obstruction. Midline incisions for bariatric surgery can result in incisional hernias in at least 15% to 20% of patients. Laparoscopic port-site hernia has also been reported. A repair is indicated if pain, obstruction, or rapid enlargement is present. Because of the Roux-en-Y configuration, internal hernias can occur at various sites including the jejunojejunostomy mesenteric defect, Petersen's space, and the transverse mesocolon defect in retrocolic gastrojejunostomies. Obstruction occurring at these areas may not result in significant abdominal distention, as these sites of obstruction are relatively proximal. A contrast swallow study with small bowel follow-through (SBFT) or a CT scan with oral contrast should be considered in a post–gastric bypass patient with abdominal pain, nausea, and vomiting. Persistent pain not explained by radiographic imaging may prompt an operative exploration looking for an etiology of the pain. Studies suggest an internal hernia can be found in up to 41% of patients explored for abdominal pain (32). Aggressive surgical treatment of patients post–gastric bypass who present with a clear picture of mechanical small bowel obstruction is indicated due to this high potential for internal and closed loop obstruction and intestinal compromise.

Vitamin and nutritional deficiencies must be carefully followed. Patients must consume between 60 and 80 g of protein per day to prevent muscle wasting and hair loss. The dietitian plays a crucial role in the day-to-day instruction and monitoring of patients, again emphasizing the importance of a comprehensive bariatric team approach. Nutritional deficiencies are extremely prevalent and require more intensive monitoring and supplementation after malabsorption operations (see Chapter 20.3).

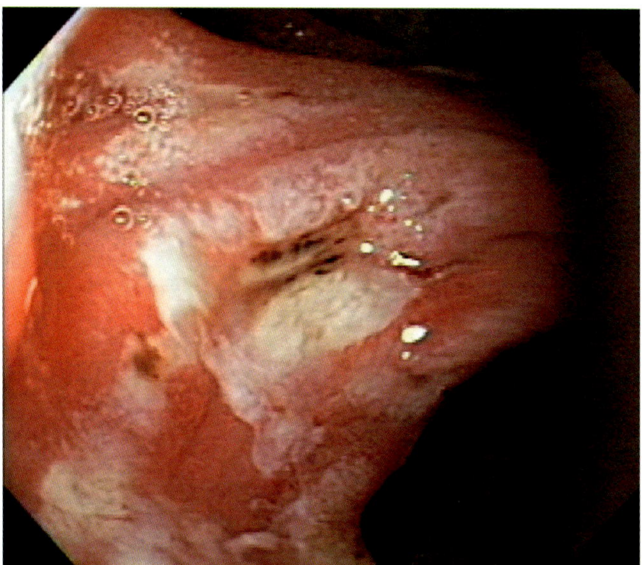

FIGURE 15-2. Endoscopic view of an anastomotic ulcer.

TABLE 15-2. Representative postoperative follow-up visit schedule

Follow-up visit	Nutritionist	Psychologist	Surgeon	Internist	Labs
3 weeks	X		X		
8 weeks	X				
3 months	X		X		X
6 months	X			X	X
1 year and annually thereafter	X	X	X	X	X

Documentation

Selection of bariatric patients should follow the National Institutes of Health (NIH) guidelines (32–35). Patient evaluation should accompany documentation of the patient's detailed medical history, diet and social history, and comorbidities to identify a suitable candidate according to the guidelines. Because bariatric procedures are not routinely covered by health insurance, this documentation is important in obtaining insurance approval. High-risk patients should undergo appropriate preoperative workups and possible treatments/prophylaxis prior to surgery.

The informed surgical consent for bariatric procedures is signed only when the patient understands the nature and the mechanism of the procedures, the proposed and realistic benefits of the surgery, and the potential major and minor complications that can occur following surgery. Thus, it is important that surgeons have several mechanisms to ensure the provision and discussion of such information, including brochures, videotapes, Web sites, support group meetings, lectures, seminars, and individual patient sessions. Bariatric surgery is in the midst of litigious medicine and the importance of allowing ample time and effort for educating the patient cannot be stressed enough. Of course, such efforts must be documented meticulously.

Operative notes should include enough details so that other surgeons and physicians involved in the patient's care can understand the exact anatomical changes made at the time of surgery. Pouch size, Roux-limb length and orientation (retro- vs. antecolic, retro- vs. antegastric), gastrojejunostomy technique (stapled vs. hand-sewn), and stomal size are some of the essential operative data that may be helpful in follow-up.

Postoperative weight loss, improvements in comorbidities, medications, exercise and dietary regimens must be carefully documented at regular intervals (Table 15-2). Use of comprehensive database software facilitates accurate documentation of detailed patient data and the treatment, and allows various outcome analyses. Unfortunately, these sophisticated databases are expensive and work-intensive to maintain, and are currently not valued by payers with reimbursement.

At all times, patient privacy has to be maintained in collecting and maintaining patient data. Bariatric surgeons should work closely with the institutional officers of the Health Insurance Portability and Accountability Act (HIPAA) to comply with the privacy laws. Any technical variation in the operation or research protocols must first obtain institutional review board (IRB) approval.

Close patient assessment, follow-up, and thorough documentation are prerequisites for improvement in surgical technique and outcomes and long-term patient care. Bariatric centers are encouraged to follow the ASBS guidelines to provide appropriate parameters within the institution to optimize care of the bariatric patient.

References

1. Cooney RN, Bryant P, Haluck R, et al. The impact of a clinical pathway for gastric bypass surgery on resource utilization. J Surg Res 2001;98:97–101.
2. Huerta S, Heber D, Sawicki MP, et al. Reduced length of stay by implementation of a clinical pathway for bariatric surgery in an academic health care center. Am Surg 2001; 67:1128–1135.
3. Dominguez-Cherit G, Gonzalez R, Borunda D, et al. Anesthesia for morbidly obese patients. World J Surg 1998;22: 969–973.
4. Huerta S, DeShields S, Shpiner R, et al. Safety and efficacy of postoperative continuous positive airway pressure to prevent pulmonary complications after Roux-en-Y gastric bypass. J Gastrointest Surg 2002;6:354–358.
5. Kyzer S, Ramadan E, Gersch M, et al. Patient-controlled analgesia following vertical gastroplasty: a comparison with intramuscular narcotics. Obes Surg 1995;5:18–21.
6. Martinotti R, Vassallo C, Ramaioli F, et al. Anesthesia with sevoflurane in bariatric surgery. Obes Surg 1999;9:180–182.
7. Bauer JJ, Gelernt IM, Salky BA, et al. Is routine postoperative nasogastric decompression really necessary? Ann Surg 1985;201:233–236.
8. Cheatham ML, Chapman WC, Key SP, et al. A meta-analysis of selective versus routine nasogastric decompression after elective laparotomy. Ann Surg 1995;221:469–476; discussion 476–478.
9. Wolff BG, Pembeton JH, van Heerden JA, et al. Elective colon and rectal surgery without nasogastric decompression. A prospective, randomized trial. Ann Surg 1989;209: 670–673.
10. Manning BJ, Winter DC, McGreal G, et al. Nasogastric intubation causes gastroesophageal reflux in patients undergoing elective laparotomy. Surgery 2001;130:788–791.

11. Huerta S, Arteaga JR, Sawicki MP, et al. Assessment of routine elimination of postoperative nasogastric decompression after Roux-en-Y gastric bypass. Surgery 2002;132:844–848.

12. Westling A, Bergqvist D, Bostrom A, et al. Incidence of deep venous thrombosis in patients undergoing obesity surgery. World J Surg 2002;26:470–473.

13. Wu EC, Barba CA. Current practices in the prophylaxis of venous thromboembolism in bariatric surgery. Obes Surg 2000;10:7–13; discussion 14.

14. Nguyen NT, Cronan M, Braley S, et al. Duplex ultrasound assessment of femoral venous flow during laparoscopic and open gastric bypass. Surg Endosc 2003;17:285–290.

15. DeMaria EJ, Sugerman HJ, Kellum JM, et al. Results of 281 consecutive total laparoscopic Roux-en-Y gastric bypasses to treat morbid obesity. Ann Surg 2002;235:640–645; discussion 645–647.

16. Higa KD, Boone KB, Ho T. Complications of the laparoscopic Roux-en-Y gastric bypass: 1,040 patients—what have we learned? Obes Surg 2000;10:509–513.

17. Schauer PR, Ikramuddin S, Gourash W, et al. Outcomes after laparoscopic Roux-en-Y gastric bypass for morbid obesity. Ann Surg 2000;232:515–529.

18. de la Torre RA, Scott JS. Laparoscopic Roux-en-Y gastric bypass: a totally intra-abdominal approach—technique and preliminary report. Obes Surg 1999;9:492–498.

19. Nguyen NT, Goldman C, Rosenquist CJ, et al. Laparoscopic versus open gastric bypass: a randomized study of outcomes, quality of life, and costs. Ann Surg 2001;234:279–289; discussion 289–291.

20. Wittgrove AC, Clark GW. Laparoscopic gastric bypass, Roux-en-Y—500 patients: technique and results, with 3–60 month follow-up. Obes Surg 2000;10:233–239.

21. Schneider BE, Villegas L, Blackburn GL, et al. Laparoscopic gastric bypass: outcomes. J Laparoendosc Adv Surg Tech 2003;13:247–255.

22. Hamilton EC, Sims TL, Hamilton TT, et al. Clinical predictors of leak after laparoscopic Roux-en-Y gastric bypass for morbid obesity. Surg Endosc 2003;17:679–684.

23. Buckwalter JA, Herbst CA, Jr. Leaks occurring after gastric bariatric operations. Surgery 1988;103:156–160.

24. Blachar A, Federle MP, Pealer KM, et al. Gastrointestinal complications of laparoscopic Roux-en-Y gastric bypass surgery: clinical and imaging findings. Radiology 2002;223:625–632.

25. Sims TL, Mullican MA, Hamilton EC, et al. Routine upper gastrointestinal/gastrograffin swallow after laparoscopic roux-en-y gastric bypass. Obes Surg 2003;13:66–72.

26. Pope GD, Goodney PP, Burchard KW, et al. Peptic/ulcer stricture after gastric bypass: a comparison of technique and acid suppression variables. Obes Surg 2002;12:30–33.

27. Levitan D, Burdick S, Schneider BE, et al. Balloon dilatation for the treatment of gastrojejunal anastomotic stricture after laparoscopic Roux-en-Y gastric bypass. Surg Endosc 2003;abstr.

28. Shiffman ML, Sugerman HJ, Kellum JM, et al. Gallstone formation after rapid weight loss: a prospective study in patients undergoing gastric bypass surgery for treatment of morbid obesity. Am J Gastroenterol 1991;86:1000–1005.

29. Sugerman HJ, Brewer WH, Shiffman ML, et al. A multicenter, placebo-controlled, randomized, double-blind, prospective trial of prophylactic ursodiol for the prevention of gallstone formation following gastric-bypass-induced rapid weight loss. Am J Surg 1995;169:91–96; discussion 96–97.

30. Villegas L, Schneider BE, Provost D, et al. Is routine cholecystectomy required during laparoscopic gastric bypass. Obesity Surg 2004;14:206–211.

31. Scott DJ, Villegas L, Sims TL, et al. Intraoperative ultrasound and prophylactic ursodiol for gallstone prevention following laparoscopic gastric bypass. Surg Endosc 2003;17:1796–1802.

32. Higa KD, Ho T, Boone KB. Internal hernias after laparoscopic Roux-en-Y gastric bypass: incidence, treatment, and prevention. Obes Surg 2003;13:350–354.

33. NIH conference: Gastrointestinal surgery for severe obesity. Consensus Development Conference Panel. Ann Intern Med 1991;115:956–961.

34. Expert Panel: Clinical Guidelines on the Identification, Evaluation, and Treatment of Overweight and Obesity in Adults: The Evidence Report, Bethesda, MD, 1998.

35. Mason EE, Amaral JF, Cowan GS Jr, et al. Guidelines for selection of patients for surgical treatment of obesity. Obes Surg 1993;3:429.

16
Bariatric Data Management

Paul E. O'Brien, Mark Stephens, and John B. Dixon

The Importance of Data Management in Bariatric Surgery

The central aim of bariatric surgery is to improve our patients' health and quality of life through control of the problem of obesity. It is a lifetime process. The weight loss may take 1 to 3 years to achieve. The maintenance of that weight loss needs to continue permanently. There is never a point in time where we can say to our patient, "The problem is solved. You are at your correct weight and you will remain there. You do not need any further help." We need an ongoing medical record for each patient. Much of the key data for a bariatric patient is numerical—weight, blood pressure, serum triglycerides, etc.—and can be managed with a paper file. But it can be better and more easily managed electronically. This chapter identifies the role of the electronic database in bariatric patient care, identifies the measures best handled in this manner, and looks at options available for implementing a database management system.

Database Functions

Tracking Outcomes: Weight, Comorbidity, Quality of Life

Weight is the most immediately important parameter of outcome to the patient and the physician. It is really just a means to an end, that being the improvement of health and quality of life, but it best reflects what is being achieved. Weight change can be expressed in several ways including weight in kilograms or pounds, excess weight, weight loss, body mass index (BMI) loss, percent of excess weight loss, and percent of excess BMI loss. Each of these has some justification. An electronic database enables any one or all of these methods to be used.

By far the most significant gain from bariatric surgery is the improvement in health, especially the control of the comorbidities of obesity through weight loss. These changes must be documented as a part of good patient care, as a method for modifying treatment of the comorbidity as change occurs and as a method for justifying the cost and invasiveness of the surgery. The management of data relating to comorbidities is often not a simple matter. Some areas, for example blood pressure or serum lipids, lend themselves to easy data management as they are expressed as numerical values. Others, such as asthma, sleep apnea, and low back pain, are more difficult to express in categorical terms. Absolute measures such as the presence of absence of symptoms or the need for specific therapy need to be used.

Improvement of quality of life (QOL) is the next most important outcome of bariatric surgery. It reflects the physical limitations caused by the size and weight; it reflects the embarrassment and loss of self-esteem and self-confidence due to obesity and it reflects the employability and the chances for promotion that are often denied to the obese. Measures of QOL provide numerical values and thus sequential changes can easily be tracked on a database.

Managing the Patient

A busy bariatric practice will have many patients, possibly thousands. We have more than 2000 patients under regular review in our clinic, with up to 150 patients reviewed in the clinic per day. A single patient might see several different physicians during the follow-up process. There is an absolute need to have a concise presentation of the patient's data readily available, summarizing all the key events and changes that have gone on before so that current status can be quickly obtained. The database provides this. We record progress notes on the screen so that they are readable, linked to the weight loss and adjustment data, and printable as a report for the family practitioner and as a hardcopy for the medical record.

Monitoring Nutritional Status

There is a permanent responsibility after bariatric surgery to ensure that patients do not develop nutritional deficiencies as a consequence of the reduced intake or the malabsorption of nutrients. This is particularly so after primary malabsorptive procedures such as biliopancreatic diversion and partial malabsorptive procedures such as gastric bypass. Protein malnutrition, as demonstrated by reduced serum albumin, iron deficiency, and folate and vitamin B_{12} deficiency are well documented. Regular measurement of these macro- and micronutrients and management of the results is best handled electronically.

Avoiding Patient Loss to Follow-Up

Permanent follow-up is essential for good bariatric patient care, and the surgeon is responsible for ensuring all possible measures are taken to avoid loss to follow-up. For adjustable procedures, such as the Lap-Band placement, optimal outcome cannot be expected to be achieved without continuing care. For procedures that are known to lead to nutritional deficiencies, such as biliopancreatic diversion (BPD) and Roux-en-Y gastric bypass (RYGBP), serious and possibly irreversible health consequences could occur in the absence of adequate monitoring. We consider a patient to be lost to follow-up if we have not reviewed the patient in 18 months and are unable to establish contact. Our database enables us to create a list of patients who have gone beyond 12 months from the last visit, and they are sought out directly or through family or friends. In a recent review of the outcomes of 700 patients, up to 6 years post Lap-Band placement, 3.6% were classified as lost to follow-up (1).

Communicating with Other Physicians

A computerized database that can generate reports facilitates efficient informing of family practitioners or medical specialists of the current status of their patients. We generate and send a summary report to the primary care physician on a regular basis with minimal effort.

Conducting Research, Audit, and Quality Control

There are three requirements for good clinical research: (1) a sufficient number of patients, (2) accurate measurement data, and (3) maintenance of data in an accessible and analyzable form. The availability of a comprehensive and accurate database is the lifeblood of clinical research. We have been able to publish extensively on the outcomes of Lap-Band placement because we have plenty of patients, we have collected the data and we have maintained a database that permits those data to be linked as needed to whatever research question is raised.

Not every staff member will be contributing to clinical research, but all should be contributing to clinical audit and quality control. All bariatric surgeons must have set up and maintained a database of relevant measures to examine if the outcomes for their group of patients are within acceptable parameters. What has been the weight loss? How many are lost to follow-up? What has been the mortality or perioperative morbidity? What is the reoperation rate? How do your outcomes compare with those of your peers? These questions can all be answered if the data are kept in an appropriate database.

The Data and Analyses Needed

There is an almost infinite range of data that could be collected. The two commonest flaws in establishing a database are attempting to collect everything in case it may be of some interest to somebody someday, and maintaining the database as an addition to, not a part of, the medical record. If you aim to collect too much information, it won't happen because the staff is too busy with other matters. If your database is independent of routine daily patient care, it won't get priority attention. Every data item stored should have a justification for being there.

We have been working with electronic databases in our bariatric practice for many years. The following key components represent our current range of data collected in our database, which is called LapBase®, and in parentheses the values calculated by the software and added to the screen:

Demographics: name; address; telephone numbers for home, work, and mobile; email address; sex; date of birth; primary care physician's name and contact details; specialists' names and contact details

Anthropometrics: weight; height (BMI, ideal weight, target weights); neck, waist, and hip circumference; blood pressure; bioimpedance (total fat mass, fat as percent of total body weight); patient photograph

Comorbidities: blood pressure, diabetes, lipids, asthma, gastroesophageal reflux, incontinence, sleep-disordered breathing, infertility, back and joint pains, heart disease, other diseases

Operations and other significant procedures: type of operation, including significant variables; for example, for RYGBP, includes length of Roux limb, type of gastrojejunostomy, etc.; date; surgeon; duration; length of stay; complications; postoperative barium meal, as small movie file

Outcomes: weight [weight change, percent excess weight loss (EWL), percent excess BMI lost], health, QOL, volume of fluid in band for laparoscopic adjustable gastric banding (LAGB) procedures, annual comorbidity reassessments

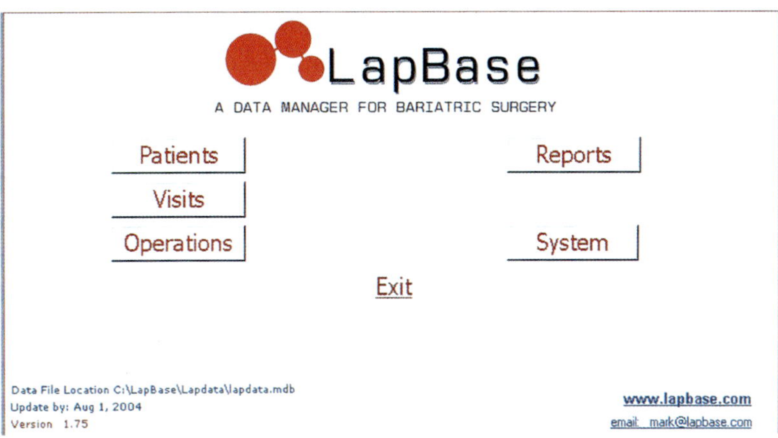

FIGURE 16-1. The Progress Notes page of the Follow-Up Details section. This page is the second of five pages and is used at each follow-up visit to document status and issues of that day. It provides a key summary of current data. For each visit, the top line provides weeks from surgery, weight, reservoir volume (RV), weight loss, percent excess weight loss (EWL), and doctor providing care on that day. The scroll bar on the right leads to all previous follow-up visits.

Progress notes are added as text statements to the page of follow-up details (Fig. 16-1). Information on repeat barium meals is filed with the follow-up data.

The Methods Available

With the input of data shown, the range of output of analyses is determined by the method of data management selected, ranging from simple text entry, mirroring the traditional medical record, to a full relational database that allows for cross-analyses among all fields.

Text (e.g., Microsoft Word)

Each patient is a file. All elements of the patient's record are entered as text statements, and the result is a medical record very similar to the paper medical record with which we are all familiar. As long as its structure is logical, all components of the record are accessible. Different patient files are accessed by alphabetical or numerical code. No analysis of data can occur unless the data are extracted from each record and separately entered into either a spreadsheet or relational database. This type of setup generally is not an improvement over using the traditional hardcopy medical records, as the effort of data entry does not yield sufficient additional information.

Spreadsheet (e.g., Microsoft Excel)

This is often described as a flat-file database. It is a simple system to set up and is ideal for storing basic lists of information. Typically each column contains a particular data point for all patients and each row contains all the data points for a particular patient. With this structure, you can summarize the data within a column, sort particular features, find values, and perform a range of mathematical and statistical analyses on individual cells or columns. However, the range of analyses is limited by the content of the columns and rows established initially.

Relational Database (e.g., Microsoft Access)

The key feature is the placement of each data point into one and only one of many tables. Each table contains the data on one defined subject. All tables are linked by a unique identifier so that any data item from any table can be linked on a form or analyzed with any other. Flexibility is the key. In Access, you create a database by first setting up tables. These are the objects that store the data. Each table stores a particular set of information. The relationships between all the tables need to be defined. Queries are then set up as the tools for extracting or combining or modifying the data from the tables. Forms are set up to let you see your information in an appropriate format. Reports are set up to provide a printed copy of data in an appropriate format. Macros provide a method for automating a series of actions on the data. LapBase is written in Microsoft Access. To make the system user friendly, the underlying program needs to be relatively complex. The current version contains 37 tables, 79 queries, 30 forms, 37 reports, and eight macros.

LapBase

LapBase (Accessmed, Melbourne; email, mark@lapbase.com; Web site, www.lapbase.com) is a relational database, using Microsoft Access, that has been specifically prepared to support the data management of bariatric patients (Fig. 16-2). It covers all current bariatric procedures. It is the result of a collaboration between a surgeon experienced in bariatric surgery (the first author of this chapter) and a gastroenterologist experienced in writing programs for medical practitioners using Microsoft Access (the second author). Some examples of the forms used are shown in Figures 16-3 to 16-6. The data that are entered have been summarized above. The outputs of the program are reviewed in the following subsections.

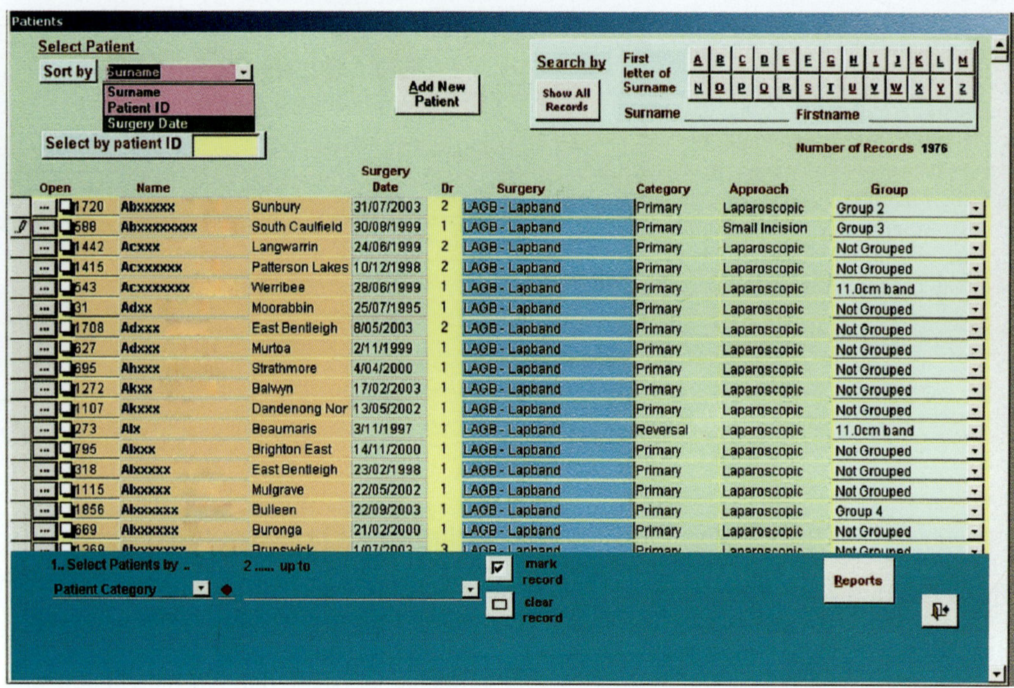

FIGURE 16-2. The main menu screen for the "LapBase" program is shown and leads to individual patient items on the left column or group data through "Reports."

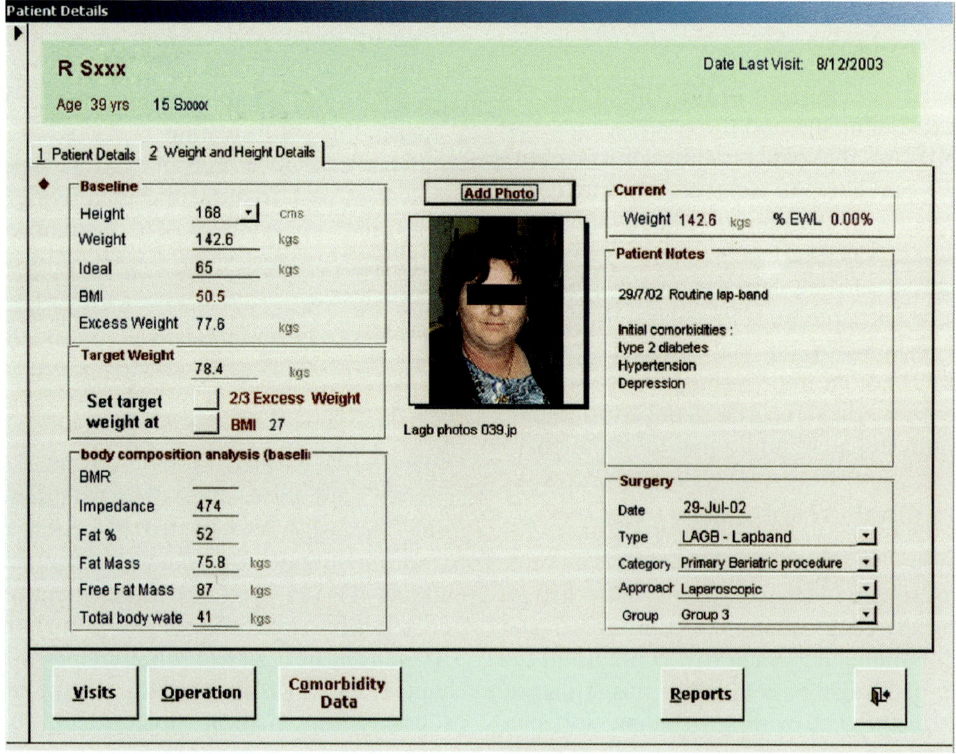

FIGURE 16-3. This is the main patient listing screen, which is opened via the "Patients" button on the main menu. It contains a listing of all patients in alphabetical order, or patient identification number or date of operation. Patients can be searched for via the alphabet, top right, or by providing part or all of surname or first name. Various other selection keys are present.

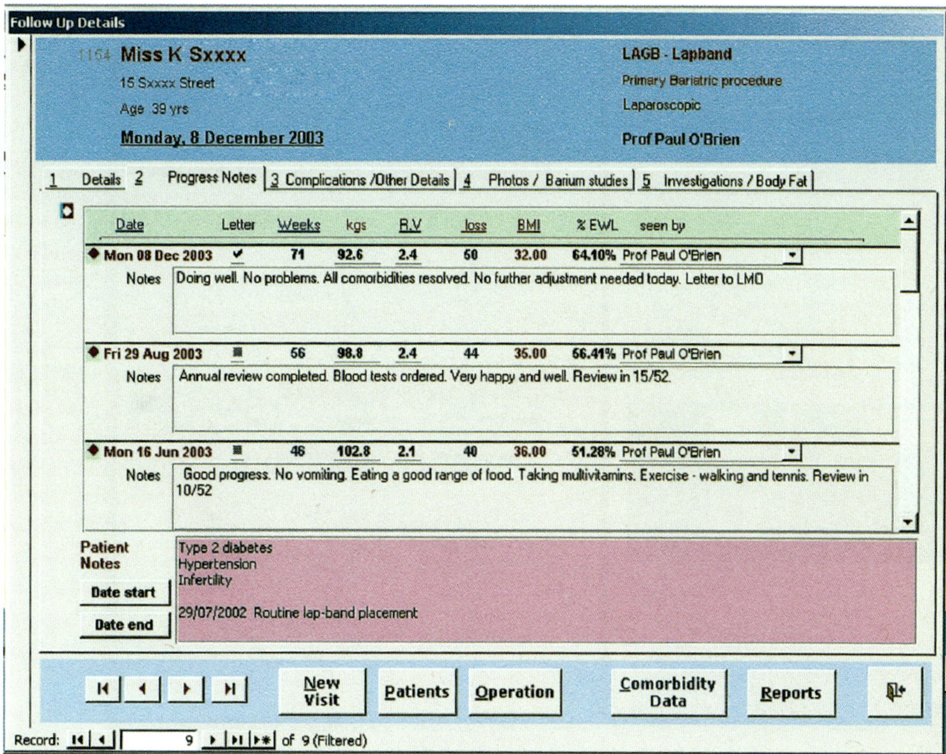

FIGURE 16-4. The second page of the Patient Details is shown. Initial weight data, target weights, body composition, notes, and key surgery data are provided.

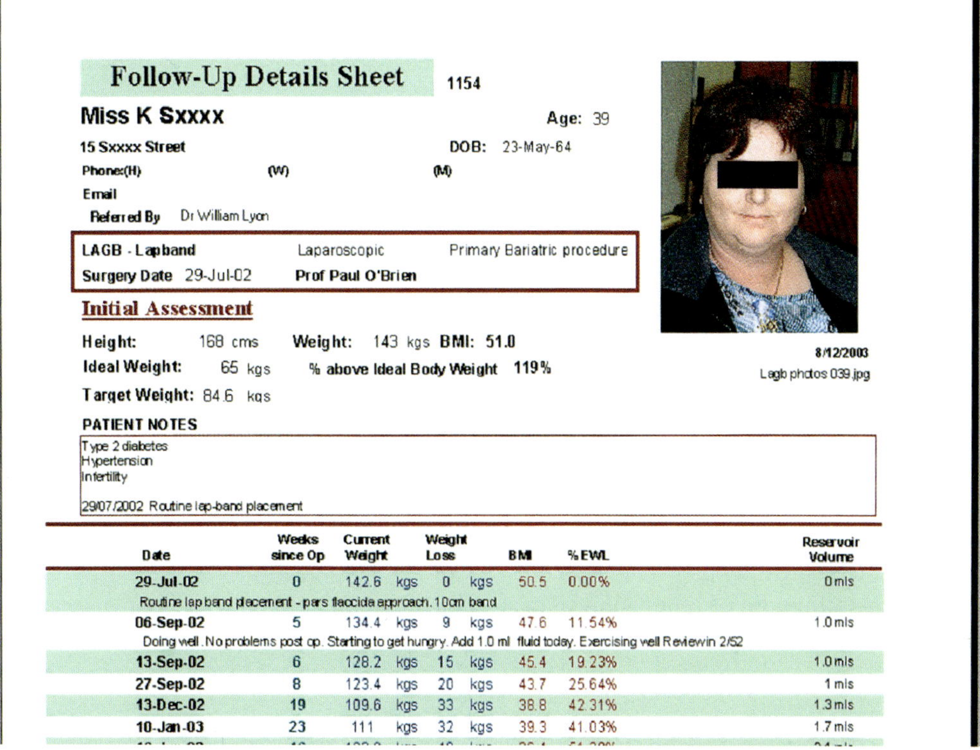

FIGURE 16-5. The Follow-Up Details Sheet provides a summary of many of the initial data at the top and then a sequential list of all follow-up data. The inclusion of the clinical notes in this summary is optional. The same data can be formatted as a letter directed to the family practitioner.

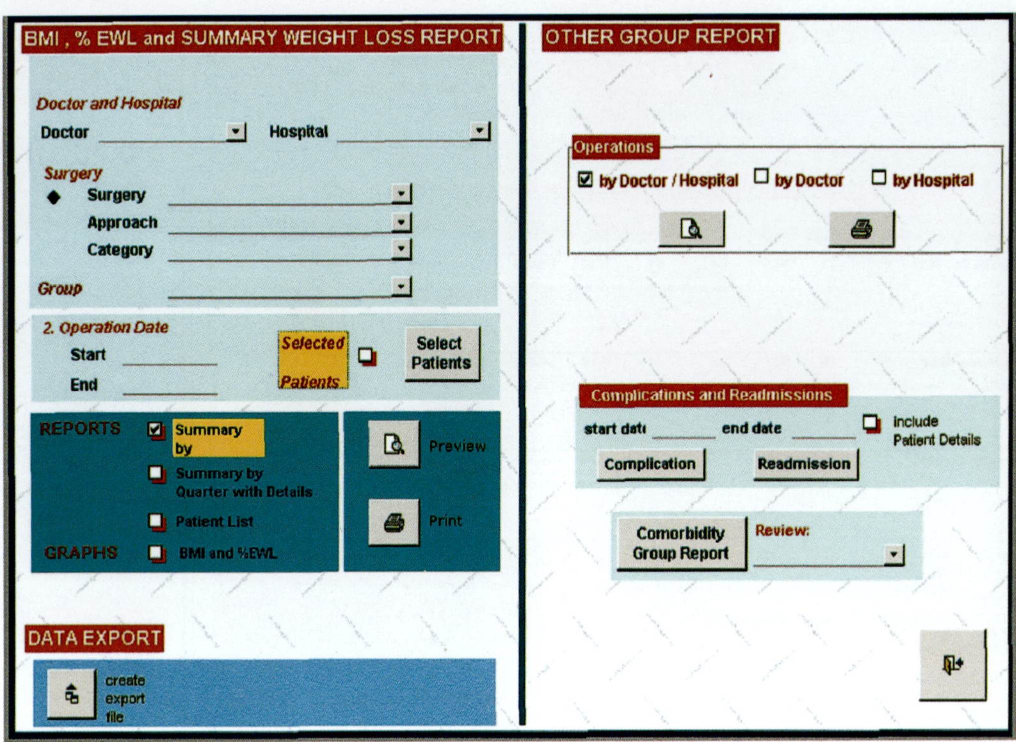

FIGURE 16-6. The "Reports" key on the Main Menu opens this page of options for generating analyses of group data. Patients for analysis can be selected in various ways and outcomes for weight loss, operations, complications, and comorbidities can be generated.

Patient Data

This is the most used area of LapBase. Initial patient entry into the database includes demographic data, weight and its related measures including target weights and body composition data, referring doctors, type and features of the operation performed, and perioperative and late complications or other events of note. All consultations are documented on screen and the key measures for assessing progress are visible in detail or in summary form. Barium studies, patient photographs, and changes in comorbidities are stored along with the relevant consultation. Referral to the hardcopy record is not needed for routine consultations. Summary data are available as reports to the family doctor or other specialist.

Group Data

The total pool of patients can be reviewed in various ways and pooled outcomes derived and printed as reports. Subgroups of the pool of patients can be identified and outcomes compared with the total pool or other subgroups.

Global Data

LapBase has the capacity to bring together in a secure and anonymous manner the data of multiple bariatric surgical groups and provide analysis of the pooled data. Bariatric surgeons will receive back a statement of their individual outcomes in comparison with global data.

Conclusion

It is strongly recommended that a relational database be established and used as an intrinsic part of all bariatric surgical practices. The use of a well-structured database is an option that should be taken up early and all data entered prospectively. It simplifies the process of patient care, permits easy but secure access to patient data by multiple practitioners and their associates, and provides the following: an overview of each patient's progress for weight loss, comorbidity change, and improvement in quality of life; reports that can be sent to the patient and the primary physicians, showing the progress that has been achieved; a summary or full details of the progress of all patients treated by the practice in the form of reports from which research or audit data can be taken directly; a mechanism whereby all of the data of the practice can be compared in a secure anonymous way with national or global norms for audit purposes; and an opportunity for better patient care and management.

Reference

1. O'Brien PE, Dixon JB, Brown W, et al. The laparoscopic adjustable gastric band (Lap-Band): a prospective study of medium-term effects on weight, health and quality of life. Obes Surg 2002;12:652–660.

17
The Current Role of Open Bariatric Surgery

Kenneth B. Jones, Jr.

Open bariatric surgery in the age of the laparoscope? You've got to be joking. Certainly I must be a dinosaur or an old dog who refuses to learn new tricks. Maybe I am afraid of the "learning curve." Or just maybe I know something others may not. Read on.

The biggest advantage of the laparoscopic approach to bariatric surgery compared to standard open procedures is the "vast improvement" in wound morbidity. As a matter of fact, the American Society for Bariatric Surgery (ASBS) and Society of American Gastrointestinal and Endoscopic Surgeons (SAGES) guidelines for laparoscopic and conventional surgical treatment of morbid obesity, under Surgical Techniques, state: "Wound complications such as infections, hernias, and dehiscences appear to be significantly reduced" (1). As usual, this statement is made based on the assumption that we are comparing laparoscopic bariatric surgery to open surgery via an upper midline incision.

Since we are not making one large incision, the assumption is that multiple small incisions produce less pain, a shorter hospital stay, which will make the laparoscopic approach more affordable, and a more rapid return to work and one's usual activities. However, I will demonstrate from my own experience with corroboration by published data that if one simply alters the open incision, that part of the question becomes moot, and other aspects of the "open" postoperative recovery period are at least equal, if not superior, to bariatric surgery done laparoscopically, for Roux-en-Y gastric bypass (RYGBP). Note that my remarks are directed toward RYGBP, the most common bariatric procedure done today, not the restrictive procedures considered elsewhere in this book.

I begin my argument by presenting my data from primary open RYGBP. In a series of over 2400 cases over a 17-year period, the excess weight loss at the 10-year follow-up was 62% (Table 17-1) (2). The most significant data are a leak rate of 0.5% in primary RYGBP, and a fatal pulmonary emboli rate of less than 0.1%, going back through my entire bariatric experience, including over 700 gastroplasty procedures beginning in 1979, totaling over 3500 primary and revision bariatric procedures at that time. The reoperation rate in this series of primary RYGBP procedures has been 1.4% ($n = 33$) due to leaks, staple line failures, incisional hernias, wound dehiscence, and definitive surgery for peptic ulcer disease. I have excluded many dermatopanniculectomies, which were done following successful weight loss, as well as a handful of cholecystectomies. I have used the following criteria for cholecystectomy at the time of bariatric surgery: (1) gallstones, (2) a strong family history of gallbladder disease, (3) a relatively strong American-Indian or Mexican-American heritage, or (4) cholesterolosis of the gallbladder at the time of surgery (3). Using these criteria, the handful of patients who have returned for laparoscopic cholecystectomy at a later date is about what one would expect from the normal population. My 10-year data of 62% excess weight loss is in line with other published series (Table 17-2) (4–6).

With this vast experience in bariatric surgery, why do I continue to do the procedure open? To put it very simply, I will demonstrate that there is usually an increased incidence of leaks and other complications using the laparoscopic approach, as well as a higher cost, and when you couple this with less wound morbidity of the left subcostal incision, I feel that there is simply no real advantage, and a significant disadvantage, to doing laparoscopic Roux-en-Y gastric bypass (LRYGBP).

Leaks and Other Complications

If one looks at the data from Schauer et al. (7), DeMaria et al. (8), and Wittgrove and Clark (9) in their published series, we see that their leak rate is almost 3%. However, Champion et al. (10), who does gastroscopy on all of their patients during surgery, have a leak rate very similar to mine, 0.4%, and Higa et al. (11), who does a double-layer hand-sewn intracorporeal anastomosis without staples at

TABLE 17-1. The author's 17-year experience with primary Roux-en-Y gastric bypass (RYGBP)

Mid-1986—April 2003: number	2421 primary RYGBPs
Average BMI	47
Height	5′4″
Weight	273 lb; 85% F
SLF	<1% since 1991
Leaks	13/2421 (0.5%)
Mortality	5 (3 PEs) 5/2421 (0.2%)
Symptomatic stomal ulcer	<2%
Splenectomy	0
EWL @ 1 year	78%
EWL @ 10 years	62%

BMI, body mass index; EWL, excess weight loss; F, female; PE, pulmonary embolism; SLF, staple line failure.

TABLE 17-3. Postoperative leaks comparing several laparoscopic RYGBP series to that of the author

Author	No. of cases	Leaks	Percent
Schauer et al. (7)	275	12	4.4
DeMaria et al. (8)	203	14	5.1
Wittgrove and Clark (9)	500	13	2.5
Champion et al. (10)	825	3	0.4
Higa et al. (11)	1040	0	0
Jones [open] (2)	2421	13	0.5

the gastrojejunostomy, and transected pouches, had no leaks in his first 1040 cases (Table 17-3).

Laparoscopic Roux-en-Y gastric bypass requires stomach transection, which in almost every series has a significantly higher incidence of leaks compared to stapling in continuity. Kirkpatrick and Zapas (6), in 212 patients in primary divided RYGBP, had 13 leaks, or 6%. Suter et al. (12), in 107 patients in primary divided Roux-en-Y gastric bypass, had a leak rate of 5%. Smith et al. (13), doing open RYGBP, had a leak rate of 1.8% compared to the combined experience of Linner (14), Yale (15), and myself (16) of 0.6% (Table 17-4).

Why should leaks occur when one transects the stomach, utilizing cutting and simultaneous stapling instruments? In my own experience I have always tried to adhere to the "1-cm rule," meaning that if the anastomosis is made incorporating the staple line, there will be some element of ischemia (Fig. 17-1). If staple lines are crossed at approximately a 90-degree angle, the risk of ischemia will be less, and if staple lines are parallel and less than 1 cm apart (the 1-cm rule), or as the crossing staple lines approach parallel (Figs. 17-1 and 17-2), there will be a higher risk of leakage (9,17). In addition, if one transects a hollow viscus, the cut ends must heal and seal. However, when stapling in continuity with no transection, healing takes place immediately, as there is no compromise of blood supply to the tissue. In my entire experience, I have had only one patient who has had a perforation along the staple line in a primary RYGBP.

This was an individual who had a previously undiagnosed insulinoma and a seizure on her fourth day postoperative, which ripped a hole in the proximal and distal pouches at the staple line, as well as causing a 180-degree disruption at the gastrojejunostomy. At reexploration there was no evidence of ischemia, with good bleeding of the edges that had perforated.

Increased Cost

The laparoscopists argue that patients get out of the hospital sooner. In several published series, this appears to be the case, that is, about 2 days rather than 3, saving approximately $1000 (7,9,18). However, I have never seen a leak that was manifested in the first 72 hours after surgery. If the patient is released in 1 or 2 days to return home several hundred miles away, a leak could be catastrophic. I compared equipment costs with laparoscopic vs. open RYGBP in one of my two hospitals, and found that laparoscopic equipment costs approximately $5200 vs. the open stapling equipment of about $1700, or a $3500 difference. Hospitals will probably double that cost to make a profit, making a difference to the patient of about $7000. When we add the added operating room (OR) time at $1250 per hour, the total charge to the patient is going to be $8000 to $10,000 more for laparoscopic RYGBP (Table 17-5).

At our Bariatric Surgery Center of the Mid South at Christus Schumpert Medical Center in Shreveport, Louisiana, an ASBS Bariatric Surgery Center of Excellence, the group that does LRYGBP actually has a length of stay virtually the same as my 3.2-day average, and an operating time almost twice as long as mine. The pain control staff has indicated there is no real difference in the pain endured by either approach. From a strictly practical

TABLE 17-2. Comparison of the author's 10-year postoperative data to other published series

Pories et al. (4)	57% EWL @ 10 years
	58% EWL @ 14 years
Sugerman et al. (5)	>50% EWL between 6 & 10 years
Kirkpatrick and Zapas (6)	15 years, mean EWL: 68%
Jones (2)	62% EWL @ 10 years

TABLE 17-4. Leaks: divided vs. stapled (intact) pouches

Author	Technique	No. leaks and patients	Percent
Smith et al. (13)	Divided	71/3855	1.8
Linner (14), Yale (15), Jones (16)	Intact	7/1186	0.6

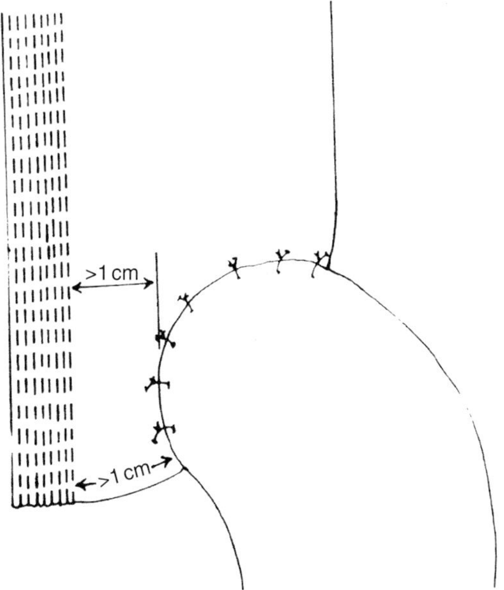

FIGURE 17-1. The "1-cm rule."

standpoint, if I am going to be spending half as much time per case in the OR as the laparoscopic group, and since there is little difference in reimbursement for either approach, I will continue to have time to have a higher volume with a significantly positive effect on my reimbursement compared to the laparoscopic group (Table 17-6).

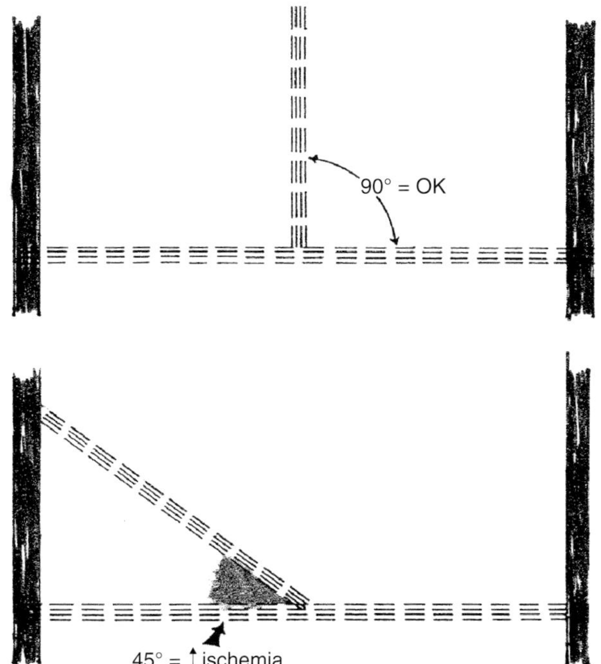

FIGURE 17-2. The narrower the angle between staple lines, the higher the risk of ischemia.

TABLE 17-5. Laparoscopic vs. open RYGBP stapling equipment cost; Doctors' Hospital, Shreveport, Louisiana

	2001	2002	2003	Approx. Difference
Laparoscopic	$4664	$4914	$5160	+$3500
Open	$1168	$1226	$1654	

The Left Subcostal Incision

Again, when we compare laparoscopic RYGBP to open, the traditional assumption is that open procedures are being done through midline incisions. However, when one compares my results as well as those of Alvarez-Cordero, using the left subcostal incision (LSI), to several other published series, it is easy to see that our incidence of incisional hernias is 38 times less than those series done through a large midline incision (18–22) (Table 17-7). Why? Simply stated, muscle has a much better blood supply than does midline fascia and it heals considerably better.

One may legitimately ask how I am so sure that my incisional hernia rate is so low, as traditionally bariatric surgical patient follow-up is so poor. I have therefore approached this question using a sampling technique. For instance, I used a portion of the patients we saw over a 4-month period in 1996, who came to the clinic for a variety of reasons, primarily for 1- to 10-year follow-up of RYGBP. We examined 173 consecutive patients and found no hernias. My incisional hernia rate was 5/1367 (0.4%), and leaks were 5/1367 (0.4%). Other wound morbidity was 2.2%. There has been very little variation from that rate (Table 17-8) (22).

If one compares the wound morbidity of several of the laparoscopic series to my LSI experience, it is easy to see that the rate of hernias and other wound morbidity is actually less than with the laparoscopic approach (7–9). I frequently tell my patients that in addition to the higher complication rate and cost of laparoscopic RYGBP, a procedure done through a single 7-inch incision or seven 1-inch incisions entails, either way, 7 inches of trauma to the abdominal wall (Table 17-9).

In addition, we should stress to our newer bariatric surgeons that they do many open cases before their first laparoscopic case. The ASBS guidelines (23) recommend 10 open cases before proceeding to laparoscopic bariatric surgery. As a preceptor for the ASBS, two of my preceptees who were quite accomplished laparoscopic bariatric surgeons initially did open RYGBP. They agreed with me that there is no real advantage and lots of potential disadvantages. In their combined series of 476 cases, their leak rate is 1.3% and their incisional hernia rate with the LSI is 1.5%, compared to mean leak and hernia rates of 3% and 7.6%, respectively, when one looks at the combined series mentioned above (18–22).

TABLE 17-6. A comparison of laparoscopic and open RYGBP at the Schumpert Bariatric Surgery Center of the Mid-South—Shreveport, Louisiana, July 1, 2002–March 31, 2003

Procedure	No.	LOS (days)	Operation time	Pain control
Laparoscopic RYGBP	56	3.5	3 hours, 38 minutes (218 minutes)	++
Open RYGBP (LSI)	101	3.1	1 hour, 40 minutes (100 minutes)	++

LOS, length of stay; LSI, left subcostal incision.

Technique

My procedure is based on a modification of the Oca-Torres procedure (24), with the following modifications: (1) an LSI; (2) the TA-90B® four-row Autosuture stapler, US Surgical, Division of Tyco, Norwalk, CT fired two times, reinforced proximally and distally with Ligaclips (Ethicon Endo-surgery, Cincinnati, OH) (Figs. 17-3 and 17-4); (3) a vertical pouch with no short gastrics being taken down and no transection of the pouch, all stapled in continuity (Fig. 17-5); (4) a retrocolic antegastric gastrojejunostomy, hand-sewn in two layers, utilizing a No. 38 bougie (13 mm in diameter) for adequate sizing; and (5) an enteroenterostomy that is done utilizing linear cutting and stapling instruments, the gastrojejunal limb being less than 150 cm, the biliopancreatic limb being less than 100 cm, depending on the patient's body mass index (BMI), according to the recommendations of Brolin et al. (25).

I pay particular attention to the following: (1) the 1-cm rule (Fig. 17-1), (2) taking care in the transection and freeing up of the jejunum and heeding the need for adequate length and freedom of the distally transected jejunum to avoid tension at the gastrojejunostomy; and (3) taking care in freeing up the esophagogastric (EG) junction to avoid perforation and ischemia. (4) I also perform a leak test; I prefer the "air bubble" test. Some prefer Methylene blue, but I believe more air pressure can be exerted with the former than with the latter. (5) I frequently use gastrostomy tubes in the bypassed stomach: in apple-shaped men; in long, hard revisions; in patients with diabetes mellitus to avoid problems with diabetic gastroparesis; with BMIs greater than 50 sometimes and always with those greater than 60; in all jejunoileal (JI) bypass conversions; and in patients with marginal pulmonary status.

Small bowel obstruction has been reported at a higher incidence with the laparoscopic approach compared to open (11,26,27), and I always take special care to make an adequate colonic mesenteric opening and secure it to the Roux limb prior to closure to prevent perijejunal herniation. I also do an adequate closure of Petersen's space as well as the potential hernia associated with the enteroenterostomy, which may be much more difficult laparoscopically. Following the discharge of patients from the hospital, I insist that they stay on a semi-soft "gooey" liquid diet for 6 weeks postoperative. In addition, I do all I can to preserve all possible blood supply, and avoid usage of the electrocautery near hollow viscera, as necrosis and leaks may follow several days later.

If one feels that it is necessary to transect the stomach in order to get adequate freedom of the proximal gastric pouch to reduce tension at the gastrojejunostomy, I have eliminated this fear by using the "Jones stitch" (Fig. 17-6), which effectively and safely pulls the pouch into the operative field. However, I readily agree that transection is sometimes necessary to get adequate length of the proximal pouch, especially with revision procedures (17).

About 15 years ago many felt that the pouch transection was necessary because of the inordinately high incidence of staple line disruption and secondary gastrogastric fistulae. Capella and Capella (28) noted that when stapled in continuity with no transection, disruption of the staples occurred in as many as 23% of patients. However, Pories's group (29) demonstrated that there was a 6% gastrogastric fistula rate when dividing pouches, and Capella and Capella also noted the same thing to be 2%.

One might ask how I know that my staple line failure rate is less than 1%. In a study done several years ago, in 650 patients, my assumption was that my staple line failure rate at that time was 0.8% with the double application of the TA-90B® four-row Autosuture stapling instrument. I came to this conclusion by upper gastrointestinal (UGI) series examination of 160 voluntary

TABLE 17-7. Incisional hernias, vertical vs. LSI

Author	No. of procedures	Hernias
Mason (18), Sugerman and McNeill (19), Amaral and Thompson (20), Alvarez-Cordero and Aragon-Virvette (21) (vertical)	1147	87 (7.6%)
Jones (22) (LSI)	2220	4 (0.2%)

TABLE 17-8. Wound complications of the left subcostal incision, January 1994–March 1997

Cases	447
Problems with wound healing	10 (2.2%)
Wound infections	4 (0.9%)
Large seromata: drainage and secondary closure in clinic	6 (1.3%)

Source: Jones (22), with permission of *Obesity Surgery.*

TABLE 17-9. Wound complications comparing laparoscopic vs. open (LSI) procedures

Author	Infections (%)	Hernias (%)
Schauer et al. (7)	5	0.7
DeMaria et al. (8)	1.5	1.8
Wittgrove and Clark (9)	5	0
Jones (open-LSI) (22)	Seromas, hematomas: <3	0.2

asymptomatic patients and found one staple line failure. In 19 symptomatic patients [gastroesophageal reflux disease (GERD) or rapid weight regain] during this period of time, their UGIs revealed four staple line failures (30). When patients have problems, they come back. I looked at this again from November 1999 to April 2003 in a series of 724 patients, in whom we did a UGI series on 62 symptomatic patients and found only five staple line failures. Again, this sampling technique indicated the staple line failure rate was less than 0.7% (5/714).

Conclusion

I hope this discussion has added something to the argument that open RYGBP is still a good, safe approach, and it may very well be better than laparoscopic RYGBP. I hope that we don't knuckle in to the pressure of our patients and industry and their perception that laparoscopic bariatric surgery is easier and better, for I have demonstrated that there is indeed a higher complication rate and greater cost with the anticipated end point virtually the same.

It is now obvious that the left subcostal incision is indeed far superior not only to midline incisions in open bariatric surgery but also to incisions made for laparoscopy. Transection of the pouches with laparoscopic RYGBP is mandatory, but has a markedly higher leak rate, and I have demonstrated that there is clearly no real advantage, and probably a significant disadvantage to transection of the pouches.

Why are we so rapidly adopting laparoscopic RYGBP? We know there is a higher risk of leaks; there is a great learning curve with a higher risk of medical malpractice exposure; there is an earlier discharge in less than 3 days, when leaks are rarely manifested before this time; there is an added expense of almost $10,000; and patients' return to work is directly proportional to their motivation, as a very small percentage of our patient population actually does such vigorous labor that they must be off for 6 weeks.

All agree that the biggest advantage of LRYGBP is the avoidance of wound morbidity. However, this argument is moot with the LSI, and the weight loss is the same with either approach. Therefore, logic dictates that I choose the safer, equally effective, less expensive approach of open RYGBP-LSI. In spite of these arguments, if one feels compelled to do LRYGBP, I would recommend the following: (1) have a basic background and considerable experience in advanced laparoscopic surgery; (2) do an open preceptorship or fellowship, which includes open as well as laparoscopic bariatric surgery; (3) participate in at least 10 open bariatric procedures; (4) take a laparoscopic bariatric surgery course if you have not done a pre-

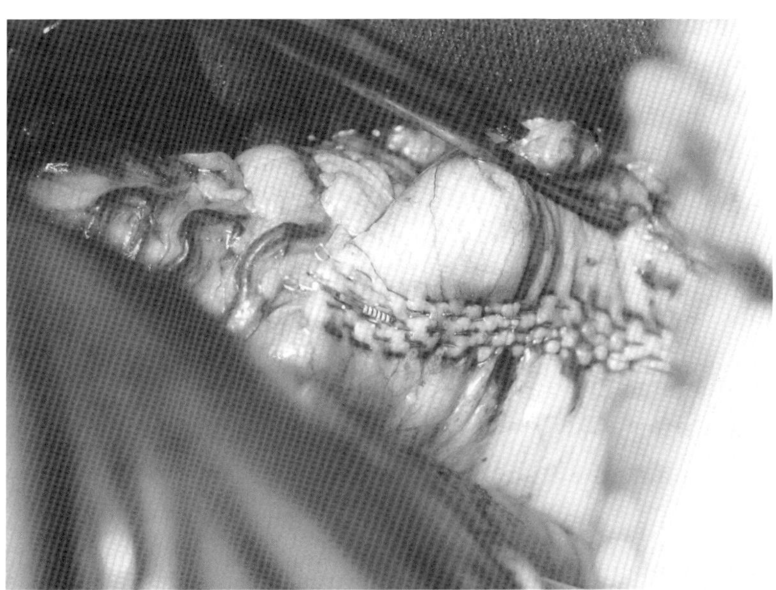

FIGURE 17-3. The distal staple line reinforced by a large Ligaclip (Ethicon Endo-surgery, Cincinnati, OH).

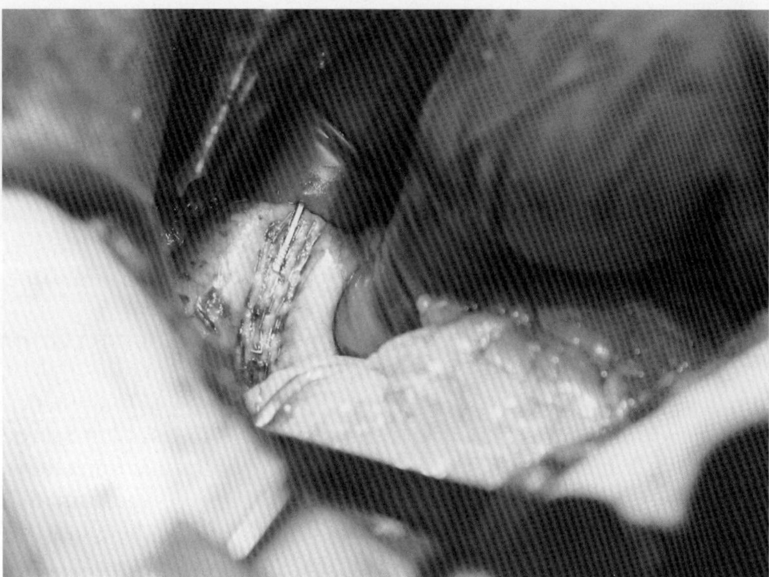

FIGURE 17-4. The proximal end of the staple line reinforced with a large Ligaclip, just adjacent to the angle of His at the esophagogastric junction. Note the inner two staple rows overlap.

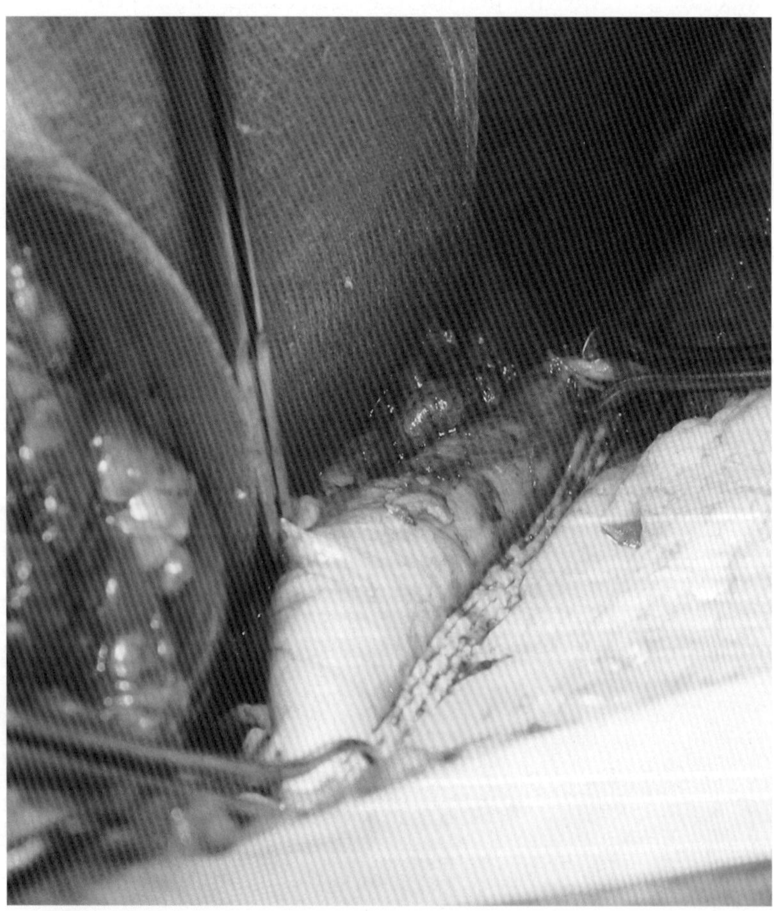

FIGURE 17-5. The 15-cc vertical pouch. The proximal (higher) end is approximately 2 cm from the esophagogastric junction.

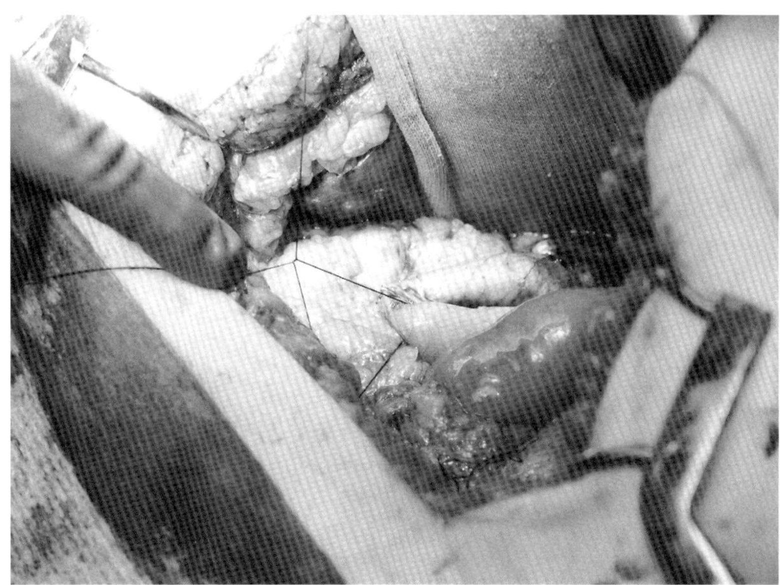

FIGURE 17-6. The "Jones stitch" attaching the distal staple line of the proximal gastric pouch to the abdominal wall fascia. The darker-appearing hollow viscus in the foreground is the proximal Roux limb ready for a tension-free anastomosis. Note the finger-size pouch.

ceptorship or had considerable training in same; (5) don't attempt revisional bariatric surgery laparoscopically until you are very comfortable with lap RYGBP; and (6) follow the Schwarz-Drew philosophy (31). They had a tremendous experience of several thousand open gastric bypass cases dating back over 20 years, starting with that of Dr. John Linner. They then took a short course in laparoscopic bariatric surgery, operated on several pigs, then did open RYGBP using laparoscopic instruments before they did their first laparoscopic bariatric surgical case, and, as one would imagine, their results have been remarkably good. Many others with large laparoscopic series reported in the literature did virtually the same thing, so it doesn't make sense for an advanced laparoscopic surgeon to jump into laparoscopic bariatric surgery without a vast experience in open bariatric surgery and all the nuances of lifelong patient follow-up.

More recently, I participated in a group study with 15 other experienced open RYGBP surgeons from throughout the United States. We compared our results of more than 25,000 open cases with the leading published laparoscopic bariatric RYGBP series in the world. We found their leak rate was five times higher, the OR time significantly longer, the monetary cost greater, small bowel obstruction about ten times higher, and the weight loss virtually the same with no difference in mortality rates, about 0.25% (32).

What is the current role of open bariatric surgery (RYGBP)? To act as the standard to which all other procedures are measured. Until LRYGBP becomes as safe and as economically feasible as open RYGBP-LSI, I'll remain a dinosaur along with many others.

Acknowledgments. The author acknowledges the contributions of Kimberly King in the technical preparation of the manuscript, Sue Wainwright and Donna Foshee for data retrieval and analysis, Steven Smith for photographic assistance, and Gary Linde for art work.

References

1. Guidelines for Laparoscopic and Open Surgical Treatment of Morbid Obesity. (Document adopted by the American Society for Bariatric Surgery and the Society of American Gastrointestinal Endoscopic Surgeons, June 2000.) Obes Surg 2000;10:378–379.
2. Jones KB. Experience with the Roux-en-Y gastric bypass, and commentary on current trends. Obes Surg 2000;10:183–185.
3. Jones KB. Simultaneous cholecystectomy: to be or not to be. Obes Surg 1995;5:52–54.
4. Pories WJ, Swanson JS, MacDonald KG, et al. Who would have thought it? An operation proves to be the most effective therapy for adult onset diabetes mellitus. Ann Surg 1995;222:339–350.
5. Sugerman HJ, Kellum JM, Engle KM. Gastric bypass for treating severe obesity. Am J Clin Nutr 1992;55(suppl 12): 560S–566S.
6. Kirkpatrick JR, Zapas JL. Divided gastric bypass: a fifteen-year experience. Am Surg 1998;64(1):62–66.
7. Schauer PR, Ikramuddin S, Gourash W, et al. Outcomes after laparoscopic Roux-en-Y Gastric Bypass for morbid obesity. Ann Surg 2000;232:515–529.
8. DeMaria EJ, Sugerman HJ, Kellum JM, et al. Results of 281 consecutive total laparoscopic Roux-en-Y gastric bypasses to treat morbid obesity. Ann Surg 2002;235:640–647.
9. Wittgrove AC, Clark GW. Laparoscopic gastric bypass, Roux-en-Y – 500 patients: technique and results, with 3–60 month follow-up. Obes Surg 2000;10:233–239.
10. Champion JK, Hunt T, DeLisle N. Role of routine intraoperative endoscopy in laparoscopic bariatric surgery. Surg Endosc 2002;16(12):1663–1665.

11. Higa KD, Bone K, Ho T. Complications of the laparoscopic Roux-en-Y gastric bypass: 1,040 patients—what have we learned? Obes Surg 2000;10:509–513.

12. Suter M, Giusti V, Heraif E. Laparoscopic Roux-en-Y gastric bypass: initial 2-year experience. Surg Endosc 2003; 17(4):603–609.

13. Smith SC, Goodman GN, Edwards LB. Roux-en-Y gastric bypass: a seven year retrospective review of 3,855 patients. Obes Surg 1995;5:314–318.

14. Linner JH. Surgery for Morbid Obesity. New York: Springer-Verlag, 1984:97.

15. Yale CE. Gastric surgery for morbid obesity. Arch Surg 1989; 124:941–946.

16. Jones KB. The double application of the TA-90B four row stapler and pouch formation: eight rows are safe and effective in roux-en-y gastric bypass. Obes Surg 1994;3:262–268.

17. Jones KB. Revisional bariatric surgery—safe and effective. Obes Surg 2001;11:183–189.

18. Mason EE. Surgical Treatment of Obesity. London: WB Saunders, 1981:340–341.

19. Sugerman HJ, McNeill PM. Continuous absorbable vs. interrupted non-absorbable suture for mid line fascial closure. Proceedings of the second annual meeting of the American Society for Bariatric Surgery, Iowa City, Iowa, 1985:153–154.

20. Amaral JF, Thompson WR. Abdominal closure in the morbidly obese. Proceedings of the third annual meeting of the American Society for Bariatric Surgery, Iowa City, Iowa, 1986:191–202.

21. Alvarez-Cordero R, Aragon-Virvette E. Incisions for obesity surgery: a brief report. Obes Surg 1991;1:409–411.

22. Jones KB. The left subcostal incision revisited. Obes Surg 1998;8:225–228.

23. American Society for Bariatric Surgery Guidelines for Granting Privileges in Bariatric Surgery. Obes Surg 2003; 13:238–239.

24. Torres JC, Oca CF, Garrison RN. Gastric bypass Roux-en-Y gastrojejunostomy from the lesser curvature. South Med J 1983;76:1217–1221.

25. Brolin RE, La Marca LB, Kenler HA, et al. Malabsorptive gastric bypass in patients with super obesity. J Gastrointest Surg 2002;6(2):195–205.

26. Higa KD, Ho T, Boone K. Internal hernias after laparoscopic roux-en-y gastric bypass: incidence, treatment and prevention. Obes Surg 2003;13: 350–354.

27. Courcoulas A, Perry Y, Buenaventuro P, et al. Comparing the outcomes after laparoscopic versus open gastric bypass: a matched paired analysis. Obes Surg 2003;13:341–346.

28. Capella JF, Capella RF. Staple disruption and marginal ulceration in gastric bypass procedures for weight reduction. Obes Surg 1996;1:44–49.

29. Cucchi SGD, Pories WJ, MacDonald KG, et al. Gastrogastric fistulas, a complication of divided gastric bypass surgery. Ann Surg 1995;221:387–391.

30. Jones KB, Homza W, Peavy P, et al. Double application of the TA-90B Four-Row Autosuture® stapling instrument: a safe, effective method of staple-line production indicated by follow-up GI series. Obes Surg 1996;6:494–499.

31. Schwartz ML, Drew RL. Laparoscopic Roux-en-Y gastric bypass: what learning curve? Obes Surg 2003;13:207abstr.

32. Jones KB, Afram JD, Benotti PN, et al. Open versus laparoscopic Roux-en-Y gastric bypass: a comparative study of over 25,000 open cases and the major laparoscopic bariatric reported series. Obes Surg 2006;16:721–727.

18
Technical Pearls of Laparoscopic Bariatric Surgery

Sayeed Ikramuddin

Surgery on the morbidly obese presents many challenges. Problematically, except for its extremes, weight or body mass index (BMI) alone does not predict the challenges that lie ahead in any bariatric procedure. Since the inception of laparoscopic bariatric surgery in 1993 all of the modern bariatric procedures have been performed laparoscopically with some modifications based on the limitations of the existing stapling equipment. The path, however, has not been without pitfalls for many surgeons. The learning curve has been steep, particularly for procedures that involve gastrointestinal tract reconstruction such as the laparoscopic Roux-en-Y gastric bypass (LRYGBP) or the biliopancreatic diversion/duodenal switch (BPD/DS) procedure. In the case of the LGB, Schauer et al. (1,2) have reported the learning curve to be as high as 100 cases. In the case of adjustable gastric banding, the technical challenges may lie less in the procedure and more in the details of band adjustment in the postoperative period. This chapter addresses some of the techniques used in bariatric surgery that facilitate the routine case as well as those that can be used to facilitate more challenging cases.

Getting Started

Patient positioning varies. Many surgeons perform the procedure with the patient in the "French position," and others perform it from the patient's right side. The latter is our preference. In principle, the surgeon should become comfortable with one approach and use it regularly, so that the operating room staff will learn the routine, which facilitates moving along with the operation. Choice of positioning will dictate the type of bed that is utilized in the operating room. The ability to sustain up to 800 pounds and still be able to provide steep reverse Trendelenburg positioning is helpful.

A common requirement of any laparoscopic surgical procedure is access to the abdomen. A fairly reliable truism is that the less the patient needs the procedure, generally the easier it is to perform. Access in these patients can be one of the most daunting parts of the procedure (see Chapter 10). Suffice it to say that despite the putative advantages of decreased vascular injuries (3), the Hasson cut down technique (4) can be quite cumbersome and time-consuming in the super-obese. One reason for this is extreme thickness of the subcutaneous adipose tissue. For this reason we have elected to establish pneumoperitoneum in the left subcostal region. We use a 150-mm Veress needle, which is commonly available. Initially we placed considerable attention on elevating the abdominal wall. This does not appear to be too important for placing the needle. Insufflation of the abdomen may require elevation in cases in which the opening pressure of the abdomen may be at the setting of maximum pressure on the insufflator. Usually an S-type retractor or a heavy suture in the skin is sufficient to facilitate this step. There are many devices on the market that promote direct entry to the peritoneal cavity either with or without the assistance of preestablished pneumoperitoneum. There is no demonstrable benefit in the case of established pneumoperitoneum. Without pneumoperitoneum there is a finite risk to the viscera or vascular structures. These devices, too, have a learning curve. It is important to be properly trained in the limitations and risks of such devices prior to using them.

Once inside the abdomen, key issues of importance include optimal port placement and retraction of the liver.

Optics

Chief among the advancements of the past decade in minimally invasive surgery is the refinement of optics, as can be seen also in the digital camera market. Use of the three-chip camera is common today. This configuration translates to enhanced color reproduction. Now with high-definition imaging even finer detail can be recognized during surgical procedures. There is no substitute for first-rate optics. Increased definition and detail may lead to increased precision in the operating room. The outcome from a missed enterotomy during a procedure can be devastating, which should be conveyed to the operating room management team. An effective bariatric program involves a team and significant resources that need to be defined at the initiation of the program.

In addition to the quality of the camera, it is important to use an angled camera in the operating room. A 45-degree angled scope is commonly used in bariatric procedures. Though it is possible to perform these procedures with 0-degree scopes, it is often not practical to do so. Use of angled scopes allows the camera assistant to keep the camera in one position while manipulating only the light cord to facilitate a wider perspective of the operative field. It is generally more disruptive to the eye to move the head of the scope rather than to move the light cord. Subtle movements of the light cord can help greatly when suturing. In addition to the traditional 10-mm scopes, it is helpful to have a 5-mm 45-degree scope to ensure adequate visualization from any port; this scope is also helpful in lysing adhesions early during the procedure or in facilitating port closure. Occasionally we will use the 45-cm bariatric laparoscope (Stryker Endoscopy, San Jose, CA). The most common indication for use is in the super-obese male patient.

During prolonged procedures the tip of the laparoscope can become fogged. In some cases this is due to leakage of carbon dioxide with cool carbon dioxide rushing past the tip of the scope. The key here is to identify the cause of the leakage. In some cases this cause is leakage in the port itself. Once identified, this is easy to remedy. If the leakage is at the level of the fascia, then sutures can be placed at the fascial level using a suture passer. In some cases it is best to minimize use of this port site, as it can make the leakage considerably worse.

Port Placement

As one becomes more comfortable with the procedure, the position of the ports can be optimized and the number of ports can be reduced. There are a number of concepts to be kept in mind while placing ports. It is generally not advisable to angle the ports for bariatric procedures. Angling the ports becomes a problem when one is working in more than one compartment of the abdomen. An example would be in the gastric bypass in which the gastric pouch would be formed in the hiatus and the jejunojejunostomy is performed in the left quadrant of the abdomen. In the case of a very thick

muscular portion of the abdominal wall, it may be necessary to angle some of the ports. One of the disadvantages of doing this is that there may be a need to place additional trocars. If the abdominal wall is simply too thick, then extra-long trocars are available. The use of these devices can be minimized by keeping the ports higher on the abdominal wall. An alternative is to enlarge the skin incision and allow the hub of the port to rest on the fascia rather than on the edge of the skin.

Camera port placement should be based on several concepts, including both the principle of triangulation and proximity. It is important to have the scope close enough to the point of surgery so there is not too acute an angle to be able to see adequately. If the scope is too close or on top of the action, then the majority of movements become paradoxical and thus more difficult to perform. For the gastric bypass we place the camera port about 20 cm below the xiphoid cartilage. Initially, it is useful to anticipate all obstacles that can hinder performing the procedure. We routinely divided the falciform ligament for our first several cases. Though we no longer do this routinely, it can often be of help in a patient with central obesity. If the surgeon is working from the patient's right side, then this maneuver facilitates sewing the gastrojejunostomy or oversewing the band.

Exposure

Adequate retraction of the liver is paramount in performing bariatric surgery. Most often the gigantic liver can be predicted in those patients, particularly females, who have tremendous central obesity with type 2 diabetes. For the past several years we have used the triangular liver retractor (Cardinal Health, Magaw, IL) to elevate the lateral segment of the liver. In some cases an additional liver retractor is necessary to elevate the left lateral segment. Another option is to insert a Nathanson liver retractor (Cook Surgical, Bloomington, IN) in the subxiphoid position. Exposure is critical to proceed with the case. To continue with creation of the gastric pouch, it is imperative that the angle of His be visualized in order to create the gastric pouch. If, using traditional maneuvers, the angle of His cannot be clearly identified, then the short gastric vessels can be taken down. This approach allows for gentle downward traction on the fundus of the stomach and eventual identification of the angle. If this does not provide the necessary exposure, then conversion to an open procedure must be considered. In the case of massive hepatomegaly in which the liver edge falls below the umbilicus, some thought should be given to abandoning the procedure. A trial of very low calorie diets and diuresis may be useful for preoperatively optimizing this situation. Another option is performing a biliopancreatic diversion, though it is necessary to inform patients ahead of time.

Staple Selection

Understanding the mechanism and limitations of staplers can prevent many potential stapler-related complications, but there is a learning curve with these devices.

Two primary types of linear staples are used today: Autosuture (Norwalk, CT) and Ethicon Endosurgery (Cincinnati, OH). Both have been used extensively to perform the gastric bypass with success. The Autosuture stapler is available in sizes up to 60 mm, with three rows of staples on either side. The stapler allows for two modes of articulation. Staple cartridges are available in 2.0-, 2.5-, 3.5-, and 4.8-mm staple heights. All staple loads can go through a 12-mm port, with the exception of the 4.8-mm green load, which requires a 15-mm port. The Autosuture stapler closes in a way that allows for tissue at the distal-most portion of the staple to be removed from the staple. This is particularly useful for the jejunojejunostomy portion of the procedure. Practically speaking there is no limitation to the number of times the stapler can be used.

The Ethicon Endosurgery staplers are also available at the same staple heights. The staple cartridges are available in two rows and three rows. The newer products include a 45-mm blue load (3.5-mm staple height), white load, and gray load. With the Ethicon device the articulation component is not part of the staple cartridge as in the case of the Autosuture product, and the articulation of the grip of the Ethicon staplers is quite firm. It is recommended to wait for up to 10 seconds once the stapler is applied in order to obtain maximal compression of the tissue to be stapled prior to firing. With this method it makes it less likely that thicker tissues will slide out of the jaw of the stapler. For example, this is particularly useful in performing a stapled linear gastrojejunostomy where tissues of variable thickness are divided. Regardless of which product is utilized, it is important to realize that both have their unique advantages once the surgeon is experienced in their use.

The Gastric Bypass

Many different approaches to the LRYGBP have been described. Major variations of the operation include the method of performing the anastomosis and the passage of the Roux limb. Anastomotic techniques include a circular stapled anastomosis, a linear stapled anastomosis, and hand-sewn anastomosis. The Roux limb can be passed in a retrogastric and retrocolic manner, antegas-

tric and antecolic manner, or retrocolic and antegastric manner, all of which appear to be successful (5,6). The LRYGBP has three critical parts: creation of the gastric pouch, the enteroenterostomy, and the gastrojejunostomy. The following subsections describe the approach we use at our center, and offer some technical pearls that we have found helpful.

The Enteroenterostomy

Many surgeons prefer to perform this part of the procedure first. The advantage is that the patient will not need repetitive changes in position. Also this approach allows for recognition of adhesions in the pelvis that may prevent the procedure from being performed laparoscopically. The table is placed in the horizontal position. The transverse colon is elevated rostrally. The omentum is flipped over the transverse colon to allow extension of the mesocolon. Appropriate triangulation of the instruments and the laparoscope is critical to facilitating this portion of the procedure. The area above the ligament of Treitz is grasped and the ligament of Treitz is clearly identified. It is not unheard of to find malrotation or nonrotation in these patients, and great care must be taken to clearly identify relevant anatomic landmarks prior to proceeding with bowel division.

The mesentery of the jejunum is inspected. In some cases we find that it is quite foreshortened. In patients with extreme central obesity, it may be best to perform the procedure in a retrocolic fashion. To perform an antecolic anastomosis, we divide the small intestine 50 cm downstream from the ligament of Treitz. We estimate the bowel length, or we use a bowel grasper with a 10-cm marker to measure the length of the bowel.

It is critical to use atraumatic instruments in running the bowel. A white staple load 60 mm in length is used to divide the small intestine. We use a gray staple cartridge approximately 2.0 mm in height along the mesentery. The best success with accurate division comes with the formation of a clear C-loop with the small intestine. This C-loop is easier to form with the transverse mesocolon retracted well rostrally (Fig. 18-1). One load will suffice for a retrocolic limb; however, two staple loads are generally needed for antecolic bowel passage, especially with a thicker mesentery. A Penrose drain is tacked to the end of the Roux limb using the Endostitch (Autosuture) device. The Roux limb is 75 cm for patients with a BMI less than 40. A 150-cm limb is used for patients with a BMI of 40 to 50. For patients who are super-obese with a BMI greater than 60, we make the Roux limb 200 cm, and for patients with a BMI of between 70 and 80, we make the Roux limb 250 cm. For patients with a BMI greater than 80, we counsel them as to the necessity of a distal Roux-en-Y gastric bypass.

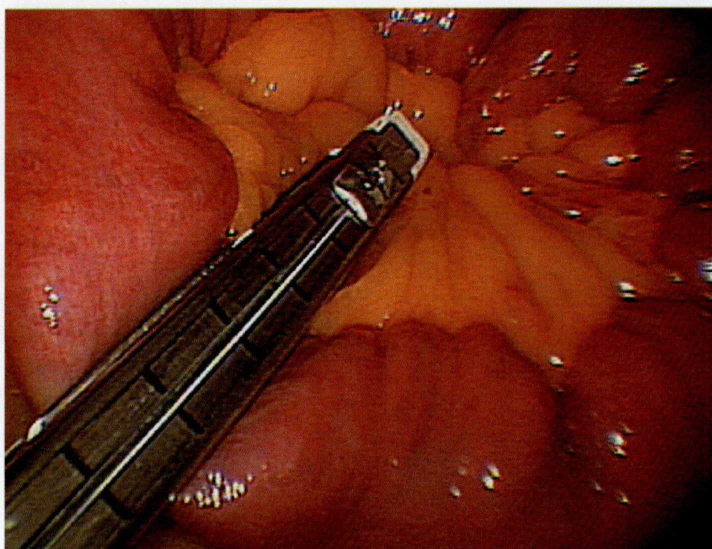

FIGURE 18-1. C-loop.

Once the length of the Roux limb is determined, we run the bowel distally. The Penrose drain points rostrally to the midtransverse colon and the mesentery points to the left side of the abdomen. The interposing small bowel is allowed to fall into the left lower quadrant as it is being run so that it does not interfere with access to the biliopancreatic limb. Following this step, we then attach the Roux limb to the biliary-pancreatic limb at its antimesenteric borders. The harmonic scalpel (Ethicon Endosurgery) is used to make enterotomies in the Roux limb and on the biliopancreatic limb. With the biliopancreatic limb it is simply a matter of excising the very top corner of the staple line with the harmonic scalpel. With the Roux limb, however, it is important to remain antimesenteric and approximately 1 cm or so proximal to the corresponding enterotomy on the biliopancreatic limb (Fig. 18-2). A white-load 60-mm stapler is inserted to its full length and fired. We place one suture at the heel of the anastomosis, and then we approximate the enterotomy at the staple line, rotate the enterotomy of the jejunojejunostomy almost 90 degrees so that the distal end of the Roux limb faces the left upper quadrant, and close it with an additional firing of a 60-mm white load. We carefully inspect the staple line to make sure there is no evidence of mucosa that is visible and that there is separation of the serosa. If there is anything visible, we use a 4–0 suture to carefully imbricate this area.

The size of the lumen is inspected externally. For a distal bypass it may be preferential to sew this enterotomy closed. Fibrin glue (Baxter, Deerfield, IL) is applied to the staple lines to minimize adhesions and to minimize bleeding. We then perform running closure of the mesenteric defect of the jejunojejunostomy beginning with an anti-obstruction stitch to prevent kinking.

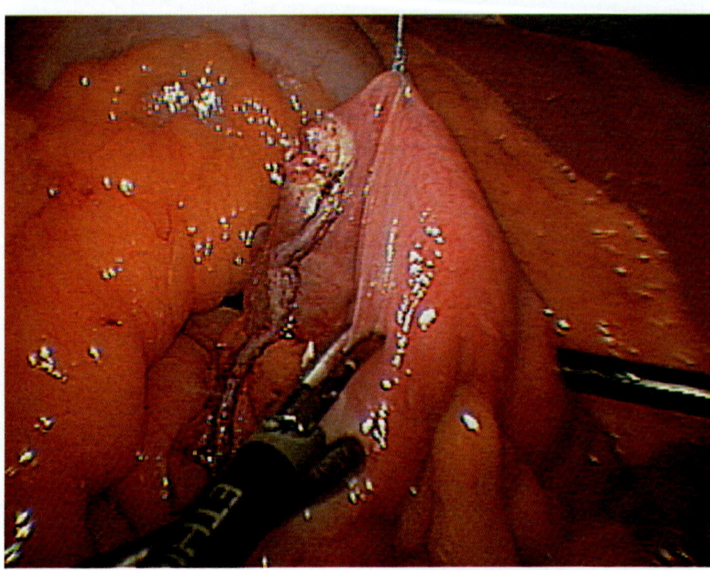

FIGURE 18-2. Enterotomies for the enteroenterostomy.

Creation of the Gastric Pouch

The patient is placed in the steep reverse Trendelenburg position. The harmonic scalpel is used to incise the hepatogastric ligament. Ideally, the caudate lobe is identified through the generally thinner hepatogastric ligament. Generally, from this dissection point it is easy to identify the left gastric artery. In some cases this anatomy can be quite apparent and a large replaced or accessory hepatic vessel can be located at this level. Care should be taken not to injure this vessel in this location, especially as it is generally not necessary to go this high in the dissection.

We begin by transecting the lesser curvature blood supply approximately 2 cm below the gastroesophageal (GE) junction on the left side below the left gastric artery. We use a white staple cartridge of 2.5-mm staple height. Bleeding from this staple line is reduced using reinforcements such as bovine pericardium. We have not found any adverse sequelae to beginning the dissection in this way, which may minimize trauma to the delicate lesser curvature of the stomach. We then transition to using a blue staple cartridge that is approximately 3.5 mm in staple height. A small lesser curvature gastric pouch approximately 15 to 20 cc in size is created. Initially we sized our pouch with a 20-cc balloon; however, this has not been necessary in our last several hundred cases. This division is carried from the lesser curvature directly up to the angle of His. Care is taken to avoid incorporation of fundus in the pouch and to ensure that there is complete division of the stomach and that no gastrogastric fistula remains. It is important to avoid tension at the crotch of the staple line, as this may result in staple separation.

Troublesome bleeding on the gastric pouch side is sometimes found; however, this can easily be controlled by a piece of Surgicel® (Johnson & Johnson, New Brunswick, NJ). If any defects are found in the staple lines, they are reinforced either using intracorporeal suturing techniques or using the Endostitch. It is important to fix corresponding defects on the gastric pouch to corresponding defects on the gastric remnant. Staple line leaks from the gastric remnant are notoriously difficult to diagnose and can be associated with significant morbidity and mortality during the postoperative period. There are often multiple adhesions posterior to the gastric remnant, which we typically do not need to take down; as in the majority of cases we perform an antecolic-antegastric Roux limb passage. In the case that retrogastric passage is anticipated, then these adhesions must be lysed. Adhesions posterior to the gastric pouch are taken down until a 1-cm area has been cleared for the gastrojejunal anastomosis.

Special considerations apply to the large sliding hiatus or paraesophageal hernia. In patients with these conditions, the hernia should be reduced with preservation of a vascular pedicle to the proximal lesser curvature of the stomach. Once the crura have been approximated, the pouch can be formed.

The Gastrojejunostomy

The greater omentum is split beginning at the midpoint of the transverse colon using the harmonic scalpel. The Penrose drain is then grasped, making sure that there is no twist of the Roux limb, and pushed up to the gastric pouch. This is best done with the patient out of the reverse Trendelenburg position to maximize mobility.

If it appears that there will be undue tension on the anastomosis, then a retrocolic-retrogastric passage is planned. Prior to beginning this passage, it is important that any remaining retrogastric adhesion be lysed using the harmonic scalpel. Once this has been confirmed, the mesentery of the colon 2 to 3 cm anterior to the ligament of Treitz is grasped and incised. The stomach is identified and pulled to the left and the Penrose drain is passed using an articulating grasper into the lesser sac. This defect must be closed judiciously at the completion of the procedure, with attention paid to closing Petersen's space. Twisting the Roux limb below the gastric remnant must be avoided.

In both approaches, the patient is slowly placed in the steep reverse Trendelenburg position. A back row of sutures beginning at the very top of the staple line of the gastric pouch (toward the angle of His) and the end of the Roux limb where the Penrose drain is attached is begun. This is continued all the way along the posterior aspect of the pouch obliquely and along the Roux limb parallel and close to the mesentery. This also serves to take tension off the anastomosis and allows for the entire gastric pouch staple line to be oversewn. Enterotomies are made at the right corner of the pouch and on a corresponding point on the Roux limb. A linear stapler is inserted to no more than 1.5 cm and fired. We use the Olympus 30 French endoscope (Olympus, Melville, NY) placed into the Roux limb and oversewn in two layers over this using the Endostitch. We place a bowel clamp and then insufflate underneath the saline to make sure there is no leakage or bubbling. A generous Petersen's defect should be closed even when performing an antecolic procedure.

Antecolic Versus Retrocolic

Though a discussion of the advantages of antecolic anastomosis over retrocolic anastomosis is beyond the scope of this chapter, there are certain technical tips that may be kept in mind when performing an antecolic anastomosis versus a retrocolic anastomosis. Both procedures can be complicated by internal hernia formation through the Petersen's space; however, in the retrocolic approach there is a mesocolic defect that additionally must be closed to prevent the occurrence of internal herniation. In patients who appear to have a very short mesentery, or for those patients with a tremendous amount or a very bulky large transverse colon mesentery, it may be beneficial to place the Roux limb retrocolically in order to avoid or diminish tension at the gastrojejunal anastomosis. In addition, there is improved access to the gastric remnant for the purpose of gastric decompression, improved access to the gastric remnant for endoscopy or endoscopic retrograde cholangiopancreatography (ERCP) in the case of choledocholithiasis, and easier removal in the case of persistent pain in the context of possible ulcer disease. In performing the procedure retrocolically, emphasis must be placed on closing the mesocolic defect. Some surgeons have recommended several interrupted sutures, but others feel that this is inadequate and perform a running suture instead.

Laparoscopic Adjustable Banding

Success and minimization of complications is contingent on accurate placement of the band in the pars flaccida position. Equally important is the technique of securing the band with gastrogastric sutures to prevent slippage and at the same time minimizing the risk of erosions. Techniques of access are identical to those in the gastric bypass. The procedure can be performed with the patient in the split-leg position with the surgeon operating between the legs. Alternatively, the patient can be in the supine position with the surgeon operating from the patient's right side. Up to six ports can be used for the procedure. Two important aspects to keep in mind are placement of the camera port and placement of the surgeon's right-hand working port. In comparison to the gastric bypass, it is possible to place the camera port much higher in the banding procedure, which facilitates the best maneuver for visualizing the angle of His and for placing gastrogastric sutures. Placement of the working port is critical. It is important that the instrument passed from this port enters the retroesophageal position at the junction of the crura. The angle of dissection basically follows that of the lower esophageal sphincter, coursing rostrally and to the left. The instrument should exit at the angle of His. Another important consideration is the minimal dissection that is needed to facilitate passage of the grasper. A small venous branch courses across the junction of the two crura, which is a reliable landmark to initiate dissection.

There are also a few issues that need to be considered in securing the band using gastrogastric sutures. Between two and four sutures are typically used. It is helpful to place the first suture proximate to the buckle of the band, leaving a good distance between the buckle and the

oversew. Using this first suture as a traction stitch pulling to the right side, it is then easy to place the additional two sutures between the fundus and the cardia of the stomach progressing to the angle of His. Generally, the smaller 9.75-cm band is suitable for smaller female patients with peripheral obesity. Males with central obesity, particularly those with a significant cardia fat pad, are best served with the larger band.

An overlooked but important component of the lap band procedure is placement of the port itself. The incidence of port and tubing related problems can be significant. In most cases these problems can be easily corrected, most often under local anesthesia. Placement of the port seems to make a difference. Early in our experience we placed the lap band port laterally usually toward the right flank. Though this is a suitable place to put the band it is not optimal. We and others have found that the best location of the port seems to be off the midline in the supraumbilical position. There is less likelihood that it will be involved in a panniculus as weight loss progresses. It is also important to make a generous incision when placing the port. The port should be clearly visible sitting flat on the rectus fascia at the end of the procedure prior to closing the skin. To minimize the risk of port twisting or flipping, four sutures should be used to tack the port into place. Deep retractors should be made available to facilitate the exposure to place these sutures.

The approach to band adjustments varies among surgeons. The primary difference is the use of fluoroscopy versus office-based adjustments. There are no good data to suggest the advantages of one over the other. One of the advantages of adjusting the band under fluoroscopy is that location and injection of the port can be facilitated. Additionally, very tight adjustment of the band can be recognized with significant reflux of barium from the pouch back into the esophagus or the development of tertiary esophageal contractions. In many cases these patients are asymptomatic. Recognition may prevent the development of maladaptive eating. Regardless of the method of adjustment, it is important not to remove the adjustment needle until confirmation that there is no complete outflow obstruction. The rationale behind this is obvious but must be learned; just because one is able to insert the needle the first time does not mean that the port can be accessed a second time. Moreover, it is important to confirm that fluid can be withdrawn from the band prior to injecting the port. In a few cases we have observed that fluid can enter and not be withdrawn, If there is any question about the integrity of the band, injection of IV contrast material into the band may identify the presence of a leak in the system. In the case of IV contrast dye allergy, simple injection of as little as 2 cc air can demonstrate free air under the right hemidiaphragm.

A detailed discussion of revisional bariatric surgery is beyond the scope of this chapter. Examples of these procedures include Nissen to gastric bypass, band to bypass, vertical banded gastroplasty to bypass, and take down of gastrogastric fistulae. In these cases, attention should be paid to the workup prior to surgery, including obtaining the previous operative note, and ordering an upper endoscopy and a radiographic evaluation of the proximal gastrointestinal tract. Reoperative laparoscopic surgery requires meticulous technique with judicious use of intraoperative endoscopy. There should be a low threshold for conversion to an open procedure. Care must be taken to choose the appropriate staple height in reoperative surgery. In some cases even the green 4.8-mm cartridge is insufficient to adequately divide the stomach. In these cases the surgeon must be comfortable with intracorporeal suturing techniques to reconstruct the gastric pouch.

Conclusion

Many techniques can facilitate performing laparoscopic bariatric surgery. There is no substitute for experience in this area. Something can be learned in every case. The dedicated bariatric surgeon should keep an open mind to learning new approaches and techniques in this ever-changing specialty.

References

1. Schauer P, Ikramuddin S, Hamad G, Gourash W. The learning curve for laparoscopic Roux-en-Y gastric bypass is 100 cases. Surg Endosc 2003;17:212–215.
2. Schauer PR, Ikramuddin S, Hamad G, et al. Laparoscopic gastric bypass surgery: current technique. J Laparoendosc Adv Surg Tech A 2003;13(4):229–239.
3. Poole GH, Frizelle FA. Modifications to the Hasson technique. Aust NZ J Surg 1996;66(11):770.
4. Molloy D, Kaloo PD, Cooper M, Nguyen TV. Laparoscopic entry: a literature review and analysis of techniques and complications of primary port entry. Aust NZ J Obstet Gynaecol 2002;42(3):246–254.
5. Wittgrove AC, Clark GW, Tremblay LJ. Laparoscopic gastric bypass, Roux-en-Y: preliminary report of five cases. Obes Surg 1994;4:353–357.
6. Higa KD, Ho T, Boone KB. Laparoscopic Roux-en-Y gastric bypass: technique and 3–year follow-up. J Laparoendosc Adv Surg Tech A 2001;11(6):377–382.

19.1
Laparoscopic Vertical Banded Gastroplasty

J.K. Champion and Michael Williams

The technique for laparoscopic vertical banded gastroplasty (VBG) arose from the open procedure in 1993, as minimally invasive surgical approaches were applied to virtually all commonly performed operations (1,2). In 1992 approximately 85% of bariatric surgeons utilized an open VBG as described by Mason at the University of Iowa, and the initial laparoscopic approaches attempted to mimic that technique (3,4). The Mason-like VBG incorporated a circular stapler to create an opening near the lesser curve, in order to insert a linear stapler vertically alongside a bougie to form a vertical pouch (Fig. 19.1-1), and the laparoscopic techniques followed that general form, but authors reported technical issues and controversies in attempting to replicate the open procedure, which will be discussed later in this chapter (3,4). In 1995 we developed a novel approach to performing a laparoscopic VBG by omitting the circular stapler and employing a totally linear stapler technique to wedge out a segment of the fundus to create a vertically oriented pouch (Fig. 19.1-2), as an alternative to the classic procedure (5).

This chapter reviews the techniques and outcomes of both the laparoscopic Mason-like circular window VBG and the wedge VBG utilizing only a linear stapler.

Technique for Laparoscopic Wedge Vertical Banded Gastroplasty

The patient is positioned supine on the table with a footboard, to allow reverse Trendelenburg tilt. The surgeon and camera operator stand to the patient's right side, with the assistant surgeon and scrub nurse positioned on the left.

The initial trocar site is for the camera and is a 12-mm incision made 15 cm below the xiphoid process, just to the left of the midline within the left rectus sheath. An Optiview trocar (Ethicon Endosurgery, Cincinnati, OH) is utilized to enter the abdomen under direct visualization using a 10-mm, 0-degree scope without insufflation. Insufflation to 15 mm is begun and the abdomen carefully inspected. The remaining five trocars are now inserted under direct visualization in the positions indicated in Figure 19.1-3. There are a total of four 5-mm ports and two 12-mm ports, with the second 12-mm port positioned in the left upper quadrant below the costal margin to utilize as the stapling port.

The patient is positioned in the reverse Trendelenburg and a 5-mm ratcheted Allis clamp is passed through the xiphoid trocar, under the left lobe of the liver and attached to the diaphragm for retraction. The fundus of the stomach is retracted laterally, and the surgeon takes down the peritoneal attachments along the left crus with monopolar electrocautery to delineate the angle of His and assist in applying the stapler for transection of the upper pouch. A measurement is then made 5 cm inferiorly from the angle of His along the lesser curve for creation of a window into the lesser sac directly alongside the gastric wall utilizing blunt dissection and electrocautery for hemostasis. This window will be used to position the band around the pouch at the end of the procedure and is used as a landmark while stapling the pouch (Fig. 19.1-4).

The dissection now proceeds horizontally from the lesser curve window to the greater curve of the stomach, and the short gastric vessels are taken down along the upper fundus all the way to the left crus and angle of His. A 50-French (F) bougie is then positioned along the lesser curve of the stomach to serve as a caliber to form the pouch during stapling. The 12-mm linear stapler (Endo GIA-2, US Surgical Corp [USSC], Norwalk, CT) with a 45-mm 3.5 load is inserted via the 12-mm port in the left subcostal position and applied transversely on the stomach beginning at the greater curve directly horizontal from the window on the lesser curve (Fig. 19.1-5). The stapler is fired horizontally until the end of the stapler touches the bougie at the lesser curve (Fig. 19.1-6). The stapler is now repositioned vertically alongside the bougie

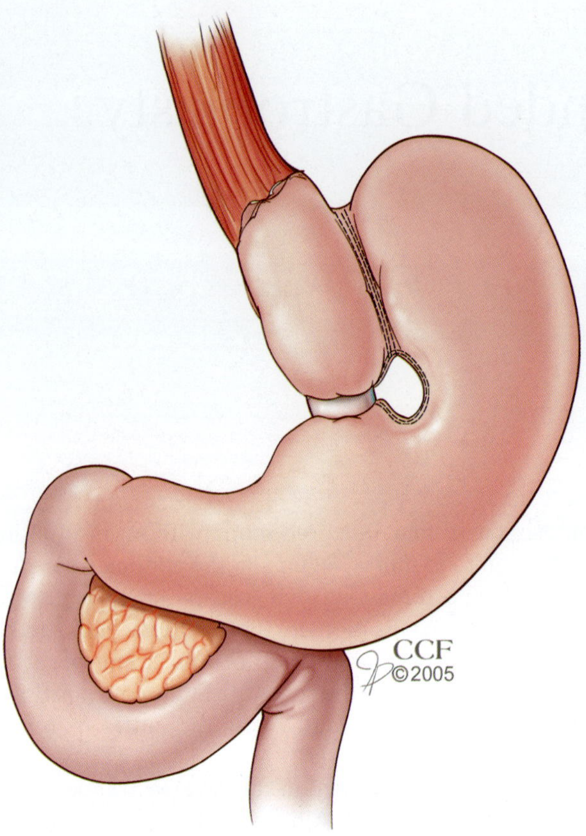

FIGURE 19.1-1. Mason-like laparoscopic vertical banded gastroplasty. (Courtesy of the Cleveland Clinic Foundation.)

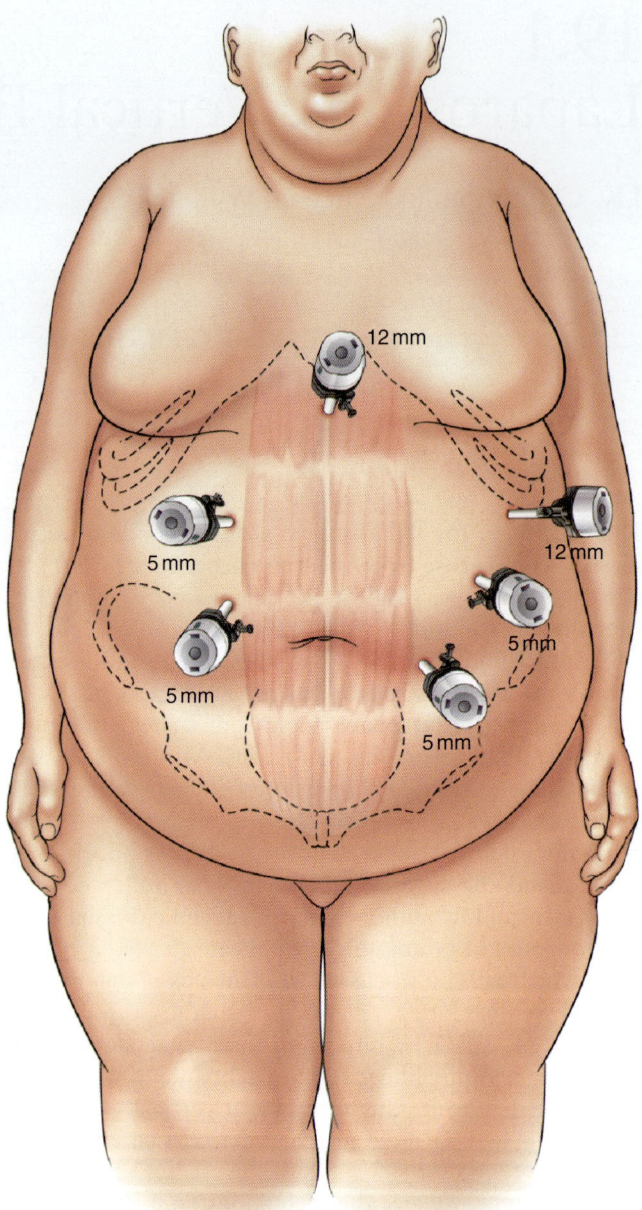

FIGURE 19.1-3. Trocar insertion sites for laparoscopic technique. (Courtesy of the Cleveland Clinic Foundation.)

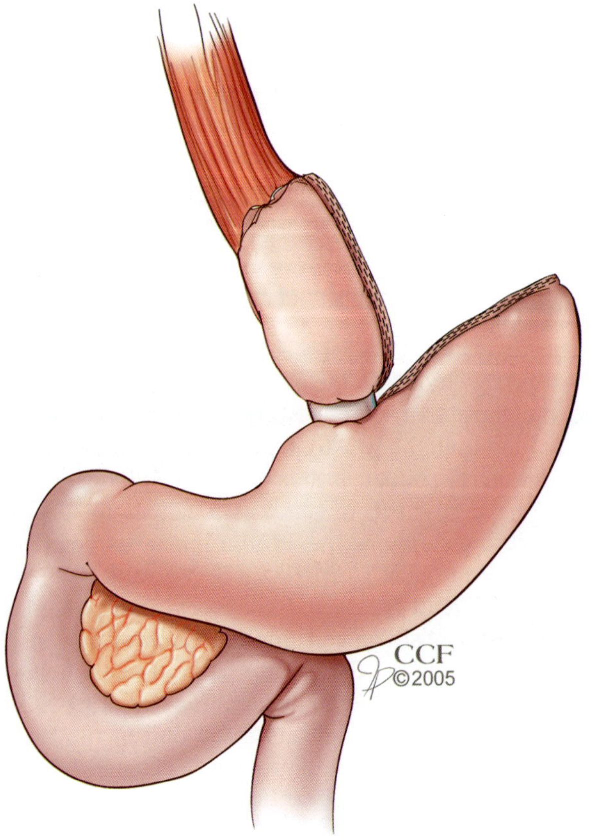

FIGURE 19.1-2. Wedge laparoscopic vertical banded gastroplasty. (Courtesy of the Cleveland Clinic Foundation.)

Figure 19.1-4. Measure 5 cm from angle of His.

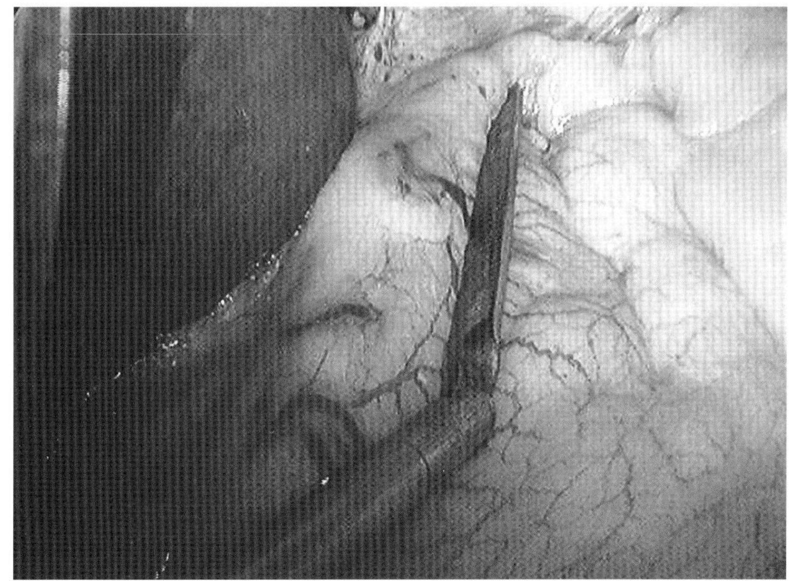

Figure 19.1-5. Stapler applied horizontally at greater curve.

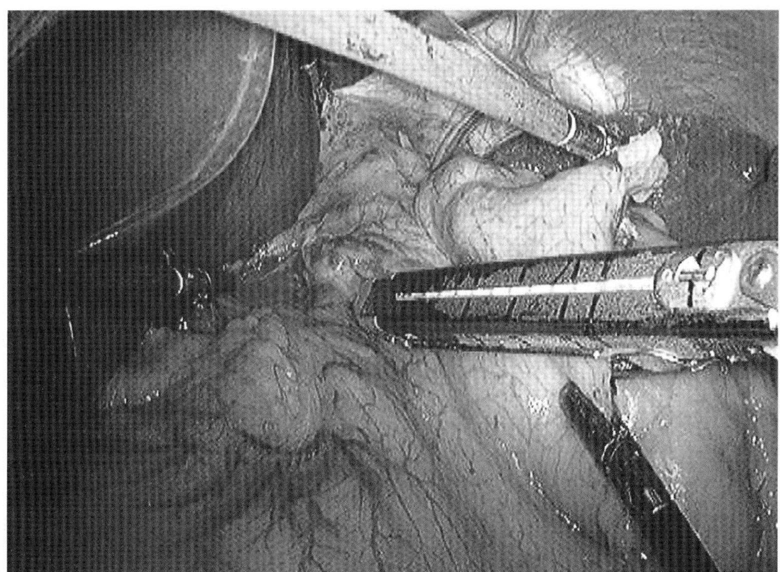

Figure 19.1-6. Stapler fired horizontally until it reaches the 54-French bougie at lesser curve.

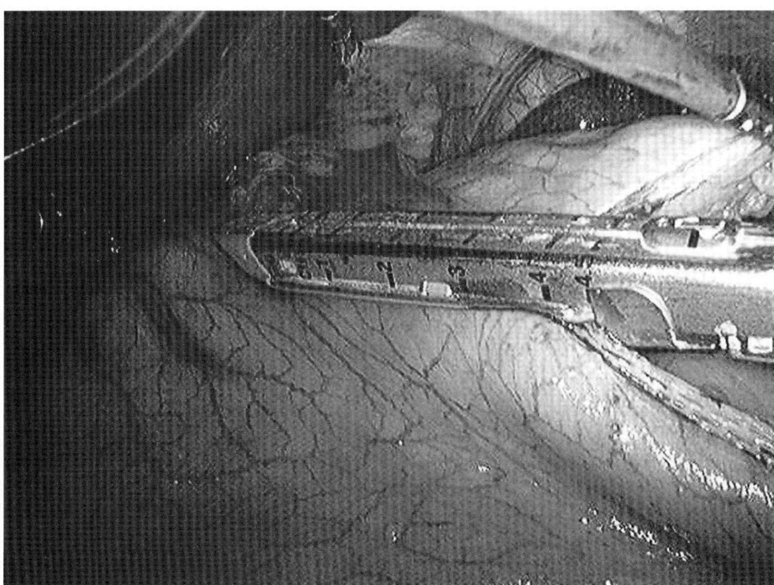

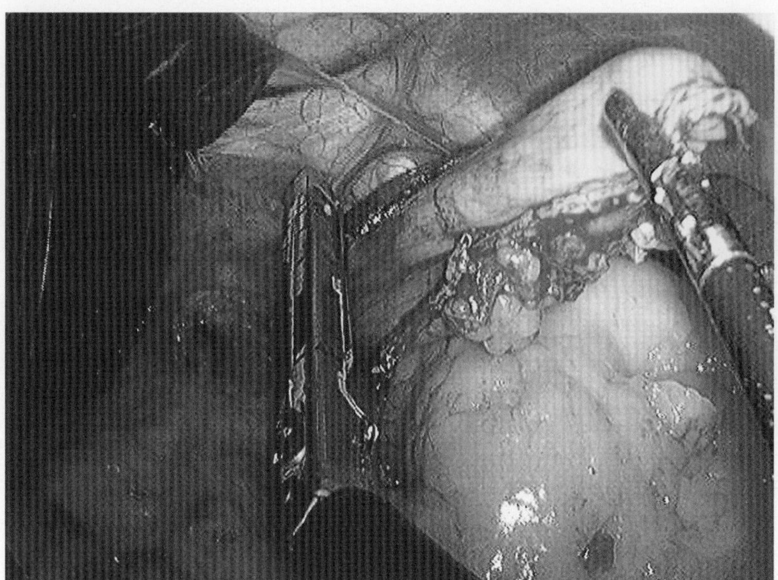

Figure 19.1-7. Stapler applied vertically along-side the bougie to wedge segment of fundus.

and fired repeatedly up through the angle of His, transecting and removing a 5 × 5 cm section of stomach (Fig. 19.1-7). The transected segment is withdrawn through the 12-mm port in the left upper abdomen (Fig. 19.1-8). If any enlargement is required, the site should be closed with a suture device at the end of the procedure. The staple line along the pouch is oversewn with a running 2-0 silk, to provide hemostasis and reinforcement of the staple line, since the patients are begun on liquids immediately postoperative and the distal band could act as a partial obstruction and increase pressure in the lumen.

A band is constructed from polypropylene mesh and is 1.5 cm by 7.0 cm. The band will be overlapped 1 cm on the ends to create a 5-cm band, so the band is marked with a stay suture 1 cm from each end to aid in placement and allow external calibration of the outlet. The band is inserted via a 12-mm port and positioned around the distal pouch through the window 5 cm below the gastroesophageal (GE) junction. A 30F bougie is carefully positioned across the outlet for closure of the band to prevent inadvertently suturing the back wall of the outlet during this process, not to calibrate the band tightness. The band is overlapped 1 cm and sutured with two horizontal mattress sutures of 0 Ethibond (Ethicon Inc., Somerville, NJ) tied extracorporeally (Fig. 19.1-9). The bougie is removed and an intraoperative esophagogastroscopy is performed to ensure proper pouch and stoma size and no leaks from the staple lines. The band is then covered anteriorly with an omental patch, which is sutured in place with a medial suture. The abdomen is

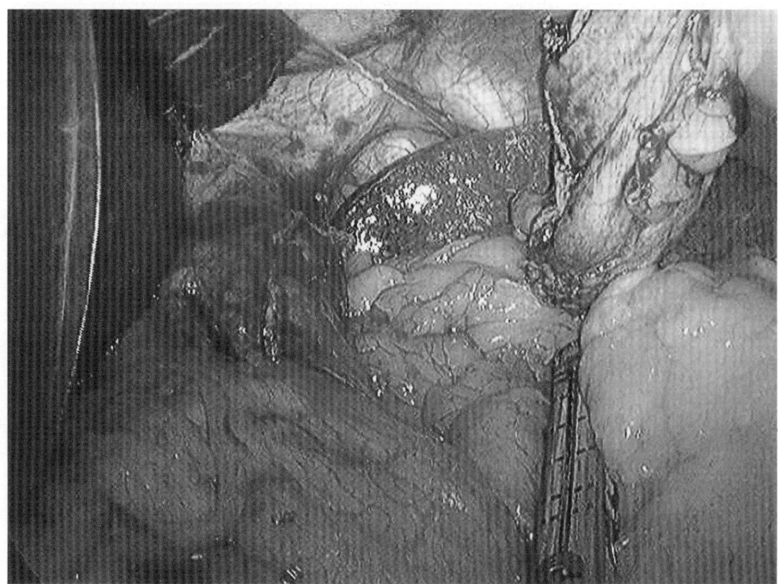

Figure 19.1-8. A 3 × 5 cm pouch formed and wedge of fundus removed.

FIGURE 19.1-9. Polypropylene band positioned and sutured at distal end of pouch.

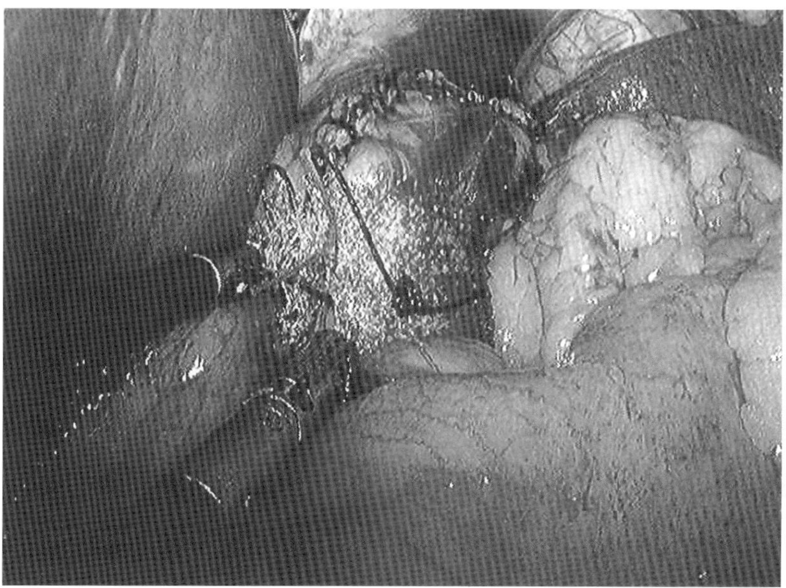

irrigated with saline, and all trocars removed under direct visualization to rule out bleeding. Trocars sites are not closed at the fascia level unless enlarged to remove the specimen. Skin incisions are closed with 3-0 plain subcuticular sutures and Steri-Strips.

Technique for Mason-Like Vertical Banded Gastroplasty

To perform the traditional technique with a circular stapler, the trocar placement is the same, except the 12-mm trocar in the left upper abdomen is replaced with a 5-mm trocar, and the lower 5-mm trocar in the right midabdomen is the site for a 12-mm trocar to apply the linear stapler. The dissection with creation of a lesser curve window 5 cm below the angle of His and mobilization of the short gastric vessels is performed as described above. The window site again serves as a landmark for pouch creation and the site for the ultimate band placement. A 50F bougie is positioned along the lesser curve, and a horizontal mattress suture is placed alongside the bougie at the level of the window to tightly reapproximate the anterior and posterior walls of the stomach and allow easier insertion of the circular stapler anvil. A 2-cm incision is made in the midclavicular line of the left upper abdomen, just below the costal margin. The anvil of a 21-mm circular stapler, with a sharp spike attached, is dropped into the abdomen via the incision. The anvil is positioned posterior to the stomach in the lesser sac, and the sharp spike and anvil shaft driven through the stomach as close as possible to the bougie at the level of the window. The spike is removed and the anvil connected to the stapler shaft by inserting it through the abdominal wall at the 2-cm anterior incision. The stapler

is closed, fired, and removed. The incision is approximated with towel clips for continued insufflation. An articulating 45-mm 3.5 linear stapler (Endo GIA-2, USSC) is inserted via the 12-mm port in the right midabdomen position through the circular window alongside the bougie vertically and fired. The firings are continued until the pouch is completely transected except for the distal outlet along the lesser curve. The staple line is oversewn with 2-0 silk suture and the distal pouch is banded as described above. The 2-cm anterior abdominal wall incision is closed with a transperitoneal suture.

Outcomes for Laparoscopic Vertical Banded Gastroplasty

Comparison of outcomes between series of laparoscopic vertical banded gastroplasties is difficult, as there are wide variations in technique, and the overall experience is small with limited follow-up.

Five-year outcomes for laparoscopic VBG from Olbers et al. (6), utilizing the Mason technique (with 109 patients pouch undivided and 30 divided), and our results with the "wedge" divided approach (7) are illustrated in Table 19.1-1. Wound morbidity was reduced in our experience, as there were no wound infections and no incisional hernias in our group; however, Olbers et al. do not comment on the incidence of wound morbidity in their series. The incidence of late reoperations was similar between laparoscopic approaches, with Olbers's group reporting an etiology of staple-line disruptions in three of 11 patients and poor weight loss in the other eight. Our reoperations were due to outlet stenosis and reflux in two of four patients, and poor weight loss in the other two. In addition, we have three pending revisions for poor weight

TABLE 19-1. Outcomes with laparoscopic vertical banded gastroplasty (VBG)

Author	Technique/band material	Leaks	SD	Revisions	%EWL/final BMI 2 years
Olbers et al., $n = 139$	Mason, 109 undivided, 30 divided, PTFE band	1 (0.07%)	3 (2%)	8%	50% 32 BMI
Champion $n = 58$	Wedge VBG polypropylene	1 (1.8%)	0	7.3%	49% 34 BMI

BMI, body mass index; EWL, excess weight loss; PTFE, polytetrafluoroethylene; SD, staple line disruption.

loss. Evaluation of our symptomatic patients or weight loss failures with a barium upper gastrointestinal series and flexible endoscopy revealed no band erosions or gastric fistulas. Olbers et al. did report one band erosion with the polytetrafluoroethylene (PTFE) band material, but did not reoperate since it was asymptomatic.

Olbers et al. reported finding pouch dilatations on radiologic exam at 6 months postoperative, and 45% of revisions for poor weight loss were due to a dilated pouch. Staple-line disruptions were responsible for another 27% of revisions, so overall 72% of revisions in their experience were secondary to technical pouch construction issues that accompany the difficulty in inserting the circular anvil close to the bougie to ensure a small pouch, or performing an undivided staple line with subsequent staple-line disruption and gastrogastric fistula. This led to the abandonment of the undivided staple line late in their series in an attempt to improve outcomes, but still ignores the difficult pouch construction issue with a laparoscopic circular stapler technique.

We had a similar early experience with the laparoscopic Mason procedure, and we were concerned with pouch volume and calibration, which Mason stressed repeatedly. We quickly abandoned the classical approach and returned to the lab to develop an alternative adaptable to the laparoscopic approach that would not compromise the operation. This led to the laparoscopic wedge VBG, which allowed us to construct an accurate pouch volume and eliminate staple line disruptions with a divided pouch. Despite the improved technical construction, our mean percent excess weight loss is similar to that of Olbers's group, with a mean percent excess weight loss of only 49%, and 43% remained morbidly obese with a body mass index (BMI) above 35. This reinforces the observation that gastric restrictive surgery, no matter what the technique, is associated with poor weight loss on average and a high incidence of revisions for poor weight loss or persistent vomiting and reflux. The technical issues are not what limit weight loss, but rather it is patient compliance.

The "holy grail" of weight-loss surgery is a method to accurately identify preoperatively the patient who is likely to succeed with pure gastric restriction versus an operation that incorporates malabsorption. This lesson should be noted by the proponents of the current in vogue modification of the VBG—adjustable gastric banding. Revisions of failed open VBGs that repair or revise back to a VBG resulted in no improvement in weight loss, so we now either reverse the failed VBG and abandon future surgical attempts at weight loss or convert to a gastric bypass (8).

In a randomized prospective trial of a Mason open versus laparoscopic VBG, Azagra et al. (9) reported a significant reduction in postoperative wound infections (10.8% vs. 3.3%, $p = .04$) and incisional hernias (15.8% vs. 0%, $p = .04$) with the minimally invasive approach. The authors reported no significant difference in percent excess weight loss or reduction in mean BMI between the two groups, but the absolute values and length of follow-up were not disclosed.

Introduction of the laparoscopic technique by either the classical Mason technique or our wedge approach, while reducing wound morbidity compared to an open approach, has failed to improve the efficacy of the procedure.

Postoperative Management and Nutritional Evaluation

Patients are admitted on the morning of surgery for a 23-hour stay, and are administered fractionated heparin and a prophylactic antibiotic preoperatively. Postoperatively they are given intravenous fluids and clear liquids overnight as tolerated, and narcotics for pain control, either intramuscular or orally. Nonsteroidal antiinflammatory drugs (NSAIDs), Cox-2 inhibitors, and aspirin are avoided due to the risk of postoperative staple-line bleeding, and the risk of ulceration or band erosion, which can occur with the medication resting in the pouch in contact with the gastric mucosa for a long period before dissolving. Patients with severe arthritis or joint pain who require NSAIDs or Cox-2 inhibitors may resume them after 6 weeks if they remain on a proton pump inhibitor, but they remain at increased risk for band erosion and pouch ulceration. Sequential compression hose, which were applied preoperatively, are continued until discharge to reduce the risk of deep venous thrombosis.

The following morning patients are discharged if they are tolerating liquids and pain medications by mouth and are clinically stable. A Gastrografin swallow is not performed routinely since the staple line was assessed in the operating room by endoscopy. However, if signs of a leak or obstruction are present, such as fever over 101°F, persistent tachycardia over 120 beats per minute, or nausea and liquid intolerance, then we perform a Gastrografin swallow.

Patients are given a prescription for an oral narcotic and a proton pump inhibitor, which is continued for 3 weeks, and they are instructed to take a multivitamin with iron and a calcium supplement daily. The postoperative diet is liquids for six meals per day for 2 weeks, then six small meals of soft food for 3 weeks, and then a regular diet of three meals per day with well-chewed small portions. Snacking and consumption of sweets or "junk" snack foods is prohibited and regular exercise encouraged. Patients are instructed to notify the office for any fever over 101°F, vomiting over 6 hours' duration, or an increase in abdominal pain.

Postoperative visits are scheduled at 3 weeks, 3 months, 6 months, 1 year, and then annually. Laboratory evaluations are routinely performed for nutritional monitoring at 6 and 12 months, and then yearly. Tests performed are a complete blood count, comprehensive chemistry, serum iron, and vitamin B_{12} level. Nutritional monitoring is required even for a VBG as the diet may not contain sufficient nutrients for good health. Patients are also required to fill out a 2-day diet journal at each visit beginning at 3 months to assess their diet. We have observed many patients consume approximately 85% carbohydrates and need to increase protein and coarse fibrous foods in their diets (10).

The major reasons for weight loss failure after laparoscopic VBG in our experience are maladaptive eating (snacking on high calorie "junk" food all day in small amounts to avoid vomiting, eating sweets or soft high carbohydrate laden foods), and failure to exercise.

Complications and Controversy with Laparoscopic Vertical Banded Gastroplasty

The laparoscopic VBG has all the traditional complications of the open gastroplasty, but also has complications as a result of a minimally invasive approach, which limits instrument motion, depth perception, and tactile sensation (11). We limit this discussion to the avoidance and management of complications from the laparoscopic approach, and the controversy associated with some technical points.

Patient selection is a factor with a laparoscopic approach, particularly early in a surgeon's experience, as not every patient is a candidate for this technique. Select patients with a BMI below 50 with a gynecoid body habitus and no prior open abdominal surgery to begin a series to minimize a conversion to an open procedure. Weight limits can be liberalized as well as accepting patients with prior open surgery once an experience of at least 100 cases is gained to work through the learning curve for this complex laparoscopic procedure (12). Conversions to an open technique usually occur due to a large liver obscuring visualization, or the instrumentation being too short to reach the top of the stomach for dissection and transection. We experienced one conversion (1.7%) to open in our series (5), and Olbers et al. (6) had six conversions (4%) due to an enlarged left lobe of the liver. This risk can be minimized by placing patients on a low-carbohydrate, high-protein diet for 10 days prior to surgery to reduce the liver size. In addition, we strongly discourage patients from having any gastric restrictive surgery for weight loss if their BMI is greater than 50, if they are "sweet eaters," diabetics, or have hyperlipidemia due to superior results with a gastric bypass for these conditions.

The incidence of a conversion to open surgery due to short instrumentation can be reduced by limiting patient size to under 400 pounds, or a BMI of 60, and utilizing 45-cm-long instruments and the new extra-long endoscopic linear staplers. In addition, to gain an extra 2 cm in length for the linear stapler, the trocar can be removed and the instrument inserted directly through the abdominal wall.

Uncontrolled intraabdominal bleeding can occur in laparoscopic bariatric cases while dividing the short gastric vessels or during the perigastric dissection particularly in the lesser sac near the base of the left crus due to a large vein that may arise from the splenic vein and perforate the posterior stomach. We have access to a second suction setup and insufflator in our operating room to address massive blood loss. Control of the bleeding is achieved with compression of the stomach with both hands and waiting at least 5 minutes before attempting ligation. If hypotension occurs or bleeding persists of more than 500 cc, we recommend conversion to an open procedure.

Pouch and stoma misconstruction and difficulty with accurate calibration are major issues and controversies with laparoscopic VBG techniques. Mason has repeatedly emphasized, after his extensive open experience, that a purely restrictive operation is dependent on a measured and calibrated pouch and outlet, and small variation can result in inadequate weight loss or morbidity from reflux and vomiting (1). Surgeons often estimate pouch size, or alter the dimensions described by Mason, and bandwidth, length, and calibration vary widely. Laparoscopy has limited depth perception with the image magnified to a varying degree depending on the distance of the lens to the tissue, and visual estimates are unacceptable. The length of the pouch should be measured with an endoscopic ruler, and the pouch width calibrated with a bougie or balloon. The band should be 1.5 cm wide and 5 cm in circumference when closed, so the outlet is externally calibrated to be approximately 12 mm. Internal calibration of the outlet around a bougie, wider bands, or smaller outlet size can increase the incidence of stoma stenosis with resulting reflux and vomiting (1).

Postoperative staple-line leaks have been reported to occur more frequently in some laparoscopic series, and can be the etiology of significant morbidity and mortality (13). To reduce this risk, we recommend a divided staple line, which reduces the incidence of staple line disruptions (6,7). We also recommend routine intraoperative endoscopy to assess the integrity of the staple and suture lines (14). Early in the surgeon's learning curve we suggest placement of a Jackson-Pratt drain and routine Gastrografin swallow on postoperative day 1 to check for leaks until the surgeon has an established track record. Gastrografin swallows have a high incidence of false negatives, and a delay in diagnosis is the usual cause of increased morbidity; therefore, we recommend immediate exploration if a patient shows signs of a possible leak such as fever, tachycardia over 120, tachypnea, or appears septic.

Conclusion

Laparoscopic VBG can be performed by two established techniques, and has been demonstrated to reduce wound morbidity compared to open procedures (9). Introduction of the laparoscopic VBG has not improved the efficacy of gastric restrictive surgery for weight loss, and the techniques are still associated with significantly less weight loss compared to a gastric bypass, and have a high incidence of revision, but are generally safer (3–7).

References

1. Mason EE, Doherty C, Cullen JJ, et al. Vertical gastroplasty: evolution of vertical banded gastroplasty. World J Surg 1998;22:919–924.
2. Buchwald H, Buchwald JN. Evolution of operative procedures for the management of morbid obesity 1950–2000. Obes Surg 2002;12:705–717.
3. Chua TY, Mendiola RM. Laparoscopic vertical banded gastroplasty: the Milwaukee experience. Obes Surg 1995;5:77–80.
4. Lonroth H, Dalenback J, Haglind E, et al. Vertical banded gastroplasty by laparoscopic technique in the treatment of morbid obesity. Surg Laparosc Endosc 1996;6:102–107.
5. Champion JK, Hunt T, Delisle N. Laparoscopic vertical banded gastroplasty and roux-en-y gastric bypass in morbid obesity. Obes Surg 1999;9:123.
6. Olbers T, Lonroth H, Dalenback J, et al. Laparoscopic vertical banded gastroplasty- an effective long-term therapy for morbid obesity patients? Obes Surg 2001;11:726–730.
7. Champion JK. Laparoscopic vertical banded gastroplasty. In: Cohen RV, Schiavon A, Schauer P, eds. Videolaparoscopic Approach to Morbid Obesity. Sao Paulo: Via Letera Medical Publishers, 2002.
8. Naslund E, Backman L, Granstrom L, et al. Seven year results of vertical banded gastroplasty for morbid obesity. Eur J Surg 1997;163:281–286.
9. Azagra JS, Goergen M, Ansay J, et al. Laparoscopic gastric reduction surgery. Surg Endosc 1999;13:555–558.
10. Champion S, Williams M, Champion JK. Importance of routine diet journals to aide in nutritional counseling for post-op bariatric patients. Obes Surg 2003;13:191–192.
11. Champion JK. Complications of laparoscopic vertical banded gastroplasty. Current Surg 2003;60:37–39.
12. Schauer P, Ikramuddin S, Hamad G, et al. The learning curve for laparoscopic Roux-en-y gastric bypass is 100 cases. Surg Endosc 2003;17:212–215.
13. Chae FH, McIntyre RC. Laparoscopic bariatric surgery. Surg Endosc 1999;13:547–549.
14. Champion JK, Hunt T, Delisle N. Role of routine intraoperative endoscopy in laparoscopic bariatric surgery. Surg Endosc 2000;16:1663–1665.

19.2
Laparoscopic Sleeve Gastrectomy

Vadim Sherman, Stacy A. Brethauer, Bipan Chand, and Philip R. Schauer

With the current epidemic of obesity spreading worldwide, surgical weight loss has been shown to be the most effective treatment. However, severely obese patients, that is, those with a body mass index (BMI) over 60, have an increased number of comorbid conditions and thus an increased operative risk. Several studies have demonstrated an increased rate of complications with weight-loss surgery in this group of patients with approximately two to three times greater risk of morbidity and mortality than the morbidly obese patient with a BMI less than 60 (1–3).

Patients with a high BMI (>60) or associated high-risk medical conditions have the greatest to gain from procedures such as the Roux-en-Y gastric bypass (RYGBP) and biliopancreatic diversion with duodenal switch (BPD-DS), but the increased risk of postoperative complications often renders them poor surgical candidates. To this end, investigators have attempted various bridging procedures designed to impart an effective weight loss and reduce the risk of complications in the subsequent, definitive weight loss procedure. These include an array of restrictive procedures such as endoscopically placed intragastric balloons, laparoscopic adjustable gastric banding (LAGB), and laparoscopic sleeve gastrectomy (LSG). The second stage would involve completion to RYGBP or BPD-DS.

The LAGB is generally performed as a primary weight loss procedure, whereas LSG has traditionally been performed as part of a BPD-DS. Indications for performing only a LSG include super-super-morbid obesity (BMI >60), high-risk comorbid conditions, increased age, unfavorable anatomy (cirrhosis, profuse visceral fat, poor exposure, extensive intraabdominal adhesions), and any combination of these factors (Table 19.2-1). The LSG has also been used in patients with inflammatory bowel disease, in whom integrity of anastomoses is a concern, and in patients with gastric nodules, in whom performance of a RYGBP would make surveillance of the gastric remnant extremely difficult.

Technique

There are minor variations of the procedure, but in general, 75% to 80% of the greater curvature is excised, leaving a tubularized stomach. We use the same port placement for LSG as we do for laparoscopic gastric bypass (see Chapter 21.4). The lesser sac is entered by opening the gastrocolic ligament. A point on the greater curve, on the antrum, is chosen as the starting point. This has previously been described as ranging from 2 to 10 cm from the pylorus. A laparoscopic stapler, with a blue load (3.5-mm staple height), is introduced and fired on the antrum, toward the angle of His. A 32- to 60-French bougie is then passed transorally into the pylorus, placed against the lesser curvature. The stapler is fired consecutively along the length of the bougie until the angle of His is reached (Fig. 19.2-1). At this point, approximately 75% to 80% of the stomach has been separated. The short gastric vessels and the greater curvature ligaments (gastrosplenic and gastrocolic) are divided with ultrasonic dissection to complete the resection (Fig. 19.2-2). The specimen may be removed by enlarging one of the 12-mm ports. A drain is then placed alongside the staple line.

Although the procedure does not involve any anastomoses, the length of the staple line still renders the patient at risk for bleeding or a leak. Several authors have described oversewing the long staple line, while others have employed buttressed staples or fibrin glue as a sealant. The potential benefits of an absorbable polyglyconate polymer staple line buttress were demonstrated in a randomized study of patients undergoing LSG with or without BPD-DS (4). Ten patients were randomized to a control group in which the LSG was performed in the conventional fashion, and the other 10 patients underwent a LSG, in which the absorbable polymer membrane was integrated into the length of the gastric staple line. Although the number of patients was small, the investigators were able to demonstrate significantly less intraoperative blood loss in the buttressed staple line group

TABLE 19.2-1. Indications for laparoscopic sleeve gastrectomy

First stage toward Roux-en-Y gastric bypass (RYGBP) or
biliopancreatic diversion with duodenal switch (BPD-DS) in
Super-super-obese (BMI >60)
Severe comorbidity
Advanced age
Combination of any of above
Poor intraoperative conditions
Extreme hepatomegaly or cirrhosis
Profuse visceral fat
Poor exposure
Extensive intraabdominal adhesions
Cardiopulmonary instability
Inflammatory bowel disease
Surveillance of gastric remnant required

(120 vs. 210 mL, $p < .05$). Furthermore, two staple line hemorrhages occurred in the control group postoperatively, but none in the buttressed staple line group. Of the 20 patients, no staple-line leaks occurred.

The LSG is a purely restrictive operation that reduces the size of the gastric reservoir to 60 to 100 mL, permitting intake of only small amounts of food and imparting a feeling of satiety earlier during a meal. More recently, studies have examined whether ghrelin levels may explain the mechanism of success of the LSG. Ghrelin, thought to be a hunger-regulating peptide hormone, is mainly produced in the fundus of the stomach. By resecting the fundus in an LSG, the majority of

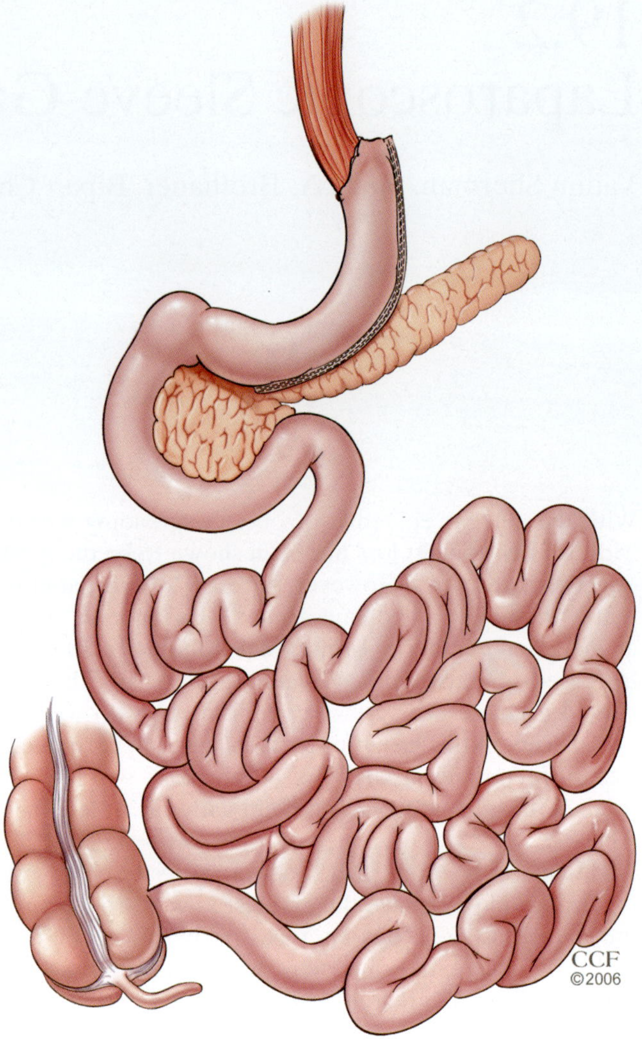

FIGURE 19.2-2. Completed sleeve gastrectomy demonstrating a tubularized stomach. (Courtesy of the Cleveland Clinic Foundation.)

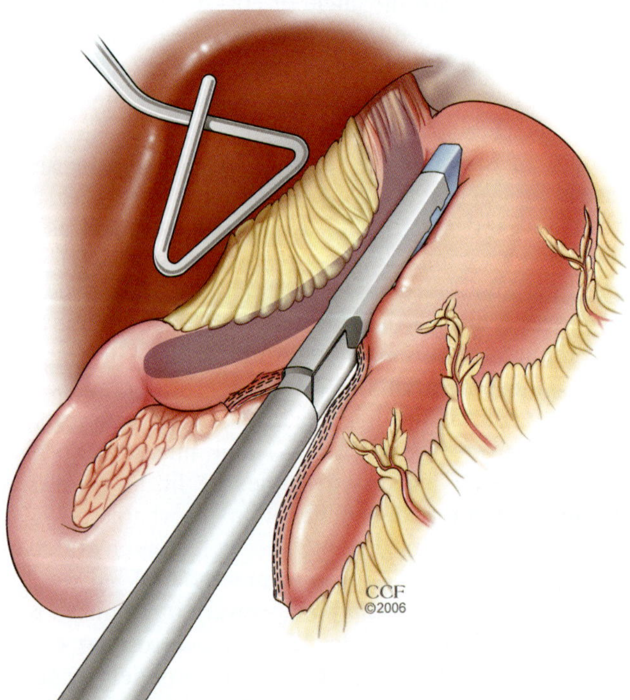

FIGURE 19.2-1. Laparoscopic sleeve gastrectomy. The stapler is fired successively from the antrum to the angle of His adjacent to an intragastric bougie. (Courtesy of the Cleveland Clinic Foundation.)

ghrelin-producing cells are removed, reducing plasma ghrelin levels and subsequently appetite.

Outcomes

In a prospective study of 20 patients, the effects of LSG on immediate and 6 months postoperative ghrelin levels were compared to that of LAGB (5). Ten patients each were randomized to undergo either LSG or LAGB. Groups were comparable at baseline, with an overall mean BMI of 45 ± 4.7. Patients who underwent LSG achieved a higher excess weight loss at 1 and 6 months postoperatively compared with the LAGB group. The LSG patients also showed a significant decrease of plasma ghrelin levels at day 1 compared to preoperatively, which remained low through 6 months. In contrast, in patients who underwent LAGB, plasma ghrelin levels did not change perioperatively and were found to significantly increase at 1 month. Although both procedures are purely restrictive in nature, the superior short-term weight loss experienced by LSG patients may be attributed to the lower ghrelin levels, which may prevent an increase in appetite as a compensatory mechanism.

These results were confirmed in a subsequent study of super-super-obese patients (6). Four female patients, with BMI ranging from 61 to 67, underwent a LSG. Weight loss and ghrelin levels were compared to a group of 15 patients (BMI 39–50) who underwent LAGB. Again, the patients who underwent LSG experienced a greater degree of weight loss compared to their LAGB counterparts (mean decrease of BMI 16.3 vs. 7.6). As well, the study confirmed that ghrelin levels were reduced after LSG, a value of 23.3% less than preoperatively (mean follow-up 6 months). Conversely, in the LAGB group, ghrelin levels had increased by 14% at a mean follow-up of 18 months. Despite the protracted decrease in ghrelin levels in the LSG patients, weight regain was noted in one patient after 1 year. Although ghrelin may be integral to the mechanism of weight loss in LSG, further studies will require larger patient groups and collection of ghrelin levels over a prolonged postoperative time course.

The safety and efficacy of LSG has been examined in a prospective study by Mognol et al. (7). The study included 10 patients, all with BMI >60 (mean 64, range 61–80), and average age of 42.7 years. Patients had an average number of 3.4 comorbidities, but 50% had hypertension and 90% had sleep apnea. Mean operative time was 120 minutes (range 90–150 minutes), and average length of stay was 7.2 days. In this small study group, there were no mortalities and no complications. At 6 months postoperatively, there was 41% excess weight loss, and average BMI had been reduced to 48. At 1 year post-LSG, excess weight loss increased to 51% and BMI further decreased to 41, although there was only 30% follow-up. Improvement of comorbidities was not reported.

Similar results were demonstrated in a retrospective study by Baltasar et al. (8) that analyzed the experience of 31 patients who underwent LSG for varying reasons. Seven patients were super-super-obese (mean BMI 65, range 61–74) and they underwent the LSG as a first stage toward completion BPD-DS. Another 23 patients had significant comorbidities or intraoperative findings that did not make the full BPD-DS advisable. One patient was converted from LAGB to LSG due to severe symptoms from the initial procedure. There were no instances of deep vein thrombosis (DVT)/pulmonary embolism (PE), leak, or pneumonia. However, there were two instances of trocar-related intraabdominal bleeding, one leading to death. Mean excess weight loss ranged from 56.1% (at 4

to 27 months) in the super-obese patients to 62.3% (3–27 month follow-up) in the lower BMI patients with significant comorbidities.

In another study, Almogy et al. (9) retrospectively examined 21 patients who underwent LSG. Indications for the procedure included high-risk patients, that is, those with severe pulmonary dysfunction, history of myocardial infarct, renal transplant, hypercoagulable state, and nephrotic syndrome. The remaining patients were initially planned for a BPD-DS, but due to intraoperative considerations (unfavorable anatomy or hemodynamic instability), only a sleeve gastrectomy was performed. Initial average BMI was 57.5 (range 53–71.5) and mean age was 44. Overall, patients had a mean number of comorbidities of 3.6, with a majority having hypertension, diabetes mellitus, venous stasis, and significant joint disease. There were no perioperative deaths, but there were two late deaths (at 3 and 6 months). Five of the 21 patients had complications (23.8%), which included postoperative hypotension, aspiration pneumonia, wound infection and sepsis, hepatic insufficiency, and a perioperative myocardial infarct. One year following LSG, patients experienced approximately 45% excess weight loss. Furthermore, hypertension, diabetes, and congestive heart failure had resolved or improved in 38%. Following sleeve gastrectomy, patients were thus able to achieve significant weight loss with an acceptable complication rate. Three patients lost enough weight to undergo subsequent spine or pelvic procedures, and two patients were able to continue on to BPD-DS, demonstrating the possibility of using LSG as an interim procedure in high-risk patients.

Debate exists as to what is the most effective initial procedure in high-risk patients. Besides LSG, options include LAGB and placement of an endoscopic intragastric balloon. Gagner's group (10) therefore compared LSG to the BioEnterics intragastric balloon (BIB) as a first-stage procedure for effective initial weight loss prior to definitive weight loss surgery. Numerous intragastric balloons have been tested and abandoned due to various complications such as erosion, ulcers, and intestinal obstruction. However, the BIB has become accepted as a viable option for weight loss outside the United States (11). The balloon is placed endoscopically and reduces the volume of the stomach, thereby acting as a restrictive procedure.

Gagner's group (10) retrospectively examined their experience in 20 LSG patients with BMI >50 to that of 57 BIB historical controls (BMI >50) described over two studies in the literature. At 6 months, the LSG group experienced a greater excess weight loss than the two BIB groups (34.9% vs. 26.1% and 21%). Baseline BMI and weight were equal between the LSG and BIB patients, but LSG patients experienced a 15.9 decrease in mean BMI versus 9.4 and 6.4 in the BIB patients.

Each patient in the LSG and BIB group demonstrated improvement in comorbidities such as hypertension, osteoarthritis, and sleep apnea. Among the 20 LSG patients, the only complication was a trocar site infection. However, 7% (four patients) in the BIB group required removal of the balloon, and one patient spontaneously eliminated the balloon in stool. Other noted complications included severe vomiting and dehydration in two patients. Both procedures, therefore, demonstrated positive results as a possible bridging procedure in the super-super-obese, although a more significant weight loss was effected with LSG, with less complications in this limited study.

The feasibility of LSG in the context of a staged procedure has also been examined. In a retrospective analysis of seven patients who underwent LSG followed by RYGBP, Pomp's group (12) demonstrated the efficacy and safety of a two-stage approach to surgical weight loss in high-risk super-super-obese patients. These patients had an average age of 43 and preoperative mean BMI of 63 (range 58–71). Mean operative time for stage I was 124 minutes and 158 minutes for stage II, with a length of stay (LOS) of 2.7 days, averaged over all 14 procedures. Following stage I, there were three complications in two patients (42.9%), which included postoperative bleeding, a urinary tract infection, and port-site hernia (discovered at stage II). Following stage II, there were two complications (28.6%), which included a gastrojejunal stricture and temporary arm nerve praxia. There were no mortalities. The second stage was performed within a mean of 11 months (range 4–22 months) and the BMI had fallen to 50 with average excess weight loss of 33%. Although follow-up for the completion RYGBP was short (average 2.5 months), patients continued to lose weight, with an average excess weight loss of 46%. Improvement or resolution of comorbidities was not reported.

The largest study of LSG to date involved 126 patients who underwent LSG as a first stage, en route to completion RYGBP (13). In the majority of the procedures (>90%), LSG had been planned preoperatively due to high BMI or severe comorbid conditions. The rest of the patients were chosen after intraoperative abdominal evaluation demonstrated unfavorable anatomy. The group of patients had a preoperative BMI of 65.4 ± 9 (range 45–91) and numerous comorbid conditions, the average number being around 9. Around 42% were American Society of Anesthesiology (ASA) I class II and 52% were ASA class IV.

Of the 126 patients, 36 patients proceeded to stage II completion RYGBP approximately 1 year post-LSG (range 4–22 months). At the time of the second stage, the mean number of comorbid conditions had decreased to 6.4 ± 3 and the percentage of patients with ASA III or IV was 44%, compared to 94% prior to stage I. The BMI had also reduced significantly to 49.5 ± 8. At stage II completion RYGBP, mean operative time for the 36 patients was 229 ± 65 minutes and mean LOS was 3 days. There were no mortalities after LSG and no mortalities after completion RYGBP. The complication rate after stage I was 14%, including five strictures, two leaks, two pulmonary embolisms, four cases of transient renal insufficiency, and five patients requiring more than 24 hours of ventilatory support.

Although the rate of complications appears elevated, the majority of complications were self-limited. Nevertheless, the marked improvement in the medical comorbidities reduced the operative risk in those patients undergoing stage II. Every patient with diabetes and almost all patients with sleep apnea showed improvement of their comorbidity prior to undergoing completion RYGBP. As well, all cases of peripheral edema resolved, and patients with degenerative joint disease showed significant improvement in activity levels prior to stage II, facilitating early ambulation postoperatively. Of the 36 patients, 6 experienced complications (17%), which included three postoperative bleeds, one leak, one acute cholecystitis, and one marginal ulcer. Although 6-month follow-up for completion RYGBP was limited to 20 patients at the time of publication, patients continued to lose weight [excess weight loss (EWL) 55%] and a clear majority had either resolution or improvement in major medical comorbidities.

The feasibility of LSG as a sole surgical weight loss option has also been examined in the Korean population (14). Due to various cultural factors, weight loss surgery is not as prevalent and this is reflected in the demographics of the low-risk population (mean BMI 37.2, range 30–56, and mean age 30, range 16–62). Although 130 patients underwent LSG, 1-year follow-up data were obtained on only 60 patients. Excess weight loss was 83.3% and BMI had decreased to 28. Preoperatively, there were an average of 2.1 comorbidities in the 60 patients and a majority of these had resolved or improved by 6 months. There was 100% resolution of fatty liver, sleep apnea, diabetes, and asthma at 6 months and 100% resolution of joint pain, reflux esophagitis, and amenorrhea at 1 year. Hypertension was resolved in 93% at 1 year, and improved in the remaining 7%. Dyslipidemia was the only comorbidity that was not fully improved at 1 year (65% resolution and 10% improvement). Of the 130 initial patients, there was one leak, one case of delayed bleeding, one case of prolonged vomiting, and two cases of atelectasis. There were no mortalities. Despite the excellent results, weight loss plateaued in the majority of patients at 1 year. Also, five of the 60 patients have been identified as requiring a secondary weight loss procedure for failure to lose adequate weight.

The LSG as a sole weight loss procedure was also examined by Langer et al. (15). The aim of the study was to evaluate the effectiveness of LSG in a mostly lower

TABLE 19.2-2. Reported case series of laparoscopic sleeve gastrectomy

	n	Age	BMI (mean)	Comorbidities per patient	OR time (min)	LOS (days)	EWL (%)	Follow-up (months)	Mortality	Complications
Cottam et al.	126	49.5	65.4	9.4	143	3	45	12	0%	14% (18/126)
Han et al.	60	30	37.2	2.1	70	—	83.3	12	0.8% (1/130)	3.1% (4/130)
Baltasar et al.	7	—	65	—	—	—	56.1	4–27	14.3% (1/7)	0%
	7	—	>40	—	—	—	33.6–90	4–16	0%	0%
	16	—	35–43	—	—	—	62.3	3–27	0%	6.3% (1/16)
Langer et al.	23	41.2	48.5	—	—	—	46	6	0%	—
							56	12		
Almogy et al.	21	44	57.5	3.6	—	7	45	6–20	9.5% (2/21)*	23.8% (5/21)
Milone et al.	20	43	68.8	3.7	—	—	34.9	6	0	5% (1/20)
Mognol et al.	10	42.7	64	3.4	120	7.2	41	6	0%	0%
							51	12		
Langer et al.	10	39.3	48.3	1.6	—	—	61.4	6	0%	0%
Regan et al.	7	43	63	3.1	124	2.7	33	11	0%	42.9% (3/7)

BMI, body mass index; EWL excess weight loss; LOS, length of stay; OR, operatingroom.
—, not reported; * outside the perioperative period.

BMI group of patients. Of the 23 patients prospectively studied, eight patients had a preoperative BMI >50 (mean BMI of the entire group was 48.5). At 6 months, mean excess weight loss among all 23 patients was 46%, and at 1 year it was 56%. No significant differences in percent EWL were demonstrated between patients with initial BMI <50 and those with BMI ≥50. Two patients required conversion to RYGBP—one patient for failure to lose weight and the other for severe gastroesophageal reflux. Partial weight regain was observed in an additional three patients in a median follow-up of 20 months. All patients underwent a contrast study on postoperative day 1, and 14 patients underwent a follow-up contrast study at 1 year. Only one patient was noted to have dilatation of the stomach (width of gastric tube >4 cm), but this patient had experienced an adequate excess weight loss of 59% and continued to experience early satiety. Weight loss from LSG was demonstrated to be very effective, even comparable to that of RYGBP; however, follow-up was limited to approximately 1 year, when long-term durability of the sleeve gastrectomy becomes an issue. Moreover, no data are provided regarding comorbidities and postoperative complications. A summary of the currently published case series utilizing LSG is shown in Table 19.2-2.

Conclusion

As the prevalence of surgical weight loss procedures continues to increase, surgeons will be faced with an increasing number of super-obese and high-risk patients. Recognizing the potential for devastating postoperative complications in this group of patients with low physiologic reserve, staging techniques such as laparoscopic sleeve gastrectomy may reduce the overall complications.

This requires a second major laparoscopic operation, which entails not only a second general anesthetic but also additional costs. However, the definitive weight loss operation can be performed when patients' anatomic factors are more reasonable and comorbid conditions have improved, thereby lessening the risk of postoperative complications.

The LSG has been shown to effect significant weight loss with a low complication rate, in addition to a beneficial impact on comorbidities. As a stand-alone procedure, excellent success has been reported in the short term. However, concerns about the longevity of the operation remain. At the present time, more long-term results are necessary to determine the durability and incidence of late complications after LSG.

References

1. Ren CJ, Patterson E, Gagner M. Early results of laparoscopic biliopancreatic diversion with duodenal switch: a case series of 40 consecutive patients. Obes Surg 2000;10(6): 514–523; discussion 524.
2. Dresel A, Kuhn JA, McCarty TM. Laparoscopic Roux-en-Y gastric bypass in morbidly obese and super morbidly obese patients. Am J Surg 2004;187(2):230–232; discussion 232.
3. Fernandez AZ Jr, Demaria EJ, Tichansky DS, et al. Multivariate analysis of risk factors for death following gastric bypass for treatment of morbid obesity. Ann Surg 2004; 239(5):698–702; discussion 702–703.
4. Consten EC, Gagner M, Pomp A, Inabnet WB. Decreased bleeding after laparoscopic sleeve gastrectomy with or without duodenal switch for morbid obesity using a stapled buttressed absorbable polymer membrane. Obes Surg 2004;14(10):1360–1366.
5. Langer FB, Reza Hoda MA, Bohdjalian A, et al. Sleeve gastrectomy and gastric banding: effects on plasma ghrelin levels. Obes Surg 2005;15(7):1024–1029.

6. Cohen R, Uzzan B, Bihan H, et al. Ghrelin levels and sleeve gastrectomy in super-super-obesity. Obes Surg 2005;15(10): 1501–1502.

7. Mognol P, Chosidow D, Marmuse JP. Laparoscopic sleeve gastrectomy as an initial bariatric operation for high-risk patients: initial results in 10 patients. Obes Surg 2005;15(7): 1030–1033.

8. Baltasar A, Serra C, Perez N, et al. Laparoscopic sleeve gastrectomy: a multi-purpose bariatric operation. Obes Surg 2005;15(8):1124–1128.

9. Almogy G, Crookes PF, Anthone GJ. Longitudinal gastrectomy as a treatment for the high-risk super-obese patient. Obes Surg 2004;14(4):492–497.

10. Milone L, Strong V, Gagner M. Laparoscopic sleeve gastrectomy is superior to endoscopic intragastric balloon as a first stage procedure for super-obese patients (BMI > or = 50). Obes Surg 2005;15(5):612–617.

11. Doldi SB, Micheletto G, Di Prisco F, et al. Intragastric balloon in obese patients. Obes Surg 2000;10(6):578–581.

12. Regan JP, Inabnet WB, Gagner M, Pomp A. Early experience with two-stage laparoscopic Roux-en-Y gastric bypass as an alternative in the super-super obese patient. Obes Surg 2003;13(6):861–864.

13. Cottam D, Qureshi F, Mattar S, et al. Laparoscopic sleeve gastrectomy as an initial weight-loss procedure for high-risk patients with morbid obesity. Surg Endosc 2006;20(6):859–863.

14. Moon Han S, Kim WW, Oh JH. Results of laparoscopic sleeve gastrectomy (LSG) at 1 year in morbidly obese Korean patients. Obes Surg 2005;15(10):1469–1475.

15. Langer FB, Bohdjalian A, Felberbauer FX, et al. Does gastric dilatation limit the success of sleeve gastrectomy as a sole operation for morbid obesity? Obes Surg 2006;16(2): 166–171.

20.1
Laparoscopic Adjustable Gastric Banding: Technique

Paul E. O'Brien and John B. Dixon

Evolution of the Technique

The laparoscopic adjustable gastric band (LAGB) was introduced in the early 1990s as a product of the rapid development of complex laparoscopic procedures after the introduction of laparoscopic cholecystectomy in 1989. The original concept of an adjustable gastric band had been developed by Szinicz and Schnapka (1) at Innsbruck, Austria in 1982. They placed a Silastic band around the upper stomach of the rabbit. An inner balloon was expanded by the injection of saline into a subcutaneous port. This original concept was used in a clinical application by Dr. Lubomyr Kusmak of New Jersey in 1986 as the adjustable silicone gastric band (ASGB) and reports of its use had been published (2). Its principal attribute of adjustability of the degree of gastric restriction was not generally recognized as a benefit in comparison with vertical banded gastroplasty, Roux-en-Y gastric bypass, and biliopancreatic diversion, which were the open surgical procedures popular at that time.

The initial LAGB, the BioEnterics Lap-Band (Inamed Health, Santa Barbara, CA) system, was developed from the ASGB to permit easier laparoscopic placement and better adjustability. The suture closure was converted to a self-locking buckle. The inner balloon was extended to cover almost the entire inner circumference, and the initial length of the device was fixed at either 9.75 or 10 cm as measured on the inner aspect. A number of LAGBs are now available commercially (Table 20.1-1). Only two are associated with any published data on safety or efficacy. The BioEnterics Lap-Band system was the first device specifically designed for laparoscopic placement, and it is supported by an extensive literature on safety and efficacy. The Swedish adjustable gastric band was originally placed by open surgery and is now placed laparoscopically without modification of the device. A more limited body of published literature is available on its safety and efficacy. In our group we have used only the Lap-Band, and this chapter addresses the technique for this device alone.

The initial placement of the Lap-Band system was performed by Dr. Mitiku Belachew at the Centre Hospitalier Hutois, Huy, Belgium, in September 1993 (3) and became available by mid-1994 to surgeons who had completed the required training program. It rapidly became widely used across Europe and across most of the developed world including South America, Mexico, Australia and New Zealand, Israel, and Saudi Arabia. The worldwide introduction of the Lap-Band has been largely completed with approval for its use in the United States being granted in June 2001.

The technique of placement of the band has evolved in a number of important ways since its inception in 1993. The technique has become easier, but the achievement of optimal results and the prevention of late complications has been found to require particular attention to detail. The technique described below is our preferred method as of early 2004. We have provided a description of the basic technique with particular emphasis on key elements or challenges.

Laparoscopic Placement

The LAGB is specifically designed for laparoscopic placement. It can be placed by open technique also and occasionally this becomes necessary, usually due to the presence of a very large, fragile liver or copious amounts of intraabdominal fat. We have found conversion to open placement to be necessary in three of our last 1400 patients. Our data and our observations indicate that the degree of visibility and therefore the accuracy of placement and fixation are much greater with laparoscopic placement. Furthermore, there are far fewer perioperative complications. We therefore do not regard open placement as an acceptable alternative. The operation requires good laparoscopic skills and prior experience with advanced laparoscopic surgery and should be undertaken

TABLE 20.1-1. Adjustable gastric bands: name, source

Name	Manufacturer
BioEnterics Lap-Band system (LAGB)	Inamed Health, U.S.
Swedish Adjustable Gastric Band (SAGB)	Ethicon Endosurgery, U.S.
Midband	Medical Innovation Development
Heliogast Band	Helioscopie, France
The A.M.I. Soft Gastric Band	Austrian Agency for Medical Innovations Ltd.
Gastrobelt II	Tyco Healthcare, Europe

therefore appear that the exact port placement is not by itself critical to good outcome and should be dictated by surgeon preference. Factors that influence that preference include prior practice of port placement especially for laparoscopic antireflux surgery, preferred instruments and ports, and the position of the surgeon, either on the patient's right side or standing between the patient's legs.

We use six ports in positions as shown in Figure 20.1-1. The number of ports used should not be regarded as an issue of great importance. Generally, the addition or subtraction of a 5-mm port is not regarded as a significant event, and certainly the safety or ease of the operation should not be compromised for such a reason. The operation could be done with just four ports, but there is no logical reason to put the patient at risk and the surgeon at difficulty just for such a dubious achievement.

only by surgeons who can reasonably expect to complete the procedure laparoscopically.

Patient Position

The surgeon stands between the patient's legs or on the patient's right side. We prefer the former as it enables a direct line for the hand–instrument interface. The patient is tipped into a steep reverse Trendelenburg position of approximately 25 degrees. A bolster is bolted to the table below the buttocks to prevent slippage. The legs are placed in well-supported, easily adjustable stirrups.

Port Numbers and Placement

There is significant variation in port placement between surgeons who otherwise do the operation in an almost identical fashion and who, at completion of the operation, have the band in exactly the same position. It would

Port 1

Port 1 is placed at the right costal margin about 6 cm lateral to the midline. This is a 5-mm port that is 150 mm long (Applied Medical, Rancho Santa, Margarita, CA). The extra length on all our 5-mm ports allows us to pass the ports on a sharp angle through the abdominal wall, heading almost directly toward the region of the esophagogastric junction. In this way there is no tension between the hand and the instrument trying to force it toward the target area. This port enters the abdomen just below the edge of the lateral segment of the left lobe of liver. This port is for the surgeon's left hand and is used for a long grasper and the left hand instrument when suturing.

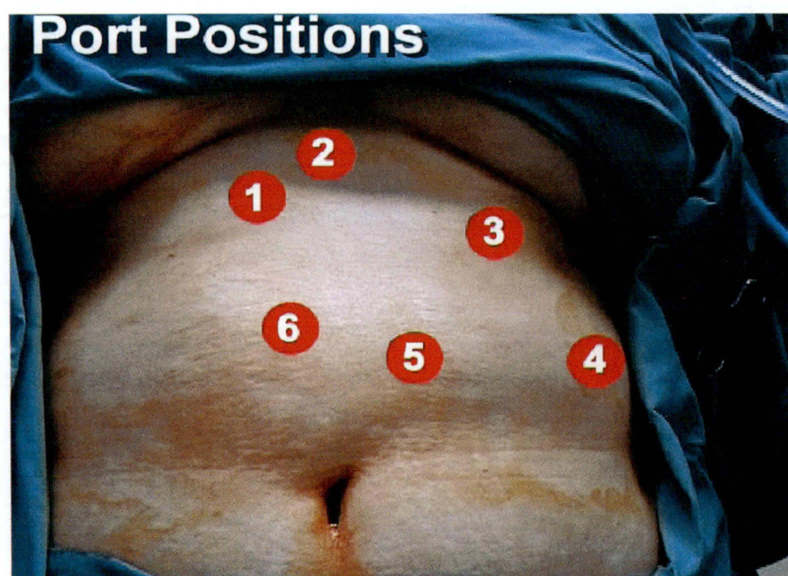

FIGURE 20.1-1. The port positions. The oval-shaped grouping with port 3 at the left costal margin and port 5 about one handbreadth below. The umbilicus is not a relevant landmark in port placement.

Port 2

A 5-mm port is passed directly into the abdomen just below the xiphisternum to make a track. It is then removed and the Nathanson liver retractor (Automated Medical Products, Edison, NJ) is passed along that track and into position to hold the liver out of the way. This method of liver retraction is by far the most effective and inexpensive method for getting this most important exposure.

Port 3

A 15-mm port (disposable, 10- to 15-mm Versiport, U.S. Surgical, Norwalk, CT) is used at this site primarily for passage of the band into the abdominal cavity. Alternatives are the 18-mm port produced by Ethicon Endosurgery (Cincinnati, OH) or placing a 10- to 12-mm port for general use and to remove that port and pass the band along the port track. This is a traumatic procedure for the patient and the band and is not recommended. The 15-mm port is used as our primary camera port for most of the operation as it is placed optimally for a 30-degree telescope to look almost directly down onto the operative field.

Port 4

Another 5-mm-diameter, 150-mm-long port is placed at the left lateral rib margin. This site is used for a grasper, for the needle holder and for the scissors.

Port 5

A 10-mm Visiport (disposable, U.S. Surgical) is our initial port and is used to achieve insufflation. The telescope remains at this site while the other ports are being placed, before being moved to port 3. Port 5 is our port for diathermy, harmonic scalpel (if used), and introducing sutures into the abdomen. The tubing exits this port site at the completion of the procedure, and the access port is placed at that site.

Port 6

A further 5 mm × 150 mm length port is placed through the right rectus muscle 3 cm from the midline at a level with port 5. This could be seen as an optional port but it serves three functions, which we find helpful. First, a grasper is used to help control the omental fat when doing the dissection at the right crus. Second, the Lap-Band placer is passed via this port. Third, the tubing is drawn out through this port to rotate the band to allow easier placement of the anterior fixation sutures.

Instruments

We use the following instruments:

Three Prestige nontoothed graspers (Aesculap, Center Valley, PA)
Nathanson liver retractor (Automated Medical Products)
Iron Intern (Automated Medical Products) for external fixation of Nathanson retractor
Zero-degree telescope for placing Visiport
Thirty-degree telescope for the remainder of the procedure
Scope warmer with hot (>55°C) saline (Applied Medical)
Lap-Band introducer (Automated Medical Products)
Lap-Band placer (Automated Medical Products)
Lap-Band closer (Automated Medical Products)
Hook diathermy
Dolphin nosed forceps
Laparoscopic scissors
Langenbeck retractors (6.5 × 2.5 cm) for access port placement

Selection of Size of Lap-Band

Three sizes are available: the 9.75-cm band; the 10-cm band; and the Vanguard, which is an 11-cm band. A judgment should be made at this stage of which band to use. We do not use the 9.75-cm band in our practice. In general, the 10-cm band is suggested for female patients, those with a body mass index (BMI) less than 45, those with gynoid type obesity, and those without copious intraabdominal fat. The Vanguard is to be preferred for the male patient, the super-obese, and those with central obesity with visible moderate to extensive intra-abdominal fat. If in doubt, use the Vanguard.

Dissection at the Angle of His

The liver is retracted up and to the right to expose the diaphragm above the esophageal hiatus. The camera is moved to port 3. The three graspers are placed through ports 1, 4, and 6. The hook diathermy is through port 5. The omental fat is drawn down and to the right by grasper at port 6. The fundus is drawn downward by the grasper at port 4. The fat pad over the esophagogastric junction is drawn to the right by the grasper at port 1. The hook diathermy is used to divide the peritoneum at the interface with the diaphragm over the left crus. The appearance at this stage is shown in Figure 20.1-2. The soft tissues are gentle teased and divided to expose the crus.

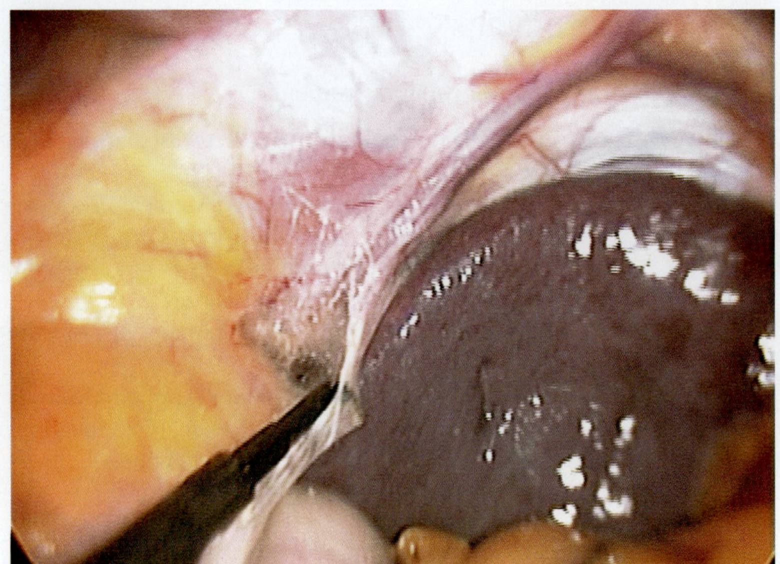

A

FIGURE 20.1-2. (A,B) Exposure of the angle of His. The lateral segment of the left lobe of liver is retracted upward. The omental fat has been retracted downward, and the fundus is drawn down and to the right. The diathermy hook is opening the peritoneum over the left crus. (B: Courtesy of the Cleveland Clinic Foundation.)

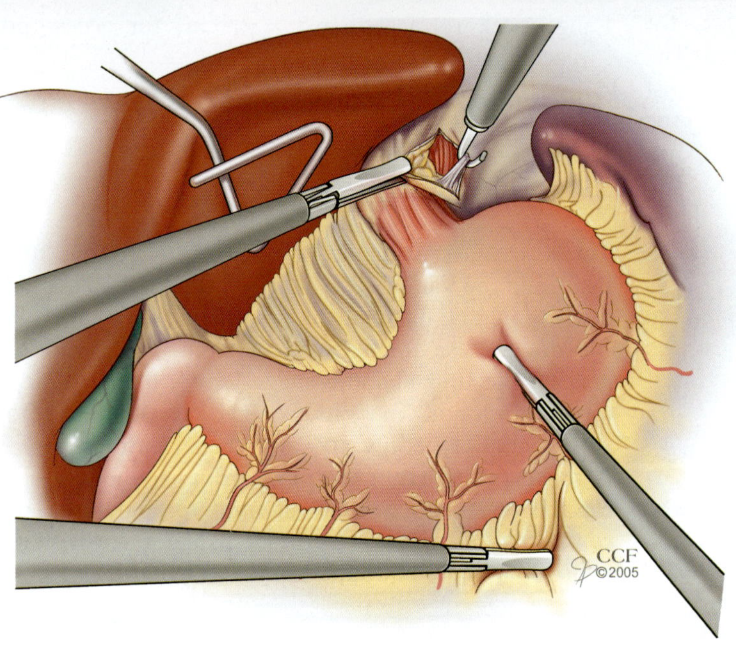

B

Dissection at the Lesser Curve

The grasper at port 6 is replaced by the Lap-Band placer. The grasper at port 4 draws the mid-lesser curve to the left. The pars flaccida of the lesser omentum is widely divided. The grasper at port 6 retracts the caudate lobe of the liver, while the grasper at port 4 retracts the fat on the posterior wall of the lesser sac to expose the anterior margin of the right crus at its lower limit (Fig. 20.1-3). This point on the right crus is recognized by the fat pad containing a significant vessel that passes across the lowest point. The inferior vena cava can be seen just to the right of the crus and should not be confused with the crus. A small opening is made in the peritoneum about 5 mm in front of the anterior margin of the right crus. The grasper in port 6 is passed into this opening and should slide without resistance along the path of the left crus (Fig. 20.1-4). The Lap-Band placer is passed along this track and allowed to spiral gently upward toward the top of the left crus with a counterclockwise rotation.

Figure 20.1-3. (A,B) Exposure of the inferior-anterior margin of the right crus. The fat pad is seen passing across toward the inferior vena cava, behind the caudate lobe of the liver. The point of dissection is onto the fat a few millimeters in front of the lowest aspect of the right crus. (B: Courtesy of the Cleveland Clinic Foundation.)

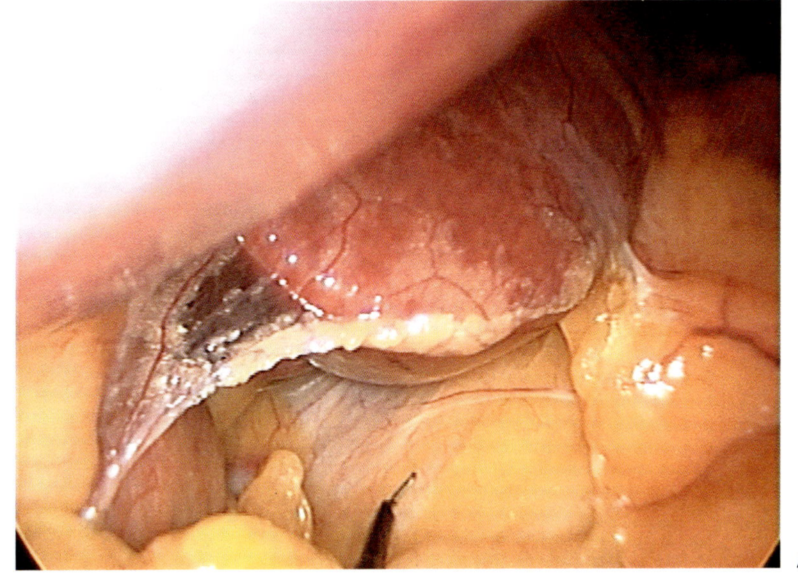

A

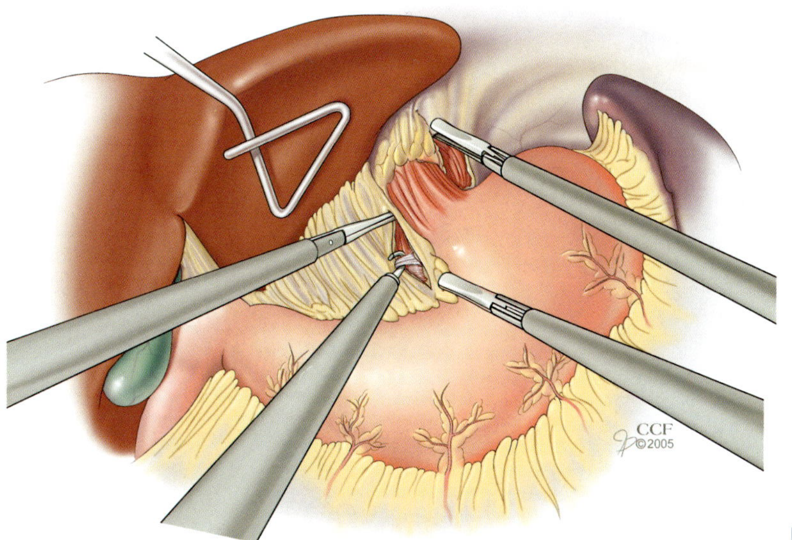

B

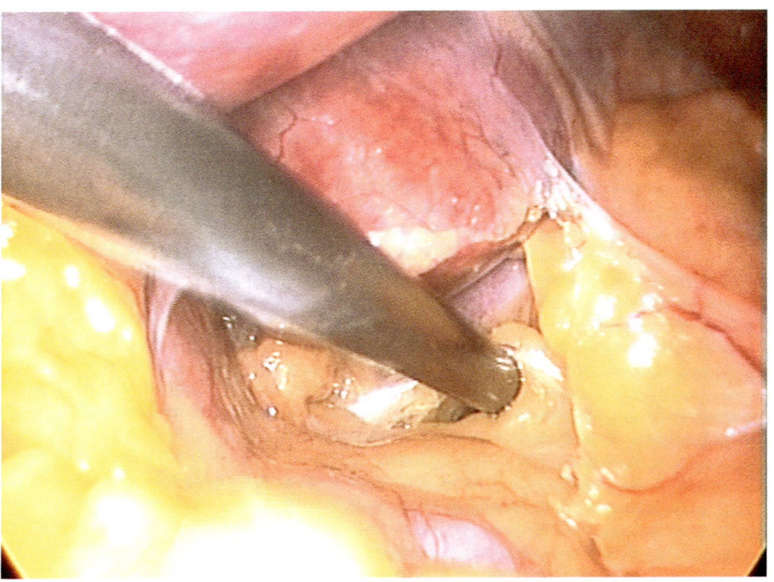

Figure 20.1-4. The peritoneum has been opened and a tunnel developed using the grasper through port 1. The Lap-Band placer is poised to pass along that path to the point of dissection on the right crus.

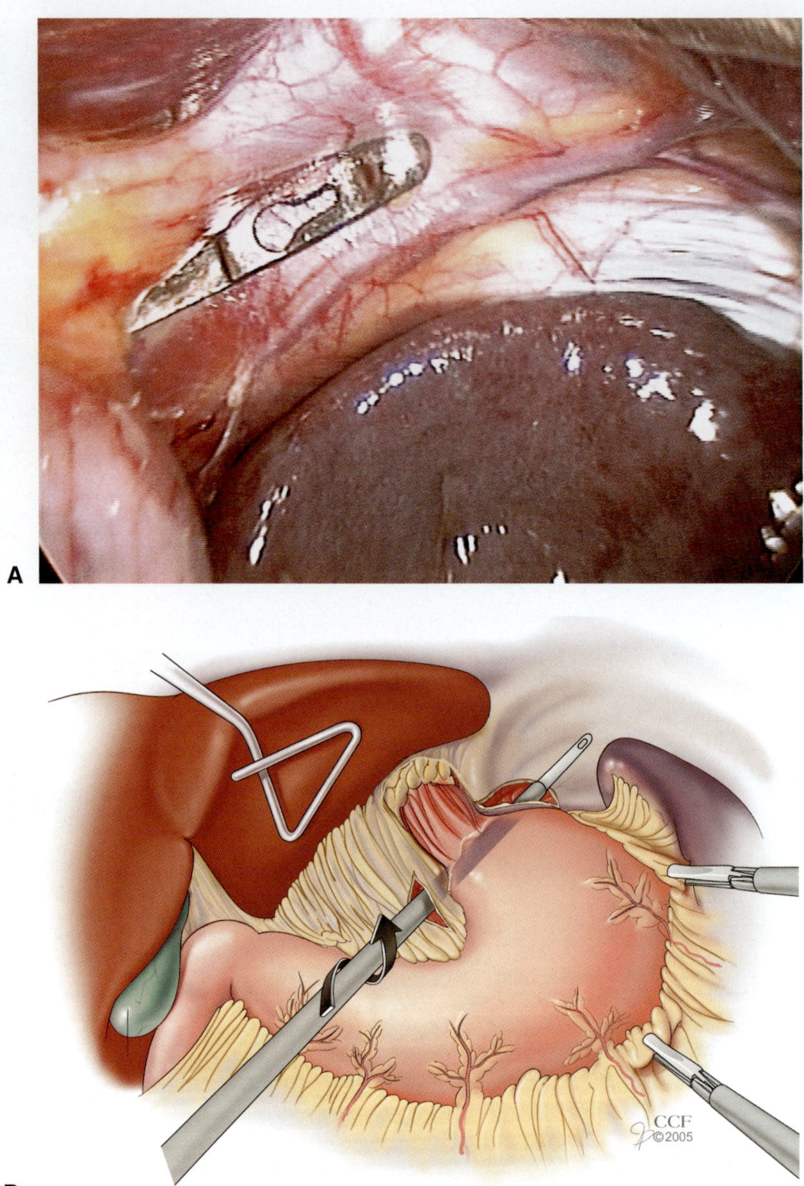

Figure 20.1-5. (A,B) The Lap-Band placer has passed along the left crus from right to left and appears at the angle of His. It is now ready to receive the tubing from the Lap-Band. (B: Courtesy of the Cleveland Clinic Foundation.)

The two graspers are moved back to the greater curve to again expose the angle of His. The tip of the Lap-Band placer is gently moved by rotation and advancement to enter the area of prior dissection. It is then advanced through the soft tissues to lie free alongside the spleen (Fig. 20.1-5). There must be no significant pressure used in passing this instrument. It is a placer and not a dissector. If there is resistance to passage, further dissection at the angle of His is indicated.

Lap-Band Placement and Calibration

The telescope is moved to port 5 and the Lap-Band, held by the introducer, is introduced into the abdomen via port 5. The telescope is returned to port 3, and 4 to 6 cm of the end of the Lap-Band tubing, which has been cut at an acute angle, is passed into the slot on the tip of the placer (Fig. 20.1-6). The placer is then withdrawn along its path to the lesser curve and the tubing retrieved. The

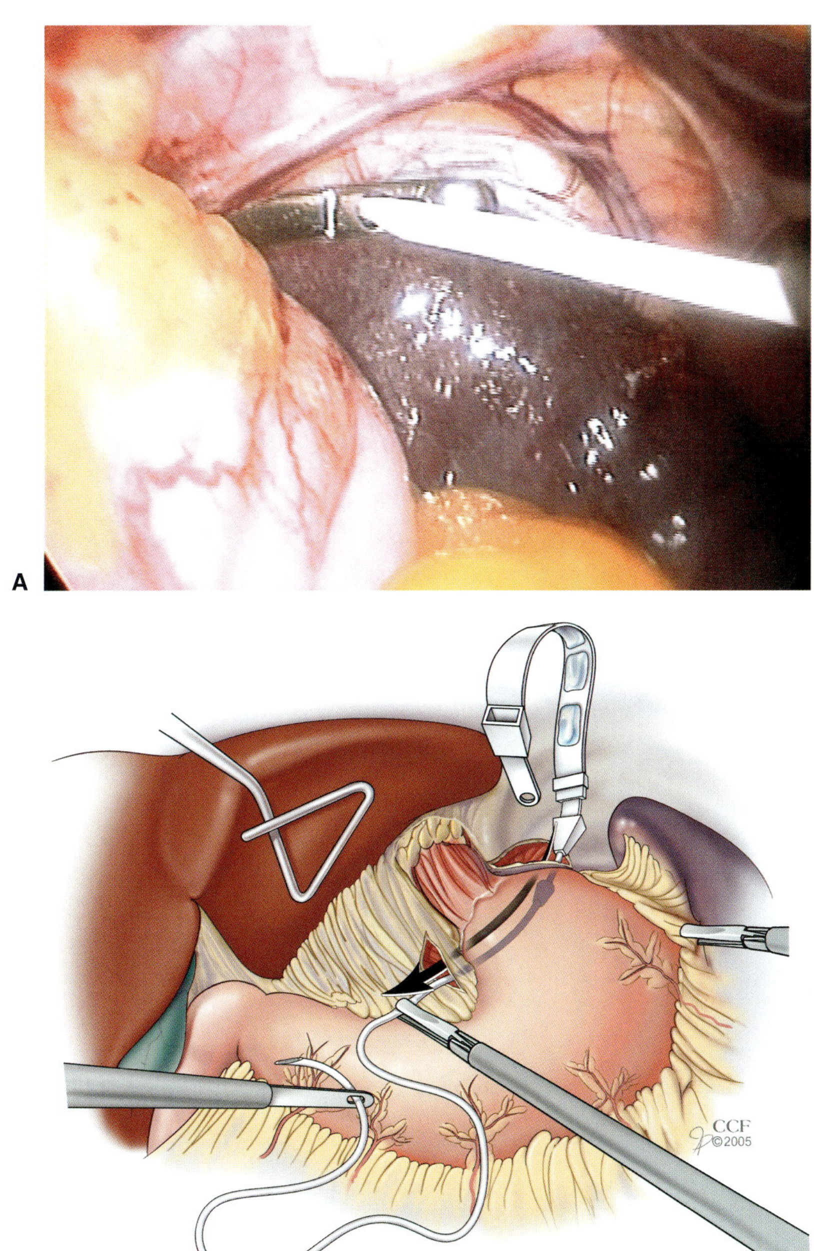

FIGURE 20.1-6. (A,B) The tubing is threaded into the Lap-Band placer, which is then withdrawn across to the lesser curve side. (B: Courtesy of the Cleveland Clinic Foundation.)

placer is removed. The tubing is drawn around until the band is in place (Fig. 20.1-7) and the buckle is then partially closed.

With the calibration tube already in place in the stomach, 25 mL of air is added to the balloon and the tube is withdrawn by the anesthetist until the balloon impacts at the esophagogastric junction. A check is made that the band would overlie the equator of the balloon. Remove the air from the calibration tube and bring the band to almost complete closure. Make an estimate if complete closure is likely to create too tight a band. If it appears tight, division of the fat of the lesser omentum along the path of the band is indicated. If it is not too tight, proceed with closure using the closure tool. Draw the tubing out of the abdomen through port 6 so as to expose the anterior surface of the band for fixation.

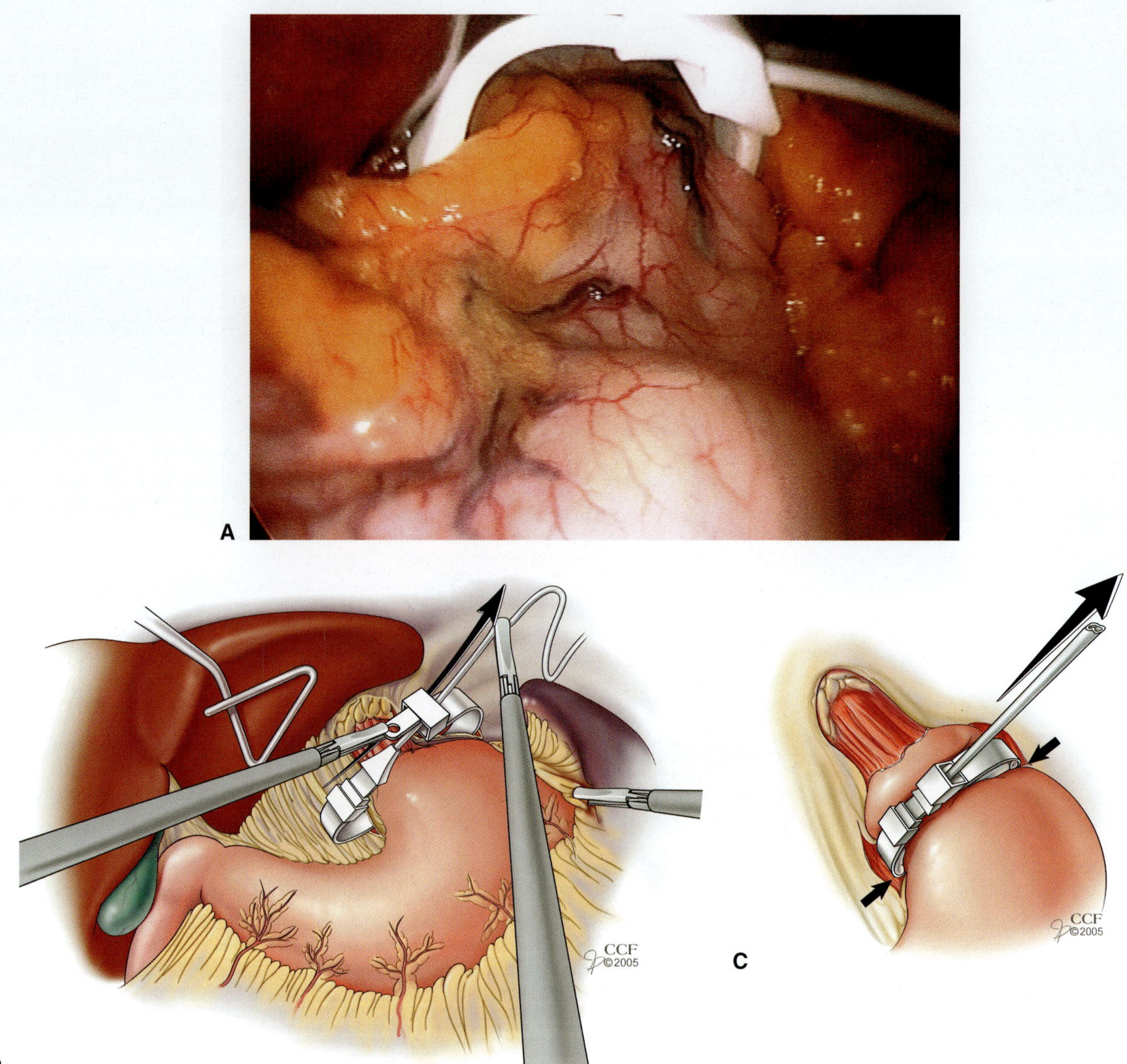

FIGURE 20.1-7. (A–C) The band is in place with the esophagogastric junction in front of the band. The calibration tube is lying with the lumen of the stomach and withdrawing of the inflated balloon against the esphagogastric junction will confirm correct positioning. (B,C: Courtesy of the Cleveland Clinic Foundation.)

Anterior Fixation

It is essential that the anterior fixation sutures are placed to hold the band across the very top of the stomach and that they securely hold those parts of the gastric wall, which could otherwise slip above the band. We place a suture (Ethibond 2/0 on 26 mm needle) though port 5 and then place a grasper through this port to select and then hold the gastric wall below and above the band that we want to include in the suture. The first suture should be near but not at the greater curve, and each suture should approximate visible gastric wall to visible gastric wall (Fig. 20.1-8). Usually three but sometimes four gastrogastric sutures are placed. We avoid bringing the anterior fixation too close to the buckle to avoid the risk of erosion through friction of the firm irregular buckle against the gastric wall (Fig. 20.1-9). The tubing is then drawn back into the abdomen and drawn out through the port 5. Insufflation is ceased, as much CO_2 as possible is released, and the port is removed.

FIGURE 20.1-8. (A,B) Sutures must approximate the stomach below the band to the stomach above the band. If gastric wall is not clearly seen above, dissection of the overlying fat and positioning with graspers may be necessary. (B: Courtesy of the Cleveland Clinic Foundation.)

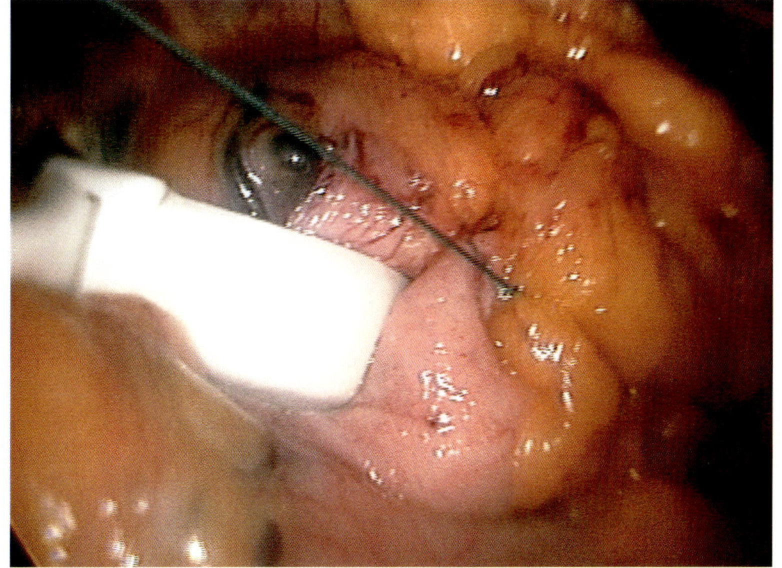

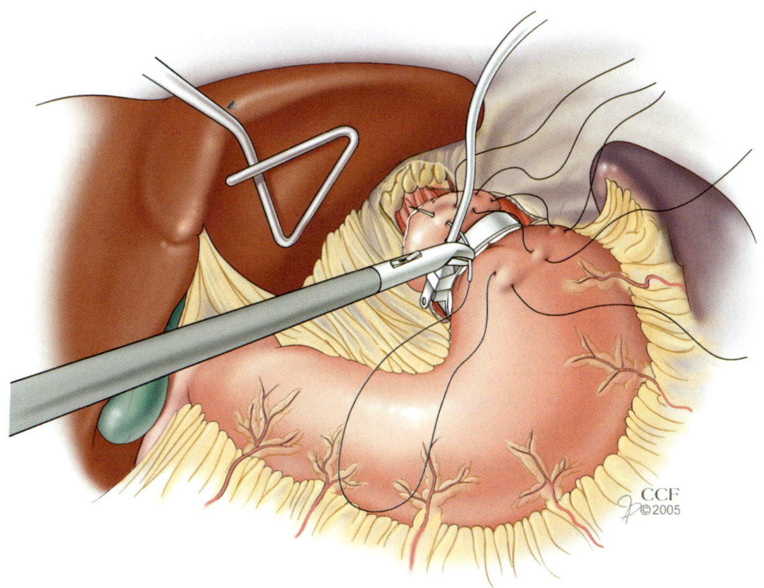

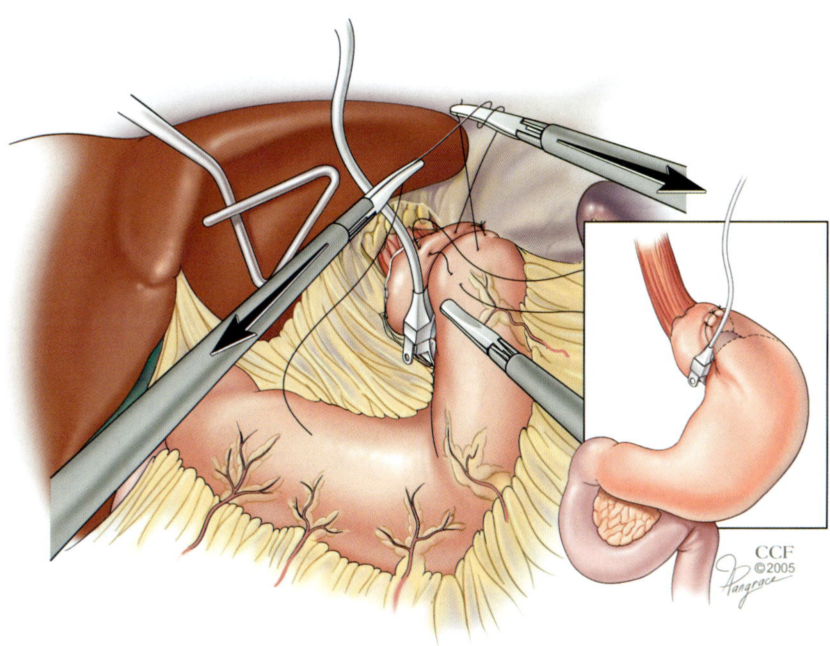

FIGURE 20.1-9. Completion of anterior fixation with avoidance of bringing the gastric wall against the buckle of the band. (Courtesy of the Cleveland Clinic Foundation.)

TABLE 20.1-2. Guidelines for adjustments to gastric banding

Consider adding fluid	Adjustment not required	Consider removing fluid
Inadequate weight loss	Adequate rate of weight loss	Vomiting, heartburn, reflux into the mouth
Rapid loss of satiety after meals	Eating reasonable range of food	Coughing spells, wheezing and choking, especially at night
Increased volume of meals	No negative symptoms	Difficulty coping with broad range of foods
Hunger between meals		Maladaptive eating behavior

Placement of the Access Port

The skin incision at port 5 is extended to 4 cm and the subcutaneous fat dissected to expose the anterior rectus sheath. Four sutures of 2-0 Prolene are placed in a square pattern about 1 cm apart. The end of the tubing from the band is trimmed and connected to the access port at the metal connector. The Prolene sutures are threaded into the port, the tubing is returned to the abdominal cavity, and the port tied into position with a smooth passage of the tubing directly into the abdomen.

Follow-Up and Adjustments

The follow-up process, including adjusting the band, is at least as important in obtaining a good result from Lap-Band placement as the operation itself, and therefore good technique for follow-up and adjustment is essential. Intrinsic to achieving a comprehensive follow-up is maintaining a database that allows tracking of each patient's progress and identifying any loss to follow-up early so that contact can be restored. A comprehensive but simple database system is reviewed in a later chapter.

Guidelines for adjustment that our group generally follows are shown in Table 20.1-2. For our standard approach of placing a 10-cm band along the pars flaccida pathway, an initial volume of 1 mL of saline is added at 5 weeks. Further additions are based on the criteria in Table 20.1-2 and generally 0.3 to 0.5 mL is added each time. For the new 11-cm band (Vanguard) we add 2.5 mL at the first adjustment, 1.0 mL at each subsequent adjustment until significant restriction is felt, and then 0.5 mL each time. As with any bariatric procedure, permanent follow-up is required. Initially we would review patients every 2 to 4 weeks, progressively stretching this out to a frequency of never greater than 12 months.

The decision to adjust the amount of fluid in the band can be made on clinical or radiologic criteria. Because of costs and logistical difficulties, we have never used the radiologic approach. Information on its use can be found in a report by Favretti et al. (4).

The level of adjustment should be sufficient to achieve a prolonged sensation of satiety in the patient. Weight loss should be steady and progressive, with the early rate of weight loss ideally being >0.5 kg but <1 kg per week. Adjustment should induce no restrictive symptoms, such as heartburn, vomiting, discomfort, or excessive difficulty with eating a normal range of food. Loss of excess weight should be planned to occur gradually over a period of 18 months to 3 years depending on the initial weight.

We consider adding additional fluid when there is inadequate weight loss, when there is rapid loss of satiety after a meal, when the patient notices increased volume of food taken at a meal, or when there is hunger between meals.

We consider removing fluid if there is vomiting, heartburn, reflux, cough spells, or wheezing and choking, especially at night, if there is difficulty in coping with a broad range of foods, or if there is maladaptive eating behavior.

When the patient is eating a reasonable range of foods, there is an adequate rate of weight loss, and there are no negative symptoms, we do not expect to adjust the volume.

Conclusion

The placement of the Lap-Band and the patient follow-up thereafter is normally a straightforward exercise and provides a safe and gradual way of achieving a major and durable loss of weight and improvement in health and quality of life. There are aspects in the details that are crucially important, making good surgeon training, continuing contact with the patient, and attendance at refresher courses important if optimal outcomes are to be achieved. With good technique for both the operation and the follow-up, the care of these patients is one of the most rewarding areas of clinical practice.

References

1. Szinicz G, Schnapka G. A new method in the surgical treatment of disease. Acta Chir Aust 1982;suppl 43.
2. Kuzmak LI, Yap IS, McGuire L, Dixon JS, Young MP. Surgery for morbid obesity. Using an inflatable gastric band. AORN J 1990;51:1307–1324.
3. Belachew M, Legrand MJ, Vincent V. History of Lap-Band: from dream to reality. Obes Surg 2001;11:297–302.
4. Favretti F, O'Brien PE, Dixon JB. Patient management after LAP-BAND placement. Am J Surg 2002;184:S38–41.

20.2
Laparoscopic Adjustable Gastric Banding: Outcomes

John B. Dixon and Paul E. O'Brien

The first laparoscopic adjustable gastric band (LAGB) was placed in 1993 (1), an event that heralded the widespread introduction of laparoscopic obesity surgery. The LAGB has become rapidly and widely accepted by bariatric surgeons and patients seeking surgical treatment for obesity. With more than 10 years of experience and more than 150,000 band placements, we are now in a good position to assess its safety and efficacy. There is now a wealth of largely observational data regarding the results of LAGB surgery. This chapter reviews the broad outcomes of LAGB surgery, with an emphasis on important outcome data that have changed techniques or expanded our knowledge regarding the treatment of severe obesity [body mass index (BMI) >35). The assessment of outcomes addresses weight loss, changes to obesity-related comorbidities, effects on quality of life and psychosocial changes, and deaths and complications.

A number of LAGB devices are now available commercially; however, as almost all the published reports relate to the BioEnterics Lap-Band System (Inamed Health, Santa Barbara, CA), and as it is the only form of LAGB approved for use in the United States, this chapter focuses on the published outcomes after Lap-Band placement. Caution must be used in simply extrapolating outcomes of the Lap-Band to that of other bands (2).

The data reviewed in this chapter have been obtained from the published literature, systematic reviews, and our prospective long-term observational studies of subjects following LAGB surgery.

Weight Loss

There is now good evidence that LAGB surgery provides significant sustained weight loss over the medium to long term with published reports extending up to 8 years (3).

Data beyond 8 years are not yet available. The results from large published series demonstrate a consistent pattern of excess weight loss of 50% to 60% by 2 years after surgery, which is maintained thereafter. There is no evidence at this time of significant weight regain, a problem often reported following gastric stapling procedures. Figure 20.2-1 presents the mean data from all studies available as of September 1, 2003, in which at least 50 patients are treated and which report weight loss as a percentage of excess weight lost (%EWL) following the LAGB. The pattern of weight loss is quite different from that seen after Roux-en-Y gastric bypass (RYGBP) surgery, in which a more rapid and extensive weight loss is experienced over the first 12 to 24 months and then some weight regain is usual. From the limited data available, the mean excess weight loss at 4 to 6 years after LAGB and RYGBP surgery is similar.

The gradual initial weight loss and medium-term durability of weight loss has been a valuable feature of LAGB surgery and has been attributed to the adjustability of the band stoma. Maintenance of the anatomic change, providing a small proximal gastric pouch above the band, seems to provide continued satiety, limiting food intake and preventing weight gain.

A recent randomized controlled trial performed at our institution evaluated the efficacy of the LAGB in mildly to moderately obese patients (BMI 30 to 35) (4). In this trial, patients were randomized to LAGB versus a program of very-low-calorie diets, pharmacotherapy, and lifestyle change for 24 months. At 2 years, the surgical group had greater excess weight loss (87.3% vs. 21.8%, $p < .001$). The metabolic syndrome was present in 15 patients in each group and resolved in all but one surgical patient and remained in eight (24%) of the nonsurgical patients ($p < .002$). Additionally, quality-of-life scores improved significantly more in the surgical group. This study represents the first trial comparing a modern bariatric procedure to medical therapy in a randomized, controlled fashion.

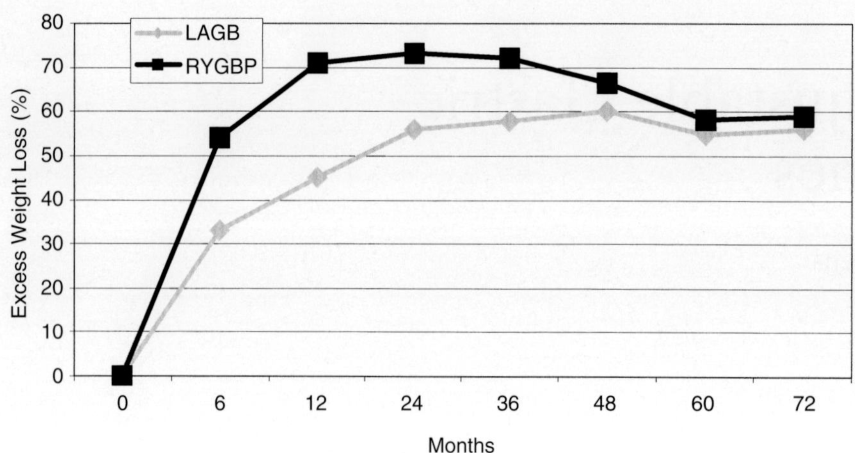

Figure 20.2-1. The percentage of excess weight loss after Lap-Band surgery and a comparison with Roux-en-y gastric bypass (RYGBP). Data include all published series with initial recruitment of at least 50 patients reporting data at 3 years or more following surgery. There were eight RYGBP studies and seven laparoscopic adjustable gastric banding (LAGB) studies.

Changes in the Comorbidities of Obesity

Obesity drives a wide range of illnesses, to the point where it could now reasonably be regarded as the worst pathogen in Western communities. One of the overwhelming features of weight loss following obesity surgery, including LAGB surgery, is the improvement or resolution of obesity-related comorbidity. A summary of some of the major health benefits follows.

The Metabolic Syndrome

Many of the health risks and problems of overweight and obesity are closely related to the metabolic syndrome. The components of this syndrome have been better defined recently and it is estimated that almost 25% of both men and women living in the United States are affected (5). The syndrome is characterized by central obesity, dyslipidemia, impaired glucose tolerance or type 2 diabetes, and hypertension. A key feature of this syndrome is impaired insulin–mediated glucose uptake or insulin resistance, but this is only one of a cascade of metabolic and inflammatory events that characterize the syndrome and contribute to increased cardiovascular risk. Other clinically significant conditions, such as non-alcoholic steatohepatitis, obstructive sleep apnea, and polycystic ovary syndrome, are also closely related to the metabolic syndrome. Sustained weight loss has a major beneficial effect on all of the components of the syndrome and significantly reduces a range of key vascular risk factors. In our randomized, controlled trial, 14 of 15 surgical patients had resolution of metabolic syndrome 2 years after Lap-Band placement compared to only six of 15 medically managed patients.

Type 2 Diabetes

Type 2 diabetes is the paradigm of an obesity-related illness, with its prevalence increasing dramatically with increasing BMI. Fifty patients were followed for 1 year after Lap-Band placement (6). There was a significant improvement in all measures of glucose metabolism, with complete remission of diabetes in 32 patients (64%), improvement of control in 13 (26%), and five (10%) were relatively unchanged. Importantly, the extent of weight loss and the time duration of diabetes were predictors of remission, indicating that early significant weight loss is indicated in the recently diagnosed diabetic. Similar impressive results have been reported following RYGBP and biliopancreatic diversion (BPD).

There are two fundamental requirements for the development of type 2 diabetes; first, insulin resistance with increased pancreatic β-cell demand, and second, inadequate β-cell response to this demand resulting in hyperglycemia. We have demonstrated that weight loss following LAGB surgery improves both insulin sensitivity and β-cell function, as measured by HOMA%S and HOMA%B, respectively, in 254 patients during the first year after placement (7). The critical factor affecting the improvement in β-cell function is the time the patient has had diabetes. This is understandable, as there is progressive irreversible β-cell damage driven by the metabolic effects of diabetes. Thus weight loss reverses basic mechanisms for the appearance and progression of type 2 diabetes.

The beneficial effects of weight loss are durable. Table 20.2-1 shows the fall in serum insulin, fasting blood glucose, glycosylated hemoglobin A_{1c}, and an index of insulin resistance over a 5-year period after LAGB placement. All measures improve by 1 year, and the improvement is sustained. Others have confirmed these beneficial effects of LAGB surgery (8,9).

TABLE 20.2-1. Changes in markers of insulin resistance with time after Lap-Band surgery

Time	n	Glucose (mmol/L)	HbA$_{1c}$ (%)	Insulin (uU/mL)	Insulin resistance index (IRI)*
Preoperative	1000	5.78	5.87	22.1	4.61
1 year postoperative	755	5.09	5.37	10.8	3.81
2 year	480	5.05	5.36	10.8	3.74
3 year	295	4.93	5.23	10.5	3.74
4 year	225	5.04	5.34	10.4	3.76
5+ year	254	4.96	5.38	11.2	3.86

* IRI is an indirect measure of insulin resistance. IRI = log$_e$ (fasting plasma glucose) + log$_e$ (fasting plasma glucose).
Note: p values calculated using analysis of variance (ANOVA) with the Tukey method of post-hoc analysis. All values are significantly lower at 1 year (p < .001 for all) and there is no significant difference between results at between 1 year and 5 years or longer.
Source: Katz A, Nambi SS, Mather K, et al. Quantitative insulin sensitivity check index: a simple, accurate method for assessing insulin sensitivity in humans. J Clin Endocrinol Metab 2000;85:2402–2410.

Dyslipidemia of Obesity

The dyslipidemia of obesity and the metabolic syndrome is characterized by high triglyceride and low high-density lipoprotein (HDL) cholesterol concentrations, with total cholesterol and low-density lipoprotein (LDL) cholesterol concentrations closer to normal ranges (10). However, in the context of central obesity, insulin resistance, high triglyceride, and low HDL cholesterol, the LDL cholesterol particles are small, dense, sticky, and easily oxidized (11,12). This highly atherogenic lipid profile is the most common pattern associated with coronary artery disease.

Weight loss following LAGB surgery is accompanied by a significant sustained fall in fasting triglyceride levels, an increase in HDL cholesterol to normal levels, and a favorable improvement in the total cholesterol to HDL cholesterol ratio (13).

Hypertension

Weight loss following LAGB surgery provides substantial falls in both systolic and diastolic blood pressure (8,14,15). Many patients present for surgery with inadequately controlled blood pressure despite medical therapy. In a consecutive series of 148 hypertensive patients, we found that 55% at 1 year had resolution of the problem (normotensive on no antihypertensive medication), 33% were improved, and 15% unchanged. We have followed blood pressure measurements at all annual postoperative follow-up visits over 5 years or longer and find that there are sustained falls in both systolic and diastolic blood pressure (Fig. 20.2-2). There appears to be a small but significant rise in both systolic and diastolic blood pressures at 4 years or longer following surgery when compared with 1 to 2 years after surgery. The Swedish Obese Subjects study found a similar rise in blood pressure, which emphasizes the need to monitor and manage this comorbidity over an extended period (16).

Other Comorbidities

Sleep Disturbance and Obstructive Sleep Apnea

There are a number of sleep disorders associated with severe obesity. Obesity increases the prevalence of the most serious of these, obstructive sleep apnea (OSA), by a factor of 10. It is also clear that weight distribution and insulin resistance are predictors of significant OSA in an obese population (17,18). Using demographic, simple anthropometric and biochemical measures, we have devised a scoring system to assess risk and therefore to help select patients for screening in overnight sleep studies (18). Excessive daytime sleepiness, which is a common, disabling, and potentially dangerous problem, is also strongly linked to obesity but not necessarily caused by OSA (17,18).

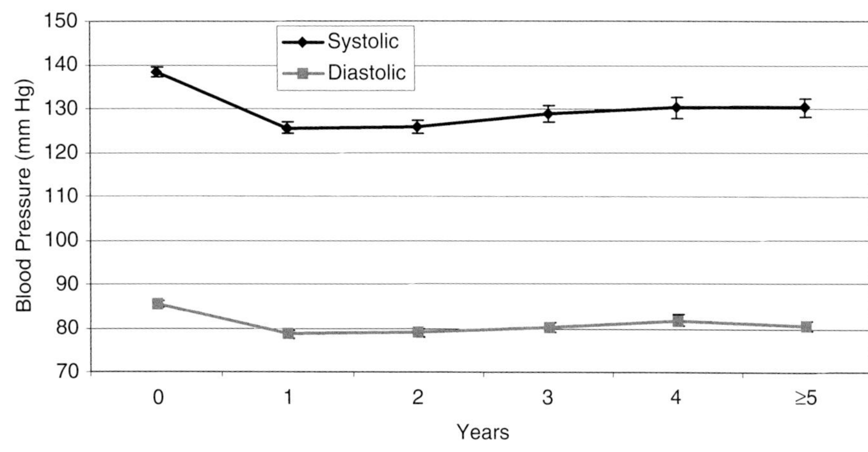

FIGURE 20.2-2. Mean ± 95% confidence intervals for blood pressure recordings at yearly follow-up visits after LAGB placement (n = 1000 at baseline). p < .001 for both; analysis of variance (ANOVA) using the Tukey method of post-hoc analysis. Measures at all yearly intervals are lower than preoperative recordings. Mean levels at 4 years or longer are significantly greater than at 1 and 2 years.

Problems associated with sleep improve dramatically with weight loss (8,19). We studied 123 consecutive patients prior to and 1 year after LAGB surgery (19). There was a high preoperative prevalence of significantly disturbed sleep in both men (59%) and women (45%). After 1 year, reported observed sleep apnea had decreased from 33% to 2%, habitual snoring from 82% to 14%, abnormal daytime sleepiness from 39% to 4%, and poor sleep quality from 39% to 2%.

Ovarian Dysfunction, Infertility, and Pregnancy

Obesity, especially central obesity, is associated with ovulatory dysfunction and infertility. Weight loss in premenopausal women lowers the active testosterone levels, largely by increasing the levels of testosterone bound to sex hormone–binding globulin, and this usually restores ovarian function and improves fertility. Women are advised to use a reliable method of contraception for 1 year following LAGB placement to reduce any fetal risk during the rapid weight loss period. Several studies have reported unplanned pregnancies in previously infertile women not long after band placement (20–22). The adjustability of the band is of particular value in the pregnant woman, enabling reduction in gastric restriction, if necessary, to allow for hyperemesis should it occur in early pregnancy, adequate fetal nutrition, healthy maternal weight gain, and reduced impact at the time of delivery and while establishing breast-feeding. Weight gain is advised in all pregnancies, and recommended weight gain can be based on the prepregnancy BMI (23). Active management of the band during pregnancy has been successful in achieving excellent maternal and infant outcomes (22). The band is then readjusted following pregnancy to help in attaining the prepregnancy weight and achieve further weight loss if necessary. Weight loss is generally safe while breast-feeding, and the postnatal period is a high-risk time for weight retention or gain in many women (24).

Asthma

There is increasing evidence of a relationship between symptoms of asthma and obesity, especially in adolescent and adult women. There is some evidence of increased bronchial reactivity and good evidence that the lung function abnormalities of severe obesity will aggravate or exacerbate asthma symptoms (25,26). There are limited data regarding the effect of weight loss on asthma in obese subjects, but all are favorable (27–29). We have demonstrated major improvements or resolution in all aspects of asthma with weight loss following LAGB surgery. Improvements include reduced symptoms, increased exercise tolerance, fewer medications including oral and inhaled corticosteroids, and fewer hospital admissions. It is possible that part of the improvement is related to the beneficial effect of an appropriately placed band on gastroesophageal reflux (30,31).

Gastroesophageal Reflux

Gastroesophageal reflux disease is more than twice as prevalent in the morbidly obese (31). A key feature of almost all currently used obesity surgery involves the creation of a small or virtual pouch of stomach just below the gastroesophageal (GE) junction. Placement of the LAGB effectively controls acid reflux (30–33). Several groups have clearly demonstrated that a correctly placed band reduces gastroesophageal reflux symptoms and lowers esophageal acid exposure (32,34). It is relevant that if the band slips and there is excessive stomach above the band, symptoms of severe gastroesophageal reflux are prominent and require investigation.

Quality of Life and Psychosocial Changes

Quality of Life

Obesity has a major negative impact on many aspects of quality of life affecting both physical and mental health (35). Studies have consistently shown major improvements in quality of life with weight loss following LAGB placement (36–40). In a large prospective study using the Medical Outcomes Trust Short Form–36, we demonstrated that patients presenting for LAGB surgery had significantly lower measures of all eight tested domains when compared with normal values. At follow-up, all eight scores improved and at 1 year following surgery were at or above those of age- and sex-matched community levels. Scores remained within the normal range over the 4-year study period (36). Similar improvements have been reported in patients having LAGB surgery for failed gastric stapling procedures (40).

Body Image

Severely obese patients generally have normal appearance orientation, that is, a normal pride or investment in their appearance or presentation (41,42), but they evaluate their appearance as being very poor. There is therefore a large discrepancy between evaluation and orientation, producing considerable psychological stress. Society's stigmatization and discrimination against severely obese subjects further compound these problems. Weight loss following LAGB surgery improves self-evaluation of appearance but does not return it to normal levels. The improvement in appearance evaluation is related to the extent of weight loss. The discrepancy between appearance orientation, which is not usually altered by weight loss, and appearance evaluation is lower with weight loss, reducing psychological stress.

Depression

The nature of the relationship between obesity and depression is becoming clearer, with most studies supporting a linear relationship rather than the "fat and jolly" hypothesis (43,44). Symptoms of depression are very common in those presenting for obesity surgery, especially younger women with very poor body image (45). Sustained weight loss following LAGB surgery is associated with a sustained reduction in the symptoms of depression, with Beck Depression Scale scores returning to normal in the majority of subjects within 12 months of surgery and remaining in the normal range over a 4-year follow-up period (45). The Swedish obesity study, utilizing largely nonadjustable gastric restrictive surgery, has provided similar results (46), but not all studies have reported sustained improvements. The Greenville group has reported only transient improvements in mental health following gastric bypass surgery (47).

Complications

Perioperative

Mortality

Safety is a major feature of LAGB surgery. A systematic review of all the published literature on safety and efficacy of LAGB compared with the gastric stapling procedures showed the perioperative mortality rate was 10 times greater for RYGBP and seven times greater for vertical banded gastroplasty (VBG) (48). In the published literature the perioperative mortality rate for LAGB is 0.05%. The minimalist nature of the surgical intervention with LAGB almost certainly explains these significant differences. In our own series of over 1600 patients there has been no perioperative mortality. While this procedure is comparatively safe, the risks associated with any bariatric surgery should not be underestimated, and before surgery is performed a well-informed risk-benefit analysis should be provided to all patients.

Morbidity

Given the relatively gentle nature of the intervention, it is not surprising that early morbidity is very low. In our series, the early complication rate is 1.8% with the commonest complication being wound infection at the subcutaneous access port site. The need to convert the laparoscopic approach to open surgery is <1% in experienced hands and is usually required if access to the operative area is restricted due to hepatomegaly or copious visceral fat. We have also treated a number of patients who have had previous gastric stapling in whom we have placed the Lap-Band by open laparotomy. Their early complication rate is higher at 17% (49). Thus, a very much reduced complication rate is seen in association with the laparoscopic approach and the lack of need to divide or open the stomach.

Late Morbidity

While early morbidity has been minimal, later complications have been of greater concern. Important late complications include band slippage or prolapse, erosion of the band into the stomach, and problems with the access port. Developments in the surgical technique and access port design have significantly reduced these late complications. Posterior band slippage has been reduced by the use of the pars-flaccida pathway for band placement, and anterior slippage has been reduced by providing careful anterior fixation. These developments have allowed the slippage rate to be dramatically reduced. In our series, the early prolapse/slippage rate was 25%, but this in now under 5% (50). Others have also reported this reduction in the incidence of prolapse with improved operative technique (3,51).

Erosion of the band into the stomach also appears to be largely preventable by avoiding tight anterior fixation especially over the buckle area (52). Anterior fixation that involved attaching the anterior gastric wall to the crus of the diaphragm also produced a high incidence of erosion. Recent design changes to the subcutaneous access port have reduced the risk of tubing breaks. Learning from the problems associated with the early use of the LAGB should provide a reliably low late complication rate, and no doubt there will be further beneficial developments. Expected prolapse, erosion, and system leakage rates should be less than 5%, 1%, and 5%, respectively.

When compared with other commonly used bariatric surgical techniques, a systematic review found an overall morbidity rate for LAGB is around 10.6% [95% confidence interval (CI) 9.5–11.6%), for VBG it is around 29.9% (CI 28.5–31.4%), and for RYGBP it is around 23.4% (22.3–24.5%). It is important to recognize that the type of morbidity is often specific to the particular surgical procedure (48).

A learning curve is important with many surgical procedures, and LAGB is no exception. A systematic review of published literature demonstrates that the incidence of complications is inversely related to the published series size (Fig. 20.2-3).

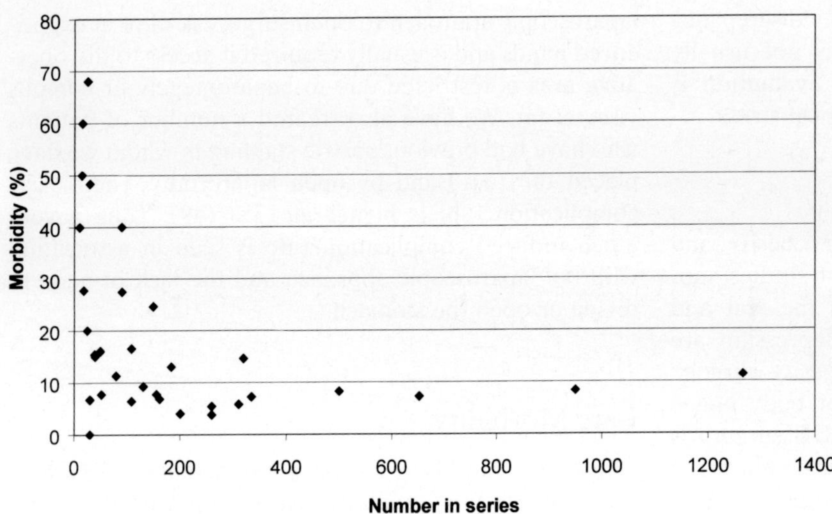

FIGURE 20.2-3. There is a significant negative relationship between series size and morbidity in series reporting the outcomes of LAGB surgery. Spearman correlation coefficient ($r = -0.62$, $p < .001$). [Adapted from data in the ASERNIP-S systematic review (48).]

Patient Selection: Outcomes

Laparoscopic adjustable gastric banding surgery is a safe, effective, and minimally invasive procedure that enables major and durable weight loss in association with improvement or resolution of a broad range of serious health problems. Its unique characteristics of adjustability and reversibility provide great flexibility for the patient both now and in the future. We have looked carefully for predictors of band effectiveness (49,53,54) and have not identified any subgroups that do not achieve a worthwhile effect from the procedure, which, based on our data, appears to be equally effective in the super-obese, in sweet eaters and non–sweet eaters, and in those with psychiatric disease or failed gastric stapling (40,53,54). However, we have not used the procedure in the mentally defective and those with malignant hyperphagia, such as Prader-Willi syndrome. To date, we have not identified any specific subgroup in which we would recommend a more invasive and higher risk procedure as a primary procedure.

References

1. Belachew M, Legrand MJ, Defechereux TH, Burtheret MP, Jacquet N. Laparoscopic adjustable silicone gastric banding in the treatment of morbid obesity. A preliminary report. Surg Endosc 1994;8:1354–1356.
2. Blanco-Engert R, Weiner S, Pomhoff I, Matkowitz R, Weiner RA. Outcome after laparoscopic adjustable gastric banding, using the Lap-Band and the Heliogast band: a prospective randomized study. Obes Surg 2003;13:776–779.
3. Weiner R, Blanco-Engert R, Weiner S, Matkowitz R, Schaefer L, Pomhoff I. Outcome after laparoscopic adjustable gastric banding—8 years experience. Obes Surg 2003;13:427–434.
4. O'Brien PE, Dixon JB, Laurie C, et al. Treatment of mild to moderate obesity with laparoscopic adjustable gastric banding or an intensive medical program: a randomized trial. Ann Intern Med 2006;144:625–633.
5. Ford ES, Giles WH, Dietz WH. Prevalence of the metabolic syndrome among US adults: findings from the third National Health and Nutrition Examination Survey. JAMA 2002;287:356–359.
6. Dixon JB, O'Brien P. Health outcomes of severely obese type 2 diabetic subjects 1 year after laparoscopic adjustable gastric banding. Diabetes Care 2002;25:358–363.
7. Dixon JB, Dixon AF, O'Brien PE. Improvements in insulin sensitivity and beta-cell function (HOMA) with weight loss in the severely obese. Diabet Med 2003;20:127–134.
8. Abu-Abeid S, Keidar A, Szold A. Resolution of chronic medical conditions after laparoscopic adjustable silicone gastric banding for the treatment of morbid obesity in the elderly. Surg Endosc 2001;15:132–134.
9. Dolan K, Bryant R, Fielding G. Treating diabetes in the morbidly obese by laparoscopic gastric banding. Obes Surg 2003;13:439–443.
10. Dixon JB, O'Brien P. A disparity between conventional lipid and insulin resistance markers at body mass index levels greater than 34kg/m(2). Int J Obes Relat Metab Disord 2001;25:793–797.
11. Despres J. The insulin resistance-dyslipidemia syndrome: the most prevalent cause of coronary artery disease. Can Med Assoc J 1993;148(8):1339–1340.
12. Koba S, Hirano T, Sakaue T, et al. Role of small dense low-density lipoprotein in coronary artery disease patients with normal plasma cholesterol levels. J Cardiol 2000;36:371–378.
13. Dixon JB, O'Brien PE. Lipid profile in the severely obese: changes with weight loss after lap-band surgery. Obes Res 2002;10:903–910.
14. Bacci V, Basso MS, Greco F, et al. Modifications of metabolic and cardiovascular risk factors after weight loss induced by laparoscopic gastric banding. Obes Surg 2002;12:77–82.
15. Dixon JB, O'Brien PE. Changes in comorbidities and improvements in quality of life after LAP-BAND placement. Am J Surg 2002;184:S51–54.

16. Sjostrom CD, Peltonen M, Wedel H, Sjostrom L. Differentiated long-term effects of intentional weight loss on diabetes and hypertension. Hypertension 2000;36:20–25.
17. Vgontzas AN, Papanicolaou DA, Bixler EO, et al. Sleep apnea and daytime sleepiness and fatigue: relation to visceral obesity, insulin resistance, and hypercytokinemia. J Clin Endocrinol Metab 2000;85:1151–1158.
18. Dixon JB, Schachter LM, O'Brien PE. Predicting sleep apnea and excessive day sleepiness in the severely obese: indicators for polysomnography. Chest 2003;123:1134–1141.
19. Dixon JB, Schachter LM, O'Brien PE. Sleep disturbance and obesity: changes following surgically induced weight loss. Arch Intern Med 2001;161:102–106.
20. Martin LF, Finigan KM, Nolan TE. Pregnancy after adjustable gastric banding. Obstet Gynecol 2000;95:927–930.
21. Weiss HG, Nehoda H, Labeck B, Hourmont K, Marth C, Aigner F. Pregnancies after adjustable gastric banding. Obes Surg 2001;11:303–306.
22. Dixon JB, Dixon ME, O'Brien PE. Pregnancy after Lap-Band surgery: management of the band to achieve healthy weight outcomes. Obes Surg 2001;11:59–65.
23. Institute of Medicine. Subcommittee on the Nutritional Status and Weight Gain During Pregnancy. Nutrition During Pregnancy. Weight Gain. Nutritional Supplements. Washington, DC: National Academy Press, 1990:1–13.
24. Lovelady CA, Garner KE, Moreno KL, Williams JP. The effect of weight loss in overweight, lactating women on the growth of their infants. N Engl J Med 2000;342:449–453.
25. Dixon J. The effects of obesity on asthma. In: Medeiros-Neto G, Halpern A, Bouchard C, eds. Progress in Obesity Research, vol 9. Montrouge, France: John Libbley Eurotext, 2003.
26. Mokdad AH, Ford ES, Bowman BA, et al. Prevalence of obesity, diabetes, and obesity-related health risk factors, 2001. JAMA 2003;289:76–79.
27. Macgregor AM, Greenberg RA. Effect of surgically induced weight loss on asthma in the morbidly obese. Obes Surg 1993;3:15–21.
28. Dixon JB, Chapman L, O'Brien P. Marked improvement in asthma after Lap-Band surgery for morbid obesity. Obes Surg 1999;9:385–389.
29. Hakala K, Stenius-Aarniala B, Sovijarvi A. Effects of weight loss on peak flow variability, airways obstruction, and lung volumes in obese patients with asthma. Chest 2000; 118:1315–1321.
30. Iovino P, Angrisani L, Tremolaterra F, et al. Abnormal esophageal acid exposure is common in morbidly obese patients and improves after a successful Lap-Band system implantation. Surg Endosc 2002;20:20.
31. Dixon JB, O'Brien PE. Gastroesophageal reflux in obesity: the effect of lap-band placement. Obes Surg 1999;9:527–531.
32. Weiss HG, Nehoda H, Labeck B, et al. Treatment of morbid obesity with laparoscopic adjustable gastric banding affects esophageal motility. Am J Surg 2000;180:479–482.
33. Schauer P, Hamad G, Ikramuddin S. Surgical management of gastroesophageal reflux disease in obese patients. Semin Laparosc Surg 2001;8:256–264.
34. Angrisani L, Iovino P, Lorenzo M, et al. Treatment of morbid obesity and gastroesophageal reflux with hiatal hernia by Lap-Band. Obes Surg 1999;9:396–398.
35. Kral JG, Sjostrom LV, Sullivan MB. Assessment of quality of life before and after surgery for severe obesity. Am J Clin Nutr 1992;55:611S–614S.
36. Dixon JB, Dixon ME, O'Brien PE. Quality of life after lap-band placement: influence of time, weight loss, and comorbidities. Obes Res 2001;9:713–721.
37. Weiner R, Datz M, Wagner D, Bockhorn H. Quality-of-life outcome after laparoscopic adjustable gastric banding for morbid obesity. Obes Surg 1999;9:539–545.
38. Horchner R, Tuinebreijer MW, Kelder PH. Quality-of-life assessment of morbidly obese patients who have undergone a Lap-Band operation: 2-year follow-up study. Is the MOS SF-36 a useful instrument to measure quality of life in morbidly obese patients? Obes Surg 2001;11:212–218; discussion 219.
39. Schok M, Geenen R, van Antwerpen T, de Wit P, Brand N, van Ramshorst B. Quality of life after laparoscopic adjustable gastric banding for severe obesity: postoperative and retrospective preoperative evaluations. Obes Surg 2000; 10:502–508.
40. O'Brien P, Brown W, Dixon J. Revisional surgery for morbid obesity—conversion to the Lap-Band system. Obes Surg 2000;10:557–563.
41. Cash TF. Body-image attitudes among obese enrollees in a commercial weight-loss program. Percept Mot Skills 1993; 77:1099–1103.
42. Dixon JB, Dixon ME, O'Brien P. Body image: appearance orientation and evaluation in the severely obese and post obese (ASBS Washington June 2001). Obes Surg 2001; 11(2):172.
43. Onyike CU, Crum RM, Lee HB, Lyketsos CG, Eaton WW. Is obesity associated with major depression? Results from the third national health and nutrition examination survey. Am J Epidemiol 2003;158:1139–1147.
44. Roberts RE, Kaplan GA, Shema SJ, Strawbridge WJ. Are the obese at greater risk for depression? Am J Epidemiol 2000;152:163–170.
45. Dixon JB, Dixon ME, O'Brien PE. Depression in association with severe obesity: changes with weight loss. Arch Intern Med 2003;163:2058–2065.
46. Karlsson J, Sjostrom L, Sullivan M. Swedish obese subjects (SOS)—an intervention study of obesity. Two-year follow-up of health related quality of life (HRQL) and eating behavior after gastric surgery for severe obesity. Int J Obes 1998;22:113–126.
47. Waters GS, Pories WJ, Swanson MS, Meelheim HD, Flickinger EG, May HJ. Long-term studies of mental health after the Greenville gastric bypass operation for morbid obesity. Am J Surg 1991;161:154–157; discussion 157–158.
48. Chapman A, Kiroff G, Game P, et al. Systematic review of laparoscopic adjustable gastric banding in the treatment of obesity. Report No. 31. Adelaide, South Australia: ASERNIP-S, 2002.
49. O'Brien P, Brown W, Dixon J. Revisional surgery for morbid obesity—conversion to the Lap-Band system. Obes Surg 2000;10:557–563.
50. O'Brien PE, Dixon JB, Brown W, et al. The laparoscopic adjustable gastric band (Lap-Band): a prospective study of medium-term effects on weight, health and quality of life. Obes Surg 2002;12:652–660.

51. Dargent J. Pouch dilatation and slippage after adjustable gastric banding: is it still an issue? Obes Surg 2003;13: 111–115.

52. O'Brien PE, Dixon JB. Weight loss and early and late complications-the international experience. Am J Surg 2002;184:S42–45.

53. Dixon JB, Dixon ME, O'Brien PE. Pre-operative predictors of weight loss at 1-year after Lap-Band surgery. Obes Surg 2001;11:200–207.

54. Hudson SM, Dixon JB, O'Brien PE. Sweet eating is not a predictor of outcome after Lap-Band placement. Can we finally bury the myth? Obes Surg 2002;12:789–794.

20.3
Laparoscopic Adjustable Gastric Banding: Postoperative Management and Nutritional Evaluation

Christine J. Ren

Experience with the nonadjustable silicone gastric band and the vertical banded gastroplasty have shown that a rigid, narrow stomal outlet leads to chronic vomiting, reflux, and subsequent weight gain due to maladaptive eating. One of the distinct advantages of laparoscopic adjustable gastric banding (LAGB) is its adjustability. This chapter discusses postoperative strategies that can maximize the efficacy of LAGB and potentially decrease the complications.

Immediate Postoperative Management

Postoperative care after LAGB is usually straightforward. Most patients are observed in a regular ward room. Patients with documented or suspected obstructive sleep apnea may require additional monitoring or a continuous positive airway pressure (CPAP) device. Prophylaxis for thromboembolism may include sequential compression devices, compression stockings, or anticoagulation therapy. Early ambulation is always encouraged.

Early postoperative retching and vomiting by the patient should be avoided. Just as in Nissen fundoplication, acute vomiting after surgery can result in an acute gastric prolapse with band slip. Anterior gastrogastric suture disruption may be a potential sequela. Aggressive antiemetic therapy should be instituted in the operating room. An intraoperative intravenous cocktail of ondansetron (Zofran)/metoclopramide (Reglan)/ketorolac (Toradol) is administered before extubation. An additional intravenous antiemetic is given liberally during the first 24 hours. Both the patient and the nursing staff are instructed on the importance of emesis prevention after surgery. Pain management involves subcutaneous injection of skin incisions with 0.25% Marcaine. Intravenous Toradol is administered as a standing order every 6 hours, with subcutaneous morphine for breakthrough pain.

Patients may be kept in the hospital overnight or discharged the same day, depending on their medical status,

pain control, and presence or absence of nausea. A postoperative esophagram documents normal, rapid esophageal emptying, no extravasation of contrast, and adequate band placement, lying in a 8 o'clock to 2 o'clock position (Fig. 20.3-1). Gastrografin is used in case a perforation is found. A gastric pouch should not be seen since the band is not filled.

If the esophagram shows delayed emptying, the normal clinical progression is for increased swelling to occur over 48 hours. These patients can usually swallow their saliva. It is advised to keep the patient NPO with intravenous hydration and antiinflammatory medication (i.e., Toradol). In contrast, complete obstruction on the film is always associated with inability to swallow saliva, and these patients do not recover with conservative measures. They must return to the operating room for laparoscopic revision. Most commonly, cutting the gastrogastric sutures, manipulating (jiggling) the band, and removing more perigastric fat give a good result. Placement of a larger band (Vanguard) may also be helpful in these circumstances. In addition, an unrecognized hiatal hernia may result in a greater amount of gastric tissue incorporated into the band, leading to obstruction. In this case, the hernia must be mobilized and reduced, the crura repaired, and the band placed in the proper position; otherwise the patient will be unable to tolerate adjustments in the future.

Patients should be kept in the hospital if there is any evidence of delayed esophageal emptying, as stomal swelling usually maximizes 24 to 48 hours after band placement. This is of particular relevance when the pars flaccida technique is used. Incorporation of perigastric fat within the band can cause external compression of the stomach and a greater likelihood of stomal narrowing. Communication with the radiologist is an important component to ensure that abnormal findings are reported. In the 959 operations performed at the New York University (NYU) Medical Center, there have been no cases of perforation, five cases of stomal obstruction, and seven cases of delayed

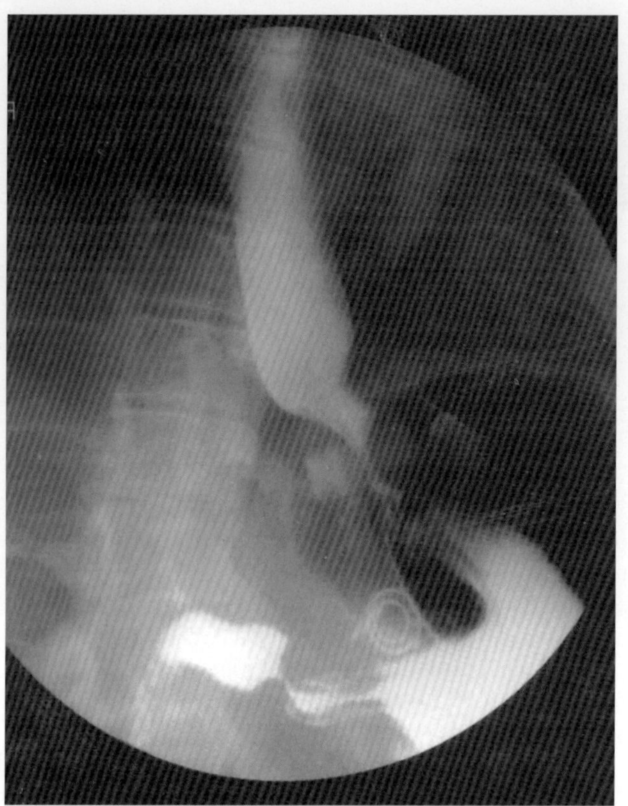

FIGURE 20.3-1. Normal postoperative esophagram.

esophageal emptying. All obstructions were symptomatic at the time of esophagraphy. Those with delayed emptying were not symptomatic until 48 hours after surgery. In addition, it provides the surgeon with a baseline esophagram to document band positioning.

Patients are seen in the office 10 to 14 days after surgery for their first follow-up, to check their wounds and reiterate dietary guidelines.

Postoperative Dietary Guidelines

Due to the possible correlation between early vomiting and gastric prolapse (1,2), patients are placed on a diet that progresses from liquids to solids over the first 6 weeks after surgery. For weeks 1 and 2 the diet is clear liquids—any fluid that is thin enough to go through a straw. For weeks 3 and 4 the diet is pureed foods—foods that do not need to be chewed, as if the patient did not have teeth. For weeks 5 and 6 the diet is soft and flaky solid foods and crunchy foods, specifically excluding chicken, steak, and bread, which tend to form a large bolus that cannot traverse through the narrow band stoma. These tough, doughy, and dry foods are poorly tolerated for 6 to 12 months by the majority of patients after gastric banding. Patients are advised not to eat and drink simultaneously, to maximize the amount of time the gastric pouch is filled with food.

Nutritional deficiencies have not been reported after LAGB, perhaps because the operation is purely restrictive. However, patients are encouraged to take a daily multivitamin. More importantly, patients should already have the nutritional knowledge and skills to make healthy food choices before any bariatric surgery, including LAGB. Patients are told that high-calorie liquids and soft foods, such as chocolate and ice cream, are physically easy to eat but will lead to weight regain or weight loss failure. At NYU, patients interested in LAGB must stop drinking all sugary caloric beverages and minimize their intake of chocolate and premium-grade ice cream at least 2 months before surgery.

The most important dietary counseling that LAGB patients need is *how* to eat—slowly and chewing thoroughly. They must learn how to put the fork down between bites. Most importantly, they must recognize when they are full, and then stop eating. This is a new skill for morbidly obese patients. Even an extra bite will make them regurgitate. Counseling on social eating and food choices is greatly appreciated by patients, since this is usually their greatest source of anxiety, particularly in young adults and teenagers as they start dating. Diurnal variation in esophageal motility may play an important role in dysphagia and appears to vary according to time of day and amount of emotional stress. Dysphagia is common when patients are eating in a stressful situation, mostly because they are typically distracted and have eaten quickly without chewing. They are counseled to have a yogurt, soup, or a protein drink during stressful times. Breakfast is sometimes difficult, and soft and pureed foods are encouraged.

Band Adjustments

The mechanisms by which LAGB works include decreasing appetite, creating satiety with a smaller amount of food, and behavior modification (3). This is a direct function of a small gastric pouch (10–15 mL) and a narrow stomal opening that slows gastric emptying (12 mm). The LAGB acts in this capacity through external constriction of the stomach, which is gradually tightened in accordance with each individual's needs. If no constriction is created, no restriction is experienced, and no weight is lost. Therefore, weight loss after LAGB is contingent on band adjustment. The band is useless if adjustments are not performed. Both patient and surgeon must understand this, otherwise weight loss will be suboptimal, the operation ineffective, and the surgery a wasted effort.

The band is left empty when initially placed. The first adjustment is performed 6 weeks postoperatively. This allows time for a capsule to form around the band and makes its position around the stomach more secure. Adjustments should be made while patients are eating solid food. The band is meant to work with solid food, specifically to maintain stretching of the gastric pouch to create an early sense of satiety. An appropriately adjusted band also acts as an appetite suppressant. A sense of hunger, increased appetite, and increased snacking are signs that the band is not appropriately tightened. Individuals who do not eat as a response to hunger (i.e., emotional eaters) may continue to eat and fail to lose weight. They may go on to graze throughout the day or choose soft high-calorie foods and beverages. Soft and liquid foods empty faster than solids, and thus more can be ingested before the feeling of satiety is reached. Thus, a band that is too tight will make solid food ingestion difficult, but easy for creamy sugary liquids. This is an example of maladaptive behavior and may necessitate band loosening.

There are two general strategies to band adjustment: in-office adjustment using a clinical algorithm, and radiographic adjustment under fluoroscopic guidance. Each has its advantages and disadvantages. In-office adjustments are quick and inexpensive, but require frequent visits due to inaccuracy of the adjustment. Radiographic adjustments are more cumbersome and expensive, but require fewer visits due to the more accurate adjustment visualized under fluoroscopy.

The maximum recommended amount of saline that a gastric band accommodates depends on the band type. The Lap-Band System (Inamed Health, Santa Barbara, CA) recommends the maximum amount of saline to be 4cc in their 9.75- and 10-cm bands. The average maximum amount of saline in a typical patient who has reached a stable weight loss is 3.0cc. The larger volume Vanguard Lap-Band holds a maximum amount of 11cm of saline.

Office-Based Adjustment

There are two aspects to band adjustments: locating the access port and determining the volume of saline to be used. When the procedure is performed in the office, the port is located by palpation. The band is adjusted by percutaneously accessing the port with a non-coring needle, and subsequently injecting sterile saline, which tightens the band. Withdrawal of saline results in band loosening with subsequent decreased restriction. The skin is cleansed with alcohol, and a non-coring needle on a 3-mL syringe filled with the desired amount of saline is introduced through the skin into the access port (Fig. 20.3-2). Successful port access is confirmed by feeling the needle hit the metal base of the access port and having free reflux of saline back into the syringe. Local anesthetic is unnecessary, as it is more painful than the needle itself. Having the patient lie on the examination table and lift his or her head up off the examination table while tensing the abdominal muscles can assist in feeling the port. Sometimes having the patient stand up will use gravity to drop the pannus and make the port more apparent.

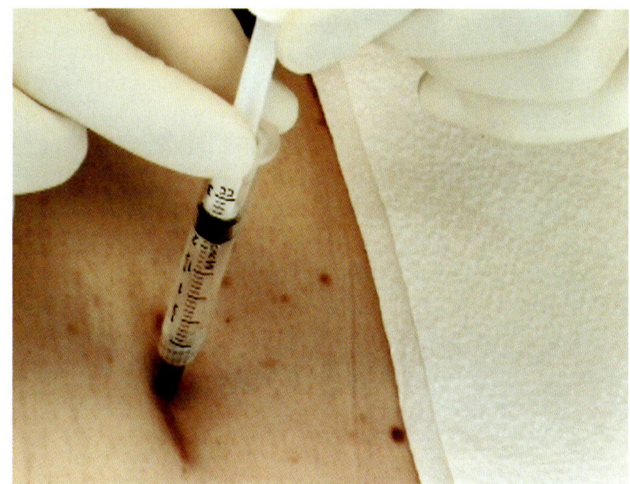

FIGURE 20.3-2. In-office percutaneous access of port (saline-filled syringe attached to non-coring needle).

Locating the port can be challenging in patients who have a large amount of subcutaneous fat, particularly women and individuals with a body mass index (BMI) greater than 60. An extra-long needle may be necessary to reach the port. An x-ray can be obtained to localize and mark the port. A port locator is available that is placed on the abdominal wall and can facilitate localization using a circular series of lights (Fig. 20.3-3). The learning curve for port localization using palpation is surprisingly long and may take up to 100 cases. Our experience has shown that on review of our first 200 consecutive Lap-Band patients (69% female, mean BMI 48.7), 660 adjustments were performed in the office (74% by a nurse practitioner, and 26% by a physician) (4). Twenty-eight (4.2%) adjustments were unsuccessfully performed by a nurse practitioner and required physician assistance. Twelve of those attempts (1.8%) on nine patients required radiographic guidance to localize the access port. All nine patients were women who were in the first 75 patients adjusted.

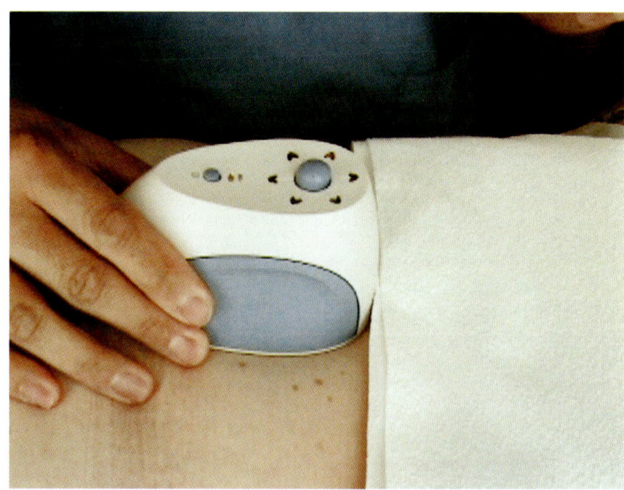

FIGURE 20.3-3. Port locator used to find access port.

If saline is already present, it can be aspirated into the syringe to document any loss of volume that may have occurred. The amount of saline to inject for each adjustment is based on three variables: hunger, weight loss, and restriction. A properly adjusted band induces the lack of hunger and appetite suppression. It should also induce a prolonged sense of satiety that lasts longer than 2 hours after a meal. Weight loss should be constant and gradual over the course of 18 to 36 months. The goal rate of weight loss is 1 to 2 lb/week or 6 to 10 lb/month. Lack of weight loss reflects too large a portion intake and suboptimal restriction, indicating the band needs tightening. Lack of restriction to tough or doughy solid foods such as steak, chicken, or bread also signals the need for band adjustment.

These signs and symptoms have been applied to a clinical algorithm that was designed at the NYU Program for Surgical Weight Loss and is used as a general guide (Fig. 20.3-4). After each adjustment, patients drink a cup of water to ensure that they do not have outlet obstruction.

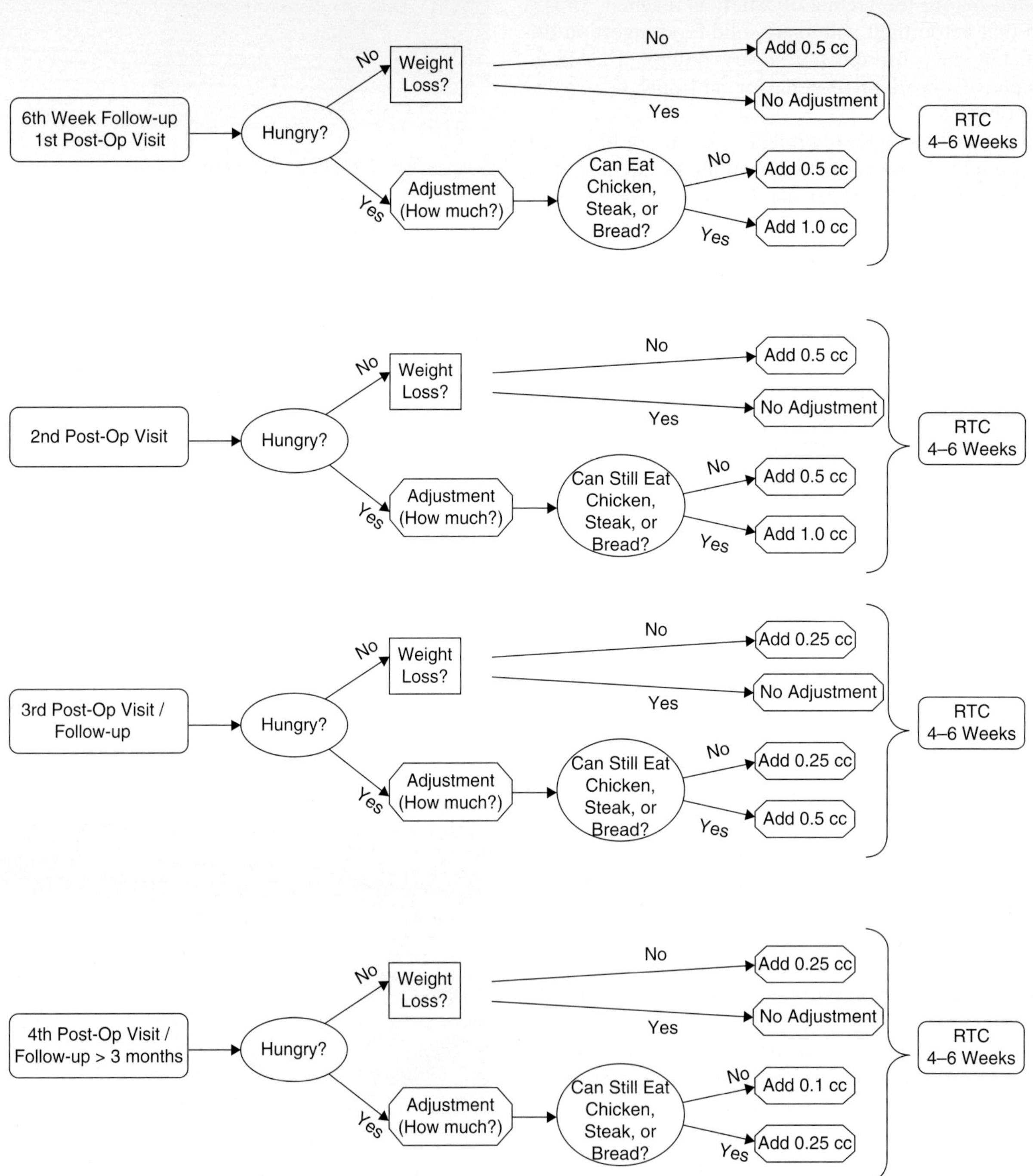

FIGURE 20.3-4. In-office adjustment algorithm. RTC, return to clinic.

Any gurgling noises will likely lead to obstruction in the next 1 to 3 days. Interestingly, we have found that the band gets slightly tighter 1 to 3 days after an adjustment. Therefore, we have our patients stay on clear liquids for 2 days, pureed foods for 2 days, and then soft solid foods by the fifth day after adjustment.

At NYU, we perform our adjustments in the office and see our patients every 4 to 6 weeks for weight and appetite evaluation. The program is structured for patients to return for regular weigh-ins, progress evaluation, adjustments, nutritional reinforcement, and behavioral counseling. We have found that frequent patient follow-up has a significant impact on percent excess weight loss (%EWL) achieved in just 1 year. Patients who return more than six times in the first year after LAGB lose an average of 50% EWL, as compared with those who return six times or less, who lose 42% EWL (5). The average number of adjustments in the first year was 4.5 and in the second year was 2. The average amount of fluid present in the band after the first year was 1.9cc. This relatively low volume may be reflective of a smaller stomal diameter achieved with the pars flaccida technique. High patient volume resulting from this postoperative follow-up regimen is accommodated with the use of a dedicated nurse practitioner. This may reflect not only utilization of the restrictive properties of the band to its full potential but also the added behavioral counseling and emotional support that patients receive with each visit.

Radiographically Guided Adjustment

Real-time fluoroscopy allows for rapid localization of the port to assist in percutaneous access. The needle can be observed simultaneously as the skin is punctured and the port accessed. Again, free reflux of saline into the syringe confirms successful access. Fluoroscopy also allows for visualization of the esophagus, gastric pouch, band, diameter of outlet, and integrity of tubing/port system. There is no standardized rate of esophageal emptying or outlet diameter that correlates with the perfect adjustment. There is also no evidence to suggest that a given outlet diameter correlates with dysphagia or clinical symptoms. Table 20.3-1 shows suggested radiographic criteria for adjustments as published by Favretti et al. (6).

However, what fluoroscopy does show is outlet obstruction, esophageal dilatation, gastric pouch dilatation or prolapse, reflux, and malfunctioning band or malpositioned band. These are situations that would require immediate intervention such as loosening the band. This may be helpful since not all of these abnormalities are necessarily reflected in clinical symptoms. Busetto et al. (7) found that in their 379 LAGB patients the average number of adjustments performed in the first year after surgery was 2.3 ± 1.7, and the mean maximum band filling after surgery was 2.8 ± 1.2 mL.

TABLE 20.3-1. Radiographic criteria for adjustment

Consider fluid removal	Consider fluid addition
Stenosis of the outlet	Wide outlet (>8mm)
Esophageal dilatation (>2×)	Immediate passage of the
Esophageal atony	barium swallow (one
Esophageal emptying of the barium	peristaltic wave)
swallow in >4–5 peristaltic waves	
Reflux	
Pouch dilatation with insufficient	
emptying	

Source: Favretti et al. (6), with permission.

Although the number of follow-up visits and adjustments are much fewer, the cost and effort required are greater. The surgeon must coordinate with a radiology facility for use of the fluoroscopy; this can be time-consuming and costly. Unless the surgeon's office has a C-arm, the average time to perform an adjustment is 15 to 20 minutes. High-volume centers can decrease this time to 10 minutes. In addition, the patient does not receive the repetitive emotional support from the caregiver.

Complaints and Symptoms

Dysphagia to solid food is the most common postoperative complaint. It usually relates to the patient's (1) eating too quickly; (2) inadvertently forgetting that he or she has a band; (3) eating food that does not break down with chewing, especially steak; (4) eating food that congeals together, such as white bread; and (5) eating while anxious or angry. Some patients simply fail to learn from these experiences and persist with these maladaptive behaviors. Chest pain from acute esophageal obstruction will occur every time. This becomes very unpleasant for the patient and can be difficult for the surgeon to manage. Figure 20.3-5 reviews recommended management of some common complaints.

Stomal obstruction from food causes pain. Initially, this severe central chest pain and salivation can be frightening. Once patients recognize it, though, they are much less concerned. The simplest course of action is to induce vomiting, which will liberate the obstructing plug. It is actually regurgitation that occurs, rather than vomiting. Immediate resolution of pain is experienced. Patients should then stay on liquids for the rest of the meal, as mucosal swelling within the band can occur. Use of carbonated drinks to free the obstructing plug is to be avoided, as the pain becomes severe when the gas expands within the obstructed esophagus.

Recurrent regurgitation or vomiting can result in local mucosal edema within the outlet; patients are advised to stay on clear liquids for the following 24 hours after any such event. If the food remains stuck, and they are unable to tolerate any liquids, even their own saliva, they must

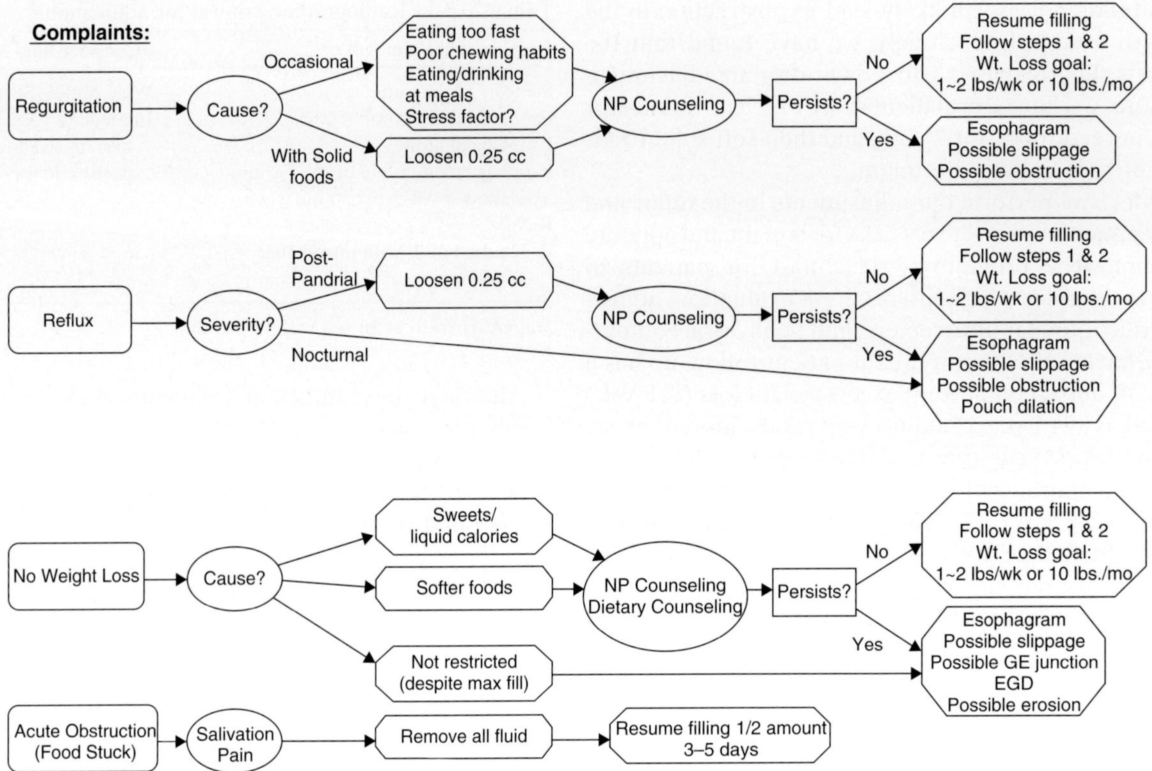

FIGURE 20.3-5. Common complaints algorithm. GE, gastroesophageal; EGD, esophagogastroduodenoscopy.

call their surgeon. The band requires immediate deflation, and all the saline must be removed to allow passage of the obstructing bolus. The band can be readjusted after 2 days.

Dysphagia and regurgitation is often worst early in the morning, improves during the day, and is rarely present in the evening. This relates to the diurnal function of esophageal motility. Many patients are best served by having a liquid breakfast, such as a cup of coffee followed by a protein shake, that they can sip slowly on the way to work. This eliminates much of the early morning stress. Explanations of these mechanisms greatly assist band patients to understand some of the difficulties they may experience and reduces the ever-present fear of failure.

Dysphagia is certainly affected by emotional issues. One very important subgroup is young people who are dating; their newfound confidence after weight loss will evaporate if they are seen to be having difficulty eating or actually vomiting. These young people need special advice: Start with an alcoholic beverage to help relax; choose foods they know they can eat, such as soup, risotto, or flaky fish; and resist pressure to eat more. Eat slowly and have a sip of wine as they eat, just as they would do normally. This allows them to fit in with their friends and to be more comfortable dating.

Reflux occurs when (1) the band is too tight, (2) there is gastric prolapse with band slip, or (3) there is an undi-agnosed hiatal hernia. These are indistinguishable clinically, but can be diagnosed by esophagraphy. Appropriate treatment entails removing fluid from the band, surgically repositioning the band, or reducing and repairing the hiatus hernia. The severe end of the spectrum is nocturnal regurgitation and reflux, often presenting as sleeplessness combined with recent-onset asthma, or even aspiration pneumonia. This is more commonly seen with gastric prolapse/band slip.

Nutritional Evaluation

Nutritional deficiencies have not been identified to be a problem after LAGB due to the purely restrictive nature of the operation. However, we check a full battery of laboratory tests including iron, folate, thiamine, vitamin B_{12}, parathyroid hormone, and calcium on an annual basis. We have found two young women to be iron deficient after 1 year, and one young woman to be low in vitamin B_{12}. The significance is unknown since preoperative iron and vitamin levels are not measured, especially in young menstruating women.

Patients who cannot tolerate the restriction of the band and adopt a maladaptive eating behavior may benefit from band removal and possible revision to a bypass procedure.

Counseling

Patients should understand that achieving weight loss requires commitment to follow-up and guidelines. They need to make changes to their nutrition and levels of activity. While LAGB is not as foolproof as Roux-en-Y gastric bypass (RYGBP), it can be just as effective in the long term. Patients must understand that they cannot have it both ways: They will not be able to eat the same way or the same things after surgery and still lose weight. The weight loss is gradual, due to the gradual nature of the restriction. A program approach is the most successful way of achieving significant maintained weight loss.

Support groups and ongoing psychotherapy can be helpful after any bariatric surgery for the patient to adjust to the loss of food, new self-image, and change in eating behavior. However, the greatest help can come from the surgeon listening to the patient and applying some of these basic principles (Table 20.3-2).

TABLE 20.3-2. Postoperative eating tips

1.	Eat when hungry
2.	If not hungry, do not eat
3.	Eat slowly
4.	Chew thoroughly
5.	Learn to put your fork down between bites
6.	Size of the meal should be the same as the palm of your hand
7.	Do not try to finish everything on the plate
8.	Do not eat and drink at the same time
9.	All beverages should have 0 calories
10.	Order an appetizer instead of an entree at a restaurant

Conclusion

The LAGB is the safest surgical tool available to assist morbidly obese patients in losing weight. The keys to its success are appropriate surgical technique, prolonged follow-up, regular adjustments, and, perhaps most importantly, an understanding of the changes that go with having a band. Its adjustability is its greatest strength. When the patient attends regularly for follow-up, and the surgeon uses adjustments wisely based on satiety, weight loss, and any other symptoms, the LAGB will deliver very satisfactory weight-loss results.

References

1. Fielding GA. Reduction in incidence of gastric herniation with LAP-BAND: experience in 620 cases. Obes Surg 2000; 10:136.
2. Dargent J. Pouch dilatation and slippage after adjustable gastric banding: is it still an issue? Obes Surg 2003;13: 111–115.
3. Dixon AF, Dixon JB, O'Brien PE. Laparoscopic adjustable gastric banding induces prolonged satiety: a randomized blind crossover study. J Clin Endocrinol Metab 2005;90(2): 813–819.
4. Dugay G, Ren CJ. Laparoscopic adjustable gastric band (Lap-Band) adjustments in the office is feasible—the first 200 cases. Obes Surg 2003;13:192(abstr).
5. Shen R, Ren CJ. Impact of patient follow-up on weight loss after bariatric surgery. Obes Surg 2003;13:537(abstr).
6. Favretti F, O'Brien PE, Dixon JB. Patient management after LAP-BAND placement. Am J Surg 2002;184:38S–41S.
7. Busetto L, Segato G, De Marchi F, et al. Postoperative management of laparoscopic gastric banding. Obes Surg 2003; 13:121–127.

20.4
Laparoscopic Adjustable Gastric Banding: Complications

Jeffrey W. Allen and Ariel Ortiz Lagardere

In the summer of 2001 the United States Food and Drug Administration approved a silicon adjustable gastric banding device for the treatment of morbid obesity (LapBand System, Inamed Health, Santa Barbara, CA) (1). This band, specifically designed for laparoscopic placement, was met with considerable enthusiasm by patients and surgeons alike, who realized the obvious potential benefits of the procedure (2). These include a short hospital stay, superior cosmesis, adjustability, and a decreased risk of malnutrition, to name a few. However, as with any surgical procedure, especially one dealing with a high-risk patient population, unexpected problems can occur. Many of the complications of gastric banding are not new; erosions, for instance, were not uncommon with vertical banded gastroplasty. Others are unique, such as gastric prolapse and tubing problems. This chapter describes the complications of laparoscopic gastric banding, their treatment, and strategies for prevention (Table 20.4-1).

Gastric Prolapse

Gastric prolapse, also known as a "slipped band," occurs when a part of the stomach below the band herniates cephalad through the band (Fig. 20.4-1). The herniated stomach is frequently the fundus, although any portion of the stomach below the band may be involved. As the herniated stomach fills with saliva and ingested materials, it becomes engorged and is pulled downward by gravity. Eventually the slipped portion of the stomach dilates and causes the band to rotate downward (Fig. 20.4-2). The result is a partial, and ultimately complete, gastric obstruction below the gastroesophageal junction and above the band.

There are three varieties of gastric prolapse: anterior, posterior, and concentric. Instances where it is the greater curve that has herniated through the band (Figs. 20.4-1 and 20.4-2) are known as an anterior slip. This appears to be more common when the band was placed initially with the pars flaccida technique. An anterior gastric prolapse generally involves the fundus of the stomach coming to rest in a plane anterior to the esophagus and the remainder of the stomach (Fig. 20.4-3). Possible technical reasons for the anterior slip include faulty gastric plication over the band due to suture failure, bites of inadequate tissue, or "hidden fundus."

The posterior slip occurs along the lesser curvature of the stomach and is more common in bands placed using the perigastric technique (Fig. 20.4-4). This is due likely to the required extra dissection that renders the stomach below the band more mobile. In some cases with the perigastric way of placing the band, the bursa is entered, which further mobilizes the posterior stomach. A posterior slip occurs when the lesser curve herniates through the band and comes to rest posterior to the remaining stomach.

A concentric slip is a somewhat controversial entity. It is characterized by excess stomach from the greater and lesser curve above the band (Fig. 20.4-5). It is unclear if this represents a true prolapse (migration of stomach from below to above the band) or a dilation of the existing stomach above the band. This condition may be due to patient noncompliance and overeating, a band that is chronically adjusted too tightly, initial placement of the band erroneously low, or an actual mechanical prolapse.

The presentation of a patient with a slipped band, regardless of the variety, is similar. Symptoms include gastroesophageal reflux, nausea, solid (and ultimately liquid) food intolerance, and back or abdominal pain. The symptoms are generally subacute in nature, and it is rare that patients present with an "acute abdomen." In this case, a perforation or other abdominal catastrophe must be considered.

The diagnosis of gastric prolapse is usually made by a contrast esophagram, although a plain abdominal radiograph occasionally will suffice. On either film the band often appears rotated to point at the patient's left hip

TABLE 20.4-1. Complications of laparoscopic adjustable gastric banding from various studies

	Gastric prolapse/pouch dilation (%)*	Esophageal dilatation (or dysmotility) (%)	Erosion (%)	Access port problems (%)
FDA trial ($n = 299$) (1)	24	10**	1	6
Belachew et al. 2002 (4) ($n = 763$)	8	NR	0.9	2.6
Cadiere et al. 2002 (5) ($n = 652$)	3.8	NR	0.3	2.7
Dargent et al. 1999 (6) ($n = 500$)	5	NR	0.6	1
Favretti et al. 2002 (7) ($n = 830$)	10	NR	0.5	11
Fielding et al. 1999 (8) ($n = 335$)	3.6***	NR	0	1.5
O'Brien et al. 1999 (9) ($n = 302$)	9	NR	NR	3.6
Vertruyen 2002 (10) ($n = 543$)	4.6	NR	1	3.0
Weiner et al. 1999 (11) ($n = 184$)	2.2***	NR	1.1	3.2

FDA, U.S. Food and Drug Administration; NR, not reported.
* Many investigators did not distinguish between true prolapse and gastric pouch dilatation; therefore, these categories are combined.
** Includes eight patients with dysmotility.
*** Prolapse only is reported. (*Note:* Not all complications shown required surgical correction.)
Source: Spivak H, Favretti F. Avoiding postoperative complications with the LAP-BAND system. Am J Surg 2002;184:31S–37S, with permission.

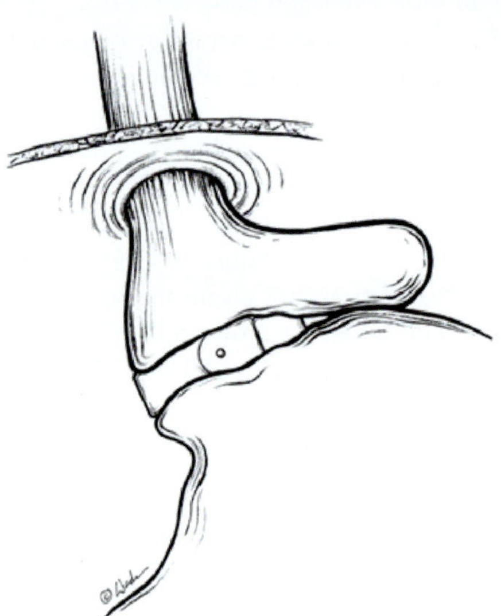

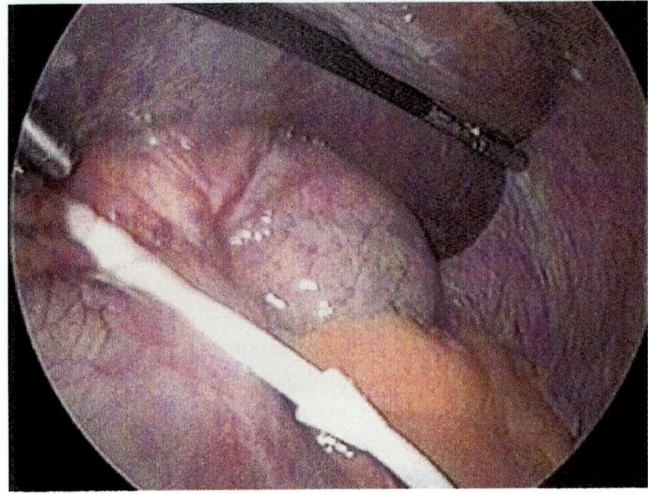

FIGURE 20.4-3 Anterior prolapse.

FIGURE 20.4-1 Gastric prolapse, also known as a "slipped band".

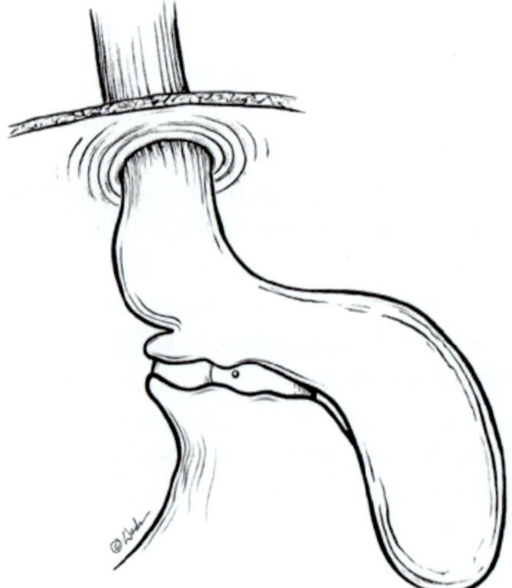

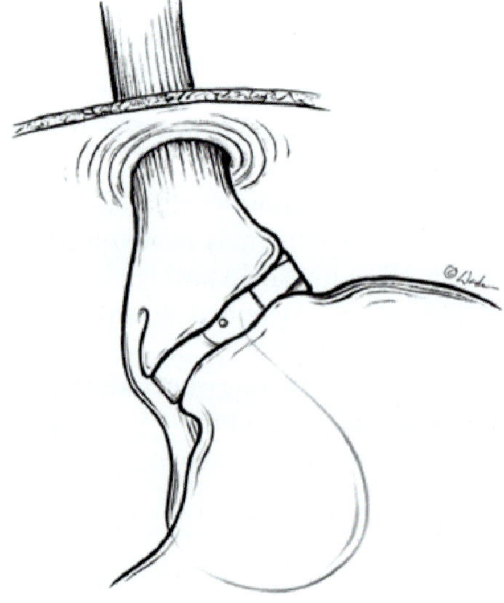

FIGURE 20.4-2 Gastric prolapse with rotation of band to transverse position

FIGURE 20.4-4 Posterior prolapse.

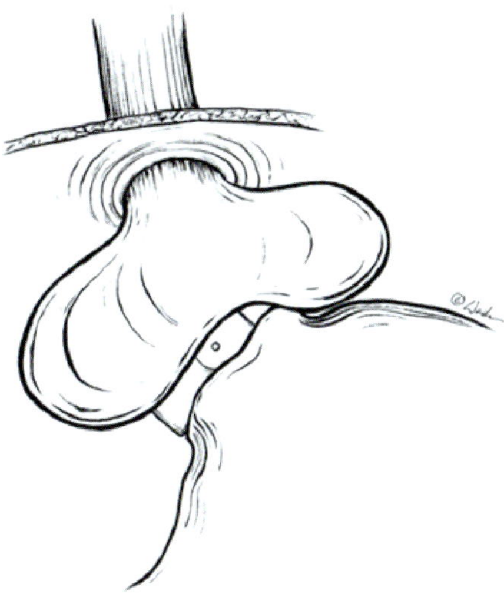

FIGURE 20.4-5 Concentric dilation.

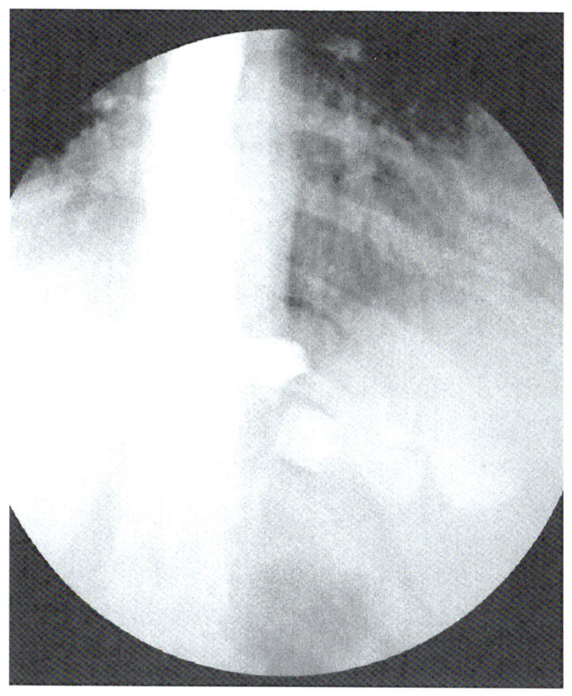

FIGURE 20.4-7 Gastric prolapse with rotation of the band to point to the patient's left hip.

instead of the normal configuration (Figs. 20.4-6 and 20.4-7). Additional radiographic features of a slip include the presence of fundus or dilated stomach above the band, an air-fluid level, the "wave sign" of fundus overhanging the band, and varying degrees of obstruction to the flow of contrast (Fig. 20.4-8). In instances where the radiograph is equivocal, an endoscopic examination may be helpful. Endoscopic evidence of gastric prolapse includes a normal band without evidence of erosion, a larger than expected amount of stomach above the band that increases with insufflation, and a fundus that hangs over the band (Fig. 20.4-9).

The treatment of gastric prolapse includes admission to the hospital, intravenous fluid resuscitation, correction of electrolytes, and operative repositioning of the band (3). Nasogastric decompression is not routinely used except in patients with complete gastric obstruction man-

ifest by intolerance of saliva. Although not generally a surgical emergency, it is preferable to perform the surgery in as timely a fashion as possible because of the possibility of aspiration or ischemic necrosis of the entrapped stomach. The development or worsening of abdominal pain may be a symptom of ischemia and should hasten the operation. In selected cases, especially when the patient has mild symptoms and equivocal radiographic findings, removal of fluid from the band and a period of outpatient nonoperative observation may be attempted.

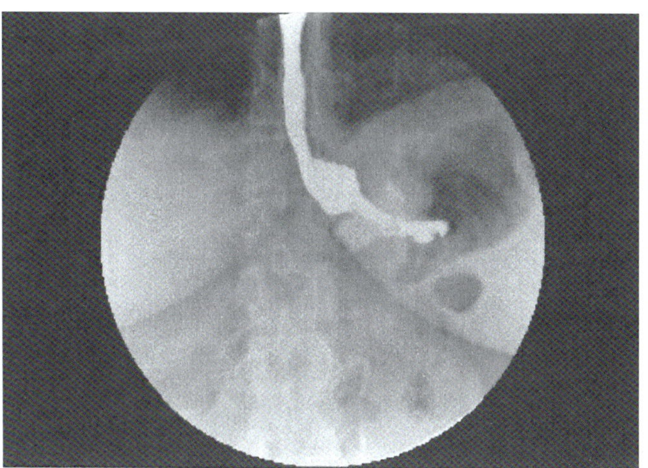

FIGURE 20.4-6 Normal position of band, pointing to patient's left shoulder.

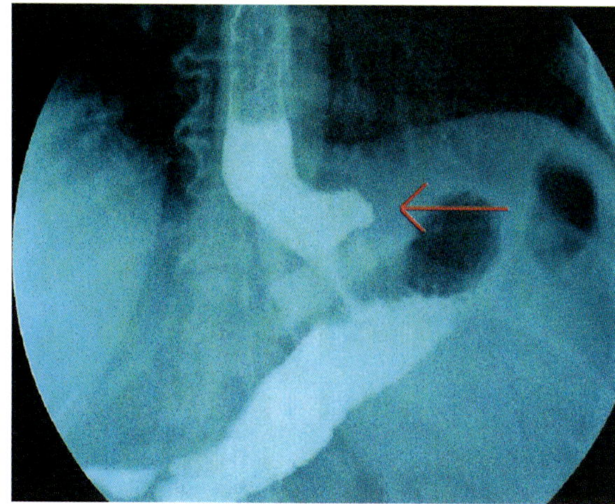

FIGURE 20.4-8 Gastric prolapse with wave sign (red arrow) as the only radiologic feature.

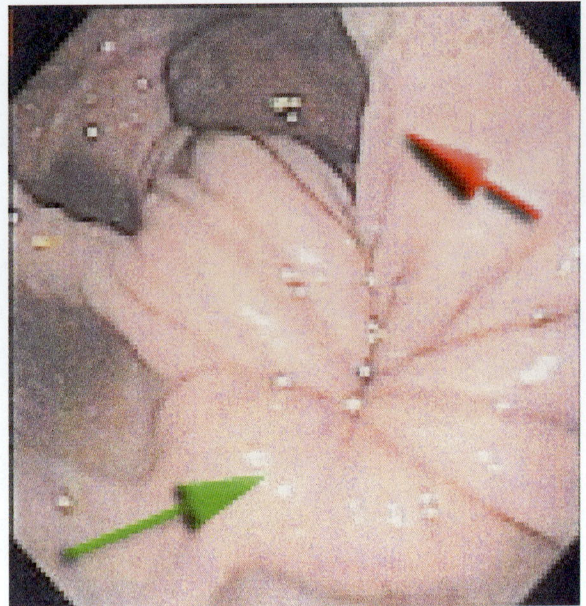

FIGURE 20.4-9 Endoscopic view of gastric prolapse. Green arrow points to normal band; red arrow points to herniated fundus hanging over band.

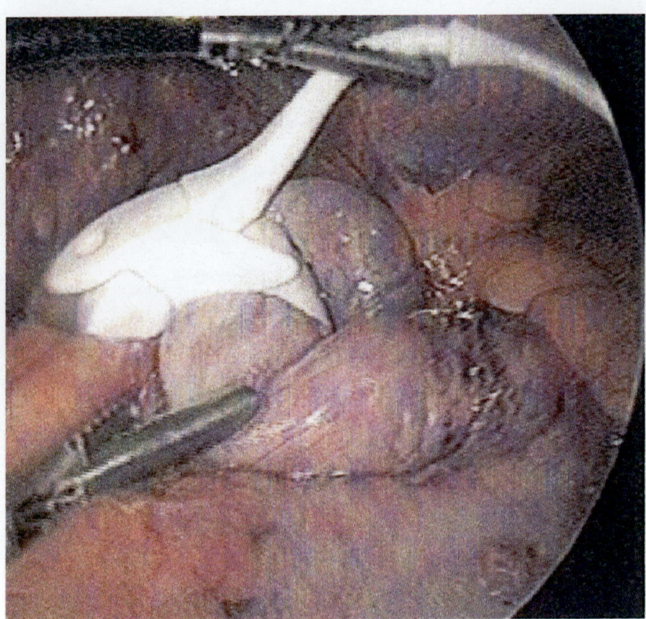

FIGURE 20.4-11 Reduction of herniated stomach.

Once in the operating room, deflation of the band and decompression of the stomach is the first step. The laparoscopic trocars should be placed in a similar configuration as in primary placement. After establishing pneumoperitoneum, the adhesions are incised and the herniated stomach identified (Fig. 20.4-10). The band is mobilized by incising the overlying capsule and taking down the previous plication. The herniated stomach is then reduced and plication is repeated (Fig. 20.4-11). If reduction of the herniated band is not possible, then the band is opened, which can be a technical challenge. A device that can be neither reduced nor opened requires removal and replacement with a new one. The old band is removed by cutting it with laparoscopic scissors. After the band is either opened or removed after cutting, the retrogastric tunnel is re-created, and the band placed as in an initial procedure. Diligent gastric plication is especially important at this time to prevent future prolapse. The postoperative course generally mimics that of the original operation, and the same nutritional plan should be used.

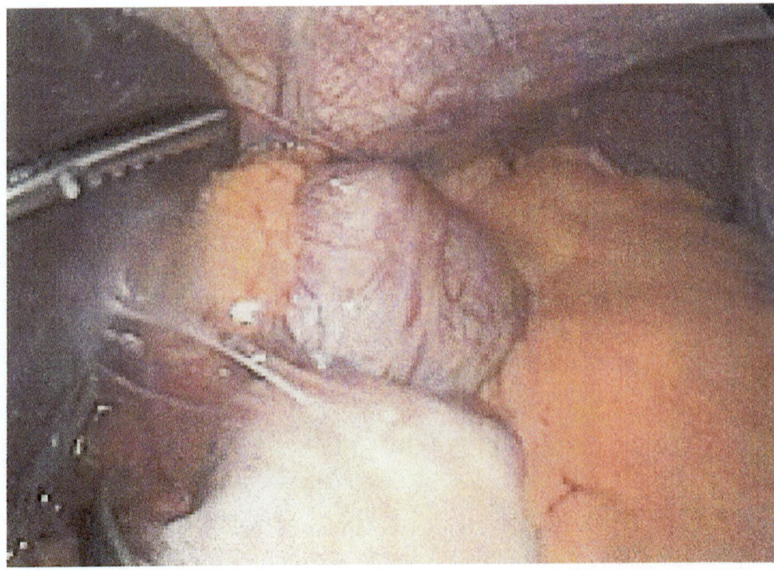

FIGURE 20.4-10 Adhesions and herniated stomach.

FIGURE 20.4-12 Erosion of tubing into the gastrointestinal tract.

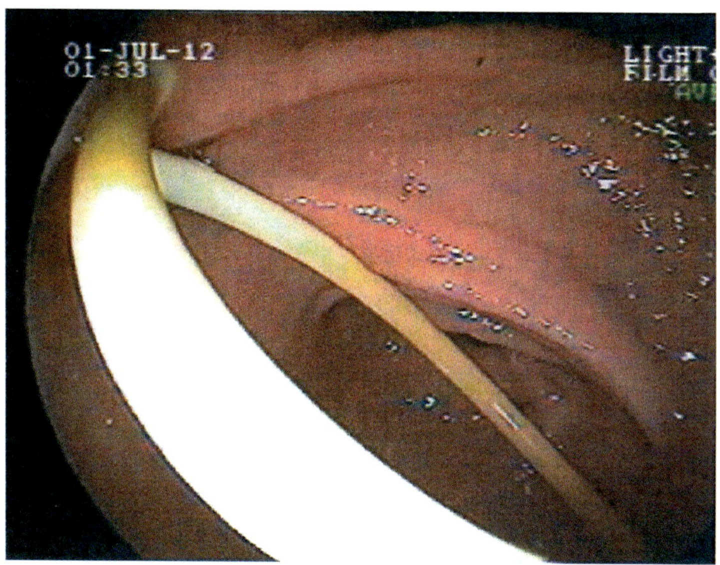

Erosion

Erosion of the band, gastric erosion, and intraluminal migration all refer to an implant that has penetrated into the lumen of the stomach. It can occur as early as a few months postoperative and is usually diagnosed during the first 2 years. A direct correlation between tension from the stomach wrap over the band and erosion has been found. In the second author's early experience, suturing over the buckle or pulling the stomach fundus over the band to the right crux was related to a higher incidence of erosion. However, the penetration of the tubing and not the band itself has also been documented and has no apparent precipitating factor (Fig. 20.4-12).

The incidence of gastric erosion varies from 1% to 4%. The true incidence can only be known if all patients were to undergo surveillance endoscopy. Routine upper endoscopy at 18 to 36 months was performed on the second author's first 600 patients, and 3.6% erosions were diagnosed. Of these, 68% had either a chronic sinus or recurrent infection at the adjustment port. Surprisingly, 32% of these erosions were asymptomatic. A total of 22 erosions were detected during routine endoscopy, with the vast majority (87%) detected during the first 24 months (Fig. 20.4-13).

A patient who has an eroded band may be symptomatic. When present, symptoms vary from mild upper gastrointestinal discomfort to recurrent or chronic port site infection or fistula. A frequent presentation is a previously asymptomatic patient who develops either reflux symptoms or a sudden change in their restriction level. This is attributable to the penetration of the implant into the lumen of the stomach with the thickening of the mucosa at the level of the stoma or the leaking of the

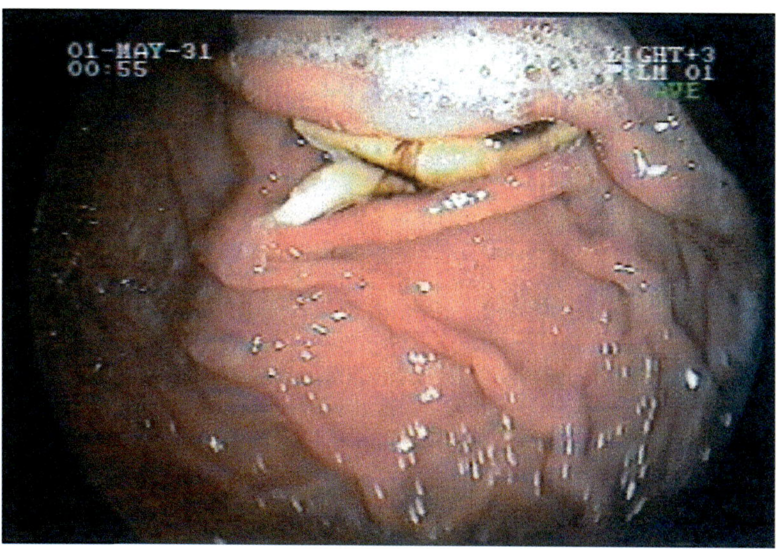

FIGURE 20.4-13 Intragastric migration of band.

inflatable part of the implant secondary to the gastric acid exposure. Another scenario is the development of symptoms months after the initial surgery, at the adjustment port site, related to either an abscess formation or a recurrent or chronic infection. There does not seem to be a common precipitating factor. Infections in this situation are often resistant to antibiotics and local treatment.

When these symptoms develop, an upper endoscopy is indicated. The visualization of the implant penetrating the lumen generally requires retroversion of the endoscope to observe the fundus and gastric plication. The band frequently penetrates into the stomach-to-stomach wrap with its outer edge penetrating first into the fundus.

The treatment of erosion is removal of the band. The surgical procedure is elective and the patient is prepared with perioperative systemic antibiotics. Operative findings can include a peritoneal reaction with medium to severe adhesions, friable tissue, and abscess formation. The technique involves following the tubing down to the implant and opening of the band is achieved by cutting the buckle open with scissors or a harmonic scalpel. Often it is not necessary to take down the previous anterior gastric wrap, which most of the time is a challenging procedure, and it increases the risk of further gastric perforation. Hydrostatic testing for a leak is performed and closure of any identified defect is accomplished. Simultaneous replacement of a gastric band has been reported, but is not widely recommended. The quality of the gastric tissue often does not permit a safe revision procedure at the time of band removal, but can be evaluated individually in each patient. Endoscopic removal of the implant has also been reported and is feasible only when the better part of the implant has penetrated the gastric lumen. It requires special endoscopic attachment to cut the device and remove it orally.

The erosion rate in the second author's patients prompted further scrutiny of the data. Video recordings of the original surgical procedures were analyzed. The common issue in all these patients was the suturing under tension over the band or over the buckle. Our technique has substantially changed since then so that all contact with the buckle of the device is eliminated during suturing and there is no tension when performing the gastric wrap. With these modifications there have been no erosions in the second author's last 400 patients.

Port Problems

The presence of the adjustment port in the subcutaneous tissue is a regular source of morbidity. Hematoma or seroma may present in the immediate postoperative period and are generally treated conservatively. The most frequently reported complications of the access component are infection and tube-port leak or break. Port-related complications, when reported, vary from 4.5% to 11%. In our experience with our first 600 patients, we reported a tube break or leak in 1%. These leaks were caused either by fatigue at the tapered end of the adjustment port (earlier model) or by needle perforation during failed adjustment sessions. All required revisions under local anesthetic for repair or replacement of the implant. It is important to mention that only a Huber-type needle should be used to access this adjustment port. The high-pressure silicone septum can tolerate up to 1000 punctures. The manufacturer of the implant (Inamed Health) has a repair kit available that includes additional tubing and a metallic connector. There is also a low-profile adjustment port that is especially useful if the patient has lost a substantial amount of weight and has less pannus to protect it.

A port can dislodge early from its sutures but will be detected upon access for adjustment. Some will be manipulated and coaxed into position for penetration, but others require fluoroscopic visualization and may require a minor surgical revision to be re-anchored. Our suggestion to avoid this problem is to observe the following guidelines.

The adjustment port should be placed distal to the entrance of the tubing into the abdomen, producing a smooth transition without any kinks or sharp angles. The adjustment port should be anchored by nonabsorbable sutures to the fascia, preferably to the anterior rectus sheath. Some surgeons have opted for a sternum or low xiphoid placement. Once placed, all the residual tubing should be directed back into the abdominal cavity. This prevents both the dislodgment of the tube through the wound early on and needle penetration during adjustments.

Kinking of the tubes can cause a valve effect; this is a rare occurrence but can be a surgical emergency when it happens. This is usually detected during adjustment sessions where saline is injected into the port but cannot be retrieved. As the injected solution accumulates in the band, the patient describes varying levels of pain from dull to intense. Immediate relief of pressure is indicated by local infiltration of anesthetic and tube manipulation through the wound near the port to relieve the valve effect and allow partial removal of the fluid.

Port-Site Infection

Infection at the port site is divided into early postoperative or late. Early infections at the port site are infrequent and generally respond to a course of oral antibiotics. Late infection, usually months after the band placement presented in 3.5% of the second author's cases as either a chronic sinus or recurrent infection. Eighty percent had an underlying gastric erosion of the band, and removal of the entire implant was necessary in all cases. It is important to rule out a gastric erosion of the implant when chronic or recurrent port-site infection is present. If no erosion is detected, 2 to 3 weeks of aggressive systemic antibiotic treatment is indicated. If the infection does not subside, port removal may be required, with subsequent replacement after the infection has completely cleared.

Intraoperative Complications

Gastric perforation is a potential technical problem during the operative placement of a gastric band. It may be due to a traction injury by a grasper or more commonly during a misadventure while creating a retrogastric tunnel for the device. The latter is potentially more dangerous because it is less likely to be recognized intraoperatively. Clues that an iatrogenic perforation may have occurred include unexplained bleeding, bile staining, particular difficulty with passage of the band through the retrogastric tunnel, and repeated false passages of the instrument used in the retrogastric position. Each situation warrants an intraoperative check consisting of passing an oral gastric tube into the stomach above the band, occlusion of the stomach distal to the band, and injection of a methylene blue solution or air. With the latter check, the abdomen should first be filled with sterile, bubble-free irrigant. Alternatively, a flexible upper endoscopy can be performed, looking for air bubbles leaking out or the transgastric passage of the band.

The discovery of a gastric perforation in the operating room is a troubling development. The safest management is to close the gastrotomy and abandon placement of the band. If the gastrotomy is not easily exposed, conversion to a laparotomy is indicated. In the case of esophageal or posterior gastric injury, consideration of a covering fundoplication is warranted. In some instances, such as partial thickness injury to the stomach or a full-thickness injury away from the banded stomach with minimal contamination, the surgeon may decide to carefully proceed with placement of the device. This is an uncommon occurrence and there are no strong data to support either decision.

An unrecognized gastric perforation is more precarious. Signs and symptoms are similar to those of a leaking gastrojejunostomy after gastric bypass and include abdominal pain, tachycardia, fever, oliguria, and hypotension. Diagnosis is by an esophagram with water-soluble contrast, although operative intervention should not be delayed for the sake of radiographic documentation, especially in a patient with a worsening clinical picture.

The treatment of a patient with a gastric perforation is removal of the band, identification and repair of the gastrotomy, and wide local drainage. In some cases, a fundoplication may be necessary to cover the perforation.

While this makes a future bariatric operation difficult or impossible, it may be the best means of damage control in a potentially life-threatening scenario.

Postoperative Obstruction

The phenomenon of postoperative obstruction is a common complication of gastric banding. This occurs when there is blockage of the outflow at the level of the band. The most frequent etiology of postoperative obstruction is a technical problem—inadequate excision of perigastric fat. Other possibilities include edema of the plicated stomach, hematoma at one of the sutures, or some form of neuropraxia. Usually this is diagnosed in an asymptomatic patient by routine contrast esophagram, which shows the band in good position and alignment, but with limited or no flow of contrast material through the band. The patient usually will vomit after the study. A common symptom of obstruction is a tightening in the chest typical of esophageal spasm.

Management of the obstruction includes continued admission to the hospital, intravenous fluids, and keeping the patient on NPO status. A nasogastric tube is seldom necessary as patients are usually able to handle their own secretions. The addition of ketorolac (Toradol) may decrease postoperative edema, but is associated with renal insufficiency so creatinine levels should be monitored with this drug.

In general, postoperative obstruction resolves with conservative management. Patients are slowly allowed to have ice chips and then clear, noncarbonated liquids as their condition improves. As soon as they are able to tolerate enough clear liquids to stay hydrated, they are discharged. A follow-up radiograph is not thought to be necessary. An upper endoscopy has not been particularly helpful in our experience in the patient with an immediate postoperative obstruction. The endoscope usually passes through the band, due to either the positive insufflation pressure or the etiology being more of a neuropraxia. However, the forward passage of the endoscope is not generally therapeutic. Failure of the obstruction to resolve is uncommon but not unheard of.

The period of waiting is not pleasing for the patient or surgeon and in the case of slow resolution (5 to 7 days) action may need to be taken. In this instance a reoperation and incision of the fat pad may relieve a mechanical obstruction. This usually may require opening the band to gain access to the adipose tissue on the lesser curve and near the angle of His. During the observation period for a postoperative obstruction, the development of severe abdominal pain, tachycardia, fever, or hypotension is indicative of a perforation above the band. This patient should undergo exploration, removal of the band, and a search for the perforation.

With experience, most surgeons are able to prevent postoperative obstruction in the majority of cases. Techniques include decreasing the bulk inside the band by excising the fat pad at the angle of His and creating a rivulet in the fat on the lesser curve. Additionally, the band should be placed as high up on the stomach as possible without abutting the esophagus. The lower the band is placed, the more bulk of stomach itself is present within the band. Finally, judicious choice of the size of the band is important. In the United States there currently are two sizes of bands available, 9.75 and 10.0cm, and the larger band is important to have on hand in patients with particularly large stomachs and excessive intraabdominal fat.

References

1. U.S. Food and Drug Administration. LAP-BAND Adjustable Gastric Banding (LAGB) System—P000008. http://www.fda.gov/cdrh/pdf/p000008.htm, Center for Devices and Radiological Health, 2002.
2. Rubenstein RB. Laparoscopic adjustable gastric banding at a U.S. center with up to 3-year follow-up. Obes Surg 2002;12(3):380–384.
3. Tran D, Rhoden DH, Cacchione RN, et al. Techniques for repair of gastric prolapse after laparoscopic gastric banding. J Laparoendosc Adv Surg Tech A 2004;14(2):117–120.
4. Belachew M, Belva PH, Desaive C. Long-term results of laparoscopic adjustable gastric banding for the treatment of morbid obesity. Obes Surg 2002;12(4):564–568.
5. Cadiere GB, Himpens J, Hainaux B, et al. Laparoscopic adjustable gastric banding. Semin Laparosc Surg 2002;9(2):105–114.
6. Dargent J. Laparoscopic adjustable gastric banding: lessons from the first 500 patients in a single institution. Obes Surg 1999;9(5):446–452.
7. Favretti F, Cadiere GB, Segato G, et al. Laparoscopic banding: selection and technique in 830 patients. Obes Surg 2002;12(3):385–390.
8. Fielding GA, Rhodes M, Nathanson LK. Laparoscopic gastric banding for morbid obesity. Surgical outcome in 335 cases. Surg Endosc 1999;13(6):550–554.
9. O'Brien PE, Brown WA, Smith A, et al. Prospective study of a laparoscopically placed, adjustable gastric band in the treatment of morbid obesity. Br J Surg 1999;86(1):113–118.
10. Vertruyen M. Experience with Lap-band System up to 7 years. Obes Surg 2002;12(4):569–572.
11. Weiner R, Wagner D, Bockhorn H. Laparoscopic gastric banding for morbid obesity. J Laparoendosc Adv Surg Tech A 1999;9(1):23–30.

20.5
Laparoscopic Adjustable Gastric Banding: Revisional Surgery

Franco Favretti, Gianni Segato, Maurizio De Luca, and Luca Busetto

Laparoscopic adjustable gastric banding (LAGB) using the Lap-Band (BioEnterics Lap-Band, Inamed Health, Santa Barbara, CA) has been performed in our institution since 1993. Adjustable gastric banding for the surgical treatment of morbid obesity originated with Kuzmak in 1986, and in 1993 was developed for laparoscopic placement. In the past 10 years the procedure has gained widespread acceptance and is now the most frequently performed bariatric procedure in many countries of the world.

Laparoscopic adjustable gastric banding brings many advantages to patient and surgeon. The procedure is completely reversible as it does not require the opening of the gastrointestinal tract or rerouting of the anatomy, and it does not rely on cutting or stapling of the stomach, so the patient does not suffer from the resultant, sometimes serious, complications. Also, LAGB has the distinction of being the only bariatric operation designed to be performed laparoscopically (operation is laparoscopically accomplished in >95% of all cases). The use of the Lap-Band, therefore, allows patients to leave the hospital much earlier than more drastic open bariatric procedures, and they can return to work and normal activity much sooner.

Even though some complications with gastric banding are unavoidable, they can be treated by laparoscopy in most cases and are rarely life threatening if managed appropriately. It is worth noting that as techniques for placement have evolved, complication rates with the Lap-Band have declined. Surgeons and patients should adopt strategies that will help avoid complications and be sensitive to any indications of their emergence.

This chapter reports the long-term outcome of a large group of morbidly obese patients treated with the Lap-Band. We focus on the complications that required revisional surgery and present our methods of diagnosis, prevention, and treatment.

Revisional Surgery

The Lap-Band operation is not without its complications, but they occur on a smaller scale and have a much lower risk profile compared with other methods currently used in obesity surgery. It is important to note that complications can usually be corrected and that the Lap-Band appears to be the lowest risk operation currently available for the treatment of morbid obesity. Another important aspect of this kind of surgery, even though it requires advanced laparoscopic experience, is that most of the complications can be corrected by laparoscopy. In case of complications our current approach is as follows:

Gastric Perforation

If the perforation is detected at surgery and if it occurs at a location distant from the band, some surgeons have repaired the stomach laparoscopically and placed the band successfully (1). But if the exposure is not satisfactory, it is advisable to postpone the placement of the band, suture the stomach wall, drain the area, and have a nasogastric tube in place. If the perforation is detected postoperatively, and gross contamination has already occurred causing peritonitis and subsequent emergency surgery, the band has to be removed and traditional surgical approaches have to be implemented.

Stomach Slippage

Different options are available for stomach slippage.

Deflation

The band system is deflated via the access port and an upper gastrointestinal (GI) radiographic series is performed. This is the only way to positively establish the cause of the symptoms and to establish whether any passage for the fluids exists through the band. In most of the cases the pouch returns to normal size and motility. After 1 month the band is gradually inflated with no more than 1.0cc at a time. After deflation, if an upper GI series still shows slippage or the contrast passes with difficulty through the band, band removal or repositioning must be performed. True stomach slippage (as opposed to gastric pouch dilatation) does not respond to the previously mentioned conservative measures and indicates the need for urgent laparoscopic or open exploration of the abdomen, especially in cases of epigastric pain.

Removal

The Lap-Band system can be removed by laparoscopy. To reach the site of the band, which is usually covered by adhesions, it is advisable to follow the connecting tube and pull it. The buckle of the band is easily identified and cut along the side of the buckle, allowing the withdrawal and removal of the device (Fig. 20.5-1). In this case another surgical procedure could be offered to the patient.

Pull-Through Technique

In the case of anterior gastric wall slippage, first the band must be deflated and exposed. At this point it is feasible to reduce the slippage, by carefully pulling the gastric wall through the band (Fig. 20.5-2). Retention sutures are applied. If the stomach above the band has become edematous or hypertrophied to the extent that reduction is not possible, the band needs to be divided and a new band

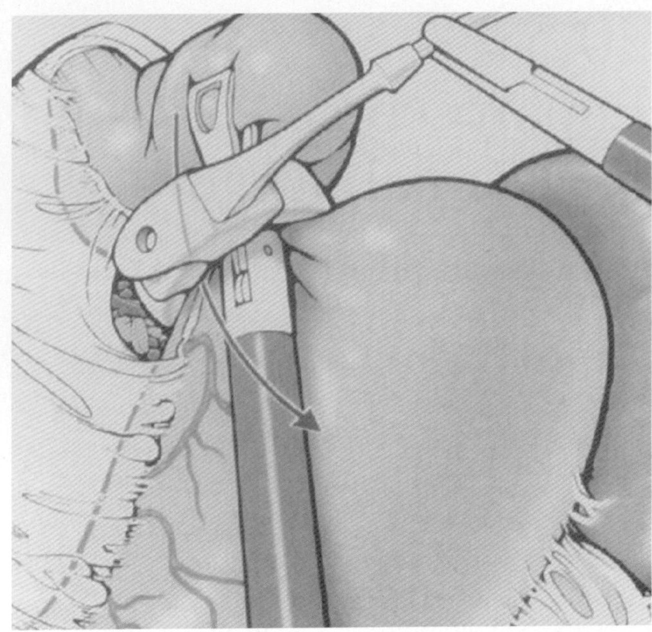

FIGURE 20.5-2. Reduction of an anterior gastric slip; pull-through technique.

placed above the enlarged gastric pouch. Of course the position of the band on the lesser curvature and the location of the retrogastric tunnel have to be checked. If they are not correct, repositioning has to be done.

Repositioning

Posterior stomach slippage is treated by removal of the band and placement of a new band higher up. The removal of the band requires just enough dissection to give access to the part of the band directly to the left of the buckle. The reference points for dissection have to be identified again to be sure that the retrogastric tunnel will be above the peritoneal reflection of the bursa omentalis. If the usual perigastric technique for dissection and creation of the retrogastric tunnel is not possible due to local adhesions, the pars flaccida technique can be easily used. The pars flaccida pathway has not been previously dissected and is therefore easy to access. In this case dissection begins directly lateral to the equator of the calibration balloon in the avascular space of the pars flaccida. After seeing the caudate lobe of the liver, blunt dissection is continued under direct visualization until the right crus is seen, followed immediately by the left crus over to the angle of His.

Stoma Obstruction

In many cases deflation of the band, a few days of liquid diet, and medical treatment with pump inhibitors can prove salutary. For patients with near-complete or partial obstruction, initial treatment can be conservative, con-

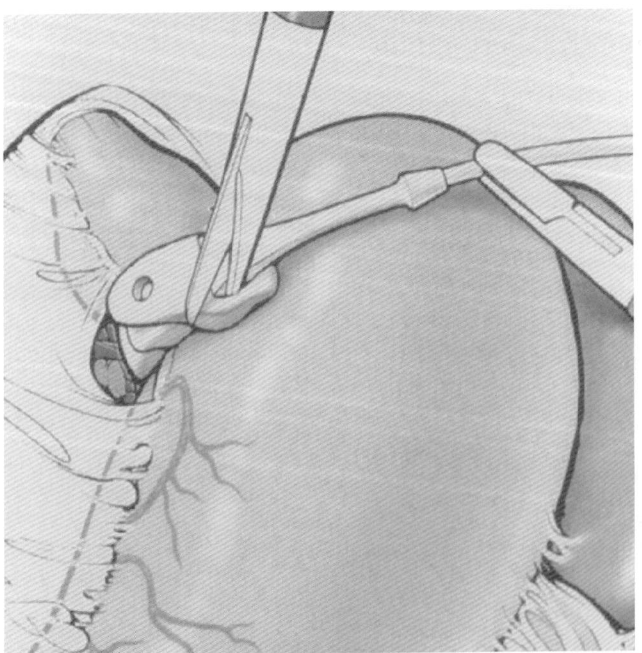

FIGURE 20.5-1. For removal, the band is cut along the side of the buckle.

sisting of rehydration and reassurance in an inpatient setting. If patients do not improve clinically and radiologically within a few days, they can be managed with exploratory laparoscopy as described earlier. If the stoma obstructions are caused by stomach slippage, pouch dilatation, or erosion, they are treated accordingly.

Esophageal and Gastric Pouch Dilatation

Its management involves complete deflation of the band and, after 2 to 3 months, slow re-inflation with the surgeon being careful not to reach the previous point of overinflation. If, after deflation, an upper gastrointestinal radiographic series shows a persisting esophageal/gastric pouch enlargement with difficult passage of the contrast medium through the deflated band, the surgeon is probably dealing with either stomach slippage or malpositioning of the band. In both cases the device is encompassing too much gastric tissue. Removal or repositioning of the band is usually required in these cases (see Stomach Slippage, below).

Erosion

The occurrence of this complication requires removal of the band. The band is removed by laparoscopy. To reach the site of the band, which is usually covered by adhesions, it is advisable to follow the connecting tube and to pull it. The buckle of the band is easily identified and a cut on its weak part permits removal of the band. A few stitches are applied to the damaged gastric wall. We usually perform a perioperative gastroscopy and a methylene blue test to confirm that there is no leak. We then insert a nasogastric tube for decompression and a perigastric drain. The surgical approach is the same even if erosion is high enough to be considered esophageal. Some authors have described techniques for band removal (usually bands other than Lap-Band) with an oral endoscope (2,3), regardless of whether or not the band is contained completely within the gastric lumen.

Gastric Necrosis

Repair of gastric necrosis requires exploratory laparotomy and implementation of traditional surgical approaches.

Tubing/Access Port Problems

If the port has to be replaced and repositioned, it can be scheduled as a day-surgery procedure. If the proximal end of the tubing is into the abdominal cavity, laparoscopy and recovery of the tubing are needed as part of the repair. Sometimes a lengthening of the tubing has to be made at the same time. With the recently improved access port design, we expect to have minimal tubing problems in the future.

Lack of Compliance/Unsatisfactory Results

If there are no technical problems with the band (slippage, pouch enlargement, erosion, and so forth) and if the patient is not satisfied with the results so far achieved, we offer to the patient, as a second choice/remedial procedure, a laparoscopic biliopancreatic diversion (BPD) with gastric preservation and proximal restriction (Fig. 20.5-3). The operation is performed by laparoscopy

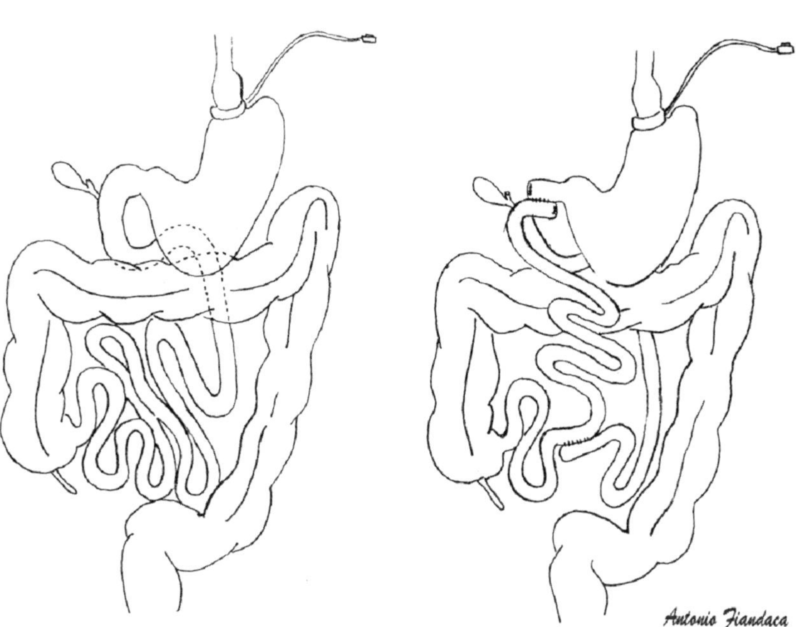

FIGURE 20.5-3. Bandinaro technique.

TABLE 20.5-1. Major complications requiring reoperation (of 1292 patients)

Complication	No. of pts.	Remedies
Early		
Gastric perforation	2	Band removed
Stomach slippage	1	Band repositioned
Late		
Stomach slippage	30	21 repositioned, 9 removed
Malpositioned band	17	16 repositioned, 1 removed
Erosion	7	7 removed
Psychological intolerance	8	8 removed
AIDS	1	Removed
Gastric necrosis	1	Gastrectomy

TABLE 20.5-2. Distribution of complications

Patient	No. of complications	Complications (%)
1–100	23	23
101–200	8	8
201–341	9	6.4
342–1177	27	3.2

(4–6), and it consists of adding a duodenal switch to the already present Lap-Band with the same lengths of Scopinaro's BPD. This procedure, being a fusion of the lap-band plus Scopinaro's BPD, is even known as *Bandinaro.*

Results

At 10 years follow-up, 95% of the 1292 patients at our institution were available for examination. Major complications requiring reoperation developed in 5.0% (65 patients). Early complications were two gastric perforations (requiring band removal) and one stomach slippage (treated by band repositioning). Late complications are shown (along with early complications) in Table 20.5-1. Thirty patients developed stomach slippage (21 repositioned, nine removed), 17 had a malpositioned band (16 repositioned, one removed), seven had erosions (all removed), eight had psychological intolerance (all removed), one had AIDS (removed), and one had gastric necrosis (gastrectomy).

In analyzing the distribution of the major complications requiring reoperation, we observed that complications were reduced with experience: from patient number 1 to 100 there were 23 (23%), from patients 101 to 200 there were eight (8%), from patients 201 to 341 there were nine (6.4%), and from patients 342 to 1177 there were 27 (3.2%) (Table 20.5-2).

Reservoir/connecting tube problems (leakages, twisting, infection) were regarded as minor complications requiring reoperation and occurred in 134 patients (11.4%). Seventy patients (6%) had stomach slippage or pouch dilatation (with or without esophageal enlargement), which responded to conservative treatment and did not require reoperation.

Weight loss expressed as body weight (BW) reduction (kg) is shown in Table 20.5-3. Weight loss expressed as body mass index (BMI) reduction is shown in Table 20.5-4. Weight loss expressed as percent excess weight loss (%EWL) is shown in Table 20.5-5. Tables 20.5-3, 20.5-4, and 20.5-5 include 1292 patients with 1- to 10-year follow-up.

TABLE 20.5-3. Weight loss expressed as body weight (BW) reduction (kg)

Postoperative year	All patients		Super-obese		Morbidly obese	
	No. of pts.	Weight	No. of pts.	Weight	No. of pts.	Weight
0	1292	128.4 ± 25.2	378	153.2 ± 23.2	914	118.2 ± 17.9
1	1129	102.9 ± 21.6	342	120.1 ± 23.4	787	96.0 ± 16.3
2	957	100.9 ± 21.8	308	116.7 ± 22.8	649	96.9 ± 18.5
3	796	101.7 ± 21.4	256	115.3 ± 22.9	540	96.1 ± 17.9
4	609	103.6 ± 22.6	179	119.4 ± 26.6	430	97.0 ± 16.9
5	451	105.6 ± 23.6	136	120.6 ± 27.9	315	99.0 ± 18.2
6	312	101.8 ± 23.1	111	115.0 ± 29.8	201	96.7 ± 17.6
7	192	98.8 ± 23.1	71	113.2 ± 30.9	121	93.6 ± 17.0
8	73	96.5 ± 25.5	18	120.8 ± 52.9	55	91.8 ± 13.8
9	19	95.9 ± 21.3	1	97.0	18	95.8 ± 23.0
10	3	84.3 ± 28.2	1	97.0	2	78.08 ± 36.8

TABLE 20.5-4. Weight loss expressed as body mass index (BMI) reduction

Postoperative year	All patients		Super-obese		Morbidly obese	
	No. of pts.	BMI	No. of pts.	BMI	No. of pts.	BMI
0	1292	46.4 ± 8.2	378	56.2 ± 5.5	914	42.4 ± 5.1
1	1129	37.4 ± 6.9	342	44.3 ± 7.1	787	34.6 ± 4.6
2	957	36.7 ± 7.0	308	42.8 ± 7.2	649	34.3 ± 5.0
3	796	37.1 ± 7.0	256	42.8 ± 7.4	540	34.7 ± 5.2
4	609	37.7 ± 7.4	179	43.7 ± 8.3	430	35.2 ± 5.3
5	451	38.2 ± 7.4	136	43.7 ± 8.4	315	35.9 ± 5.6
6	312	37.2 ± 7.6	111	41.9 ± 9.4	201	35.3 ± 5.5
7	192	36.9 ± 8.1	71	42.5 ± 10.8	121	34.8 ± 5.7
8	73	36.2 ± 9.6	18	45.8 ± 19.6	55	34.4 ± 4.7
9	19	35.0 ± 6.3	1	41.4	18	34.1 ± 6.2
10	3	33.8 ± 10.8	1	41.4	2	30.1 ± 11.5

Discussion

Lap-Band surgery has become the most commonly performed bariatric operation outside the United States, particularly in Europe, Australia, and Latin America. Approximately 125,000 patients underwent this procedure worldwide, and it has been our operation of choice since September 1993.

Suitability for this surgery must be determined by a multidisciplinary team (internist, dietitian, psychologist, and surgeon). Results can be optimized by adequate multidisciplinary follow-up as well. The surgical technique has been gradually modified and standardized such that we have been able to reduce our operating time significantly and to report a morbidity (major complications requiring reoperation) of 5.0% with zero mortality for the entire study. There is a striking difference between our results and the results reported by Oria (7), who has not performed this procedure, in his literature review.

Key steps of the perigastric technique, standardized by our team and that of the Free University of Bruxelles, were (1) reference points for dissection (inflated balloon equator and left crus), (2) retrogastric tunnel above the bursa omentalis, (3) embedment or imbrication of the band, and (4) virtual pouch (8,9).

The Lap-Band procedure produces less weight loss than gastric bypass and other malabsorptive procedures. However, in the long run (up to 10 years) our weight-loss curves are stable in time, with morbidly obese patients losing as an average 30 kg, 8 points on the BMI, and 45% EWL while the super-obese lost 40 kg, 12 points of BMI, and 44% EWL. The Lap-Band operation is not without its complications, but these occur on a smaller scale and have a much lower risk profile compared with other methods currently used in obesity surgery. It is important to note that complications can usually be corrected and that the Lap-Band appears to be the lowest risk operation currently available for the treatment of morbid obesity. Another important aspect of this kind of surgery, even though it requires advanced laparoscopic experience, is that most of the complications can be corrected by laparoscopy. The emergence of many problems can be minimized with proper operative technique and close postoperative management and follow-up. Some points for their prevention are detailed in the following section.

TABLE 20.5-5. Weight loss expressed as percent excess weight loss (%EWL)

Postoperative year	All patients		Super-obese		Morbidly obese	
	No. of pts.	%EWL	No. of pts.	%EWL	No. of pts.	%EWL
0	1292	—	378	—	914	—
1	1129	41.3 ± 19.4	342	36.4 ± 16.5	787	43.3 ± 20.1
2	957	44.0 ± 22.3	308	41.4 ± 18.4	649	45.0 ± 23.0
3	796	41.8 ± 24.0	256	40.2 ± 20.0	540	42.5 ± 25.4
4	609	39.4 ± 29.5	179	38.0 ± 21.5	430	40.0 ± 25.6
5	451	36.8 ± 26.5	136	38.2 ± 21.8	315	36.2 ± 28.2
6	312	39.4 ± 26.3	111	42.8 ± 25.7	201	38.1 ± 26.5
7	192	40.9 ± 26.3	71	41.1 ± 27.1	121	40.9 ± 26.2
8	73	42.9 ± 27.4	18	43.7 ± 34.8	55	42.7 ± 26.6
9	19	43.5 ± 30.2	1	42.9	18	43.6 ± 32.7
10	3	53.0 ± 49.6	1	42.9	2	58.1 ± 69.0

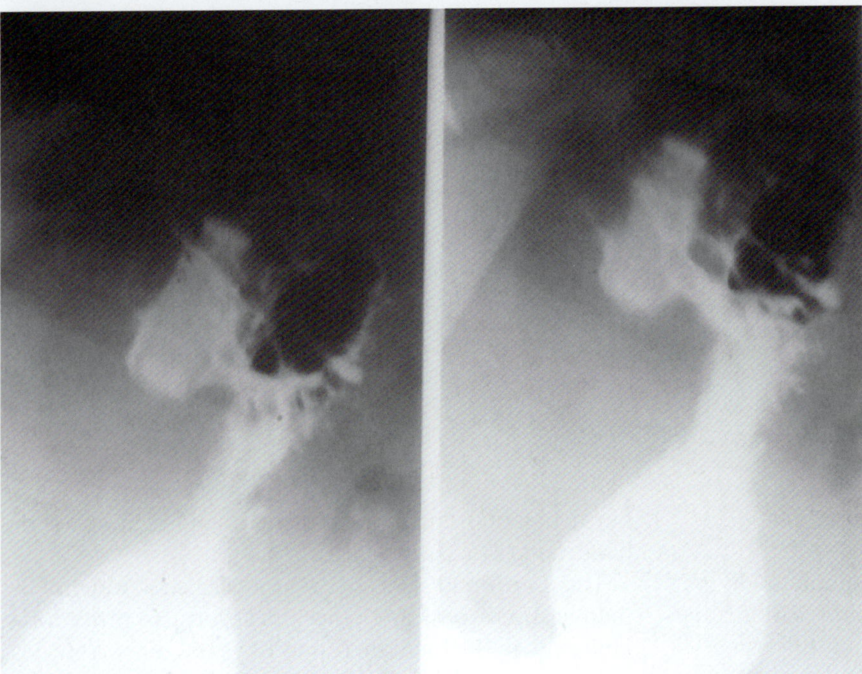

FIGURE 20.5-4. Gastric perforation: Gastrografin swallow on postoperative day 1 may show a leak.

Prevention of Problems

Gastric Perforation

The stomach may be perforated during surgery mainly at the creation of the retrogastric tunnel. This step can be difficult in patients with very high BMI, visceral obesity, and especially in male subjects.

Causes and Incidence

The relationship of this gastric perforation to the surgical procedure is evident, and emergency surgery is indicated. Most surgeons have reported one or two stomach perforations, primarily during the learning curve period (10–15), with a gastric perforation rate ranging from 0.2% (16) to 3.5% (17).

Symptoms

Gastric perforation is characterized by free leakage of gastric contents into the peritoneum similar to when perforation of the gastric lining leads to peritonitis.

Diagnosis

This complication can be detected easily during surgery by inflating the stomach with a methylene blue solution once the band tubing has been pulled into the retrogastric tunnel. Using the methylene blue after the band has been positioned and locked could be useless. In fact, the band might completely fill the perforation and not show any leakage. An upper GI x-ray series with Gastrografin, done routinely on the first postoperative day, can show the perforation (Fig. 20.5-4).

How to Avoid It

During the creation of the retrogastric tunnel, there is a blind area. If we want to avoid this complication, the area can be reduced by a wider downward exposition of the left crus and by a wider dissection along the lesser curvature. This is a consideration if the perigastric dissection path is used. To avoid gastric wall injuries, the calibration tube must be withdrawn during dissection, which should be undertaken perpendicularly so as not to enter the inferior mediastinum along the esophagus. We have found that the articulating dissector (Fig. 20.5-5) (Automated Medical, Edison, NJ) is atraumatic enough to avoid damaging the gastric wall. Good surgical technique with adequate

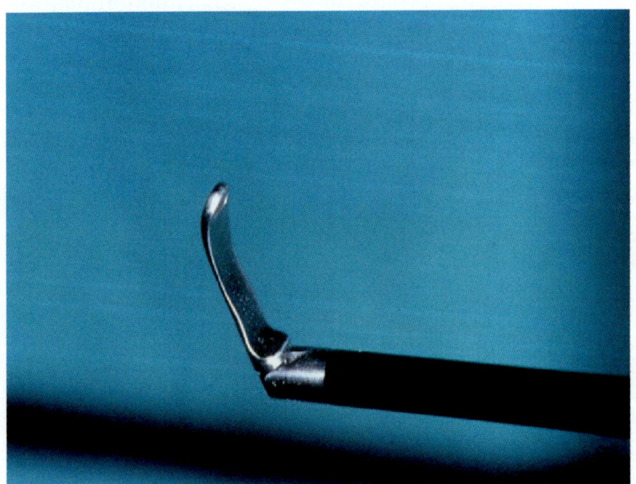

FIGURE 20.5-5. Articulating dissector (Courtesy of Automated Medical Products, Corp., Edison, NJ.)

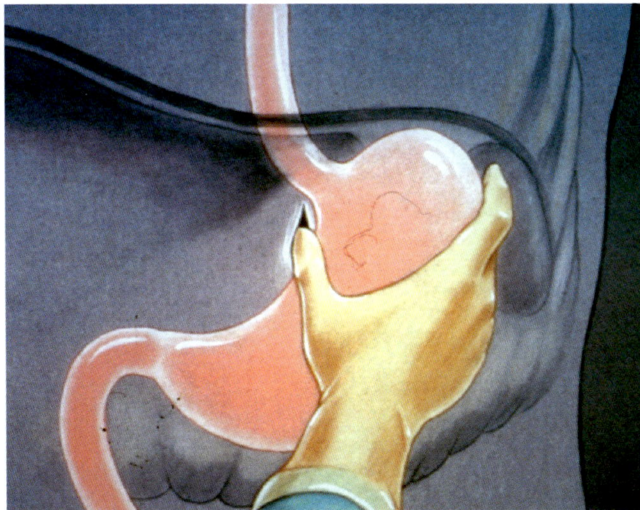

FIGURE 20.5-6. Video hand-assisted technique may be used in case of difficult dissections.

exposure and use of appropriate instruments can reduce the incidence of this serious complication (14).

If the retrogastric dissection turns out to be risky, a valuable option is the video hand-assisted technique. The right hand of the surgeon is introduced into the abdomen through a mini-laparotomy (Fig. 20.5-6). The perigastric dissection is undertaken digitally using the in-place calibration tube as a reference. The articulating instrument is put in place, the mini-laparotomy is closed, and the rest of the operation is completed, usually by laparoscopy.

Stomach Slippage

Stomach slippage is the postoperative development of an overly large upper gastric pouch. Often referred to as gastric prolapse and often confused with pouch dilatation, this complication can occur anteriorly or posteriorly.

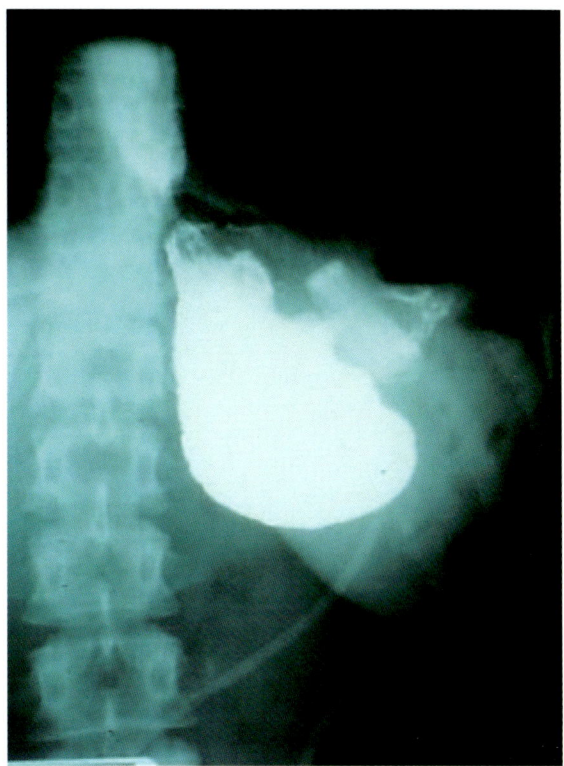

FIGURE 20.5-7. Posterior stomach slippage radiograph.

Causes

Posterior gastric slippage is the most common type. The posterior gastric wall moves through the band, resulting in the creation of a large posterior pouch (Fig. 20.5-7). The band rotates to a vertical position, or even rotates beyond the vertical, with the inferior aspect of the band lying more to the left. This problem is principally a consequence of placing the band across the apex of the lesser sac (Fig. 20.5-8) rather

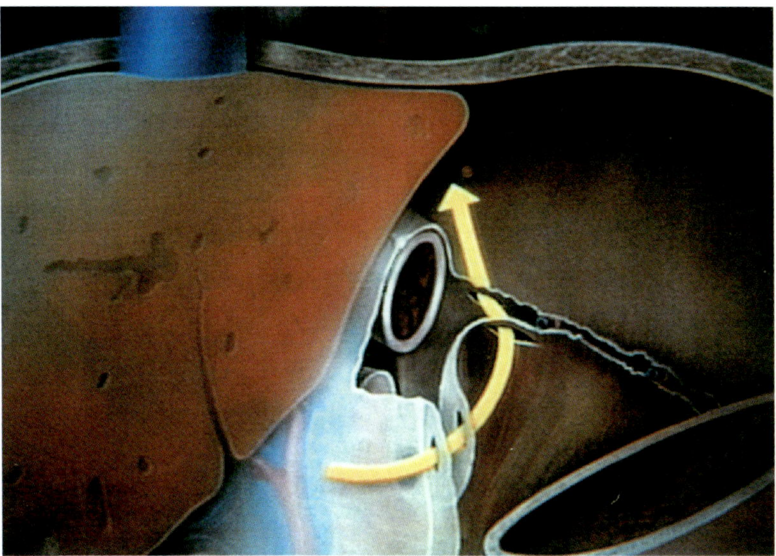

FIGURE 20.5-8. Retrogastric tunnel incorrectly created across the lesser sac.

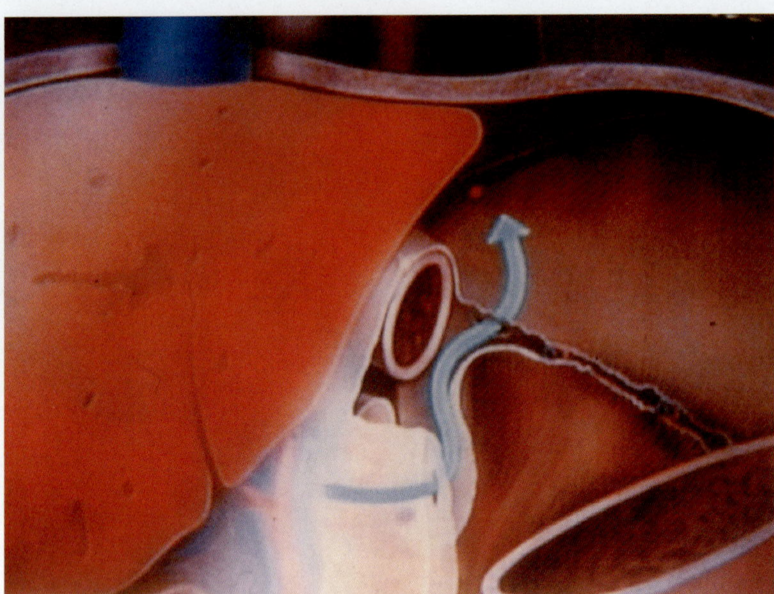

FIGURE 20.5-9. Retrogastric tunnel created above peritoneal reflection of the bursa omentalis.

than through the tissue above the lesser sac (Fig. 20.5-9).

Anterior gastric slippage results from failure of the anterior fixation (retention sutures). The band moves to a horizontal position, and the enlarged proximal stomach overlies the left side of the band. The sutures may be placed in a way that fails to fix the lateral (greater curvature) aspect. They may be insufficient in number to give full fixation or they may be inserted above the band into the fat pad overlying the esophagogastric junction rather than into the upper gastric wall so they subsequently tear out. Both posterior and anterior pouch dilatation lead to excessive stomach tissue inside the band and to obstruction between the upper pouch and the lower stomach.

Incidence

This is the most frequent complication associated with the Lap-Band procedure. Its incidence has been dramatically reduced over the years (from as high as 22% down to less than 5%) (18) by a better understanding of the anatomy of the gastroesophageal junction (GEJ) and by the evolution of the surgical technique.

Three techniques for the positioning of the Lap-Band have been described: (1) the perigastric method (8,19) (Fig. 20.5-10); (2) the pars flaccida method (20) (Fig. 20.5-11); and (3) the pars flaccida to perigastric technique (21) (Fig. 20.5-12).

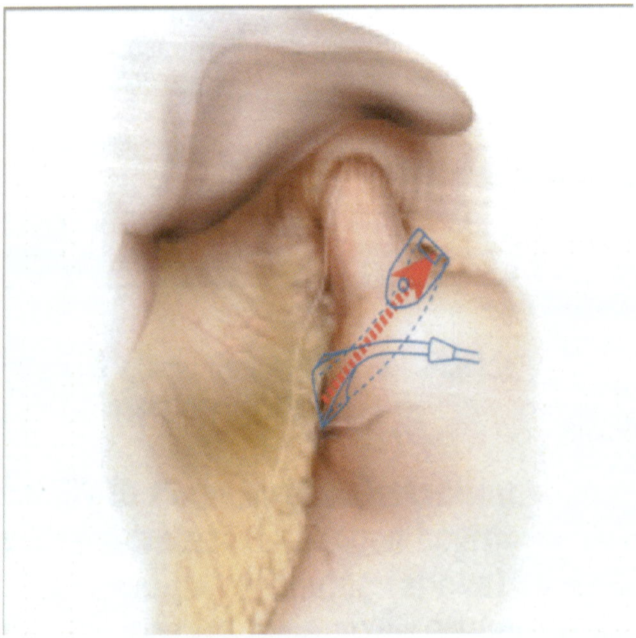

FIGURE 20.5-10. The perigastric dissection technique.

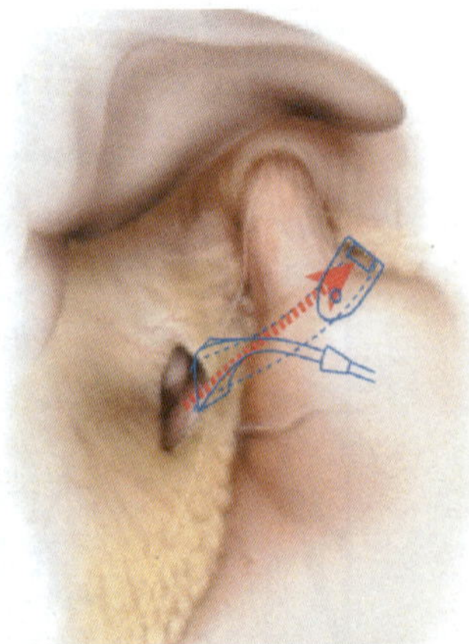

FIGURE 20.5-11. The pars flaccida dissection technique.

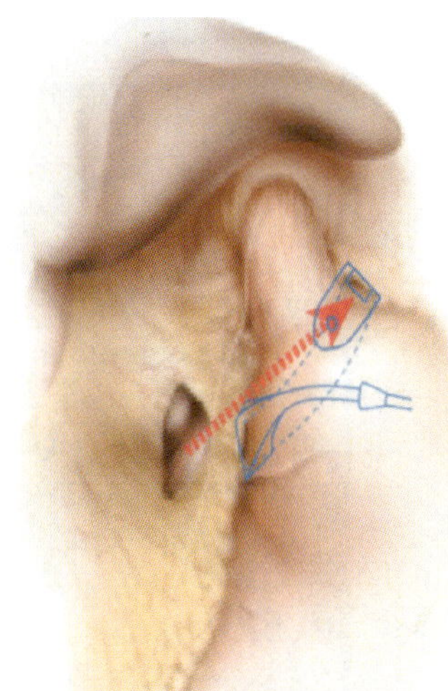

FIGURE 20.5-12. The pars flaccida to the perigastric dissection technique; the second step.

Of these, the perigastric technique may have the highest rate of slippages (20), probably because it is more difficult to master. But in fact, the perigastric technique, properly performed, has a very low incidence of slippage, 10% in our series, of whom 1.9% required reoperation (22).

Symptoms

Stomach slippage should be suspected when patients who have had a normal postoperative period begin to experience changes in their eating habits. The symptoms of slippage are the symptoms of partial or complete obstruction and of fluid stasis in the lower esophagus and upper distended gastric pouch. These symptoms include heartburn, vomiting, free reflux of fluid into the mouth, dysphagia, coughing and choking spells (particularly at night), wheezing, and ability to tolerate only fluids.

The problem is usually chronic. Nevertheless, the patient can develop significant dehydration with electrolyte imbalance and ischemia of the upper stomach. Ischemic lesions are particularly dreadful since they can lead to gastric necrosis.

Diagnosis

Investigation and management depend on the severity and acuteness of symptoms. No patient should have the aforementioned symptoms as a normal part of the post Lap-Band process. Therefore, the onset of these symptoms indicates that either the band has been set too tightly or there is some slippage present. An upper gastrointestinal x-ray series is diagnostic.

How to Avoid It

To avoid this complication, it is important to correctly select the sites for dissection along the lesser curvature and into the phrenogastric ligament. A reliable reference point for dissection is the equator of the balloon (calibration tube inflated with 25 cc of air and withdrawn to the gastroesophageal junction), which, on the phrenogastric ligament, corresponds to the left crus.

The retrogastric tunnel is created by joining the reference points. The dissection has to be perpendicular and has to aim at the left crus. The bursa omentalis should not be entered and the dissection has to be performed into the phrenogastric ligament above the peritoneal reflection of the bursa omentalis. Once the Lap-Band has been positioned, an anterior embedment is carried out with a few retention sutures applied from the greater toward the lesser curvature. Following these steps, it is unlikely that either the band or the stomach walls can slip.

It is unquestionable that the lower reported incidence of stomach slippage (18,23) is due to the following factors: (1) the creation of a "virtual" pouch, as the smaller pouch has less ability to stretch and pull the gastric fundus from below the band; (2) the sound placement of retention gastrogastric sutures; and (3) the posterior positioning of the band very high and in close proximity to the gastroesophageal junction. This anatomic tendency for high posterior position is clearly evident in the pars flaccida and combined pars flaccida to perigastric techniques. However, surgeons experienced with the perigastric technique have always recommended a high posterior position as well (22).

Stoma Obstruction

Stoma obstruction is defined as an obstruction to the passage of food from the gastric pouch to the rest of the stomach. Stomas obstruction can happen any time, early or late in the postoperative period.

Symptoms

Symptoms include sialorrhea, vomiting, dysphagia, epigastric/retrosternal and chest pain, inability to swallow, new onset of reflux, and repeated aspiration and pulmonary complications in severe cases.

Causes

Stoma obstruction in the early postoperative period has a number of possible causes, all of which serve to narrow the stoma and simulate the effect of an overtight band. After band placement using the pars flaccida approach, stoma obstruction is most often associated with smaller bands applied over a thick GEJ area or too distal from the GEJ.

After band placement using the perigastric or the pars flaccida to perigastric approach, stoma obstruction is usually caused by the incorporation of too much tissue inside the band. In most of the cases, in fact, the band is

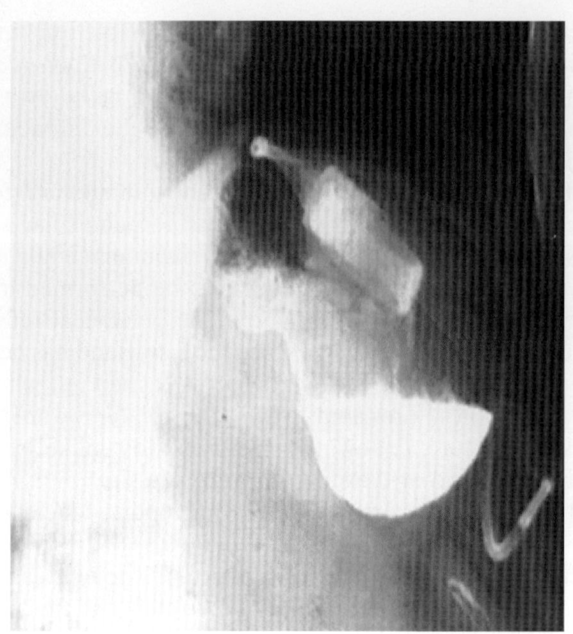

FIGURE 20.5-13. Early complete stoma obstruction due to a malpositioned band.

positioned too distally from the GEJ, causing a large amount of fundus and stomach wall to be encompassed by the band. Because the circumference of the band is fixed, obstruction results (Fig. 20.5-13).

In other cases, especially in heavy male patients with thick GEJ areas, the 9.75- or 10-cm bands may be placed around too much tissue. The surgeon can perform a delicate dissection, thinning out the area where the band is to be placed.

If a band still appears too tight just prior to locking, then consider using the two-step dissection option (21). When the pars flaccida technique has been used and when a band appears to be too tight just prior to locking

the buckle, then stop, unthread the band tubing, and back the band out of the retrogastric space. Leave the tubing in position behind the stomach and inflate the calibration tube to 25 cc. Pull the tube back so the balloon is firmly stopped against the bottom of the GEJ. Select a point at the equator (midline) of the inflated balloon on the edge of the lesser curve (as would be done to start the perigastric dissection). Deflate the balloon and pull the calibration tube back into the esophagus. Bluntly dissect straight down (anteroposterior) alongside the lesser curve. Do not follow the stomach wall behind the stomach, just dissect straight downward until the band tubing is found in the pars flaccida pathway. Pull the band tubing up through the new perigastric window and rethread the buckle. Just before locking all the way, confirm that the band now fits loosely. If not, excise fat tissue on the anterior gastric wall as needed to avoid the band's being overtight.

Postoperative edema of the area incorporated by the band due to hematoma or postoperative reaction may also lead to stomal obstruction. Late stoma obstructions are usually related to gastric pouch dilation, stomach slippage, erosion, pouchitis, or esophagitis caused by bad eating habits (Fig. 20.5-14). Figure 20.5-15, which shows the same patient is seen as in Figure 20.5-14, demonstrates with resolution of dilatation with a 2-cc deflation of the band.

Diagnosis

In most of the previously mentioned cases, a postoperative contrast study with Gastrografin (always to be done on the first postoperative day) often reveals complete obstruction or near-complete obstruction with minimal flow from the esophagus and gastric pouch to the portion of the stomach below the band. Tertiary esophageal contractions (uncoordinated contractions) are usually evident.

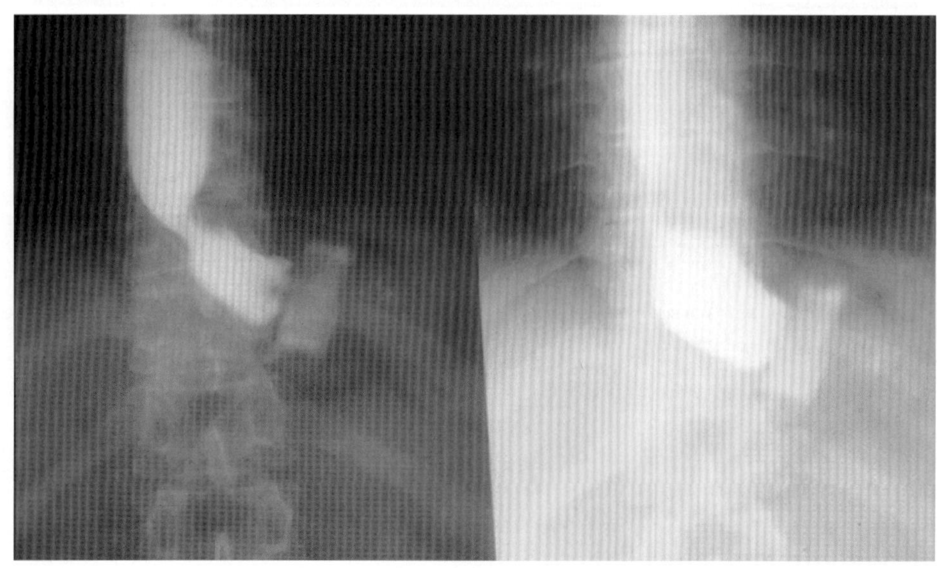

FIGURE 20.5-14. Nine months postoperative stoma obstruction; pouchitis/esophagitis due to bad eating habits.

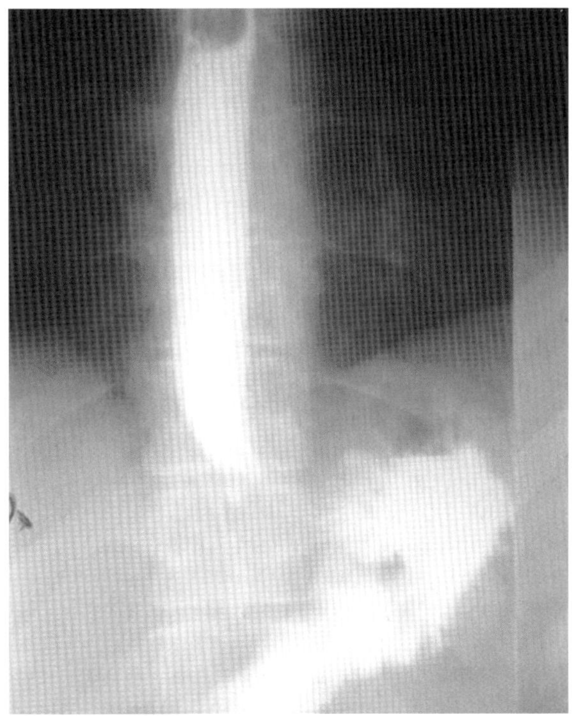

FIGURE 20.5-15. Resolution of dilatation with 2 cc deflation of band; same patient as in Figure 20.5-14.

Esophageal and Gastric Pouch Dilatation

Esophageal and gastric pouch dilatation without stomach slippage has been reported (24).

Incidence

Esophageal dilatation is a debatable complication, having been observed and reported at essentially only one site in the U.S. Food and Drug Administration (FDA) clinical trial (25). In our series of 830 patients, 92 cases (11%) of esophageal and gastric pouch dilatation were reported. Of these 92 cases, 83 (90%) were caused by gastric slippage and 9 (0.9%) were caused by malposition of the band (22). It is our observation that esophageal dilatation is a transient clinical *finding* indicative of an overtightened band or a chronic outlet obstruction due to band malposition or slippage.

Causes

Even though the two entities, stomach slippage and gastric pouch dilatation, are different from an etiopathogenic point of view, they sometimes overlap; in a few cases the actual cause could be debatable. When this type of pouch enlargement occurs it is most likely caused by overinflation of the band, resulting in a mechanically severe outlet obstruction, creation of an oversized pouch during surgery (band placed too low or malpositioned), or patient's lack of compliance regarding oral intake

(inappropriate food intake, insufficient chewing of food, and overeating causing vomiting).

All these factors can stress and stretch the new small gastric pouch. Eventually the pouch and even the esophagus may dilate, as occurs in other restrictive procedures. Failure to address the issue will result in an atonic pouch and large atonic esophagus.

Symptoms

Symptoms are indistinguishable from those previously described for stomach slippage.

Diagnosis

Periodic esophageal imaging may help detect dilatation and therefore should be conducted at least once in the first postoperative year or at the time of adjustment.

How to Avoid It

Creating a small upper pouch (15 mL or, even better, virtual pouch) has been demonstrated to be vital to the success of surgery. There is a dramatic decrease in pouch enlargement problems when the initial pouch size is no more than 15 mL or virtual. The size of the pouch and the dissection points for the retrogastric passage of the band have to be accurately determined with the use of the calibration tube/balloon supplied with each Lap-Band system.

Apart from the cases caused by an overinflated band (Fig. 20.5-16), we believe most of the reported cases are

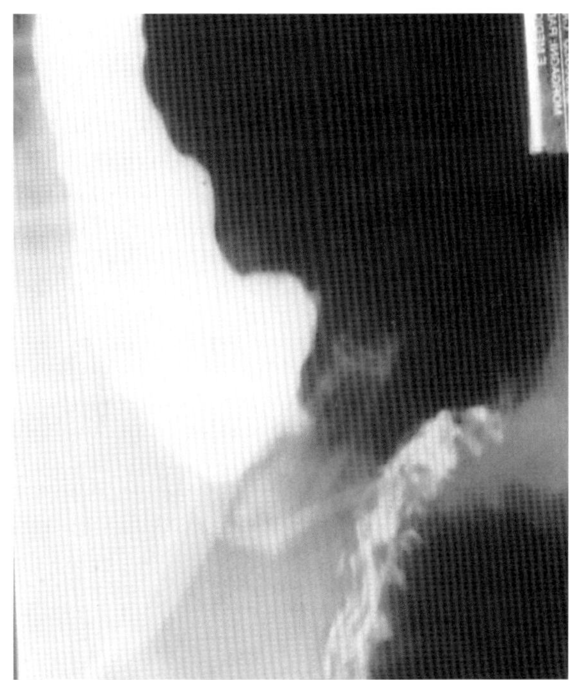

FIGURE 20.5-16. Esophageal dilatation due to overinflated band, resolved with deflation.

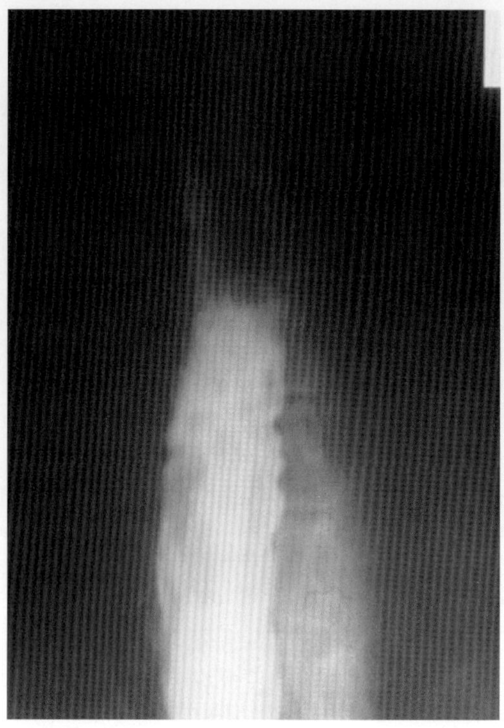

FIGURE 20.5-17. Esophageal dilatation due to malpositioned band, ultimately required removal.

due either to stomach slippage (see previous discussion) or to malpositioning of the band (Fig. 20.5-17). We avoid this complication by respecting the reference points for dissection and carrying out the retrogastric dissection as previously described. While creating the pouch, avoid any cul-de-sac that could cause further enlargement of the pouch, leading to *food intolerance*. The cul-de-sac is avoided by removing the calibration tube and by applying the retention sutures from below upward. To reduce the incidence of early food intolerance we recommend that the Lap-Band stoma initially be kept large (band uninflated) after surgery. A more open stoma may help accommodate any postoperative edema or patient difficulty in compliance while learning new eating habits.

Erosion

Band erosion, defined as the partial or complete movement of a synthetic band into the gastric lumen of the stomach, is also known as *migration, gastric incorporation,* and *gastric inclusion.* It exists as a possible complication following bariatric surgical procedures in which synthetic materials (silicone, Marlex, Dacron, and so forth) are used to create the gastric stoma. Band erosion may occur following vertical banded gastroplasty and gastric bypass as well as Lap-Band system surgery. The occurrence of this complication renders any weight loss procedure ineffective and requires removal of the band, generally via surgery.

Incidence

This complication occurred in 1% of the patients of the Lap-Band FDA clinical trial (25). Omitting series in the international literature that include a large number of revision procedures and those performed during the learning curve, the Lap-Band system erosion rate is well below 1% (9,16,22,26–28).

Causes

The level of laparoscopic expertise and the extent of Lap-Band system experience affect the surgeon's ability to avoid complications. The incidence of erosion is attributed to one or to a combination of the following: small, undetected injuries to the gastric wall that occur during band placement; necrosis due to pressure of the band; and access port infection.

There is some disagreement among surgeons regarding the actual evolution of this process. While some believe that first the access port becomes infected, and then the infection travels down the tubing to the band causing erosion (29), most believe that the infection of the port is a symptom of an already-present erosion (30).

Symptoms

Most symptoms of erosion are of benign nature, nonurgent, and not life threatening. There is rarely ileus or sepsis found associated with the onset of erosions. Erosions may go unnoticed for a considerable period of time because the capsule seals off the band from the peritoneal cavity, and the band gradually transitions into the lumen without leakage or sepsis developing. Surgeons have observed a variety of (usually clinically benign) symptoms that may serve as indicators of band erosion (31–34). Many of these symptoms may be seen in combination, and patients may present with weight gain without apparent cause, feeling of lack of restriction/satiety, ineffectiveness of band adjustments, passage of contrast medium through and around the band shown on x-ray, and chronic and persistent port infection (port site infection may be the first symptom of erosion, usually due to migration of bacteria from the stomach to the port site area along the tubing).

Diagnosis

An erosion can be diagnosed by an upper GI x-ray series, by esophagogastroduodenoscopy (EGD) (Fig. 20.5-18), and by fistulography.

How to Avoid It

A meticulous, gentle, and careful operative dissection may avoid at least some of these erosion problems. If the

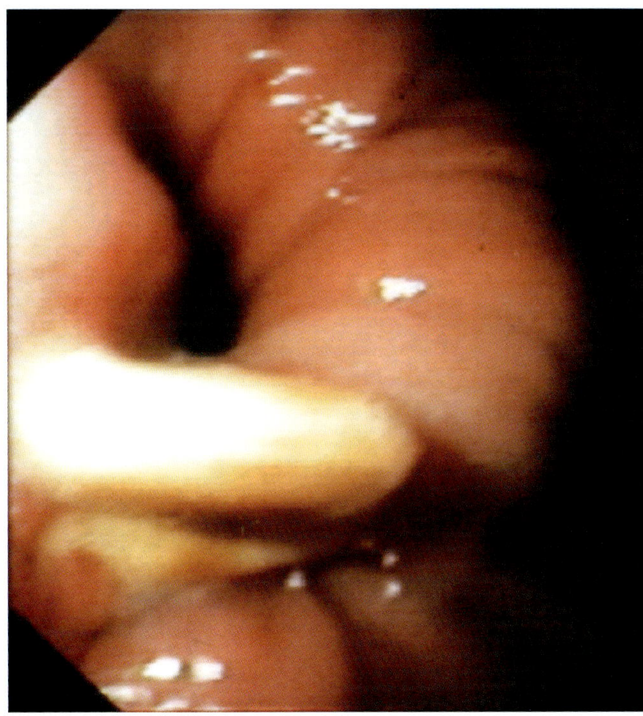

FIGURE 20.5-18. Gastric erosion; endoscopic view of band inside gastric lumen.

surgeon suspects that an injury to or perforation of the lumen has occurred during surgery, the injury should be addressed and serious consideration should be given to whether placement should proceed at that time. During surgery, placement of gastrogastric sutures over the locking mechanism (buckle) should be avoided. This area protrudes and can cause pressure necrosis to the gastric wall that covers it. Instead, all retention sutures should be placed to the left side of the locking mechanism.

Gastric Necrosis

By gastric necrosis we mean the necrosis of the upper gastric pouch.

Incidence

Necrosis is very rare. In one series of 400 patients only one case (0.25%) was reported (35). In our own series of 1292 patients we recently experienced our first case as well. This patient, complaining of symptoms suggesting either gastric slippage or a gastric pouch dilatation, was hospitalized at her local hospital. Despite our suggestions about the need for referral and for prompt appropriate treatment, she was kept there for a number of days under conservative treatment. Finally, due to the onset of exacerbating abdominal tenderness and peritonitis, she underwent exploratory laparotomy and gastric resection.

Causes

Gastric necrosis may occur early in the postoperative period or later when it is likely the result of a long-term undetected stomach slippage. Stomach slippage or gastric pouch dilatation can cause the band to exert continuous pressure against the gastric wall, which, in turn, may decrease the blood supply to the fundus. This pressure may also result from overinflation of the band. The combination of decreased blood supply and continuous pressure may lead to necrosis of the gastric wall. Even in the absence of stomach slippage, an overdistended gastric pouch by itself can impair blood supply and progressively lead to gastric wall necrosis. The theoretical link between stomach slippage and necrosis is the reason stomach slippage should be considered a surgical emergency.

Symptoms

We have to consider that stomach slippage and pouch dilatation, if not diagnosed and treated accordingly, can lead to gastric necrosis. The typical symptoms are abdominal tenderness and peritonitis. Abdominal pain is a herald, a sign that must be responded to immediately.

Diagnosis

If the symptoms are not considered diagnostic, an upper GI x-ray series with Gastrografin and an EGD can be done.

Tubing/Access Port Problems

The access port is an essential component of the Lap-Band system, and its placement requires careful attention.

Incidence and Causes

In our own series we had tubing and port problems in 11% of the cases. The complication is fairly common in most series (36,37). In part, these problems can be linked to design features at the interface between the access port and the tubing, and in part they can be linked to the method of placement of the port.

Symptoms

The patient is fully asymptomatic or complains of some discomfort at the port site. There might be difficulties in accessing the port for adjustment. Often the patient complains of a sudden loss in sensation of satiety and of an increase in body weight.

Diagnosis

Absence of fluid in the system indicates that something is wrong. There should be no normal loss of fluid. A plain

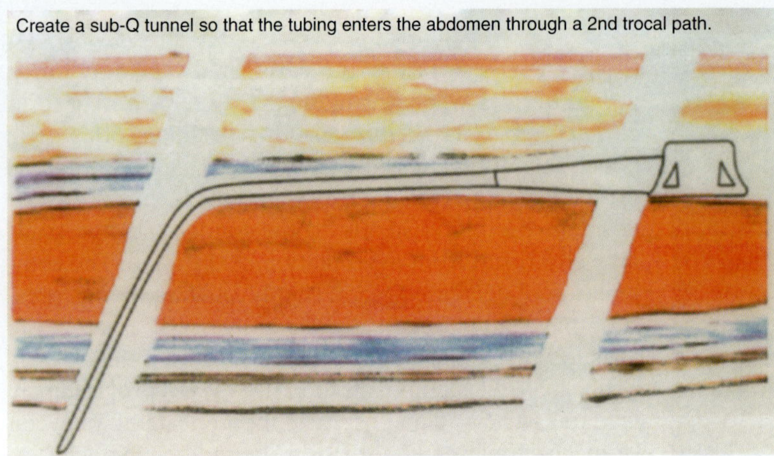

FIGURE 20.5-19. Access port placement option using a second trocar path.

x-ray of the abdomen is appropriate to see if there has been complete detachment of the tubing with movement of the proximal end back into the abdomen. When in doubt, injection of contrast medium (Conray) into the system shows the leakage in most cases. Very small leaks in the tubing, especially those due to needle sticks, may not be obvious. Contrast media can flow along the tubing and pool around the band.

How to Avoid It

The access port should be placed lateral to the trocar opening. A pocket must be created for the port so it is placed far enough from the trocar path to avoid abrupt kinking of the tubing (Fig. 20.5-19). Alternatively, a smooth arching path without sharp turns or bends may be created either with a 5-mm trocar or a hemostat to provide a gradual entry path into the abdominal cavity (Fig. 20.5-20) or creating a subcutaneous tunnel so that the tubing enters the abdomen through a second trocar path. The port is usually positioned in the left hypochondrium, and sutured to the rectus fascia with four Prolene sutures; its optimal orientation is shown in Figure 20.5-21.

With the recently improved access port design, we expect to have minimal tubing problems in the future.

Lack of Compliance/Unsatisfactory Results

In case of unsatisfactory results or lack of compliance, we offer to the patient, as a second choice/remedial surgery, the bandinaro procedure (6) (see Fig. 20.5-3). It consists of adding a duodenal switch to the already present Lap-Band with the same lengths of Scopinaro's BPD.

Incidence and Causes

It is estimated that 25% of patients fail to maintain long-term weight loss after adjustable gastric banding (22). Once the presence of slippage, pouch enlargement, erosion, or tubing/port problems have been excluded, the main reason for unsatisfactory results is the patient's lack of compliance with the Lap-Band system.

Symptoms

Patients are asymptomatic, except for the unsatisfactory weight loss, a couple of years after the original Lap-Band

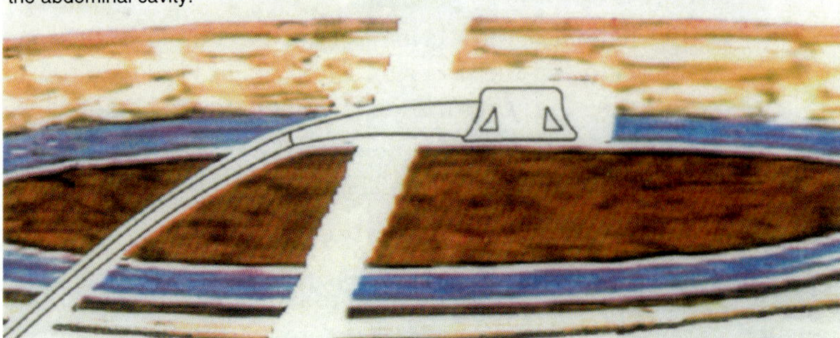

FIGURE 20.5-20. Correct access port placement option to prevent kinking of the tubing.

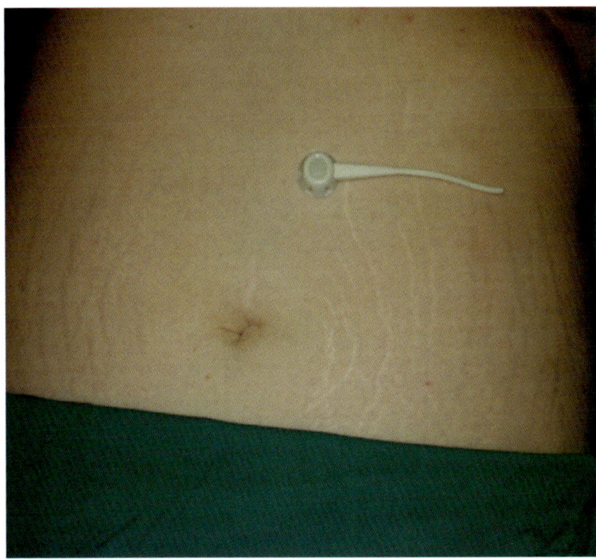

FIGURE 20.5-21. Horizontal orientation of the access port.

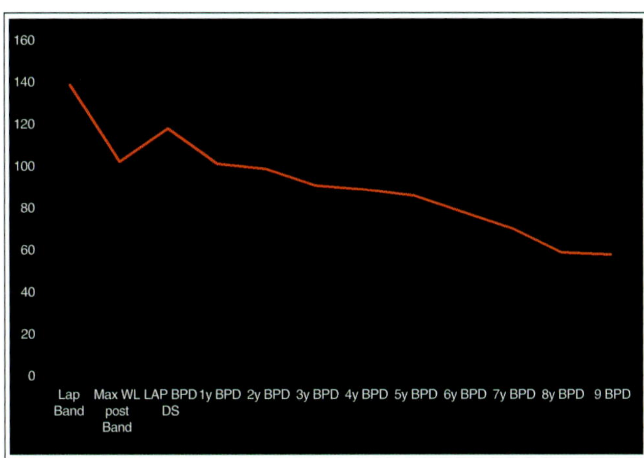

FIGURE 20.5-22. Bandinaro weight loss in kilograms.

procedure. They have been unable to change their eating habits in accordance with the new gastric restrictive situation.

Diagnosis

An upper GI x-ray series and an EGDS have to be done in order to exclude problems at the level of the band.

Rationale

Vassallo et al. (4) proposed in 1997 a duodenal switch done by laparotomy, in addition to a transitory gastroplasty or an absorbable band of polydioxanone, preserving the stomach entirely. In this series the patients experienced no diarrhea or protein deficiency. Sleeve gastrectomy was added to the duodenal switch (5) to reduce the marginal ulcer incidence and to add some sort of restriction. The work of De Meester has demonstrated that the preservation of 3 to 4 cm of viable duodenum is enough to greatly reduce the incidence of marginal ulcers. Moreover, a restriction can be achieved by applying a Lap-Band, therefore avoiding a sleeve gastric resection with its irreversibility, risk of bleeding, leakage, and stenosis.

Results

From 1994 to June 2003, 40 patients underwent a bandinaro at our institutions as a second choice/remedial surgery after failed gastric restrictive procedures [four had a previous open vertical banded gastroplasty (VBG), 22 an open adjustable silicone gastric banding, and 14 a laparoscopic Lap-Band]. In 12 cases the bandinaro procedure was done by laparoscopy. The morbidity in the open group has been one case of pancreatitis and one case of internal hernia, both requiring reoperation. In the laparoscopic group we had two duodeno-ileal fistulas, which underwent successful conservative treatment. The weight loss was very satisfactory, and it is shown in Figures 20.5-22 and 20.5-23. In fact, these patients lose an average of more than 60 kg, and reach in excess of 75% EWL.

Conversion to Another Bariatric Procedure

Failure of restrictive procedures can also be treated with conversion to a gastric bypass or a purely malabsorptive procedure. Failed VBG and adjustable gastric banding can effectively be treated with conversion to gastric bypass (38,39). Though these procedures are technically

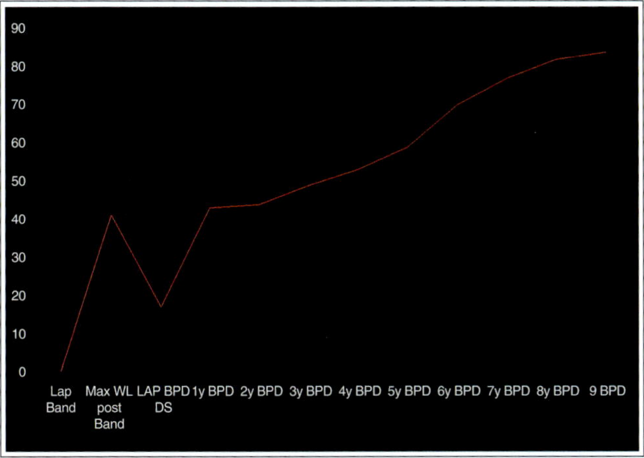

FIGURE 20.5-23. Bandinaro weight loss in percent excess weight loss.

demanding, several series have reported the safety and efficacy of this approach to treat failed weight loss or complications related to the Lap-Band (38–44). In a series of 70 patients who underwent conversion of LAGB to laparoscopic Roux-en-Y gastric bypass (LRYGBP), the early complication rate was 14%, the late major complication rate was 9%, and there was no perioperative mortality. Three patients were converted to an open procedure due to extensive adhesions. The indications for conversion to gastric bypass were inadequate weight loss (25%) or weight regain (49%), symptomatic pouch dilation (20%), erosion (5%), and psychological intolerance of the band in one patient. The mean operative time was 240 minutes. At 18 months of follow-up, mean EWL was 70%, and 60% of the patients achieved a BMI <33 during that time (41). Weber et al. (44) retrospectively reviewed 62 patients who failed LAGB and underwent either rebanding (n = 30) or LRYGBP (n = 32) over a 7-year period. Both procedures were performed with low complication rates and mortality was absent. One year after revision, the mean BMI in the LRYGBP group had decreased from 42 to 32 while the BMI in the re-banding group had remained unchanged at 38. These authors concluded that gastric bypass is the rescue therapy of choice after failed LAGB.

Conversion to BPD after failed Lap-Band is another option in this group of patients. In a series by Dolan and Fielding including 1439 LAGB patients, band removal was performed in 85 patients, and the most common reasons for removal were persistent dysphagia (29%), recurrent slippage (28%), failure to lose weight (16%), and intolerance (14%). Erosion occurred in six patients (7% of removals). A total of 79 patients underwent band removal with simultaneous conversion to BPD or BPD and duodenal switch (BPD-DS) (open or laparoscopic). The average BMI at the time of revision was 46. Thirty-eight patients had synchronous band removal and laparoscopic BPD. There were no major complications in this group. Excess weight loss at 1 year was 37%, less than is seen with primary BPD, and eight patients (21% of lap BPD patients) failed to lose weight after laparoscopic BPD and required shortening of their common channel. Laparoscopic BPD-DS was performed with band removal in 21 patients. There was one gastric staple line leak, and %EWL at 12 months was 28%. Six of these patients (18%) required shortening of the common channel to 40cm. Despite shortening the common channel after laparoscopic BPD or BPD-DS in 14 patients who failed to lose weight initially, five continued to have minimal or no weight loss.

Removal of the band with simultaneous conversion to a malabsorptive procedure can be performed safely in experienced hands. As evidenced by Dolan's study, though, a small subset of patients will be refractory to any bariatric procedure. Laparoscopic conversion from Lap-Band to gastric bypass is also an effective option for patients who have failed the gastric banding. As more experience is gained with these conversion procedures, the optimal approach for a failed Lap-Band will become more clearly defined.

Conclusion

The Lap-Band has proven to be remarkably safe. Given the anesthetic and operative risk status of these patients, it is difficult to think of any surgical procedure that could have a better safety record than Lap-Band placement. The minimally invasive nature of the procedure—no cutting, stapling, or alteration of the anatomy—tends to keep the complication rate down, especially serious complications.

There are some clear requirements for the successful use of the Lap-Band. Though these requirements are not difficult or unusual, they are essential. The surgeon needs to have good laparoscopic skill and bariatric experience. Reasonable competence and experience can be achieved with good, specifically oriented training and proctoring. There must be a commitment to the patients, to their education and support, to their ongoing routine care and problems. This commitment is best realized by a multidisciplinary support team (dietitian, psychologist, internist, and surgeon).

Because of the ability to adjust the degree of restriction, the weight loss is achieved in a gradual way. Ideally, it occurs slowly over 2 years or longer and should not be associated with symptoms of severe restriction or vomiting, but rather with a sense of satiety before eating and an early sense of fullness after eating small amounts.

The Lap-Band is the only bariatric surgical procedure that is entirely reversible. Patients are not trapped permanently into a state of distorted anatomy that can only be undone with difficulty. It is comforting for both the patient and the surgeon that, should the need arise, the band can easily be removed and the stomach allowed to return to normal.

Most Lap-Band complications are not life threatening and, when they do occur, many can be remedied laparoscopically.

The evolution of the procedure, with modifications to the device and the technique, has served to greatly reduce the incidence of complications. And, of course, avoiding complications in the first place is always the best complication management strategy. When complications and failed weight loss do occur after Lap-Band, revisional surgery may be required. Addition of a malabsorptive procedure (our approach) or conversion to laparoscopic gastric bypass, BPD, or BPD-DS can be accomplished safely with excellent results for most patients.

References

1. Forestieri P, Meucci L, De Luca M, Formato A, De Werra C, Chiacchio C. Two years of practice in adjustable silicone gastric banding (Lap-Band): evaluation of variations of body mass index, percentage ideal body weight and percentage excess body weight. Obes Surg 1998;8:49–52.

2. Mittermair RP, Weiss H, Nehoda H, Aigner F. Uncommon intragastric migration of the Swedish adjustable gastric band. Obes Surg 2002;12:372–375.

3. Baldinger R, Mluench R, Steffen R, et al. Conservative management of intragastric migration of the Swedish adjustable gastric band by endoscopic retrieval. Gastrointest Endosc 2001;53:98–101.

4. Vassallo C, Negri L, Della Valle A, et al. Biliopancreatic diversion with transitory gastroplasty preserving the duodenal bulb: 3 year experience. Obes Surg 1997;7:30–33.

5. Hess DS, Hess DW. Biliopancreatic diversion with duodenal switch. Obes Surg 1998;8:267–282.

6. Cadiere GB, Favretti F, Himpens J, Segato G, Capelluto E. Anneau gastrique et derivation bilio-pancreatique par laproscopie. J Coelio Chir 2001;38:33–35.

7. Oria HE. Silicone adjustable gastric banding for morbid obesity. Systematic review update, January 1999–May 2000. Obes Surg 2000;10:322–323.

8. Chelala E, Cadiére GB, Favretti F, et al. Conversions and complications in 185 laparoscopic adjustable silicone gastric banding cases. Surg Endosc 1997;11:268–271.

9. O'Brien P, Brown W, Smith A, et al. The Lap-Band provides effective control of morbid obesity—a prospective study of 350 patients followed for up to 4 years. Obes Surg 1998; 8:398.

10. Belva PH, Takieddine M, Lefebvre JC, Vaneukem P. Laparoscopic lap-band gastroplasty: European results. Obes Surg 1998;8:364.

11. Castillo Gonzáles A, Wiella GR, Cordero AR. Banda gastrica ajustable para el tratamiento de la obesidad severa: comunicacion preliminar. Cirujano Gen 1996;18(4):324–329.

12. Favretti F, Cadiére GB, Segato G, et al. Laparoscopic adjustable silicone gastric banding (Lap-Band®): how to avoid complications. Obes Surg 1997;7:352–358.

13. Natalini G, Carloni G, Cappelletti S, et al. Laparoscopic adjustable silicone gastric banding (LASGB) for treatment of morbid obesity. Obes Surg 1997;7:310.

14. Dargent J. Laparoscopic adjustable gastric banding: lessons from the first 500 patients in a single institution. Obes Surg 1999;9:446–452.

15. Biesheuvel TH, Sintenie JB, Pels Rijcken TH, Hoitsma HFW. Laparoscopic adjustable silicone gastric banding for treating morbid obesity in the centre of Amsterdam. Obes Surg 1998;8:360.

16. Spivak H, Favretti F. Avoiding postoperative complications with the Lap-Band system. Am J Surg 2002;184:31S–37S.

17. Belachew M, Legrand MJ, Defechereux TH, Burtheret MP, Jacquet N. Laparoscopic adjustable silicone gastric banding in the treatment of morbid obesity, a preliminary report. Surg Endosc 1994;8:1354–1356.

18. Cadière GB, Favretti F, Bruyns J, Himpens J, Lise M. Gastroplastie par coelio-videoscopie: technique. J Coelio Chir 1994;10:27–31.

19. Fielding G, Allen J. A step-by-step guide to placement of the Lap-Band adjustable gastric banding system. Am J Surg 2002;184:26S–31S.

20. Weiner R, Bockhorn H, Rosenthal R, Wagner D. A prospective randomized trial of different laparoscopic gastric banding techniques for morbid obesity. Surg Endosc 2001;15: 63–68.

21. Favretti F, Cadiere GB, Segato G, et al. Laparoscopic banding: selection and technique in 830 patients. Obes Surg 2002; 12:385–390.

22. Belachew M, Zimmermann J-M. Evolution of a paradigm for laparoscopic adjustable gastric banding. Am J Surg 2002;184:21S–25S.

23. Niville E, Dams A. Late pouch dilation after laparoscopic adjustable gastric and esophagogastric banding: incidence, treatment and outcome. Obes Surg 1999;9:381–384.

24. U.S. Food and Drug Administration, Center for Devices and Radiological Health. Lap-Band Adjustable Gastric Banding (LAGB) System-P000008. http:www.fda.gov/cdrh/pdf/p000008.htm.

25. Belachew M, Belva PH, Desaive C. Long-term results of laparoscopic adjustable gastric banding for the treatment of morbid obesity. Obes Surg 2002;12:564–568.

26. Cadiere GB, Himpens J, Vertruyen M, et al. Laparoscopic gastroplasty (adjustable silicone gastric banding). Semin Laparosc Surg 2000;7:55–65.

27. Fielding GA, Rhodes M, Nathanson LK. Laparoscopic gastric banding for morbid obesity: surgical outcome in 335 cases. Surg Endosc 1999;13:550–554.

28. Vertruyen M. Experience with Lap-Band system up to 7 years. Obes Surg 2002;12:569–572.

29. Turicchia G, Grandi U, Giusti E, Stancanelli V. Laparoscopic adjustable silicone gastric banding (LASGB) for morbid obesity: preliminary experience. Obes Surg 1995; 5:259.

30. Carbajo Caballero MA, Martin del Olmo JC, Blanco Alvarez JI, et al. Intragastric migration of laparoscopic adjustable gastric band (Lap-Band) for morbid obesity. J Laparoendosc Adv Surg Tech 1998;8(4):241–244.

31. Abu-Abeid S. LAGB erosions. Presented to the American Society for Bariatric Surgery, Memphis, June 2000.

32. Meir E, Van Baden M. Adjustable silicone gastric banding (ASGB) and band erosion (BE). Obes Surg 1998;8: 385.

33. De Jong ICDYM, Tan KG, Oostenbroek RJ. Adjustable silicone gastric banding: a series with three cases of band erosion. Obes Surg 2000;10:26–32.

34. Meir E, Van Baden M. Adjustable silicone gastric banding and band erosion: personal experience and hypotheses. Obes Surg 1999;9:191–193.

35. Chevallier JM, Zinzindohoue F, Elian N, et al. Adjustable gastric banding in a public university hospital: prospective analysis of 400 patients. Obes Surg 2002;12:93–99.

36. Susmallian S, Ezri T, Charuzi I. Laparoscopic repair of access port site hernia after Lap-Band® system implantation. Obes Surg 2002;12:682–684.

37. Fabry H, Van Hee R, Hendrickx L, Totté E. A technique for prevention of port complications after laparoscopic

adjustable silicone gastric banding. Obes Surg 2002;12: 285–288.

38. Gonzalez R, Gallagher SF, Haines K, Murr MM. Operative technique for converting a failed vertical banded gastroplasty to Roux-en-Y gastric bypass. J Am Coll Surg 2005; 201(3):366–374.

39. Westling A, Ohrvall M, Gustavsson S. Roux-en-Y gastric bypass after previous unsuccessful gastric restrictive surgery. J Gastrointest Surg 2002;6(2):206–211.

40. Kothari SN, DeMaria EJ, Sugerman HJ, et al. Lap-band failures: conversion to gastric bypass and their preliminary outcomes. Surgery 2002;131(6):625–629.

41. Mognol P, Chosidow D, Marmuse JP. Laparoscopic conversion of laparoscopic gastric banding to Roux-en-Y gastric bypass: a review of 70 patients. Obes Surg 2004;14(10): 1349–1353.

42. van Wageningen B, Berends FJ, Van Ramshorst B, Janssen IF. Revision of failed laparoscopic adjustable gastric banding to Roux-en-Y gastric bypass. Obes Surg 2006;16(2): 137–141.

43. Calmes JM, Giusti V, Suter M. Reoperative laparoscopic Roux-en-Y gastric bypass: an experience with 49 cases. Obes Surg 2005;15(3):316–322.

44. Weber M, Muller MK, Michel JM, et al. Laparoscopic Roux-en-Y gastric bypass, but not rebanding, should be proposed as rescue procedure for patients with failed laparoscopic gastric banding. Ann Surg 2003;238(6):827–833; discussion 833–834.

20.6
Laparoscopic Adjustable Gastric Banding: Controversies

Mohammad K. Jamal, Eric J. DeMaria, and Ricardo Cohen

Background

Laparoscopic adjustable gastric banding (LAGB) has been proposed as a treatment of choice for morbid obesity by many bariatric surgeons around the world. It has been the most commonly performed bariatric procedure in Australia and Europe since the early 1990s (1). After its approval in 2001 in the United States by the Food and Drug Administration (FDA), the use of the Lap-Band has increased and has provided patients with an alternative treatment to the Roux-en-Y gastric bypass (RYGBP). The LAGB is a purely restrictive procedure like the vertical banded gastroplasty (VBG), thereby excluding any bowel anastomosis, staple line complications, or risk of leaks. As evident from the long-term follow-up of purely restrictive procedures like VBG, excess weight loss and consequent cure of comorbidities may be modest when compared to other procedures such as the RYGBP or combined restrictive and malabsorptive procedures. Furthermore, minimal long-term weight loss benefits of VBG have suggested that this procedure is not durable.

Initial trials with the LAGB in the United States were disappointing. Thirty-six patients underwent placement of the Lap-Band at the Medical College of Virginia Hospitals between March 1996 and May 1998 as part of the A trial of the device in the United States under an Investigational Device Exemption from the FDA (2). All patients accepted for Lap-Band placement included those specifically requesting the procedure, patients with a preoperative body mass index (BMI) less than 50, patients with no or limited previous abdominal operations, and patients in whom dietary screening did not reveal a significant calorie intake in the form of sweets. The Lap-Band was placed using a standard laparoscopic technique (3).

To date 18 of 36 (50%) Lap-Bands have been removed. Indications for removal and conversions included failed weight loss (defined as loss of <50% of excess weight or a BMI >35), failed weight loss with esophageal dilatation, failed weight loss with leaking band, and esophageal dilatation with frequent emesis. Fourteen of 18 were converted to a gastric bypass involving either laparoscopic ($n = 8$) or open ($n = 5$) techniques. Overall mean percentage excess weight loss (%EWL) was 62% (range 29–106%); 43% of the weight loss was after conversion to a gastric bypass, whereas only 19% was after Lap-Band placement. Similar resolution of comorbid conditions was only seen after conversion to RYGBP (Table 20.6-1). African-American patients demonstrated very poor weight loss as compared to Caucasians following LAGB. The two groups demonstrated no significant differences in preoperative body weight, percent of ideal body weight (%IBW), or BMI. However, the postoperative percentage decreases in excess body weight and weight lost in kilograms was lower in African Americans at 12-, 24-, and 36-month follow-up. Of the 18 patients with the Lap-Band in place, the mean percentage of excess weight loss was only 32%.

In another study, Angrissani et al. (4) reported the results of the Italian Collaborative Study Group for the Lap-Band system. The LAGB was performed on 1863 patients recruited in the study with a mean BMI of 43.7. Weight loss was evaluated at 6, 12, 24, 36, 48, 60, and 72 months, at which times the BMI was 37.9, 33.7, 34.8, 34.1, 32.7, 34.8, and 32, respectively. The overall mortality was 0.53%, whereas the open conversion rate was 3.1%, being higher in super-obese (BMI $\geq$50) than in morbidly obese patients (BMI <50). Most common complications reported were tube-port failure, gastric pouch dilatation, and gastric erosion. No data on resolution of obesity-related comorbidities were provided in this study. The data from several studies show only a modest decline in BMI after placement of the Lap Band (Table 20.6-2).

More recent data suggests that weight loss after LAGB in the U.S. studies averages 41% at 1-year follow-up which is inferior to the 53% to 64% EWL reported in most European studies. Resolution of comorbidities after

TABLE 20.6-1. Resolution of comorbid conditions

Comorbidity	n	Resolution with Lap-Band	Resolution after conversion to gastric bypass
Diabetes	4	0	3
Stress urinary incontinence	5	2	2
Degenerative joint disease	10	1	3
Gastroesophageal reflux	5*	1	4

* Three additional patients developed reflux only after placement of Lap-Band. These three patients had resolution after conversion to gastric bypass.

LAGB is also modest, with a reported resolution of type 2 diabetes mellitus in 64% of patients, with a slight improvement in insulin sensitivity and β-cell function (5).

It has been claimed lately that LAGB is less "aggressive" than the other laparoscopic procedures. That may be true if the surgical technique and anatomic/physiologic changes are taken into consideration. However, it is important to stress that obesity is currently the second largest cause of preventable death in the United States and a devastating disease, with its incidence and associated complication rate rising exponentially every year. Surgery is currently the most effective proven treatment to control this epidemic, and the RYGBP is the gold-standard operation. Hence, the evaluation of any other surgical treatment should be based on comparison with the RYGBP, in terms of EWL, resolution of comorbid conditions, long-term benefits, and low morbidity and mortality. An operation like the gastric bypass, performed by experts, cannot be classified as overtly aggressive if its results are good or even excellent regarding weight loss and cure of comorbidities, if it carries a low risk of morbidity and mortality, and if it can be done using minimally invasive techniques. Can the operative mortality from gastric bypass be compared to deaths secondary to undertreated morbid obesity? The answer is yes—morbid obesity and its associated conditions are more aggressive and lethal than morbidity from proven effective surgical treatments such as the laparoscopic RYGBP (LRYGBP).

As shown by several studies, LAGB is characterized by a lack of cure of comorbid conditions secondary to non-efficient weight loss, with deaths occurring due to persistent obesity and associated illnesses, and complications occurring related to the device itself, to the injection port, and to other reasons (3,6–8). One should not forget that LAGB may result in a higher incidence of vomiting and possible corruption of eating behavior, resulting in a poor quality of life.

There are many controversial topics in the field of bariatric surgery today. One of the points of current debate is the choice of the best bariatric procedure. The proponents of LAGB claim that it is currently the best approach to treat morbidly and super-obese patients, but this claim is controversial. The main goal of a successful bariatric surgeon is to provide the best weight loss surgical option for the patient. The LAGB may be technically easier, but there are a considerable number of topics that need to be addressed, an important one being proper patient selection.

Patient Selection

Several studies have shown that patients with sweet-eating behavior are not suitable candidates for pure restrictive procedures. But how easy is it to identify them? Do obese patients regularly tell surgeons or dieti-

TABLE 20.6-2. Summary of recent Lap-Band results in the literature

Author	Year	n	BMI pre/post (1-year follow-up)	Complication rate (%)	Reoperation rate
Angrissani	2003	1863	44/34	10.2	N/I
O'Brien	2002	709	45/35	19	19
Angrissani	1999	40	45/33	20	10
Furbetta	1999	201	43/35	4.4	4.4
Angrissani	1999	31	45/29	26	23
Foresteiri	1998	62	50/38	N/I	3.3
Favretti	2002	830	46/37	15	3.9
Abu-Abeid	1999	391	43/31	4.1	6.6
Miller	1999	158	44/34	8.2	7
DeMaria	2001	36	45/36	N/I	41
Ponce	2005	1014	48/37	5.5	4.8

BMI, body mass index; N/I, not identified on review.

tians that they are sweet or binge eaters? What is the successful screening rate of those patients? Surely, the incidence of sweet-eaters is greater than we think, and consequently, improper screening of such candidates will lead to poor outcomes. Furthermore, it is always possible for patients to change their food choices, especially after a bariatric procedure (e.g., by increasing carbohydrate intake), rendering the procedure unsuccessful. Many screening tests have been proposed, but all have severe limitations. If this factor is taken into account, the number of appropriate candidates for an LAGB will decrease dramatically. Other consequences of bad judgment in selecting patients for LAGB, in addition to poor weight loss, are discussed later in this chapter.

Surgical Technique

The LAGB is a technically easier laparoscopic procedure than the laparoscopic RYGBP (LRYGBP) or the laparoscopic biliopancreatic diversion (LBPD). Pars flaccida or perigastric dissection and band positioning have been widely discussed in the literature, and there is general agreement that the first approach is the best as it has fewer complications, such as posterior gastric perforation and band prolapse. Several studies support the pars flaccida approach and more authors seem to favor and recommend this technique (9–11).

The question of whether the LAGB is easy enough to be performed by novice bariatric/laparoscopic surgeons in a patient possessing multiple comorbidities remains unanswered. Should the guidelines for performing this procedure be stricter and more specific for morbidly obese patients? Is it necessary to verify that the surgeon can identify a complication or failure of the method and be ready to perform a revision? All we know is that the learning curve for performing the LAGB is probably less steep than for the LRYGBP. The answers to these questions are perhaps as varied as the number of bariatric surgeons themselves.

Operative time, which was a major point that used to favor gastric banding, is no longer an issue today. Skilled and well-trained bariatric surgeons are performing the LRYGBP safely in the same time it takes to place a Lap-Band.

Adjustments

The strategies for band adjustment are as varied as the number of surgeons performing the procedure. Some advocate that this adjustability is the major factor that could differentiate LAGB results from the past bad outcomes of VBG. The following questions arise in the minds of surgeons performing LAGB adjustments: Is sterile technique required? Is fluoroscopic guidance necessary? Is the swallow test after the adjustment enough to determine if the band's inflation was sufficient? What is the best period for adjustment? What time interval should be allowed between adjustments?

It is recommended that the first adjustment should be performed no less than 1 month after surgery to avoid a higher incidence of vomiting and band prolapse. Most authors recommend placing patients on a liquid diet for at least 6 weeks, after which graduated inflation of the balloon should be undertaken. This should be guided by clinical evaluation of symptoms and weight loss at follow-up. The Swedish manufacturer of the gastric band (SAGB, AB Obtech, Sweden) recommended that patients leave the operating room with the band adjusted with 1 mL of saline, claiming that no higher rates of complications occurred and weight loss was more effective. This claim was not made by the other major band manufacturer.

In our experience with the Lap-Band (the FDA A trial), saline was added to the band reservoir under fluoroscopic guidance based on the patient's weight loss and satiety. Serial upper gastrointestinal studies, as mandated by the trial, were obtained during the follow-up period. More recent data suggest that serial upper gastrointestinal series and gastroscopy should be limited to patients with suspected complications or inadequate weight loss. These adjustments generally can be made in an outpatient clinic setting using sterile technique. Recent reports of dynamic radioisotope scintigraphy (DRS) using technetium (Tc)-99-phytate–labeled plain yogurt for band adjustment have emerged in the bariatric surgical literature. Long-term data to support the widespread use of this technique are lacking.

Postoperative Follow-Up

Follow-up is an interesting point of controversy. The LRYGBP patients need much less follow-up than do LAGB patients. The latter patients' bands need to be adjusted, and they have a higher incidence of vomiting, discomfort, and initial lack of weight loss than do the LRYGB or the LBPD patients. A few years ago we had more than five times the number of LRYGBP patients than LAGB patients, but we took five times more calls from the latter patients.

The almost complete absence of nutritional complications is balanced by the adaptation of eating habits that may be deleterious in some patients. It has been frequently reported that many patients develop sweet-eating behaviors when faced with postoperative limitations of oral intake quantity. Dietary counseling may help to prevent such oral indiscretions. More commonly, patients who act on their craving for sweets either fail to lose weight or regain their lost weight.

Complications

Chevallier et al. (12) reported his experience with over 1000 patients who underwent LAGB. In their series, intraoperative complications included gastric and esophageal perforations ($n = 3$), liver injuries ($n = 4$), failure to insert the band ($n = 7$), and conversion to an open procedure ($n = 12$). Their more notable postoperative complications included slippage of the band ($n = 104$), band migration ($n = 3$), and esophageal dilatation ($n = 5$). Complications specific to the port occurred in 57 patients and included infection, disruption, leakage of the tube, and rotation.

In another series reported by Favretti et al. (13), the records of 830 consecutive patients undergoing laparoscopic placement of the adjustable band were reviewed. Major complications requiring reoperation occurred in 4% (36 patients) including one gastric perforation, early (one case) and late (17 cases) gastric prolapse, nine malpositionings, four gastric erosions, three cases of psychological intolerance, and one HIV conversion (band removed). Overall, their data revealed that 142 of 479 patients (30%) experienced poor weight loss (<30% reduction in excess weight) over 3 years of follow-up, although the report incorrectly suggests this figure to be 20%. Clearly, reoperation for complications and failure of laparoscopic banding procedures will become increasingly common as more of these procedures are done in the United States. Some of the more notable complications are discussed in the following subsections.

Esophageal Dilatation

Few surgeons described any routine contrast studies of the gastrointestinal tract in the follow-up of LAGB unless patients present with a complaint indicating a complication. In the United States, the FDA-sponsored A trial contrast studies were mandatory and showed surprising results, with about 50% of patients having radiologically confirmed esophageal dilatation, with the consequent symptoms of reflux and vomiting. Once the diagnosis of esophageal dilatation was made, band deflation was undertaken. But esophageal dilatation and dysmotility symptoms persisted, requiring conversion to a gastric bypass procedure in five patients. In 2002, a new technique was described that placed the band around the distal esophagus. The research group is convinced that a forced achalasia with dysphagia is very important as a weight loss mechanism, and that the absence of these symptoms will frequently lead to poor results.

Why are these findings not being reported by surgeons with large LAGB numbers? Are symptoms not recorded or not considered important? Is dysphagia an important tool used by surgeons in the process of re-education of eating habits? Are contrast studies almost never being performed, so esophageal dysmotility/dilatation is not diagnosed? The topic of esophageal dysmotility is one of the major controversies regarding gastric banding, only second to differences in weight loss. How important is it? Is deflating the band the only measure to control it? Is it really reversible? Or similar to Chagas' disease, is it a progressive myoelectrical pathology secondary to the presence of a foreign body around the gastroesophageal junction that at a given point will be irreversible? Only long-term follow-up will answer these questions and provide the crucial information about the problems of esophageal dilatation and dysphagia.

Reflux

This is another point of controversy with many viewpoints. Some authors, including Overbo et al. (14) and Doherty et al. (15), described an increased incidence of acid regurgitation, vomiting, and reflux after placing the LAGB. It is described with a high incidence of food intolerance unresponsive to band deflation. What could be the possible mechanism? Stomal stenosis and pouch dilatation were the probable causes. However, there is no correlation, at least documented, that esophageal dysmotility could play an important role in the etiology of severe reflux.

On the other hand, O'Brien et al. (9), and Favretti et al. (13) do not even list reflux as an important factor in the poor quality of life in the follow-up of band patients. Gastroesophageal reflux disease (GERD) with or without a hiatal hernia (regardless of the severity) diagnosed in the preoperative screening is not considered a contraindication for LAGB by these authors. In fact, Favretti and Cadiere et al. (11) reported a 55% improvement in GERD after LAGB. In 2002, Schauer's group (16) reported that the best surgical approach to morbidly obese patients with GERD is the laparoscopic gastric bypass. These different approaches to morbidly obese patients by different authors are confusing, and their treatment remains unclear. Theoretically, the logic behind the improvement of GERD after LAGB is difficult to explain. How is a prosthesis, placed close to the gastroesophageal (GE) junction and tightened gradually to provide slow, graded emptying with anatomic and physiologic continuity (like normal acid production), different from the small gastric reservoir performed during the LRYGBP? This question remains unanswered.

The fact is, if one follows band and bypass patients closely and compares their gastrointestinal complaints, the first group will have more symptoms such as dysphagia to solids, vomiting, and heartburn. It is probable that long-term follow-up can shed light on such differences between surgical results regarding issues of esophageal dysmotility, GERD, and vomiting after LAGB.

Gastric Pouch Dilatation and Band Slippage

One of the common indications for reoperation after LAGB is gastric pouch dilatation (GPD) (6,7), with an incidence ranging from 3% to 20% in different series. This may occur with or without band slippage. The diagnosis of GPD is based on clinical symptoms of food intolerance and esophagitis and confirmed by radiologic studies showing obstruction of the proximal pouch without transit through the band. Suter (8) attributed the pouch dilatation to initial malpositioning of the gastric band. The GPD is of limited significance in most cases, but large or asymmetrical dilatations are ultimately associated with slippage of the band and a subsequent change in its axis. This may lead initially to a progressive increase in food intake, dysphagia, and ultimately weight gain. In Suter's series of 272 patients who underwent LAGB, 20 (7.4%) developed pouch dilatation or slippage. Nineteen of them required reoperation because of severe reflux, failure to lose weight, weight regain, or a combination of these factors. Nine patients underwent laparoscopic band repositioning, whereas the rest underwent band change (n = 4) or conversion to a vertical band gastroplasty (n = 2) or RYGBP (n = 4). The initial mean weight was 129 kg with a mean BMI of 44.5. The mean maximal weight loss since gastric banding was 38.7 kg, the mean BMI was 32.6, and the mean body weight was 95 kg. The average time between initial gastric banding and reoperation was 20 months. The results following laparoscopic repositioning were described as good in two patients, satisfactory in one, and poor in six patients. Further reoperations in this group consisted of band removal in three patients and LRYGBP in two patients.

Risk factors for GPD may include early consumption of solid food, early inflation of the band, consumption of carbonated beverages, and vomiting, but band location is likely the most important. In the early experience with LAGB, the band was placed within the lesser sac on the posterior stomach wall, creating a larger pouch (up to 25 mL), with a high incidence of pouch dilatation and slippage (17–22). The incidence of this complication has been lower with the Swedish adjustable gastric band (SAGB) device, which has been placed above the lesser sac, resulting in a smaller pouch (15 mL). Many series show that pouch dilatation and band slippage can be dramatically reduced by creating a "virtual" tiny pouch above the lesser sac, with band fixation using anterior gastrogastric sutures near the cardioesophageal junction.

If band deflation fails as a first-line conservative measure to treat GPD and slippage, surgery is indicated, usually in the form of band removal/replacement or conversion to a procedure like RYGBP or biliopancreatic diversion with duodenal switch.

Weight Loss and Resolution of Comorbidities

It is clear that LAGB produces less weight loss when compared to the LRYGBP or other malabsorptive procedures. Though restrictive procedures may not lead to significant nutritional consequences, they are generally not as effective in weight reduction or maintenance. The LAGB patients might develop maladaptive eating behaviors, such as eating concentrated sweets, and a strict preoperative screening process to weed out sweet-eaters cannot prevent this from happening. This may be the major cause of weight-loss failure in purely restrictive procedures like the LAGB.

The other issue is whether surgeons are satisfied or not with their results. O'Brien from Australia considers success to be an excess weight loss (EWL) of at least 25% in a 2-year follow-up. This percentage of EWL is usually achieved by the fourth or fifth month in LRYGBP patients. Most authors consider surgery a failure if less than 50% of EWL is obtained. The average EWL in large LAGB series in a 5-year follow-up is about 55%, whereas the mean EWL in LRYGBP series varies from 68% to 75% in the same period of follow-up.

It was already reported that even a small weight loss could bring major improvements in comorbidities. A cure of the high rates of type 2 diabetes mellitus (85–95%), hypertension (65–75%), and sleep apnea (95–100%), easily reproduced in most RYGBP series, is not achieved with LAGB in any published series. An alternative viewpoint would suggest that 30% to 50% improvement in comorbidities would be better than none! Another important and interesting aspect reported in the A trial was the poor weight loss seen in African-American patients and minimal improvement in associated illnesses. Similar results were found in Brazil, where Caucasians had a better weight loss.

Reversibility and Reoperations

The LAGB procedure results in a lack of adhesions and it is easily reversible. If slippage is found, the prosthesis can be repositioned, as advocated by some, or simply taken out if necessary. But if any other problem appears, such as erosion, posterior slippage or intraabdominal sepsis without gastric/esophageal perforation, treatment is difficult. Adhesions are often found, as is scar tissue over the gastric wall and surrounding tissues that makes further surgical intervention or revision to another procedure difficult.

The view that placement of the Lap–Band is a minor and nontraumatic step to treat morbid obesity is not well based on scientific evidence. The LAGB fails more often than any other bariatric procedure due to only modest weight loss and a small improvement in associated illnesses. This results in the need for patients to undergo high-risk revisional surgery that in itself is fraught with complications and high leak rates. Considering that there are many sources of complications, such as port problems, tube leakages or failures, and other device-related issues, the incidence of reoperations, even if described as minor, is much higher than in bypass/malabsorptive procedures (15–27% compared with 1.5–4%). Reoperations to revise the injection port/tube may be done as outpatient procedures, but they entail direct and indirect costs.

Conclusion

Because there are other successful bariatric operations, such as the LRYGBP and LBPD, which have well-proven results, the LAGB must demonstrate satisfactory long-term outcomes in terms of excess weight loss with acceptable morbidity and mortality. In addition, it should also show comparable resolution of comorbid conditions just as the other procedures provide in severely obese patients. The LRYGBP has similar results in different surgical practices in different countries, and the mean EWL, cure of comorbidities, and quality of life assessment are comparable and reproducible. That is not true in LAGB studies worldwide, with some groups reporting formidable results, while others report disappointing outcomes. The issues of esophageal dysmotility, reflux, inappropriate eating behavior, and inadequate weight loss must be clarified as LAGB gains wider utilization.

References

1. Martikainen T, Pirinen E, Alhava E, et al. Long-term results, late complications and quality of life in a series of adjustable gastric banding. Obes Surg 2004;14:648–654.
2. Kothari S, DeMaria E, Sugerman H, Kellum J. Lap-Band failures: Conversion to gastric bypass and their preliminary outcomes. Surgery 2002;131:625–629.
3. DeMaria E, Sugerman H, Meador J, et al. High failure rate after laparoscopic adjustable gastric banding for treatment of morbid obesity. Ann Surg 2001;233:809–818.
4. Angrissani L, Furbetta F, Doldi B, et al. Lap Band adjustable gastric banding system: the Italian experience with 1863 patients operated on 6 years. Surg Endosc 2003;17:409–412.
5. Ren C. J. Controversies in bariatric surgery: Evidence-based discussions on laparoscopic adjustable gastric banding. J Gastrointest Surg 2004;8:396–397.
6. Belachew M, Legrand M, Vincent V, et al. Laparoscopic adjustable gastric banding. World J Surg 1998;22:955–963.
7. Weiner R, Wagner D, Bockhorn H. Laparoscopic gastric banding for morbid obesity. J Laparoendosc Adv Surg Tech 1999;9:23–30.
8. Suter M. Laparoscopic band repositioning for pouch dilatation/slippage after gastric banding: disappointing results. Obes Surg 2001;11:507–512.
9. O'Brien PE, Brown WA, Smith A, et al. Prospective study of a laparoscopically-placed adjustable gastric band in the treatment of morbid obesity. Br J Surg 1999;86:113–118.
10. Dargent J. Laparoscopic adjustable gastric banding: lessons from the first 500 patients in a single institution. Obes Surg 1999;9:446–452.
11. Favretti F, Cadiere GB, Segato G, et al. Laparoscopic adjustable silicon gastric banding (Lap-Band®): How to avoid complications. Obes Surg 1997;7:352–358.
12. Chevallier JM, Zinzindohoué F, Douard R. Complications after laparoscopic adjustable gastric banding for morbid obesity: experience with 1,000 patients over 7 years. Obes Surg 2004;14:407–414.
13. Favretti, F, Cadiere, GB, Segato, G, et al. Laparoscopic banding: Selection and techniques in 830 patients. Obes Surg 2002;12:385–390.
14. Overbo KK, Hatlebakk JG, Viste A, et al. Gastroesophageal reflux in morbidly obese patients treated with gastric banding and vertical banded gastroplasty. Ann Surg 1999;228:51–58.
15. Doherty C, Maher JW, Heitshusen DS. Prospective investigation of complications, re-operations and sustained weight loss with an adjustable gastric banding device for treatment of morbid obesity. J Gastrointest Surg 1998;2:102–108.
16. Frezza EE, Ikramuddin S, Gourash W, et al. Symptomatic improvement in gastroesophageal reflux disease (GERD) following laparoscopic Roux-en-Y gastric bypass. Surg Endosc 2002;16(7):1027–1031.
17. Miller K, Hell E. Laparoscopic adjustable gastric banding: a prospective 4-year follow-up study. Obes Surg 1999;9:183–187.
18. Suter M, Giusti V, Heraief E, et al. Early results of laparoscopic gastric banding compared with open vertical banded gastroplasty. Obes Surg 1999;9:374–380.
19. Belachew M, Legrand M, Vincent V, et al. L'approche coelioscopique dans le traitement de la chirurgie de l'obesite morbide. Technique et resultants. Ann Chir 1997;51:165–172.
20. Suter M, Bettschart V, Giusti V, et al. A three-year experience with gastric banding. Surg Endosc 2000;14:532–536.
21. Berrevoet F, Pattyn P, Cardon A, et al. Retrospective analysis of laparoscopic gastric banding technique: short-term and mid-term follow-up. Obes Surg 1999;9:272–275.
22. Chelala E, Cadiere GB, Favretti F, et al. Conversions and complication in 185 laparoscopic adjustable silicon gastric banding cases. Surg Endosc 1997;11:268–271.

21.1
Circular Stapler Technique for Gastroenterostomy

Alan Wittgrove and Tomasz Rogula

In 1993, the first author of this chapter developed the laparoscopic gastric bypass, and in 1994 the technique was first reported with results (1). In this operation, the gastroenterostomy was created with a 21-mm circular stapling device. The technique of stapler anvil placement involves pulling the anvil down from the mouth to the stomach pouch with a wire being placed percutaneously. This technique was derived from the method used in the percutaneous endoscopic gastrostomy tube placement. The key step was the development of the Endopath Stealth endoscopic/conventional circular stapler, 21 mm, by Ethicon Endosurgery (Cincinnati, OH) (2). We used the 21-mm stapler because it creates a uniform and reproducible 12-mm anastomosis and that was the size of the gastroenterostomy we used for over 6 years as we performed the operation via an open laparotomy. This also preserved the minimal gastric pouch, which is essential to long-term weight control (3). We had tried several methods of anvil placement as we were developing the concept of the laparoscopic gastric bypass in nonhuman models. We settled on the transoral placement because we had extensive experience in placing percutaneous endoscopic gastrostomy (PEG) catheters and it was a relatively easy adaptation. No esophageal injury was noted in the first 1400 patients on whom this technique was done as confirmed by endoscopy in every case (1).

Some concerns were reported on possible esophageal injuries and the size of an anvil. To avoid complications, surgeons should adhere to the basic guidelines and use the correct device, as available circular staplers are not generically equivalent. Any forcing maneuvers and pushing of the anvil from above may lead to problems. Also, elevation of the angle of the jaw during traction of the wire from below, and deflation of the endotracheal tube (at times), are important technical details. A stuck anvil is very rare but can be retrieved using endoscopic techniques (3).

Evolution of Laparoscopic Gastric Bypass Technique

The gastric bypass operation has evolved with many variations since the loop gastric bypass was described by Mason and Ito (4) in 1969. Due to many complications such as alkaline gastritis and esophagitis, this operation was abandoned, and the Roux-en-Y technique was developed and refined. Laparoscopic Roux-en-Y gastric bypass was first described in 1994 by Wittgrove et al. (1). The technique involves creation of 15- to 30-mL isolated gastric pouch; a 21-mm stapled circular anastomosis; a 75-cm retrocolic, retrogastric Roux limb, and stapled side-to-side jejunojejunostomy. Wittgrove et al. employ a transoral pull-wire technique to advance the anvil into the small gastric pouch. Many surgeons currently follow this technique; however, some prefer to extend the Roux-limb length to 150 cm or more for super-obese patients. Gagner and colleagues use an antecolic, antegastric Roux limb. It avoids the creation of the retrocolic tunnel, though there are suggestions that it may create tension and increase the risk of stricture at the gastroenterostomy. Champion and Williams (6) describe the gastrojejunal anastomosis using end-side connection with the linear stapling device. Higa et al. (7) successfully perform a hand-sewn gastrojejunostomy. Most surgeons agree that mesenteric defects, including Petersen's defect, should be routinely closed in some fashion. Internal hernias and bowel obstructions have been reported, which have prompted surgeons to begin closing all mesenteric defects or at least trying to better ensure adhesion formation in these locations in some manner.

As outlined above there continues to be debate concerning the formation of the gastrojejunostomy in the Roux-en-Y gastric bypass (RYGBP). Before the laparoscopic era, the gastric anastomosis was commonly performed in a hand-sewn fashion. In general, there are three approaches to the laparoscopic techniques: the circular stapler, the linear stapler, and hand sewn. Some feel the third technique is more technically demanding as described by Higa. Despite the controversies, most agree that the selection of a particular technique mainly depends on surgeons' preferences, their familiarity with the technique, and their expertise. None of these approaches is considered a "gold standard" in laparoscopic bariatric surgery, but it is recommended that surgeons select one technique as their primary procedure. This facilitates developing comfort and expertise in the procedure and presenting the results in the patients as a single series.

Each technique has possible complications, among which gastrointestinal anastomosis leak remains one of the most important. It is considered prudent to check the gastrojejunostomy for leaks before closing the incision. Several methods are described. Many authors place methylene blue solution in the gastric pouch and look for any coloring around the anastomosis. Our technique is to use the endoscope to insufflate air into the gastric pouch, with the small bowel cross-clamped several centimeters distal to the anastomosis. We then observe the anastomosis while it is under irrigation fluid to see if air bubbles escape. This technique allows immediate evaluation of the anastomosis, especially in regard to possible technical errors or bleeding.

Technique for Circular Stapler Gastroenterostomy

The patient is placed in the standard supine position on the operating table (Fig. 21.1-1). Pneumoperitoneum is induced by inserting a Veress needle in the left upper abdominal quadrant, just below the rib margin. The initial operating port is inserted at the umbilicus with the assistance of the laparoscope, and subsequent cannulas are introduced under direct laparoscopic vision. The trocars at

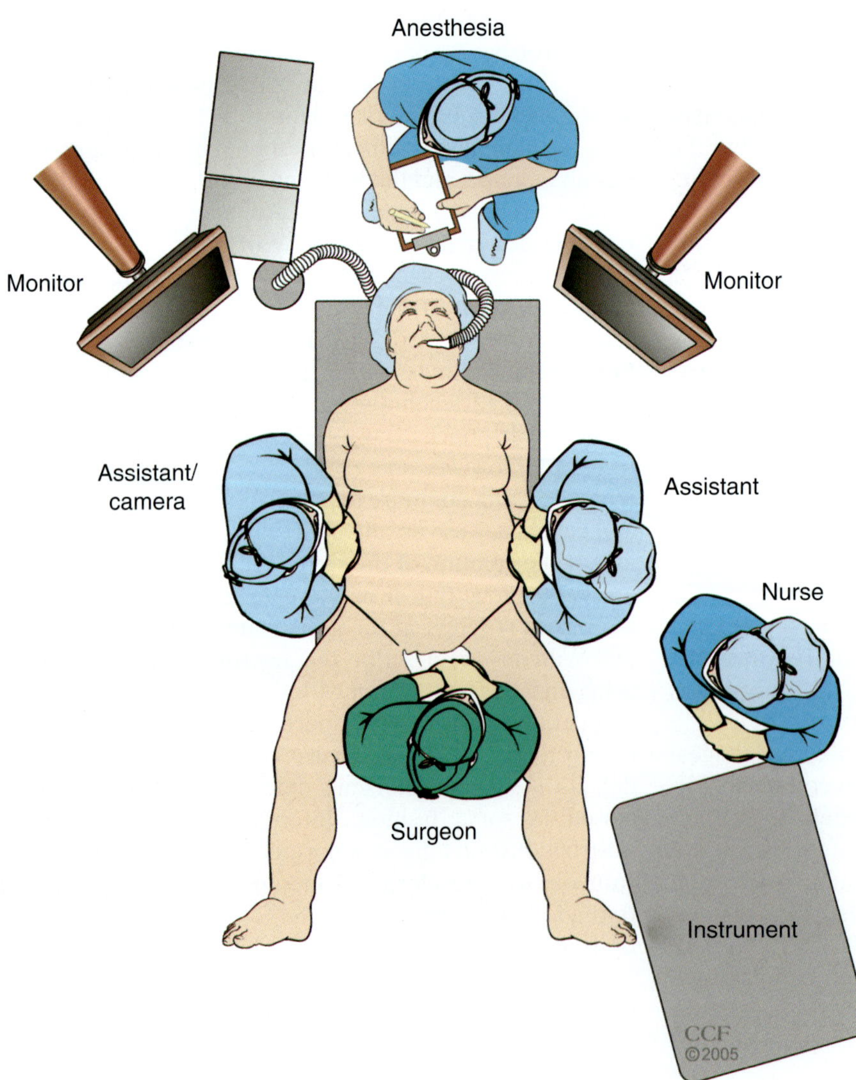

FIGURE 21.1-1. Patient positioning and operating team positions. (Courtesy of the Cleveland Clinic Foundation.)

FIGURE 21.1-2. Creating the gastric pouch with a linear stapler. (Courtesy of the Cleveland Clinic Foundation.)

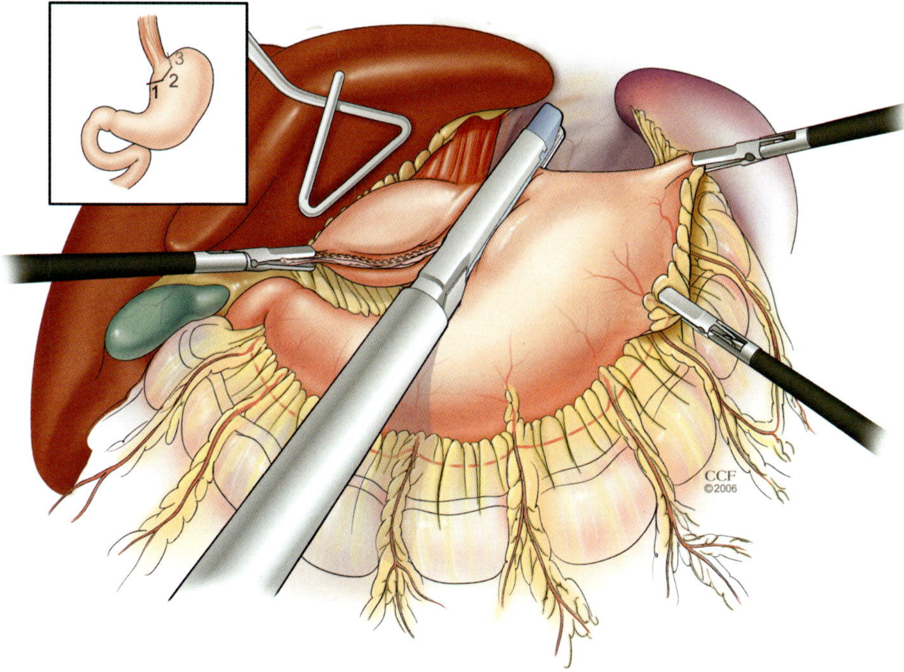

the umbilicus, right upper quadrants and left upper quadrants are 10 to 12 mm in size. We use smooth cannulas but there are ridged cannulas available if the ports come out with repeated instrument movement. A 5-mm port is placed at the subxiphoid area for the liver retractor.

A 5-mm toothed grasper is placed through the subxiphoid port and attached to the diaphragm near the esophagus, to retract the liver. The esophagus is verified and the cardioesophageal junction (angle of His) is identified as the adhesions are taken down under direct visualization. A balloon catheter, such as a Baker jejunostomy tube, is inflated in the body of the stomach and snuggled into the esophagogastric junction. The dissection is begun along the lower edge of the balloon, along the lesser curvature, directly on the gastric wall. The anterior wall of the stomach is elevated for countertraction, and a tunnel is created adjacent to the gastric wall, around the lesser curvature and extending along the posterior gastric wall. An initial application of the linear (45 or 60 mm) stapling device is then made in a horizontal orientation. The dissection is then continued, and the direction of the transection line is turned vertically, aiming for the angle of His (Fig. 21.1-2) and the upper pole of the spleen. Care should be taken to remove the balloon catheter before the stapling device is fired so as to limit the risk of transfixing these catheters in the staple lines.

The pouch should be vertically oriented and of sufficient in size to admit the anvil of the 21-mm circular stapler (about 15 cc). Two to four applications of the 45-mm linear stapler are sufficient to create the proper-sized gastric pouch.

The endoscopist then performs flexible endoscopy of the gastric pouch, and a percutaneous venous cannula is used to introduce a loop suture into the gastric lumen, where it is grasped by the endoscopist and retrieved through the mouth (Fig. 21.1-3). The loop is easily passed through the stem of the Stealth anvil and is then used to draw the anvil, stem-first, through the oropharynx and

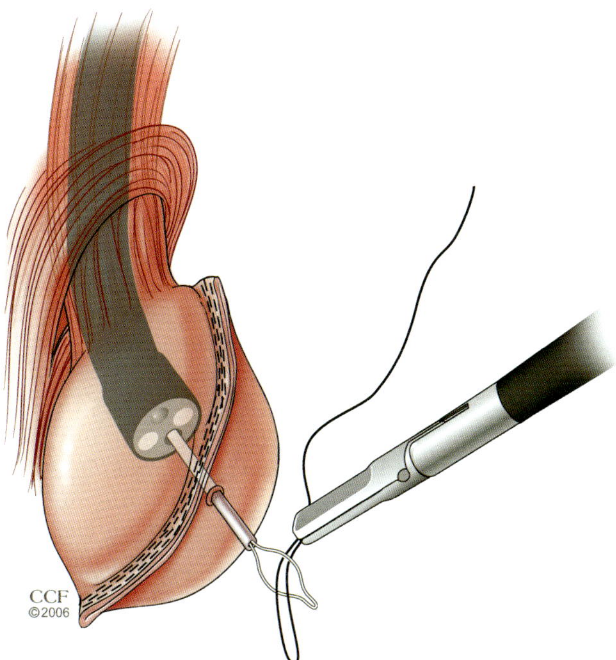

FIGURE 21.1-3. An endoscope is passed into the gastric pouch. A snare is passed through a small posterior gastrotomy and used to pull the guidewire out of the patient's mouth in a retrograde fashion. (Courtesy of the Cleveland Clinic Foundation.)

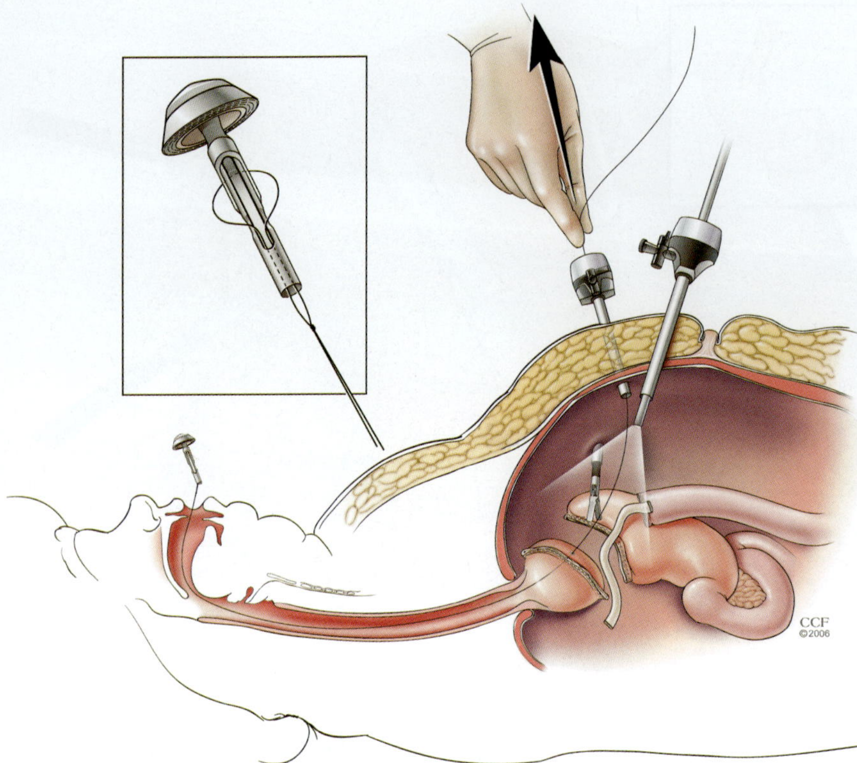

FIGURE 21.1-4. The anvil of the circular stapler is attached to the anvil and is then pulled antegrade into the gastric pouch. (Courtesy of the Cleveland Clinic Foundation.)

esophagus into the stomach pouch (Fig. 21.1-4). The narrowest area of the anvil's transit is at the level of the balloon on the endotracheal tube. If there is difficulty pulling the anvil down the esophagus, momentary deflation of the balloon of the endotracheal tube may be necessary, to allow the anvil into the distal esophagus. The anesthesiologist should maintain control of the endotracheal tube during this maneuver. The anvil is placed under tension, and gentle manipulation is applied to create an opening just large enough to bring the stem through the wall of the stomach pouch. Cautery may be used if the loop is a pull "wire"; however, we use a loop "suture," and cautery should be avoided. The anvil is generally placed through the gastric wall posterior to the staple line. The suture on the anvil serves to elevate the gastric pouch and retract it anteriorly, which tends to facilitate the completion of the gastroenterostomy.

The hepatogastric omentum is opened into the lesser sac and a Penrose drain is placed behind the stomach. This is used to bring the small bowel into the upper abdomen after the enteroenterostomy is completed.

The omentum is retracted into the upper abdomen. The colon is retracted anteriorly and cephalad, and a peritoneal incision is made anterior and to the left of the ligament of Treitz (Fig. 21.1-5). Dissection at this location leads to ready penetration of the mesocolon into the lesser peritoneal sac. A blunt grasping forceps, or reticulating forceps, is then passed behind the colon and stomach into the lesser sac, and a portion of the Penrose drain is grasped and drawn back into the lower abdominal field.

The small bowel is examined, and the proximal jejunum is identified at the ligament of Treitz. The peritoneal reflection must be clearly demonstrated, to avoid misidentification. The small bowel is followed distally for approximately 10 to 12 cm, to reach a comfortable length of small bowel and mesentery. The small bowel is then transected using the linear 45-mm stapling device with minimal transection of the small bowel mesentery, and the proximal end is immediately grasped by the assistant surgeon for identification. The distal end of the transected small bowel is then used to construct the 75-cm Roux limb. A side-to-side enteroenterostomy is then constructed. This is accomplished with two applications of the 35-mm linear stapling device, and the opening for the introduction of the 35-mm stapler is closed with the linear 45-mm (or 60-mm) stapler.

The Penrose drain is then sutured to the distal portion of the previously transected small bowel, and a sufficient length of small bowel, approximately 10 cm, is drawn into the upper abdomen (Fig. 21.1-6). A longitudinal incision is made on the antimesenteric aspect on the small bowel, 5 to 6 cm from the stapled end. The 21-mm circular

FIGURE 21.1-5. An opening is created in the transverse mesocolon for passage of the Roux limb in the retrocolic, retrogastric space. (Courtesy of the Cleveland Clinic Foundation.)

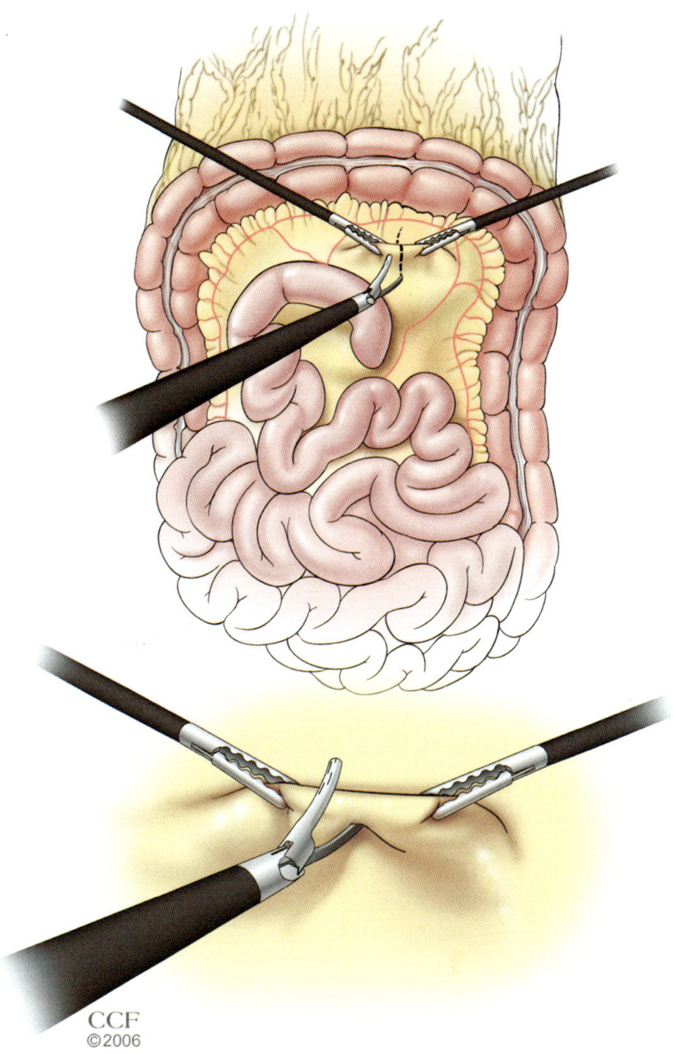

stapler is then inserted directly through the skin at the lower port site on the left. The stapler is introduced into the lumen of the small bowel through the enterotomy and advanced to the stapled end. The stem of the anvil is grasped, using the anvil grasping forceps, through the upper right lateral port. The penetrator of the stapler is then extended, and united with the anvil stem (Fig. 21.1-7). The orientation of the bowel is observed and maintained as the stapler is closed and discharged. The stapler is withdrawn, and the enterotomy is closed with an application of the linear stapling device. Three sutures are placed from the small bowel to the pouch to involute the gastroenterostomy. This closes any potential crossed staple lines and buttresses any potential ischemic gastric tissue between the two staple lines. The small bowel is then cross-clamped, and it is at this point that we perform our final endoscopy with air insufflation.

The small bowel is then returned below the mesocolon, without excess tension, so that the staple line of the closed enterotomy rests at the transverse colon mesentery. This helps to fixate the small bowel and obliterate the potential internal hernia space. We additionally place a suture from the small bowel to the mesentery on the patient's left side to further fixate and close this space. The small bowel mesentery is then closed to minimize internal hernias at the enteroenterostomy site as well.

A drain is placed in the sulcus of the liver and diaphragm, cephalad to the gastroenterostomy and into the subdiaphragmatic space on the left (Fig. 21.1-8). We close the fascia of the left lower port site, where the circular stapler was placed. The fascia at the remaining port sites is not closed. We then place a percutaneous "pain pump" catheter under direct laparoscopic visualization just lateral to the left lower port site, just anterior to the peritoneum.

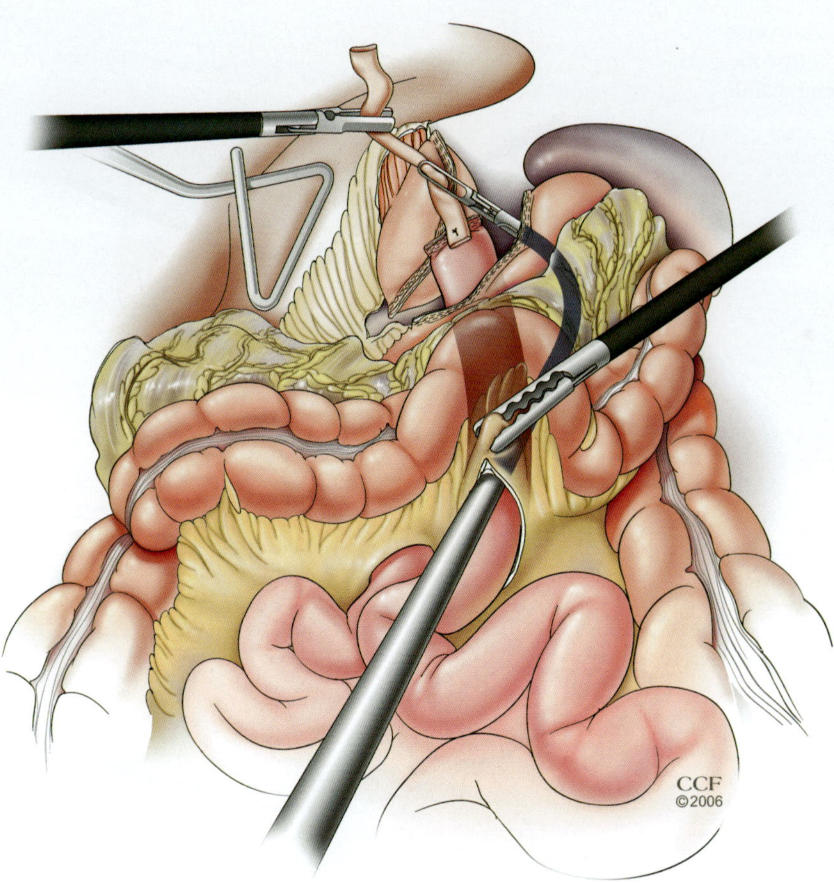

FIGURE 21.1-6. The Roux limb is delivered to the gastric pouch through the retrocolic, retrogastric space using a Penrose drain. (Courtesy of the Cleveland Clinic Foundation.)

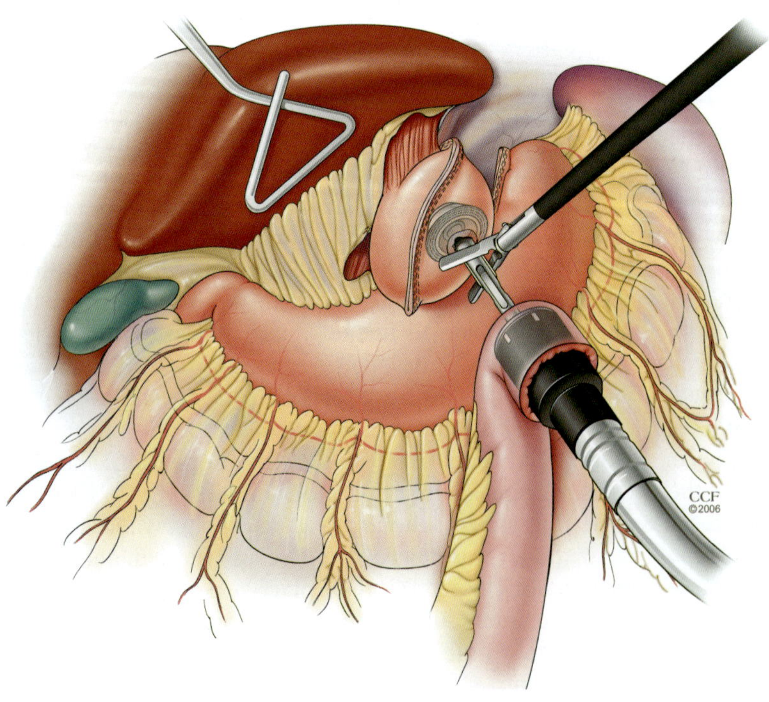

FIGURE 21.1-7. The stapler is placed into the lumen of the Roux limb and joined with the anvil. The Roux limb can be placed in the retrocolic, retrogastric position or the antecolic, antegastric position (shown here) using this technique. (Courtesy of the Cleveland Clinic Foundation.)

FIGURE 21.1-8. The completed circular stapled anastomosis. (Courtesy of the Cleveland Clinic Foundation.)

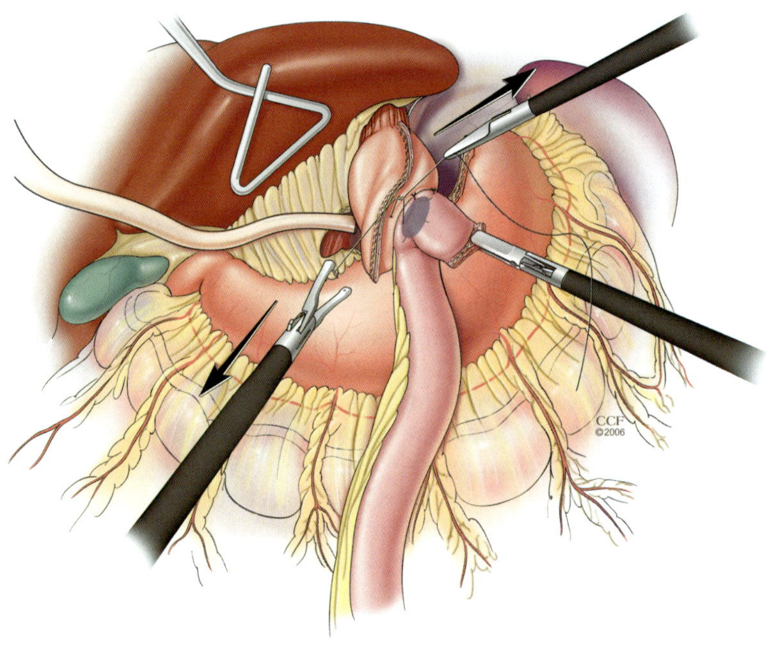

Postoperative Care

No nasogastric suction is employed postoperatively. Minimal narcotic use is required postoperatively and the "pain pump" catheter administers local anesthetic to the most uncomfortable port site for the first 48 hours. Water, broth, and sugar-free Jell-O are generally allowed on the first postoperative day. An upper gastrointestinal (GI) radiologic examination with a water-soluble contrast is performed on the second postoperative morning. Most patients are discharged on water, broth, and sugar-free Jell-O on the second postoperative day.

Learning Curve

Initially, the procedures are usually lengthy; however, as experience accumulates, operating time is usually reduced to 1 to 2 hours. The literature now defines the learning curve as roughly the first 100 cases. An increased rate of early complications is anticipated during this period. Protocols are being developed to shorten the curve and minimize the complications during that time to decrease the patient's risk. Adequate experience and skill in advanced laparoscopy are essential. The operative technique can be challenging at best and more challenging in males or as the body mass index (BMI) increases. It is important for surgeons early in their experience to operate on patients with lower weights who are less seriously medically compromised. Early in the laparoscopic bariatric experience there were significant limitations in the instrumentation, both in functionality and length. This made it especially difficult operating on the super-

obese patients, with a BMI exceeding 50 (5). The instrument manufacturers have responded to this need by producing excellent products that now facilitate our work, laparoscopically and endoscopically.

Modifications of the Stapling Technique

Since the initial laparoscopic gastric bypass we did in 1993, there have been several minor modifications.

The size of the gastric pouch continues to be 15 cc, sized each time with a sizing balloon. Endoscopy, for introduction of the 21-mm circular stapler anvil, can be performed immediately after gastric division, or just prior to the gastroenterostomy. The pull wire is grasped by the endoscopic snare either intragastrically or by allowing the snare to penetrate the gastric wall and grasp the loop as the snare is in the intraperitoneal space.

As noted above, currently we place more sutures in the mesentery to close the defects instead of the technique we used for the first 1000 cases.

The proximal Roux limb is passed retrocolic and retrogastric, at the base of the transverse mesocolon. This approach shortens the path of the Roux limb to the proximal gastric pouch and reduces bowel tension. This pull-through technique is facilitated by using a length of Penrose drain. The Penrose drain is retrieved through the clear area of the lesser omentum, near the caudate lobe of the liver, and the small bowel limb is drawn into the upper abdominal space in close proximity to the proximal gastric pouch. We have used several different techniques for this maneuver but we find this easy and efficient.

Intraoperative endoscopy, upon completion of the gastroenterostomy, with the proximal small bowel cross-clamped, helps with the early detection of air leakage while the bowel wall is distended with air from the endoscope (5). Here again, we have tried several different techniques, but we find this quite effective and we believe there is benefit in performing an endoscopic evaluation intraoperatively.

The most significant change in technique was placing the circular stapler directly through the skin incision rather than placing it through a 33-mm trocar, as was originally described. As we first discarded the port, we found our wound infection rate increased. We tried several methods of protecting the wound from the potentially contaminated anvil of the circular stapler. The method that proved to be most effective was simply using the plastic sheath already on the instrument. We loosen the plastic as we are ready to remove the instrument and slide the plastic down over the end of the stapler, into the subcutaneous tissue. With this maneuver our wound infection rate dropped to less than 1%.

Our most recent modification is the use of the ON Q pain catheter (I-Flow Corp., Lake Forest, CA) to infiltrate local anesthetic into the area of most discomfort to minimize the need for narcotics. Our group has discontinued the use of routine patient-controlled analgesia (PCA) narcotics with the insertion of this catheter. Patients are generally more awake and alert and certainly have less risk of aggravating their sleep apnea.

Results

Weight loss is often emphasized as the primary result by many physicians and lay people, but in reality the main result is an improvement in the comorbid conditions such as diabetes, obstructive sleep apnea, and hypertension. The laparoscopic gastric bypass is not a cosmetic operation; however, most patients do lose weight as they gain their health. Significant, graded, comorbidities were reduced or completely resolved in over 95% of patients. Gastroesophageal reflux disease resolved in 98% of patients. Diabetes mellitus resolved completely in 98%, and was reduced in the remaining 2% of patients. Sleep apnea was eliminated in 97% of the afflicted patients. Of 118 hypertensive patients, 91% experienced clinical remission; 10 patients remained mildly hypertensive on medication. There was a greater than 50% excess weight loss (EWL) within 6 months of surgery, and this rises steadily to an average 80% EWL at 18 months (5).

In the first 1000 of the first author's cases, the complications were as follows: Leak that required reoperation occurred in 0.8% of patients. Hemorrhage requiring transfusion occurred in 0.6%. Wound infection occurred in 6.9% and prompted us to change the way we sheathed the circular stapler, as noted above. Stricture requiring dilation occurred in 3.8% and small bowel obstruction occurred in 0.8%.

Various techniques of the construction of the gastrojejunostomy were described by many authors with the intention of decreasing complications, but they appear more operator dependent than technique dependent. Among both early and late complications, anastomotic leaks remain the most significant, if not in number then in prolonged hospital stay, overall cost, morbidity, and possible death. Current literature on gastric bypass reports a range of up to 2% to 5% incidence of leaks. Carrasquilla et al. (8) reports a very low incidence of leaks: 0.1% (one in 1000 cases). Their technique involves the antecolic and antegastric approach and the use of a circular stapler for the gastroenterostomy.

Stenosis of the gastroenterostomy after laparoscopic Roux-en-Y gastric bypass (LRYGBP) is another situation that occurs after either stapled or hand-sewn anastomoses. Prospective analysis of 1000 patients who underwent LRYGBP with the gastroenterostomy constructed with a linear stapler revealed a 3.2% stricture rate (9). The majority of strictures occur within the first 4 to 6 weeks after surgery. Some strictures occur later and are generally related to smoking or medication usage. In our series, endoscopic dilation was quite effective in treating the strictures at the gastroenterostomy. An experienced endoscopist is needed to dilate the stricture, as there is the potential for perforation and overdilation. In our personal series, all early strictures responded to dilation and there were no reoperations. Some series show dilation to be less effective and emphasize the need for surgical revision (9).

Nguyen et al. (10) analyzed the frequency of anastomotic stricture following laparoscopic gastric bypass (GBP) using a 21-mm vs. a 25-mm circular stapler for construction of the gastrojejunostomy, and the safety and efficacy of endoscopic balloon dilation in the management of anastomotic stricture. Anastomotic stricture occurred more frequently with the use of the 21-mm compared to the 25-mm circular stapler. Symptoms of stricture are usually presented within 6 weeks after the primary operation. Recurrent stricture developed in 17% of patients. The EWL at 1 year for patients in whom the 21-mm circular stapler was used for creation of the gastrojejunostomy was similar to that for patients in whom the 25-mm circular stapler was used (10). Long-term results are needed to assess if there are significant differences with the use of the various sizes of stapling devices.

Early gastrointestinal hemorrhage after gastric bypass is an infrequent complication. Nguyen et al. reported that 3.2% of patients who underwent LRYGBP with creation of the gastrojejunostomy using a circular stapler, developed postoperative hemorrhage in 24 hours after surgery. Clinical presentations may include hematemesis, bright red blood per rectum, melena, and hypotension. Nuclear scintigraphy is rarely required for identification of the hemorrhage site. Conservative management is usually sufficient; however, patients with hemodynamic instability and patients with early onset of hemorrhage may require operative intervention for control of hemorrhage. The sites of hemorrhage include not only the gastrojejunostomy but also the gastric remnant staple lines (11).

Alternative Surgical Techniques

Most of the technical modifications of circular stapler gastroenterostomy concern anvil placement. Although there are very few reports describing pharyngeal or esophageal injuries, the risk of such injuries and of difficulties in maneuvering the anvil from the pharynx to the proximal part of the stomach is still a potential concern. A case of hypopharyngeal perforation after an attempted transoral insertion of an anvil was reported by Nguyen and Wolfe (12). In an effort to overcome this potential risk and to obviate the need for intraoperative endoscopy, alternative techniques of anvil placement have been described. Placement is achieved by attaching the anvil to a suture and directing it toward a chosen site, in the soon to be gastric pouch, through a distal gastrotomy. These techniques require pushing the anvil penetrating needle across gastric mucosa to position the anvil in the desired site (13). Similarly, good results were reported by Murr and Gallagher (14), who described a technique for introducing the anvil of the circular stapler using a totally transabdominal approach. Some optional techniques avoid upper endoscopy for the transoral introduction of the circular stapler anvil down to the gastric pouch (15). Gagner (personal communication, 2004) popularized an approach using a nasogastric tube connected to the anvil and introducing the anvil transorally (Fig. 21.1-9). No endoscopic control is necessary with these techniques. The integrity of the gastroenterostomy is verified with the injection of methylene blue into the gastric pouch.

A modification described by Gould et al. (16) involves the creation of a gastrostomy for transgastric placement of the anvil. All of these techniques are technically challenging and require experienced laparoscopic surgeons to obtain excellent results and low complication rates. Their surgical technique involves the antecolic, antegastric placement of the Roux limb while using a 21-mm circular stapler to create the gastrojejunostomy. Among the reported complications were two gastrogastric fistulas and late stenosis of the gastrojejunostomy of almost 14%. These strictures were often associated with other complications such as leak or marginal ulcer, and required endoscopic dilation.

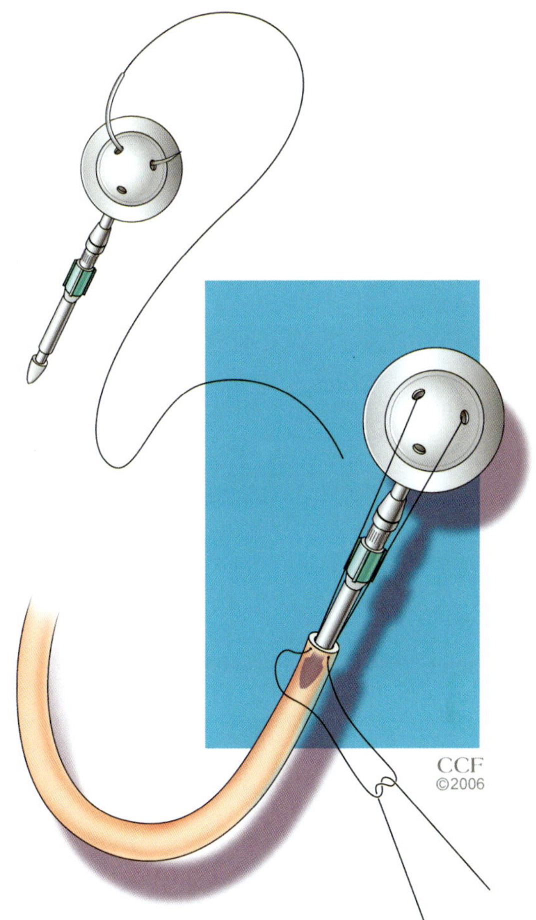

FIGURE 21.1-9. The anvil can be sewn into the cut end of a nasogastric tube to facilitate passage into the gastric pouch. This avoids the need for an endoscopic guidewire. Using this technique, the nasogastric tube is passed transorally and delivered through a gastrotomy in the pouch. The entire tube is pulled through the pouch to place the anvil in the proper position. The suture is then cut and the tube removed through an abdominal trocar. (Courtesy of the Cleveland Clinic Foundation.)

There continues to be some discussion regarding the optimal approach to the gastroenterostomy. The three options are hand sewn, circular stapled, and linear stapled. The hand-sewn technique as compared to stapled approaches is technically more demanding and possibly more time-consuming; however, there is generally a savings in instrument costs. Gonzales et al. (17) reported that in their experience, anastomotic stricture and wound infection rates were higher after circular stapling. These findings may reflect the learning curve and indicate the role of intensive laparoscopic training with new instruments and techniques.

Shope et al. (18) compared the results of two laparoscopic techniques for gastroenterostomies: circular end-to-end and linear cutting staplers. Operative time was shorter for the linear stapler; few anastomotic leaks following the linear technique required early reoperations, and the incidence of wound infection was increased following the circular technique. No important differences in EWL, length of hospital stay, total hospital costs, and operating-room costs were noted. The authors suggest that selection of anastomotic technique should mainly be based on the surgeon's preference.

Hand-assisted RYGBP, at times, is treated as an initial step in the introduction of a fully laparoscopic access. With increasing experience, the surgical approach can be changed from hand-assisted to the laparoscopic Roux-en-Y (19).

References

1. Wittgrove AC, Clark GW, Tremblay LJ. Laparoscopic gastric bypass, Roux-en-Y: preliminary report of five cases. Obes Surg 1994;14(4):353–357.
2. Wittgrove AC, Clark GW. Combined laparoscopic/endoscopic anvil placement for the performance of the gastroenterostomy. Obes Surg 2001;11(5):565–569.
3. Wittgrove AC, Clark GW. Laparoscopic gastric bypass: Endostapler transoral or transabdominal anvil placement. Obes Surg 2000;10(4):376–377.
4. Mason EE, Ito C. Gastric bypass. Ann Surg 1969;170(3):329–339.
5. Wittgrove AC, Clark GW, Schubert KR. Laparoscopic gastric bypass, Roux-en-Y: technique and results in 75 patients with 3–30 months follow-up. Obes Surg 1996;6(6):500–504.
6. Champion JK, Williams MD. Prospective randomized comparison of linear staplers during laparoscopic Roux-en-Y gastric bypass. Obes Surg 2003;13(6):855–859; discussion 860.
7. Higa KD, et al. Laparoscopic Roux-en-Y gastric bypass for morbid obesity: technique and preliminary results of our first 400 patients. Arch Surg 2000;135(9):1029–1033; discussion 1033–1034.
8. Carrasquilla C, et al. Total stapled, total intra-abdominal (TSTI) laparoscopic Roux-en-Y gastric bypass: one leak in 1000 cases. Obes Surg 2004;14(5):613–617.
9. Schwartz ML, et al. Stenosis of the gastroenterostomy after laparoscopic gastric bypass. Obes Surg 2004;14(4):484–491.
10. Nguyen NT, Stevens CM, Wolfe BM. Incidence and outcome of anastomotic stricture after laparoscopic gastric bypass. J Gastrointest Surg 2003;7(8):997–1003; discussion 1003.
11. Nguyen NT, Rivers R, Wolfe BM. Early gastrointestinal hemorrhage after laparoscopic gastric bypass. Obes Surg 2003;13(1):62–65.
12. Nguyen NT, Wolfe BM. Hypopharyngeal perforation during laparoscopic Roux-en-Y gastric bypass. Obes Surg 2000;10(1):64–67.
13. de la Torre RA, Scott JS. Laparoscopic Roux-en-Y gastric bypass: a totally intra-abdominal approach—technique and preliminary report. Obes Surg 1999;9(5):492–498.
14. Murr MM, Gallagher SF. Technical considerations for transabdominal loading of the circular stapler in laparoscopic Roux-en-Y gastric bypass. Am J Surg 2003;185(6):585–588.
15. Borao FJ, Thomas TA, Steichen FM. Alternative operative techniques in laparoscopic Roux-en-Y gastric bypass for morbid obesity. JSLS 2001;5(2):123–129.
16. Gould JC, Garren MJ, Starling JR. Lessons learned from the first 100 cases in a new minimally invasive bariatric surgery program. Obes Surg 2004;14(5):618–625.
17. Gonzalez R, et al. Gastrojejunostomy during laparoscopic gastric bypass: analysis of 3 techniques. Arch Surg 2003;138(2):181–184.
18. Shope TR, et al. Early results after laparoscopic gastric bypass: EEA vs GIA stapled gastrojejunal anastomosis. Obes Surg 2003;13(3):355–359.
19. Gould JC, et al. Evolution of minimally invasive bariatric surgery. Surgery 2002;132(4):565–571; discussion 571–572.

21.2
Circular Stapled Transabdominal Technique

Benjamin E. Schneider and Daniel B. Jones

Since the first description of laparoscopic Roux-en-Y gastric bypass in 1994, surgeons have performed the gastrojejunal anastomosis using a circular end-to-end anastomosis (EEA) stapled technique. The circular stapled method may be favored as it allows for construction of a very small gastric pouch and represents a safe, consistent, and relatively simple method of anastomosis.

Initially, the gastrojejunostomy was created by a transoral technique in which the circular stapler anvil was introduced orally using endoscopic guidance (1,2). This technique required an experienced endoscopist to advance the endoscope into the gastric pouch. Next, a venous catheter was used to pass a guidewire into the gastric pouch for endoscopic retrieval. The pull wire was then attached to the EEA anvil and advanced in an antegrade fashion from the mouth through the esophagus and into the gastric pouch in a technique similar to that used to perform a percutaneous endoscopic gastrostomy (PEG) tube. This required temporary deflation of the balloon of the endotracheal tube and lifting the patient's head and jaw anteriorly to allow the anvil to pass into the distal esophagus. Although large series have reported no anvil-related complications, other surgeons have noted significant injuries associated with the transoral technique (3,4). Proprietary differences among EEA manufacturers may prevent universal application of the transoral approach.

It has been suggested that various anvil stem lengths and the use of a spiked anvil may contribute to difficulty passing the EEA anvil and to esophageal injury (3). Trouble navigating the anvil at the level of the cricopharyngeus muscle as well as complications including esophageal perforation and gastric wall injuries have led surgeons to develop a transgastric technique for anvil placement (5–8). In addition to safety, other potential advantages of the transgastric technique include obviating the need for the surgeon to perform endoscopy, avoidance of wound contamination with oral flora, and reduced risk of inadvertent endotracheal tube migration or dislodgment during manipulation of the anvil through the esophagus.

A number of transgastric techniques have evolved. Among the alternatives, transgastric anvil placement may be performed either by using a balloon cholangiogram catheter to position the anvil as described by de la Torre (6) and Scott et al. (5), or by first creating the gastric pouch and opening the end (6,8). The anvil with an attached suture may then be inserted directly into the pouch. The needle of the attached suture is passed from within the stomach to a selected site on the gastric pouch. The suture is then used to pull the anvil through the pouch wall and the pouch-gastrotomy is closed.

In a simplified technique, the intended gastric pouch is first sized by inflating a 15-mL gastric balloon at the level of the gastroesophageal junction (Fig. 21.2-1). A gastrotomy is performed on the anterior wall of the stomach. A 21-mm EEA anvil with an attached looped suture is placed within the abdominal cavity through one of the port sites. The suture is then held with a 45-cm, modified Maryland grasper (Jones Perforator, Stryker Endoscopy, San Jose, CA) and advanced through the gastrotomy (Fig. 21.2-2) (9). Using the tip of the grasper to penetrate the gastric wall, the suture is advanced at the selected anastomotic site within the area of the proposed gastric pouch. The suture is pulled anteriorly to allow the anvil spike to advance through the gastric wall. Next, the pouch is fashioned using several firings of a laparoscopic gastrointestinal anastomosis (GIA) stapler (Endo-GIA 60mm, 3.5mm staples, US Surgical, Division of Tyco, Princeton, NJ) (Fig. 21.2-3). Care must be taken to ensure that no tubes remain within the stomach before creating the pouch, as they are at risk for division by the GIA stapler. Such an oversight may result in staple line disruption, leak, and retained tube fragment.

The gastrotomy is approximated with three tacking sutures and closed with an application of the GIA stapler. Finally, the EEA is placed through a port site and once within the Roux limb it is mated with the anvil

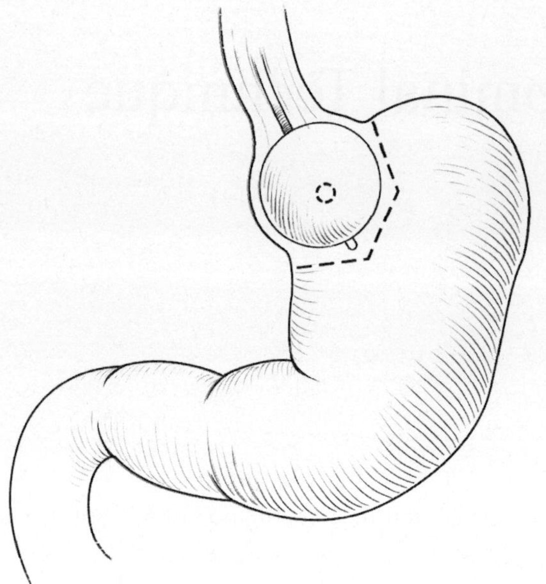

FIGURE 21.2-1. Sizing the pouch, and the intragastric balloon.

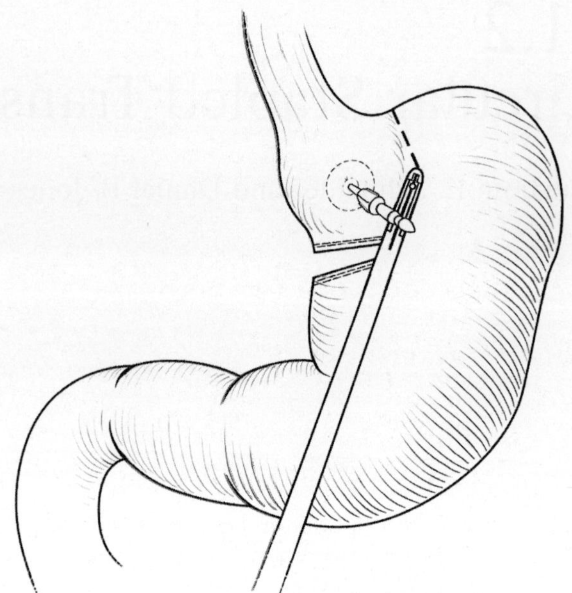

FIGURE 21.2-3. Gastric division.

(Fig. 21.2-4). Before deploying the EEA, the mesentery of the Roux limb should be inspected to ensure that it is oriented properly. The EEA is fired and removed. The open end of the Roux limb is then excised using a 2.5-mm GIA linear stapler (Fig. 21.2-5). The anastomosis is reinforced with several absorbable horizontal mattress sutures in order to decrease tension. The gastrojejunostomy is then tested for leak by insufflating saline with or without methylene blue via a nasogastric tube. Alternatively, endoscopic insufflation may be performed, evaluating the anastomosis by air leak test. On postoperative day 1, an upper gastrointestinal (UGI) contrast study may be obtained to help ensure that no leak is present (10,11).

Success with either the transgastric or transoral technique should be expected to be comparable as they result in a technically similar gastroenteric anastomosis. Series data suggest outcomes following circular stapled gastroenteric anastomosis are similar to those after hand sewn or linear stapled anastomosis. Using the EEA, anastomotic leak rates following gastric bypass have ranged from 1.3% to 2.2% (2,12). The leak rate among studies

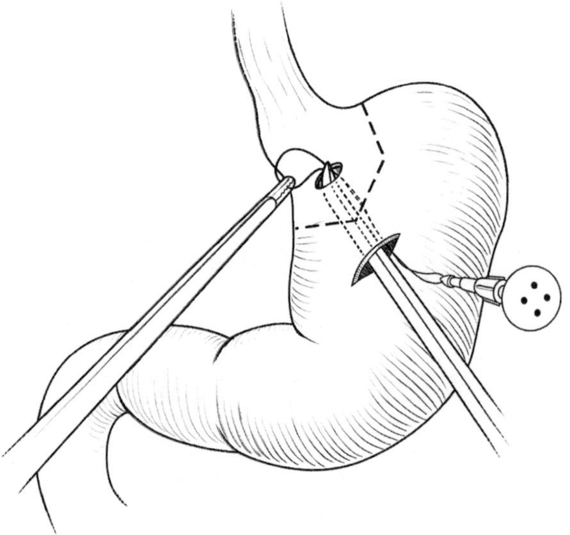

FIGURE 21.2-2. Transgastric end-to-end anastomosis (EEA) anvil placement.

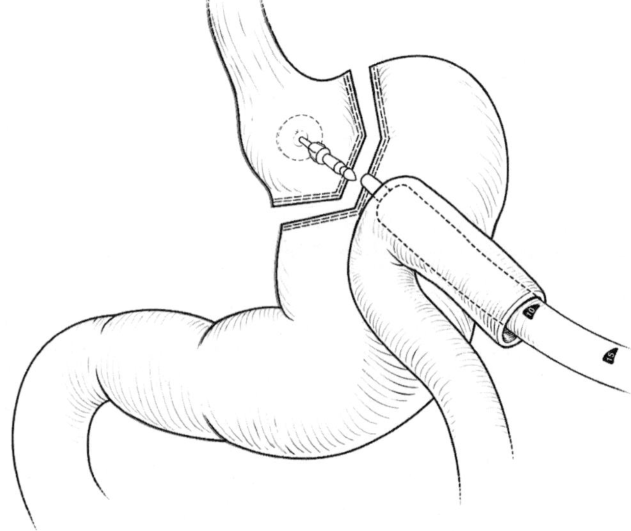

FIGURE 21.2-4. EEA placement.

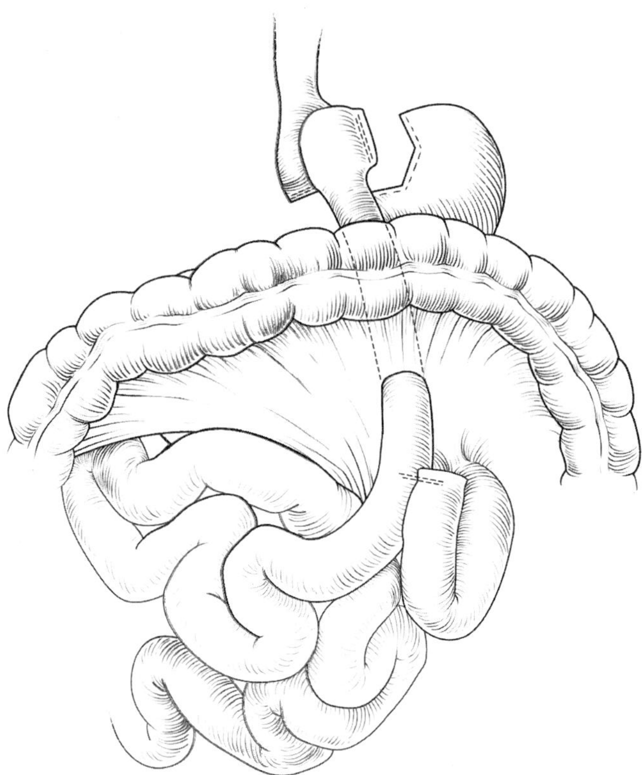

FIGURE 21.2-5. Completed gastric bypass.

employing hand-sewn and linear stapled gastroenteric anastomosis have been similar (2–5.1%) (13–15). Anastomotic stricture may result from local ischemia, undue tension, or a technically narrow anastomosis. Although some reports suggest a higher incidence of gastrojejunal stricture following circular stapled anastomosis, larger series have demonstrated acceptable rates of stenosis (1.6–6.9%) (2,16). Such strictures may be managed safely with either pneumatic balloon or bougie dilation, thus averting the need for further surgical intervention (17). Although these reports are anecdotal, wound infection rates following circular stapled anastomosis may be lower with a transgastric route by avoiding wound contamination with oropharyngeal flora from either extracted tissues or the EEA tip.

Despite reported success, transoral anvil placement may not be universally applied by all surgeons using the various available EEA devices. The transgastric approach allows for direct placement of the anvil at the intended anastomotic site without endangering the esophagus or requiring endoscopy (18).

References

1. Wittgrove AC, Clark GW, Tremblay LJ. Laparoscopic gastric bypass, Roux-en-Y: preliminary report of five cases. Obes Surg 1994;4:353–357.

2. Wittgrove AC, Clark GW. Laparoscopic gastric bypass, Roux-en-Y 500 patients: technique and results, with 3–60 month follow-up. Obes Surg 2000;10:233–239.

3. Wittgrove AC, Clark GW. Laparoscopic gastric bypass: Endostapler transoral or transabdominal anvil placement. Obes Surg 2000;10:376.

4. Wittgrove AC, Clark GW. Combined laparoscopic/endoscopic anvil placement for the performance of the gastroenterostomy. Obes Surg 2001;11:565–569.

5. Scott DJ, Provost PD, Jones DB. Laparoscopic Roux-en-Y gastric bypass: transoral or transgastric anvil placement? Obes Surg 2000;10:361–365.

6. de la Torre RA, Scott JS. Laparoscopic Roux-en-Y gastric bypass: a totally intra-abdominal approach - technique and preliminary report. Obes Surg 1999;9:492–498.

7. Nguyen NT, Wolfe BM. Hypopharyngeal perforation during laparoscopic Roux-en-Y gastric bypass. Obes Surg 2000;10:64–67.

8. Teixeira JA, Borao FJ, Thomas TA, Cerabona T, Artuso D. An alternative technique for creating the gastrojejunostomy in laparoscopic Roux-en-Y gastric bypass: experience with 28 consecutive patients. Obes Surg 2000;10:240–244.

9. Schneider BE, Provost PD, Jones DJ. Obesity surgery—laparoscopic Roux-en-Y and gastric banding procedures. In: Jones D, Wu JS, Soper NJ, eds. Laparoscopic Surgery: Principles and Procedures. St. Louis: Quality Medical Publishing, 2004.

10. Sims TL, Mullican MA, Hamilton EC, Provost DA, Jones DB. Routine upper gastrointestinal Gastrografin swallow after laparoscopic Roux-en-Y gastric bypass. Obes Surg 2003;13:66–72.

11. Hamilton EC, Sims TL, Hamilton TT, Mullican MA, Jones DB, Provost DA. Clinical predictors of leak after Roux-en-Y gastric bypass. Surg Endosc 2003;17:679–684.

12. Nguyen NT, Goldman C, Rosenquist CJ, et al. Laparoscopic versus open gastric bypass: a randomized study of outcomes, quality of life, and costs. Ann Surg 2001;234:279–291.

13. Higa KD, Boone K, Ho T. Complications of the laparoscopic Roux-en-Y gastric bypass: 1,040 patients: what have we learned? Obes Surg 2000;10:509–513.

14. De Maria EJ, Sugerman HJ, Kellum JM, Meador JG, Wolfe LG. Results of 281 consecutive total laparoscopic Roux-en-Y gastric bypass to treat morbid obesity. Ann Surg 2002;235:640–647.

15. Schauer PR, Ikramuddin S, Gourash W, Ramanathan R, Luketich J. Outcomes after laparoscopic Roux-en-Y gastric bypass for morbid obesity. Ann Surg 2000;232:515–529.

16. Gonzalez R, Lin E, Venkatesh KR, Bowers SP, Smith CD. Gastrojejunostomy during laparoscopic gastric bypass: analysis of 3 techniques. Arch Surg 2003;138:181–184.

17. Barba CA, BM, Lorenzo M, Newman R. Endoscopic dilation of gastroesophageal anastomosis stricture after gastric bypass. Surg Endosc 2003;17:416–420.

18. Jones DB, Maithel SK, Schneider BE. Roux-en-Y gastric bypass. In: Atlas of Minimally Invasive Surgery. Cine-Med, Inc.: Woodbury, CT, 2006:298–332.

21.3
Laparoscopic Roux-en-Y Gastric Bypass: Hand-Sewn Gastrojejunostomy Technique

Kelvin Higa

The current popularity of bariatric surgery is attributable, in part, to the minimally invasive solutions developed in the 1990s. In previous decades, although surgeons had demonstrated excellent results and low complication rates, medical professionals, third-party payers, and the public showed little acceptance of these procedures. Currently, the limitations of medical management and the exponential rise in obesity rates have contributed to a demand that far outweighs the supply of bariatric surgeons. It was estimated in 2001 that there may be as many as 20,000 prospective patients per bariatric surgeon (1). Therefore, it is important that surgeons maintain or improve operative efficiency when adopting new techniques while more surgeons are trained in this specialty.

The minimally invasive revolution began in 1993 when Wittgrove, Clark, and Tremblay first performed a proximal gastric bypass laparoscopically (2). Later, they were able to show that this technique was viable and produced weight loss and reduction in comorbidities equal to or better than many *open* series (3). Discussed elsewhere in this text, the laparoscopic/endoscopic anvil placement technique for creation of the gastrojejunal anastomosis was the foundation for most other procedures that followed. Initial anastomotic leakage rates of up to 5% were observed (4), however the rates decreased with experience (5).

In 1999, de la Torre and Scott (6) published a series of laparoscopic Roux-en-Y gastric bypass procedures using a totally intraabdominal approach for the formation of the gastrojejunal anastomosis with a circular stapler (6). Champion, and later Schauer et al. (7) developed the linear cutter technique that obviates the need for transoral passage of instrumentation, thus avoiding the potential for esophageal injury, while creating a stable, calibrated anastomosis.

In 1996 my group began development of the hand-sutured technique because of our concerns regarding failure rates of stapled anastomoses; we performed our first procedure in 1998 (8). The design of the procedure paralleled the open Roux-en-Y procedures that we were performing. Based on this experience and extrapolation of theories of gastric pouch formation (9), we adopted the basic configuration described by MacLean et al. (10). Knowing that small changes in anatomy or technique might have pronounced effects in short- and long-term results and complications, it was important for us to emulate the open configuration as closely as possible, given the limitations of available laparoscopic instrumentation at that time.

The basis for this technique is the formation of a linear, vertically oriented pouch excluding the distensible fundus of the stomach. This provides a serviceable platform for which a hand-sewn anastomosis to the Roux limb can be performed. This technique has been reproduced and adopted by many centers, but is not as popular as the stapled techniques. The long learning curve and inexperience with advanced laparoscopic suturing are the major drawbacks. However, once mastered, these techniques enable the surgeon to resolve almost all complications related to bariatric surgery, or other complex foregut surgery for that matter, laparoscopically, and with a greater degree of precision. This technique also allows the surgeon to achieve an operative efficiency that surpasses the open equivalent (Table 21.3-1).

Indications and Selection Criteria for Surgery

We follow the National Institutes of Health (NIH) Consensus Development Conference Statement (11) guidelines regarding gastrointestinal surgery for severe obesity (Table 21.3-2), in association with the American Society for Bariatric Surgery (ASBS) and the Society of American Gastrointestinal Endoscopic Surgeons (SAGES) recommendations for surgical intervention (Table 21.3-3).

TABLE 21.3-1. Advantages and disadvantages of hand-sewn technique

Disadvantages
• Long learning curve

Advantages
• Low leak rate in "open" series when surgeons are familiar/comfortable with the technique
• Complications, including stenosis, decreased
• Less expensive than stapled anastomosis
• Does not require endoscopy equipment
• Does not require enlargement of port or incur increased infections due to contamination of port site by endomechanical device
• Allows for a small, linear gastric pouch
• Can be performed by a single surgeon without a skilled surgeon as assistant
• Avoids esophageal instrumentation
• Enables secondary or revision surgery
• Allows surgeon to develop important skills necessary to resolve complications

Contraindications for the laparoscopic approach are relatively few in our center (Table 21.3-4). Larger patients may be more challenging, but the added benefits of avoiding the morbidity of a large incision make this approach worthwhile. Likewise, patients who had previous open surgery benefit from mobilizing adhesions laparoscopically rather than lengthening an already extensive incision. The role of bariatric surgery in adolescents (age <18 years) and the elderly (age >60 years) has not been well defined, but evolving experience indicates similar results to other age groups (12). Similarly,

TABLE 21.3-2. Summary of National Institutes of Health (NIH) Consensus Development Conference Statement for Gastrointestinal Surgery for Severe Obesity, 1991

• Patients whose body mass index (BMI) exceeds 40 are potential candidates for surgery if they strongly desire substantial weight loss.
• In certain instances, less severely obese patients (BMI 35–40) may be considered for surgery in the presence of high-risk comorbid conditions such as diabetes mellitus or sleep apnea. Also included are obesity-related physical problems interfering with lifestyle such as employment, family function, and ambulation.
• Patients seeking therapy for severe obesity for the first time should be considered for treatment in a nonsurgical program with integrated components of a dietary regimen, appropriate exercise, and behavioral modification and support.
• Gastric restrictive or bypass procedures could be considered for well-informed and motivated patients with acceptable operative risks.
• Patients who are candidates for surgical procedures should be selected carefully after evaluation by a multidisciplinary team with medical, surgical, psychiatric, and nutritional expertise.
• The operation should be performed by a surgeon substantially experienced with the appropriate procedures and working in a clinical setting with adequate support for all aspects of management and assessment.
• Lifelong medical surveillance after surgical therapy is a necessity.

TABLE 21.3-3. Guidelines for laparoscopic and open surgical treatment of morbid obesity adopted by the American Society for Bariatric Surgery (ASBS) and Society of American Gastrointestinal and Endoscopic Surgeons (SAGES), June 2000

Surgical therapy should be considered for individuals who:
• Have a body mass index (BMI) of 35 to 40 and have obesity-related comorbidities.

Or
• Have a BMI of greater than 40 without comorbidities if the weight adversely affects their life

And
• Can show that dietary attempts at weight control have been ineffective.

ethnic and cultural differences as related to outcomes are currently being evaluated.

Preparation for Surgery

The treatment of morbid obesity requires a dedicated multidisciplinary team consisting of a surgeon, psychologist, nutritionist, physical therapist, anesthesiologist, and others. More importantly, the patient must be an active participant in the bariatric surgical program if optimal outcomes are to be achieved. Optimization of preoperative nutrition and cardiopulmonary performance is advisable and can help to limit one of the major causes of laparoscopic conversions—hepatic enlargement limiting visualization of the proximal stomach. Medical weight reduction, although limited in long-term management alone, may be quite helpful in decreasing the size of the liver and the amount of intraperitoneal fat preoperatively, thus enabling the surgeon to safely perform the procedure laparoscopically while establishing sound nutritional and exercise habits beneficial after surgery.

Bowel preparation is unnecessary. A liquid diet 24 hours before surgery will prevent the possibility of retained food in the stomach from obstructing the jejunojejunal anastomosis immediately after surgery, a potential cause of acute gastric distention (13).

TABLE 21.3-4. Contraindications for laparoscopic bariatric surgery

• Unsuitable candidate for bariatric surgery in general, e.g., inadequate cardiopulmonary reserve to tolerate the procedure, uncontrolled drug or alcohol dependency, impaired intellectual capacity, and so forth
• Presence of large incisional hernias that would require repair at the time of bariatric procedure
• Presence of intraabdominal adhesions preventing laparoscopic visualization and dissection in general
• Abdominal compartment syndrome or potential for inadequate pneumoperitoneum

Bariatric patients are at moderate risk for perioperative venous thromboembolism (14). Prophylaxis in the form of mechanical (sequential compression boots and early ambulation) and pharmacologic (subcutaneous fractionated or unfractionated heparin) is advised. Traditional parenteral antibiotic prophylaxis is standard.

Positioning of the patient in the operating room must include attention to the prevention of pressure sores and neuropathy. Dedicated operative tables must be weight-rated appropriately with lateral extensions to accommodate the larger patients. Protocols for patient transfer and other safety issues should be included as part of a hospital-wide awareness program.

Surgical Procedure

Optimal port placement allows for dissection of the small bowel without compromising the exposure of the proximal stomach. Extremes of size can be challenging: adequate space to allow the formation of the Roux limb in smaller patients can be as problematic as the inadequate length of instrumentation and difficulties associated with visualization of the proximal stomach in larger patients. Interestingly, authors describe various approaches and port locations to solve these issues while maintaining the critical nature of their particular port placement. We use five ports (Fig. 21.3-1). This arrangement also allows for concomitant cholecystectomy if indicated.

Initial entry is performed without insufflation using a nonbladed optical trocar system. The camera is placed midline, 8 to 12 cm from the xiphoid, while other ports are placed to allow creation of the Roux limb, formation of the gastric pouch, and performance of the gastrojejunal anastomosis. Attention to the angle of entry of the port can reduce the resistance of the abdominal wall to the instrumentation, allowing for a more precise and less fatiguing operation. The ports can be *redirected* by creation of a new fascial pathway, preserving the original skin entry site. These specific ports do require fascial closure, which greatly improves operative efficiency and also reduces a potential source of postoperative pain.

The omentum is displaced cephalad to expose the ligament of Treitz. In patients whose omentum is adherent to pelvic structures or involved in an incarcerated ventral hernia, we prefer to incise the gastrocolic omentum and open the transverse mesocolon from above, thus exposing the ligament of Treitz directly. Ventral hernias are repaired at a later date when optimal weight loss and nutrition ensure a greater degree of primary success and the use of prosthetic mesh is not compromised by contamination of enteric contents.

The proximal jejunum is transected with a 2.5-mm linear stapler, and the mesentery is divided with another

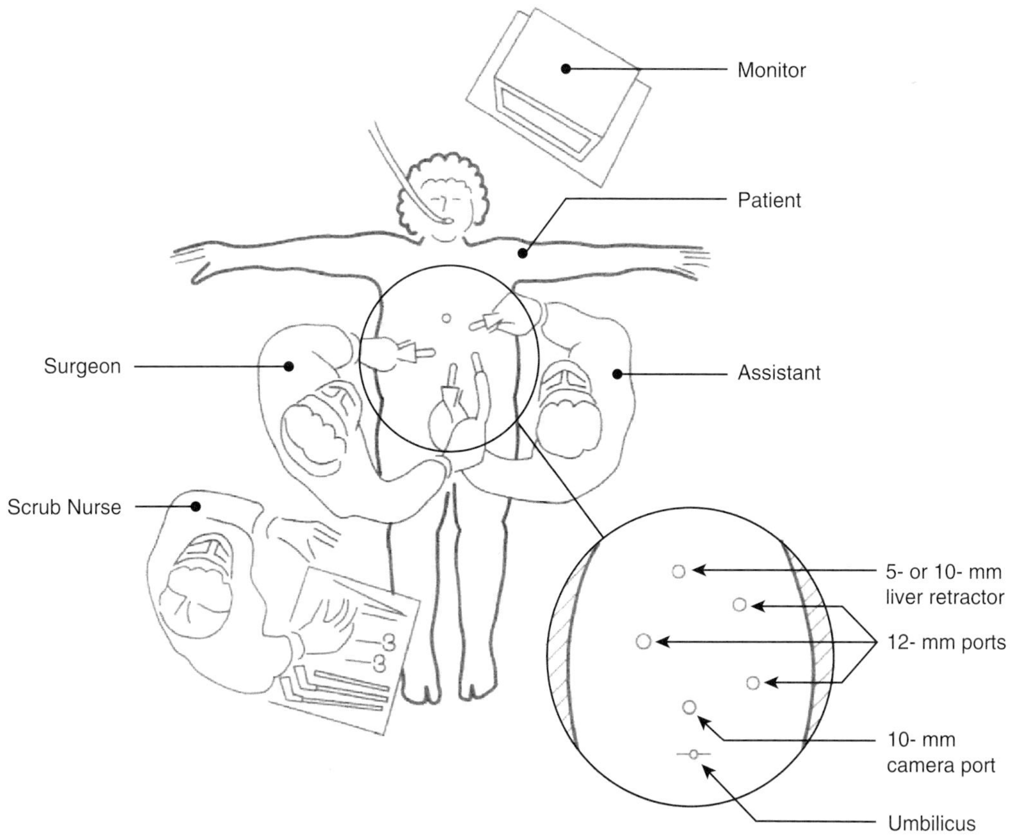

FIGURE 21.3-1. Position and port placement.

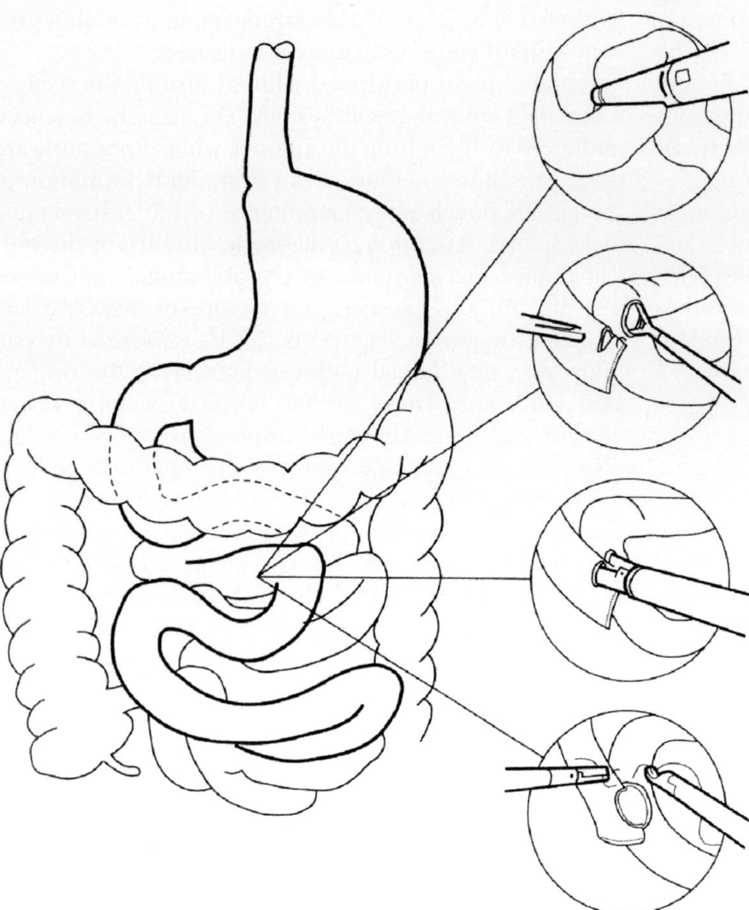

firing of the instrument or with the harmonic scalpel. The Roux limb is measured and a side-to-side linear anastomosis is performed (Fig. 21.3-2). Typically, the length of the Roux limb can be up to 150 cm without an associated increased incidence of malabsorptive complications (15). The enterotomy is closed with a single layer of absorbable suture. The mesenteric defect must be closed with a continuous, nonabsorbable suture to limit the possibility of internal herniation.

The Roux limb is passed through a retrocolic tunnel and fixed to the transverse mesocolon with nonabsorbable sutures, which also includes closing the Petersen's space, again, to help prevent possible internal herniation. Alternatively, some surgeons prefer an antecolic route for the Roux limb, claiming a lower incidence of postoperative bowel obstructions (16).

There are times when the mesocolon is uncomfortably short and will not allow for the safe passage of a retrocolic Roux limb. In these rare instances, the decision to route the Roux limb antecolic must be made before the transection of the jejunum. This site must be more distal from the ligament of Treitz, typically 50 to 100 cm, to limit the tension on the gastrojejunal anastomosis. By lengthening the biliopancreatic limb, iron and calcium absorption may be less efficient, and the incidence of these deficiencies may be theoretically increased or more difficult to manage with oral supplementation alone.

Controversy exists as to whether the large resultant Petersen's space associated with an antecolic Roux limb requires closure. Clearly, these patients are still at risk for intestinal volvulous (17). Therefore, our philosophy is to eliminate the risk of postoperative bowel obstruction rather than simply settling for a reduction in the incidence. However, the long-term stability of suture closure of these defects is still to be determined.

The liver retractor is now placed to allow dissection of the proximal stomach. Occasionally, a very large liver will not allow for sufficient visualization—an indication for open conversion. However, displacement of the liver to the right, rather than anterior, will allow sufficient exposure in the largest of patients. Alternatively, the surgeon may decide to abort the procedure, evaluate the cause of hepatic enlargement (usually steatosis), and institute therapy (medical weight reduction) in anticipation of performing the procedure at a later time under more ideal circumstances. In this way, surgical restraint and proper judgment may reduce the morbidity associated with these operations.

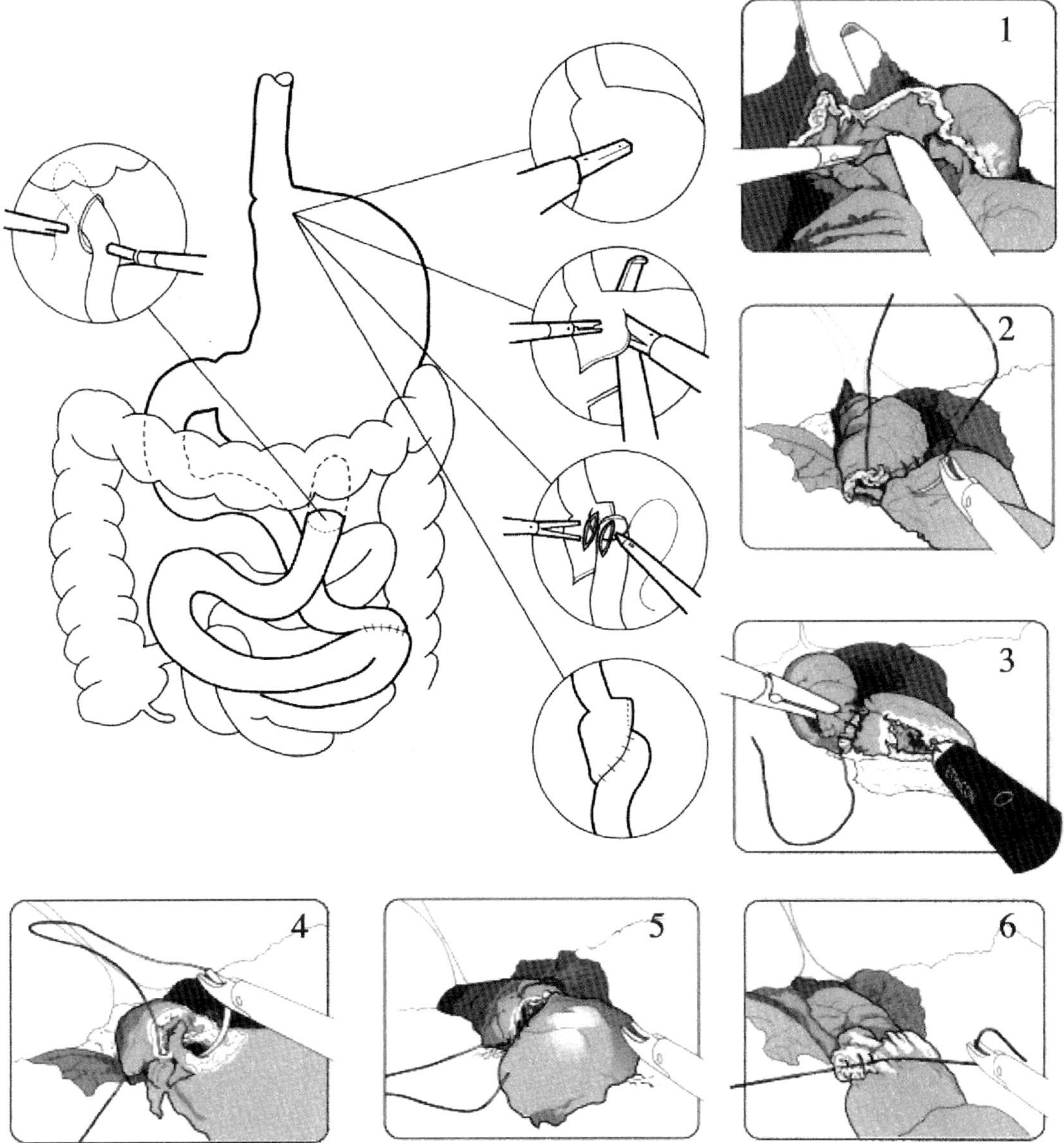

FIGURE 21.3-3. Formation of the gastric pouch and gastrojejunostomy.

Perigastric dissection along the lesser curve of the stomach is performed 3 to 5 cm distal to the gastroesophageal junction and continues until the retrogastric space is reached. At times, dense adhesions to the pancreas are encountered. Visualization is enhanced by opening a gastrocolic window and approaching this area from behind the stomach. Care is taken to avoid thermal injury to the adjacent viscera and vagus nerves.

A six-row, 3.5-mm linear cutter stapler is used to form the lesser curve based, proximal gastric pouch (Fig. 21.3-3). Four-row staplers have been unreliable, in our experience, without suture reinforcement to prevent failure (10). It is essential to exclude the distensible gastric fundus to obtain optimal long-term weight management. This requires meticulous dissection behind the stomach at the level of the angle of His and also helps to prevent injury to the esophagus or spleen. A gastric pouch of no more than 20 cc is optimal (18).

The inferior aspect of the pouch is determined with the first horizontal stapler brought in via the right upper quadrant (RUQ) port. All subsequent firings are vertically oriented through the left upper quadrant (LUQ) port. High, subcostal placement of this port allows the standard-length stapling instrument to reach the angle of His in every instance. It is preferable to divide the fat pad at the hiatus to better visualize the gastroesophageal junction before stapling. Occasionally, a 4.5-mm stapler is required for exceptionally thick tissue.

The 34-French (F) orogastric tube is advanced into the stomach after the first horizontal stapling and assists in the estimation of pouch size and prevents inadvertent transection or impingement of staples on the esophagus.

The retrocolic Roux limb is brought anterior to the gastric remnant to lie in close approximation to the newly formed gastric pouch. Although some surgeons prefer a retrogastric route, subsequent access and visualization of the anastomosis is more difficult if revision surgery is necessary. A two-layer, hand-sewn anastomosis completes intestinal continuity.

The formation of the gastrojejunostomy begins with a running posterior, exterior layer of 3-0 polyglactin (Vicryl) sutures. Beginning distally and sewing proximally, the antimesenteric side of the Roux limb is approximated to the inferior staple line of the gastric pouch, incorporating the staples in the suture line. Enterotomies are performed on the gastric pouch and Roux limb adjacent to the suture line. A second posterior, full-thickness, running suture line is performed and continued anterior beyond the termination of the first posterior suture.

Two anterior suture lines are run from the distal anterior aspect of the enterotomy, the first being full thickness and the second seromuscular. Before completion of the anastomosis, the 34F tube is carefully inserted across the anastomosis to help calibrate the opening as well as providing assurance of a patent anastomosis. The anterior sutures are tied with their respective posterior counterparts.

The anastomosis and proximal staple lines can be tested with blue dye, air insufflation via the orogastric tube, or operative endoscopy. However, we do not employ routine testing or drainage of the anastomosis unless dictated by clinical suspicion. The port sites are inspected for bleeding on withdrawal of the trocars and the skin is closed with simple absorbable monofilament sutures.

Postoperative Management

Perioperative antibiotic is continued for 24 hours, while thromboembolism prophylaxis continues until the patient is discharged. Analgesia is in the form of patient-controlled narcotic delivery systems and intravenous ketorolac. Oral narcotics are offered when clear liquids are tolerated. Metoclopramide is administered routinely and a variety of antiemetic pharmacologic agents are available for nurses to use at their discretion.

TABLE 21.3-5. Serum nutritional parameters

CBC
Liver profile
Lipid profile
Folate
Iron studies
Parathyroid hormone
B_{12}
B_6
Calcium

Routine postoperative contrast studies add little to the management of these patients and serve only to delay discharge secondary to nausea (19). A normal postoperative upper gastrointestinal (UGI) study should not preclude the surgeon's intervening based on clinical suspicion of a leak (20).

Patients are started on clear liquids the day of surgery and are required to ambulate with assistance. Preoperative oral medications can be resumed as soon as the patient can tolerate clear liquids. Most patients are discharged by the second postoperative day.

Patients are continued on a clear liquid diet for 1 week and slowly advanced to solids over a 3- to 4-week period. Patients are instructed to take either an H2-blocker or proton pump inhibitor for 30 days. Routine follow-up visits are at 1 week, 3 weeks, and quarterly for the first year, and then on a yearly basis. Ongoing nutritional, emotional, exercise counseling, and support groups are provided. Complete nutritional assessment occurs on a yearly basis or when symptoms or clinical suspicion dictates (Table 21.3-5).

Results

Wittgrove et al.'s (5) 8-year data suggest long-term weight loss equivalent to or better than 5-year data for open gastric bypass reported by MacLean et al. (21) and 14-year data reported by Pories et al. (22) (Table 21.3-6). Our 5-year data suggest the same (Fig. 21.3-4). More importantly, reduction in medical morbidities is quite remarkable, underscoring the impact and importance of surgical weight reduction in health care maintenance.

Early complication rates and operative times suffer from a very steep learning curve. This is dependent not

TABLE 21.3-6. Comparison of published data

Technique	Transoral Circular Stapler	Linear Cutter		Hand-Sewn
Author	Wittgrove and Clark	Schauer	Champion	Higa, Boone, and Ho
Patients (n)	500	275	63	1500
Leak (G-J) (%)	2.2	1.5	3.0	0
Stenosis (%)	1.6	4.7	6.3	4.9
Excess weight loss (EWL)	73%	77%	82%	69%
Hospital stay (days)	2.6	2.6	2.5	1.6
Early complications (%)	10.4	3.3	3.7	7.5
Late complications (%)	2.2	27.0	6.3	7.5

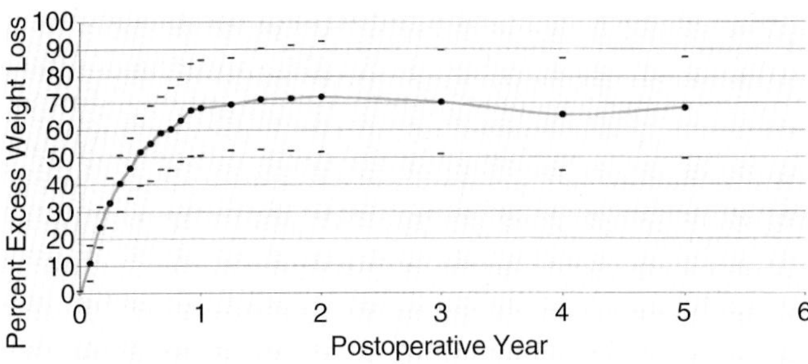

FIGURE 21.3-4. Percent excess weight loss over time with the laparoscopic Roux-en-Y gastric bypass.

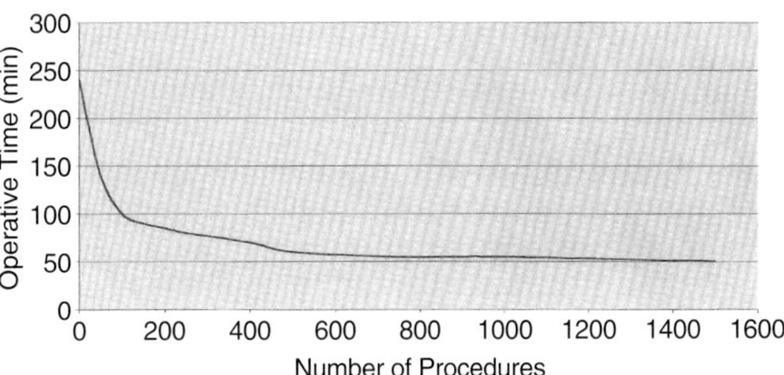

FIGURE 21.3-5. The learning curve of a primary physician for the laparoscopic Roux-en-Y gastric bypass.

only on the initial experience of the surgeon but also on the surgeon's ability to organize a systematic method of approaching this complex operation. Efficiency as a result of preparedness of the operative team is critical. Our data suggest that performing more than 100 procedures as the primary surgeon may be necessary for this learning process (Fig. 21.3-5), which correlates with the experience of others (23).

Short-term percent excess weight loss (%EWL), reduction in medical comorbidities, and improvement in quality of life have been well documented for the open as well as the laparoscopic gastric bypass. However, and just as

importantly, definitive 5- to 10-year data are lacking for all but a few selective series. Interestingly, short-term data appear to be superior to that from open standard gastric bypass series, suggesting a subtle difference in the anatomic construct of the laparoscopic procedures.

Management of Early Complications

The most common complication in our series is stenosis of the gastrojejunal anastomosis. This has remained constant at 4.9% to 5.21% (Table 21.3-7) and responds well

TABLE 21.3-7. Complications (2805 patients)

Type	Complication	n	Male	Female	Percent*
Anastomotic stenosis	Gastrojejunostomy	146	33	113	5.21
	Mesocolon	15	1	14	0.53
	Jejunojejunostomy	2	0	2	0.07
					Total 5.81
Hernia	Trocar	4	3	1	0.14
	Internal	128	—	—	4.6
					Total 4.7
Leaks	Staple line	21	9	12	0.75
	Gastrojejunostomy	2	0	2	0.07
	Jejunojejunostomy	1	0	1	0.04
					Total 0.86
Infection (nonleak)	Wound	3	1	2	0.11
	Pneumonia	2	1	1	0.07
	Hepatic abscess	1	1	0	0.04
					Total 0.21
Bleeding	Intervention required	13	7	6	0.46
	Transfusion only	11	1	10	0.39
	Observation	7	1	6	0.25
					Total 1.1
Thromboembolic	Pulmonary embolism	5	0	5	0.18
	Deep venous thrombosis	2	1	1	0.07
					Total 0.25
Biliary	Gallstones	77	7	70	2.75
	Acalculous cholecystitis	5	0	5	0.18
					Total 2.92
Marginal ulcer	Treated medically	17	3	14	0.61
	Perforation	9	0	9	0.32
	Revision required	3	0	3	0.11
					Total 1.03
Death	Perioperative	4	1	3	0.14
Total		478/2805			17

* Some total percents are not exact sums of the above percents due to rounding.

TABLE 21.3-8. Incidence of gastrojejunal stenosis

Author	n	Stenosis: n (%)
Wittgrove et al., 2002 (5)	1000	40 (4.0)
Schauer et al., 2000 (7)	275	13 (4.7)
Higa et al., 2001 (29)	1500	73 (4.9)
Champion et al., 1999 (30)	63	4 (6.3)
DeMaria et al., 2002 (31)	281	18 (6.6)

to endoscopic balloon dilation. Patients complain of regression or intolerance of diet advancement at about the third postoperative week. The etiology of this phenomenon is unclear and appears unrelated to the method of gastrojejunostomy (Table 21.3-8). Rarely does it occur at the level of the mesocolon or jejunojejunostomy. These locations do not respond to endoscopic dilation and must be repaired operatively. At times, a recurrent gastrojejunal stenosis also requires operative attention.

The second most common complication in our series is that of internal hernias and bowel obstructions (Table 21.3-9). These may occur immediately postoperatively or many years after the procedure. Primarily due to migration of bowel through an open mesenteric defect, this phenomenon can be difficult to detect in the absence of overt bowel obstruction. Often patients complain of intermittent, severe, postprandial abdominal pain, but noninvasive radiographic studies are completely normal in at least 50% of cases. Diagnostic laparoscopy must be performed based on clinical suspicion, and reduction and repair of the defects are straightforward (24).

The prevention of internal hernias requires meticulous closure of all potential defects with nonabsorbable suture material. Some surgeons have brought the Roux limb antecolic in hopes that the most common cause of small bowel obstruction, that of transmesocolic herniation, is eliminated. However, the large resulting Petersen's space and the jejunal mesentery defects are still potential sites that need to be addressed (25). We have not observed an internal hernia since we adopted the mesenteric closure techniques as suggested by Sugerman and DeMaria.

Proximal anastomotic leaks or staple-line disruptions are tolerated poorly by the bariatric patient. Leaks are often subtle in their initial presentation; the only indication may be sustained tachycardia (>120/min). Typical symptoms of abdominal pain, fever, or leukocytosis can be indistinguishable from cardiac events, pulmonary

TABLE 21.3-9. Internal hernia data (2805 patients)

Location	n	Percent
Mesocolon	61	2.2
Jejunojejunostomy	41	1.5
Petersen's	13	0.5
Multiple sites	13	0.5
Total	128	4.6

embolism, acute gastric distention, or hemorrhagic shock. Morbidly obese patients have little cardiopulmonary reserve; therefore, time to treatment is critical. Workup and evaluation must be expeditious and directed by clinical suspicion. If a leak is suspected, reexploration, usually laparoscopically, is the only definitive method to rule it out.

At surgery, there should be an attempt to identify and repair the defect knowing that it will sometimes fail. Operative endoscopy is often helpful in identifying the leak and evaluating the repair. Drainage is essential, and enteric access via a gastrostomy tube in the gastric remnant can be established at this time. This prevents gastric distention and can later be used as a conduit for nutritional support.

Venous thromboembolism is the primary cause of death in most series. Surprisingly, given the physical attributes of the patient population, comorbid conditions, and nature of the operation (position, prolonged operative times, and so forth), this is a rare occurrence. The use of both mechanical and pharmacologic prophylaxis along with early mobilization made possible by elimination of incisional pain likely contributes to these outcomes. The use of prophylactic vena cava filters should be limited to patients with previous pulmonary embolism or significant pulmonary hypertension.

Management of Late Complications

The use of tobacco or nonsteroidal analgesic agents contributes to marginal ulceration. Patients present with abdominal pain, dyspepsia, and occasionally bleeding. The diagnosis can be made radiographically, but endoscopy is often required for evaluation and treatment of an associated gastrojejunal stenosis or for control of bleeding.

Perforated marginal ulcers are amenable to laparoscopic intervention. The absence of significant intraabdominal adhesions and the anterior location of the anastomosis allows for a relatively simple closure and omental patch. Operative endoscopy is helpful in these cases to rule out gastrogastric fistulas and to evaluate the gastrojejunal anastomosis and repair.

Protein malabsorption/malnutrition is uncommon in proximal gastric bypass procedures. Still, patients should consume between 60 and 80g of protein daily and the levels should be monitored appropriately. Often, patients do not tolerate meat initially and tend to avoid it. Rarely, protein supplementation is necessary. Vitamin and mineral deficiency can occur in up to 30% of patients (26). Ongoing nutritional evaluation and counseling along with oral multivitamin, calcium, and B_{12} supplementation are recommended.

Our data do not support routine cholecystectomy. However, no complications were observed as a result of removing the gallbladder at the time of the Roux-en-Y. Still, our approach is to consider concomitant cholecystectomy for known gallstones, but only if technically straightforward given the patient's individual anatomy. In other words, if the dissection or identification of the cystic duct/common bile duct junction appears problematic, then it is advisable to wait until the patient has lost significant weight after gastric bypass before advising cholecystectomy. This approach helps to ensure more favorable anatomy and lower the risk of bile duct injury. The trocar sites of the gastric bypass can be used for the subsequent cholecystectomy as adhesions are rarely encountered.

The causes of inadequate initial weight loss and weight regain are multifactorial. It has been observed that participation in support groups by patients and follow-up with the surgeon may yield superior results. However, as the pathophysiology of surgical weight loss is poorly understood, the patients are often blamed for poor performance. This adds to the frustration shared by the patient and physician.

Clearly, the concept of obesity as a chronic disease should mandate a multidisciplinary and lifelong approach to therapy. This includes the possibility of secondary surgical procedures for selected patients who do not achieve correction or stabilization of medical comorbid conditions. These considerations would take the form of a higher degree of restriction or malabsorption or both. Unfortunately, revision procedures are associated with at least double the morbidity of the primary operation with unknown long-term results and therefore must be performed only by surgeons with a great deal of experience and interest in this area.

Conclusion

The laparoscopic gastric bypass is one of the most challenging surgical procedures performed today. The distortion and obscuration of anatomy by intraabdominal fat in combination with limitations of instrumentation has led to many ingenious solutions in an attempt to emulate proven, standard techniques. Although current endomechanical staplers have proven to be reliable, initial designs were less forgiving in this application. Despite reliable anastomotic stapling techniques, experts agree that advanced laparoscopic suturing skills are still required to perform this operation safely.

Current procedural refinements have allowed for operative efficiencies surpassing the open gastric bypass. The patient benefits of minimally invasive surgery in terms of wound morbidity, cardiovascular compromise, and immune function have been demonstrated (27,28). However, the learning curve entails a long and tedious endeavor. In addition, the bariatric patient presents more

than just a technical challenge. Ultimately, the treatment of obesity requires a multidisciplinary team dedicated to lifelong management of this serious disease process. Morbid obesity, unlike its associated comorbidities, cannot be cured—only controlled. Surgeons unable to appreciate the management of obesity beyond just the surgical procedure should not venture into this specialty. However, there is no more powerful therapy for the treatment and prevention of disease than weight reduction. There is no more effective a method of initial weight reduction and long-term weight control than bariatric surgery. The laparoscopic Roux-en-Y gastric bypass with hand-sewn gastrojejunostomy has proven itself in this regard.

References

1. Health Care Advisory Board. Bariatric surgery programs: Clinical innovation profile. Marketing and Planning Leadership Council, 2002.
2. Wittgrove AC, Clark GW, Tremblay LJ. Laparoscopic gastric bypass, Roux-en-Y: preliminary report of five cases. Obes Surg 1994;4:353–357.
3. Wittgrove AC, Clark GW. Laparoscopic gastric bypass: a five-year prospective study of 500 patients followed from 3–60 months. Obes Surg 1999;9:123–143.
4. Wittgrove AC, Clark GW, Schubert KR. Laparoscopic gastric bypass, Roux-en-Y: technique and results in 75 patients with 3–30 month follow-up. Obes Surg 1996;6:500–504.
5. Wittgrove AC, Endres JE, Davis M, et al. Perioperative complications in a single surgeon's experience with 1,000 consecutive laparoscopic Roux-en-Y gastric bypass operations for morbid obesity. Obes Surg 2002;12:457–458(abstr L4).
6. de la Torre RA, Scott JS. Laparoscopic Roux-en-Y gastric bypass: a totally intra-abdominal approach: technique and preliminary report. Obes Surg 1999;9:492–498.
7. Schauer PR, Ikramuddin S, Gourash W, et al. Outcomes after laparoscopic Roux-en-Y gastric bypass for morbid obesity. Ann Surg 2000;232:515–529.
8. Higa KD, Boone KB, Ho T, et al. Laparoscopic Roux-en-Y gastric bypass for morbid obesity: technique and preliminary results of our first 400 patients. Arch Surg 2000;9:1029–1033.
9. Mason EE, Maher JW, Scott DH, et al. Ten years of vertical banded gastroplasty for severe obesity. In: Mason EE, guest editor; Nyhus LM, editor-in-chief. Surgical Treatment of Morbid Obesity. Problems in General Surgery Series, vol 9. Philadelphia: Lippincott, 1992:280–289.
10. MacLean LD, Rhode BM, Forse RA. Surgery for obesity: an update of a randomized trial. Obes Surg 1995;5:145–150.
11. Gastrointestinal surgery for severe obesity. National Institutes of Health Consensus Development Conference Draft Statement. Obes Surg 1991;1:257–266.
12. Capella RF. Bariatric surgery in adolescents: is this the best age to operate? Obes Surg 2002;12:196(abstr 13).
13. Higa KD, Boone KB, Ho T. Complications of the laparoscopic Roux-en-Y gastric bypass: 1,040 patients—what have we learned? Obes Surg 2000;10:509–513.

14. Westling A, Bergvist D, Bostrom A, et al. Incidence of deep venous thrombosis in patients undergoing obesity surgery. World J Surg 2000;26:470–473.
15. Brolin RE, Kenler HA, Gorman JH, Cody RP. Long-limb gastric bypass in the super obese: a prospective randomized trial. Ann Surg 1991;215:387–395.
16. Champion JK. Small bowl obstruction after laparoscopic Roux-en-Y gastric bypass. Obes Surg 2002;12:197–198 (abstr 17).
17. Khanna A, Newman B, Reyes J, Fung JJ, Todo S, Starzl TL. Internal hernia and volvulus of the small bowel following liver transplantation. Transplant Int 1997;10(2):133.
18. MacLean LD, Rhode BM, Nohr CW. Late outcome of isolated gastric bypass. Ann Surg 2000;231:524–528.
19. Singh R, Fisher B. Sensitivity and specificity of postoperative upper GI series following gastric bypass. Obes Surg 2003;13:73–75.
20. Sims TL, Mullican MA, Hamilton EC, et al. Routine upper gastrointestinal Gastrografin swallow after laparoscopic Roux-en-Y gastric bypass. Obes Surg 2003;13:66–72.
21. MacLean LD, Rhode BM, Forse RA. Results of the surgical treatment of obesity. Am J Surg 1993;165:155–162.
22. Poires WJ, Swanson MS, MacDonald KG. Who would have thought it? An operation proves to be the most effective therapy for adult-onset diabetes mellitus. Ann Surg 1995;222:339–352.
23. Schauer PR, Ikramuddin S, Hammad G, et al. The learning curve for laparoscopic Roux-en-Y gastric bypass in 100 cases. Surg Endosc 2003;17:212–215.
24. Higa K, Ho T, Boone K. Internal hernias after laparoscopic Roux-en-Y gastric bypass: incidence, treatment and prevention. Obes Surg 2003;13:350–354.
25. Schweitzer MA, DeMaria EJ, Broderick TJ, Sugerman HJ. Laparoscopic closure of mesenteric defects after Roux-en-Y gastric bypass. J Laparoendosc Adv Surg Tech A 2000;10(3):173–175.
26. Rhode BM, MacLean LD. Vitamin and mineral supplementation after gastric bypass. In: Deitel M, Cowan G, eds. Update: Surgery for the Morbidly Obese Patient. Toronto, Ontario: FD-Communications, 2000.
27. Schauer PR. Physiologic consequences of laparoscopic surgery. In: Eubanks WS, Soper NJ, Swanstrom LL, eds. Mastery of Endoscopic Surgery and Laparoscopic Surgery. Philadelphia: Lippincott Williams & Wilkins, 2000:22–38.
28. Nguyen NT, Lee SL, Goldman C, et al. Comparison of pulmonary function and postoperative pain after laparoscopic vs open gastric bypass: a randomized trial. J Am Coll Surg 2001;192:469–476.
29. Higa K, Ho T, Boone K. Laparoscopic Roux-en-Y gastric bypass; technique and 3–year follow-up. J Laparoendosc Adv Surg Tech 2001;11:377–382.
30. Champion JK, Hunt T, DeLisle N. Laparoscopic vertical banded gastroplasty and Roux-en-Y gastric bypass in morbid obesity. Obes Surg 1999;9:123–144.
31. DeMaria EJ, Sugerman HJ, Kellum JM, et al. Results of 281 consecutive total laparoscopic Roux-en-Y gastric bypasses to treat morbid obesity. Ann Surg 2002;235:640–647.

21.4
Linear Stapled Technique for Gastrojejunal Anastomosis

Paul A. Thodiyil, Tomasz Rogula, and Philip R. Schauer

Since its first description by Dr. Allan Wittgrove et al. (1) in 1994, the technique of laparoscopic Roux-en-Y gastric bypass has undergone a number of modifications. In the original description, the gastrojejunostomy was created with a 21-mm circular stapler, with the anvil introduced transorally. While there were no esophageal injuries in the first 1400 patients (2), there has been some concern about esophageal injuries and a reported higher incidence of gastrojejunal anastomotic strictures (3).

Alternative techniques of hand sewn anastomosis (4,5) or a linear stapled anastomosis (6,7) have been championed by several authors. Despite the controversies, the choice of the anastomotic technique should depend for the most part, based on present evidence, on the surgeon's preferences and expertise.

Technique of Laparoscopic Roux-en-Y Gastric Bypass

The patient is placed in the supine position with the surgeon on the right and assistant on the left (Fig. 21.4-1). Abdominal access is obtained in the left upper quadrant with an optical viewing trocar (Endopath XL, Ethicon Endosurgery, Cincinnati, OH), and the abdomen is insufflated to 15 mm Hg. Trocar positions are shown in Figure 21.4-2.

We create the Roux limb and jejunojejunostomy first. The ligament of Treitz is identified and the proximal jejunum is placed in a C configuration (Fig. 21.4-3). The jejunum is measured 30 to 50 cm from the ligament of Treitz and divided with a linear stapler (Echelon 60, Ethicon Endosurgery). One or two more firings of the linear stapler with a white load are used to divide the small bowel mesentery and provide additional mobility for the Roux limb (Fig. 21.4-4). After the jejunum has been divided, a Penrose drain is sewn to the distal limb (the Roux limb) and the Roux limb is measured 75 cm from the drain (Fig. 21.4-5). The Roux limb is measured

to 150 cm for patients with a body mass index (BMI) >50. The Roux limb and biliopancreatic limb are then approximated with a stay suture, and adjacent enterotomies are created. The linear stapler is placed into each lumen and fired to create a side-to-side, functional end-to-end anastomosis (Fig. 21.4-6). The common enterotomy is closed with another firing of the linear stapler and two more stitches are placed. One is placed at the "crotch" of the anastomosis to relieve tension at the end of the staple line and the other, the "Brolin stitch," approximates the end of the biliopancreatic limb and the Roux limb. The mesenteric defect is closed with nonabsorbable suture (Fig. 21.4-7).

After the creation of the jejunojejunostomy and the Roux limb, the patient is placed in the reverse Trendelenburg position to allow better exposure of the upper abdomen.

The omentum is split down the middle using the Harmonic Scalpel (Ethicon Endosurgery) to reduce tension on the Roux limb in the antecolic position. The omentum is divided to the level of the transverse colon to provide a path for the Roux limb. The Roux limb is then advanced in an antecolic, antegastric fashion up toward the stomach (Fig. 21.4-8).

The patient is placed in a full reverse Trendelenburg position. The left lobe of the liver is retracted anteriorly with a 5-mm liver retractor. A window is created in the gastrohepatic ligament with ultrasonic scalpel. After the anesthesiologist has removed all intragastric devices, a white load (60 mm, 2.8-mm stapler) is fired across the mesentery of the lesser curvature. Blue loads (45 mm, 3.5-mm stapler) are then fired across the gastric cardia, 1 to 2 cm below the fat pad, to create a 15-mL gastric pouch (Fig. 21.4-9). The angle of His is mobilized and a tunnel created between the lesser and greater sacs at this point. This facilitates placement of the last staple load while excluding the fundus from the pouch. Staple lines on both sides are examined for hemostasis and integrity. The gastric pouch is then mobilized off of the left crus to

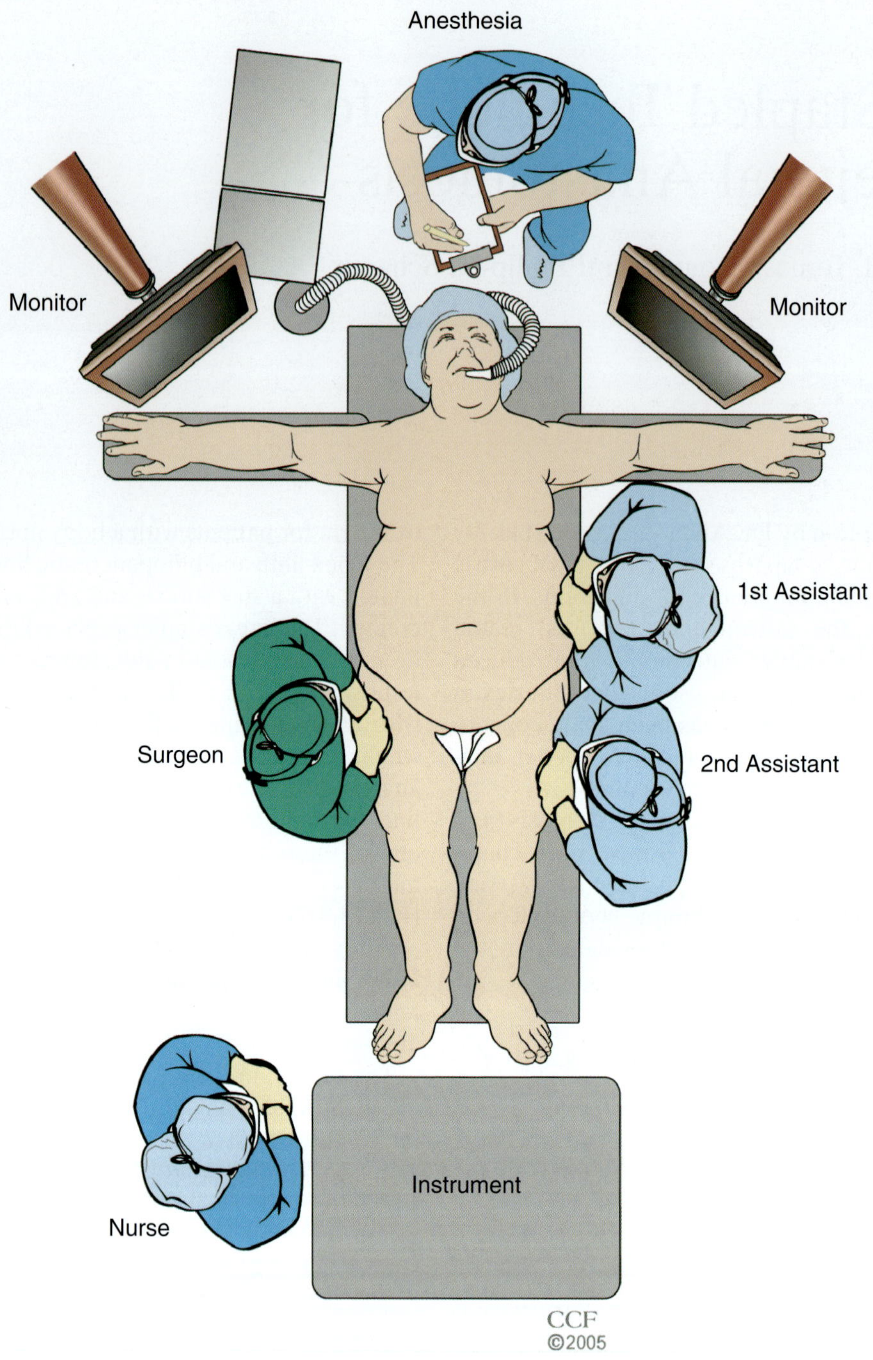

FIGURE 21.4-1. Patient positioning and position of the surgical team for the laparoscopic gastric bypass. (Courtesy of the Cleveland Clinic Foundation.)

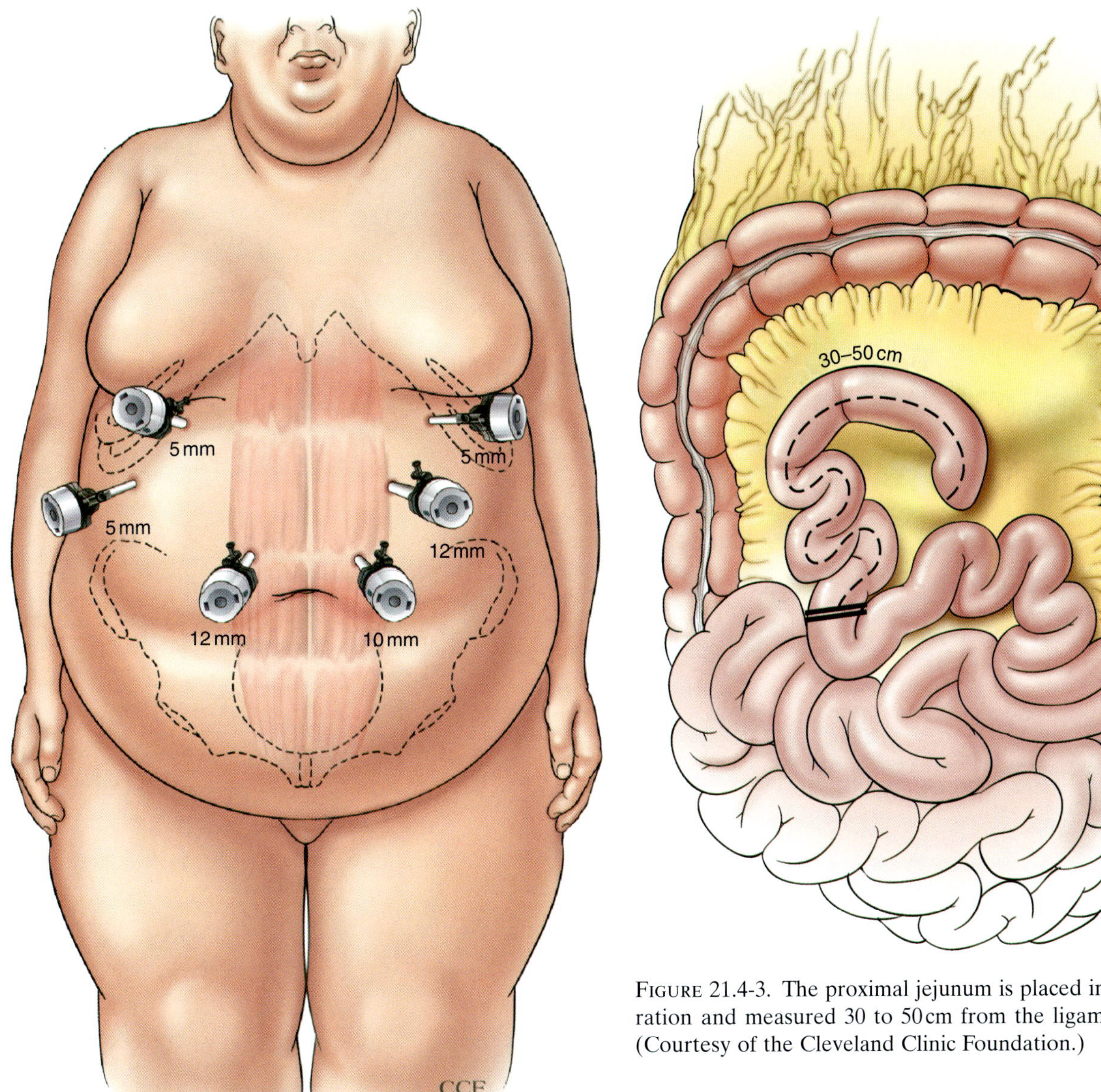

FIGURE 21.4-3. The proximal jejunum is placed in a C configuration and measured 30 to 50 cm from the ligament of Treitz. (Courtesy of the Cleveland Clinic Foundation.)

FIGURE 21.4-2. Port placement for laparoscopic gastric bypass using the linear stapled technique for the gastrojejunostomy. (Courtesy of the Cleveland Clinic Foundation.)

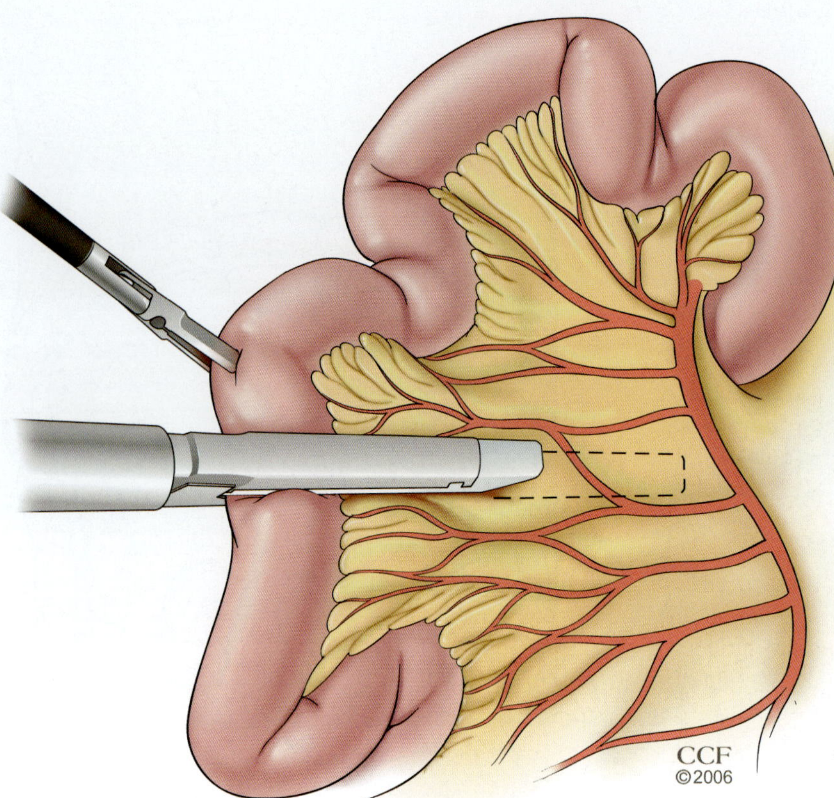

FIGURE 21.4-4. The jejunum is divided with a linear stapler. Two more firings of the stapler are used to divide the mesentery. This provides additional mobility for the Roux limb. (Courtesy of the Cleveland Clinic Foundation.)

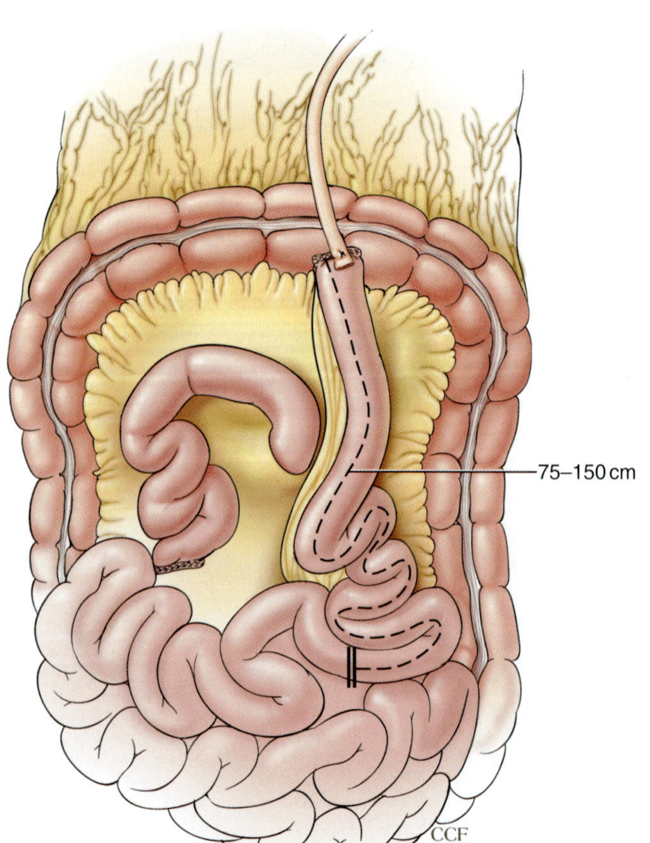

FIGURE 21.4-5. A Penrose drain is sewn to the distal segment and the bowel is measured 75 cm [150 cm for patients with a body mass index (BMI) >50] from the Penrose drain. (Courtesy of the Cleveland Clinic Foundation.)

FIGURE 21.4-6. After the Roux limb is measured, it is approximated to the biliopancreatic limb. Enterotomies are made using ultrasonic shears and a linear stapler is used to create the anastomosis. (Courtesy of the Cleveland Clinic Foundation.)

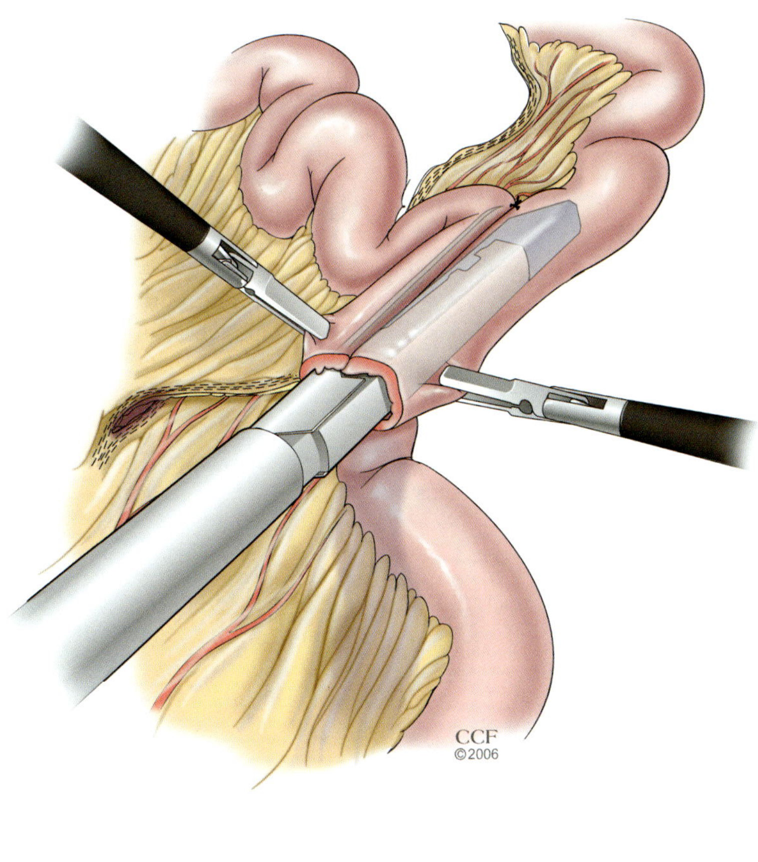

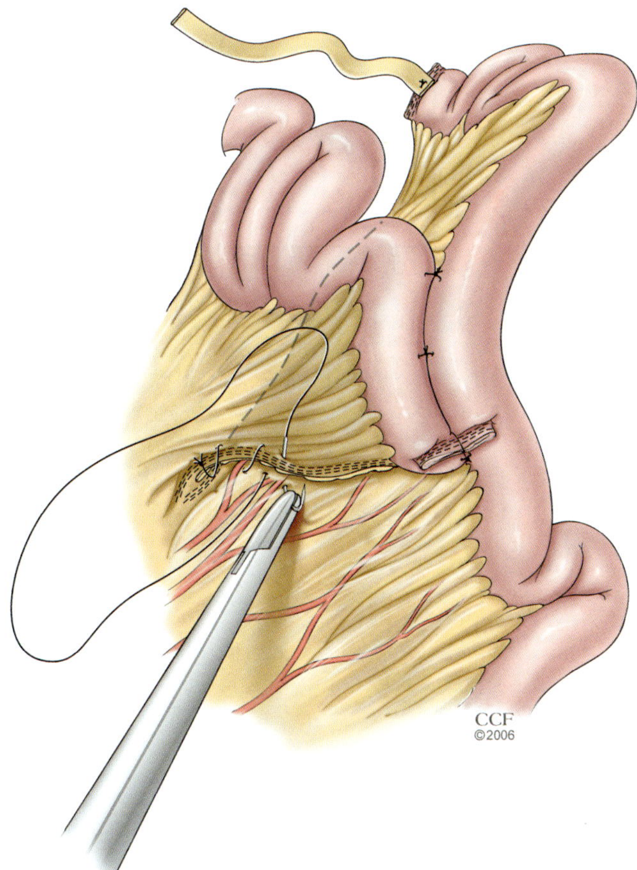

FIGURE 21.4-7. The common enterotomy is closed with a linear stapler. A "crotch" stitch is placed at the confluence of the two bowel limbs and a "Brolin" stitch is placed to approximate the end of the biliopancreatic limb to the side of the Roux limb. The mesenteric defect is closed with nonabsorbable suture. (Courtesy of the Cleveland Clinic Foundation.)

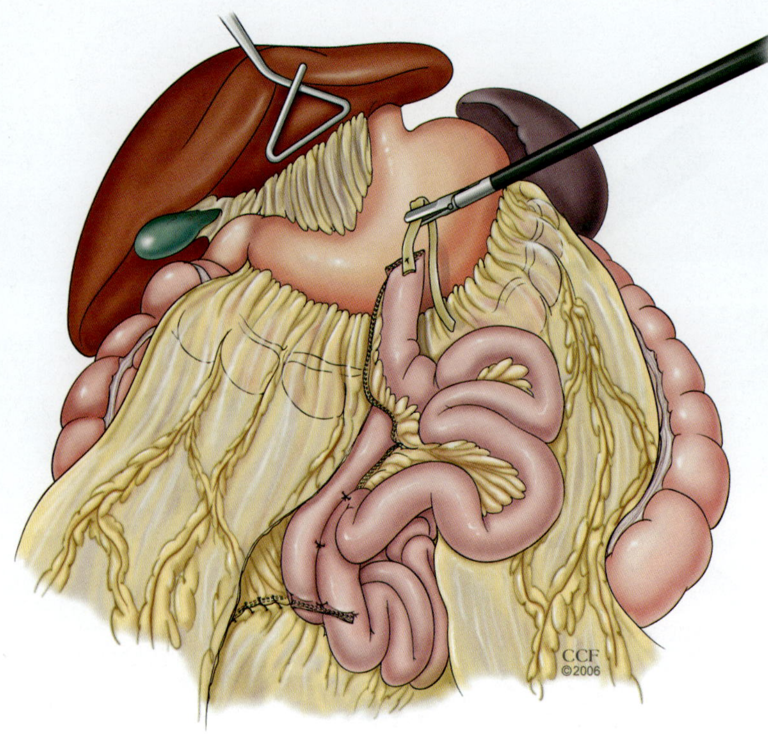

FIGURE 21.4-8. The omentum is divided to the level of the transverse colon, and the Roux limb is delivered to the stomach in the antecolic, antegastric position. (Courtesy of the Cleveland Clinic Foundation.)

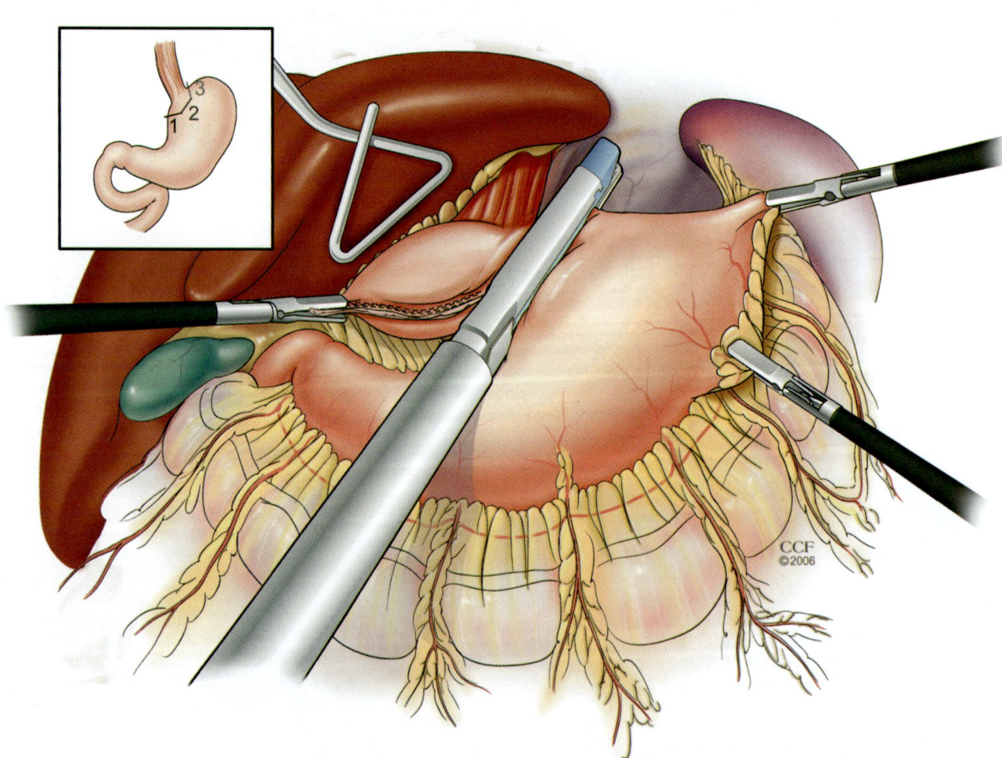

FIGURE 21.4-9. The gastric pouch is created using the linear stapler. The lesser omentum is divided first and the stomach is divided horizontally 1 to 2 cm below the esophageal fat pad. Three or four firings of the stapler are used to create a 15- to 20-mL vertical gastric pouch (inset). (Courtesy of the Cleveland Clinic Foundation.)

provide additional separation from the gastric remnant and to provide additional mobility for creation of the gastrojejunostomy.

The end of the Roux limb is sutured to the posterior aspect of the gastric pouch using 2-0 Surgidac (U.S. Surgical, Division of Tycon, Princeton, NJ) (Fig. 21.4-10). Enterotomies are made in the gastric pouch and in the Roux limb with the ultrasonic scalpel. A blue load is inserted approximately 1.5 cm into the pouch and applied to create a stapled end-to-side gastrojejunostomy (Figs. 21.4-11 and 21.4-12). The residual enterotomy is closed in two layers, with the first in running fashion starting in both corners using 2-0 Polysorb. Prior to tying the two suture ends in the middle, a flexible endoscope is passed down the esophagus through the anastomosis and into the Roux limb. This allows closure of the enterotomy with the endoscope acting as a stent (Fig. 21.4-13). The second anterior layer of 2-0 Surgidac is placed, approximating the Roux limb and encompassing the gastric pouch staple line starting from the greater curvature side to the lesser curvature side.

With the endoscope in place, a soft bowel clamp is placed across the Roux limb just distal to the endoscope. An air–water test is done with air insufflation while the anastomosis is submerged in water. If a leak

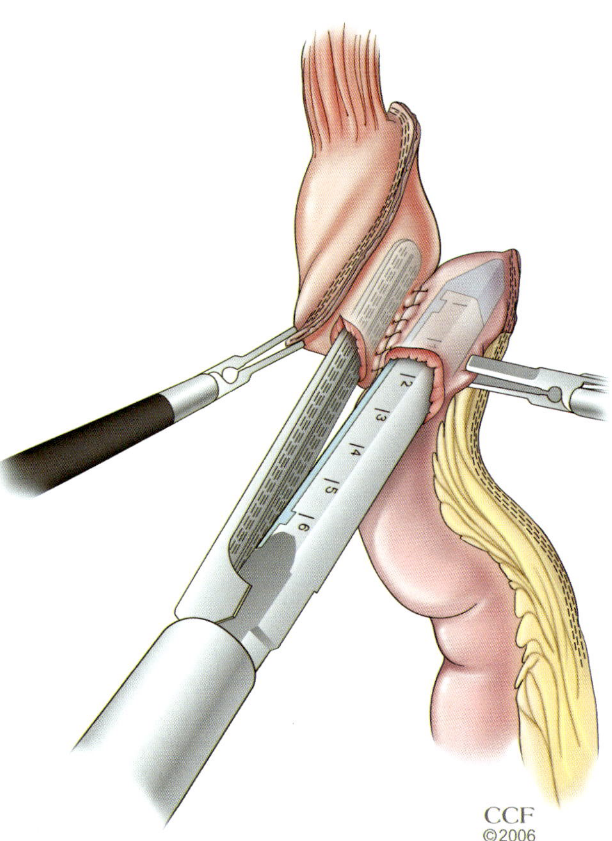

FIGURE 21.4-11. An enterotomy and a gastrotomy are created, and 1.5 cm of the linear stapler is placed into each lumen. (Courtesy of the Cleveland Clinic Foundation.)

is present, the site is localized and suture repaired. The area is further reinforced with application of fibrin tissue glue (Tisseel, Baxter, Deerfield, IL). An omental patch is placed over the anastomosis and is secured with 2-0 Surgidac. A 15-French round, Jackson-Pratt bulb suction drain is placed posterior to the anastomosis and brought out through the right upper quadrant port site. The completed Roux-en-Y gastric bypass is shown in Figure 21.4-14.

Postoperative Management

The patient remains nil per oral (NPO) on the day of surgery. Nasogastric tubes are not routinely employed. On the first postoperative day, an upper gastrointestinal contrast study using Gastrografin and dilute barium is performed. In the absence of leaks or obstruction, the patient is commenced on a clear liquid diet at 30 mL every half hour that is progressed in amount over the next 24 hours. The patient is discharged on the second

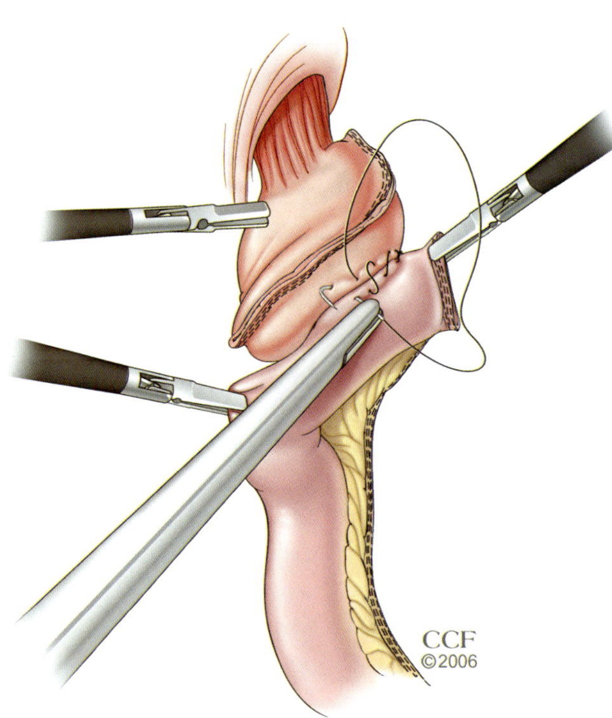

FIGURE 21.4-10. The Roux limb is approximated to the posterior wall of the gastric pouch using nonabsorbable sutures. (Courtesy of the Cleveland Clinic Foundation.)

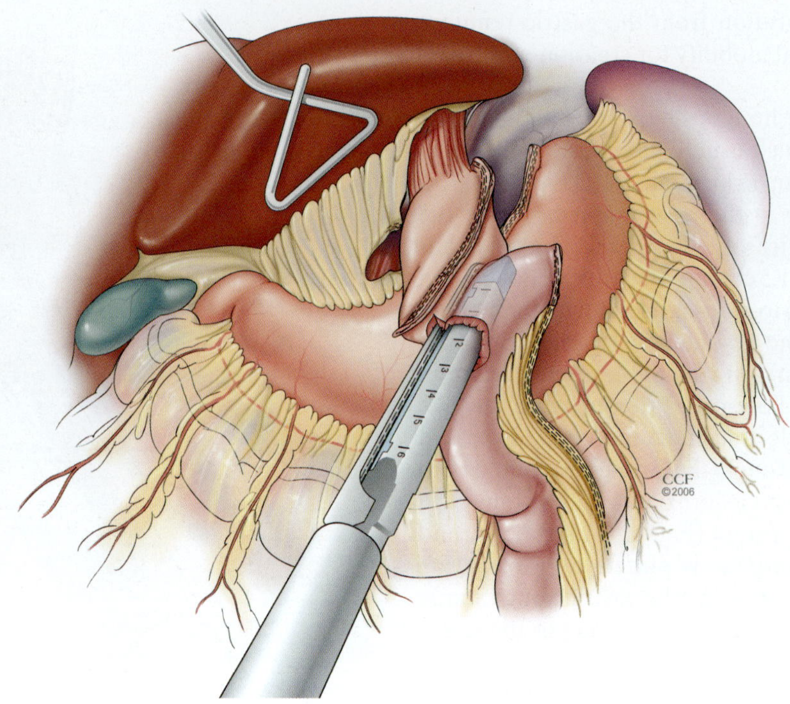

FIGURE 21.4-12. The linear stapler is fired to create the anastomosis. (Courtesy of the Cleveland Clinic Foundation.)

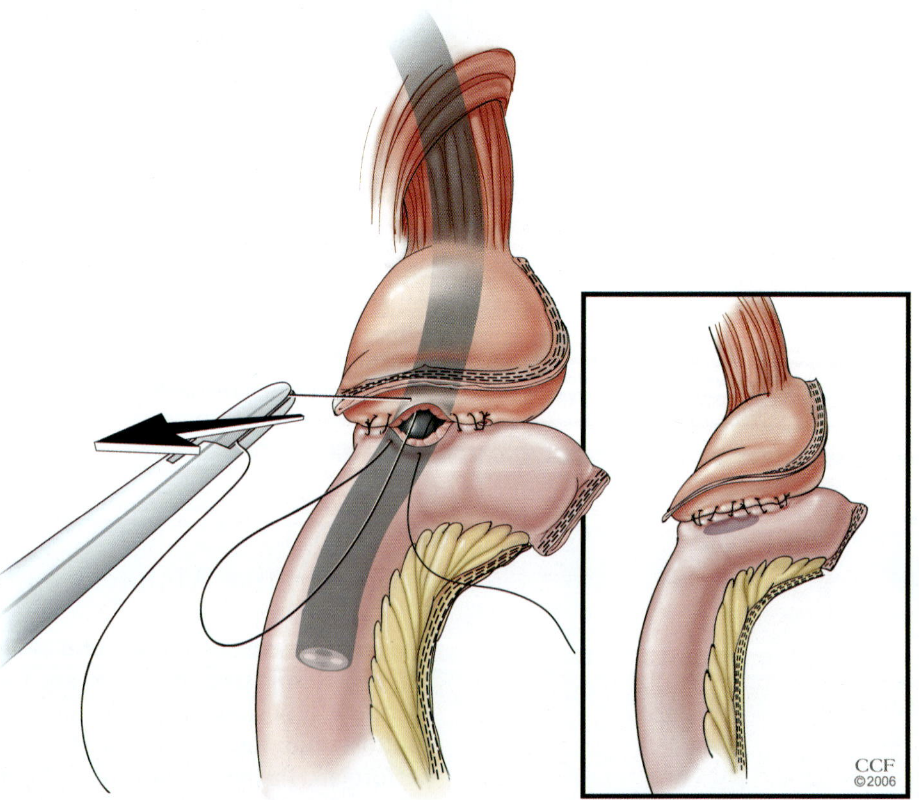

FIGURE 21.4-13. Nonabsorbable sutures are used to close the common opening from each end. An endoscope is passed into the Roux limb to size the anastomosis. A second layer of non-absorbable suture is placed to complete the anastomosis. The endoscope is used to check the anastomosis for leaks and bleeding. (Courtesy of the Cleveland Clinic Foundation.)

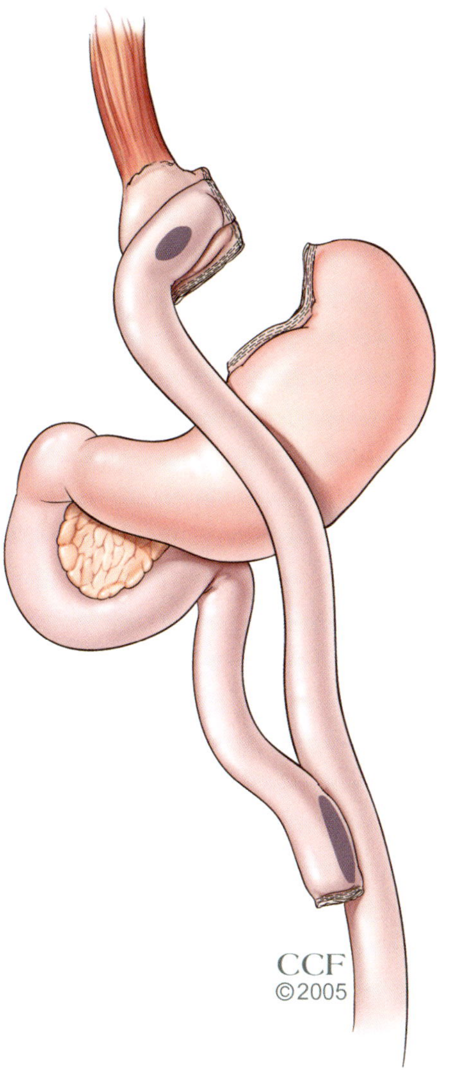

FIGURE 21.4-14. Completed Roux-en-Y gastric bypass. (Courtesy of the Cleveland Clinic Foundation.)

postoperative day. The Jackson-Pratt drain is removed when the patient is seen in the clinic at 1 week, assuming there is no abnormality either in the volume or character of the drain output.

Technical Cautions

In revision gastric bypass surgery, the gastric wall may be of such thickness as to prevent application of this technique with the blue staple load. A mucosa-to-mucosa anastomosis will be difficult to ensure and a blue load may be of inadequate staple height. In this situation, a hand-sewn anastomosis with the endoscope acting as a guide to the true gastric lumen will facilitate the safe creation of a gastrojejunostomy.

Complications

Anastomotic leaks, strictures, and marginal ulceration are the three most common complications associated with the gastrojejunostomy (8,9). There is clearly a leaning curve associated with this technique. Our first 250 patients had a radiologic leak rate of 3.3%, falling to 1% with our most recent 250 patients, after over 3000 patients. The literature reports a 2% to 5% incidence of leaks.

Stricture of the gastroenterostomy after laparoscopic Roux-en-Y gastric bypass (LRYGBP) can complicate stapled and hand-sewn anastomoses. A prospective study of 1000 patients undergoing LRYGBP with the gastrojejunal anastomosis made with a linear stapler revealed 3.2% patients with stenosis at the gastroenterostomy. Strictures typically develop within a year after surgery. While endoscopic dilation is effective initial therapy, over 50% of patients require multiple dilations. Failure to achieve durable dilatation after five or more attempts may point to ischemia as contributory factor, and these patients may require surgical revision (10).

Alternative Anastomotic Techniques

Shope et al. (11) compared the results of two laparoscopic techniques for gastrojejunal anastomosis: circular end-to-end anastomosis (EEA) and linear cutting gastrointestinal anastomosis (GIA) staplers. Operative time was shorter for the GIA; few anastomotic leaks following GIA technique were serious and required early reoperations; the incidence of wound infections was increased following the EEA technique. No important differences in excess weight loss, length of hospital stay, total hospital costs, and operating-room costs were noted. The authors suggest that selection of the anastomotic technique should mainly be based on surgeon preference (11).

References

1. Wittgrove AC, Clark GW, Tremblay LJ. Laparoscopic gastric bypass, Roux-en-Y: preliminary report of five cases. Obes Surg 1994;4:353–357.
2. Wittgrove AC, Clark GW. Combined laparoscopic/endoscopic anvil placement for the performance of the gastroenterostomy. Obes Surg 2001;11:565–569.
3. Gonzalez R, Lin E, Venkatesh KR, Bowers SP, Smith CD. Gastrojejunostomy during laparoscopic gastric bypass: analysis of 3 techniques. Arch Surg 2003;138:181–184.
4. Higa KD, Boone KB, Ho T, Davies OG. Laparoscopic Roux-en-Y gastric bypass for morbid obesity: technique and preliminary results of our first 400 patients. Arch Surg 2000;135:1029–1033; discussion 1033–1034.
5. Higa KD, Ho T, Boone KB. Laparoscopic Roux-en-Y gastric bypass: technique and 3-year follow-up. J Laparoendosc Adv Surg Tech A 2001;11:377–382.

6. Champion JK, Williams MD. Prospective randomized comparison of linear staplers during laparoscopic Roux-en-Y gastric bypass. Obes Surg 2003;13:855–859; discussion 860.

7. Korenkov M, Goh P, Yucel N, Troidl H. Laparoscopic gastric bypass for morbid obesity with linear gastroenterostomy. Obes Surg 2003;13:360–363.

8. Nguyen NT, Stevens CM, Wolfe BM. Incidence and outcome of anastomotic stricture after laparoscopic gastric bypass. J Gastrointest Surg 2003;7:997–1003; discussion 1003.

9. Nguyen NT, Rivers R, Wolfe BM. Early gastrointestinal hemorrhage after laparoscopic gastric bypass. Obes Surg 2003;13:62–65.

10. Schwartz ML, Drew RL, Roiger RW, Ketover SR, Chazin-Caldie M. Stenosis of the gastroenterostomy after laparoscopic gastric bypass. Obes Surg 2004;14:484–491.

11. Shope TR, Cooney RN, McLeod J, Miller CA, Haluck RS. Early results after laparoscopic gastric bypass: EEA vs GIA stapled gastrojejunal anastomosis. Obes Surg 2003;13:355–359.

21.5
Laparoscopic Roux-en-Y Gastric Bypass: Outcomes

Tomasz Rogula, Paul A. Thodiyil, Stacy A. Brethauer, and Philip R. Schauer

Obesity is a rapidly growing health problem that contributes to numerous life-threatening or disabling problems including type 2 diabetes mellitus, hyperlipidemia, degenerative joint disease, and obstructive sleep apnea. Significant weight reduction in the morbidly obese patient improves or reverses associated illness and benefits the patient's general well-being. The resolution of comorbidities following surgically induced weight loss is well established. Type 2 diabetes mellitus resolves in 82% to 98.8% of patients, hypertension in 52% to 91.5%, gastroesophageal reflux in 72%–97.8%, hypercholesterolemia in 63% to 97%, sleep apnea in 74% to 97.8%, stress urinary incontinence in 44% to 97%, arthritis in 41% to 90.3%, and migraine headache in 57% (1–5). Superior outcomes are expected with increasing experience, perfection of operative technique, and refinements in postoperative care.

Various complications, including anastomotic leaks, pulmonary embolism, hemorrhage, stenosis of the gastrojejunal anastomosis, and wound infections correlate less with body habitus than with the operative experience of the surgeon (6). An experience of more than 75 laparoscopic Roux-en-Y gastric bypasses (LRYGBPs) also decreases operative time and length of hospital stay (7). In experienced hands, conversion to an open operation is seldom necessary and usually occurs in the super-obese patient with a massively enlarged liver or excessive intraperitoneal fat that prohibits a safe laparoscopic operation.

The type and frequency of complications have changed with the development of laparoscopic technique. The rate of some complications has increased with laparoscopic gastric bypass whereas others have almost disappeared due to the smaller access incision. Specifically, significantly fewer abdominal wall complications such as wound infections and incisional hernias are seen after laparoscopic gastric bypass. There is an increased rate of bowel obstruction, gastrointestinal tract hemorrhage, and stomal stenosis in laparoscopic patients; however, anastomotic leaks and pulmonary embolisms occur with similar rates with both approaches (8). Length of hospital stay and return to normal activities are improved in laparoscopic gastric bypass. Excessive weight loss in early postoperative follow-up after LRYGBP is greater than in open gastric bypass (9).

Recent data on outcomes of bariatric surgery lead to the conclusion that, despite the change in the types of complications that can occur in laparoscopic versus open gastric bypass, the numerous advantages of laparoscopy make this the preferable approach for the treatment of morbidly obese patients (10).

Resolution of Comorbidities

Metabolic Syndrome

The cluster of cardiovascular risk factors referred to as the metabolic syndrome consists of abdominal obesity, atherogenic dyslipidemia, elevated blood pressure, insulin resistance or glucose intolerance, a proinflammatory state, and a prothrombotic state. Obesity is thought to be a necessary factor for the development of the metabolic syndrome, but many obese people do not develop the metabolic syndrome. The rate of metabolic syndrome has been reported as high as 52% in patients seeking bariatric surgery (11).

Bariatric surgery results in the simultaneous improvement of all the components of the metabolic syndrome. In a study by Mattar et al. (12), the incidence of metabolic syndrome decreased from 70% to 14% 15 months after bariatric surgery [with 60% excess weight loss (EWL)] and Lee et al. (13) demonstrated 95.6% resolution of the metabolic syndrome in 337 patients 1 year after LRYGBP.

Type 2 Diabetes Mellitus

Laparoscopic Roux-en-Y gastric bypass for morbid obesity leads to impressive improvement in patients with type 2 diabetes mellitus. Fasting plasma glucose and glycosylated hemoglobin concentrations return to normal levels in over 80% of patients. A significant reduction in the use of oral antidiabetic agents and insulin is seen in 80% of patients. In a meta-analysis that included 3625 patients with diabetes or impaired glucose tolerance, diabetes resolved in 99% of patients after biliopancreatic diversion (BPD), 84% after gastric bypass, 72% after gastroplasty, and 48% after gastric banding (14). Large series of laparoscopic gastric bypass report resolution of diabetes in 83% to 98% of patients (1,5,15). Patients with a shorter duration of diabetes, less severe diabetes, and the greatest weight loss after surgery have the highest rates of biochemical normalization after LRYGBP (15). Improved glucose control with concomitant reduced serum insulin levels occurs immediately following surgery prior to massive weight loss. This may be due to alterations of specific gut hormones that stimulate β-cell function or improved peripheral glucose uptake following weight loss after gastric bypass surgery (16). Another possible mechanism includes reduced caloric intake with concomitant reversal of insulin resistance in muscle (17). Diabetes mellitus may be associated with poorer postoperative weight loss in some patients (18).

Hypertension

The incidence of hypertension in the bariatric surgery population ranges from 35% to 51% (14,19). In Buchwald et al.'s (14) meta-analysis that included open Roux-en-Y gastric bypass and LRYGBP, 75% of patients had resolution of their hypertension after bariatric surgery and an additional 12% improved. Hypertension resolved in 52% to 92% of patients after laparoscopic gastric bypass in large series (1,5,15). Sugerman et al. (19) studied the relationship among diabetes, hypertension, and severe obesity and found that the longer a person remains severely obese, the higher the likelihood of developing diabetes, hypertension, or both. In this study, 75% of patients with diabetes also had hypertension. Excess weight loss of 59% at 5 to 7 years resulted in resolution of hypertension in 66% of patients and diabetes in 86% (19).

Hyperlipidemia

Dyslipidemia and hypercholesterolemia are common in the bariatric surgery population. Bariatric surgery improves serum lipid profiles in 79% of patients and thereby decreases cardiovascular risk. The highest rates of change occur with malabsorptive BPD or gastric bypass procedures with improvement in hyperlipidemia in over 96% of patients. Schauer et al. (20) demonstrated resolution of hyperlipidemia in 63% of patients undergoing LRYGBP.

Obstructive Sleep Apnea and Pulmonary Dysfunction

Surgically induced weight loss greatly reduces sleep apnea symptoms in the majority of patients. Excellent results were reported despite the type of surgical approach (21). Laparoscopic Roux-en-Y gastric bypass very effectively controls sleep apnea. In long-term follow-up, 93% of patients demonstrated significant improvement (22). Results are usually confirmed with repeated polysomnography that reveals considerable improvement or even a complete recovery of disordered breathing during sleep and normalization of sleep structure (23). Atrial and ventricular arrhythmias are frequently observed in association with apneic episodes, and these are also ameliorated after gastric bypass surgery (24). Recurrence of sleep apnea has been reported after an initial response to surgically induced weight loss, despite the fact that the weight was not regained (25).

Another problem in severe obese patients is decreased ventilation secondary to abdominal fat impeding the movement of the diaphragm as wells as adipose tissue in and around the thorax. Such hypoventilation leads to hypercarbia and daytime somnolence. This condition, called pickwickian syndrome, leads to severe problems including prolonged hospitalization, complications secondary to extended intubation and mechanical ventilation, pneumothorax, adult respiratory distress syndrome, and pneumonia. The only effective cure is substantial weight loss (26). Patients with pickwickian syndrome are at higher risk of operative mortality; however, the overall risk-benefit ratio generally favors surgery (27).

Altered intraoperative pulmonary mechanics are better tolerated by obese patients without concomitant pulmonary dysfunction (28). Additionally, patients undergoing laparoscopic gastric bypass have significantly fewer pulmonary problems than open gastric bypass patients at the early postoperative stage; for example, segmental atelectasis occurs ten times less often after laparoscopic gastric bypass (29).

Gastroesophageal Reflux

Many patients referred for bariatric surgery have evidence of chronic gastroesophageal reflux disease (GERD). Laparoscopic Roux-en-Y gastric bypass is very effective treatment for GERD, leading to complete resolution or significant improvement of symptoms and decreased medication use. Three laparoscopic gastric bypass studies report resolution of GERD in 72% to 98% of patients (14,20). Long-term follow-up confirmed very good control of GERD in morbidly obese patients within 3 years (30). The LRYGBP simultaneously treats GERD and results in weight loss and comorbidity reduction and should be offered as the primary procedure for these patients instead of fundoplication (31). The LRYGBP can also be used for recalcitrant GERD in morbidly obese patients who have previously undergone an antireflux procedure with poor results (9). Vertical banded gastroplasty is not an effective procedure in GERD patients and frequently causes reflux symptoms, and malabsorption operations have no proven efficacy against GERD (32).

Arthritis and Back Pain

Overweight and obesity cause more rapid deterioration of weight-bearing joints, such as the knees, ankles, and hips. The pathogenesis of osteoarthritis involves a dual process of catabolism and repair at the weight-bearing joints. Obesity is associated with an increase in symptomatic osteoarthritis of the knee, hip, and the lumbar spine (32). Weight loss surgery is the only therapeutic intervention that has been shown to slow the progression of damage in joints that are already involved, or reverse pathologic changes. The resolution of weight-induced degenerative joint disease is reported in 41% to 90% of patients (1,5,20). Improvement or complete resolution is measured by self-esteem quality of life assessment and the need for antiinflammatory and analgesic medication.

Morbidly obese individuals with severe degenerative joint disease who are initially considered unsuitable for arthroplasty because of their weight should be considered for bariatric surgery. Total joint arthroplasty after surgical treatment of obesity has an excellent outcome with an acceptable complication rate. In this patient population, the majority of prostheses are stable with no evidence of radiographic loosening or wear at final surveillance (33).

Urinary Incontinence

Urinary incontinence not caused by autonomic neuropathy responds very quickly to weight loss (34). Stress urinary incontinence completely resolves or significantly improves in 44% to 97% of patients following LRYGBP (1,5,20). First, this is a result of a decrease in the volume of liquid that can be consumed. Second, there is a decrease in intraabdominal pressure from the decrease in bulk food consumed and a reduction in abdominal fat. These factors result in less pressure on the urethral sphincter and improvement in incontinence (19,35). As abdominal weight continues to decrease, the incidence of incontinence diminishes. Improvement is usually evaluated subjectively by quality-of-life questionnaires. Objectively, improvement can be measured by changes in vesical pressure, the increase in bladder pressure with coughing, bladder-to-urethra pressure transmission with cough, urethral axial mobility, number of incontinence episodes, and the need to use absorptive pads (36).

Thyroid Disorders

Hypothyroidism is often associated with increased body weight. Hypothyroidism improves in more than 40% of patients following gastric bypass surgery. Reduction of thyroxine requirements is most likely the result of the decrease in the body mass index (BMI) (37). Obese patients with subnormal thyroid function who are euthyroid on replacement therapy prior to bariatric surgery have short-term weight loss similar to obese patients who have normal thyroid function (38).

Nonalcoholic Fatty Liver Disease

Nonalcoholic fatty liver disease (NAFLD) includes a spectrum of disease that begins with fatty infiltration of the liver and progresses to fibrosis and ultimately to cirrhosis in 25% of patients (39). The prevalence of NAFLD in morbidly obese patients ranges from 20% to 40%, and surgical weight loss has a significant impact on this disease. In a study by Mattar et al. (13), 70 patients who underwent laparoscopic bariatric surgery had pre- and postoperative liver biopsies. After surgical weight loss of 59% EWL, there was marked improvement in liver steatosis (from 88% to 8%), inflammation (from 23% to 2%), and fibrosis (from 31% to 13%) with an interval of 15 ± 9 months between biopsies. Inflammation and fibrosis resolved in 37% and 20% of patients, respectively, corresponding to improvement of 82% in grade and 39% in stage of liver disease (13). Similar improvement of fatty liver disease and metabolic syndrome have been demonstrated after biliopancreatic diversion (40) and laparoscopic adjustable gastric banding (41).

Cirrhosis

The safety and efficacy of bariatric surgery in patients with liver diseases is one of the major concerns in bariatric surgery. It is estimated that about 1.5% of patients who undergo LRYGBP have cirrhosis. The diagnosis of cirrhosis is usually made intraoperatively. In large series, cirrhotic patients undergoing LRYGBP have an acceptable complication rate and achieve satisfactory early weight loss that is similar to that in noncirrhotic patients (42). It is unclear whether pneumoperitoneum created during laparoscopic gastric bypass reduces hepatic portal blood flow and alters postoperative hepatic function in cirrhotic patients. After LRYGBP, alanine aminotransferase (ALT) and aspartate aminotransferase (AST) only transiently increase and return to baseline levels at 72 hours. Interestingly, a similar transient increase is also seen in open gastric bypass (43).

Clinical Outcomes

Weight Loss

Laparoscopic Roux-en-Y gastric bypass produces significant weight loss in patients with clinically severe obesity. The LRYGBP was introduced by Wittgrove et al. (44) in 1993, and it is now the most commonly performed bariatric procedure worldwide (45). Initial randomized prospective studies comparing results of LRYGBP with open bypass suggest better EWL for LRYGBP at 3 and 6 months. However, by 12 months excess weight loss was equivalent (68% vs. 62%) (46). Further experience reported in case series confirmed excellent weight loss following LRYGBP with 68% to 85% EWL 1 to 5 years after surgery (1–4). Longer follow-up after RYGBP reveals some weight regain with 60% to 70% EWL at 5 years. Fourteen-year follow-up of open RYGBP demonstrates EWL of 49% (17). Similar long-term weight loss data are not yet available for LRYGBP.

Operative Time

Operative time generally ranges from less than 2 hours to up to 4 hours and appears to increase with increasing BMI and decrease with experience. The learning curve for laparoscopic gastric bypass is long and more demanding than with many other minimally invasive operations (47). With extensive experience, operative times for LRYGBP can be reduced significantly and are comparable to open gastric bypass operative times regardless of BMI (2).

Length of Hospital Stay

The length of hospital stay after laparoscopic gastric bypass is typically 2 to 3 days. Although some centers report similar length of hospital stay for both open and laparoscopic gastric bypass patients, the majority report a shorter length of stay in the hospital after laparoscopic gastric bypass, usually 2 to 3 days versus 4 to 5 days (48,49). Despite the surgical approach, full return to gastrointestinal function and sustained oral intake usually takes 1 to 2 days if the patient does not require extra pain medication and no complications occur.

Postoperative Pain and Pulmonary Function

The degree of postoperative pain after open gastric is clearly related to the length of the surgical incision, the extent of intraabdominal dissection, and overall trauma to the abdomen from surgical retraction. Laparoscopic gastric bypass patients require less self-administered pain medication and have lower visual analog scale pain scores on the first postoperative day compared to open RYGBP patients (29).

Pulmonary complications occur after open and laparoscopic RYGBP, but there was no significant difference in rates of postoperative pneumonia in a large review of the literature (0.33% open, 0.14% laparoscopic). A randomized trial by Nguyen and colleagues (29) did show significant advantages in early postoperative pulmonary function with the laparoscopic approach.

Recovery and Quality of Life

Recovery measured by the number of days between the operation and the patient's return to activities of daily living and work is significantly improved after laparoscopic gastric bypass when compared to open gastric bypass (46). The average time of return to normal activity is 21 days after laparoscopic gastric bypass surgery (50).

Quality-of-life, general well-being, health distress, and perceived attractiveness are significantly impaired in morbidly obese patients (51). Although the long-term quality of life following laparoscopic gastric bypass does not differ from that after open gastric bypass, laparoscopic gastric bypass patients have more interest in sexual activity and are able to work more than open gastric bypass patients 3 months postoperatively (46).

Complications

Conversion to Open Operation

With adequate surgeon experience, conversion in laparoscopic gastric bypass is rare and occurs in fewer than 5% of cases. The reasons for conversion to laparotomy include difficulty in initiating pneumoperitoneum, enlarged liver causing difficulty in obtaining exposure, extensive abdominal adhesions, and failure to make progress. Conversion rate is also influenced by the fact that many experienced surgeons operate on complicated cases, such as revisional procedures. In a large series of more than 1200 patients, the conversion rate was 3%. In this report, the cause of conversion included technical difficulties in 80%, intraoperative bleeding in 10%, and an enlarged liver obstructing access to the operative field in 10% (52).

Anastomotic Intestinal Leak

Anastomotic intestinal leaks are associated with significant mortality and morbidity. Gastrointestinal leak is usually diagnosed clinically, based on physical parameters such as tachycardia, respiratory distress, fever, peritonitis, decreased urine output, and hypotension (53).

In the majority of reports, the incidence of leaks varies from 0% to 5%. Beyond the end of the learning curve

(75 to 100 cases), the likelihood of gastrointestinal leak may be significantly reduced (0% to 1.6%) (1,5,46, 47,54–56). Studies also show that older, heavier men with multiple comorbid conditions are at increased risk for leak and mortality. Surgeons early in their learning curve should avoid these high-risk patients to reduce complications (57). Randomized studies comparing laparoscopic and open gastric bypass demonstrated no significant difference in the occurrence of leak (1.3% vs. 2.6%) (58). In some reports, the antecolic and antegastric technique of gastric bypass resulted in a considerable improvement in the incidence of leaks (2). Modifications in stapling technologies, in particular using biologic buttressing materials, may further reduce the risk of postoperative anastomotic leak (46). Fibrin sealant applied to the gastrointestinal anastomosis site appears to eliminate anastomotic leaks in some series (59).

Anastomotic Stricture

Gastrojejunal anastomotic strictures are one of the most common complication of LRYGBP, occurring in 4% to 28% of patients (60). A randomized comparative study comparing laparoscopic and open bypass revealed a higher incidence of stricture following LRYGBP (11.4% vs. 2.6%) (6). A hand-sewn gastroenteric anastomosis appears to decrease the incidence of strictures; however, this is not confirmed in prospective randomized studies (6). For circular stapling technique, the 25-mm circular stapler results in a significantly lower stricture rate compared to the 21-mm stapler without compromising weight loss (61). Stenosis most commonly occurs 1 to 3 months after surgery but rarely can occur years later. Gastrojejunal anastomotic strictures are successfully treated with one or two endoscopic dilations in the majority of cases.

Thromboembolism

Despite many efforts taken for perioperative prophylaxis against low venous thrombosis (62–64), pulmonary thromboembolism is the leading cause of mortality following gastric bypass (65). Theoretically, laparoscopic surgery increases the risk of thromboembolism due to diminished venous return induced by the pneumoperitoneum and Trendelenburg positioning (1,2,4). Despite these potential risks, many studies have demonstrated an incidence of pulmonary embolus following laparoscopic gastric bypass of 0% to 1.1% and these rates are similar to the open series (2,4,5,29,57,66–68). The mortality rate due to pulmonary embolism following LRYGBP ranges from 0% to 0.4% (2,46,49). Although extremely rare, acute mesenteric venous thrombosis following Roux-en-Y gastric bypass is a severe and life-threatening complication that requires early exploration and anticoagulation (46).

Blood Loss

Intraoperative blood loss for LRYGBP is less when compared to open gastric bypass (137 vs. 395 mL) (2,70). The most common location of postoperative bleeding is the staple line of the gastric remnant or gastrojejunostomy, or less frequently at the jejunojejunostomy. Overall, the incidence of gastrointestinal bleeding following LRYGBP is low, ranging from 0.6% to 3.3% (1,2,20, 46,71), but a review of the open and laparoscopic gastric bypass literature revealed that the incidence is higher in the laparoscopic group (1.9% vs. 0.6%) (8).

Two thirds of patients who bleed postoperatively develop intraluminal bleeding, manifested by a drop in hematocrit, tachycardia, and melena. About 15% of patients with intraluminal bleeding can be unstable and require urgent reoperation. The majority of these patients can be observed and transfused if necessary with resolution of the intraluminal bleeding. The diagnosis and treatment of acute intraluminal bleeding after LRYGBP is difficult due to the inaccessibility of the bypassed stomach and the jejunojejunostomy and the risks associated with early postoperative endoscopy (72).

Marginal Ulceration

Vomiting, epigastric pain, and gastrointestinal bleeding may be symptomatic for marginal ulcer following gastric bypass. The reported incidence of marginal ulceration following LRYGBP (0.7% to 10%) is similar to that reported in open series (0.49% to 16%) (3,4,46,73–78). Ulceration may be due to local ischemia, foreign body, gastric acid secretion, anastomotic tension, *Helicobacter pylori* infection, gastrogastric fistula, or nonsteroidal antiinflammatory drugs. Conservative management with acid-suppression medication and sucralfate is successful in majority of patients (79). Surgical revision may be needed for treatment of gastrogastric fistula.

Incisional and Internal Hernias

The decreased rate of incisional hernias after LRYGBP is one of the most significant advantages of this approach. After open gastric bypass, incisional hernia can occur in up to 24% of patients at 14 years (79). Internal hernia following Roux-en-Y gastric bypass may occur at the mesenteric defect of the jejunojejunostomy, at the transverse mesocolic window, or through the space between the mesentery of the Roux limb and the transverse mesocolon (Petersen defect). The incidence of internal hernias ranges from 0.7% to 2.5% of patients (79). Initially, numerous studies reported a higher incidence of internal hernia and bowel obstruction following LRYGBP. Introduction of several technical modifications, including closure of defects with nonabsorbable suture and placement of an antiobstruction stitch adjacent to the small bowel anastomosis, has led to a reduction in internal hernia formation (80). Higa et al. (79), in their experience of 1040 patients, reported a 50% reduction in the hernia rate after introduction of a nonabsorbable suture to close the mesocolic defects. The incidence of small bowel obstruction due to internal hernias reaches 2% in a large series of laparoscopic gastric bypass patients, and is usually associated with a high morbidity. A significant decrease in occurrence was found after adoption of antecolic placement of the Roux limb (81).

Wound Infection

Wound infection is a significant problem following open gastric bypass and occurs in up to 25% of patients (82). The incidence of wound infections has drastically dropped in laparoscopic series (0.1% to 8.7%) (1,2,81). Randomized studies on open and LRYGBP support this benefit of laparoscopic surgery, showing infection rates of 10.5% in open gastric bypass and 1.3% in the laparoscopic patients (83).

Cholelithiasis

Cholelithiasis is relatively common in patients who rapidly lose weight after gastric bypass. Following this surgery, gallstones may be sonographically detectable within 6 months after surgery in 38% of patients, with 41% of these becoming symptomatic (84). The incidence of symptomatic cholelithiasis following LRYGBP reaches 1.4% to 5.4% (19,54,85,86). In the past, the increased risk for gallstones led to routine prophylactic cholecystectomy in patients undergoing gastric bypass (47,87). The prophylactic use of oral ursodiol at 600 mg daily for the first 6 months after LRYGBP significantly reduces the incidence of gallstone formation (2% vs. 32% in placebo, $p < .01$) (72). Therefore, the indication for routine cholecystectomy became questionable, and many surgeons now perform concomitant cholecystectomy only for patients with symptomatic gallstones. Combining these two procedures significantly increases operative time and nearly doubles the hospital stay (56). Another rational approach involves routine intraoperative sonography and selective cholecystectomy in nonsymptomatic patients with close follow-up (46).

Nutritional Deficiencies

Iron, vitamin B_{12}, and other micronutrient deficiencies can occur after standard gastric bypass (88). Taking a single multivitamin tablet alone is usually insufficient to prevent iron and vitamin B_{12} deficiencies after LRYGBP. Iron deficiency occurs in 13% to 52% of patients (2 to 5 years after surgery) despite supplementation with a mul-

tivitamin and iron (for menstruating women). Vitamin B_{12} deficiency occurs in up to 37% of patients who are prescribed a multivitamin after surgery. Once a specific deficiency is identified during follow-up, additional supplementation is indicated.

Calcium absorption in the duodenum and jejunum and vitamin D absorption in the jejunum and ileum are impaired after RYGBP as well. These deficiencies can occur in up to 10% and 51%, respectively, and occur more frequently with long-limb gastric bypass (88). These deficiencies can lead to secondary hyperparathyroidism and can result in increased bone turnover and decreased bone mass as early as 3 to 9 months after surgery (89).

Mortality

Mortality rates after laparoscopic gastric bypass range from 0% to 2%, and there was no difference in mortality rates between open and laparoscopic gastric bypass in three randomized trails (46,68,90). The mortality rate for gastric bypass (open and laparoscopic) in Buchwald et al.'s (13) meta-analysis was 0.5% (5644 patients).

Mortality in large cases series is low. Higa et al. (2) reported an overall mortality rate of 0.5% in 1040 patients, and Wittgrove et al. (1) reported no mortality in their series of 500 laparoscopic gastric bypass operations. Schauer et al. (20) reported one death in their series of 275 LRYGBP patients (0.4%) secondary to a pulmonary embolism. In LRYGBP series with >100 patients, the mortality rate ranges from 0% to 0.9% (1,2,5,20,91).

The risk factors associated with perioperative death include male sex, advanced age, anastomotic leak, pulmonary embolus, preoperative weight, and hypertension. The access method, open versus laparoscopic, is not predictive of death, but the operation type, proximal versus long limb, is predictive (77).

Flum et al. (92) reported advancing age and surgeon volume were associated with mortality after bariatric surgery. In this study, Medicare patients older than 65 had a significantly higher risk of death after bariatric surgery than did younger patients. All-cause 30-day and 90-day mortality for 16,155 Medicare patients who underwent bariatric surgery (81% RYGBP, open and laparoscopic) was 2% and 2.8%, respectively. Patients older than 65 had 4.8% 30-day and 6.9% 90-day mortality rates. The risk of early death after surgery was associated with lower surgeon volume, which has been demonstrated in other studies as well (93). A larger review of 60,077 patients who underwent open and laparoscopic gastric bypass surgery in California reported mortality rates more consistent with those seen in large case series. In this review, in-hospital mortality was 0.18%, 30-day mortality was 0.33%, and 1-year mortality was 0.91% (94).

Severely obese individuals have a decreased life expectancy, and there is evidence that bariatric surgery can improve the life span of obese patients. In an observational cohort study comparing bariatric surgery patients to matched controls, the 5-year mortality in patients undergoing bariatric surgery was 0.68% compared to 16.2% in the medically managed obese patients (89% relative risk reduction) (95). In this study, 81.4% of the 1035 patients underwent gastric bypass, but only 21 were performed laparoscopically.

Flum and colleagues (96) evaluated survival after gastric bypass in a retrospective cohort study and found a 27% reduction in 15-year mortality in morbidly obese patients who underwent gastric bypass versus those who did not. After the surgical patients reached the first postoperative year, the long-term survival advantage increased to 33%.

Outcomes in Super-Obese Patients

Laparoscopic Roux-en-Y gastric bypass has been shown to be safe and effective for patients with BMI ≥50. Resolution or improvement of comorbidities is noted in the majority of patients 1 year after surgery. Short-term excess weight loss is slightly lower than EWL in patients who are not super-obese. Excess weight loss after LRYGBP in patients with BMI >50 ranges from 51% to 69% 1 to 3 years after surgery (97–99). In one series comparing 167 LRYGBP patients with BMI <60 to 46 patients with BMI ≥60, the mean EWL at 1 year in patients with BMI <60 was 64% versus 53% in patients with BMI ≥60 (98).

Conversion rates are similar to those for operations done for less heavy patients; however, operative time for the patients with BMI ≥60 is longer, and major complications (infectious complications and gastrointestinal leak) tend to occur more often in heavy patients (84,100). Studies also indicate increased mortality rate in super-obese patients (5% for super-obese vs. 0.4% for obese) (101). Increasing the length of the Roux limb to 150 cm in Roux-en-Y gastric bypass effectively increases excess weight loss in super-obese patients. However, extending the Roux limb length did not significantly improve weight loss outcome in patients with a BMI <50 (86).

Cost Analysis

Operative costs of the procedure are higher for laparoscopic gastric bypass compared to open. The difference between the laparoscopic and open gastric bypass operations is the expense of the disposable instruments required by laparoscopic procedure. The direct operative costs are 37% to 58% greater for laparoscopic gastric bypass than for open gastric bypass (46,102). These costs may be partially compensated by the hospital service,

which is 33% less expensive after laparoscopic gastric bypass than after open gastric bypass. Differences are evident in terms of direct operative cost (LRYGBP $4922 vs. open $3591) and are attributable to higher equipment charges ($4098 vs. $2788) and longer operative time (225 vs. 195 minutes). This difference is often offset by increased nursing and pharmaceutical costs for the open surgery (46). The total (direct and indirect) cost, however, is similar for the two operations ($14,087 vs. $14,098) (46). Although the total costs are similar, LRYGBP might have the advantage if intangible costs such as pain, lost work days, and patient well-being and satisfaction are considered. Potential cost savings may be achieved with the increased use of reusable laparoscopic instruments and the reduced operative time.

Conclusion

A decade of experience has demonstrated excellent outcomes of the laparoscopic Roux-en-Y gastric bypass. Minimally invasive techniques are extremely helpful for morbidly obese patients, particularly as a means to reduce or eliminate cardiopulmonary and wound-related complications. Most series have a mean follow-up of less than 2 years but consistently demonstrate a favorable EWL of 65% to 80%. Most authors report that major life-threatening comorbidities either resolve or improve with significant weight loss. Complication rates for open and laparoscopic RYGBP are similar, but the types of complications differ according to the technique used. Operating time, conversion rates, and anastomotic leak rates improve with increasing surgeon experience. The mean hospital stay (including complications) is typically 2 to 3 days. There are currently no long-term studies (>5 years) evaluating the efficacy of LRYGBP. Durability has been demonstrated with the open RYGBP, though, and given the identical anatomic changes, it is reasonable to expect similar long-term outcomes with the laparoscopic approach.

References

1. Wittgrove AC, Clark GW. Laparoscopic gastric bypass, Roux-en-Y—500 patients: technique and results, with 3–60 month follow-up. Obes Surg 2000;10(3):233–239.
2. Higa KD, Boone KB, Ho T. Complications of the laparoscopic Roux-en-Y gastric bypass: 1,040 patients—what have we learned? Obes Surg 2000;10(6):509–513.
3. Higa KD, Ho T, Boone KB. Laparoscopic Roux-en-Y gastric bypass: technique and 3-year follow-up. J Laparoendosc Adv Surg Tech A 2001;11(6):377–382.
4. Schauer PR, Ikramuddin S, Gourash W, et al. Outcomes after laparoscopic Roux-en-Y gastric bypass for morbid obesity. Ann Surg 2000;232(4):515–529.

5. DeMaria EJ, Sugerman HJ, Kellum JM, et al. Results of 281 consecutive total laparoscopic Roux-en-Y gastric bypasses to treat morbid obesity. Ann Surg 2002;235(5): 640–645; discussion 645–647.

6. Shepherd MF, Rosborough TK, Schwartz ML. Heparin thromboprophylaxis in gastric bypass surgery. Obes Surg 2003;13(2):249–253.

7. Nguyen NT, Rivers R, Wolfe BM. Factors associated with operative outcomes in laparoscopic gastric bypass. J Am Coll Surg 2003;197(4):548–555; discussion 555–557.

8. Podnos YD, Jimenez JC, Wilson SE, et al. Complications after laparoscopic gastric bypass: a review of 3464 cases. Arch Surg 2003;138(9):957–961.

9. Courcoulas A, Perry Y, Buenaventura P, Luketich J. Comparing the outcomes after laparoscopic versus open gastric bypass: a matched paired analysis. Obes Surg 2003;13(3):341–346.

10. Jones DB, Provost DA, DeMaria EJ, et al. Optimal management of the morbidly obese patient SAGES appropriateness conference statement. Surg Endosc 2004.

11. Grundy SM, Brewer HB Jr, Cleeman JI, et al. Definition of metabolic syndrome: Report of the National Heart, Lung, and Blood Institute/American Heart Association conference on scientific issues related to definition. Circulation 2004;109(3):433–438.

12. Mattar SG, Velcu LM, Rabinovitz M, et al. Surgically-induced weight loss significantly improves nonalcoholic fatty liver disease and the metabolic syndrome. Ann Surg 2005;242(4):610–617; discussion 618–620.

13. Lew WJ, Yu PJ, Wang W et al. Laparoscopic Roux-en-Y versus mini-gastric bypass for the treatment of morbid obsity: a prospective randomized controlled clinical trial. Ann Surg 2005;242:20–28.

14. Buchwald H, Avidor Y, Braunwald E, et al. Bariatric surgery: a systematic review and meta-analysis. JAMA 2004;292(14):1724–1737.

15. Schauer PR, Burguera B, Ikramuddin S, et al. Effect of laparoscopic Roux-en Y gastric bypass on type 2 diabetes mellitus. Ann Surg 2003;238(4):467–484; discussion 484–485.

16. Friedman JE, Dohm GL, Leggett-Frazier N, et al. Restoration of insulin responsiveness in skeletal muscle of morbidly obese patients after weight loss. Effect on muscle glucose transport and glucose transporter GLUT4. J Clin Invest 1992;89(2):701–705.

17. Pories WJ, Swanson MS, MacDonald KG, et al. Who would have thought it? An operation proves to be the most effective therapy for adult-onset diabetes mellitus. Ann Surg 1995;222(3):339–350; discussion 350–352.

18. Perugini RA, Mason R, Czerniach DR, et al. Predictors of complication and suboptimal weight loss after laparoscopic Roux-en-Y gastric bypass: a series of 188 patients. Arch Surg 2003;138(5):541–545; discussion 545–546.

19. Sugerman HJ, Sugerman EL, DeMaria EJ, et al. Bariatric surgery for severely obese adolescents. J Gastrointest Surg 2003;7(1):102–107; discussion 107–108.

20. Schauer PR, Ikramuddin S, Gourash W, et al. Outcomes after laparoscopic Roux-en-Y gastric bypass for morbid obesity. 2000;232(4):515–529.

21. Scheuller M, Weider D. Bariatric surgery for treatment of sleep apnea syndrome in 15 morbidly obese patients: long-term results. Otolaryngol Head Neck Surg 2001;125(4):299–302.

22. Charuzi I, Lavie P, Peiser J, Peled R. Bariatric surgery in morbidly obese sleep-apnea patients: short- and long-term follow-up. Am J Clin Nutr 1992;55(2 suppl):594S–596S.

23. Charuzi I, Ovnat A, Peiser J, et al. The effect of surgical weight reduction on sleep quality in obesity-related sleep apnea syndrome. Surgery 1985;97(5):535–538.

24. Peiser J, Ovnat A, Uwyyed K, et al. Cardiac arrhythmias during sleep in morbidly obese sleep-apneic patients before and after gastric bypass surgery. Clin Cardiol 1985; 8(10):519–521.

25. Pillar G, Peled R, Lavie P. Recurrence of sleep apnea without concomitant weight increase 7.5 years after weight reduction surgery. Chest 1994;106(6):1702–1704.

26. Kessler R, Chaouat A, Schinkewitch P, et al. The obesity-hypoventilation syndrome revisited: a prospective study of 34 consecutive cases. Chest 2001;120(2):369–376.

27. Sugerman HJ, Fairman RP, Sood RK, et al. Long-term effects of gastric surgery for treating respiratory insufficiency of obesity. Am J Clin Nutr 1992;55(2 suppl):597S–601S.

28. Nguyen NT, Anderson JT, Budd M, et al. Effects of pneumoperitoneum on intraoperative pulmonary mechanics and gas exchange during laparoscopic gastric bypass. Surg Endosc 2004;18(1):64–71.

29. Nguyen NT, Lee SL, Goldman C, et al. Comparison of pulmonary function and postoperative pain after laparoscopic versus open gastric bypass: a randomized trial. J Am Coll Surg 2001;192(4):469–476; discussion 476–477.

30. Frezza EE, Ikramuddin S, Gourash W, et al. Symptomatic improvement in gastroesophageal reflux disease (GERD) following laparoscopic Roux-en-Y gastric bypass. Surg Endosc 2002;16(7):1027–1031.

31. Schauer P, Hamad G, Ikramuddin S. Surgical management of gastroesophageal reflux disease in obese patients. Semin Laparosc Surg 2001;8(4):256–264.

32. Scapinelli R. [Obesity and articular tropho-mechanic disorders]. Clin Ortop 1975;26:97–108.

33. Parvizi J, Trousdale RT, Sarr MG. Total joint arthroplasty in patients surgically treated for morbid obesity. J Arthroplasty 2000;15(8):1003–1008.

34. Cummings JM, Rodning CB. Urinary stress incontinence among obese women: review of pathophysiology therapy. Int Urogynecol J Pelvic Floor Dysfunct 2000;11(1):41–44.

35. Noblett KL, Jensen JK, Ostergard DR. The relationship of body mass index to intra-abdominal pressure as measured by multichannel cystometry. Int Urogynecol J Pelvic Floor Dysfunct 1997;8(6):323–326.

36. Bump RC, Sugerman HJ, Fantl JA, McClish DK. Obesity and lower urinary tract function in women: effect of surgically induced weight loss. Am J Obstet Gynecol 1992; 167(2):392–397; discussion 397–399.

37. Raftopoulos Y, Gagne DJ, Papasavas P, et al. Improvement of hypothyroidism after laparoscopic Roux-en-Y gastric bypass for morbid obesity. Obes Surg 2004;14(4):509–513.

38. Chousleb E, Szomstein S, Podkameni D, et al. Routine abdominal drains after laparoscopic Roux-en-Y gastric bypass: a retrospective review of 593 patients. Obes Surg 2004;14(9):1203–1207.

39. Youssef WI, McCullough AJ. Steatohepatitis in obese individuals. Best Pract Res Clin Gastroenterol 2002;16(5): 733–747.

40. Marceau P, Kaufman D, Biron S, et al. Outcome of pregnancies after biliopancreatic diversion. Obes Surg 2004; 14(3):318–324.

41. Dixon JB, Bhathal PS, Hughes NR, O'Brien PE. Nonalcoholic fatty liver disease: improvement in liver histological analysis with weight loss. Hepatology 2004;39(6):1647–1654.

42. Dallal RM, Mattar SG, Lord JL, et al. Results of laparoscopic gastric bypass in patients with cirrhosis. Obes Surg 2004;14(1):47–53.

43. Nguyen NT, Braley S, Fleming NW, et al. Comparison of postoperative hepatic function after laparoscopic versus open gastric bypass. Am J Surg 2003;186(1):40–44.

44. Wittgrove AC, Clark GW, Tremblay LJ. Laparoscopic gastric bypass, Roux-en-Y: preliminary report of five cases. Obes Surg 1994;4(4):353–357.

45. Buchwald H, Williams SE. Bariatric surgery worldwide 2003. Obes Surg 2004;14(9):1157–1164.

46. Nguyen NT, Goldman C, Rosenquist CJ, et al. Laparoscopic versus open gastric bypass: a randomized study of outcomes, quality of life, and costs. Ann Surg 2001;234(3): 279–289; discussion 289–291.

47. Schauer P, Ikramuddin S, Hamad G, Gourash W. The learning curve for laparoscopic Roux-en-Y gastric bypass is 100 cases. Surg Endosc 2003;17(2):212–215.

48. Spanos C, Salzman E, Triglio CM, Shikora SA. A comparative study in percentage of weight loss between laparoscopic and open Roux-en-Y gastric bypass. Obes Surg 2001;11:384.

49. Eagon CJ, Marin D. Laparoscopic gastric bypass has shorter length of stay and less complications but is more costly compared with open gastric bypass. Surg Endosc 2001;15:S120.

50. Fisher BL. Comparison of recovery time after open and laparoscopic gastric bypass and laparoscopic adjustable banding. Obes Surg 2004;14(1):67–72.

51. Mathus-Vliegen EM, Tytgat GN. Intragastric balloons for morbid obesity: results, patient tolerance and balloon life span. Br J Surg 1990;77(1):76–79.

52. Felix EL, Swartz DE. Conversion of laparoscopic Roux-en-Y gastric bypass. Am J Surg 2003;186(6):648–651.

53. Hamilton EC, Sims TL, Hamilton TT, et al. Clinical predictors of leak after laparoscopic Roux-en-Y gastric bypass for morbid obesity. Surg Endosc 2003;17(5):679–684.

54. Oliak D, Ballantyne GH, Davies RJ, et al. Short-term results of laparoscopic gastric bypass in patients with BMI > or = 60. Obes Surg 2002;12(5):643–647.

55. Fernandez AZ Jr, DeMaria EJ, Tichansky DS, et al. Experience with over 3,000 open and laparoscopic bariatric procedures: multivariate analysis of factors related to leak and resultant mortality. Surg Endosc 2004;18(2):193–197.

56. Oliak D, Owens M, Schmidt HJ. Impact of fellowship training on the learning curve for laparoscopic gastric bypass. Obes Surg 2004;14(2):197–200.

57. Shikora SA, Kim JJ, Tarnoff ME. Reinforcing gastric staple-lines with bovine pericardial strips may decrease the likelihood of gastric leak after laparoscopic Roux-en-Y gastric bypass. Obes Surg 2003;13(1):37–44.

58. Sapala JA, Wood MH, Schuhknecht MP. Anastomotic leak prophylaxis using a vapor-heated fibrin sealant: report on 738 gastric bypass patients. Obes Surg 2004;14(1):35–42.

59. Gonzalez R, Lin E, Venkatesh KR, et al. Gastrojejunostomy during laparoscopic gastric bypass: analysis of 3 techniques. Arch Surg 2003;138(2):181–184.

60. Nguyen NT, Stevens CM, Wolfe BM. Incidence and outcome of anastomotic stricture after laparoscopic gastric bypass. J Gastrointest Surg 2003;7(8):997–1003; discussion 1003.

61. Ahmad J, Martin J, Ikramuddin S, et al. Endoscopic balloon dilation of gastroenteric anastomotic stricture after laparoscopic gastric bypass. Endoscopy 2003;35(9): 725–728.

62. Griffen WO Jr, Bivins BA, Bell RM, Jackson KA. Gastric bypass for morbid obesity. World J Surg 1981;5(6):817–822.

63. Fobi MA, Lee H, Holness R, Cabinda D. Gastric bypass operation for obesity. World J Surg 1998;22(9):925–935.

64. Hall JC, Watts JM, O'Brien PE, et al. Gastric surgery for morbid obesity. The Adelaide Study. Ann Surg 1990; 211(4):419–427.

65. Nguyen NT, Cronan M, Braley S, et al. Duplex ultrasound assessment of femoral venous flow during laparoscopic and open gastric bypass. Surg Endosc 2003;17(2):285–290.

66. Szomstein S, Avital S, Brasesco O, et al. Laparoscopic gastric bypass in patients on thyroid replacement therapy for subnormal thyroid function—prevalence and short-term outcome. Obes Surg 2004;14(1):95–97.

67. Sapala JA, Wood MH, Sapala MA, Flake TM Jr. Marginal ulcer after gastric bypass: a prospective 3-year study of 173 patients. Obes Surg 1998;8(5):505–516.

68. Westling A, Gustavsson S. Laparoscopic vs open Roux-en-Y gastric bypass: a prospective, randomized trial. Obes Surg 2001;11(3):284–292.

69. Sanyal AJ, Sugerman HJ, Kellum JM, et al. Stomal complications of gastric bypass: incidence and outcome of therapy. Am J Gastroenterol 1992;87(9):1165–1169.

70. Champion JK, Williams M. Small bowel obstruction and internal hernias after laparoscopic Roux-en-Y gastric bypass. Obes Surg 2003;13(4):596–600.

71. Westling A, Ohrvall M, Gustavsson S. Roux-en-Y gastric bypass after previous unsuccessful gastric restrictive surgery. J Gastrointest Surg 2002;6(2):206–211.

72. Sugerman HJ, Brewer WH, Shiffman ML, et al. A multicenter, placebo-controlled, randomized, double-blind, prospective trial of prophylactic ursodiol for the prevention of gallstone formation following gastric-bypass-induced rapid weight loss. Am J Surg 1995;169(1):91–96; discussion 96–97.

73. de la Torre RA, Scott JS. Laparoscopic Roux-en-Y gastric bypass: a totally intra-abdominal approach—technique and preliminary report. Obes Surg 1999;9(5):492–498.

74. Fobi M, Lee H, Igwe D, et al. Prophylactic cholecystectomy with gastric bypass operation: incidence of gallbladder disease. Obes Surg 2002;12(3):350–353.

75. Amaral JF, Thompson WR. Gallbladder disease in the morbidly obese. Am J Surg 1985;149(4):551–557.

76. Hamad GG, Ikramuddin S, Gourash WF, Schauer PR. Elective cholecystectomy during laparoscopic Roux-en-Y gastric bypass: is it worth the wait? Obes Surg 2003;13(1): 76–81.

77. Schneider BE, Villegas L, Blackburn GL, et al. Laparoscopic gastric bypass surgery: outcomes. J Laparoendosc Adv Surg Tech A 2003;13(4):247–255.

78. Nguyen NT, Huerta S, Gelfand D, et al. Bowel obstruction after laparoscopic Roux-en-Y gastric bypass. Obes Surg 2004;14(2):190–196.

79. Higa KD, Ho T, Boone KB. Internal hernias after laparoscopic Roux-en-Y gastric bypass: incidence, treatment and prevention. Obes Surg 2003;13(3):350–354.

80. Felsher J, Brodsky J, Brody F. Small bowel obstruction after laparoscopic Roux-en-Y gastric bypass. Surgery 2003; 134(3):501–505.

81. Mognol P, Vignes S, Chosidow D, Marmuse JP. Rhabdomyolysis after laparoscopic bariatric surgery. Obes Surg 2004;14(1):91–94.

82. Khurana RN, Baudendistel TE, Morgan EF, et al. Postoperative rhabdomyolysis following laparoscopic gastric bypass in the morbidly obese. Arch Surg 2004;139(1): 73–76.

83. Nguyen NT, Goldman CD, Ho HS, et al. Systemic stress response after laparoscopic and open gastric bypass. J Am Coll Surg 2002;194(5):557–566; discussion 566–567.

84. Moose D, Lourie D, Powell W, et al. Laparoscopic Roux-en-Y gastric bypass: minimally invasive bariatric surgery for the superobese in the community hospital setting. Am Surg 2003;69(11):930–932.

85. Kreitz K, Rovito PF. Laparoscopic Roux-en-Y gastric bypass in the "megaobese." Arch Surg 2003;138(7):707–709; discussion 710.

86. Feng JJ, Gagner M. Laparoscopic biliopancreatic diversion with duodenal switch. Semin Laparosc Surg 2002;9(2): 125–129.

87. Kligman MD, Thomas C, Saxe J. Effect of the learning curve on the early outcomes of laparoscopic Roux-en-Y gastric bypass. Am Surg 2003;69(4):304–309; discussion 309–310.

88. Bloomberg RD, Fleishman A, Nalle JE, et al. Nutritional deficiencies following bariatric surgery: what have we learned? Obes Surg 2005;15(2):145–154.

89. Coates PS, Fernstrom JD, Fernstrom MH, et al. Gastric bypass surgery for morbid obesity leads to an increase in bone turnover and a decrease in bone mass. J Clin Endocrinol Metab 2004;89(3):1061–1065.

90. Lujan JA, Frutos MD, Hernandez Q, et al. Laparoscopic versus open gastric bypass in the treatment of morbid obesity: a randomized prospective study. Ann Surg 2004; 239(4):433–437.

91. Papasavas PK, Hayetian FD, Caushaj PF, et al. Outcome analysis of laparoscopic Roux-en-Y gastric bypass for morbid obesity. The first 116 cases. Surg Endosc 2002; 16(12):1653–1657.

92. Flum DR, Salem L, Elrod JA, et al. Early mortality among Medicare beneficiaries undergoing bariatric surgical procedures. JAMA 2005;294(15):1903–1908.

93. Nguyen NT, Paya M, Stevens CM, et al. The relationship between hospital volume and outcome in bariatric surgery at academic medical centers. Ann Surg 2004;240(4): 586–593; discussion 593–594.

94. Zingmond DS, McGory ML, Ko CY. Hospitalization before and after gastric bypass surgery. JAMA 2005; 294(15):1918–1924.

95. Christou NV, Sampalis JS, Liberman M, et al. Surgery decreases long-term mortality, morbidity, and health care use in morbidly obese patients. Ann Surg 2004;240(3): 416–423; discussion 423–424.

96. Flum DR, Dellinger EP. Impact of gastric bypass operation on survival: a population-based analysis. J Am Coll Surg 2004;199(4):543–551.

97. Biertho L, Steffen R, Ricklin T, et al. Laparoscopic gastric bypass versus laparoscopic adjustable gastric banding: a comparative study of 1,200 cases. J Am Coll Surg 2003;197(4):536–544; discussion 544–545.

98. Farkas DT, Vemulapalli P, Haider A, et al. Laparoscopic Roux-en-Y gastric bypass is safe and effective in patients with a BMI > or = 60. Obes Surg 2005;15(4):486–493.

99. Parikh MS, Shen R, Weiner M, et al. Laparoscopic bariatric surgery in super-obese patients (BMI > 50) is safe and effective: a review of 332 patients. Obes Surg 2005;15(6): 858–863.

100. Dresel A, Kuhn JA, McCarty TM. Laparoscopic Roux-en-Y gastric bypass in morbidly obese and super morbidly obese patients. Am J Surg 2004;187(2):230–232; discussion 232.

101. Fernandez AZ Jr, Demaria EJ, Tichansky DS, et al. Multivariate analysis of risk factors for death following gastric bypass for treatment of morbid obesity. Ann Surg 2004; 239(5):698–702; discussion 702–703.

102. Liu C. Cost-analysis of laparoscopic versus open Roux-en-Y gastric bypass for morbid obesity. Obes Surg 2001;11:165.

21.6
Laparoscopic Roux-en-Y Gastric Bypass: Postoperative Management and Nutritional Evaluation

Tomasz Rogula and Giselle Hamad

Gastric bypass surgery requires ongoing patient effort and commitment to attaining and maintaining the appropriate body weight and a healthy lifestyle. Surgery helps limit the food intake, whereas patients should attempt to improve their eating habits and dietary practice. This requirement should be made clear to prospective patients and continually emphasized during pre- and postoperative counseling. For maintaining the desired weight, patients need to learn how to make the right food selections and comply with all nutrient supplementations. The Roux-en-Y gastric bypass procedure involves bypassing a large part of the stomach and the duodenum, and a variable length of the proximal jejunum. Consequently, patients are at risk for developing various deficiencies, in particular protein, iron, vitamin B_{12}, folate, calcium, and other macro- and micronutrients. With proper supplementation these deficiencies are largely avoidable.

This chapter provides practical guidance on postoperative management in patients undergoing laparoscopic Roux-en-Y gastric bypass. Extensive experience with more than 3000 operations proved these recommendations to be worthwhile.

Nutrient Deficiencies Following Gastric Bypass

Protein

Protein is always at the center of any weight-loss approach. Inadequate protein intake is a major concern following Roux-en-Y gastric bypass. The small gastric pouch and bypassed portion of the jejunum may lead to insufficient protein intake and absorption. It has been suggested that patients who underwent Roux-en-Y gastric bypass consume insufficient amounts of protein, possibly mediated by protein intolerance (1). Patients having gastric reduction operations are at risk of having the outlet of the pouch made too small, thus limiting their ability to ingest foods and liquids; however, the major concern in these patients is prolonged vomiting (Table 21.6-1). The most severe consequence on such starvation injury includes sudden death from protein malnutrition (2). In rare cases, patients may develop a myopathy in the setting of malnutrition following Roux-en-Y gastric bypass with no concomitant vitamin or electrolyte deficiencies (3).

Protein constitutes the lean body mass that needs to be retained after gastric bypass, whereas excess body fat is lost (4). Because the body tends to break down protein and convert it to sugar, the preferred source of energy production, protein must be replenished and protected in all weight-loss procedures and diets. Protein consumption must be of high quality, that is, it must contain all of the essential amino acids. Sources of high-quality protein include milk, cheese, whey, soy, eggs, fish, and meat. They all must be low fat or fat free (5). Measuring the serum prealbumin and changes in body composition helps assess the patient's protein intake (4). Malnutrition can be defined as the ratio of total exchangeable sodium (Na_e) to total exchangeable potassium (K_e). Also multiple isotope dilution technique is useful in assessing nutritional status (6).

Micronutrient Deficiencies

The Roux-en-Y gastric bypass operation for weight reduction functionally resembles a subtotal gastrectomy, with some nutritional deficiencies similar to those seen in major gastric resections for various conditions. Gastric bypass patients often develop micronutrient deficiencies despite close medical follow-up (7). The most frequent problems are the combined iron and vitamin B_{12} deficiencies (8). These deficiencies may develop at any time following surgery. Iron deficiency may arise as early as the first 6 months, and is usually followed by vitamin B_{12} deficiency. Iron, vitamin B_{12}, and folic acid status are determined by measuring hemoglobin, red blood cell mean corpuscular volume (MCV), and folate levels (9).

TABLE 21.6-1. Postoperative complaints and complications and suggested nutritional solutions

Problems	Solutions
Nausea and vomiting	Advise the patient to wait several days before introducing again the particular food causing troubles. It may be necessary to return to liquids or pureed foods temporarily. Eating/drinking too fast or too much, or insufficient chewing, may also cause nausea or vomiting. Advise the patient to avoid cold beverages and those with caffeine or carbonation.
Dumping syndrome	Advise the patient to avoid all sweetened foods and beverages and high fatty foods. Fluids should not be drunk with meals: patient should wait a half hour to 1 hour before drinking beverages after meals. If dumping syndrome occurs, advise the patient to lie down for 20 to 30 minutes.
Lactose intolerance/diarrhea	Prescribe lactase-treated milk and lactase enzyme tablets; try Lactaid 100% or Dairy Ease 100%.
Constipation	Constipation may occur temporarily during the first postoperative month but generally resolves with adaptation to changes in volume of food. The regular use of fruits and fruit juices reduces the risk of recurrent constipation. Low-calorie fluids should be taken regularly.
Diarrhea	Advise the patient to limit the following foods: high fiber; greasy; milk and milk products; and very hot or cold foods. Advise the patient to eat smaller meals. Fluids should be taken between meals.
Heartburn	Advise the patient to avoid carbonated beverages and not use a straw.
Bloating	Advise the patient to limit liquids to 2 oz at one time and to drink slowly.
Partial obstruction of the anastomosis	The gastrointestinal anastomosis may be temporarily blocked if foods with large particle size are eaten without thorough chewing. Advise the patient not to progress to solid foods until a full diagnosis is made.
Rupture of the staple line	Advise the patient that eating an excessive quantity of food at one time should be avoided.
Stretching of the stomach pouch and dilation of the gastrojejunostomy	Advise the patient that the risk of stretching the stomach pouch can be reduced by avoiding large portions of food at one time and by modifying the texture of foods only gradually in the early postoperative weeks. Advise the patient to follow the recommendations for advancing the diet to prevent this stretching.
Weight gain or no further weight loss	High calorie foods or beverages must be excluded from the diet. Patients are advised to keep a record of all foods, beverages and snacks consumed to determine the exact reason for this happening. Portion sizes should be measured. Advise the patient to drink only low calorie beverages in addition to skim milk.

Nutrient deficiencies following gastric bypass may be a consequence of inadequate body reserves preoperatively, low nutrient intakes, insufficient supplementation, and noncompliance in taking vitamins (10). Patients after gastric bypass are at risk of malabsorption of iron, B vitamins, calcium, and vitamin A, because the major sites of their absorption, the duodenum and the upper jejunum, are bypassed. Diminished gastric acid secretion from the small pouch additionally decreases absorption of iron, B_{12} vitamin, calcium, and folic acid (11,12). Micronutrients deficiency is relatively common, although the clinically evident level of deficiency is sporadically seen in the American population. Morbidly obese patients are usually at greater risk for micronutrient deficiency, as they usually have several nutrient deficits before surgery (13).

Vitamin B_{12}

One of the most significant effects of gastric bypass is decreased absorption of protein-bound vitamin B_{12}. Vitamin B_{12} deficiency occurs when a portion of the stomach is removed or separated from ingested food. Gastric acid secretion from the gastric pouch is negligible after gastric bypass, and food-bound vitamin B_{12} is maldigested and subsequently malabsorbed, presumably due to pouch achlorhydria (11). Intrinsic factor, produced in the stomach, binds to B_{12}, allowing its absorption in the small intestine. One strategy in preventing vitamin B_{12} deficiency after gastric bypass is to give high doses of B_{12} orally and hope that enough of the binding protein will eventually reach the B_{12}, enabling it to be absorbed in the intestine and into the bloodstream. Another strategy is intramuscular injecting of vitamin B_{12}, which goes into the bloodstream and does not need the binding protein. Also, oral drugs containing both vitamin B_{12} and intrinsic protein are available. Multivitamins formulations contain a form of vitamin B_{12} that can be absorbed into the bloodstream through the oral mucosa. Sublingual tablets containing vitamin B_{12} are also useful. Measuring B_{12} levels in the serum is helpful in evaluating the effectiveness of vitamin B_{12} supplementation. The vast majority of patients reach normal level during oral B_{12} therapy and only a small number require monthly parenteral injections of B_{12} (14).

Folate

Folate deficiency is less common than vitamin B_{12} deficiency, and occurs secondary to decreased intake of folate-rich foods. Folic acid can mask an underlying vitamin B_{12} deficiency; therefore, folic acid supplementation should always include vitamin B_{12}. Folic acid cures the macrocytic anemia; however, it does not prevent the neurologic symptoms and neural tube defects caused by vitamin B_{12} deficiency (15). Postoperative supplementation of vitamin B_{12} should exceed the amount of folic acid given after gastric bypass because of the tendency of lower serum vitamin B_{12} levels in these patients. Vitamin C taken concomitantly with vitamin B_{12} decreases its activity.

Iron

Iron is transferred to the liver, spleen, and bone marrow, where it is stored. The typical requirements are 30 to 35 mg/day. The normal diet provides 15 to 30 mg/day, and iron must be in the ferrous form. The daily loss of iron for men is 1.0 to 1.5 pg/day, and it is 2 to 3 pg/day for women of menstrual age. Iron-deficiency anemia may be present in up to 50% of patients 2 years after gastric bypass surgery (16). Patients are frequently anemic in the early postoperative period, especially menstruating women. Prophylactic oral iron supplementation prevents iron deficiency in menstruating women after Roux-en-Y gastric bypass; however, it may not protect these women from developing anemia (9). The causes of iron-deficiency anemia include some operative blood loss, the reduced intake of iron as a consequence of necessary dietary restrictions, the decreased absorption of iron from the lack of gastric acidity, and continued losses in menstruating women. Other causes include new or continuing blood loss from the gastrointestinal tract that usually occurs at the anastomoses.

None of the available forms of iron supplementation is ideal. However, the gluconate form of iron is absorbed better than the sulfate form in a low to no acid environment and should be routinely prescribed for patients after gastric bypass. Taking iron orally causes constipation and nausea. Iron injections are painful and difficult to administer. Liquid forms stain the teeth. Measuring serum iron levels, blood counts, and reticulocyte counts helps assess the effectiveness of iron supplementation. If the patient is gradually improving it may be prudent not to prescribe an iron supplement. If significant anemia persists, then further iron supplementation should be prescribed. Iron tablets are better tolerated when taken immediately after a meal. It has been suggested that iron status should be corrected immediately after gastric bypass surgery, especially in menstruating women (9). The intensity of the treatment should be matched to the severity of the anemia. Iron-deficiency anemia should be differentiated from other anemias, including normochromic, normocytic anemia, often resulting from severe protein-calorie malnutrition. In such cases, resolution results from continued improvement in protein intake and nutritional balance over time. In a case of true iron-deficiency anemia, iron supplementation is continued until serum ferritin values increase, reaching the normal range. Excess iron supplementation may cause iron toxicity.

Weight loss in patients with a body mass index (BMI) ≥50 has been problematic after conventional Roux-en-Y gastric bypass (RYGBP). Some surgeons use a distal RYGBP in which the Roux-en-Y anastomosis is performed 75 cm proximal to the ileocecal junction to facilitate greater malabsorption and thus weight loss. Initial results show that the Roux limb length is correlated with weight loss in super-obese patients. However, the greater incidence of metabolic sequelae after this surgery should be considered. Anemia is significantly more common after this modification of gastric bypass compared to conventional procedure (17). In other studies, there was no difference in either calorie intake or incidence of iron and vitamin B_{12} deficiency between long limb and conventional RYGBP. No metabolic sequelae or diarrhea was noted following this modification of RYGBP (18).

Calcium and Magnesium

Studies of the effects on the skeleton of laparoscopic Roux-en-Y gastric bypass surgery have shown elevated levels of markers of bone turnover. The total hip, trochanter, and total body bone mineral density are decreased significantly, with significant decreases in bone mineral content at these sites. Within 3 to 9 months after surgery, morbidly obese patients have an increase in bone resorption associated with a decrease in bone mass (19). Calcium supplementation after gastric bypass is essential. Calcium and magnesium should be supplemented in a 2:1 proportion. Patients taking magnesium in a 1:1 ratio to calcium may complain of excessive diarrhea. Vitamin D deficiency has been well documented following gastric bypass surgery; however, hypovitaminosis D, when it is found in post–bariatric surgery patients, may not be caused by the surgery since it may have been present to some degree preoperatively (13). Vitamin D should be taken with calcium supplements to promote absorption. Vitamin D supplementation should be diminished or withheld in patients who regularly consume vitamin D–fortified foods. Postmenopausal women who underwent Roux-en-Y gastric bypass may show evidence of secondary hyperparathyroidism, elevated bone resorption, and patterns of bone loss. It has been suggested that greater dietary supplementation may be beneficial for these patients (20).

Other Vitamins and Micronutrients

Other vitamins and minerals can be deficient in the diet or not well absorbed after gastric bypass surgery. Fat-soluble vitamins A and D are occasionally supplemented in gastric bypass, especially if the patient is unable to reduce fat intake and has significant diarrhea. Magnesium or zinc may be deficient because of decreased intake and increased loss by the kidneys. Zinc is essential to utilize vitamins A and B, whereas vitamin P is vital for vitamin C absorption. Utilization of vitamin B, production of sex hormones, and blood cell formation are supported by magnesium.

The Wernicke-Korsakoff syndrome and peripheral neuropathy are uncommon in bariatric surgical practice. This complication tends to strike patients eating unbalanced diets or undergoing rapid weight loss. Thiamine-related neurologic derangements usually respond very well to vitamin B_1 replenishment. A high degree of clinical suspicion in bariatric patients and urgent therapeutic intervention is necessary whenever postoperative vomiting persists for several days (21,22). The possibility of metabolic problems must be also considered as a result of the patient's alcoholism, poor compliance with the prescribed micronutrient intake, poor oral intake, and the decreased absorptive ability of the small bowel (23).

Dosing and Interactions

The supplementation dosing should guarantee 24-hour coverage with nutrients (Table 21.6-2). It is advisable to break the supplement in half and take half in the morning and the other half 8 hours later. B-complex vitamins should be taken early in the day to prevent sleep difficulties at night. Most patients take their supplementation with meals, which facilitates the absorption and tolerance of oral intake, particularly iron. Water-soluble vitamins remain in the circulation for 2 to 3 hours after ingestion, while fat-soluble vitamins are stored for about 24 hours, mainly in the liver.

Commonly used medications can decrease absorption and utilization of nutrients. Some patients may require the H2-receptor blockers for prevention or gastroduodenal ulcers after gastric bypass. This medication interferes with vitamin B_{12} absorption. These patients may require an increased dose of vitamins to compensate for this effect. B vitamin complex may be washed out with a large volume of coffee, soft drink, or sugar intake.

Oral or Injectable Preparations?

The vitamin and micronutrient supplementation can be taken orally or parenterally. Oral vitamin therapy is more reliable, less troublesome for patients, and less costly than the parenteral form. Patients who do not comply with oral management, or show diminished intestinal absorption, require parenteral iron or vitamin B_{12} supplementation. Subcutaneous administration of vitamin B_{12} is suggested for severely depleted patients who are unable to take oral vitamin B_{12}. Intramuscular iron supplementation administered weekly has proved to be effective in patients with iron-deficiency anemia who are resistant to oral therapy.

TABLE 21.6-2. Dosage, rationale, administration, and interactions of vitamins and mineral supplements

Supplement	Mandatory or optional	Dosage	Rationale	Administration	Interactions
Multivitamin	Mandatory	1 pill a day or 2 pills of children's chewable	Provides complete micronutrient supplementation	A.M., with meals	None
Calcium	Mandatory	500 mg 2–3 times a day calcium citrate	Improves calcium turnover and bone mineralization	A.M., with meals	Caffeinated products, spinach, and whole wheat products may decrease absorption; calcium decreases iron absorption
Vitamin B_{12}	Mandatory	500 µg/day tablets or sublingual; 1000 µg/month injectable	Prevents macrocytic anemia and nervous system problems	A.M. tablets or injectable	None
Iron (gastric bypass)	Mandatory	Ferogon (tablet); 300 mg Slow FE 160 mg; Fergan 240 mg; Niferex 150 mg	Prevents microcytic anemia	2 to 3 times daily with meals	Should be taken at different time than calcium
Iron (gastric banding)	Mandatory	Feosol 325 mg (tablet) or 10 mL (elixir); Slow FE 160 mg; Fergan 240 mg; Niferex 150 mg	Prevents microcytic anemia	P.M., with vitamin C	Should be taken at different time than calcium
Zinc	Optional	10–20 mg	Supports immune system and wound healing; hair loss may represent zinc deficiency	A.M.	Overdosing may interfere with absorption of other nutrients
Stool softeners	Optional	As needed	Improve bowel movements	As needed	None

Caloric Balance

Dietary fat contributes more than twice as many calories (9 calories/g) as equal amounts of either protein or carbohydrate (each 4 calories/g). The greater caloric value of fats compared with other macronutrients should be related to the reduction in the level of fats in the postoperative diet. Food volume reduction is not enough to compensate for the increased energy provided by the high-fat diet. The Food and Nutrition Board's Committee on Diet and Health recommends that no more than 30% of caloric intake come from fats (24).

Modifying the patient's diet should reduce the intake of calories. In particular, easily absorbable sugars are not recommended. They lead to large calorie intake without a sufficient feeling of satiety. Generally, the natural sugars in fresh fruit, dairy products, and vegetables are well tolerated. Patients should be instructed to avoid juice, sugar-containing beverages, and concentrated sweets, and to be careful with condiments and sauces that contain sugar, such as ketchup and honey-mustard dressing. Nutritional counseling should be supplemented with written materials on label reading and recognizing high-fat foods, types of fat and cholesterol, serving sizes, meal planning, and low-fat cooking (25,26).

In addition to great caloric ingestion with sugars, the dumping syndrome is another important consideration. Dumping syndrome is characterized by a set of symptoms, including a shaky, sweaty, and dizzy sensation accompanied by a rapid heart rate and, often, severe diarrhea. When sugar is consumed, it is dumped into the small intestine, causing an osmotic load, which results in a fluid shift from the blood into the intestine. The insulin response causes symptoms of hypoglycemia. The influx of fluid into the intestine, due to the osmotic load, can lead to a watery diarrhea. Patients experiencing the dumping syndrome should avoid sugar (27).

Lactose, the natural sugar in milk, can cause bloating and excessive gas production. The malabsorptive process can cause inadequate lactose production, either short- or long-term, leading to diarrhea, bloating, and gas after milk intake. If this is problematic, soy milk, which is lactose-free, or Lactaid-treated milk can be used (28).

Generally, the caloric intake of lipids and dextrose does not meet the patient's caloric needs for weight maintenance after bariatric surgery. Recommendations include administering of hypocaloric feeding, with adequate protein (29). It is suggested to estimate nonprotein calories at 15 to 20 calories per kilogram of adjusted body weight. Adjusted body weight is calculated as follows: current weight — ideal body weight × 25% + ideal body weight. Because of the high dextrose load and the frequency of diabetes or impaired glucose tolerance in the obese population, often insulin has to be added to control elevated blood sugar levels (28).

Studies on morbidly obese patients who had undergone gastric bypass surgery have shown a significant decrease in the average total caloric intake in immediate and long-term postoperative follow-up (30). Fat, carbohydrate, and protein intake decrease equally for the first 12 months, at which time fat intake reaches a plateau while carbohydrate and protein intake continue to rise. Weight reduction after gastric bypass surgery is related to decreased caloric intake, predominantly in the fat component (31).

Nutrition Management After Roux-en-Y Gastric Bypass

Nutrition Review

The bariatric program team should include a dietitian who is experienced in the management of morbidly obese patients. The anatomy and physiology of the gastrointestinal system is radically changed after gastric bypass, and patients require individual dietetic supervision. Patients should be seen by the dietitian at each postoperative visit to review their compliance with dietary instructions, including estimated intake of protein and calories, problems with ingestion of various foods, and liquid intake. The dietitian should then determine if further discussion or additional instruction is needed. The physician should be alerted to any significant deficiencies or problems the patient is having in adapting to their procedure.

Protein

Several protein-rich foods should be introduced early, as the diet advances after surgery. We recommend skim milk throughout the day. In some patients milk causes bloating or nausea, and should be replaced with milk with lactase, such as Lactaid. Patients' meals should start with protein, which should include the maximum tolerated amount. Meat, poultry, fish, dairy products, and eggs contain the necessary amount of protein. When preparing foods, frying should be avoided as much as possible, as it may add extra fat, causing discomfort. Strained low-fat creamy soups, low-fat cottage cheese, ricotta, and light yogurt are recommended during the initial diet phase. Meals may also include pureeing low-fat cuts of meat, poultry, or fish or baby food with pureed meats, scrambled eggs, or Egg Beaters.

As the diet advances further, high-protein foods should be continued, including skim milk throughout the day. Patients having trouble tolerating milk or other protein sources may want to use a protein powder preparation (i.e., Met-Rx Protein Plus, Optimum Nutrition 100% Whey Protein) to increase protein intake. These products are easily available in pharmacies, nutrition stores, or supermarkets. Some protein supplements may contain large amounts of other substances (e.g., caffeine, hidden sugars) or they may interact with medications (e.g., herbs). Plant proteins are not complete proteins. A complete protein is one food that contains all of the essential amino acids. The plant proteins should be used together with animal protein sources to provide all the amino acids (5,32).

After surgery, patients start their initial diet (phase I). The dietitian reviews the phase I diet with the patient and answers any questions that may arise. Additional follow-up appointments should be scheduled upon request. The team should be available for consultation and questions during office hours.

Vitamins and Micronutrients

Multivitamins

Multiple vitamins (e.g., Theragram, Centrum, or equivalent) are taken in liquid form or tablets. In the first month after surgery, the dosing should not exceed once per day. After 1 month, the patient may take any reasonably sized multiple vitamin pills or capsules, usually in the morning, before breakfast. Taking multivitamin supplements results in a lower incidence of folate deficiency but does not prevent iron or vitamin B_{12} deficiency (8).

Vitamin B_{12}

Vitamin B_{12} is taken as one $500\mu g$ pill per day or injection of $1000\mu g$ each month, usually in the morning (5,33).

Iron

Iron deficiency is secondary to decreased intake of heme iron, and the decreased acid in the pouch does not allow the ferrous iron to be converted to the more absorbable form of ferric iron. Also, iron is absorbed in the duodenum, which is bypassed.

We recommend oral administration, twice daily with meals for patients after gastric bypass. Once a day supplementation taken with vitamin C is appropriate for patients after gastric banding. The sulfate form of iron is appropriate for banding patients, whereas the gluconate form of iron is best for patients after gastric bypass.

Iron tablets may be taken with juice (e.g., orange juice) or water, but not with milk or antacids. Some foods, such as yogurt, cheese, eggs, milk, whole-grain breads and cereals, tea, and coffee, may impair oral iron absorption. Some patients may experience staining of teeth, especially when tablets are crushed.

Vitamin C

Vitamin C enhances absorption of iron for banding patients and maintains intracellular cement substance, with preservation of capillary integrity. It also promotes wound healing, reduces liability to infection, and is essential for production of connective tissue. Vitamin C is administrated at the dose of 500 to 1500 mg per day with iron for banding patients. Gastric bypass patients do not normally need supplemental vitamin C beyond that obtained from diet and multivitamins. Due to drug interactions with antacids, cholestyramine resin, cimetidine, fluoroquinolones, and vitamin E, separate dosing is recommended when possible (5).

Calcium

Calcium plays an important role in tooth and bone formation, stimulates collagen formation and tissue repair, and plays a part in oxidation-reduction reactions. Calcium is taken in the dose of 500 mg twice a day, 1 hour apart from all other vitamins and medications. Patients who have had gastric bypass will absorb the citrate form of calcium much better than the carbonate form. Oral calcium should be taken 1 to $1\frac{1}{2}$ hours after meals. Oxalic acid (found in rhubarb and spinach), phytic acid (in bran and whole cereals), and phosphorus (in dairy products) should be avoided in the meal preceding calcium consumption; these substances may interfere with calcium absorption. Calcium decreases iron absorption, and thus simultaneous administration should be avoided (5).

Zinc

Zinc is administrated optionally in the postoperative phase. It participates in synthesis and stabilization of proteins and nucleic acids in cellular and membrane transport systems. Zinc is taken in a dose of 10 to 20 mg per day (5).

Stool Softeners

Stool softeners are optional for patients who have problems with bowel movements postoperatively. In some patients iron causes constipation. Softeners are usually taken one to two times per day or every other day. Only stool softeners without laxative additives can be used (5).

Dietary Guidance for Gastric Bypass Surgery

Nutrition

The diet administrated at the early postoperative stage is designed to restrict caloric intake to produce the desired weight loss, to help develop appropriate eating habits, and to prevent disruption of staple lines and obstruction of the stoma. General principles include the following: (1) Appropriate fluid intake is essential to maintain suitable hydration. Patients are instructed to drink 64 ounces of fluid per day. They should drink one cup of liquid over the course of an hour and stop within 30 to 60 minutes of a meal. Beverages are swallowed slowly, without using a straw. (2) Adequate protein intake is essential. (3) Mineral supplements should be prescribed to meet recommended daily allowances. (4) Multivitamins, vitamin B_{12}, iron, and calcium are required daily. (5) High-calorie foods, beverages, and snacks should be avoided. (6) Patients are instructed to chew foods thoroughly to prevent obstruction of the stoma. (7) The diet is prescribed gradually, depending on tolerance (5).

In general, patients are instructed to eat three small meals per day and stop eating as soon as they feel full. A meal should take at least 20 minutes, but no longer than 30 minutes. High-calorie beverages such as soda, shakes, alcoholic beverages, fruit drinks, sweetened iced teas, or sweetened waters should be avoided. Similarly, high-calorie sweets such as candy, cake, cookies, ice cream, and snack foods such as chips and nuts must be removed from the patients' diet. Protein foods at each meal help maximize protein intake. Commercial protein powders or dried milk powder, such as Pro Performance, Whey Protein, Met-Rx Protein Plus, or Challenge Protein 95, may be added to skim milk to increase protein intake. Exercise should be gradually introduced as soon as the patient's condition allows. Appropriate hydration is essential; patients are advised to carry a bottle of water with them (5).

Diet Progression

The diet progresses in the following sequence:

Phase I: Postoperative/Clear Liquids (<1 Week)

The most important goal of the first 1 to 2 weeks after surgery is to keep the patient well hydrated. The patient should aim for 64 ounces of water per day by constantly sipping liquids. It may be necessary to dilute fruit juices in order to avoid nausea or diarrhea, but patients should gradually be able to tolerate full-strength juices. It is not uncommon for patients to experience nausea or vomiting in this phase, but it should not cause hydration discontinuity.

For phase I of the postoperative diet, clear liquids are suggested, such as apple, cranberry, and pulp-free orange juice (half strength), and clear beef, chicken, and vegetable broths are recommended. Unsweetened coffee or tea (sugar substitutes may be added), sugar-free jelly, sugar-free popsicles, sugar-free frozen juice bars, Gatorade, all sport drinks, flavored waters (noncarbonated), and Crystal Light water are good alternatives.

Phase II: Pureed (2–3 days—1 Month)

After patients gradually start to tolerate clear liquids, they can try foods of a more solid consistency. This phase involves eating pureed foods, which should be the consistency of baby food to facilitate chewing and ingestion. The rate at which patients are able to tolerate the diet progression differs from person to person.

The key goals of this phase are as follows:

1. Incorporate high-protein foods into the diet.
2. Start taking the chewable vitamin supplements with minerals.
3. Continue hydration with at least 64 ounces of liquids per day.

The protein portion of the meal should be eaten first. Some examples of high-protein foods that can be introduced at this phase include cottage cheese, ricotta cheese, scrambled eggs or Egg Beaters, pureed beef, chicken, turkey, fish (not shellfish), and baby food meats. Fish and chicken are usually more readily tolerated than beef.

Liquids should be stopped at least a half hour before meals and not be resumed until a half hour to 1 hour after meals. Suggested fluids between meals include skim milk, fruit juices, broths, unsweetened coffee or tea, sugar-free jelly, and sugar-free popsicles (as in the previous stage.)

It is very important that the patient chew all foods thoroughly to avoid blockage or nausea. Therefore, liquids are introduced first as they are tolerated, and then gradually solids are introduced. Again, the progression in this phase varies among patients.

Phase III: Adaptive/Soft Food (1–2 Months)

The goal of this phase is to progress to more solid food. This may include soft foods such as tuna fish, mashed potatoes, oatmeal (unstrained), cooked vegetables, and canned fruits. The patients should be able to eat the whole portion of protein food, fruit, vegetable, and starch.

In general, in this phase we recommend the following: (1) Continue to incorporate high protein foods into the diet. (2) Continue to take chewable vitamin supplements with minerals. (3) Continue to hydrate with fluids (64 ounces per day). (4) Add a variety of low-fat, low-calorie starches, fruits, and vegetables to the diet as tolerated.

Patients are advised to stop eating when they feel full. All foods must be cooked without added fat. Meat, fish, or poultry should be baked, boiled, or broiled. Fat can be replaced with vegetables seasoned with herbs. Patients who do not tolerate milk may try yogurt, cottage cheese, or an egg as a source of protein.

Phase IV: Stabilization/Food of Regular Consistency (After 2 Months)

During this phase, patients are able to eat foods of a regular consistency. However, this does not mean that they should return to their old eating patterns. Patients are advised to continue to eat three balanced meals a day, which contain nutrient-rich foods such as meat, poultry, pork, dairy products, vegetables, fruits, and starch. These foods contain an adequate portion of protein, vitamins, and minerals. Since patients will only be able to tolerate limited amounts of food at a time, it is very important to eat nutrient-dense foods, rather than foods that are high in sugar or fat content but do not contain protein, vitamins, or minerals.

Even when eating vitamin- and mineral-rich foods, it is still important to continue to take vitamin and mineral supplements to meet the patient's total needs, since the amount of food is restricted.

Patients at this phase should eat three well-balanced, nutritious meals each day with adequate amounts of protein and fluid as well as a vitamin and mineral supplement. Again, it is important to advise patients to stop eating as soon as they feel full and not to eat longer than 30 minutes for each meal. All foods must be cooked without added fat, which can be replaced with vegetables seasoned with herbs or spices.

Foods to Avoid After Gastric Bypass

Some foods are difficult to tolerate during phase I. Most of these foods are better tolerated in phase IV. Meats, starches, fruits, and vegetables are gradually introduced as tolerated. Large quantities of sweetened foods, high-fat foods, and high-calorie beverages may cause weight gain and possible digestive problems. Patients may have difficulties with ingesting meat and meat substitutes: steak; hamburger; tough, gristly meat like pork chops; fried or fatty meat; poultry; or fish. Also, some starches, such as bran, bran cereals, granola, popcorn, whole-grain or white bread (nontoasted), whole-grain cereal, and chunky soups (with vegetables or noodles) may not be well tolerated. Foods that should be generally avoided include fibrous vegetables (dried beans, peas, celery, cabbage), raw vegetables, mushrooms, French fries, potato chips, tortillas, highly seasoned and spicy food, pickles, and seeds. Patients should not eat dried fruits, coconut, or orange and grapefruit membranes. Carbonated sweetened beverages, candies, desserts, jam, and jelly should be excluded from the patient's diet.

Caffeine is a stimulant and is naturally found in more than 60 plants, including cocoa, tea, and coffee. Caffeine is also added to soft drinks and is often a component of many over-the-counter medications and dietary supplements including certain protein powders and drinks. Caffeine temporarily increases heart rate and acts as a diuretic. As a result, caffeine can cause dehydration if these drinks are the main source of fluid intake. The recommended intake of caffeine is 300 mg or no more than 3 to 5 ounces of coffee. Caffeine intake should be decreased gradually to avoid the headaches caused by withdrawal.

Conclusion

The goal of postoperative management is to help the patient lose adequate excess weight, a consequence of which is the reduction of many comorbidities and an improved quality of life. This goal can be achieved by teaching the patient to eat a healthy diet and to perform regular physical activity. Education is essential for any well-established bariatric program, often with help of support groups and a knowledgeable staff.

To minimize the long-term problems from protein loss, the adequate intake of protein must be stressed, with adequate counseling to help the patient find a source of palatable and affordable protein. Gastric bypass patients are given a prophylactic multivitamin/mineral supplement containing vitamin B_{12}, iron, and calcium to compensate for malabsorption of nutrients. Some essential nutrients do not have established recommended daily allowances and are considered optional. Through nutrition counseling and support, patients will be able to implement dietary changes and meet their nutritional needs.

References

1. Moize V, Geliebter A, Gluck ME, et al. Obese patients have inadequate protein intake related to protein intolerance up to 1 year following Roux-en-Y gastric bypass. Obes Surg 2003;13(1):23–28.
2. Mason EE. Starvation injury after gastric reduction for obesity. World J Surg 1998;22(9):1002–1007.
3. Hsia AW, Hattab EM, Katz JS. Malnutrition-induced myopathy following Roux-en-Y gastric bypass. Muscle Nerve 2001; 24(12):1692–1694.
4. Gordon M. Metabolic changes after Roux-en-Y gastric bypass: a preliminary report. Obes Surg 1993;3(4):425–428.
5. Schauer PR, Eid GM, Hamad GG, Mattar SG, Ramanathan RC. Preoperative Teaching Handbook. Bariatric Surgery. Pittsburgh: University of Pittsburgh Physicians, Department of Surgery, Minimally Invasive Surgery, 2003:33–58.
6. MacLean LD, Rhode BM, Shizgal HM. Nutrition following gastric operations for morbid obesity. Ann Surg 1983; 198(3):347–355.
7. Halverson JD. Metabolic risk of obesity surgery and long-term follow-up. Am J Clin Nutr 1992;55(2 suppl):602S–605S.
8. Brolin RE, Gorman JH, Gorman RC, et al. Are vitamin B12 and folate deficiency clinically important after Roux-en-Y gastric bypass? J Gastrointest Surg 1998;2(5):436–442.
9. Brolin RE, Gorman JH, Gorman RC, et al. Prophylactic iron supplementation after Roux-en-Y gastric bypass: a prospective, double-blind, randomized study. Arch Surg 1998;133(7): 740–744.

10. Boylan LM, Sugerman HJ, Driskell JA. Vitamin E, vitamin B-6, vitamin B-12, and folate status of gastric bypass surgery patients. J Am Diet Assoc 1988;88(5):579–585.
11. Behrns KE, Smith CD, Sarr MG. Prospective evaluation of gastric acid secretion and cobalamin absorption following gastric bypass for clinically severe obesity. Dig Dis Sci 1994; 39(2):315–320.
12. Recker RR. Calcium absorption and achlorhydria. N Engl J Med 1985;313(2):70–73.
13. Buffington C, Walker B, Cowan GS Jr, Scruggs D. Vitamin D deficiency in the morbidly obese. Obes Surg 1993;3(4): 421–424.
14. Provenzale D, Reinhold RB, Golner B, et al. Evidence for diminished B12 absorption after gastric bypass: oral supplementation does not prevent low plasma B12 levels in bypass patients. J Am Coll Nutr 1992;11(1):29–35.
15. Haddow JE, Hill LE, Kloza EM, Thanhauser D. Neural tube defects after gastric bypass. Lancet 1986;1(8493):1330.
16. Rhode BM, Shustik C, Christou NV, MacLean LD. Iron absorption and therapy after gastric bypass. Obes Surg 1999;9(1):17–21.
17. Brolin RE, LaMarca LB, Kenler HA, Cody RP. Malabsorptive gastric bypass in patients with superobesity. J Gastrointest Surg 2002;6(2):195–203; discussion 204–205.
18. Brolin RE, Kenler HA, Gorman JH, Cody RP. Long-limb gastric bypass in the superobese. A prospective randomized study. Ann Surg 1992;215(4):387–395.
19. Coates PS, Fernstrom JD, Fernstrom MH, Schauer PR, Greenspan SL. Gastric bypass surgery for morbid obesity leads to an increase in bone turnover and a decrease in bone mass. J Clin Endocrinol Metab 2004;89(3):1061–1065.
20. Goode LR, Brolin RE, Chowdhury HA, Shapses SA. Bone and gastric bypass surgery: effects of dietary calcium and vitamin D. Obes Res 2004;12(1):40–47.
21. Chaves LC, Faintuch J, Kahwage S, de Alencar FA. A cluster of polyneuropathy and Wernicke-Korsakoff syndrome in a bariatric unit. Obes Surg 2002;12(3):328–334.
22. Loh Y, Watson WD, Verma A, Chang ST, Stocker DJ, Labutta RJ. Acute Wernicke's encephalopathy following bariatric surgery: clinical course and MRI correlation. Obes Surg 2004;14(1):129–132.
23. Grace DM, Alfieri MA, Leung FY. Alcohol and poor compliance as factors in Wernicke's encephalopathy diagnosed 13 years after gastric bypass. Can J Surg 1998;41(5):389–392.
24. Council NR. Diet and Health: Implications for Reducing Chronic Disease Risk. Report of the Committee on Diet and Health, Food and Nutrition Board. National Academy Press, 1989.
25. Mallory G. Maximum nutrition, minimum calories. Obes Surg 1992;2(4):375–378.
26. Kendall A, Levitsky DA, Strupp BJ, Lissner L. Weight loss on a low-fat diet: consequence of the imprecision of the control of food intake in humans. Am J Clin Nutr 1991; 53(5):1124–1129.
27. Eagon JC, Miedema BW, Kelly KA. Postgastrectomy syndromes. Surg Clin North Am 1992;72(2):445–465.
28. Elliot K. Nutritional considerations after bariatric surgery. Crit Care Nurs Q 2003;26(2):133–138.
29. Kushner RF, Wall-Alonso E, Alverdy J. Obesity. Silver Spring, MD: A.S.P.E.N. Nutrition Support Practice Manual, 1988.
30. Naslund I, Jarnmark I, Andersson H. Dietary intake before and after gastric bypass and gastroplasty for morbid obesity in women. Int J Obes 1988;12(6):503–513.
31. Coughlin K, Bell RM, Bivins BA, Wrobel S, Griffen WO Jr. Preoperative and postoperative assessment of nutrient intakes in patients who have undergone gastric bypass surgery. Arch Surg 1983;118(7):813–816.
32. Marcason W. What are the dietary guidelines following bariatric surgery? J Am Diet Assoc 2004;104(3):487–488.
33. Rhode BM, Tamin H, Gilfix BM, Sampalis JS, Nohr C, MacLean LD. Treatment of vitamin B12 deficiency after gastric surgery for severe obesity. Obes Surg 1995;5(2): 154–158.

21.7
Laparoscopic Roux-en-Y Gastric Bypass: Complications

Kelvin Higa and Keith Boone

There is little debate as to the metabolic, health, and economic issues related to morbid obesity. In 2000, it was estimated that 47 million Americans have metabolic syndrome (1). A middle-aged morbidly obese white man faces a 22% reduction in life expectancy compared with a man with a normal body mass index (BMI) (2). Disability and loss of work time contribute to an estimated economic impact of over $100 billion/year (3). Bariatric surgical intervention has been shown to have a positive impact, not only in controlling or eliminating medical comorbid conditions, but also on life expectancy (4).

Critics of bariatric surgery often cite complication rates that may seem excessive in the context of elective procedures. Mortality statistics are often quoted as high as 1.9%, ignoring the mortality of the untreated patient (5). Critics of minimally invasive surgery claim lower perioperative complication rates, ignoring the long-term wound consequences and intraabdominal effects of open, traditional surgery. Clearly, subsequent operations for complications or unrelated conditions are invariably more complex after open surgery due to dense adhesions as well as incisional considerations. Although comparative studies are few, outcomes and patient preferences favor the laparoscopic approach (6,7).

This chapter focuses on surgical complications of the laparoscopic gastric bypass. Technically, these operations are among the most challenging of all minimally invasive procedures (8). In addition, the metabolic and cardiopulmonary consequences of obesity add to the complexity and incidence of complications related to surgical intervention. Yet, most large series continue to report a relatively low perioperative mortality of less than 0.5% (9). Complications cannot be entirely eliminated, but early recognition and intervention can greatly improve the outcomes.

However, morbidly obese patients often do not exhibit the normal physiologic response to intraabdominal sepsis, such as fever or pain. This, combined with the ergonomic difficulties involved with doing the physical examination or imaging studies, can lead to delays in diagnosis and treatment. By staying vigilant and working with a specialized team focusing on prevention and early recognition of complications, the bariatric surgeon can limit the incidence and severity of these inevitable problems in this patient population.

Intraoperative

Intraoperative complications result from a lapse in judgment, technical error, or both. Judgment is related to the surgeon's personal experience and expertise, command of the current literature, and knowledge of physiologic principles and anatomy as applied to the individual patient. Judgment also relates to proper selection and preparation of the patient and knowing one's limitations. Conversion from laparoscopic to an open procedure should not be considered a complication, especially early in the learning curve. However, a high percentage of conversions or prolonged operative times indicates the need for additional supervision or training.

Technical errors will occur regardless of the surgeon's experience, ability, or expertise. Ironically, because of the video documentation available today, surgeons are beginning to understand how technical errors can occur even with the most experienced individuals. It is postulated that altered perception and flawed interpretation of visual cues contributes to these occurrences (10). Therefore, it is incumbent on institutions to provide surgeons with the best in optical resolution and work environment to reduce the risk of technical complications.

As in all laparoscopic procedures, initial abdominal access can be associated with visceral or vascular injury (11). The choice of the Veress needle, open Hasson, or optical trocar technique is a matter of surgeon preference. There appears to be no demonstrable advantage of one technique over another. However, it is generally agreed that fascial defects greater than 12 mm in diameter should be closed to prevent possible herniation. This does not seem to be the case when using non-bladed trocars (12).

Among the most devastating intraoperative complications are those that are not recognized at the time of surgery. Injury to viscera out of the visual field due to direct or thermal injury, twisting or kinking of the intestine, or devascularization will often present early in the postoperative period and can be missed by routine upper gastrointestinal (UGI) series. Computed tomography (CT) scanning may be more sensitive in this setting. However, in these circumstances, it is important that the surgeon be willing to act solely on clinical indications and reexplore the patient early rather than waiting for radiographic confirmation.

Bleeding

Intraluminal bleeding is a rare occurrence but can be frustrating to manage. Initially, the patient presents with signs of hypovolemia that may be indistinguishable from a gastrointestinal leak, pulmonary embolism, or cardiac event. Tachycardia, low urine output, and hypotension often precede hematochezia. A complete blood count (CBC), arterial blood gas (ABG), and electrocardiogram (ECG) will aid in differentiating this entity from the other life-threatening events.

Volume expansion with possible transfusion is advised along with stopping all forms of coagulation inhibition such as deep vein thrombosis (DVT) prophylaxis or ketorolac analgesia injections. A coagulation panel and serial hemoglobin (Hgb) studies help to determine if further intervention is required.

A continued drop in hemoglobin or the inability to stabilize intravascular volume requires urgent attention. Possible sources of bleeding include any of several staple lines or anastomoses, or rarely, preexisting, unrelated entities such as an arteriovenous (AV) malformation or duodenal ulcer.

Nuclear medicine bleeding scans can be helpful in delineating the source, but more often an upper endoscopy will diagnose and treat the most common source of bleeding: the gastrojejunal anastomosis. Bleeding from the gastric remnant staple line can present with acute gastric distention, or obstruction of the jejunojejunostomy due to clot. These patients do not present with hematochezia initially; however, an enlarged gastric remnant is seen on abdominal CT scanning. Immediate operative intervention with oversewing of the staple line and a gastrostomy tube is required in these cases.

Staple-line reinforcement with primary sutures or prosthetic material may provide an increased level of hemostasis, but there are no controlled studies that substantiate this. The use of the correct staple height for the given tissue is the most effective means to limit this complication. Regardless, most forms of intraluminal bleeding are self-limited and rarely require intervention.

Extraluminal hemorrhage often presents more dramatically with a precipitous episode of hypovolemic shock requiring urgent resuscitation. Differentiating extraluminal hemorrhage from pulmonary emboli or a cardiac event is crucial. However, the differentiation from an anastomotic leak is not essential preoperatively, as both require immediate surgical intervention.

Despite the urgency of the situation, there is almost always time to restore intravascular volume so that laparoscopic exploration is possible. Inducing anesthesia before resuscitation can lead to immediate circulatory collapse. Communication between the surgeon and anesthesiologist is important to properly manage these patients.

Leaks

Leaks due to anastomotic or stapler failure often present early, usually within 24 hours of surgery. The typical scenario of abdominal pain, fever, sustained tachycardia, and the perception of "impending doom" are not always present in this patient population. In fact, unexplained tachycardia by itself warrants further investigation.

The most common source of an anastomotic leak is the gastrojejunostomy. This can be evaluated with fluoroscopy, but false negatives have been reported (13,14). A CT scan appears to have a greater degree of sensitivity and is also useful in evaluating the defunctionalized stomach as well as other possible causes of abdominal pain.

Noninvasive studies should only be used as an adjunct to clinical suspicion in borderline cases. If a leak is truly suspected, immediate reexploration is advised rather than waiting for a confirmatory study (15). One of the great advantages of laparoscopic surgery is the ease with which this can be accomplished without the additional stress of reopening a large incision.

The surgeon has three goals at reexploration:

1. Identify and close the leak.
2. Provide directed drainage.
3. Provide enteral access for decompression and/or feeding (gastrostomy tube).

Operative endoscopy is often helpful in delineating the leak as well as testing the stability of the repair. The repair will sometimes fail, resulting in a controlled enterocutaneous fistula; hence the need for enteral feeding while waiting for the fistula to close.

A delay in diagnosis or intervention can result in prolonged illness secondary to multisystem organ failure and may lead to death. Early consultation with the appropriate medical specialists assists in the management of these complex patients. Access to an intensive care unit (ICU) with proper nursing and respiratory care is essential to the survival of these patients.

Mechanical stapling devices cannot accommodate a large degree of variance among tissue thickness and are often pushed to their design limits in the obese patient population (Fig. 21.7-1). The surgeon must use caution,

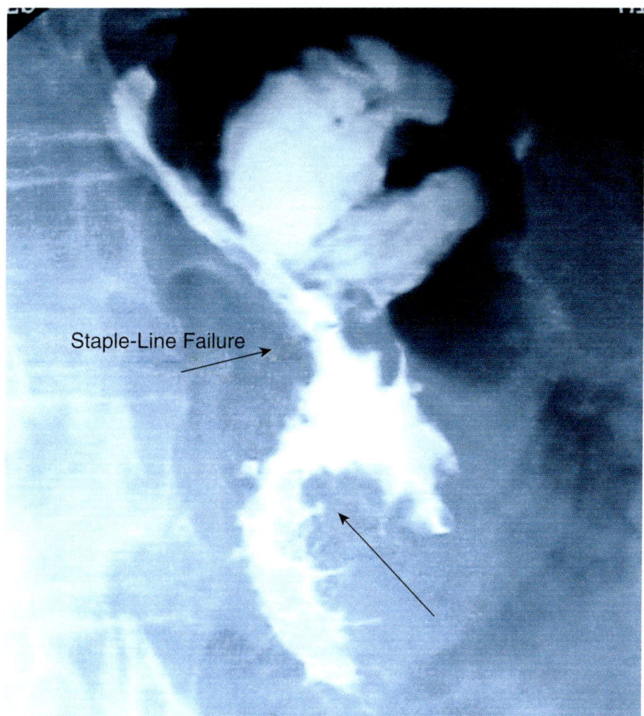

FIGURE 21.7-1. Upper gastrointestinal (UGI) leak.

choosing the appropriate instrument for each application. Developing stapling and anastomotic technologies may improve the reliability of the devices and improve future outcomes. However, all mechanical devices will fail with a certain frequency; the surgeon must be prepared to deal with that situation whether it occurs at the time of surgery or in the postoperative period.

Leaks discovered late, usually 5 to 7 days after surgery, often present in a blunted, subacute fashion. Patients have been home for a number of days and present with fever, pain, or general malaise. Localized left-upper-quadrant tenderness may be minimal. Decreased breath sounds of the left lung base often correspond to the atelectasis and sympathetic pleural effusion seen on chest x-ray. Computed tomography often delineates a well-formed abscess. The decision for operative or radiographic drainage depends on the surgeon, the reliability and skill of the invasive radiologist, the location of the abscess cavity in relation to other abdominal organs, and the overall condition of the patient.

Interestingly, most leaks when properly drained will ultimately close, provided there is no obstruction distally. Nutrition is provided by the intravenous or enteric route if access has been established. Broad-spectrum antibiotics, prevention of pressure sores, DVT, and ongoing psychological counseling constitute further treatment while the patient recovers.

In summary, leaks are a serious consequence of gastrointestinal surgery. Their incidence can be reduced (but not totally eliminated) by careful application of endomechanical devices and meticulous attention to detail. Expe-

dient evaluation and treatment can limit the physiologic and infective consequences of the leak, while delays in treatment will result in disaster. Paramount in the management of leaks is the establishment of effective drainage and, if possible, enteric access for nutrition.

Marginal Ulcer

Marginal ulcers can present anytime in the postoperative course of the Roux-en-Y patient. They are more often seen in patients who use tobacco or nonsteroidal analgesic agents. Typical symptoms are pain and bleeding, and patients sometimes present with a frank perforation. It has been shown that acid-producing parietal cells are present in the gastric pouch after gastric bypass (16). Therefore, treatment includes active acid reduction, eradication of *Helicobacter pylori*, if present, and determining if a gastric pouch to stomach fistula exists. The occasional perforated marginal ulcer is usually anterior and is amenable to laparoscopic repair and drainage.

Upper endoscopy is useful in diagnosing a marginal ulcer, treating active bleeding, and documenting resolution after treatment. Chronic ulcers may be due to ischemia, an undiagnosed gastric pouch, or a native stomach fistula, and may require operative revision. Fistulas can be difficult to diagnose and may not be detectable by contrast studies or endoscopy.

The incidence of marginal ulcer varies from 0.7% to 1.0% (17), and, similarly to gastrojejunal stenosis, does not correlate with the method of anastomosis, whether stapled—circular or linear—or hand-sewn.

Stenosis and Obstruction

Bowel obstruction is most often secondary to stenosis of the gastrojejunal anastomosis. Incidence is variable, but usually occurs after the third week of surgery and does not seem to be related to individual technique (Table 21.7-1). Typical symptoms are of progressive dysphagia without abdominal pain. The absence of pain helps to distinguish this entity from other forms of bowel obstruction, such as that due to internal herniation. A UGI series is diagnostic but often unnecessary. Given the classical clinical presentation, patients can be referred immediately for endoscopic evaluation and treatment. Fortunately, this entity is amenable to endoscopic balloon dilation and rarely requires revision (18). Recurrent stenosis sometimes requires repeat dilations.

Stenosis of the mesocolon in the case of retrocolic routing of the Roux limb is extremely rare, variable in its presentation after surgery, and indistinguishable from gastrojejunal stenosis clinically (Fig. 21.7-2). A UGI series can diagnose this entity; however, a second area of narrowing beyond the gastrojejunostomy is often discovered at the time of initial endoscopy. This entity does not

TABLE 21.7-1. Incidence of stomal stenosis

Author	n	Stenosis n (%)
Wittgrove et al., 2002 (30)	1000	40 (4.0)
Schauer et al., 2000 (31)	275	13 (4.7)
Higa et al., 2001 (32)	2805	146 (5.2)
Champion et al., 1999 (33)	63	4 (6.3)
DeMaria et al., 2002 (34)	281	18 (6.4)
Spaulding et al., 1997 (35)	Review of open series	9–20

respond to endoscopic dilation and requires operative intervention. Findings at the time of surgery are of a dense cicatrix surrounding the Roux limb at the mesocolon. This can be easily transected using the hook cautery or harmonic scalpel. The etiology is unclear, but may be related to the individual inflammatory reaction to various suture materials.

Kinks of the bowel often present early, usually at the level of the jejunojejunostomy, where the relatively fixed staple line intersects the mobile Roux limb (Fig. 21.7-3). This allows the Roux limb to fold back on itself, creating an obstruction that is accentuated with increasing distention (19). This can lead to rapid gastric remnant dilation and should be treated urgently to prevent perforation of the gastric remnant or failure of the gastric staple line. Fixation of the bowel as described by Brolin (20) helps straighten out the Roux limb as it approaches the biliopancreatic limb and prevents this occurrence (Fig. 21.7-4).

A 360-degree twist of the bowel, usually the Roux limb, is discovered only after formation of the gastrojejunostomy (Fig. 21.7-5). Obviously, complete revision of the anastomosis is necessary and can be difficult if the gastric pouch is appropriately small. Hand-sewn anastomoses are easier to revise under these circumstances, but prevention, by routine visualization of the course of the Roux limb prior to performing the anastomosis, is advised.

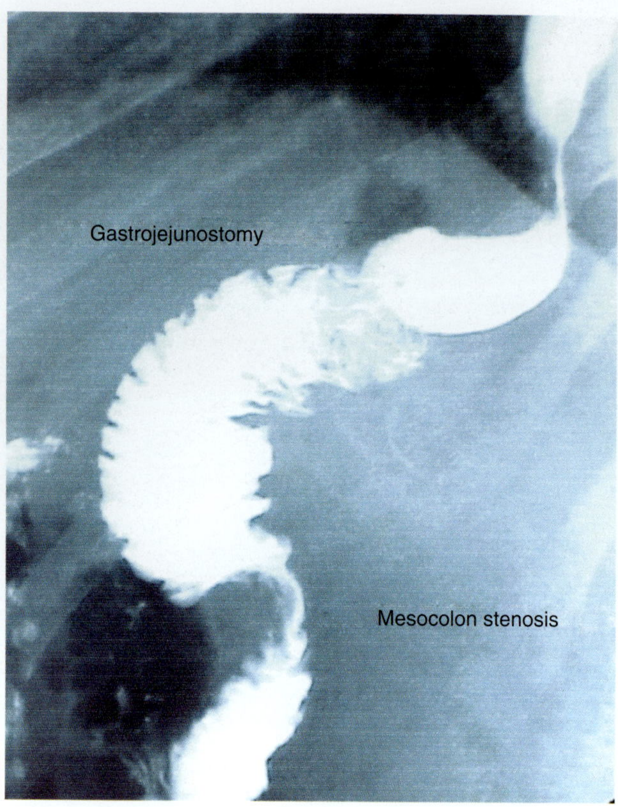

FIGURE 21.7-2. UGI mesocolon stenosis.

Small bowel obstructions due to adhesions can occur after any procedure that violates the peritoneal cavity. These are indistinguishable from small bowel obstructions due to internal hernias clinically. The treatment of small bowel obstructions in gastric bypass patients requires more aggressive attention because of the inability to decompress the gastric remnant without operative intervention (12).

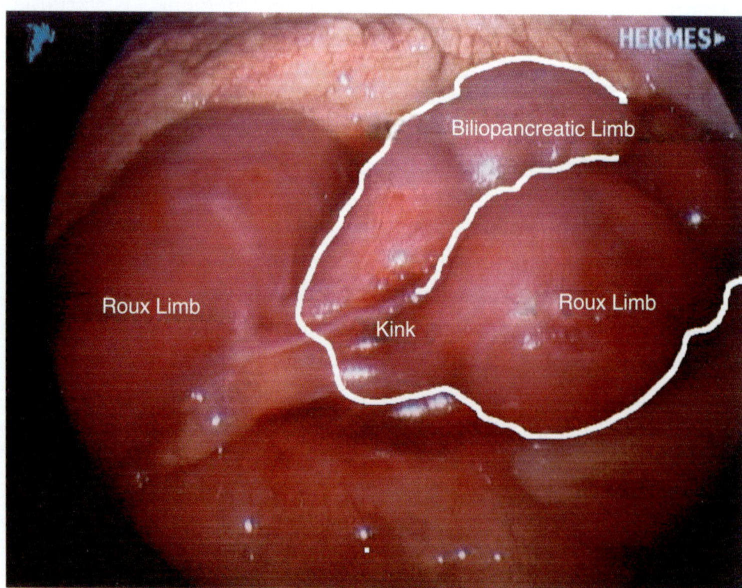

FIGURE 21.7-3. Kink at jejunojejunostomy.

FIGURE 21.7-4. Straightening out the kink.

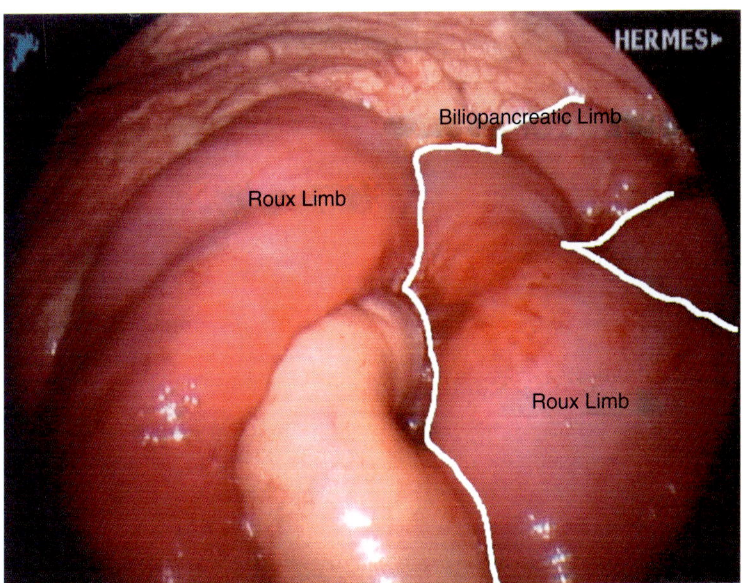

Exploration can be performed laparoscopically if abdominal distention is not severe. The source of obstruction, whether due to an internal hernia or adhesions, is identified and repaired. A gastrostomy tube placed in the gastric remnant for decompression is often advisable.

Internal hernias can occur through any mesenteric defect (Fig. 21.7-6). The most common source of small bowel obstruction due to an internal hernia is through the mesocolic defect in a retrocolic Roux limb position. Defects in the jejunal mesentery or Petersen's space are also at risk, but are less likely to cause an obstruction. Volvulus can occur around an antecolic Roux limb as well (21). Therefore, patients are at lifelong risk for small bowel obstruction as long as there is the potential for intestinal entrapment. Most series underreport the incidence because of the limited time of study.

Internal hernias can be present in the absence of small bowel obstruction. Patients presenting with intermittent, postprandial abdominal pain after gastric bypass should be evaluated for typical causes such as biliary tract disease or marginal ulceration (Fig. 21.7-7). We have observed that at least 20% of these patients have no radiographic evidence of an internal hernia on retrospective review (22). In fact, more than half of the symptomatic internal hernias are currently repaired on the basis of intermittent pain without evidence of small bowel obstruction. Therefore, we conclude that all patients who present with unexplained, severe abdominal pain after gastric bypass require exploration (laparoscopic) as part of their workup. The only way to prevent internal hernia potential is by the meticulous closure of all mesenteric defects whether the Roux limb is retro- or antecolic (Table 21.7-2).

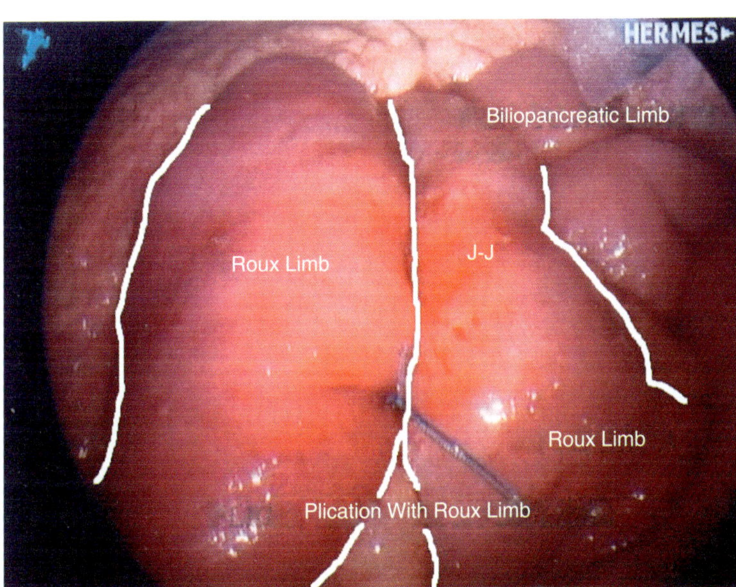

FIGURE 21.7-5. Plication of a kink with the Roux limb.

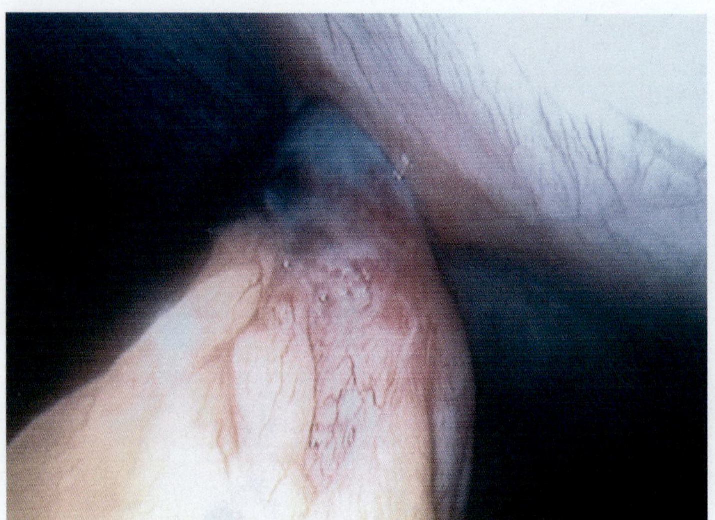

FIGURE 21.7-6. Richter's hernia at port site.

Wound Issues

Serious wound complications are rare and are due to either infections or herniation. Fascial closure of 12-mm or larger defects produced by traditional bladed trocars is advised to prevent incisional hernias. However, in our experience, the "non-bladed," separating-type trocars do not require fascial closure routinely.

Wound infections respond readily to oral antibiotics and are more an issue in techniques that pass an intraluminal, circular, stapling device directly through the unprotected abdominal wall. Wound protection with plastic sleeves can limit this problem. Bleeding from trocar sites is almost always self-limited, although the resultant ecchymosis can be quite dramatic, especially to patients.

Thromboembolic Events

Although rare, thromboembolic events are responsible for the majority of perioperative deaths in most large series (23). Prevention by preoperative evaluation of potential hypercoagulable syndromes when indicated, along with perioperative chemical and mechanical prophylaxis, is advised. Vena cava filters, especially removable ones, may be indicated in patients who have a prior history of pulmonary emboli or significant pulmonary hypertension.

Biliary Tract Disease

Clearly, the incidence of gallstones is elevated with surgical or medical weight loss. Shiffman et al. (24) noted an

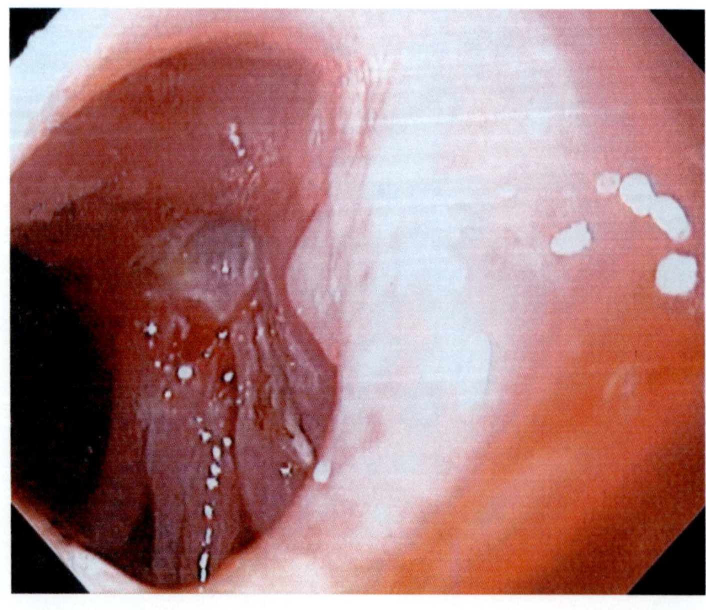

FIGURE 21.7-7. Marginal ulceration at gastrojejunostomy.

TABLE 21.7-2. Incidence of small bowel obstruction (SBO)/internal hernia

Series	Schauer 2000	DeMaria 2002	Champion 2003	Higa 2003	Nguyen 2003
Incidence	1/275	5/281	6/711	63/2000	2/225
Percent	0.4%	1.8%	0.8%	3.2%	0.9%
Includes internal hernia without SBO	No	No	No	Yes	No

incidence of 36% after surgery. Villegas et al. (25) discovered that 30% of their patients developed gallstones or sludge in the gallbladder 6 months after laparoscopic gastric bypass, but only 7% were symptomatic. Although routine use of ursodiol after surgery has been shown to significantly reduce the incidence of gallstones, compliance with this medication has been an issue due to side effects and the cost of the medication (26,27).

Hamad et al. (28) have shown that cholecystectomy at the time of laparoscopic bypass significantly increased hospitalization and operative time. However, overall complication rates did not change compared with laparoscopic bypass alone. Concomitant cholecystectomy presents technical challenges due to suboptimal port placement as well as anatomic issues common in the obese patient. Although development of gallstones is more common after rapid weight loss, cholecystectomy is subsequently easier to perform because of the reduction in intraabdominal fat, and is not complicated by the presence of adhesions as it is in traditional, open surgery.

Occasionally, common bile duct stones are encountered postoperatively. Although it is possible for experienced endoscopists to perform an endoscopic retrograde cholangiopancreatography (ERCP) after proximal gastric bypass, common bile duct exploration, either laparoscopic or open, should be within the capabilities of most bariatric surgeons (Fig. 21.7-8).

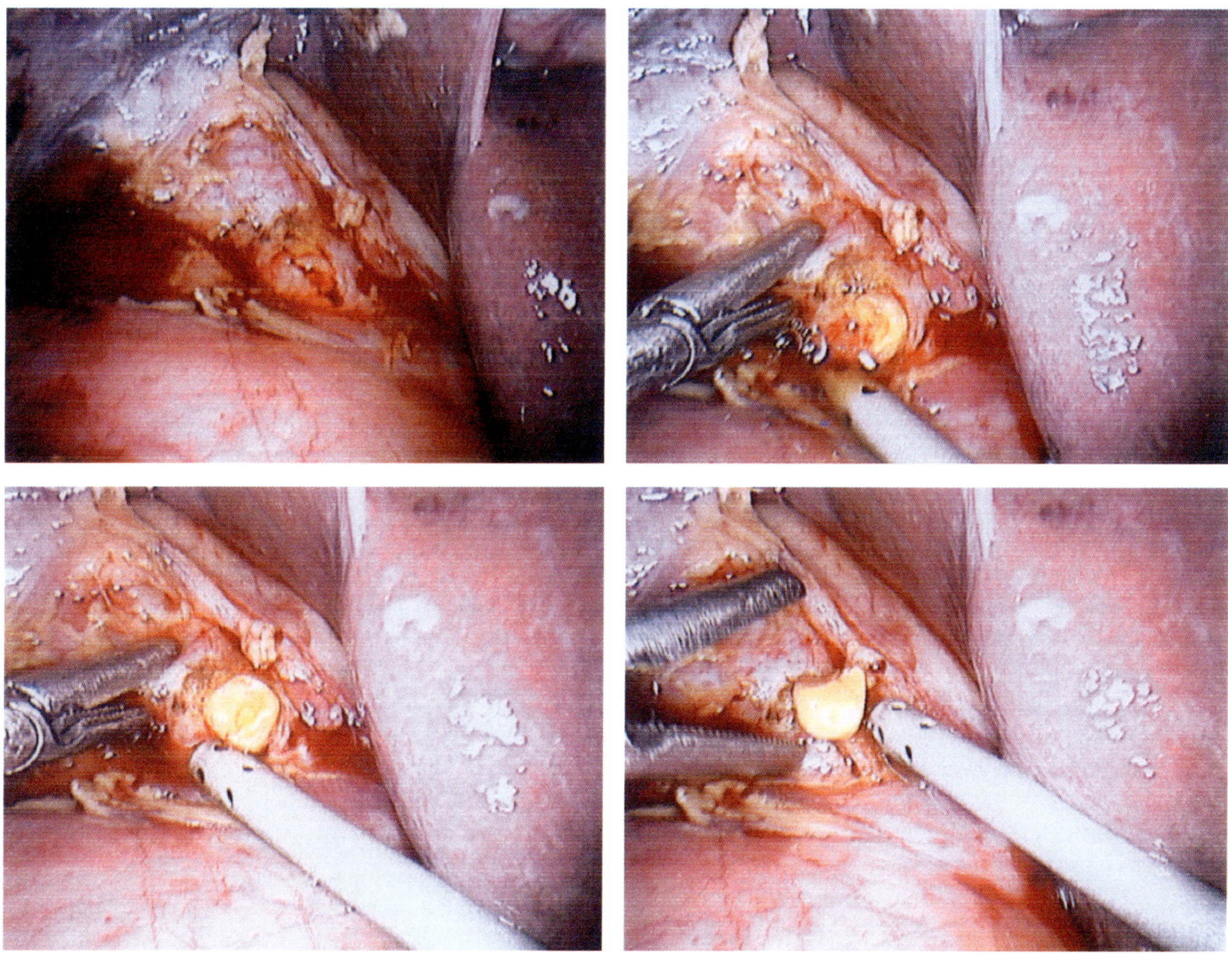

FIGURE 21.7-8. Common bile exploration after Roux-en-Y gastric bypass.

Nutritional Issues

Malnutrition due to dysfunctional eating influenced by psychological or anatomic derangements brought on by surgery can be acute, such as thiamine deficiency, or chronic, in the case of iron or calcium depletion. Routine oral vitamin and calcium supplementation and education with respect to proper dietary choices will prevent most deficiency syndromes. However, interval nutritional evaluation is recommended as part of routine health care maintenance after surgery.

Excessive Weight Loss

Excessive weight loss to the point of BMI reduction below 18.5 or under ideal body weight as determined by the New York Life Insurance Company table analysis requires investigation as to dysfunctional eating patterns or psychological issues. Excessive weight loss may also indicate cross-addiction to alcohol or drugs (29).

Consideration should be given to reversal of the procedure, establishment of an enteral route for dietary supplementation, psychological counseling, or detoxification as determined by the clinical setting.

Death

The low death rates achieved by most experienced programs is commendable, considering the number and severity of comorbid conditions associated with the morbidly obese patient. Mortality is most often due to cardiopulmonary events such as pulmonary emboli, although prolonged illness from sepsis and intestinal leaks can be a contributing factor.

Most large published series quote a mortality rate of less than 0.5%. This may not accurately represent statistics outside these major centers. Flum analyzed hospital data from the Washington state area for 30-day hospital mortality as well as mortality after hospitalization. The rate for in-hospital mortality was 1.1%, while overall mortality associated with all bariatric procedures was 1.9%. The learning curve was an issue, as the mortality for surgeons with less than a 25-case experience averaged 5%, while surgeons with over a 250-case experience had almost a 0% mortality.

Outcomes data dependent on surgeon experience is not unique to bariatric surgery. However, as this specialty has become more publicized, accurate mortality, complication, and ultimately weight loss data play an increasingly important role in identifying centers of excellence.

Conclusion

Primary bariatric surgery is always elective. Therefore, it is incumbent on the surgeon to properly optimize all medical conditions prior to surgery. The surgeon must have a low threshold to actively evaluate and improve cardiac performance, and optimize blood pressure, glucose control, and sleep apnea. This, along with psychological preparedness, can minimize potential complications.

Reducing the incidence and severity of complications requires more than a knowledgeable surgeon. It requires a team of highly trained professionals working together. Included are institutions willing to provide the tools and services required of this demanding specialty beyond that of the operating room and an efficient billing service. Central to this team is the bariatric surgeon coordinating care provided by cardiologists, pulmonologists, medical intensivists, radiologists, endocrinologists, psychologists, nutritionists, anesthesiologists, and nursing staff all dedicated to treat this multisystem disease.

Comprehensive bariatric surgical programs offer the vast majority of morbidly obese patients the only hope for long-term weight control. Despite the long learning curve involved with many minimally invasive approaches, the overall advantages as opposed to traditional open surgery should not be overlooked.

References

1. Ford ES, Giles WH, Dietz WH. Prevalence of the metabolic syndrome among US adults: findings from the third National Health and Nutrition Examination Survey. JAMA 2002;287:356–359.
2. Fontaine KR, Redden DT, Wang C, et al. Years of life lost due to obesity. JAMA 2003;289(2):287–293.
3. Wolf A, Colditz G. Current estimates of the economic cost of obesity in the United States. Obes Res 1998;6(2):97–106.
4. Torgerson JS. Effects of long-term weight loss maintenance on health-related quality of life and obesity related costs. The Swedish Obese Subjects (SOS) Study. In: Progress in Obesity Research, vol 9. Montrouge: John Libbey, Eurotext, 2003.
5. Flum DR, Dellinger EP. The impact of gastric bypass surgery on survival: a population-based analysis. Presented at the American College of Surgeons Clinical Congress, JACS 2004;199:543–551.
6. Courcoulas A, Perry Y, Buenaventura P, Luketich J. Comparing the outcomes after laparoscopic versus open gastric bypass: a matched paired analysis. Obes Surg 2003;13(3):341–346.
7. Nguyen NT, Ho HS, Palmer LS, Wolfe BM. A comparison study of laparoscopic versus open gastric bypass for morbid obesity. J Am Coll Surg 2000;191(2):149–155; discussion 155–157.
8. Schauer PR, Ikramuddin S. Laparoscopic surgery for morbid obesity. Surg Clin North Am 2001;81:1145–1179.

9. Podnos YD, Jimenez JC, Wilson SE, Stevens CM, Nguyen NT. Complications after laparoscopic gastric bypass. A review of 3464 cases. Arch Surg 2003;138:957–961.

10. Way LW, Stewart L, Gantert W, et al. Causes and prevention of laparoscopic bile duct injuries: analysis of 252 cases from a human factors and cognitive psychology perspective. Ann Surg 2003;237:460–469.

11. Philips P, Amaral J. Abdominal access complications in laparoscopic surgery. J Am Coll Surg 2001;192:525–536.

12. Serra C, Baltasar A, Bou R, Miró J, Cipagauta LA. Internal hernias and gastric perforation after a laparoscopic gastric bypass. Obes Surg 1999;9:546–549.

13. Singh R, Fisher BL. Sensitivity and specificity of postoperative upper GI series following gastric bypass. Obes surg 2003;13:73–75.

14. Ganci-Cerrud G, Herrera MF. Role of radiologic contrast studies in the early postoperative period after bariatric surgery. Obes Surg 1999;9:532–534.

15. Sims TL, Mullican MA, Hamilton EC, Provost DA, Jones DB. Routine upper gastrointestinal Gastrografin swallow after laparoscopic Roux-En-Y gastric bypass. Obes Surg 2003;13:66–67.

16. Schauer PR, Matter SG, Martin J, et al. Objective evidence of persistent acid reflux after Roux-en-Y gastric bypass for morbid obesity. In press.

17. Cameron. Current surgical therapy laparoscopic gastric bypass. In press.

18. Nguyen NT, Stevens CM, Wolfe BM. Incidence and outcome of anastomotic stricture after laparoscopic gastric bypass. J Gastrointest Surg 2003;7:997–1003.

19. Nguyen NT, Huerta S, Gelfand D, Stevens CM, Jim J. Bowel obstruction after laparoscopic Roux-en-Y gastric bypass. Obes Surg 2004;14:190–196.

20. Brolin RE. The antiobstruction stitch in stapled Roux-en-Y enteroenterostomy. Am J Surg 1995;169(3):355–357.

21. Champion JK, Williams M. Small bowel obstruction and internal hernias after laparoscopic Roux-en-Y gastric bypass. Obes Surg 2003;13(4):596–600.

22. Higa KD, Ho T, Boone KB. Internal hernias after laparoscopic Roux-en-Y gastric bypass: incidence, treatment and prevention. Obes Surg 2003;13(3):350–354.

23. Wu EC, Barba CA. Current practices in the prophylaxis of venous thromboembolism in bariatric surgery. Obes Surg 2000;10:7–13.

24. Shiffman ML, Sugerman HJ, Kellum JM, et al. Gallstone formation after rapid weight loss: a prospective study in patients undergoing gastric bypass surgery for treatment of morbid obesity. Am J Gastroenterol 1991;86:1000–1005.

25. Villegas L, Schneider B, Provost D, et al. Is routine cholecystectomy required during laparoscopic gastric bypass? Obes Surg 2004;14:60–66.

26. Sugerman HJ, Brewer WH, Shiffman ML, et al. A multicenter, placebo-controlled, randomized, double-blind, prospective trial of prophylactic ursodiol for the prevention of gallstone formation following gastric-bypass induced rapid weight loss. Am J Surg 1995;169:91–96; discussion 96–97.

27. Wudel LJ Jr, Wright JK, Debelak JP, et al. Prevention of gallstone formation in morbidly obese patients undergoing rapid weight loss: results of a randomized controlled pilot study. J Surg Res 2002;102:50–56.

28. Hamad GG, Ikramuddin S, Gourash WF, Schauer PR. Elective cholecystectomy during laparoscopic Roux-en-Y gastric bypass: is it worth the wait? Obes Surg 2003;13:76–81.

29. Higa KD, Ho T, Boone KB, Roubicek MC. Narcotic withdrawal syndrome following gastric bypass—a difficult diagnosis. Obes Surg 2001;11:631–634.

30. Wittgrove AC, Endres JE, Davis M, et al. Perioperative complications in a single surgeon's experience with 1,000 consecutive laparoscopic Roux-en-Y gastric bypass operations for morbid obesity. Obes Surg 2002;12:457–458(abstr L4).

31. Schauer PR, Ikramuddin S, Gourash W, et al. Outcomes after laparoscopic Roux-en-Y gastric bypass for morbid obesity. Ann Surg 2000;232:515–529.

32. Higa K, Ho T, Boone K. Laparoscopic Roux-en-Y gastric bypass; technique and 3–year follow-up. J Laparoendosc Adv Surg Tech 2001;11:377–382.

33. Champion JK, Hunt T, DeLisle N. Laparoscopic vertical banded gastroplasty and Roux-en-Y gastric bypass in morbid obesity. Obes Surg 1999;9:123–144.

34. DeMaria EJ, Sugerman HJ, Kellum JM, et al. Results of 281 consecutive total laparoscopic Roux-en-Y gastric bypasses to treat morbid obesity. Ann Surg 2002;235:640–647.

35. Spaulding L. The incidence of small bowel resection on the incidence of stomal stenosis and marginal ulcer after gastric bypass. Obes Surg 1997;7:485–487.

21.8
Gastric Bypass as a Revisional Procedure

Rodrigo Gonzalez, Scott F. Gallagher, Michael G. Sarr, and Michel M. Murr

In most experienced bariatric centers, revisional procedures comprise 10% to 15% of the operations performed, most of which are referred from other bariatric surgeons. The need for revisional surgery has been reported in 5% to 36% of patients undergoing vertical banded gastroplasty (VBG) and from 5% to 23% of patients undergoing Roux-en-Y gastric bypass (RYGBP) (1,2). This chapter discusses RYGBP as a revisional procedure for failed bariatric procedures. Although the number of revisional procedures done laparoscopically is very small, there is a growing body of evidence that supports its safety and feasibility (3–6). Yet, it is important to remember that the principles of evaluating failed bariatric procedures and the rationale for revisional surgery are not dictated by the method of accessing the abdominal cavity but rather are governed by lessons learned from the cumulative experience of an evidence-based approach and a tertiary, bariatric practice.

General Preoperative Considerations

Traditionally, a bariatric operation is considered to be successful when more than 50% of excess body weight is lost and maintained after long-term follow-up. Recently, the control and improvement of comorbidities has been recognized to be as important an end point as weight loss and is more frequently reported. Another important factor to consider when analyzing outcomes of bariatric procedures is the improvement in quality of life.

It is imperative that the surgeon fully understand the reason for failure of the previous weight-loss operation and not simply blame it on overeating. Endoscopy, barium swallow, and computed tomography (CT) scan should be used liberally, and not only as diagnostic tools. It is also important to educate the patient about the relatively higher operative risks and relatively less expected long-term weight loss, compared to the initial weight-loss operation. In addition, the often technically demanding revisional procedure should only be undertaken by well-trained and experienced bariatric surgeons.

Who Should Perform Revisional Bariatric Operations?

The International Federation of Surgery of Obesity states, "Reoperative bariatric surgery is an intricately complex and demanding area which requires considerable primary bariatric experience. The bariatric surgeon, who is early in his/her experience, should refer back to, confer with, or otherwise work with one or more bariatric surgical colleagues" who have extensive experience in reoperative bariatric surgery and a multidisciplinary approach, which are critical for successful long-term outcomes and patient satisfaction.

General Technical Considerations

Vertical Banded Gastroplasty (VBG)

The VBG was the operation of choice of many bariatric surgeons during the 1980s. However, it has fallen out of favor because of unsatisfactory weight loss and a relatively high incidence of long-term adverse outcomes such as emesis, maladaptive eating syndrome, and gastroesophageal reflux disease (GERD) (2). We recommend revising a failed VBG to RYGBP, to eliminate the untoward effects (e.g., band erosion, stomal stenosis, esophageal reflux, and maladaptive eating behavior) while inducing a durable and sustainable weight loss.

Patients with staple-line disruption at the time of diagnosis will have a greater than anticipated eating capacity, and will perhaps complain of weight gain. Meanwhile, patients with pouch obstruction usually have weight loss exceeding normal parameters. The latter group of patients is content with their weight loss and may object to a revision of the operation, knowing that they may regain some of the weight, as they are able to eat normally again.

Unsatisfactory Weight Loss

In the absence of staple-line disruption (Fig. 21.8-1), excessive intake of energy-dense foods (soda, ice cream, potato chips, etc.) that annul the restrictive function of the procedure is the primary cause of poor weight loss after VBG. Another cause of weight gain following VBG is disruption of the vertical staple line, allowing patients to ingest greater quantities of food; this complication has been reported to occur in up to 50% of patients (Fig. 21.8-2) (1,2,7).

Stomal Stenosis

There are two varieties of symptomatic stomal stenosis: mechanical and functional. The pathogenesis of mechanical stomal stenosis is not clear, but it may result from ulceration of the stomal canal or from a fibrosing reaction to the band (Fig. 21.8-1). We have encountered patients with functional obstruction of the stoma due to the lack of propulsive contractile activity in an atonic pouch, or a tilting of the external band that narrows the functional, luminal diameter of the stoma (7,8). The clinical presentation of stomal stenosis is often misinterpreted as overeating, which also correlates with patients' symptoms of emesis, GERD, or narcotic addiction; hence, an upper gastrointestinal (UGI) study and endoscopy are crucial to making the correct diagnosis. Endoscopic dilations of stenotic stomas provide temporary relief until a definitive procedure can be undertaken.

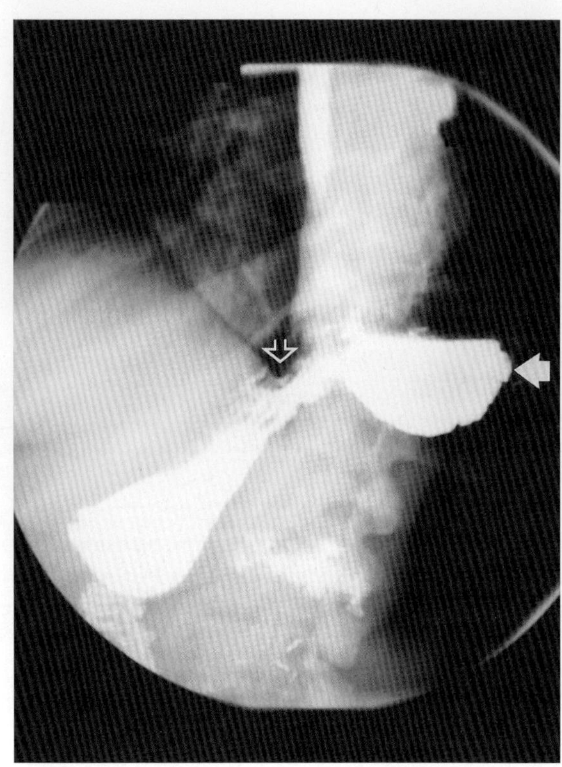

FIGURE 21.8-2. Radiograph of a patient after vertical banded gastroplasty (VBG) with subsequent unsatisfactory weight loss and maladaptive eating behavior. The pouch (solid arrow) is markedly distended secondary to stenosis at the banded stoma (open arrow). The vertical staple line is intact.

Band Erosion

The incidence of band erosion has been reported between 1% and 7%, usually occurring between 1 and 3 years after surgery (1,2,9). Erosion of the band can result in bleeding, nonhealing ulceration, mechanical obstruction, and rarely perforation. Therefore, patients initially present with emesis, upper gastrointestinal hemorrhage, abdominal discomfort, or even an acute abdomen. Endoscopic removal of eroded bands has been described to be successful in selected patients.

Gastroesophageal Reflux Disease

Symptoms of GERD are common after VBG and may result from postprandial esophageal loading or true reflux from the distal stomach. It has been suggested that pouch emptying is disrupted by the vertical partitioning of the stomach, thereby inducing pouch-esophageal reflux. In addition, larger pouches may include acid-secreting mucosa. The presence of Barrett's esophagus alone as an indication for conversion of VBG to RYGBP remains unproven; however, if symptoms persist, conversion to RYGBP should be pursued.

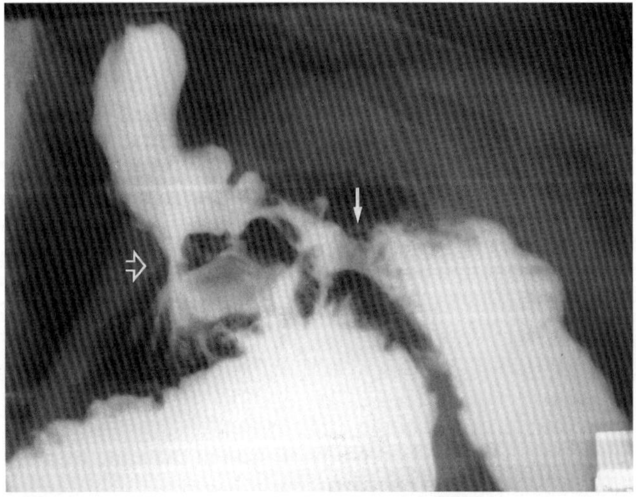

FIGURE 21.8-1. Radiograph of a patient after VBG that demonstrates the contrast entering the pouch and then preferentially filling the fundus and body of the stomach instead of through the band indicating a staple-line dehiscence (solid arrow). The pouch outlet is stenotic (open arrow).

Operative Technique

The aim of operative intervention should be revision of the VBG (and other gastroplasties) to a vertical, disconnected RYGBP. We have recently described our operative technique for converting a failed VBG to a RYGBP (7). We recommend cholecystectomy, if not previously done, as in all of our primary procedures. Locating the band is facilitated by dissecting the left lobe of the liver, which is usually firmly adherent to the band, or by entering the lesser sac to localize the left gastric artery bundle posteriorly.

Subsequently, dissecting the overlying, redundant dilated pouch of the proximal stomach helps localize the vertical staple line. The angle of His is then dissected free, and a window is made cephalad to the neurovascular bundle and the lesser curvature several centimeters proximal to the VBG stoma in order to facilitate passage of the linear stapler (Fig. 21.8-3A). The band can be removed at this point. The dilated pouch can be entered through a gastrotomy at the band site. This maneuver permits examination of the staple line, allowing retrograde insertion of the anvil of the circular stapler in preparation for the gastrojejunostomy (10). If the proximal pouch is not dilated, it is technically easier to insert the anvil of the circular stapler via a gastrotomy in the newly created gastric pouch and to secure it with purse-string sutures. The distal portion of the VBG pouch, including its stoma, is distal to this second application of the stapler, and drains into the distal stomach either through the stoma or, when present, through a dehiscence in the vertical staple line. When the stoma is stenotic and

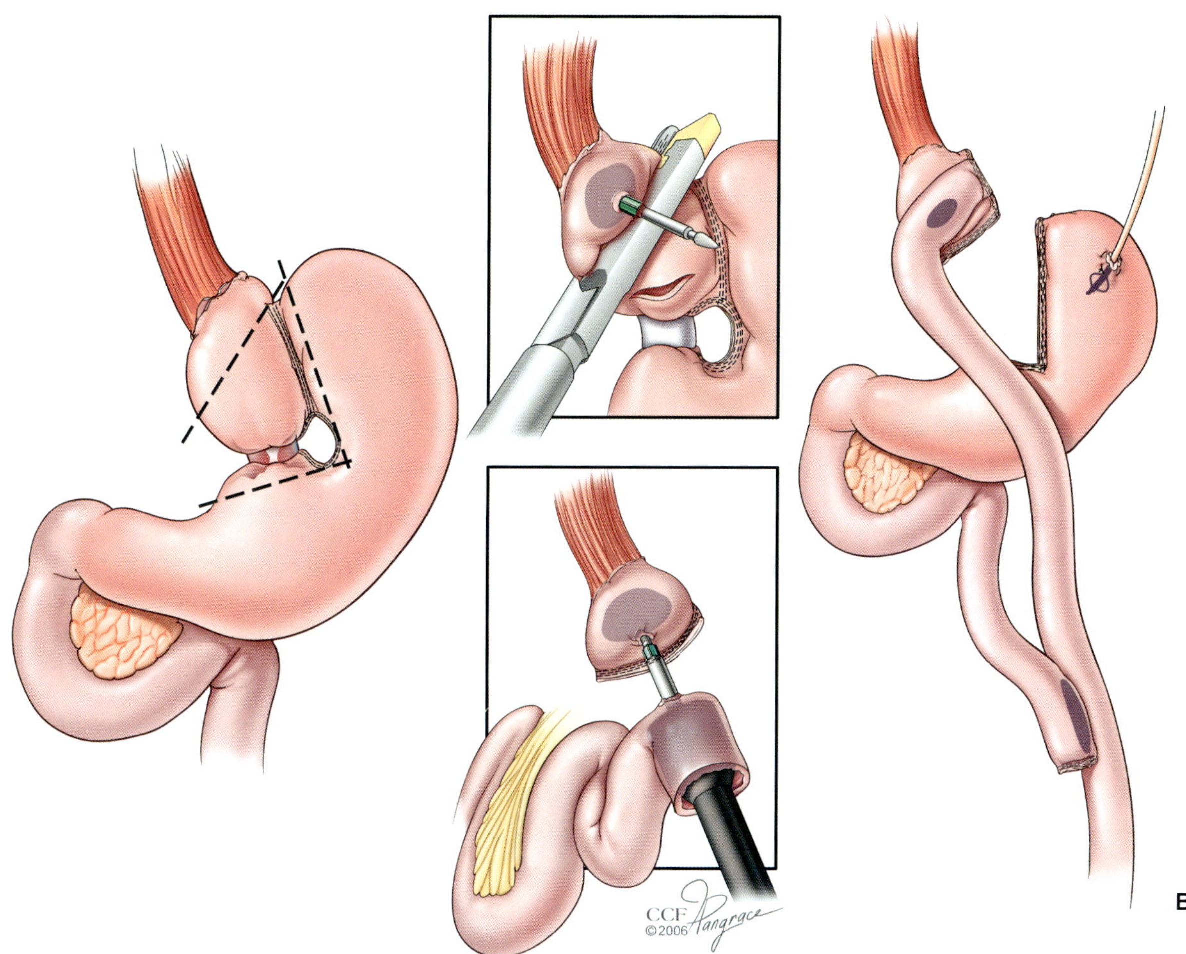

FIGURE 21.8-3. (A) Vertical banded gastroplasty with dilated pouch and stenotic stoma. Lines of transection for revision to Roux-en-Y gastric bypass are shown. Dissection is completed at the angle of His and along the lesser curvature. The anvil is introduced into the pouch through a gastrotomy at the band site and exteriorized through the anterior wall of the cardia (inset, top). Once the divided gastric pouch is created around the anvil, the band and old vertical staple line are resected and a circular stapled anastomosis is completed (inset, bottom). (B) Completed revision of vertical banded gastroplasty to Roux-en-Y gastric bypass. A gastrostomy tube placed in the excluded stomach for all revisional bariatric surgery. (Courtesy of the Cleveland Clinic Foundation.)

the staple line is intact, a gastrogastrostomy is necessary to ensure drainage into the distal stomach.

In patients in whom the band has eroded into the stomach, the second 90-mm linear stapler is applied distal to the first staple line in such a manner as to include the entire vertical staple line of the VBG. The stomach between the two staple lines including the stoma is then resected. A gastrostomy tube is routinely placed in the defunctionalized excluded stomach (Fig. 21.8-3B).

The gastrostomy tube serves two important functions. It decompresses the defunctionalized stomach while relieving pressure from the staples/resection lines and provides eternal access if a complication arises following this complex reoperative procedure. When constructing the gastrojejunostomy, we prefer to use a 21-mm circular stapler similar to constructing a primary RYGBP. For super-obese patients [body mass index (BMI) > 59] undergoing revision for a failed VBG, we recommend the very, very long RYGBP, to incorporate a more malabsorptive component to the procedure (11). We have abandoned the partial pancreaticobiliary bypass for super-obese patients because of unsatisfactory results (11).

Results of Vertical Banded Gastroplasty Reversal

Simple removal of the band results in weight gain; re-stapling the stomach pouch for staple-line disruption and gastric pouch dilatation has resulted in poor outcomes. Sustained and durable weight loss after conversion from VBG to RYGBP has also been well documented (12,13). In a series of 25 patients with GERD requiring conversion from VBG to RYGBP, we found a complete or near-complete resolution of heartburn in 96% of patients and no progression to severe dysplasia in patients with Barrett's esophagus. However, postoperative complications were somewhat increased, which is consistent with previous reports in the literature (12).

Jejunoileal Bypass

The overwhelming metabolic consequences have relegated jejunoileal bypass (JIB) to the history books among bariatric surgeons. The complications include liver damage (i.e., cirrhosis), severe electrolyte abnormalities, oxalate nephrolithiasis and nephropathy, autoimmune migratory polyarthritis, cholelithiasis, and enteropathies (pseudo-obstruction bypass enteritis, bacterial overgrowth, and intussusception) (14–16). Overall mortality rates in the first 2 years have been reported as high as 4% and are most commonly a consequence of liver failure (14,16). It is estimated that 25% to 40% of patients will require takedown and reversal of the JIB for metabolic complications (14–19). Asymptomatic patients without clinically apparent cirrhosis or other metabolic complications should be closely monitored and may not require reversal of their JIB.

When JIB takedown is clinically indicated, we recommend undertaking a concomitant RYGBP, since 90% of patients will regain their weight when the intestinal anatomy is reversed to normal without a concomitant bariatric procedure (19). It is important to counsel patients about meal-volume restrictions after RYGBP since many are quite satisfied with their weight loss despite the onset of JIB-related complications and typically prefer to maintain their ability to eat a full-size meal.

Operative Technique

The operation should begin with delineation of the intestinal anatomy as well as a liver biopsy to document any preexisting liver disease. We carry out a cholecystectomy at this stage if not done previously, because of the increased incidence of gallstones. The functional bowel should be readily apparent because of a two- to threefold increase in the lumen size and a markedly thickened wall. The bypassed jejunum and ileum are universally of much smaller caliber and a shorter mesentery. However, the most distal end of the bypassed segment, where it is anastomosed to the colon or ileum, can be easily recognized due to its characteristic dilatation. At this stage, the stomach is prepared for the concomitant gastric bypass as described previously (10). Subsequently, the jejunoileal anastomosis is disconnected, and a side-to-side ileoileostomy is constructed with a linear mechanical stapler or is hand-sewn. A side-to-end anastomosis is preferable if the lumen of the ileum is narrow. Similarly, a jejunojejunostomy is done to connect the bypassed stomach to the Roux limb (bypassed jejunum).

In preparation for incorporating the bypassed proximal jejunum as the Roux limb, the mesentery is divided for a distance of 5 to 10 cm to allow for a tension-free gastrojejunostomy. After occluding the jejunum 20 cm distal to the cut edge of the Roux limb, air is injected into the lumen in an attempt to enlarge its lumen and facilitate introducing the circular stapling device. It is not uncommon that a 21-mm circular stapler will not fit within the proximal jejunum, mandating a hand-sewn anastomosis. A gastrostomy tube is routinely inserted into the bypassed stomach until the bypassed and atrophied small bowel regains its function.

Results of Jejunoileal Bypass Reversal

Improvement or complete resolution of diarrhea, hepatic inflammation and fibrosis, and oxalosis and renal function is uniform after JIB reversal (14,18,20). However, reversal has no impact on cirrhosis. Although JIB-related metabolic complications were corrected following conversion to RYGBP, 67% of patients were unsatisfied because of restrictions in eating habits or weight gain (8).

Loop Gastric Bypass

The current RYGBP anatomy was developed from the original loop gastric bypass in order to eliminate persistent bile reflux (21). Recently, the loop gastric bypass was reintroduced laparoscopically as the mini-gastric bypass (Fig. 21.8-4). Although it may achieve adequate weight loss, it predisposes the patient to the risk of unrelenting bile gastritis and esophagitis. The most common indications for revisional surgery after loop gastric bypass are bile reflux with or without associated complications (e.g., esophagitis, Barrett's esophagus, aspiration pneumonia) and unsatisfactory weight loss. When necessary, we recommend converting the loop gastric bypass to a RYGBP.

Operative Technique

The bypass anatomy can be readily identified by the afferent and efferent limbs (Fig. 21.8-5A). If the pouch is large, as is usually the case, the gastrojejunostomy is taken down, and the efferent limb is used as the Roux

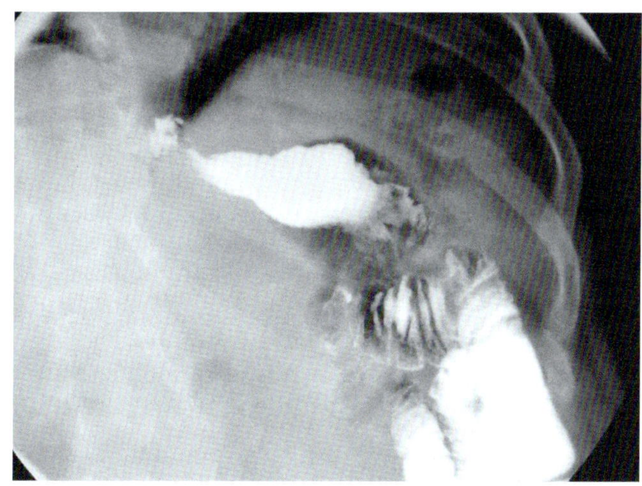

FIGURE 21.8-4. Radiograph of a patient after loop gastric bypass (or the so-called mini–gastric bypass) with an anastomotic, bleeding ulcer. The afferent limb (left) is mildly opacified by contrast retrograde; the efferent limb (right) fills antegrade and is opacified by denser contrast.

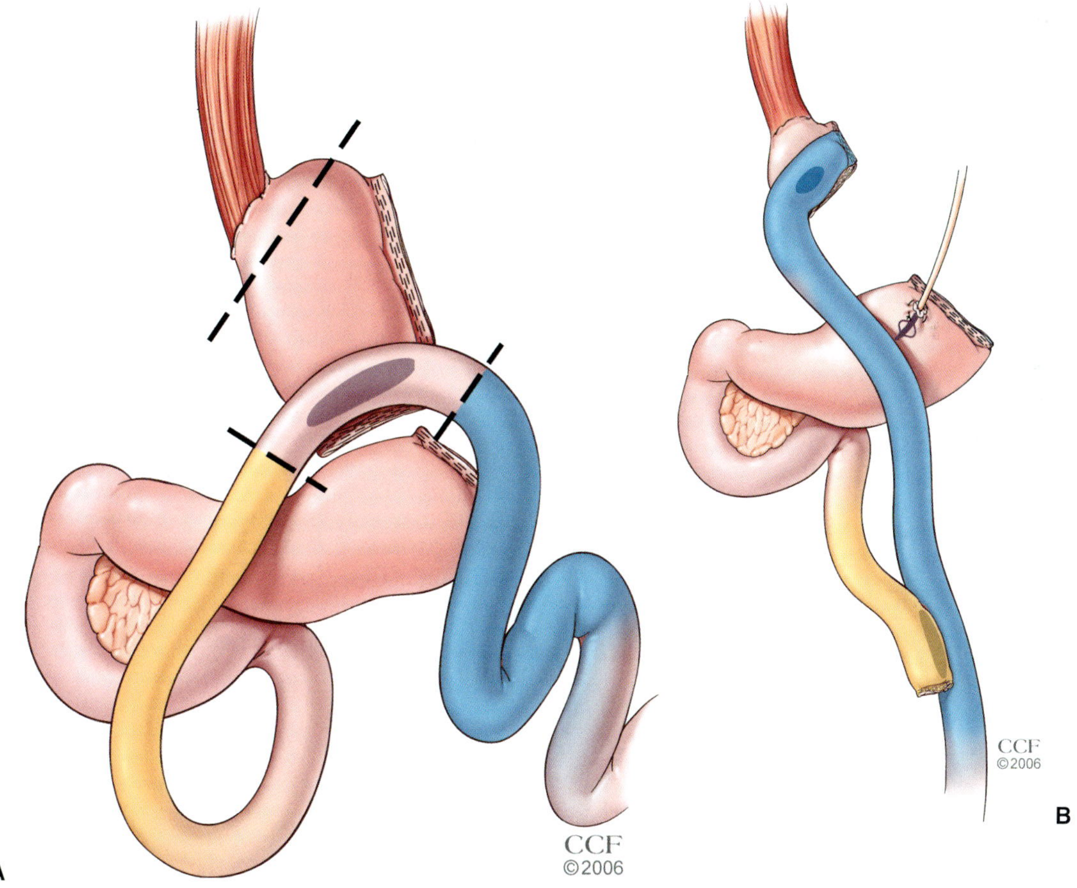

FIGURE 21.8-5. (A) Anatomy of the loop, or mini–, gastric bypass. The dotted lines represent the lines of transection to convert the loop gastric bypass to a Roux-en-Y gastric bypass. The lesser curvature and angle of His are dissected and a retrogastric tunnel created. The linear stapler is used to create a small gastric pouch. An anvil can be placed in the gastric pouch through a gastrostomy if a circular stapled gastrojejunostomy is planned. The afferent and efferent loops are identified and divided on either side of the large gastric pouch. The efferent limb is used as the Roux limb and the afferent limb is the biliopancreatic limb. (B) The completed revision with placement of a gastrostomy tube in the gastric remnant. (Courtesy of the Cleveland Clinic Foundation.)

limb and the afferent limb is anastomosed to the Roux limb 100 to 150 cm distal to the transection (Fig. 21.8-5B). After taking down the greater curvature at the gastrojejunostomy, a vertically oriented pouch is fashioned in the usual manner for a RYGBP by preserving the neurovascular bundle and dividing the stomach using linear staples. The segment of stomach remaining between the newly divided pouch and the distal staple line of the original pouch can be resected or anastomosed using a gastrogastrostomy. A gastrostomy tube is usually included to decompress the excluded stomach. On the rare occasion when the proximal gastric pouch is small and it is certain that the previous gastric partition is intact, a simple conversion from a loop to a Roux anatomy can be considered.

Results of Loop Gastric Bypass Reversal

After conversion to RYGBP, patients note virtually immediate resolution of the associated bile reflux. Pulmonary sequelae of the reflux as well as anastomotic complications are also significantly diminished.

Roux-en-Y Gastric Bypass

Approximately 15% of patients undergoing RYGBP have unsatisfactory weight loss. Complications are the most common indication for RYGBP revision. Although relatively less frequent, excessive weight loss may also be an indication for revision.

Pouch Dilation

An enlarged pouch appears to be a common reason for unsatisfactory weight loss or weight gain after RYGBP. The tendency for a pouch enlargement is most likely a consequence of a horizontal partitioning of the stomach, thereby including the fundus that exhibits receptive relaxation.

Gastrojejunostomy Stricture

Most commonly nonpeptic strictures are secondary to nonsteroidal antiinflammatory drugs (NSAIDs) generally used by patients for relief of obesity-related joint pain. Anastomotic strictures can also be related to ischemia at the gastrojejunostomy, resulting from tension at the anastomosis or excessive mobilization of the Roux limb mesentery. Ischemic strictures usually occur within 90 days of the operation and are more frequent following circular-stapled than hand-sewn anastomosis (22). Peptic strictures are often accompanied by anastomotic ulcers that can be refractory to medical treatment and may result in significant bleeding. The treatment involves discontinuation of all NSAIDs and endoscopic balloon dilatation. Operative revision is reserved for strictures that are refractory to repeated dilation or chronic strictures accompanied by fibrotic reaction extending beyond the anastomosis. Operative revision of strictures involves a complete takedown and reconstruction of the anastomosis.

A less common cause of stricture is peptic ulceration. Ulceration occurs from an enlarged proximal pouch containing parietal cells, staple-line disruption, or a gastrogastric fistula, which allows for acid reflux from the distal stomach into the pouch. GERD after RYGBP has been a controversial issue and is discussed in Chapter 31. Most experts advise downsizing a large pouch or re-stapling to correct the gastrogastric fistula.

Staple-Line Disruption

Staple-line breakdown occurs in 5% to 10% of patients with a nondisconnected RYGBP. Most commonly, staple-line dehiscence results in weight gain and possibly symptoms of reflux and ulcers in the Roux limb or anastomosis. These gastrogastric fistulas that may develop subsequent to a leak can increase in size and eliminate the restrictive component of RYGBP.

Bile Reflux Esophagitis

Theoretically this complication should not occur; however, bile reflux esophagitis may develop from a staple line dehiscence or from a Roux limb that is functionally too short. We recommend making the Roux limb at least 100 cm in length at the time of the primary operation and least 150 cm from the gastrojejunostomy in revisional procedures for bile reflux, especially when associated with unsatisfactory weight loss.

Diarrhea/Steatorrhea

Chronic diarrhea or steatorrhea can induce a severe protein and fat malabsorption after a distal RYGBP. These patients must first be resuscitated with parenteral nutrition. Operative intervention then follows to lengthen the ileal common channel. A tube gastrostomy or jejunostomy is often inserted to allow further enteral nutrition.

Gastrogastric Fistula

These fistulas are rare and occur in <1% of patients as a consequence of a leak on incomplete division of the stomach staple line. There are few data regarding operative treatment of these fistulas for unsatisfactory weight loss or nonhealing stomal ulcers.

Unsatisfactory Weight Loss

In the absence of a mechanical, anatomical cause, these patients require intense psychological counseling to control their detrimental and hazardous eating habits. Once all other potential, underlying anatomic causes are identified or eliminated, patients should be evaluated by an interdisciplinary team. It is our observation that many of these patients with unsatisfactory weight loss and an anatomically intact RYGBP have switched to eating energy-dense foods. In selected cases, the addition of a malabsorptive procedure such as the very, very long RYGBP (11), as opposed to reinforcing the stoma with a band, may be beneficial, yet there is little evidence to recommend this approach. The treatment of some patients with an unsatisfactory weight loss despite significant steatorrhea and the distal RYGBP remains an enigma.

Operative Technique

When the proximal pouch is too large, the gastrojejunostomy should be taken down and the pouch markedly reduced in volume by stapling-off and excluding any residual fundus (Fig. 21.8-6). In the case of a staple-line dehiscence, the stomach should be disconnected from the pouch using linear staples with interposition of omentum or a loop of jejunum. Revisions for anastomotic strictures can be difficult due to the associated serosal and perigastric inflammation, and revision to an esophagojejunostomy may be necessary.

Results of Roux-en-Y Gastric Bypass Revision

The results of revising an anatomically intact RYGBP for unsatisfactory weight loss have been disappointing. Revisions for anatomic complications of RYGBP uniformly resolve the associated symptoms and maintain weight loss.

Lap-Band

As of yet none of the authors of this chapter have had any significant experience with revision or conversion of a failed Lap Band. However, we anticipate that the size of the stomach between the esophagogastric junction and the band may dictate the type of revisional procedure

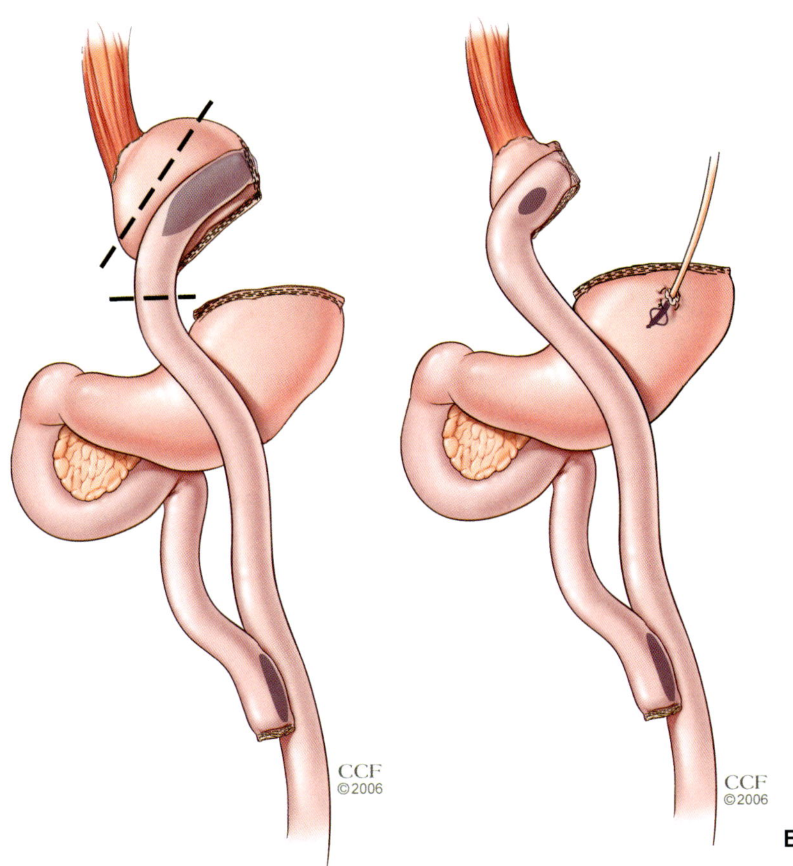

FIGURES 21.8-6. (A) Revision of a failed Roux-en-Y gastric bypass involves reduction of the pouch size and revision of the gastrojejunal anastomosis. The dotted lines represent the lines of transection to create a smaller gastric pouch and to resect the dilated or strictured anastomosis. (B) Completed revision with a 15-mL vertically oriented pouch. A gastrostomy tube is placed to provide decompression of the gastric remnant and feeding access if necessary. (Courtesy of the Cleveland Clinic Foundation.)

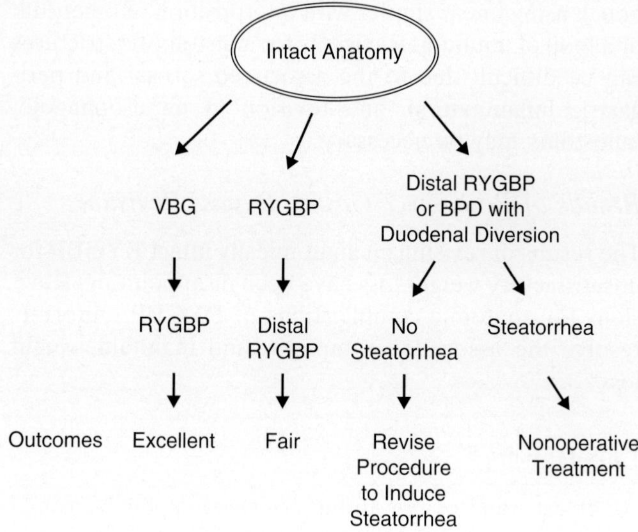

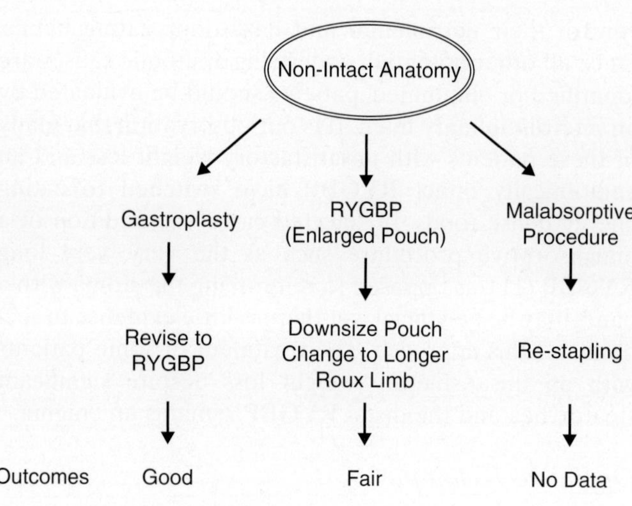

FIGURE 21.8-8. Revisional operation algorithm for unsatisfactory weight loss with non-intact anatomy.

FIGURE 21.8-7. Revisional operation algorithm for unsatisfactory weight loss with intact anatomy. BPD, biliopancreatic diversion; VBG, vertical banded gastroplasty; RYGBP, Roux-en-Y gastric bypass.

eventually required. The most common reasons for revision of a gastric banding procedure are insufficient weight loss (62%), partial or complete obstruction (13%), pouch dilation (9%), band erosion (6%), necrosis of the stomach (4%), reflux esophagitis (2%), and perforation of the stomach (2%) (23,24). Conversion to a RYGBP biliopancreatic diversion with duodenal switch, rather than rebanding, is considered the procedure of choice of most bariatric surgeons (24) for unsatisfactory weight loss. Operative intervention may be designed with a similar approach to that of reoperative surgery for a failed VBG.

Treatment Algorithms

Figures 21.8-7 to 21.8-10 outline common scenarios based on symptoms or complications of specific bariatric procedures. They are intended as a guideline that should be tailored to the patient's complaints and symptoms.

We recommend RYGBP as the revisional procedure of choice for failed restrictive bariatric procedures, specifically VBG and gastric banding. Concerns about technical feasibility of RYGBP after the Lap-Band may be overstated. Although rare, we have reversed or "taken

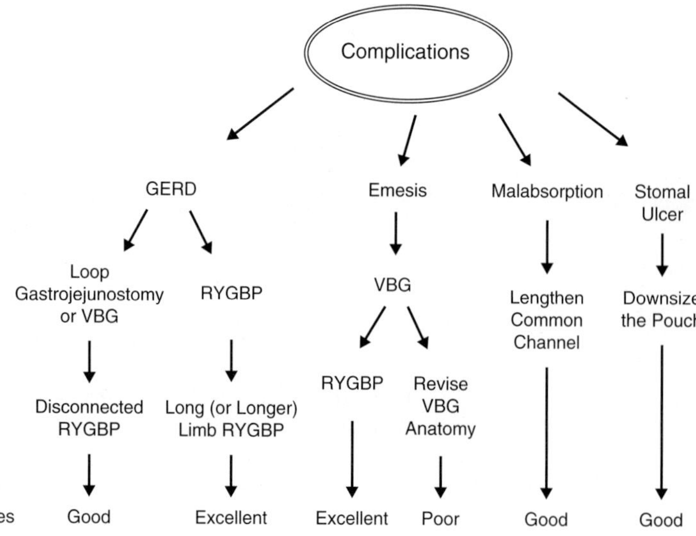

FIGURE 21.8-9. Revisional operation algorithm for postoperative complications. GERD, gastroesophageal reflux disease.

FIGURE 21.8-10. Revisional operation algorithm for jejunoileal bypass (JIB) complications.

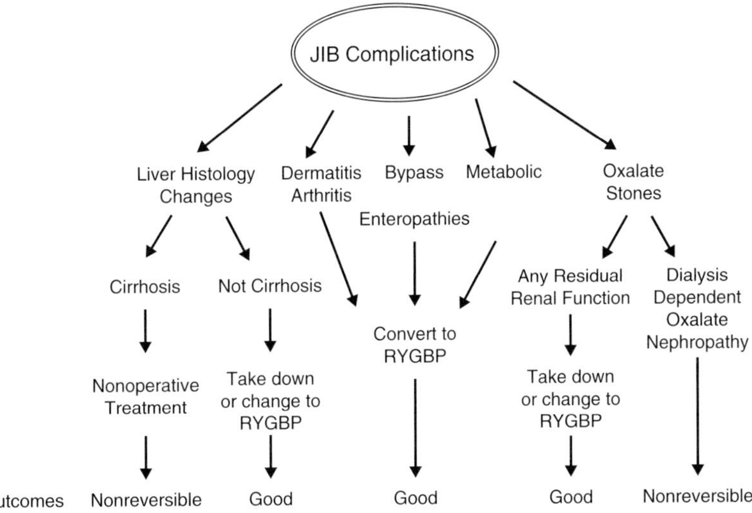

down" failed JIB, RYGBP, Lap-Band, or an RYGBP without a concomitant corrective bariatric procedure based on patient's discretion and full understanding of the eventual weight regain.

Revision of RYGBP for unsatisfactory weight loss in the absence of a markedly enlarged pouch by lengthening the Roux Limb and thereby shortening the common channel is associated with modest success because of the underlying dietary indiscretion. Similarly, reports of successful weight loss after banding a failed RYGBP are anecdotal.

More commonly, we are treating an increasing number of patients with severe protein calorie anastomotic secondary to high-grade strictures, short common channel, or short bowel syndrome; we aggressively pursue parenteral nutrition in the initial phase of nutritional resuscitation and then proceed with enteral feedings via a nasoenteric tube or a gastrostomy tube into the excluded stomach. Revisional surgery to address the underlying anatomic problem can be safely undertaken after normalization of nutritional parameters.

Conclusion

A flat and long learning curve is associated with primary bariatric surgery. Unsatisfactory results are frequently reported during this period, especially in patients with obesity-related comorbidities. It is therefore reasonable to expect that revisional surgery will be even more difficult to master, and therefore it should be undertaken only by an experienced bariatric surgeon in conjunction with a multidisciplinary team with adequate experience and adequate facilities for managing obese patients. Revisional bariatric surgery is associated with favorable outcomes in a select group of patients; the mortality and morbidity of revisional bariatric surgery is considerably higher than that of primary bariatric procedures.

References

1. MacLean LD, Rhode BM, Samplis J, et al. Results of the surgical treatment of obesity. Am J Surg 1993;165:155–162.
2. del Almo DA, Diez MM, Guedea ME, Diago VA. Vertical banded gastroplasty: is it a durable operation for morbid obesity? Obes Surg 2004;14:536–538.
3. McCormick JT, Papasavas PK, Caushaj PF, Gagne DJ. Laparoscopic revision of failed open bariatric procedures. Surg Endosc 2003;17:413–415.
4. Khaitan L, van Sickle K, Gonzalez R, Lin E, Ramshaw B, Smith CD. Laparoscopic revision of bariatric procedures: Is it feasible? Am Surg 2005;71:6–12.
5. Cohen R, Pinheiro JS, Correa JL, Schiavon C. Laparoscopic revisional bariatric surgery. Myths and facts. Surg Endosc 2005;19:822–825.
6. de Csepel J, Nahouraii R, Gagner M. Laparoscopic gastric bypass as a reoperative bariatric surgery for failed open restrictive procedures. Surg Endosc 2001;15:393–397.
7. Gonzalez R, Gallagher SF, Haines K, Murr MM. Operative technique for converting a failed vertical banded gastroplasty to Roux-en-Y gastric bypass. J Am Coll Surg 2005;201:366–374.
8. Behrns KE, Smith CD, Kelly KA, et al. Reoperative bariatric surgery. Lessons learned to improve patient selection and results. Ann Surg 1993;218:646–653.
9. Moreno P, Alastrué A, Rull M, et al. Band erosion in patients who have undergone vertical banded gastroplasty. Incidence and technical solutions. Arch Surg 1998;133:189–193.
10. Murr MM, Gallagher SF. Technical considerations for transabdominal loading of the circular stapler in laparoscopic Roux-en-Y gastric bypass. Am J Surg 2003;185:585–588.
11. Murr MM, Balsiger BM, Kennedy FP, Mai JL, Sarr MG. Malabsorptive procedures for severe obesity: comparison of pancreatico-biliary bypass and very very long Roux-en-Y gastric bypass. J Gastrointest Surg 1999;3:607–612.

12. Sugerman HJ, Kellum JM Jr, DeMaria EJ, Reines HD. Conversion of failed or complicated vertical banded gastroplasty to gastric bypass in morbid obesity. Am J Surg 1996; 171:263–269.
13. Balsiger BM, Murr MM, Mai J, Sarr MG. Gastroesophageal reflux after intact vertical banded gastroplasty: correction by conversion to Roux-en-Y gastric bypass. J Gastrointest Surg 2000;4:276–281.
14. Requarth JA, Burchard MD, Collachio TA, et al. Long-term morbidity following jejunoileal bypass: the continuing potential need for surgical reversal. Arch Surg 1995;130:318–325.
15. Kirkpatrick JR. Jejunoileal bypass: a legacy of late complications. Arch Surg 1987;122:610–614.
16. Hocking MP, Duerson MC, O'Leary JP, Woodward ER. Jejunoileal bypass for morbid obesity: late follow-up in 100 cases. N Engl J Med 1983;308:995–999.
17. Dean P, Joshi S, Kaminski DL. Jejunoileal bypass: can the mistake by corrected? Gastroenterology 1990;98:1710–1719.
18. Våge V, Solhaug JH, Berstad A, et al. Jejunoileal bypass in the treatment of morbid obesity: a 25-year follow-up study of 36 patients. Obes Surg 2002;12:312–318.
19. Frandsen J, Pedersen SB, Richelsen B. Long term follow up of patients who underwent jejunoileal bypass for morbid obesity. Eur J Surg 1998;164:281–286.
20. Styblo T, Martin S, Kaminski DL. The effects of reversal of jejunoileal bypass operations on hepatic triglyceride content and hepatic morphology. Surgery 1984;96:632–640.
21. Brown RG, O'Leary JP, Woodward ER. Hepatic effects of jejunoileal bypass for morbid obesity. Am J Surg 1974;127:53–58.
22. Gonzalez R, Lin E, Venkatesh KR, et al. Gastrojejunostomy during laparoscopic gastric bypass. Analysis of 3 techniques. Arch Surg 2003;138:181–184.
23. van Wageningen B, Berends FJ, van Ramshorst B, Janssen IFM. Revision of failed laparoscopic adjustable gastric banding to Roux-en-Y gastric bypass. Obes Surg 2006;16:137–141.
24. Weber M, Muller MK, Michael JM, Belal R, Horber F, Hauser R, Clavien PA. Laparoscopic Roux-en-Y gastric bypass, but not rebanding, should be proposed as rescue procedure for patients with failed laparoscopic gastric banding. Ann Surg 2003;6:827–834.

21.9
Laparoscopic Roux-en-Y Gastric Bypass: Controversies

J.K. Champion and Sayeed Ikramuddin

The characterization of the Roux-en-y gastric bypass as the "gold standard" for bariatric surgery has been misleading because there is no standard technique employed by the majority of surgeons (1). The laparoscopic gastric bypass has followed in the footsteps of the open approach and varies widely in construction (2–6). Controversies exist over the ideal methods to maximize outcomes and minimize complications, which are the goals of every surgical procedure. This chapter explores several of the current controversies about the laparoscopic gastric bypass technique.

Enhancement of Weight Loss

There have been countless modifications of the gastric bypass, most of which were designed to enhance weight loss, and include variation in the size of the pouch, stoma, and Roux-limb length. Further modifications include banding of the pouch or the anastomosis to prevent dilatation. Most of these modifications were reported anecdotally and the analysis of results was retrospective. There are a few circumstances where prospective evidence exists to substantiate the techniques employed.

The principal idea is to preclude the need for revisional surgery due to failure of weight loss, because revisional bariatric surgery is time-consuming, carries a higher risk, and in general has less impressive weight loss than is seen with primary surgery. Steps should be taken at the first operation to minimize the need for reoperative surgery. Unfortunately, little is known about the effect of these procedural variations. Some of the changes made in the evolution of the procedure have minimized the need for reoperative surgery. The original gastric bypass utilized a loop gastrojejunostomy, which resulted in a high rate of alkaline reflux, necessitating conversion to a Roux anatomy. Another change is a stapled gastric pouch rather than an "isolated" or divided gastric bypass. In more recent practice surgeons utilize a divided stomach and thus the chance of staple-line breakdown with gastrogastric fistula is somewhat diminished. The only way to perform the procedure laparoscopically is to transect the gastric pouch from its distal remnant, which still must be ruled out, however, in the presence of a recalcitrant marginal ulcer.

Regain of weight following the gastric bypass has been attributed to both enlargement of the stoma and enlargement of the gastric pouch (7). It is also important to note that it is likely that many patients with an enlarged stoma and pouch have an excellent result postoperatively. On the other hand, all surgeons who perform revisional bariatric surgery have seen patients with a perfect anatomic gastric bypass with a small pouch and narrow stoma who have regained all of their weight. Revision of the gastric bypass in cases of moderate pouch dilatation in an attempt to produce further restriction has sometimes proved unsuccessful (8). In these cases a standard proximal gastric bypass will be converted to a distal gastric bypass to produce a mild to moderate weight loss at best (9).

In response to late failures following the gastric bypass, some authors have advocated the need for reinforcement of the stoma or the pouch. This can be accomplished using a Silastic ring (10) or a small segment of tensor fascia lata. The latter can be applied to both the gastric pouch or to the anastomosis itself. Fobi et al. (9) described a combined vertical banded gastroplasty using a 5.5-cm Silastic ring in conjunction with the gastric bypass. They have reported results at 2 years and at 6 years. More than 90% of patients have greater than 40% excess weight loss (EWL). These studies are not controlled, and reinforcement of the pouch is not without complications including erosions of the band or food intolerance. This technique of pouch reinforcement can also be duplicated laparoscopically. Bessler et al. (10) recently presented their experience of a randomized prospective double-blind study of a polypropylene band around the gastric pouch versus no band. At 1 year there was no difference in weight loss or complication rates. Long-term data are pending (11). Sapala et al. (12) have suggested the use of the "micropouch" to decrease the incidence of marginal ulceration as well as to maximize weight loss. Results have shown weight loss comparable to established techniques.

Limitation of absorption is another approach to augment weight loss. There are three ways this can be accomplished: by elongating the Roux or alimentary limb, by decreasing the length of the common channel, and by increasing the length of the biliopancreatic limb. A detailed description of this anatomy was provided in earlier chapters.

Except for passive diffusion, there will be little absorption of nutrients in the absence of bile and pancreatic juices through the Roux limb. The length of the Roux limb is defined as the distance from the gastrojejunal anastomosis to the anastomosis with the biliopancreatic limb. For routine gastrointestinal surgery the Roux limb is 40 cm as a minimum in order to minimize the risk of alkaline gastritis. In many cases the standard Roux limb is considered to be 75 cm. An extended or long limb bypass is considered to be 150 cm. A distal bypass, in contrast, describes a connection of the alimentary (Roux limb) with the biliopancreatic limb 50 to 100 cm from the ileocecal valve. Though this represents a nice way to categorize patients, this approach does not take into account that the length of the small bowel can vary greatly with the body mass index (BMI) of the patient (13); thus subtle differences in small bowel bypass length may not be relevant.

Perhaps the intervention that seems to have the strongest evidence in accentuating weight loss in the short term, particularly in the super-obese, is lengthening of the Roux limb. Torres (14) first suggested the role of the distal bypass. Brolin et al. (15) in 1992 reported the results of a prospective randomized study comparing the effect of a 75-cm Roux limb with that of a 150-cm Roux limb with a constant length biliopancreatic limb in the super-obese (BMI > 50). Patients were followed up to 4 years postoperatively. By 12 months after surgery there was a significant difference in weight loss in the longer Roux limb group. This difference persisted for about 36 months and then appeared to diminish. Several years later, Brolin et al. (16) compared these patients with patients having a true distal bypass to the short and long bypass groups. Weight loss was greatest in the distal bypass group at maximal follow-up. Most notable was the incidence of some form of metabolic sequelae in all of the distal bypass patients. Thus for patients who are super-obese there appears to be some advantage to having some degree of malabsorption. For patients with a BMI of less than 50 there probably does not appear to be an advantage to the longer bypass.

These findings were supported by MacLean et al. (7). In a retrospective study, the authors attempted to determine whether longer limb length affected weight loss following gastric bypass in patients who were morbidly obese (BMI ≤ 50) or super-obese (BMI > 50). They followed a total of 242 patients for a mean of 5.5 years. The short limb operation was a Roux-en-Y gastric bypass with a 40-cm Roux limb and a 10-cm afferent limb. The long-limb operation had a 100-cm Roux limb and a 100-cm afferent limb. Only the super-obese patients (mean BMI of 56) benefited from a long-limb bypass. Final BMI was 35.8 ± 6.7 in the short-limb patients and 32.7 ± 5.1 in the long-limb patients ($p = .049$). Patients with a BMI > 60 benefited the most from long-limb bypass. In contrast to the Brolin et al. report, no macronutritional side effects unique to the long-limb bypass were encountered (7).

Choba and Flancbaum (17) attempted to define the effect of Roux limb length on weight loss following the gastric bypass in a randomized prospective study. There were no significant differences in age, sex, race, initial BMI, or excess weight between patients within each weight category. When the number of patients achieving 50% EWL was evaluated, there was no difference between groups with a BMI < 50; however, among patients with a BMI > 50, a significantly greater percentage of those having a 250-cm limb achieved >50% EWL at 18 months postoperatively. This difference did not persist at 24 and 36 months.

Location of the gastrojejunal anastomosis on the gastric pouch has been considered a possible variable in weight loss. Classically there are two types of pouches used in the gastric bypass operation: vertical or horizontal. In the horizontally based gastric pouch the gastrojejunal anastomosis is placed high along the angle of His. A TA-type stapler is typically passed from the greater curvature to the lesser curvature following the ligation and division of a few short gastric vessels. A theoretical disadvantage of this approach is a slight increase in the risk of gastric pouch dilatation. The vertically based lesser curve pouch is the one most commonly used in the laparoscopic gastric bypass. This has a potential advantage of decreased pouch dilatation as the lesser curve is less likely to stretch. There have been some reports of increased marginal ulceration in using a pouch of this type (12).

Approaches to the Super-Obese and High Risk

An emerging area of controversy is the operative approach in the super-obese and in patients who are high risk. Patients considered in the super-risk group are those with advanced age, male gender, and central obesity with a BMI >50. These patients tend to have a higher perioperative complication rate (18). Patients who are super-obese typically have not enjoyed the same overall weight loss benefits that have been seen in patients who are not super-obese (19).

The sleeve gastrectomy has been proposed as an interim weight-loss step for this population of patients. This technique of Magenstrasse and Mill was originally described as an alternative to the vertical banded gastroplasty (20). Laparoscopically, this procedure was described in 1999 by McMahon. These procedures have been designed to develop a simpler and more physiologic type of gastroplasty. The weight loss from this procedure can be used to facilitate more malabsorptive procedures several months from the initial postoperative period. The idea is that patients who are in the category of high risk based on weight or comorbid conditions would not undergo a full gastric bypass procedure or duodenal switch until they reached their maximum weight loss following a sleeve gastrectomy.

In this procedure, the gastrectomy is performed by beginning gastric division approximately 6 cm proximal to the pylorus around a 36-French bougie using a linear staple cartridge. The division is taken up to the angle of His. Patients are then encouraged to lose weight over a period of 6 months to 1 year and then present for reoperative bariatric surgery. In theory this is a rational approach for the treatment of obesity in this population. However, certain issues need to be kept in mind: patients need to have a dual anesthetic, the insurance coverage for these procedures needs to be determined, and there is always a risk of failure of weight loss. The overall risk of leakage from the gastrectomy staple line is less when compared to a procedure in which a complex gastrojejunal anastomosis and an enteroenterostomy need to be performed. But there is still a definite risk. Initial weight loss data in these patients have been presented by a number of authors. Short-term results show weight loss that is nearly equivalent, and not statistically different, for weight loss in this patient population following gastric bypass (21). Long-term data are pending. Many issues remain unresolved with this approach; however, it may represent a promising alternative to those patients in high-risk categories. Certainly, the risks, the alternatives, and the potential risk for no insurance coverage for the second procedure need to be discussed in detail with the patient when contemplating this approach.

Antecolic Versus Retrocolic Roux Limb Placement

Controversy exists about whether the antecolic or the retrocolic placement of the Roux limb is better in laparoscopic gastric bypass. Proponents of the retrocolic approach claim it is the shortest distance for passage of the Roux limb to the gastric pouch and will result in less tension on the gastrojejunostomy anastomosis, and therefore will result in fewer leaks and strictures (2). The disadvantages include a longer operating time and the creation of a mesenteric defect in the transverse mesocolon that has potential to stenose, or if too wide can result in an internal hernia, both of which result in a small bowel obstruction and the need for reoperation (22). The longer operating time is the result of maneuvers to pass the limb blindly behind the colon and the time required to suture the mesenteric defect to attempt to prevent internal hernias.

Proponents of the antecolic approach argue that the longer distance to pass the limb proximally was clinically insignificant in the vast majority of patients, and the technique, with improved visualization, was simpler and quicker to perform, did not result in an increase in stenosis or leaks at the gastrojejunostomy site, and in fact reduced the incidence of internal hernias and small bowel obstruction (22–24).

Many surgeons have presented data that document that the antecolic approach has significant advantages over a retrocolic placement (22–24). The first author of this chapter published results comparing laparoscopic gastric bypass in 246 retrocolic procedures and 465 antecolic procedures and demonstrated a significant reduction ($p = .006$) in the incidence of small bowel obstruction in the antecolic group (0.43% in antecolic group vs. 4.5% in retrocolic group) and no increase in leaks or stoma stenosis (22). Similar outcomes with the antecolic approach compared to the retrocolic technique have been reported independently by Felix and Brown (23) (1.5% vs. 5.0%) in a series of 736 patients and by Schauer et al. (24) (0.4% vs. 2.0%) in a series of 726 patients.

Surgeons who adopt the antecolic technique as their approach need to be aware that the Roux limb will occasionally not reach the gastric pouch if the small bowel mesentery is short, and therefore they may have to employ a retrocolic placement, so they must be competent in both techniques.

Preventing Internal Hernias

Internal hernias are a known complication of the Roux-en-Y gastric bypass whether performed as an open procedure or laparoscopically (25). They may occur at one of three sites: the transverse mesocolon window, Petersen's space, and the mesenteric defect at the enteroenterostomy site. It was initially believed the incidence of small bowel obstruction would be less with a laparoscopic approach, but this has been demonstrated not to be the case. The initial incidence of internal hernias was higher in the laparoscopic technique, which was theorized as probably due to fewer adhesions with a minimally invasive approach, and failure to close the mesenteric defects (26). Many open surgeons don't close the defects, so a controversy exists about whether closure reduces the incidence of internal hernias after laparoscopic gastric bypass, and if so, what is the appropriate method for closure.

Suture closure of the three mesenteric defects has been demonstrated to reduce the incidence of internal hernias after laparoscopic gastric bypass, but it has not eliminated the complication (22,26). The first author of this chapter compared the incidence of internal hernias in a group of 246 laparoscopic retrocolic gastric bypass patients of whom 149 did not have the defects sutured and in 97 who underwent suture closure with a permanent continuous suture (22). The incidence of internal hernias was reduced, but not eliminated, and the overall incidence of small bowel obstruction was similar (4.0% vs. 3.7%, $p = .70$) between groups. While internal hernias were reduced with suture closure, the incidence of adhesive obstructions increased, keeping the overall incidence of small bowel obstruction and reoperation similar, but with different etiologies. In addition, we have been observing late internal hernias (around 3 years postoperative) presenting in patients who underwent suture closure of defects at the initial operation after losing a great deal of weight. Based on the results reported in the literature a strong argument can be made that the best method to reduce the incidence of internal hernias is to adopt an antecolic approach, and it is not necessary to close the mesenteric defects with this approach. Internal hernias can occur with any technique, even the antecolic approach, but the antecolic technique does eliminate the mesocolon defect and the remaining defects are more open, which allows the bowel to slide freely through the opening, and may be the reason that fewer problems have been observed. Small tight defects, such as occur with a retrocolic passage of the Roux limb, appear to have the greatest potential for entrapment and obstruction.

For surgeons who perform the retrocolic technique, the question arises as to whether there is a method of mesenteric defect closure that has been demonstrated to offer an advantage compared to other methods. The defects can be closed with an interrupted or continuous suture technique, and with absorbable or permanent suture. Higa et al. (5) has reported better results with a permanent continuous technique, compared to interrupted or absorbable suturing. The first author of this chapter had a similar early experience when we attempted closure with interrupted suture, and even the laparoscopic hernia stapler, which left defects between the ligatures, did not reduce our incidence of internal hernias. We quickly adopted a continuous silk suture technique, which produced the best outcomes in our experience, and our rec-ommendation is to utilize a permanent continuous suture technique. The addition of fibrin glue may provide staple-line hemostasis and reinforcement but has not been demonstrated to add anything but expense to the technique for suture closure of the mesenteric defects.

Preventing Leaks After Laparoscopic Gastric Bypass

Leaks are a known complication of laparoscopic gastric bypass and can be a significant etiology of postoperative morbidity and mortality. Therefore, methods to reduce this dreaded complication are welcomed by bariatric surgeons (3–5). Opinions vary widely in regard to the influence of anastomotic technique, the utility of intraoperative testing and drains, and the role of postoperative radiologic evaluations.

Current anastomotic techniques for the gastrojejunostomy include the circular stapler, the linear stapler, or the hand-sewn approach (3–6). While each approach has its advocates, there remains controversy over whether one technique offers an advantage or reduced leak rate compared to the others. Leak rates appear to be similar between techniques as long as they are done correctly by experienced surgeons who have appropriate laparoscopic suturing skills (27). Certain principles have emerged from early reports that demonstrated a higher leak rate with purely stapled anastomosis, linear or circular, which didn't involve suture reinforcement of the staple line at some site. The addition of suture reinforcement of the circular anastomosis or linear stapler technique was associated with a reduction in leak rates (4). The suture reinforcement varies from a total oversewing of the entire staple line, effectively creating a two-layer anastomosis, to simple one-layer closure of the enterotomy site for insertion of the linear stapler to form the anastomosis. The hand-sewn technique can apparently be accomplished equally well by a one- or two-layer technique (5,27). There is no information to suggest the choice of permanent versus absorbable suture makes a difference in leak rates.

Reinforcement of staple lines and anastomotic sites has been proposed to reduce the incidence of leaks by utilizing either fibrin glue or buttress strips (28–31). Experience with fibrin glue has been reported in two series to reduce the incidence of leaks, compared with historical reports and with internal and external case controls for comparison, but the studies did not include randomization. Increased operating room costs were reported. The routine utilization of fibrin sealant should be considered premature until additional prospective randomized trials justify the expense. Buttress strips were reported by Shikora et al. (31) to increase staple-line burst pressure in an animal model and to reduce staple-line leaks in their clinical bariatric practice compared to a historical control. This study was flawed in that the authors compared their last 250 laparoscopic gastric bypass cases with buttress strips to their first 100 cases during the learning curve, which is an unfair comparison. Buttress strips also cost approximately $1000 per case, which is a consideration with the reimbursement rates that most facilities receive under managed care. Buttress strips are an unproven technology at present and require further study before adoption into a bariatric practice.

There are considerable differences of opinion over the utilization of intraoperative testing for leaks, regarding both whether it is necessary and if so, which technique is best. Current techniques include simple inspection, intraoperative esophagogastroduodenoscopy (EGD), instillation of methylene blue via a nasogastric tube, or instillation of air or oxygen via a gastric tube (32).

The most sensitive test appears to be intraoperative EGD with instillation of air via the gastroscope, with a Glassman clamp occluding the small bowel and the staple lines placed under saline irrigation. Champion et al. (32) reported identifying 29 staple-line leaks intraoperatively in 825 laparoscopic bariatric procedures that underwent concomitant suture repair, and resulted in only three leaks (0.36%) postoperative. Similarly, Ramanathan et al. (33) identified a 10% incidence of air leaks in 182 laparoscopic gastric bypass patients intraoperatively by EGD, but only 3.8% of patients experienced leaks postoperatively. Critics of the EGD technique state that forceful instillation of air under pressure with the gastroscope is too strenuous a test and it results in too many false-positive tests; also, the technique is technically more complex and it increases costs. Some surgeons, however, lack privileges for intraoperative gastroscopy or fear alienating the gastroenterologist if they perform the test themselves, so they rationalize reasons to forgo the exam.

Instillation of methylene blue via a gastric tube positioned in the gastric pouch appears to be not as sensitive as an EGD in a study comparing intraoperative EGD with methylene blue as reported by Schauer et al. (3). No studies have compared all three techniques directly or have compared air instillation alone to EGD.

Utilization of drains varies widely among published reports (2–6). There are reports of routine utilization of drains in every case, selective usage for indications, and avoidance of drains after laparoscopic gastric bypass. In addition, the timing of removal of the drain varies, with some surgeons removing the drain before discharge and some waiting for 10 days postoperative when the patient returns for follow-up. Proponents of drains acknowledge they don't prevent leaks, but may allow management of leaks while avoiding a repeat operation. Late removal of drains appears to be associated with an increased "clinical leak" rate, which probably represents an infected drain path or staple erosion secondary to irritation

caused by the drain. Opponents of drains state they add needless expense and lull surgeons into conservative management of leaks, which can be disastrous in certain clinical situations. This is particularly true for leaks at the enteroenterostomy, which will not be apparent with an upper abdominal drain, and delay in surgery is more likely to be fatal. The presence of a drain with a clinical leak does not mean it can be managed conservatively; sound judgment is required in assessing the condition of the patient. Sepsis mandates a surgical exploration immediately, regardless of an existing drain. Ironically, some surgeons utilize drains for their laparoscopic gastric bypasses but not for open surgery (4).

Doing a routine postoperative gastrointestinal series with contrast has been advocated early in a surgeon's learning curve to aid in assessment for leaks. This is probably appropriate for the first 100 cases until the learning curve has been completed. The water-soluble contrast studies have a definite false-negative and false-positive rate and must be interpreted based on clinical findings in the patient (34). Signs of possible leakage include tachycardia, tachypnea, fever, and leukocytosis. Multiple reports have established that selective utilization of a postoperative upper gastrointestinal series is appropriate based on the patient's clinical course, and have led to a marked reduction in needless expense (35,36).

Conclusion

There has been a great deal of discussion about the technical specifications of the gastric bypass. But relatively little is understood about the operation and its mechanism of action. We do understand that the operation does work. Efforts to standardize the procedure with a goal of minimizing complications and facilitating uniform reporting of outcomes are the key to resolution of controversial issues with the Roux-en-Y gastric bypass.

References

1. Talieh J, Kirgan D, Fisher BL. Gastric bypass for morbid obesity: a standard surgical technique by consensus. Obes Surg 1997;7:198–202.
2. Wittgrove AC, Clark GW. Laparoscopic gastric bypass, Roux-en-Y—500 patients: technique and results, with 3–60 month follow-up. Obes Surg 2000;10:233–239.
3. Schauer PR, Ikramuddin S, Gourash W, et al. Outcomes after laparoscopic Roux-en-Y gastric bypass for morbid obesity. Ann Surg 2000;232:515–529.
4. DeMaria EJ, Sugerman HJ, Kellum JM, et al. Results of 281 consecutive total laparoscopic Roux-en-Y gastric bypasses to treat morbid obesity. Ann Surg 2002;235:640–647.
5. Higa KD, Boone KB, Ho T. Complications of the laparoscopic Roux-en-Y gastric bypass: 1040 patients—what have we learned? Obes Surg 2000;10:509–513.

6. Nguyen NT, Goldman C, Rosenquist CJ, et al. Laparoscopic versus open gastric bypass: a randomized study of outcomes, quality of life, and costs. Ann Surg 2001;234:279–291.

7. MacLean LD, Rhode BM, Nohr CW. Long-or short-limb gastric bypass? J Gastrointest Surg 2001;5:525–530.

8. Halverson JD, Koehler RE. Gastric bypass: analysis of weight loss and factors determining success. Surgery 1981; 90(3):446–455.

9. Fobi MAL, Lee H, Igwe D, et al. Revision of failed gastric bypass to distal Roux-en-Y gastric bypass: a review of 65 cases. Obes Surg 2001;11:190–195.

10. Bessler MD, Daud A, Olivero-Rivera D, DiGiorgi M. Prospective randomized double blinded trial of banded versus standard gastric bypass in patients with malignant obesity. Presented at the 21st annual meeting of the American Society for Bariatric Surgery, 2004.

11. Fobi MAL, Lee H, Igwe D, Malgorzatam S, Tambi J. Prospective Comparison of Stapled versus transected Silastic ring gastric bypass: 6-year follow-up. Obes Surg 2001;11:18–24.

12. Sapala JA, Wood MH, Sapala MA, Schuhknecht MP, Flake TM. The Micropouch gastric bypass: technical considerations in primary and revisionary operations. Obes Surg 2001; 11:3–17.

13. Hess DS, Hess DW. Biliopancreatic diversion with a duodenal switch. Obes Surg 1998;8(3):267–282.

14. Torres CJ. Why I prefer gastric bypass distal Roux-en-Y gastroileostomy. Obes Surg 1991;1:189–194.

15. Brolin RE, Kenler HA, Gorman JH, et al. Long limb gastric bypass in the superobese, a prospective randomized. Ann Surg 1992;215:387–395.

16. Brolin RE, La Marca LB, Kenler HA, et al. Malabsorptive gastric bypass in patients with superobesity. J Gastrointest Surg 2002;6:195–205.

17. Choban P, Flancbaum L. The effect of Roux limb length on outcome after Roux-en-Y gastric bypass: a randomized prospective clinical trial. Obes Surg 2002;12:540–545.

18. Livingston EH, Huerta S, Arthur D, Lee S, DeShields S, Heber D. Male gender is a predictor of morbidity and age a predictor of mortality for patients undergoing gastric bypass surgery. Ann Surg 2002;236:576–582.

19. Marceau S, Biron S, Lagace M, et al. Biliopancreatic diversion, with distal gastrectomy, 250 cm and 50 cm limbs: long-term results. Obes Surg 1995;5:302–307.

20. Johnston D, Dachtler J, Sue-Ling HM, King RF, Martin G. The Magenstrase and Mill operation for morbid obesity [see comment]. Obes Surg 2003;13(1):10–16.

21. Lee C, Cirangle PT, Feng JJ, Jossart GH. Comparison of BMI matched patients undergoing isolated laparoscopic sleeve gastrectomy versus the laparoscopic Roux-en-Y gastric bypass. Presented at the 21st annual meeting of the American Society for Bariatric Surgery, 2004.

22. Champion JK, Williams M. Small bowel obstruction and internal hernias after laparoscopic Roux-en-Y gastric bypass. Obes Surg 2003;13:596–600.

23. Felix E, Brown JE. Preventing small bowel obstruction after laparoscopic Roux-en-Y gastric bypass. Obes Surg 2002;12:197.

24. Schauer PR, Ikramuddin S, Hamad G, et al. Ante-colic versus retro-colic laparoscopic Roux-en-Y gastric bypass. Surg Endosc 2003;17:S188.

25. Schweitzer MA, DeMaria EJ, Broderick TJ, et al. Laparoscopic closure of mesenteric defects after Roux-en-Y gastric bypass. J Laproendosc Adv Surg Tech 2000;10:173–175.

26. Higa KD, Ho T, Boone KB. Internal hernias after laparoscopic Roux-en-Y gastric bypass: incidence, treatment and prevention. Obes Surg 2003;13:350–354.

27. Gonzalez R, Lin E, Venkatesh KR, et al. Gastrojejunostomy during laparoscopic gastric bypass. Arch Surg 2003; 138:181–184.

28. Liu CD, Glantz GJ, Livingston EH. Fibrin glue as a sealant for high risk anastomosis in surgery for morbid obesity. Obes Surg 2003;13:45–49.

29. Sapala JA, Wood MH. Prevention of anastomotic leaks using a vapor heated fibrin sealant: an analysis of 738 gastric bypass patients. Obes Surg 2003;13:211–212.

30. Arnold W, Shikora SA. Comparing seam burst pressure: buttressed versus non-buttressed linear cutting staple devices in a porcine model. Obes Surg 2002;12:208.

31. Shikora SA, Kim J, Tarnoff ME. Reinforcing gastric staple lines with bovine pericardial strips may decrease the likelihood of gastric leak after laparoscopic roux-en-y gastric bypass. Obes Surg 2003;13:37–44.

32. Champion JK, Hunt T, Delisle N. Role of routine intraoperative endoscopy in laparoscopic bariatric surgery. Surg Endosc 2002;16:1663–1665.

33. Ramanathan R, Ikramuddin S, Gourash W, et al. The value of intra-operative endoscopy during laparoscopic roux-en-y gastric bypass. Surg Endosc 2000;14:S212.

34. Hamilton EC, Sims TL, Hamilton TT, et al. Clinical predictors of leak after laparoscopic roux-en-y gastric bypass for morbid obesity. Surg Endosc 2003;17:679–684.

35. Hawthorne A, Kuhn J, McCarty T. The role of routine upper GI series following Roux-en-Y gastric bypass. Obes Surg 2003;13:222–223.

36. Singh R, Fisher BL. Sensitivity and specificity of post-op GI series following gastric bypass for morbid obesity. Obes Surg 2002;12:195–196.

22.1
Laparoscopic Biliopancreatic Diversion with Duodenal Switch

Ronald Matteotti and Michel Gagner

The jejunoileal bypass was the first malabsorptive procedure performed and the only available bariatric procedure in earlier times. First performed in 1953 by Varco and Kremen, it dominated the bariatric field over 20 years (1). The procedure consisted of an end-to-end jejunoileostomy with a separate ileocecostomy for drainage of the bypassed segment. Excellent weight loss was seen, but major complications such as gas-bloat syndrome, diarrhea, changes in electrolytes, impaired mental status, nephrolithiasis, eruptive integument lesions, and hepatic fibrosis and failure occurred. Because of these serious complications, this procedure was not used routinely (1).

In 1963, results of massive intestinal bypass, bypassing nearly the entire small intestine, the right ascending colon, and half of the transverse colon were published by Payne et al. (2). The series consisted of 10 morbidly obese female patients in whom the intestinal continuity was restored performing a T-shaped end-to-end anastomosis of the proximal 37.5 cm of the jejunum to the middle part of the transverse colon. The clinical pattern showed uncontrolled diarrhea, changes in electrolytes, and liver failure. Initially this procedure was designed as a two-stage operation. The primary goal was uncontrolled weight loss followed by a second operation to restore additional length of intestine once the ideal body weight was attained. However, all patients in this series gained their original weight after the second intervention (3).

In 1969 Payne and DeWind (3) deleted the radical colonic anastomosis and proposed restoring the intestinal continuity by performing an end-to-side jejunoileostomy proximal to the ileocecal junction. The primary goal of this modified procedure was to achieve a balance between caloric intake and caloric needs of the body and to avoid a second procedure to restore additional intestinal length after appropriate weight loss was seen.

In the next few years a few attempts were made to develop a less radical approach in order to avoid major complications (4,5). Payne and DeWind totally abandoned the bypass to the colon. The same surgical group published in 1969 a series of 80 morbidly obese patients in whom they anastomosed the proximal 35 cm of jejunum to the distal ileum, creating a common channel of 10 cm. This operation was designed as a one-step procedure demonstrating significant weight loss and moderate long-term side effects.

In the following years this operation was the most commonly performed procedure in the United States. This classic jejunoileal bypass was widely adopted, but nearly 10% of the patients did not lose weight as predicted, most probably due to a reflux of nutrients into the bypassed ileum (4). Therefore, to avoid this reflux of nutrients, some groups (6–8) returned to the previous described procedure of Varco and Kremen and started again to perform an end-to-end procedure, attaching the jejunal stump to the transverse colon or cecum to avoid intussusception. In all these cases, the ileocecal valve was preserved to decrease postoperative diarrhea and to avoid electrolyte loss. In the next few years different variations were done, especially variations in the length of the remaining ileum. In a series reported by Buchwald and Varco (8) in 1971, 40 cm of jejunum were anastomosed to 4 cm of ileum and the bypassed bowel was drained into the cecum. This modification produced significant weight loss; in addition, a remarkable decrease in cholesterol and triglycerides was observed. To avoid nutrient reflux, some surgical groups (9–13) tried different modifications of the jejunoileal anastomosis, such as an ileogastrostomy for drainage of the bypassed segment of intestine or shortening the proximal intestinal segment back to the ligament of Treitz. However, these procedures did not gain acceptance in larger series and were almost exclusively performed by the surgeons who developed them.

From this past experience, major lessons were learned to avoid major complications, such as that no limb of the small intestine should be left without flow through it. Therefore, modifications were performed, such as creating an alimentary limb, containing the flow of food, and creating a biliopancreatic limb, containing either bile or bile and pancreatic juice. In 1978, Lavorato et al. (14) performed a standard end-to-side jejunoileal bypass and anastomosed the proximal end of the bypassed segment of small intestine to the gallbladder with the aim of diverting the bile into the bypassed limb. In 1981, a similar operation was described but was not widely performed (15).

The modern era of malabsorptive procedures started in Italy, with Scopinaro and his group (16) performing a classical biliopancreatic diversion (BPD). They reported their first series in 1979. This procedure consisted of a horizontal distal gastrectomy with a proximal gastric pouch of approximately 200 to 500 mL, with closure of the duodenal stump, gastroileostomy with a 250-cm limb of distal ileum, and a biliopancreatic limb anastomosed to the distal ileum, 50 cm proximal to the ileocecal valve, creating an extremely short common channel. In 1993, this prototype of a BPD was modified by Marceau et al. (17) to a duodenal switch. They created a lesser curvature tube with a greater curvature gastric resection, preserved the pylorus, anastomosed the enteric limb to the proximal duodenum, and cross-stapled the duodenum distally without dividing it. However, these patients showed disruption of this staple line, because the duodenum does not tolerate cross-stapling.

In 1998 Hess and Hess (18) modified this procedure, anastomosing the enteric limb to the postpyloric duodenum after dividing the duodenum distal to the pylorus and closing this distal duodenal stump. This procedure is called the biliopancreatic diversion with the duodenal switch (BPD-DS) and is rapidly gaining worldwide acceptance. Following the creation of this modern malabsorptive procedure, a major innovation was performing this procedure laparoscopically thus combining this operation with all the benefits of a laparoscopic approach. This was first done by Gagner in early July 1999, and it was published in 2001 (19).

Technique

Several steps are included in this procedure. As a first step, the duodenum is divided distal to the pylorus, followed by a pylorus-preserving sleeve gastrectomy. In the next step, a duodenoenterostomy, the alimentary limb is created. The common channel is now measured and the biliopancreatic limb anastomosed to the distal ileum.

Operative Setup

All patients undergo general anesthesia and endotracheal intubation. The patient wears pneumatic compression boots (20,21) and is placed in the French position, with legs abducted and the surgeon standing between the legs. Two monitors are used, one on each side of the patient's head. Usually the procedure is done with two assistants, one on either side (Fig. 22.1-1). Using an open technique, the peritoneal cavity is entered at the umbilicus and pneumoperitoneum is attained with 15 mm Hg of CO_2. A combination of 5-, 10-, and 12-mm trocars are needed for each procedure. Usually seven trocars are enough but up to nine can be used.

Division of the Duodenum and Sleeve Gastrectomy

A self-retraining liver retractor is inserted to better expose the greater curve of the stomach, and dissection is done with 5-mm harmonic shears (Ethicon, New Brunswick, NJ). Using an angled endoscope (10 mm, 30 to 45 degrees) greatly facilitates the exposure of the angle of His. A linear stapler, 45 mm/3.5 mm (Tyco, U.S. Surgical Corp., Norwalk, CT) is used to divide the duodenum, usually 2 cm distal to the pylorus. A 60-French bougie is passed into the stomach and aligned along the lesser curvature.

Sequential stapler firings along this inserted bougie are then used to create a sleeve gastrectomy (Fig. 22.1-2). The staplers used in this part of the operation are 60 mm/ 4.8 mm, covered with bioabsorbable Seamguard (W.L. Gore & Associates, Medical Products Division, 3750 West Kiltie Lane, Flagstaff, AZ) to prevent bleeding and to diminish the rate of leakage. The remaining gastric pouch usually measures approximately 150 to 200 mL.

Creation of a Duodenoenterostomy: The Alimentary Limb

The remaining gastric pouch is anastomosed to the distal 250 cm of divided ileum to perform the alimentary limb. No biliopancreatic secretion runs through this part of the intestine. This anastomosis is performed with a linear stapler, a 2-cm circular stapler, or a hand-sewn technique. The anastomosis itself is placed antecolic. If a linear stapler approach is used, great care must be taken to open the duodenum with the harmonic scalpel posterior to the stapler line, so that the entire staple line can be incorporated in the following running silk 2-0 suture closure. If a circular stapler is used, then an anvil of a 25-mm circular end-to-end anastomosis stapler (CEEA, U.S. Surgical Corp.) is placed into the proximal duodenal stump using a purse-string suture of 3-0 Prolene. Alternatively, the anvil can be sutured into the cut end of a nasogastric tube and delivered transorally through an opening in the duodenum (Fig. 22.1-3). The circular stapler itself is brought in transabdominally, advancing it into the lumen of the distal ileum and attaching it to the anvil previously placed in the duodenal stump (Fig. 22.1-4). The remaining defect is closed using a running silk 2-0 suture. To remove the

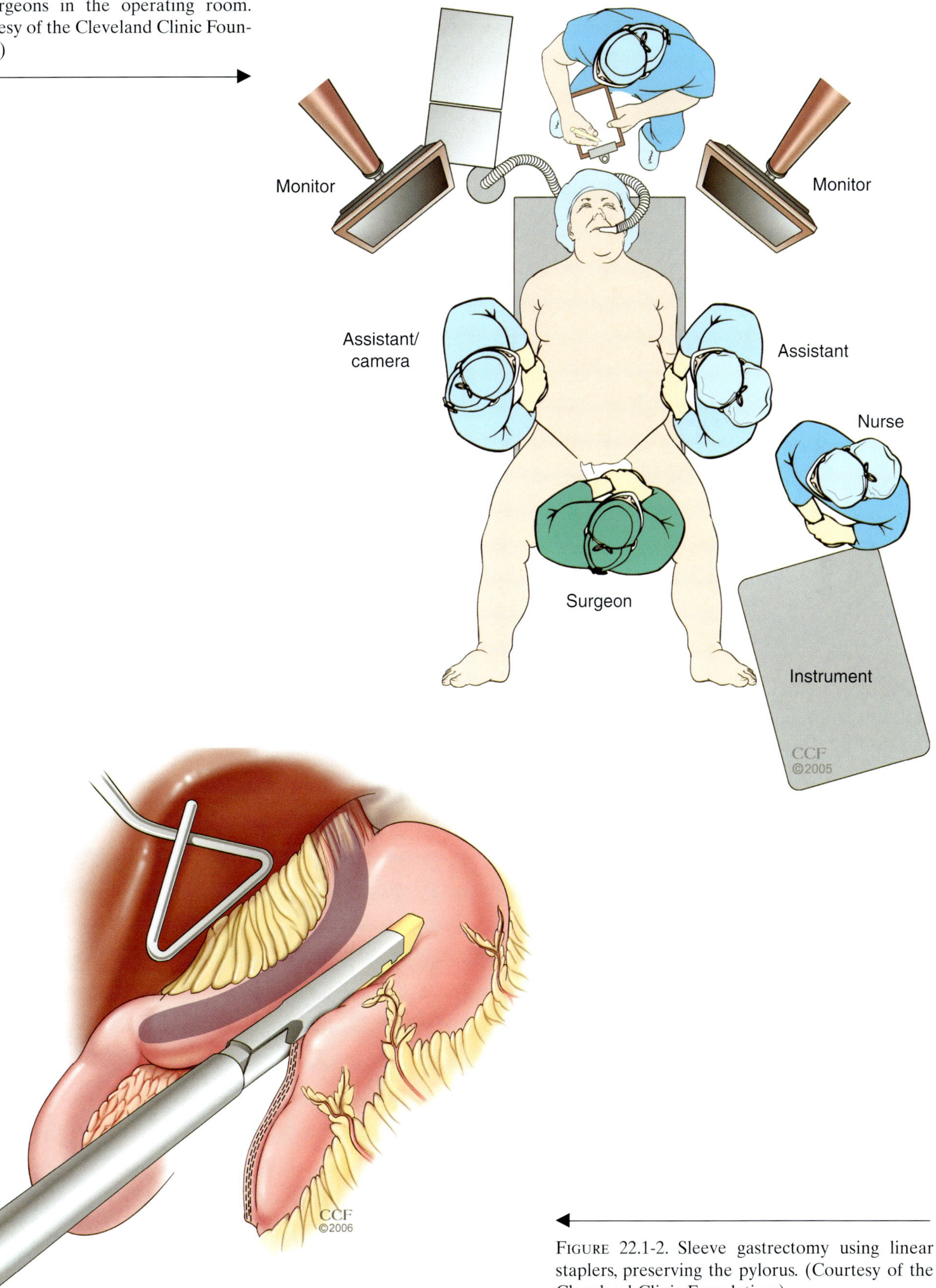

FIGURE 22.1-1. Setup and positioning of the surgeons in the operating room. (Courtesy of the Cleveland Clinic Foundation.)

FIGURE 22.1-2. Sleeve gastrectomy using linear staplers, preserving the pylorus. (Courtesy of the Cleveland Clinic Foundation.)

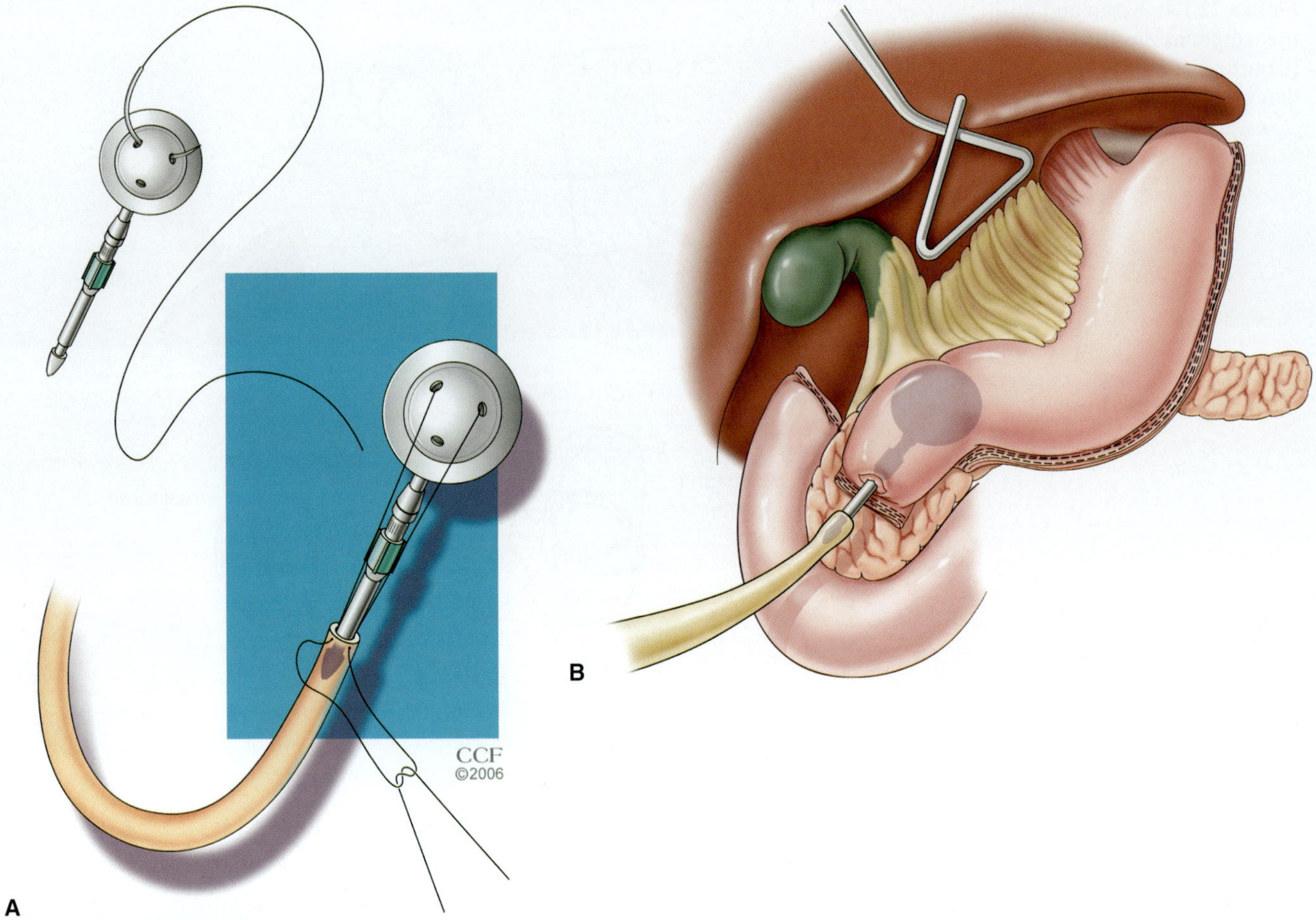

FIGURE 22.1-3. Transoral placement of the end-to-end anastomosis (EEA) circular stapler anvil through the duodenum. (A) The anvil is prepared by connecting it to an 18-French nasogastric tube and securing it with a Prolene suture in the flexed position. (B) After passing the nasogastric tube through the gastric sleeve, the shaft of the anvil is pulled through a small duodenotomy. (Courtesy of the Cleveland Clinic Foundation.)

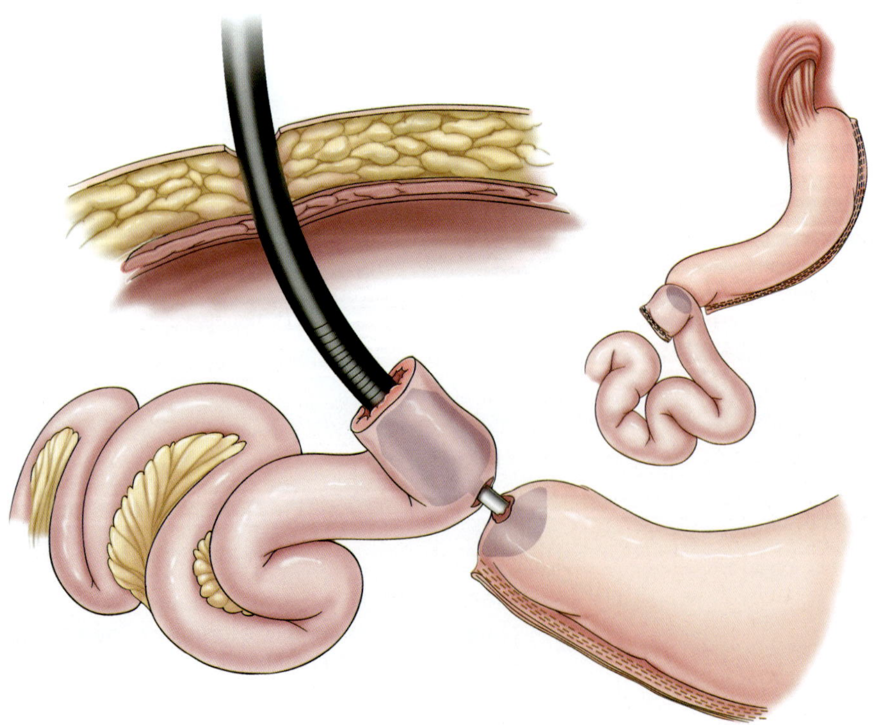

FIGURE 22.1-4. Formation of the duodenoileostomy using a circular stapler. (Courtesy of the Cleveland Clinic Foundation.)

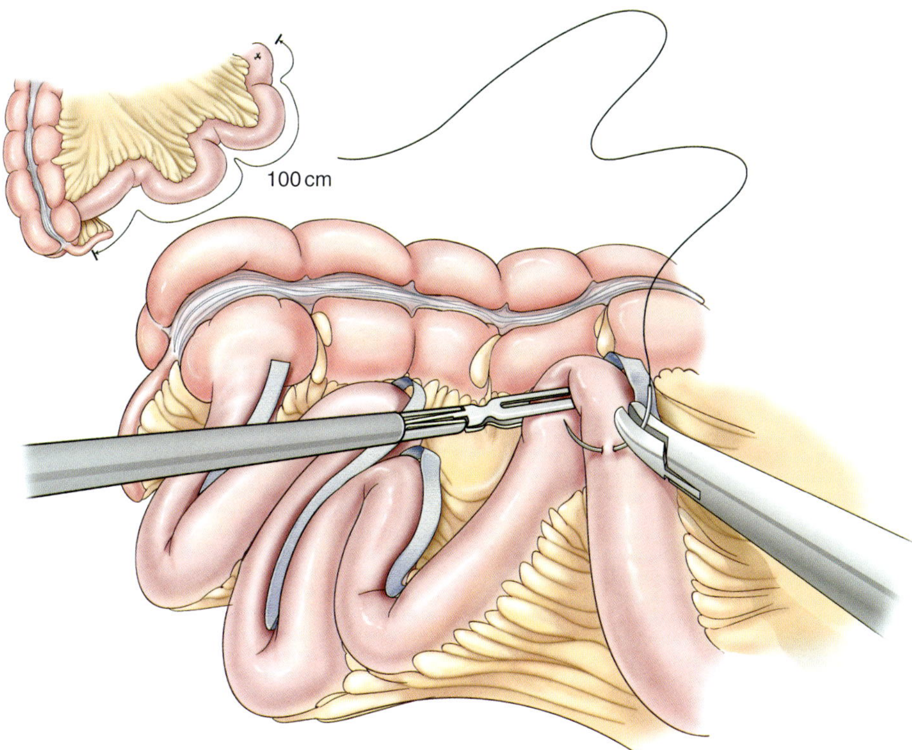

FIGURE 22.1-5. The 100-cm common channel is measured back from the ileocecal valve and marked with a stitch. (Courtesy of the Cleveland Clinic Foundation.)

contaminated device, a camera drape secured around the circular stapler is used as a wound protector. A methylene blue test is performed to assess the integrity of this anastomotic site. The size of the gastric pouch is approximated by the volume of methylene blue required to distend the pouch. Some surgical groups use a total hand-sewn technique to perform this proximal anastomosis (22).

Measurement of the Common Channel

The common channel is measured under medium stretch, after identifying the ileocecal junction using a flexible cotton band and defined as 100 cm long. A single silk 2-0 suture is placed at this location to mark its beginning (Fig. 22.1-5).

Distal Ileoenteric Anastomosis: The Biliopancreatic Limb

The biliopancreatic limb is totally excluded from digestive continuity, bypassing the duodenum, jejunum, and proximal ileum. This anastomosis is done using linear staplers (Fig. 22.1-6), oversewing the remaining defect with a running silk 2-0 suture (Fig. 22.1-7). The small bowel mesentery and mesocolon is closed as well with a running 2-0 silk suture. This space is usually referred to as Petersen's space. After this step, the gastric specimen, previously placed in the left upper quadrant, is removed using a nonpermeable retrieval bag through one of the trocar sites, which usually has to be slightly enlarged. Fascial closure of all trocar sites >5 mm is done using a suture-passing device. A cholecystectomy is performed only when stones or sludge are present. The completed procedure (Fig. 22.1-8) shows an alimentary limb of 150 cm and a common channel of 100 cm.

Postoperative Care

On the first postoperative day a water-soluble (Gastrografin) upper gastrointestinal contrast study is performed selectively. The patient is allowed to have clear liquids and oral analgesics, and the feeding regimen is continued with a pureed diet on the second postoperative day. Follow-up appointments are scheduled for 3 weeks, 3 months, 6 months, 12 months, and annually thereafter. All patients receive follow-up nutritional counseling for a protein-enriched diet (80 to 100 g/day), and multivitamins, oral calcium supplements (500 mg/day), iron, and fat-soluble vitamins (D, E, A, and K) are given on a daily basis. If the gallbladder is still in place, the patient is prescribed ursodiol (Actigall, Ciba-Geigy, Summit, NJ) 300 mg twice a day for gallstone prophylaxis. Beginning at 3

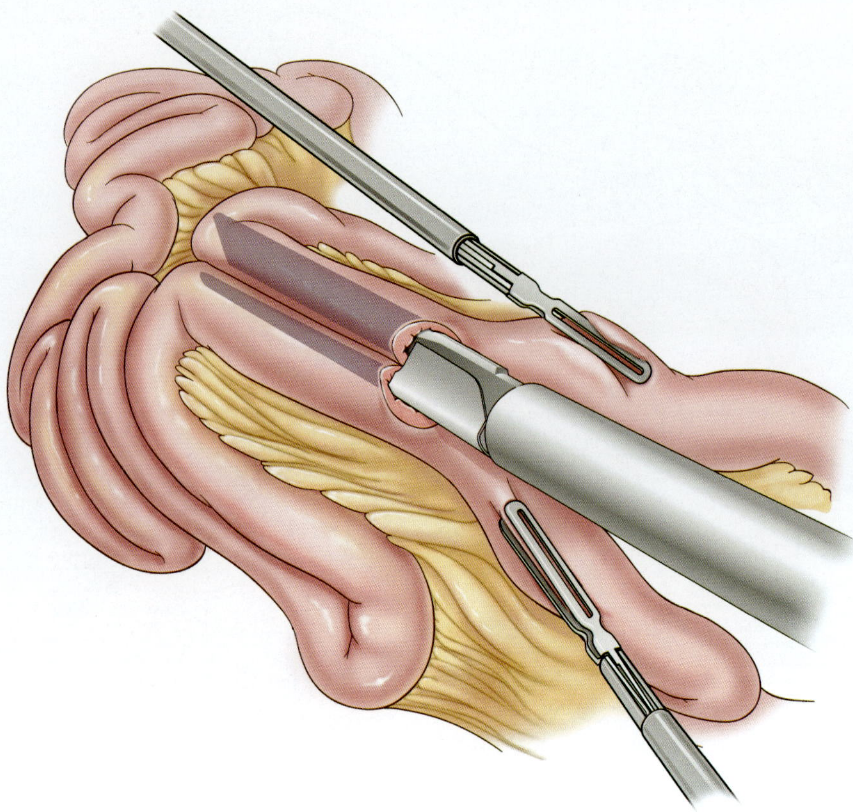

Figure 22.1-6. Ileoileostomy side-to-side, functional end-to-end anastomosis using a linear stapler. (Courtesy of the Cleveland Clinic Foundation.)

months, laboratory evaluation for nutritional deficiencies is performed at each visit, including iron, ferritin, B_{12}, folate, albumin, parathyroid hormone (PTH), calcium, phosphorus, alkaline phosphatase, zinc, selenium, lipid profile, triglycerides, electrolytes, complete blood count, vitamin D, and vitamin A. Patients are encouraged to join a monthly support group that may include a surgeon, nutritionist, clinical nurse coordinator, and social worker.

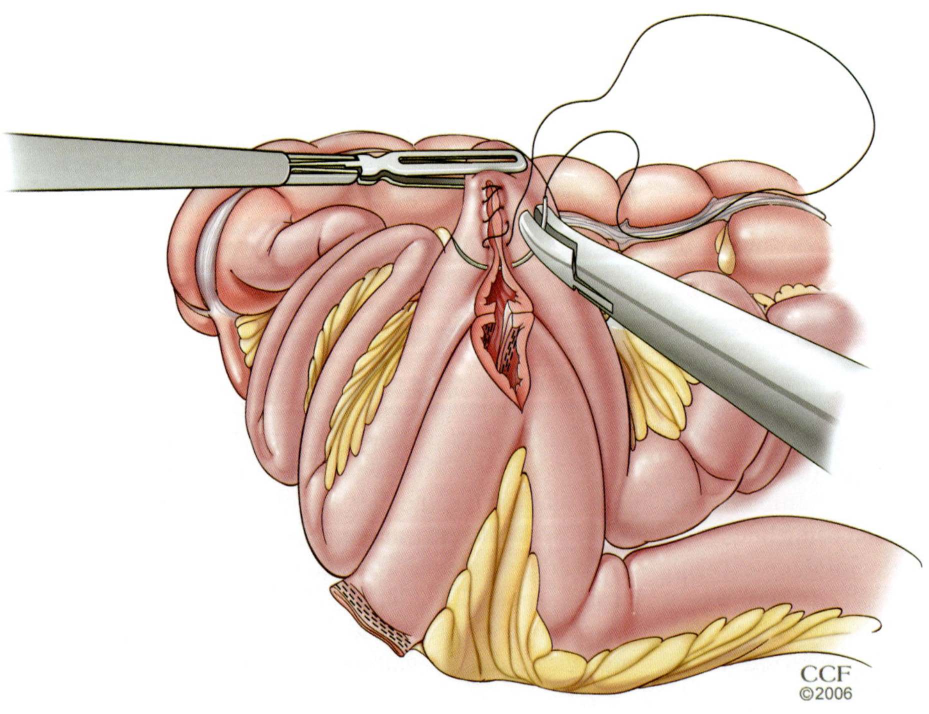

Figure 22.1-7. The common enterotomy at the small bowel anastomosis is closed using the hand-sewn technique. (Courtesy of the Cleveland Clinic Foundation.)

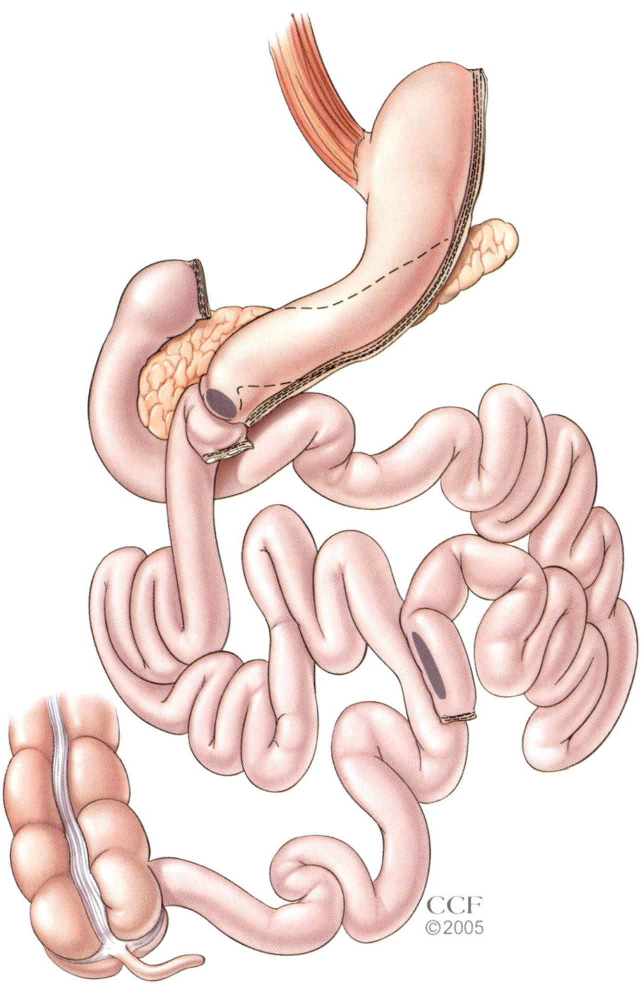

FIGURE 22.1-8. The completed procedure. (Courtesy of the Cleveland Clinic Foundation.)

Results and Other Approaches

Results of the latest series published in the literature are reported in Tables 22.1-1, 22.1-2, and 22.1-3. Following modern malabsorptive procedures in 1979 by Scopinaro and his group (16), and abandoning the jejunoileal bypass with all its sometimes fatal consequences, a major innovation led to the now performed biliopancreatic diversion with duodenal switch.

Food intake is restricted from a sleeve gastrectomy and food absorption decreased from a biliopancreatic limb. This was first done by Marceau et al. (17) in 1993 and was later modified to its definitive technique by Hess and Hess (18) in 1998. The key point in this final modification was dividing the proximal duodenum with closure of the duodenal stump, not just cross-stapling it, which was not well tolerated by patients. This operation, called the duodenal switch, preserves the antropyloric pump and leaves the vagal innervation undisturbed, and the sleeve gastrectomy itself minimizes the ulcerogenicity of the duodenal switch by reducing the parietal cell mass (23).

After years of performing BPD the open way, mostly done in Italy by Scopinaro, a logical next step was performing this technically challenging operation laparoscopically. The primary goal was not only to demonstrate its technical feasibility but also to add all benefits of a laparoscopic approach to this high-risk patient group, and to minimize wound and cardiopulmonary complications. In 2001 de Csepel et al. (19) published for the first time the feasibility of using a laparoscopic approach to perform a BPD-DS in a porcine model, and after positive results started to use this procedure as well in humans. Only a few surgical groups now perform this operation laparoscopically (20,22,24–30). These procedures are complex and technically difficult to perform (23,24). All studies (Table 22.1-1) are retrospective and no prospec-

TABLE 22.1-1. Laparoscopic biliopancreatic diversion (BPD) or duodenal switch (DS): patient characteristics

Author	Year of publication	Study type	Patients (n)	Age	Female (%)	BMI (preop)	Comorbidities (%)
Gagner et al. (20)	2000	Retrospective	40	43	70	60	75
Paiva et al. (24)	2002	Retrospective	40	39	72	43.6	95
Scopinaro et al. (25)	2002	Retrospective	26	36	73	43	NR
Baltasar et al. (22)	2002	Retrospective	16	36.5	16	>40	NR
Rabkin et al. (26)*	2003	Retrospective	345	43	86.6	50	NR
Dolan and Fielding (27)	2004	Retrospective	38[a]	42[a]	93.7	37[a]	NR
			21[b]	41[b]		34[b]	NR
Resa et al. (28)	2004	Retrospective	65	45.3	69.2	48.4	100
Slater and Fielding (29)	2004	Retrospective	11	45	81.8	45.3	NR
Weiner et al. (30)	2004	Retrospective	63	40.2	88.8	55.8	[x]
Total/mean	—	—	685	41.1	72.3	45.7	—

NR, not recorded.

[a] BPD.

[b] DS.

* Hand-assisted series.

[x] Existent, but no overall reported.

TABLE 22.1-2 Laparoscopic BPD or DS: operative data

Study	Operation type: BPD or DS	Conversion (%)	Operation time (min)	Upper anastomosis circular/linear/hand-sewn	Pouch (mL)	Reop (%)	App.	Cho.	Liver biopsy
Gagner et al. (20)	DS	2.5	210	Circular	175	7.5	NR	No	NR
Paiva et al. (24)	BPD	0	210	Linear (circular)	350	0	NR	Yes	NR
Scopinaro et al. (25)	BPD	26	240	Linear (circular)	300	NR	NR	NR	NR
Baltasar et al. (22)	DS	NR	232	Hand-sewn (circular)	NR	12.5	NR	NR	NR
Rabkin et al. (26)*	DS	2	201	Circular	124	4	Yes	Yes	Yes
Dolan and Fielding (27)	BPD DS	3.3	NR	NR	NR	13.5	NR	NR	NR
Resa et al. (28)	BPD	4.6	176	Linear	200	3	NR	NR	NR
Slater and Fielding (29)	DS	36.3	51	Linear	**	NR	NR	NR	NR
Weiner et al. (30)	DS	0	207	Circular Linear Hand-sewn	NR	5.8	Yes	Yes	NR
Total/mean		9.3	190.8	—	229.8	6.6	—	—	—

NR, not recorded; App., appendectomy; Cho., cholecystectomy.
[a] BPD.
[b] DS.
* Hand-assisted series.
** No pouch created; revision operation with Lap-Band® in situ.

tive randomized study is available that compares laparoscopic gastric bypass and BPD or BPD-DS.

The literature to date reports a total of 685 patients, and a little more than half, exactly 345, were performed using a hand-assisted technique (26). This approach is likely to be abandoned for a complete laparoscopic approach, as performed by Gagner and his group. The mean age in all these studies is 41.1 years, and 72.3% are female. The preoperative mean body mass index was 45.7. Four of these nine studies reported a high percentage of associated comorbidities, such as hypertension, diabetes mellitus, degenerative joint disease, and sleep apnea (20,24). If we look at the operative data (Table 22.1-2), there is heterogeneity as well. Two groups (24,25) perform a BPD using a classical distal gastrectomy instead of preserving the pylorus, which is a main goal of DS (20,22,26). The conversion rate varies widely and is highest in the series of Slater and Fielding (29), with 26%, whereas a mean of 9.3% is reported. This high conversion rate in the series of Slater and Fielding is due to a small number of patients in their cohort and due to the fact that all their operations were revisions after failed primary bariatric surgery.

If we look at the proximal anastomosis, there is a wide range of technical possibilities. While Gagner and his group proposed using a 25-mm circular stapler in their first cases and now use a 21-mm stapler (CEEA, U.S. Surgical Corp.) to perform the proximal anastomosis, other groups are performing the gastro- or duodenoileostomy using linear staplers or even a hand-sewn technique. They switched to the linear stapler performance after initial experience with the circular stapler, which entailed technical difficulties in introducing the 25-mm CEEA into the ileal stump or had a high rate of stenosis (25). The 21-mm CEEA is now preferred. Note that performance of this technically challenging anastomosis is highly correlated

TABLE 22.1-3 Laparoscopic BPD or DS: follow-up data

Study	Follow-up (months)	LOS (days)	Complications, early (%)	Deaths (%)	EWL (%)
Gagner et al. (20)	9	4	15	5	58
Paiva et al. (24)	NR	4.3	12.5	2.5	NR
Scopinaro et al. (25)	12	NR	NR	0	68
Baltasar et al. (22)	NR	5.8	NR	0	NR
Rabkin et al. (26)*	24	3	2.6	0	91
Dolan and Fielding (27)	36[a]	5[a]	11.9	0	38[a]
	12[b]	6[b]			28[b]
Resa et al. (28)	36	7.8	12.3	0.65	81.82
Slater and Fielding (29)	6	2.5	NR	0	**
Weiner et al. (30)	12	6.5	10	NR	NR
Total/mean	18.3	5	10.7	1	60.8

NR, not recorded; LOS, length of stay; EWL, excessive weight loss.
[a] BPD.
[b] DS.
* Hand-assisted series.
** Body mass index <30.

with the experience of the surgeon. Some groups change their technique over time based on their level of experience and on the complications they encountered. This is very well demonstrated in the series of Dolan and Fielding (27), who performed a circular anastomosis, a linear stapled one in combination with oversewing the front part, or a total hand-sewn technique.

Another point that is not sufficiently addressed in the literature is the performance of a cholecystectomy to prevent gallstones, to remove the appendix, and to take a liver biopsy to assess the initial damage of this organ. If we look at the reports available, only Paiva et al. (24), Rabkin et al. (26), and Weiner et al. (30) are performing a cholecystectomy routinely, while Rabkin et al. and Weiner et al. remove the appendix as well but only Rabkin et al. takes a liver biopsy.

Looking at the postoperative course of these patients (Table 22.1-3) we see a mean excessive weight loss of 60.8% during a mean follow-up of 18.3 months. Rabkin et al. (26) reports in their series, during a follow-up of 24 months, a mean excessive weight loss of 91%. The mean excessive weight loss is lowest in the series of Dolan and Fielding (27), which could give a wrong impression about the effectiveness of this procedure. They experienced in their group a weight loss of 38% in patients undergoing a BPD and 28% in patients undergoing a DS. This cohort consisted of patients after failed laparoscopic adjustable gastric banding. The mean reoperation rate of 6.6% is acceptable, and the early complication rate of 10.7% is in the range for these high-risk patients. The mean length of hospital stay using a laparoscopic approach is 5 days, compared to a minimum of 5 days in a larger series of 701 patients using the open procedure (31). The overall mortality was only reported by three groups as 5%, 2.5%, and 0.65% (20,28,32).

Conclusion

These preliminary results demonstrate the technical feasibility of this procedure, especially knowing that it is typically used for the super-obese population, which is at higher risk than the normal obese population. Future studies with a larger number of patients should be able to demonstrate the effectiveness of this procedure in reducing weight and reducing the resumption of comorbidities such as hyperlipidemia, sleep apnea, hypertension, and diabetes mellitus. We recommend using a laparoscopic approach to perform this procedure to minimize local and systemic complications in these high-risk patients. In the series of Dolan and Fielding (27) and Slater and Fielding (29) we see an interesting trend for the future, and it seems that performing a BPD or BPD-DS has the potential to serve as "the bariatric solution" to failed weight-loss surgery of any kind.

References

1. Buchwald H, Rucker RD. The rise and fall of jejunoileal bypass. Norwalk, CT: Appleton Century Croft, 1987.
2. Payne JH, DeWind LT, Commons RR. Metabolic observations in patients with jejunocolic shunts. Am J Surg 1986; 106:272-289.
3. Payne JH, DeWind LT. Surgical treatment of obesity. Am J Surg 1969;118(2):141–147.
4. Deitel M. Jejunocolic and jejunoileal bypass: an historical perspective. In: Deitel M, ed. Surgery for the Morbidly Obese Patient. Philadelphia: Lea & Febiger, 1998:81–89.
5. Lewis LA, Turnbull RB Jr, Page IH. Effects of jejunocolic shunt on obesity, serum lipoproteins, lipids, and electrolytes. Arch Intern Med 1966;117(1):4–16.
6. Scott HW Jr, Sandstead HH, Brill AB, Burko H, Younger RK. Experience with a new technic of intestinal bypass in the treatment of morbid obesity. Ann Surg 1971;174(4):560–572.
7. Salmon PA. The results of small intestine bypass operations for the treatment of obesity. Surg Gynecol Obstet 1971; 132(6):965–979.
8. Buchwald H, Varco RL. A bypass operation for obese hyperlipidemic patients. Surgery 1971;70(1):62–70.
9. Palmer JA. The present status of surgical operation for obesity. In: Deitel M, ed. Nutrition in Clinical Surgery. Baltimore: Williams & Wilkins, 1980:281–292.
10. Kral JG. Duodenoileal bypass. In: Deitel M, ed. Surgery for the Morbidly Obese Patient. Philadelphia: Lea & Febiger, 1998:99–103.
11. Cleator IG, Gourlay RH. Ileogastrostomy for morbid obesity. Can J Surg 1988;31(2):114–116.
12. Forestierie P, DeLuca L, Bucci L. Surgical treatment of high degree obesity. Our own criteria to choose the appropriate type of jejuno-ileal bypass: a modified Payne technique. Chir Gastroenterol 1977;11:401–408.
13. Starkloff GB, Stothert JC, Sundaram M. Intestinal bypass: a modification. Ann Surg 1978;188(5):697–700.
14. Lavorato F, Doldi SB, Scaramella R. Evoluzione storica della terapia chirurgica della grande obesita. Minerva Med 1978;69:3847–3857.
15. Eriksson F. Biliointestinal bypass. Int J Obes 1981;5(4): 437–447.
16. Scopinaro N, Gianetta E, Civalleri D, Bonalumi U, Bachi V. Bilio-pancreatic bypass for obesity: II. Initial experience in man. Br J Surg 1979;66(9):618–620.
17. Marceau P, Biron S, Bourque RA, Potvin M, Hould FS, Simard S. Biliopancreatic diversion with a new type of gastrectomy. Obes Surg 1993;3(1):29–35.
18. Hess DS, Hess DW. Biliopancreatic diversion with a duodenal switch. Obes Surg 1998;8:267–282.
19. de Csepel J, Burpee S, Jossart G, et al. Laparoscopic biliopancreatic diversion with a duodenal switch for morbid obesity: a feasibility study in pigs. J Laparoendosc Adv Surg Tech A 2001;11(2):79–83.
20. Ren CJ, Patterson E, Gagner M. Early results of laparoscopic biliopancreatic diversion with duodenal switch: a case series of 40 consecutive patients. Obes Surg 2000;10(6):514–523; discussion 524.

21. Kim WW, Gagner M, Kini S, et al. Laparoscopic vs. open biliopancreatic diversion with duodenal switch: a comparative study. J Gastrointest Surg 2003;7(4):552–557.
22. Baltasar A, Bou R, Miro J, Bengochea M, Serra C, Perez N. Laparoscopic biliopancreatic diversion with duodenal switch: technique and initial experience. Obes Surg 2002; 12(2):245–248.
23. Marceau P, Hould FS, Simard S, et al. Biliopancreatic diversion with duodenal switch. World J Surg 1998;22(9):947–954.
24. Paiva D, Bernardes L, Suretti L. Laparoscopic biliopancreatic diversion: technique and initial results. Obes Surg 2002;12(3):358–361.
25. Scopinaro N, Marinari GM, Camerini G. Laparoscopic standard biliopancreatic diversion: technique and preliminary results. Obes Surg 2002;12(3):362–365.
26. Rabkin RA, Rabkin JM, Metcalf B, Lazo M, Rossi M, Lehmanbecker LB. Laparoscopic technique for performing duodenal switch with gastric reduction. Obes Surg 2003; 13(2):263–268.
27. Dolan K, Fielding G. Bilio pancreatic diversion following failure of laparoscopic adjustable gastric banding. Surg Endosc 2004;18(1):60–63.
28. Resa JJ, Solano J, Fatas JA, et al. Laparoscopic biliopancreatic diversion: technical aspects and results of our protocol. Obes Surg 2004;14(3):329–333; discussion 333.
29. Slater GH, Fielding GA. Combining laparoscopic adjustable gastric banding and biliopancreatic diversion after failed bariatric surgery. Obes Surg 2004;14(5):677–682.
30. Weiner RA, Blanco-Engert R, Weiner S, Pomhoff I, Schramm M. Laparoscopic biliopancreatic diversion with duodenal switch: three different duodeno-ileal anastomotic techniques and initial experience. Obes Surg 2004;14(3): 334–340.
31. Anthone GJ, Lord RV, DeMeester TR, Crookes PF. The duodenal switch operation for the treatment of morbid obesity. Ann Surg 2003;238(4):618–627; discussion 627–628.
32. Paiva D, Bernardes L, Suretti L. Laparoscopic biliopancreatic diversion for the treatment of morbid obesity: initial experience. Obes Surg 2001;11(5):619–622.

22.2
Laparoscopic Malabsorption Procedures: The Technique of Biliopancreatic Diversion

George A. Fielding

Scopinaro's lifelong commitment to biliopancreatic diversion (BPD) has demonstrated its effectiveness as a tool offering sustained weight loss (1). Scopinaro's initial technique really has not changed much since the 1970s. The procedure offers a two-pronged attack: initial restriction and then maintenance by malabsorption (2). Benefits derived from laparoscopic techniques applied to abdominal procedures relate to elimination of wound complications, namely pain and suffering, and delayed complications from the incision itself. The greatest benefit has come in those procedures where the morbidity was almost entirely related to the wound, particularly cholecystectomy, fundoplication, and splenectomy in the upper abdomen and inguinal hernia and colectomy in the lower abdomen (3–6).

Bariatric surgery has a foot in both camps. The size of the wound in our patients has implications for infection, the incidence of pneumonic complications, and the very high rate of incisional hernia (7,8). However, the most feared complication is intestinal leak. This has not been eliminated by laparoscopic techniques. In fact, they were increased for a time until the techniques were mastered in obese patients. Due to the sometimes formidable technical challenge of making a Roux loop, and then bringing it high in the abdomen to the esophagogastric angle, various methods have evolved to form that anastomosis. These include circular stapler, side-to-side stapling, and hand sewn (9–12).

Both open and laparoscopic BPD is performed much less frequently than laparoscopic Roux-en-Y bypass. However, the same principles apply to BPD. During the 1990s it became evident that the safest and most effective way to perform advanced laparoscopic procedures was to replicate the open procedure that has stood the test of time. The operation described here replicates open BPD as described by Scopinaro et al. (13).

Procedure

This procedure is performed with the surgeon standing at the side of the patient (Fig. 22.2-1). Upper abdominal laparoscopic surgery in Europe started with the surgeon standing between the patient's legs with a central camera and the surgeon operating with hands to either side of the camera. The same exposure can be gained with the legs flat and together. It is a simpler setup, less stressful to the patient, reduces the risk of deep vein thrombosis, and is much easier for nursing and ancillary staff in the operating room. There is no need to insert a Foley catheter as one is operating in the upper abdomen. Catheterization of morbidly obese patients can be a technical challenge in itself, and confers no conceivable benefit. The Nathanson Liver Retractor (Cook), a fixed retractor inserted through a subxiphoid port and attached to the table, is the most effective means of liver retraction. It does not require an assistant, does not move, does not tear the liver, and greatly facilitates the view in the upper abdomen. Ports are introduced toward the right iliac fossa for the development of the Roux limb and then removed and reinserted through the same skin incision to point to the upper abdomen for the gastric part of the procedure. Where possible, muscle spreading ports such as the Optiview (Ethicon, New Brunswick, NJ) should be used to reduce the size of the port incision, so that port hole suturing is unnecessary. Cholecystectomy is not performed. If the patient develops biliary colic at a later date, laparoscopic cholecystectomy is performed in a much slimmer patient with a much smaller liver.

Pneumoperitoneum is achieved using an Optiview (Ethicon) inserted laterally in the left subcostal region, the thinnest part of the abdominal wall in the morbidly obese patient. This eliminates tedious dissection at the umbilicus, or the inherent danger that exists with a Veress

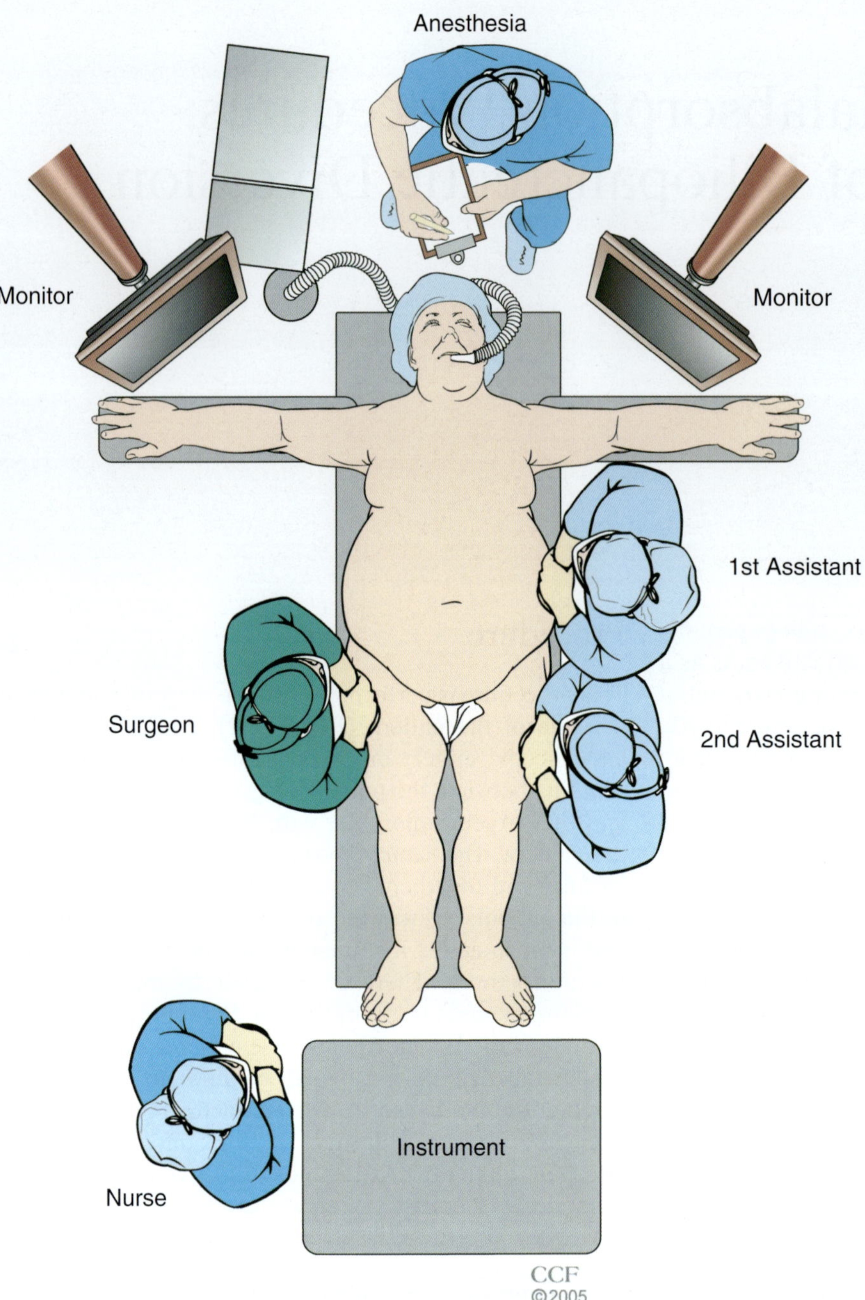

FIGURE 22.2-1. Positioning of surgeon and assistants for biliopancreatic diversion. (Courtesy of the Cleveland Clinic Foundation.)

needle. The great benefit is that at the end of the procedure it leaves only a 4- to 5-mm defect that does not require suturing. Lateral positioning under the left subcostal region gives great vision of the greater curvature of the stomach. It is also an excellent position to give a broad view of the right iliac fossa, with the hands then able to be placed on either side for mobilization and creation of the Roux limb.

Trocar Positions

Port placement is shown in Figure 22.2-2. Trocar 1 is the insufflation Optiview port in the left subcostal region, lat-erally. Trocar 2 is in the left iliac fossa, midway between the umbilicus and the anterior/superior iliac spine. This trocar assists in creation of the Roux limb. Trocar 3 is a subxiphoid, 5-mm entry point for the Nathanson liver retractor. Trocar 4 is in the midline, midway between the xyphoid and the umbilicus. First, this serves to create the Roux limb and second, when turned the other way, this is an excellent position when one is performing the anastomosis to the stomach. Trocar 5 is in the right subcostal region, toward the midaxillary line. A 12-mm Optiview is initially used for the stapling of the Roux limb and then turned, cephalad, to be used to divide the duodenum. An optional sixth port can be used between

Creation of Biliopancreatic Diversion

The telescope is placed in the left subcostal port. A 50-cm tape and a 6-inch 3-0 PDS polydioxanone suture are inserted into the abdomen and left lying in the right upper quadrant on the ascending colon.

The ileocecal junction is identified, cecal adhesions are divided using the harmonic shears through the midline port, and the caecum is mobilized. This is particularly beneficial in the super-obese male patient when there is often difficulty bringing a distally based Roux limb to the stomach.

The measuring tape measures 50 cm along the terminal ileum, which is then marked with a suture, and then a further 200 cm (Fig. 22.2-3). At this second point, the bowel is stretched between two bowel graspers, and the linear 60 mm stapler with a white cartridge is fired directly across the intestine and down onto the mesentery. A second firing of the white 60-mm cartridge is applied across the mesentery.

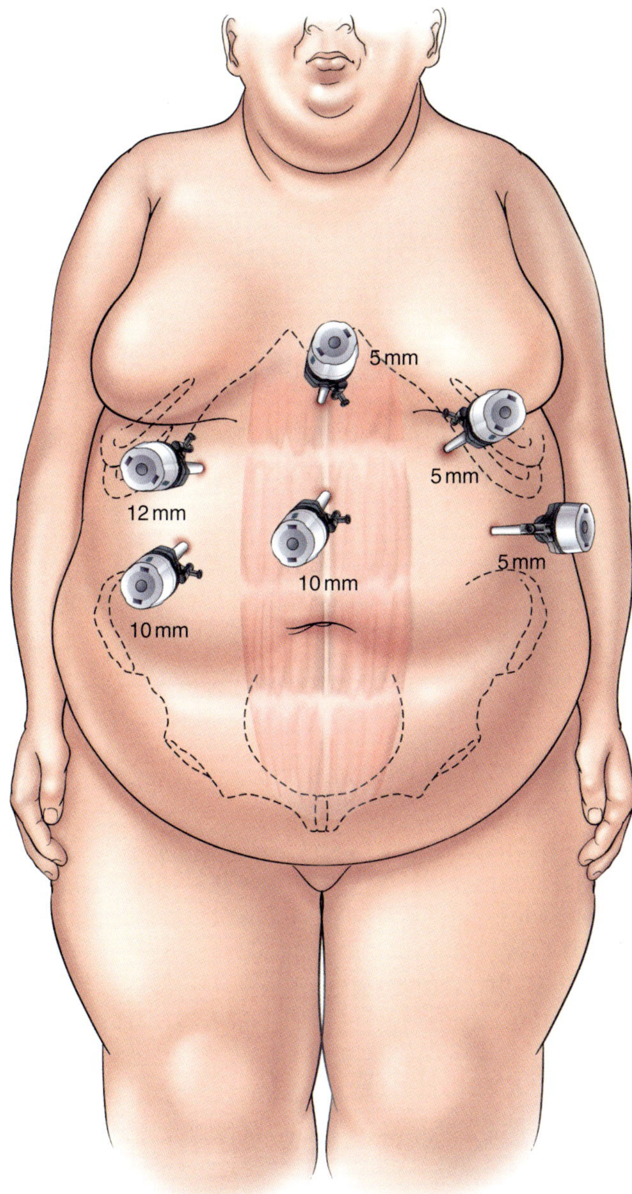

FIGURE 22.2-2. Trocar positions for laparoscopic biliopancreatic diversion. (Courtesy of the Cleveland Clinic Foundation.)

trocars 4 and 5, at a slightly lower level. This is sometimes required to dissect the duodenum, if it is more difficult to lift off the pancreas.

The standard Scopinaro biliopancreatic diversion is performed by this laparoscopic technique—distal gastrectomy to create a 250-mL stomach, which is then anastomosed to a 200-cm alimentary limb, joining a 50-cm common channel.

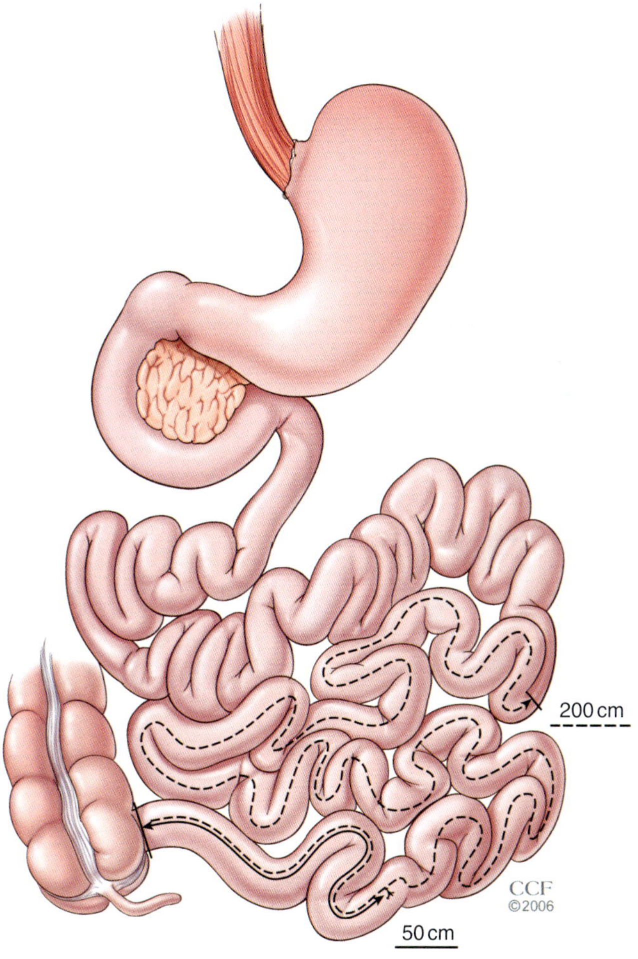

FIGURE 22.2-3. Measurements for the common channel (50 cm from the ileocecal valve) and division of the small bowel (200 cm from the ileocecal valve). (Courtesy of the Cleveland Clinic Foundation.)

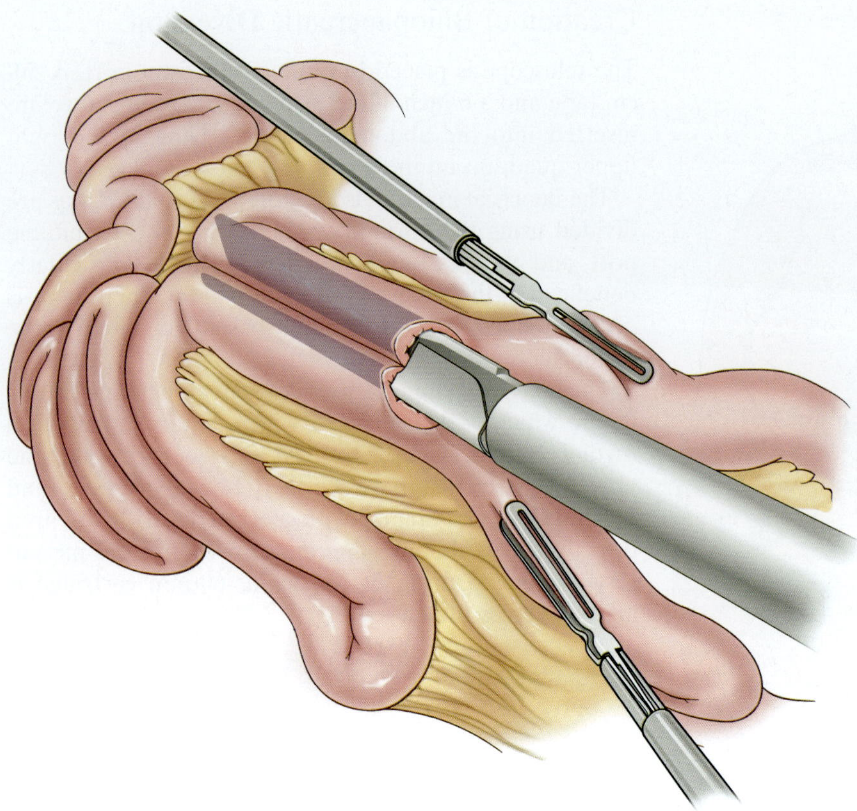

FIGURE 22.2-4. Stapled side-to-side small bowel anastomosis 50cm from the ileocecal valve. (Courtesy of the Cleveland Clinic Foundation.)

The proximal end of the division is then brought down to the marked point at 50cm. Correct orientation of the bowel is confirmed, as it is surprisingly easy to have the bowel twisted or to be bringing the wrong end down. Failure to check can result in the creation of a Roux-en-O—a potential catastrophe (14) The linear stapler, using a white cartridge, makes a side-to-side anastomosis (Fig. 22.2-4). The staple defect is hand-sewn using 3–0 PDS in a continuous fashion (Fig. 22.2-5). The apex of the staple line is oversewn. The mesentery defect is sutured with a continuous 3-0 PDS suture.

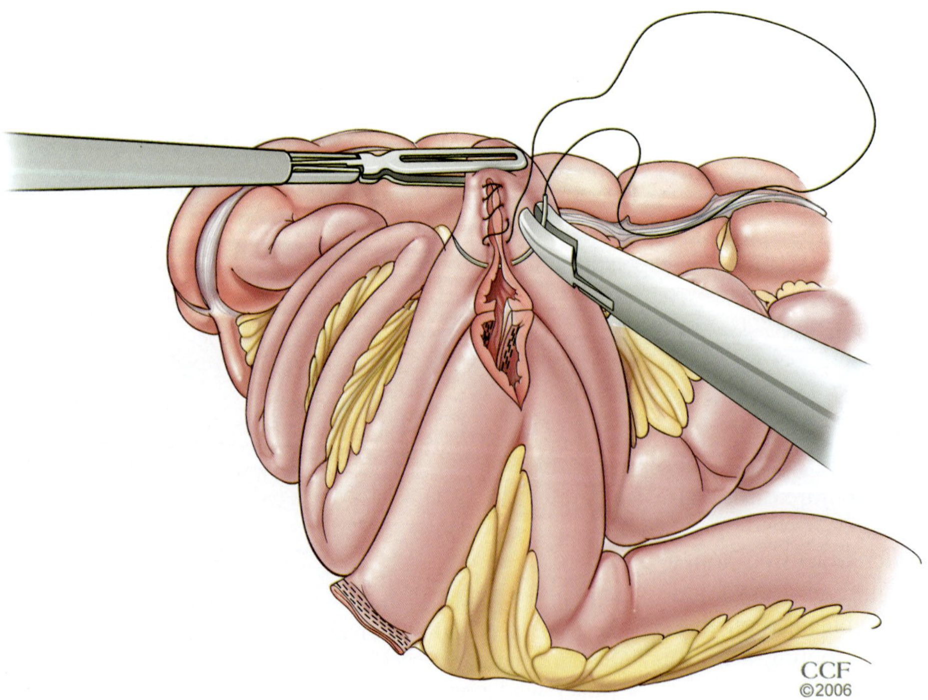

FIGURE 22.2-5. Hand-sewn closure of the common enterotomy after creating the stapled anastomosis. (Courtesy of the Cleveland Clinic Foundation.)

The ports are then withdrawn through the fascia, and reinserted pointing cephalad. The liver retractor is inserted through the subxiphoid port. The camera is left in the left subcostal port, as this provides a beautiful view of the greater curve of the stomach.

Gastrectomy

Gastric division starts just distal to the origin of the left gastric artery, across to a point on the greater curvature, 12 to 15 cm down from the angle of His (Fig. 22.2-6). It is important to perform an adequate gastric resection. The omentum is freed from the stomach using harmonic shears. The greater curvature is skeletonized along its length around the pylorus down to the first part of the duodenum. This dissection can be performed by the surgeon using a two-handed technique, with the camera in the left subcostal port, with minimal assistance.

The camera is moved to the midline port, to allow a direct view across the duodenum. Because the pylorus has been skeletonized and the blood supply is inconsequential, it is a straightforward matter to elevate the first part of the duodenum and divide it with linear stapler white cartridge. One needs to be aware of the path of the common bile duct.

The right gastric artery is taken close to the duodenum, usually with the harmonic scalpel; the linear stapler vascular cartridge is then reinserted and fired along the lesser curve, dividing the supply to the lesser curve. The origin of the left gastric artery is identified, and division of the stomach is performed about 2 cm distal to that. My preference is to do the division from the lesser curve side across, once again using the right subcostal port to insert the stapler. This approach seems to take a nice angle across the stomach. I use a blue 60-mm cartridge usually requiring two, and sometimes three, firings.

Anastomosis

The anastomosis is created to the posterior wall of the stomach. The Roux limb is placed in an anticolic position. A pulley stitch facilitates this step. A suture is placed through the stomach, and then through the antimesenteric border of the alimentary limb. It is brought up and placed through the stomach again and back through the alimentary limb, so there is a double throw on both the bowel and stomach. This suture is tied approximating the stomach and the bowel without undue focal pressure on either point.

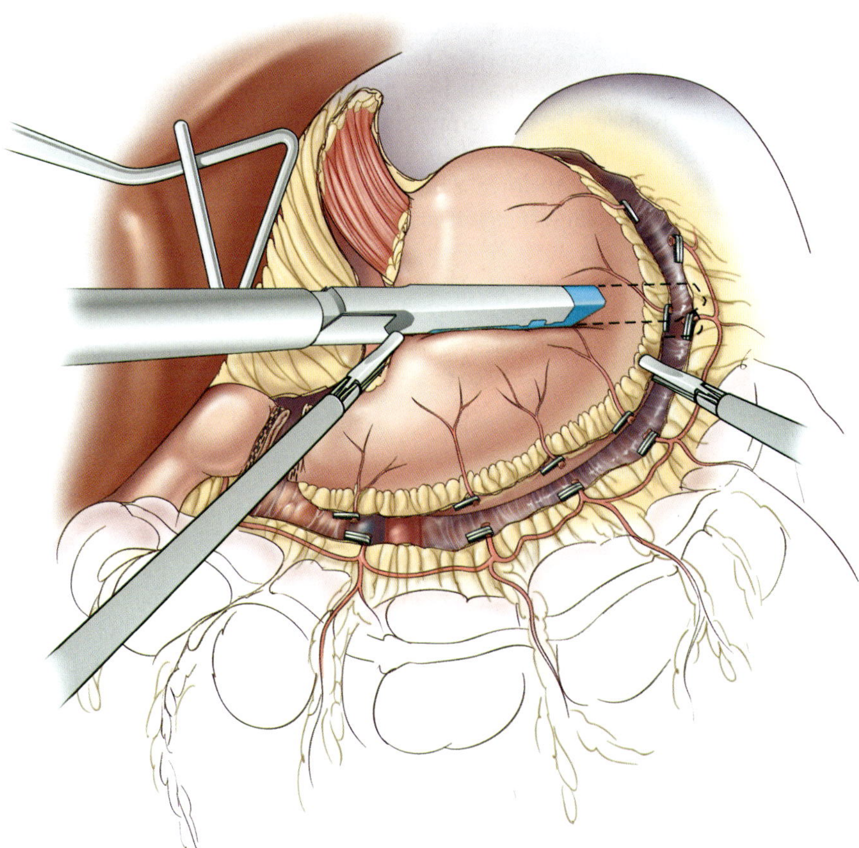

FIGURE 22.2-6. The stomach is divided from the origin of the left gastric artery to a point on the greater curvature 15 cm from the angle of His. The short gastric vessels and gastroepiploic branches are divided. The first portion of the duodenum and lesser omentum are divided with staplers to complete the resection. (Courtesy of the Cleveland Clinic Foundation.)

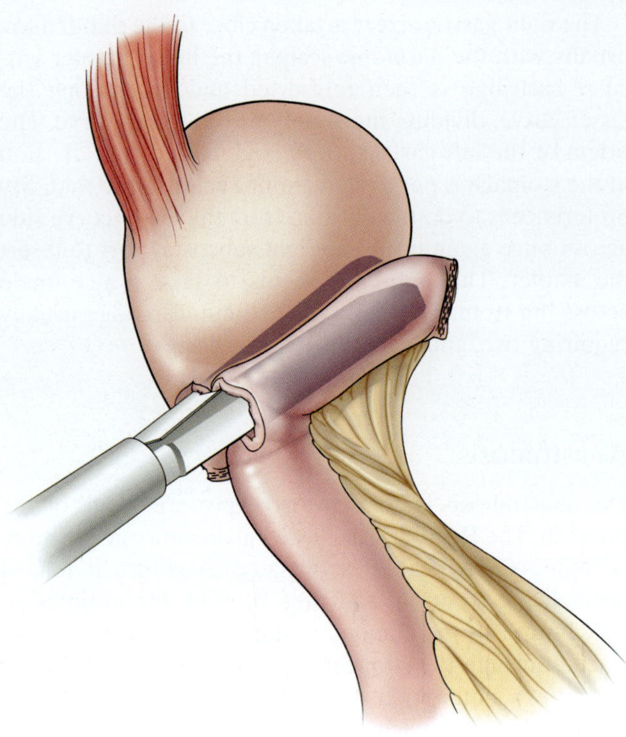

FIGURE 22.2-7. A side-to-side linear stapled anastomosis is completed between the proximal stomach and the alimentary limb. (Courtesy of the Cleveland Clinic Foundation.)

The camera is then placed in the midline port, the harmonic scalpel is inserted through the subcostal port, and incisions are made in the stomach and antimesenteric border of the alimentary limb. The linear stapler with a white 60 cartridge is inserted through the left subcostal port, in an optimal line to perform a side-to-side anastomosis (Fig. 22.2-7). The camera is left in the midline port and the defect is sutured with 3-0 PDS in a continuous fashion.

The apex of the staple line is reinforced, which helps relieve tension. Although the anastomosis is performed significantly further down the stomach than with the Roux bypass, the limb is very distally based. It can be as difficult to bring the limb of bowel to this point as it is to bring a proximally based limb to a Roux-en-Y anastomosis.

The anastomosis is tested with an "air and water test." The gastrectomy specimen is placed in a specimen bag and withdrawn through the left subcostal incision (Fig. 22.2-8), which is usually extended by 1 inch to allow this to be done easily. A drain is inserted to lie beside the duodenal stump, up under the liver across toward the gastric anastomosis. There is no need to suture any of the trocar defects with the ports used. The completed procedure is shown in Figure 22.2-9.

Postoperative Care

All patients have lower limb compression pumps, stockings, subcutaneous heparin, and early mobilization. Patients commence oral fluids once intestinal activity returns. They remain on a light diet for 2 weeks and then resume normal meals. Dietitian and surgical review is linked in a full bariatric team setting. Follow-up is scheduled for every 6 weeks for the first year, and then every 3 months thereafter. Baseline nutritional supplements include multivitamins, iron, folate, and calcium, with vitamin D. Blood work is done every 3 months, and trace elements and fat-soluble vitamins added as necessary.

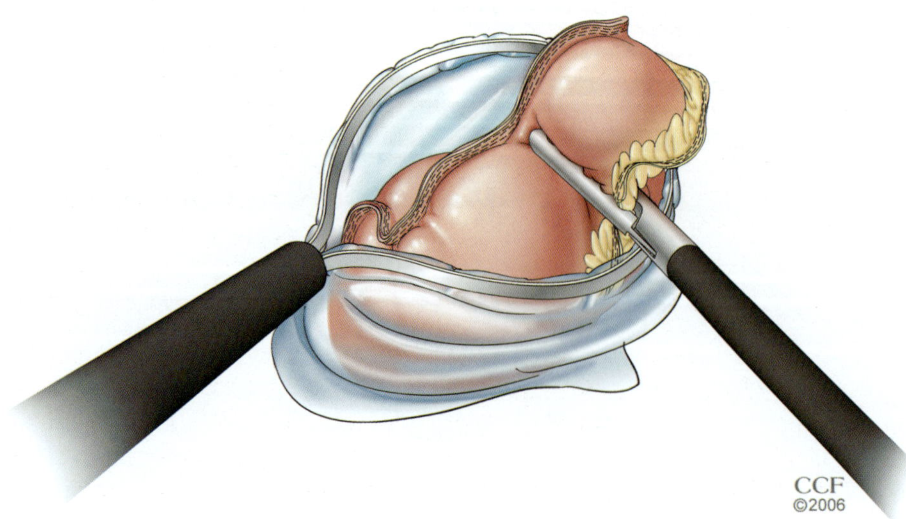

FIGURE 22.2-8. The resected stomach is placed in a specimen bag and removed through the left subcostal incision. (Courtesy of the Cleveland Clinic Foundation.)

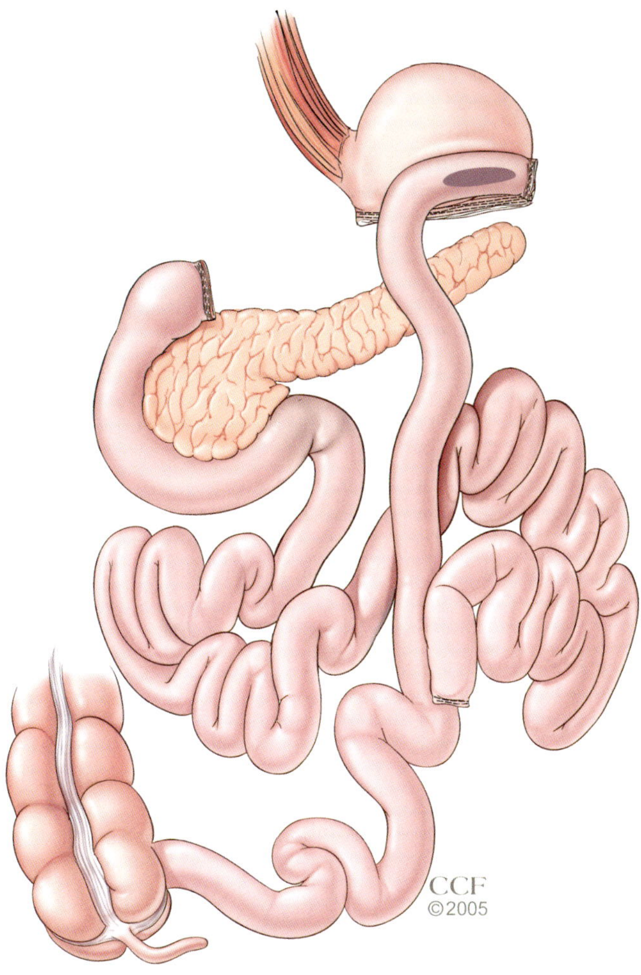

FIGURE 22.2-9. The completed laparoscopic biliopancreatic diversion. (Courtesy of the Cleveland Clinic Foundation.)

Results

Between July 1998 and October 2002 the author performed 255 BPDs and BPDs with a duodenal switch (DS). The first 59 BPDs were open procedures. The first 14 laparoscopic BPDs, with at least 3-year mean follow-up, are available for review (15). These first 14 patients (12 female and two male) had a mean age of 41 years (range, 28 to 57) and a mean body mass index (BMI) of 44.8 (range, 30.1 to 63). Five were revision of failed lap bands. The mean operating time was 169 minutes (range, 140 to 239), compared to a mean operating time of 134 minutes (range, 83 to 290) for the 59 open BPDs performed prior to this group. Mean hospital stay was 6 days (range, 5 to 16) compared to 8.5 days (range, 4 to 72) for open. There was no major morbidity or mortality.

Mean follow-up occurred for 41 months (range, 30 to 45). The BMI had fallen from the mean of 44.8 (see above) to 30.9 (range, 22.1 to 38.5) at 36 months. The percent of excess weight loss (EWL%) was 54.1% (range, 8.5% to 125.8%) at 12 months and 69% (range, 34.2% to 120%) at 36 months. There is no difference in BMI or EWL with open BPD. At follow-up at 41 months, one patient has required common channel shortening due to inadequate loss and one has needed common channel lengthening due to malnutrition.

During the same time, 30 laparoscopic BPD-DSs were performed. These patients had a mean BMI of 45.5 (range, 30 to 67). Mean operation time was 181 minutes (range, 92 to 315); mean hospital stay was 7 days (range, 4 to 146). Follow-up was shorter at a mean of 30 months (range, 10 to 39). Three years after the procedure these patients had a mean BMI of 32 (range, 30.4 to 39.5) and mean EWL% of 65.9 (range, 27 to 79).

Discussion

There are many steps in a laparoscopic BPD. The concentration, effort, and level of skill required are not to be underestimated. However, if the surgeon is adequately skilled and works with a good team, this is a relatively straightforward advanced laparoscopic surgical technique. It is certainly less formidable than a sleeve gastrectomy with a duodenal switch. This is purely because the duodenum is divided under direct vision, having been devascularized, rather than having to make a difficult dissection in the tight plane between the pancreas and duodenum while maintaining duodenal blood supply.

Paiva et al. (16) have presented 40 patients with laparoscopic BPD between July 2000 and April 2001. The patients had average BMI of 43.6 (range, 38 to 65), and 35% were super-obese. Their procedure included cholecystectomy. There was one death due to a pulmonary embolus. Average operating time was 210 minutes, with a hospital stay of 4.3 days. There was 12.5% major complication rate, with two pulmonary emboli, two bleeding staple lines, and one leak, with one death from a pulmonary embolus (2.5%). Their patients had very substantial weight loss, as one would expect with a BPD. Four patients with 6-month follow-up had a 48% EWL, and a further four at 10 months had a 91% EWL.

Scopinaro et al. (17) presented 26 patients operated in this manner, including cholecystectomy. Five of the 26 were converted due to technical difficulties. There were two cases of postoperative anastomotic stenosis. As with Paiva et al., weight loss was very satisfactory. The seven patients with 12-month follow-up had a 68% EWL.

Both surgeons performed the procedure with the patient in the legs-up position, with the surgeon standing between the legs, and used hand-held liver retraction. This requires a second assistant and a lot more maneuvering around the table. The sequence was somewhat different when the gastrectomy was performed first: the

Roux limb was made and then the gastric anastomosis was performed. Ergonomics are vitally important in laparoscopic surgery, specifically to reduce exhaustion in these long, complex procedures. If the Roux limb is created first, the ports and vision can then be directed cephalad and remain there until the end of the procedure so that mobilization of the stomach, gastrectomy, and gastrointestinal anastomosis are performed in one sitting.

Creation of the Roux limb is the most tedious part of this procedure. The constant mobility of the small bowel can be awkward. It is important to complete this task first, when the surgeon is feeling most alert, rather than as fatigue sets in and concentration is reduced. The gastric resection is much easier, as the stomach is a fixed organ. A steady ergonomic flow to the completion of the operation with the major step at the end is easier for the surgeon and assistants.

The final major difference is that both surgeons reported using a retrocolic approach. I have found no need for this. It provides no advantage from a functional point of view; it is necessary only if the Roux limb does not reach the divided stomach without tension. Mobilization of the cecum to allow the base of the Roux limb to be moved cephalad improves Roux limb mobility. Based on these results, and those of Paiva and Scopinaro, there is good evidence that the functional outcome of laparoscopic BPD is the same as with the open procedure, as one would expect it to be.

References

1. Scopinaro N, Adami GF, Marinari GM, et al. Biliopancreatic diversion. World J Surg 1998;22(9):936–946.
2. Scopinaro N, Gianette E, Cavalleri D. Biliopancreatic bypass for obesity: II. Initial experiences in man. Br J Surg 1979;66:618–620.
3. Martin IJ, Bailey IS, Rhodes M, et al. Towards T-tube free laparoscopic bile duct exploration: a methodologic evolution during 300 consecutive procedures. Ann Surg 1998; 228(1):29–34.
4. Stevenson AR, Stitz RW, Lumley JW, et al. Laparoscopically assisted anterior resection for diverticular disease: follow-up of 100 consecutive patients. Ann Surg 1998; 227(3):335–342.
5. Rhodes M, Rudd M, O'Rourke N, et al. Laparoscopic splenectomy and lymph node biopsy for hematologic disorders. Ann Surg 1995;222(1):43–46.
6. Bessell Jr, Finch R, Gotley DC, et al. Chronic dysphagia following laparoscopic fundoplication. Br J Surg 2000;87(10): 1341–1345.
7. Sarr MG, Felty CL, Hilmer DM, et al. Technical and practical considerations involved in operations on patients weighing more than 270 kg. Arch Surg 1995;130(1): L102–105.
8. Fernandez AZ, DeMaria EJ, Tichansky DS, et al. Experience with over 3000 open and laparoscopic bariatric procedures: multivariate analysis of factors related to mortality and leak. Surg Endosc 2003;17(suppl).
9. Oliak D, Ballantyne GH, Davies RJ. Short-term results of laparoscopic gastric bypass in patients with BMI $\geq$60. Obes Surg 2002;12:643–647.
10. Gibbs K, White N, Vaimakis S, et al. Laparoscopic gastric bypass in the "massive superobese." Obes Surg 2003;13: 221–222.
11. Schauer PR, Ikramuddin S, Gourash W, et al. Outcomes after laparoscopic Roux-en-Y gastric bypass for morbid obesity. Ann Surg 2000;232:515–529.
12. DeMaria EJ, Sugerman HJ, Kellum JM, et al. Results of 281 consecutive total laparoscopic Roux-en-Y gastric bypasses to treat morbid obesity. Ann Surg 2002;235:640–647.
13. Scopinaro N, Adami GF, Marinari GM, et al. Biliopancreatic diversion. World J Surg 1998;22(9):936–946.
14. Mitchell MT, Pizzitola VJ, Knuttinen MG, et al. Atypical complications of gastric bypass surgery. Eur J Radiol 2005;53:366–373.
15. Dolan K, Hatzifotis M, Newbury L, et al. A nutritional and weight loss comparison between pancreatico-biliary diversion and duodenal switch. Ann Surg 2004;240(1):51–56.
16. Paiva D, Bernardes L, Suretti L. Laparoscopic biliopancreatic diversion: technique and initial results. Obes Surg 2002; 12(3):358–361.
17. Scopinaro N, Marinari GM, Camerini G. Laparoscopic standard biliopancreatic diversion: technique and preliminary results. Obes Surg 2002;12(3):362–365.

22.3
Laparoscopic Malabsorption Procedures: Outcomes

Jay C. Jan and Emma J. Patterson

Malabsorption procedures for surgical weight reduction were initially described 50 years ago (1). The jejunoileal bypass and other early forms of intestinal bypass relied on malabsorption of nutrients to induce weight loss. However, the jejunoileal bypass was associated with significant metabolic complications due to the defunctionalized bypassed intestine. Complications, such as severe diarrhea, electrolyte disturbances, hyperoxaluria, nephrolithiasis, anemia, arthritis, liver dysfunction, and even liver failure, eventually led to the abandonment of these first-generation malabsorption procedures by the 1980s. The current malabsorption procedures are based on the biliopancreatic diversion (BPD), which was introduced by Scopinaro in 1976 (2). Unlike the original malabsorption procedures, no blind or defunctionalized segment of small intestine is created, and as a result many of the significant complications of the jejunoileal bypass are avoided. Advantages of the biliopancreatic diversion over other bariatric procedures include fewer dietary restrictions with more normal eating behavior, no excluded gastric remnant that is relatively inaccessible endoscopically, and excellent long-term weight loss. Malabsorption procedures have been slow to gain widespread popularity, perhaps due to concerns regarding the morbidity and mortality compared with other procedures, specifically early complications, such as staple line leakage, bleeding, or pancreatitis, and late complications such as nutritional deficiencies. Recently, the laparoscopic approach to malabsorption procedures has been reported.

History and Outcomes of Open Biliopancreatic Diversion

The biliopancreatic diversion is a hybrid procedure combining modest short-term gastric restriction with long-term intestinal malabsorption. Scopinaro's technique consists of a horizontal distal gastrectomy, which creates a 200- to 500-mL proximal gastric pouch and a long-limb Roux-en-Y intestinal reconstruction (3). The small intestine is divided 250 cm proximal to the ileocecal junction. The proximal small intestine becomes the biliopancreatic limb and the distal small intestine becomes the alimentary limb. The biliopancreatic limb is anastomosed to the alimentary limb 50 cm proximal to the ileocecal junction, creating a common digestive channel. Shortening the functional alimentary tract to 250 cm decreases the absorptive surface of the gut for ingested nutrients. Diverting bile and pancreatic secretions distally to the ileum delays the mixing of food with bile and pancreatic secretions and decreases fat absorption.

To reduce the incidence of marginal ulceration and dumping while maintaining the weight loss results of the biliopancreatic diversion with distal gastrectomy (BPD-DG), Marceau et al. (4) and Hess and Hess (5) modified the Scopinaro procedure. They replaced the distal gastrectomy with a vertical two-thirds *sleeve* gastrectomy, in which the greater curvature of the stomach is resected, and they added the duodenal switch. The duodenal switch was originally described by DeMeester et al. (6) in 1987 as an operation for bile reflux gastritis. Using a canine model, DeMeester et al. found that the suprapapillary duodenojejunal anastomosis resulted in a lower incidence of marginal ulceration compared to gastrojejunostomy. In the biliopancreatic diversion with duodenal switch (BPD-DS), a duodenoileostomy is performed, preserving the pylorus and a short segment of duodenum in the alimentary stream. The presence of a portion of duodenum adds protection against peptic ulcer via the secretion of bicarbonate and inhibition of gastric acid secretion. In an effort to reduce the incidence of protein deficiency and the severity of steatorrhea, Marceau et al. also lengthened the common digestive channel from 50 to 100 cm.

Long-term outcomes with BPD-DG and BPD-DS have been reported in several large series (Table 22.3-1). Perioperative morbidity ranged from 2% to 16% with

TABLE 22.3-1. Open biliopancreatic diversion series

Reference	No. of patients	Type of procedure	Age (years)	Female (%)	Preoperative BMI	Early complication rate (%)	Length of follow-up (years)	EWL (%)	Revision rate (%)	Perioperative mortality (%)
Scopinaro et al. (3,7)	2241	BPD-DG	37	69	47	1.7	12	78	4	0.4
Marceau et al. (4)	252	BPD-DG	37	80	46	16.7	8	61	1.7*	1.6
Marceau et al. (4)	465	BPD-DS	37	80	47	16.3	4	73	0.1*	1.9
Hess and Hess (5)	440	BPD-DS	40	78	50	7.0	8	70	3.9	0.5
Baltasar et al. (9)	125	BPD-DS	37	77	50	NR	5	81	2.5	1.6
Anthone et al. (8)	701	BPD-DS	42	78	53	2.9	5	66	5.7	1.4

BPD-DG, biliopancreatic diversion with distal gastrectomy; BPD-DS, biliopancreatic diversion with duodenal switch; BMI, body mass index; EWL, excess weight loss; NR, not reported.
* Yearly revision rate.

0% to 1.9% perioperative mortality. Weight loss ranged from 66% to 80% of excess body weight. In 1998, Scopinaro et al. (7) reported a 21-year experience with BPD-DG in 2241 patients. In this large series, excellent weight loss results were obtained with low morbidity and mortality. Patients lost 74% of excess weight at 2 years and 78% at 12 years of follow-up. Biliopancreatic diversion was effective in treating obesity-related comorbid conditions; hypercholesterolemia and diabetes resolved in 100% of patients and hypertension improved in the majority in Scopinaro's series. Specific long-term complications included anemia, stomal ulcers, and protein malnutrition. Anemia initially occurred in 35% to 40%, but decreased to less than 5% with iron supplementation. Stomal ulcers occurred in up to 15% of patients, but the incidence decreased to 3.2% with H2-blocker oral prophylaxis postoperatively. Protein malnutrition, characterized by hypoalbuminemia, anemia, edema, weakness, and alopecia, is the most serious complication of biliopancreatic diversion and typically requires hospitalization with parenteral nutrition (3). Protein malnutrition occurred in 11.9% of patients; however, the incidence was reduced to 3.2% with increasing the gastric pouch size and lengthening the alimentary limb (3,7).

More recently, Anthone et al. (8) described a 10-year experience with open BPD-DS with 701 patients. Significant perioperative morbidity such as staple line or anastomotic leak, bleeding, bowel obstruction, sepsis, gluteal rhabdomyolysis, or wound dehiscence occurred in 2.9%, and perioperative mortality was 1.4%. Patients lost 66% of excess body weight at 5 years of follow-up. Late complications included hypoalbuminemia in 1.7% of patients, hypocalcemia in 29.3%, and anemia in 48.3%. Biliopancreatic diversion patients generally have two to four daily bowel movements, characterized as soft and malodorous (steatorrhea) (3,4,9). Up to 5.7% of patients require surgical revision due to protein malnutrition or persistent diarrhea. This is usually a procedure aimed at lengthening the common channel. Because of the long-term risk of nutritional deficiencies, patients require vitamin and mineral supplementation and close lifelong follow-up.

In comparison to the Roux-en-Y gastric bypass, the most commonly performed bariatric procedure in the United States, malabsorption procedures offer several putative advantages. Biliopancreatic diversion permits better dietary quality with normal eating behavior. Marceau et al. (4) noted that most patients ate without restriction and exhibited decreased appetite. Anthone et al. (8) reported that at 3 years from surgery patients consumed approximately two thirds of their preoperative dietary volume without specific food intolerances, whereas Scopinaro et al. (3) reported increased food intake postoperatively. Both gastric bypass and biliopancreatic diversion result in substantial weight loss and improvement in obesity-related comorbid conditions. However, weight loss generally peaks between 12 and 18 months postoperatively after gastric bypass; most patients exhibit some regain of weight 3 to 5 years after surgery.

Pories et al. (10) published long-term follow-up data for a series of 608 open gastric bypass patients over 14 years. These patients had a nadir weight loss of 70% excess body weight at 2 years, with gradual weight regain over the ensuing years, for a mean weight loss of 49% of excess body weight at 14 years of follow-up. Scopinaro's (3) series of BPD-DG patients maintained 72% excess weight loss at 18 years of follow-up, the longest sustained weight loss reported in bariatric literature. Furthermore, the difference in weight loss is more pronounced in superobese patients, with a body mass index (BMI) ≥50. Anthone reported 82% of patients undergoing BPD-DS were considered to have successful results (loss of greater than 50% of excess body weight) at 5 years of follow-up, including 95% of patient with BMI <50 and 73.3% of patients with BMI ≥50. Similar observations have been made by Hess and Hess (5) and Baltasar et al. (9). These results compare favorably with the success rate of 93% in patients with BMI <50 and only 57% in patients with BMI ≥50 reported in MacLean's (11) series of gastric bypass patients at 5.5 years of follow-up.

TABLE 22.3-2. Laparoscopic biliopancreatic diversion series

Reference	No. of patients	Type of procedure	Age (years)	Female (%)	Preoperative BMI	Length of OR time (minutes)	Length of hospital stay (days)	Conversion rate (%)	Early complication rate (%)	Mortality (%)	Length of follow-up (months)	EWL (%)
Ren et al. (13)	40	BPD-DS	43	70	60	210	4	2.5	15	5.0	9	58
Paiva et al. (15)	40	BPD-DG	39	73	43.6	210	4.3	0	12.5	2.5	10	90
Scopinaro et al. (14)	26	BPD-DG	36	73	43	NR	NR	26	7.7	0	12	68
Baltasar et al. (19)	16	BPD-DS	23–50	88	43–56	195–270	5–8	0	37.5	0	NR	NR
Rabkin et al. (12)	345	BPD-DS*	43	87	50	201	3	2	10	0	24	91

BPD-DG, biliopancreatic diversion with distal gastrectomy; BPD-DS, biliopancreatic diversion with duodenal switch; BMI, body mass index; OR, operating room; EWL, excess weight loss; NR, not reported.
* Laparoscopy-assisted or hand-assisted.

History and Outcomes of Laparoscopic Biliopancreatic Diversion

The application of laparoscopic techniques to malabsorption procedures has been reported in several series. As with other laparoscopic bariatric procedures, the goals were to improve perioperative morbidity, decrease pain, prevent wound-related complications, and allow earlier return to work. By maintaining the fundamental technical principles of the open procedures, similar weight loss outcomes are anticipated with laparoscopic operations. Five series of laparoscopic malabsorption procedures have been published to date (Table 22.3-2). Two describe a totally laparoscopic approach to BPD-DG; two describe a totally laparoscopic approach to BPD-DS. The largest series, that of Rabkin et al. (12), describes the application of laparoscopy-assisted and hand-assisted laparoscopic techniques to BPD-DS. Perioperative morbidity ranged from 7.7% to 37.5% and perioperative mortality ranged from 0% to 5%. The conversion rates and operative times varied widely. Ren et al. (13) noted that operative time increased with higher BMI. When looking at major morbidity, mortality, and conversion rate, patients with BMI ≥65 had a higher rate of complications than those with BMI <65 (38% vs. 8.3%). The available short-term follow-up data demonstrate that weight loss is comparable to open series of biliopancreatic diversion (12–15).

In the only comparison between open and laparoscopic malabsorption procedures, Kim et al. (16) retrospectively evaluated 54 super-obese (BMI ≥50) patients who underwent either open or laparoscopic BPD-DS (Table 22.3-3). No significant difference was noted in operative time, blood loss, length of hospital stay, perioperative morbidity and mortality, and weight loss. These studies demonstrate that a minimally invasive approach to malabsorption procedures is technically feasible in the morbidly obese and super-obese, but may be associated with prohibitive risks in the super-super obese (BMI ≥60). A less invasive procedure, such as laparoscopic adjustable gastric banding or Roux-en-Y gastric bypass, may be preferable in this higher risk subcategory of patients.

As a result of the increased perioperative morbidity in the super-super-obese population with laparoscopic BPD-DS, some centers have proposed a two-stage procedure in order to decrease perioperative morbidity and mortality (17,18). The first-stage consists of a simple sleeve gastrectomy. The theory is to allow a safer initial procedure to induce weight loss such that the second stage, the duodenal switch, may be performed with reduced risk. Questions remain regarding patient selection, timing of the two-stage approach, and short- and

TABLE 22.3-3. Comparison of laparoscopic vs. open biliopancreatic diversion with duodenal switch

Outcome measure	Laparoscopic BPD-DS ($n = 28$)	Open BPD-DS ($n = 28$)	p value
Median operative time (min)	210	259	NS
Median estimated blood loss (mL)	100	300	NS
Median length of hospital stay (days)	4	5	NS
Perioperative complications (%)	23	17	NS
Perioperative mortality (%)	7.6	3.5	NS
Median excess weight loss at 12 months (kg)	76.7	56.8	NS

BPD-DS, biliopancreatic diversion with duodenal switch.
Source: Kim et al. (16), with permission.

long-term outcomes compared with single-stage procedures. Another novel two-stage approach to laparoscopic malabsorption procedures is the *Bandinaro*. Laparoscopic adjustable gastric banding is performed as a first stage and a duodenal switch as a second stage, if necessary. The possible advantage of this approach is that only patients who fail a less invasive procedure, gastric banding, progress to a more complex and higher risk procedure, biliopancreatic diversion.

Conclusion

The biliopancreatic diversion, with or without duodenal switch, produces excellent long-term weight loss and improves obesity-related comorbid conditions. The experience with the laparoscopic approach, however, has been limited, and the approach is technically challenging in expert hands. Early reports demonstrate that the laparoscopic approach is feasible, with acceptable morbidity and mortality in the appropriate patient population. Long-term weight loss is expected to be similar to the results from series of open malabsorption procedures since the technical aspects of open and laparoscopic approaches are similar. The relative risks and benefits of laparoscopic malabsorption procedures versus with open malabsorption procedures are comparable to other bariatric procedures, such as Roux-en-Y gastric bypass and adjustable gastric banding, but these procedures have not been studied prospectively.

References

1. Kremen AJ, Linner JH, Nelson CH. An experimental evaluation of the nutritional importance of proximal and distal small intestine. Ann Surg 1954;140(3):439–448.
2. Scopinaro N, Gianetta E, Civalleri D, Bonalumi U, Bachi V. Bilio-pancreatic bypass for obesity: II. Initial experience in man. Br J Surg 1979;66(9):618–620.
3. Scopinaro N, Gianetta E, Adami GF, et al. Biliopancreatic diversion for obesity at eighteen years. Surgery 1996;119(3): 261–268.
4. Marceau P, Hould FS, Simard S, et al. Biliopancreatic diversion with duodenal switch. World J Surg 1998;22(9):947–954.
5. Hess DS, Hess DW. Biliopancreatic diversion with a duodenal switch. Obes Surg 1998;8(3):267–282.
6. DeMeester TR, Fuchs KH, Ball CS, Albertucci M, Smyrk TC, Marcus JN. Experimental and clinical results with proximal end-to-end duodenojejunostomy for pathologic duodenogastric reflux. Ann Surg 1987;206(4):414–426.
7. Scopinaro N, Adami GF, Marinari GM, et al. Biliopancreatic diversion. World J Surg 1998;22(9):936–946.
8. Anthone GJ, Lord RV, DeMeester TR, Crookes PF. The duodenal switch operation for the treatment of morbid obesity. Ann Surg 2003;238(4):618–628.
9. Baltasar A, Bou R, Bengochea M, et al. Duodenal switch: an effective therapy for morbid obesity—intermediate results. Obes Surg 2001;11(1):54–58.
10. Pories WJ, Swanson MS, Macdonald KG, et al. Who would have thought it? An operation proves to be the most effective therapy for adult-onset diabetes mellitus. Ann Surg 1995;222(3):339–350.
11. MacLean LD, Rhode BM, Nohr CW. Late outcome of isolated gastric bypass. Ann Surg 2000;231(4):524–528.
12. Rabkin RA, Rabkin JM, Metcalf B, Lazo M, Rossi M, Lehmanbecker LB. Laparoscopic technique for performing duodenal switch with gastric reduction. Obes Surg 2003; 13(2):263–268.
13. Ren CJ, Patterson E, Gagner M. Early results of laparoscopic biliopancreatic diversion with duodenal switch: a case series of 40 consecutive patients. Obes Surg 2000;10(6):514–523.
14. Scopinaro N, Marinari GM, Camerini G. Laparoscopic standard biliopancreatic diversion: technique and preliminary results. Obes Surg 2002;12(2):241–244.
15. Paiva D, Bernardes L, Suretti L. Laparoscopic biliopancreatic diversion: technique and initial results. Obes Surg 2002;12(3):358–361.
16. Kim WW, Gagner M, Kini S, et al. Laparoscopic vs. open biliopancreatic diversion with duodenal switch: a comparative study. J Gastrointest Surg 2003;7(4):552–557.
17. Crookes PF, Almogy G, Hamoui N, Anthone GJ. Isolated sleeve gastrectomy for high risk morbidly obese patients. Obes Surg 2003;13(4):534(abstr).
18. Himpens J, Vleugels T, Sonneville T. Isolated sleeve gastrectomy for morbid obesity. Obes Surg 2003;13(4):562 (abstr).
19. Baltasar A, Bou R, Miro J, Bengochea M, Serra C, Perez N. Laparoscopic biliopancreatic diversion with duodenal switch: technique and initial experience. Obes Surg 2002; 12(2):245–248.

22.4
Laparoscopic Malabsorption Procedures: Postoperative Management and Nutritional Evaluation

Dennis Hong and Emma J. Patterson

Minimally invasive malabsorptive procedures such as the biliopancreatic diversion, developed by Scopinaro et al. (1), and duodenal switch, popularized by Marceau et al. (2) and Hess (3), are effective surgical procedures to produce permanent weight loss. However, they are technically more complex with morbidity and mortality that may exceed those seen with laparoscopic adjustable gastric band or Roux-en-Y gastric bypass (4). In addition, malabsorptive procedures carry a higher risk of nutritional abnormalities such as protein and vitamin deficiencies. Because of higher risks associated with malabsorptive procedures, the postoperative management and nutritional assessment in these patients is a lifelong commitment for both patient and surgeon.

Minimally invasive malabsorptive procedures are a recent development with limited long-term follow-up. However, the data from large series of open malabsorptive procedures illustrate that nutritional and vitamin deficiencies can be a devastating complication for the patient. Thus, the surgeon must be vigilant in following these patients. This chapter describes our routine postoperative management of patients who undergo minimally invasive malabsorptive procedures.

Inpatient Postoperative Management

Due to the complexity and the devastating consequences of early complications in this patient population, careful postoperative monitoring and management is critical to ensuring an acceptable outcome. Routine hospital care is outlined in Table 22.4-1. Patients are instructed to bring their continuous positive airway pressure (CPAP) machines to the hospital on the day of surgery, and this is used in the postanesthetic care unit (PACU). Once fully awake and stable, patients are sent to a regular surgical ward staffed by nurses experienced in dealing with morbidly obese patients following bariatric surgery. Another acceptable alternative, more frequently follow-

ing open bariatric surgery, is to monitor the patient in an intensive care unit the first postoperative night. Patient-controlled analgesia (usually morphine or Dilaudid) is prescribed for the first 12 hours following surgery. Three doses of Toradol (Roche Laboratories) are given intravenously during the first 24 hours postoperatively. Oral pain medication is begun once the patient tolerates an oral diet. Aggressive antiemetics, typically Zofran (Glaxo, Smith and Kline), are used to avoid nausea and retching. We encourage early ambulation and use an intermittent pneumatic compressive device for prophylaxis against deep venous thromboembolism.

A survey of the American Society of Bariatric Surgeons reported that 50% of surgeons used unfractionated heparin, 33% used pneumatic compressive devices, 13% used low-molecular-weight heparin, and 38% used a combination of methods (5). Despite this survey, we believe there is no compelling evidence to support the routine use of heparin or multimodal therapy. In addition to early ambulation, we insist patients use CPAP postoperatively when suffering from sleep apnea to decrease their risk of pulmonary complications. This has not been adopted universally because of the theoretical risk of blowing pressurized air into the gastric pouch and small bowel, thus increasing anastomotic leaks. Most studies have suggested this not to be the case (6). We do not use nasogastric tubes or intraabdominal drains routinely, although some surgeons do. Evidence regarding these practices is conflicting, with no clear consensus among surgeons (7,8).

On postoperative day 1, the Foley catheter is removed in the morning if the patient is stable. A water-soluble contrast study is obtained early in the morning to rule out anastomotic leaks. The evidence on routine radiologic studies following bariatric surgery is conflicting. Some investigators suggest routine radiologic examinations to detect early postoperative complications following bariatric surgery and modify the clinical approach (9,10). Others contend that routine radiologic studies are not beneficial and recommend them only when clinically

TABLE 22.4-1. Routine inpatient postoperative management following malabsorptive procedures

Postoperative period	Management
Day 0	1. Nothing by mouth 2. Maintenance intravenous fluids 3. Pneumatic antiembolic compressive stockings 4. Foley catheterization 5. Patient-controlled analgesic (morphine or Dilaudid) and Toradol 6. Antiemetics (IV Zofran) 7. Ambulation 8. Incentive spirometry and CPAP (if indicated)
Day 1	1. Water-soluble UGI contrast study: if normal, start stage 1 bariatric diet (see text) 2. Routine blood work: CBC, electrolytes, renal function 3. Removal of Foley catheter 4. Switch to oral analgesics (crushed or liquid) 5. Resume patient's normal medications (crush pills if appropriate) 6. Ambulation 7. Continue incentive spirometry and CPAP (if indicated)
Day 2	1. Advance to stage 2 bariatric diet 2. Dietitian pre-discharge counseling 3. Discharge home if tolerates oral diet and pain controlled

CBC, complete blood count; CPAP, continuous positive airway pressure; UGI, upper gastrointestinal.

indicated (11). Our experience has been that routine contrast studies are helpful to rule out leaks and serve as a baseline for potential future contrast studies.

Once the water-soluble contrast is confirmed to be normal, a clear liquid diet is started. Analgesics are switched to an oral route. All oral medications are crushed. We selectively obtain a pharmacology consult to instruct patients on which medications they are safely able to crush. Frequent ambulation is continually stressed to the patient.

On postoperative day 2, the patient is advanced to a pureed diet. Our inpatient dietitian does postoperative dietary counseling with each patient prior to discharge, to reinforce appropriate eating habits and food choices following a malabsorptive procedure and the importance of taking all of the vitamins. Maintaining adequate hydration is emphasized (aiming for a minimum consumption of 60 ounces of fluid per day). The importance of a very high protein diet is also stressed; patients are instructed to consume 60 to 80 g of protein per day initially, and later to aim for 80 to 100 g per day. Most patients are discharged on the second day with oral pain medications. They are instructed to maintain a pureed diet for 3 weeks until the first follow-up visit.

Outpatient Postoperative Management and Nutritional Assessment

Table 22.4-2 illustrates our outpatient management in patients following malabsorptive procedures. The potential complications and negative metabolic sequelae warrant close and lifelong follow-up. Frequent follow-up office visits are required in the first 2 years following surgery because of the increased rate of anatomic and metabolic complications within this time period. Unique complications more commonly found following malabsorptive procedures concern potential deficiencies in protein and vitamins. At each follow-up, we carefully screen for any nutritional deficiencies via a thorough history and physical and laboratory tests.

Protein Deficiency

Protein deficiency, characterized by hypoalbuminemia, anemia, edema, asthenia, and alopecia, is the most serious complication following malabsorptive procedures. The critical period is the initial 6 months following surgery when the prevalence of hypoalbuminemia can be as high as 20% (12). This is usually the result of inadequate protein intake prior to intestinal compensation. We strongly recommend that patients increase their daily protein intake to a minimum of 80 g of protein by 3 weeks after their surgery.

The rate of protein deficiency reported in the literature varies depending on the malabsorptive procedure. Brolin et al. (13) reported 13% (five of 39) of patients following

TABLE 22.4-2. Routine outpatient postoperative management following malabsorptive procedures

Postoperative period	Management
3 weeks	1. Assess wound 2. Advance to high protein mechanical soft diet, then advance texture as tolerated 3. Start vitamin supplementation: multivitamin once daily; Niferex forte 150 mg BID; Citracal 2 tabs b.i.d.; B_{12} 100 μg o.d. 4. If gallbladder present, start ursodiol, 300 mg b.i.d. for 6 months
Every 3 months up to year 1	1. Routine laboratory work: CBC, comprehensive chemistry panel, hepatic function, lipid profile, TSH, ferritin, B_{12}, folate, total protein, albumin, PTH, calcium, vitamin D-25 level 2. Bone densitometry scan at 1 year and yearly thereafter
Every 6 months up to year 2	See above
Yearly follow-up	See above

PTH, parathyroid hormone; TSH, thyroid-stimulating hormone.

distal Roux-en-Y gastric bypass (common channel 75 cm) developed low albumin levels. Two of the five patients required hospitalization for parenteral nutritional support. Baltasar et al. (14) reported three of 60 patients with hypoalbuminemia following a biliopancreatic-duodenal switch, all successfully treated on an outpatient basis. Scopinaro et al. (15) reported 114 of 958 patients (11.9%) who developed protein malnutrition after a minimum follow-up of 2 years following BPD (50 cm common channel). Thirty-nine patients (1.7%) required elongation of the common limb or restoration of small bowel anatomy.

Protein deficiency years following surgery can be problematic. Thus vigilant and lifelong follow-up is needed, with serum albumin and total protein levels at every follow-up visit (Table 22.4-2). Mild hypoalbuminemia is initially treated with increasing the daily protein to a minimum of 100 g per day. Patients are encouraged to keep food logs, consult the dietitian regularly, and return for repeat testing in 3 weeks for repeat albumin and pre-albumin levels. Scopinaro et al. (16) demonstrated that there is a positive relationship between intestinal protein absorption and intake. Therefore, increasing protein intake should correct most mild and moderate protein deficiencies. Hospitalization for protein malnutrition refractory to increases in oral intake may be necessary. If severe protein deficiency is present, then hospitalization is indicated for initiation of enteral tube feeding or intravenous hyperalimentation. Yearly rates of hospitalization for parenteral nutrition have been reported to be as high as 1% after duodenal switch (12). In some severe cases, refractory protein malnutrition may require lengthening the common channel or reestablishing normal small bowel anatomy.

Vitamin Deficiencies

Vitamin malabsorption is caused by two main factors: (1) the duodenum and proximal jejunum, where the majority of vitamins are usually absorbed, is no longer available; and (2) a decrease in fat absorption that occurs after a malabsorptive procedure. These two factors can lead to deficiencies in fat-soluble vitamins such as A, D, E, and K and non–fat-soluble vitamins such as calcium, iron, and B_{12}. Oral supplementation of these vitamins and minerals is recommended to prevent potential deficiencies (Table 22.4-2).

Iron deficiency is the most common abnormality following a malabsorptive procedure. This is particularly important in menstruating women. Iron deficiency is manifested by decreased levels of iron, ferritin, and microcytic anemia. Oral supplementation is required and increased if laboratory levels are abnormal. Up to 10% of patients may require parenteral iron supplementation for severe iron deficiency (17).

Disturbances in calcium and vitamin D absorption may increase the risk of postoperative bone disease. All patients, especially postmenopausal women, should understand the importance of daily calcium and vitamin D supplementation. At each follow-up visit parathyroid hormone (PTH), calcium, and vitamin D-25 levels are checked. One of the earliest abnormalities of calcium deficiency is an increased PTH level. In addition, yearly bone density scans are performed to detect osteopenia or osteoporosis. Despite these risks, bone seems to be relatively tolerant to metabolic changes following malabsorptive procedures. In a prospective study of 33 patients followed for 10 years, Marceau et al. (18) found overall bone mineral density was unchanged at the hip and was decreased by 4% at the lumbar spine. Overall fracture risk was unchanged.

Deficiencies in vitamins A, D, E, and K may occur due to the abnormalities in fat absorption following malabsorptive procedures. The most common reported deficiency is vitamin D with rates approaching 50% (13). Routine supplementation of all four lipid-soluble vitamins is recommended, and vitamin D-25 levels should be monitored because of its association with bone mineralization. We do not measure vitamin E, carotene (for vitamin A), or international normalized ratio (INR) (for vitamin K) unless clinically indicated.

Less common deficiencies such as zinc and thiamine have also been reported. Experimental animal models have suggested that pancreatic secretions may be instrumental for zinc absorption (19). However, Scopinaro's group (20) found no difference in serum or hair zinc levels of 14 patients who underwent biliopancreatic diversion compared with a control morbidly obese group after a minimum 1-year follow-up.

Deficiencies in thiamine can also be problematic following malabsorptive procedures, especially in patients with chronic vomiting and minimal food intake following surgery. Symptoms of Wernicke-Korsakoff disease, typically seen in chronic alcoholics, have been reported to occur in 0.18% of patients following biliopancreatic diversion (21). Although rare in occurrence, thiamine deficiency can be devastating if not properly diagnosed and treated.

Although malabsorptive procedures have been performed for over 20 years, there remain no guidelines for vitamin supplementation. In a survey of 24 surgeons who performed biliopancreatic diversion, 95% prescribed a multivitamin, 95% calcium, 67% iron, 42% B_{12}, 58% vitamin A, and 67% vitamin D (22). Similarly, there was no consensus on the frequency of ordering laboratory tests. Forty-six percent order laboratory tests every 3 months, 33% every 6 months, 16% every year, and, surprisingly, 5% did not order laboratory tests routinely. We follow these patients every 3 months for the first year, every 6 months the second year, and yearly thereafter,

TABLE 22.4-3. Potential vitamin deficiencies following malabsorptive procedures

Vitamin deficiency	Symptoms/signs of deficiency
Not fat-soluble	
Ca^{2+}	*Acute:* neuromuscular irritability, paresthesias, Chvostek's and Trousseau's signs, laryngospasm, tetany, prolonged QT interval on ECG *Chronic:* muscle cramps, mental retardation, pseudopapilledema, extrapyramidal signs, personality disturbances, dry rough skin, alopecia, abnormal dentition, osteoporosis
Fe^{2+}	Hypochromic microcytic anemia
B_{12} (cobalamin)	Megaloblastic anemia, jaundice, sore tongue, anorexia, diarrhea, numbness and paresthesia in extremities, weakness, ataxia, positive Romberg and Babinski signs, disturbances of mentation, psychosis
Thiamine	*Early stage:* anorexia, irritability, apathy, generalized weakness *Chronic deficiency:* Wernicke's encephalopathy —horizontal nystagmus, ophthalmoplegia, cerebellar ataxia, mental impairment; Wernicke-Korsakoff syndrome—Wernicke's encephalopathy and loss of memory, confabulatory psychosis
Zinc	Immune deficiency, delayed wound healing, dermatoses, glossitis, photophobia, alopecia, diarrhea, mental lethargy
Fat-soluble	
D	Signs and symptoms of hypocalcemia and hypophosphatemia, rickets (children), osteomalacia
E	Areflexia, ataxic gait, decreased vibration and position sensations, ophthalmoplegia, skeletal myopathy, pigmented retinopathy
A	Hyperkeratotic skin lesions, night blindness, dryness of eyes, xerosis, Bitot spots
K	Coagulation abnormalities

provided there are no complications, and more frequently if there are (Table 22.4-2). At each visit, the patient's recent progress is reviewed, symptoms or signs of vitamin deficiencies are assessed (Table 22.4-3), and routine laboratory tests are performed (Table 22.4-2).

Conclusion

Postoperative management and nutritional assessment following minimally invasive malabsorptive procedures is critical to the ultimate success of these procedures. Because of the potential for severe protein and vitamin deficiencies, malabsorptive procedures have not gained widespread acceptance. We recommend selecting patients who are committed to long-term follow-up and complying with vitamin supplementations.

References

1. Scopinaro N, Gianetta E, Friedman D, Adami GF, Traverso E, Bachi V. Evoluation of biliopancreatic bypass. Clin Nutr 1986;137–146.
2. Marceau P, Hould FS, Simard S, et al. Biliopancreatic diversion with duodenal switch. World J Surg 1998;22:947–954.
3. Hess DS. Bilio-pancreatic bypass with a duodenal switch procedure. Obes Surg 1994;4:106(abstr).
4. Ren C, Patterson E, Gagner M. Early results of laparoscopic biliopancreatic diversion with duodenal switch: a case series of 40 consecutive patients. Obes Surg 2000;10:514–523.
5. Wu EC, Barba CA. Current practices in the prophylaxis of venous thromboembolism in bariatric surgery. Obes Surg 2000;10(1):7–13.
6. Huerta S, Deshields S, Shpiner R, et al. Safety and efficacy of postoperative continuous positive airway pressure to prevent pulmonary complications after Roux-en-Y gastric bypass. J Gastrointest Surg 2002;6(3):354–358.
7. Huerta S, Arteaga JR, Sawicki MP, et al. Assessment of routine elimination of postoperative nasogastric decompression after Roux-en-Y gastric bypass. Surgery 2002;132(5):844–848.
8. Serafini F, Anderson W, Ghassemi P, et al. The utility of contrast studies and drains in the management of patients after Roux-en-Y gastric bypass. Obes Surg 2002;12(1):34–38.
9. Toppino M, Cesarani F, Comba A, et al. The role of early radiological studies after gastric bariatric surgery. Obes Surg 2001;11(4):447–454.
10. Sims TL, Mullican MA, Hamilton EC, et al. Routine upper gastrointestinal Gastrografin swallow after laparoscopic Roux-en-Y gastric bypass. Obes Surg 2003;13(1):66–72.
11. Singh R, Fisher BL. Sensitivity and specificity of postoperative upper GI series following gastric bypass. Obes Surg 2003;13(1):73–75.
12. Marceau P, Hould FS, Lebel S, et al. Malabsorptive Obesity Surgery. Surg Clin North Am 2001;81(5):1113–1127.
13. Brolin RE, LaMarca LB, Kenler HA, Cody RP. Malabsorptive Gastric Bypass in patients with superobesity. J Gastrointest Surg 2002;6:195–205.
14. Baltasar A, del Rio J, Escriva C, et al. Preliminary results of the duodenal switch. Obes Surg 1997;7;500–504.
15. Scopinaro N, Gianetta E, Adami GF, et al. Biliopancreatic diversion for obesity at eighteen years. Surgery 1996;119:261–268.
16. Scopinaro N, Marinari GM, Camerini G, et al. Energy and nitrogen absorption after Biliopancreatic diversion. Obes Surg 2000;10:436–441.
17. Baltasar A, Bou R, Bengochea M, et al. Duodenal switch: an effective therapy for morbid obesity—intermediate results. Obes Surg 2001;11:54–58.
18. Marceau P, Biron S, Lebel S, et al. Does bone change after biliopancreatic diversion? J Gastrointest Surg 2002;6:690–698.
19. Adamama-Moraitou K, Rallis T, Papasteriadis A, et al. Iron, zinc and copper concentration in serum, various organs, and

hair of dogs with experimentally induced exocrine pancreatic insufficiency. Dig Dis Sci 2001;46(7):1444–1457.

20. Vanderhoof JA, Scopinaro N, Tuma DJ, et al. Hair and plasma zinc levels following exclusion of biliopancreatic secretions from functioning gastrointestinal tract in humans. Dig Disc Sci 1983;29(4):300–305.

21. Primavera A, Brusa G, Novello P, et al. Wernicke-Korsakoff Encephalopathy following biliopancreatic diversion. Obes Surg 1993;3(2):175–177.

22. Brolin RE, Leung M. Survey of vitamin and mineral supplementation after gastric bypass and biliopancreatic diversion for morbid obesity. Obes Surg 1999;9:150–154.

22.5
Laparoscopic Malabsorption Procedures: Complications

Christine J. Ren

Biliopancreatic diversion (BPD), without or with duodenal switch (BPD-DS), limits nutrient absorption regardless of intake. These procedures carry significant risk due to increased operative risk of the obese patient, the complexity of the operation, and subsequent nutritional derangements.

Laparotomy in the morbidly obese is associated with significant complications, and operative mortality for open malabsorptive operations ranges from 0% to 1.7% (1–13). Laparoscopy has its greatest impact on wound and cardiopulmonary complications, which are the complications that are most frequent in morbidly obese patients. The development of advanced laparoscopic techniques coincided with increased demand for less morbid bariatric surgery. However, minimally invasive techniques carry their own set of complications, and mortality was higher (2.5%) in the early experience of laparoscopic malabsorption operations (10,14–18). For this reason, laparoscopic BPD and BPD-DS are operations that should be undertaken only by surgeons who are experienced with advanced laparoscopic techniques and aware of the multidisciplinary demands of bariatric surgery. This chapter discusses the surgical and nutritional complications specific to laparoscopic biliopancreatic diversion with and without duodenal switch (Table 22.5-1).

General Postoperative Complications

Obesity is a risk factor in itself. There are special challenges to successful preoperative, intraoperative, and postoperative management of these patients. Comorbidities may impact their perioperative course, and differential diagnosis, administration of anesthesia, and performance of technical procedures are more difficult.

Tables 22.5-2 to 22.5-5 review the major complications after open and laparoscopic BPD and BPD-DS as published in the literature. Three coexisting variables appear to correlate with poor postoperative recovery after laparoscopic malabsorptive surgery: body mass index (BMI) >65, android body morphology, and revisional surgery.

Ren et al. (16), in a series of 40 patients undergoing laparoscopic BPD-DS (75% of whom had BMI >50), found 50% complication rate (major morbidity, mortality, and conversion) in patients with BMI >65, as compared with 8% in those patients with BMI <65. This correlates with increased complications with increased weight in open nonbariatric surgery. Prem et al. (19) found higher mortality in women weighing over 300 lb (20%), as compared with those weighing less than 300 lb (2%), who underwent surgery for uterine neoplasm. Similarly, higher BMI is correlated with increased rate of anastomotic leak and mortality in Roux-en-Y gastric bypass, even in experienced surgical hands (20). This has led some laparoscopic bariatric surgeons to seek safer surgical options for those patients considered superobese, by performing complex operations in stages. The first operation is a purely restrictive operation such as a laparoscopic adjustable gastric band or a laparoscopic sleeve gastrectomy, which carries a low morbidity. After a significant weight loss, which lowers the operative risk, the patient undergoes a second operation, the duodenal switch, to add malabsorption to the existing restrictive component.

The morphology of the obese patient plays an important role in surgical access. Android morphology, with truncal distribution of fat, has been associated with an increased risk of hypertension and heart disease, especially in men. The android shape makes laparoscopic access more difficult due to the torque created on the instruments, resulting in limited range of motion. This is particularly true in a patient with grade 4 or 5 pannus (pannus below the thigh). These patients might fare better with an open technique. In contrast, the gynecoid-type patient, with body fat distribution around the hips and thighs, would benefit from a laparoscopic technique.

TABLE 22.5-1. Surgical complications after laparoscopic malabsorptive procedures

1. Surgical and acute postoperative complications
   a. Pulmonary embolus
   b. Intraabdominal leak
   c. Hemorrhage
2. Delayed postoperative complications
   a. Gastrointestinal
      i. Marginal ulcer
      ii. Gastric outlet obstruction
      iii. Intestinal obstruction
      iv. Intestinal bacterial overgrowth
   b. Nutritional
      i. Protein malnutrition
      ii. Anemia
      iii. Metabolic bone disease
      iv. Fat-soluble vitamin deficiencies

TABLE 22.5-2. Open and laparoscopic biliopancreatic diversion

First author, year	n	BMI	Female (%)	Follow-up max months (range)	Mortality (%, 30-day)	Early Complications: n (%)	Late Complications: n (%)
Open BPD							
Michielson, 1996	33	49.5	70	36	0	21	63
Nanni, 1997	59	48.6	91.5	24	1.7	5.1	23.7
Scopinaro, 1998	1356	47	68	155	0.4 (0.7*)	2.8	—
Marceau, 1998	252	46	80	156	1.6	16.7	—
Noya, 1998	50	50.7	50	24	2	10	30
Rabkin, 1998	32	45	81	48	0	—	—
Totte, 1999	180	48.8	80	36	0	16	30.6
Murr, 1999	11	64	30	108	0 (10*)	20	—
Bajardi, 2000	142	—	—	24	—	14.8	—
Dolan, 2003	59	45	79	53	0	21	19
Laparoscopic BPD							
Paiva, 2002	40	43.6	80	10	2.5	25	12.5
Scopinaro, 2002	26	43	73	12	0	7.7	—
Dolan, 2003	14	45	86	38	0	7	21

n, number of patients; BMI, body mass index; —, not reported.
* Late mortality occurring after 30 days.

TABLE 22.5-3. Complications of open and laparoscopic biliopancreatic diversion

First author, year	PE (%)	Leak (%)	Bleeding (%)	Pancreatitis (%)	Delayed gastric emptying (%)	Wound infection/dehiscence (%)	Marginal ulcer (%)	Stomal stenosis (%)	Incisional hernia (%)	Revision for protein malnutrition (%)
Open BPD										
Michielson, 1996	0	—	—	—	—	15	15	—	15	—
Nanni, 1997	1.7	—	—	—	—	—	2	—	17	—
Scopinaro, 1998	0.7	0.2	0.2	—	—	1.7	8.3 (*3.2)	—	15	7.1
Marceau, 1998	0.4	1.6	—	1.6	9.1	0.8	—	—	—	1.7% per year
Noya, 1998	0	2	—	—	6	—	10	2	12	1.7
Totte, 1999	0.6	1.1	—	0.6	6.1	5	11	—	17.8	3
Murr, 1999	0	10	10	0	—	—	—	—	—	—
Dolan, 2003	0	3	0	0	—	11	0	0	—	—
Laparoscopic BPD										
Paiva, 2002	5	2.5	5	—	—	2.5	—	—	—	—
Scopinaro, 2002						7.7**		7.7	0	—
Dolan, 2003	0	7	0	0	0	0	0	0	0	—

BMI, body mass index; —, not reported.
* On H2 blockers.
** Occurred in four conversions.

TABLE 22.5-4. Open and laparoscopic biliopancreatic diversion with duodenal switch

First author, year	n	BMI	Female (%)	Follow-up max months (range)	Mortality (%, 30-day)	Early complications: n (%)	Late complications: n (%)
Open BPD-DS							
Marceau, 1998	465	47	80	49	2	16.3	—
Hess, 1998	440	50	78	108	0.5	9	—
Rabkin, 1998	37	—	—	48	0	16	40.5
Baltasar, 2001	125*	50	77	60	1.6	8.8	4
Anthone, 2003	701	53	78	120	1.4	2.9	—
Dolan, 2003	31	44	71	37	0	35†	—
Laparoscopic BPD-DS							
Ren, 2000	40	60	70	12	2.5 (2.5)	15	—
Baltasar, 2002	16	>40	88	18	0	43.8	—
Rabkin, 2003**	345	50	87	24	0	7.2	7.8
Dolan, 2003	30	46	67	39	3.3	23.3†	—

* 102 primary BPD-DS.
** Laparoscopically and hand-assisted combined.
† Complications include both early and late.

Malabsorption operations as revisions for failed primary bariatric operations carry a higher complication rate due to the increased incidence of staple line leak. In 125 BPD-DS patients, Baltasar et al. (12) found that the two deaths and four of five leaks occurred in patients who were undergoing revisions from vertical banded gastroplasty (VBG). Dolan and Fielding (21) similarly found that four of five major complications (80%) in their series of 79 BPD patients occurred in revisions.

Surgical and Acute Postoperative Complications

The three most serious and potentially life-threatening surgical complications after malabsorptive operations are (1) pulmonary embolus (PE), (2) intraabdominal leak, and (3) bleeding.

Pulmonary Embolus

Obesity, prolonged operative time, and postoperative immobilization increase the risk of thromboembolic disease. Other factors that increase the risk of thromboembolism in these patients are the use of exogenous estrogen, hypoxia, previous history of thromboembolic event, venous stasis disease, and genetic predispositions to hypercoagulability. Therefore, an extensive operative time for the sake of completing the operation laparoscopically places the patient at undue risk for PE and should be avoided. In a recent survey of American Society for Bariatric Surgery (ASBS) members in which 95% of the operations performed were open gastric surgery for morbid obesity, the incidence of deep venous thrombosis (DVT) was found to be 2.6% and the incidence of PE to be 0.95% (22).

Interestingly, the incidence of thromboembolism is slightly lower in the laparoscopic bariatric literature. In

TABLE 22.5-5. Complications of open and laparoscopic biliopancreatic diversion with duodenal switch

First author, year	PE (%)	Leak (%)	Bleeding (%)	Pancreatitis (%)	Delayed gastric emptying (%)	Wound infection/ dehiscence (%)	Marginal ulcer (%)	Stomal stenosis (%)	Incisional hernia (%)	Revisions for protein malnutrition (%)
Open BPD-DS										
Marceau, 1998	0.7	4.9	—	1.7	6.2	1	0	—	—	0.1% per year
Hess, 1998	0.5	4	1.4	—	—	—	0	—	—	2.3
Rabkin, 1998	5.4	5.4	—	2.7	—	5.4	—	—	24	12.2
Baltasar, 2001	0.8	4	1.6	0	—	0.8	—	—	5.8	2.4
Anthone, 2003	0.6	0.7	0.7*	—	—	0.7	—	—	—	5.7
Dolan, 2003	0	6.5	0	0	0	8	—	—	0	—
Laparoscopic BPD-DS										
Ren, 2000	0	2.5	10	0	0	0	—	—	—	—
Baltasar, 2002	0	0	6.3	—	6.3	18.8	—	—	—	—
Rabkin, 2003*	0.9	4.3	—	—	—	—	—	1.7	—	—
Dolan, 2003	0	6.6	6.6	3.3	0	—	—	0	—	—

* Includes three splenectomies.

large series of laparoscopic Roux-en-Y gastric bypass (RYGBP), the incidence of DVT and PE both ranged from 0% to 0.3% (23,24). The BPD and BPD-DS literature reflects an incidence of PE ranging from 0% to 5.4% (Tables 22.5-3 and 22.5-5).

As already mentioned, early ambulation is the most effective component to DVT prophylaxis and is facilitated by laparoscopy. Sequential compression devices and subcutaneous heparin should be routinely used as prophylaxis.

Intraabdominal Leak

Peritonitis is extremely difficult to recognize in the morbidly obese patient. The high mortality after intraabdominal leak is due to a delay in diagnosis. The most important determinant of patient survival is a high index of suspicion and early detection.

Anastomotic leaks can occur at any staple or suture line. The extensive resection and reconstruction involved in the BPD and BPD-DS lend themselves to surgical complications, which can involve the (1) proximal gastroenterostomy or duodenoenterostomy, (2) gastric pouch staple line, (3) duodenal stump, and (4) distal enteroenterostomy. Leak rates have been slightly higher for laparoscopic approaches due to individual surgical learning curves, coupled with the complexity of the operation. Leak rates are higher in BPD-DS as compared with BPD due to the long sleeve gastrectomy staple line.

Anastomotic or gastric leak after open bariatric surgery is associated with up to 55% mortality. Peritonitis must be suspected in any morbidly obese patient with acute respiratory failure. Clinical symptoms and signs are similar to a massive pulmonary embolus: severe tachypnea, tachycardia (heart rate >120), and sudden hypotension. The acute onset of respiratory failure is likely secondary to sepsis-induced adult respiratory distress syndrome (ARDS). Occasionally, bile or clear frothy fluid will be evident in the closed-suction drains.

Upper gastrointestinal (GI) radiographic contrast study with water-soluble agent such as diatrizoate meglumine (Gastrografin) can be diagnostic. Similarly, if drains are still present, the patient can be given diluted methylene blue to drink with subsequent monitoring of the drain output. Leaks at the duodenal stump or from the distal jejunojejunostomy are not reliably accessible to any radiographic contrast study and will not be evident on examination. The only test that may provide insight to a large stump leak would be a nuclear hepatobiliary scan (hepatic 2,6-dimethyliminodiacetic acid, HIDA) demonstrating bile flow through the biliopancreatic limb and out into the peritoneal cavity. However, it is highly nonspecific and usually difficult to read. Laboratory values are usually normal, with the exception of an occasionally elevated white blood cell count. Laboratory analysis can be performed on the drain fluid to measure amylase and bilirubin. If the patient's clinical status is deteriorating, intraabdominal leak must be suspected and immediate surgical exploration by laparoscopy or laparotomy performed, even in the face of a normal radiographic contrast study or laboratory results.

The treatment of an intraabdominal leak is dependent on the size of the leak and, more importantly, on the clinical status of the patient. A small radiographic leak from the proximal anastomosis can be successfully treated conservatively with drains, antibiotics, and parenteral nutrition. However, if the leak is large, persists, or worsens, or if the patient's clinical status deteriorates, surgical repair or diversion is indicated. Concomitant placement of a feeding jejunostomy tube into the biliopancreatic limb facilitates enteral feeding while the patient remains without oral intake. Surgical repair and drainage can be accomplished laparoscopically or by laparotomy. Duodenal stump leaks are more evasive to diagnose and more treacherous to treat. Simple oversewing of the stump typically is insufficient to prevent breakdown. In large leaks, a lateral duodenostomy tube may be indicated.

Hemorrhage

Postoperative bleeding causes tachycardia, hypotension, oliguria, a decrease in hematocrit, and possibly blood in the drains, hematemesis, or hematochezia. It occurs in up to 10% of open and laparoscopic BPD and BPD-DS operations. The extensive staple line on the vascular stomach along the sleeve gastrectomy in BPD-DS is prone to bleeding, which is exacerbated by subcutaneous heparin. Linear staplers using 3.5-mm cartridge are recommended for safe gastric resection. Larger sized cartridges always result in bleeding. Oozing from the staple line can be controlled with clips, suturing, or ultrasonic scalpel. Some surgeons have used reinforcing agents such as fibrin glue or bovine pericardial strips. Staple-line bleeding is usually self-limited.

Hematemesis suggests staple line bleeding at the mucosa, into the lumen of the alimentary tract. Upper endoscopy enables direct visualization and coagulation of the bleeding, with either epinephrine or cautery. Although most surgeons feel uncomfortable performing endoscopy with a fresh anastomosis, we have been successful with esophagogastroduodenoscopy (EGD) and coagulation of a staple-line bleed as early as several hours after the operation, with no adverse sequelae. Transfusion is reserved for older and symptomatic patients.

The only true diagnostic test for bleeding is exploration, by laparoscopy or laparotomy. Patients who are hemodynamically unstable or have a persistent drop in hematocrit must return to the operating room. Treatment is dependent on the cause of hemorrhage.

Delayed Postoperative Complications

Delayed postoperative gastrointestinal or nutritional complications after laparoscopic malabsorption operations are similar to those found in open surgery.

Gastrointestinal Complications

Marginal Ulcer

Scopinaro et al. (3) initially reported a 12.5% incidence of marginal ulcer. This decreased to 8.3% after resecting more of the distal stomach, and even further to 3.2% with prophylactic use of H2-blockers after surgery. Marginal ulceration after BPD-DS has essentially been eliminated with the duodenal switch modification. Many surgeons believe that the majority of acid-producing mucosa is removed with the sleeve gastrectomy, and that preservation of a duodenal cuff provides mucosal protection for the ileum. No series comparing BPD with DS report marginal ulcers in either group (4,10), but this may be explained by small sample size. However, it is recommended that all patients should be on lifelong H2 blockers.

Gastric Outlet Obstruction

Gastric emptying depends on both the size of the outlet and the propulsive activity of the stomach. Mechanical and functional derangements of the stomach after surgery can lead to obstruction. Proximal anastomotic stenosis can occur after both the BPD and BPD-DS. Immediate postoperative gastric obstruction is usually due to edema and will resolve in several days. Prolonged gastric outlet obstruction then may be due to mechanical or functional causes. Narrowing of the stoma secondary to technical error is more likely to occur after BPD-DS because of the smaller lumen duodenum. The patient has intolerance to all oral intake, including liquids. Barium swallow documents obstruction, and upper endoscopy shows stomal narrowing. Surgical revision of the anastomosis is necessary.

Gastroparesis after gastric resection is well described in the ulcer surgery literature. In fact, 27% incidence of delayed gastric emptying can occur after distal gastrectomy with Roux-en-Y reconstruction (25). It is also more common after pylorus-preservation than pylorus resection when performing pancreaticoduodenectomy (26). An upper GI study using dilute liquid barium typically shows a dilated gastric pouch with a normal stoma but no emptying. Patients typically are intolerant to solid food but can drink liquids. Upper endoscopy confirms the patency of the anastomosis. Gastric motility usually returns after 4 to 6 weeks of bowel rest and total parenteral nutrition (TPN).

Delayed stomal stenosis, which arises 4 to 6 weeks after surgery, can be attributed to several variables: suture material, ischemia, and leak. Sutures may cause inflammatory reaction, and thus fibrosis. Ischemia may be caused by tension on the anastomosis, devascularization of the pouch during division of the stomach, or devascularization of the ileum after division of the mesentery. A subclinical localized contained leak often leads to peristomal inflammation and fibrosis. In addition, fibrosis from marginal ulcer can cause stenosis. Delayed stomal stenosis due to fibrosis may be more common after BPD due to the reactive nature of the stomach and may be avoided by making the gastroenterostomy no less than 6 cm long.

Intestinal Obstruction

Causes of postoperative bowel obstruction after laparoscopic bariatric surgery include (1) adhesions, (2) internal hernia, (3) stenosis of the small bowel, and (4) incorrect bowel limb anastomosis.

In the open procedure literature, bowel obstruction was most commonly caused by adhesions, occurring at a rate of 3% to 4%. Laparoscopic techniques create less adhesions postoperatively and decrease the risk of adhesive obstruction to 0.3% (24). Although postoperative adhesions are minimal after laparoscopy, there can still be other causes of small bowel obstruction: (1) adhesions already present from prior surgery, especially if performed by laparotomy; (2) adhesion of bowel or omentum to anterior abdominal wall at a trocar site; or (3) adhesions caused by a missed or subclinical postoperative leak.

No current effective treatment exists to prevent adhesive bowel obstruction. However, bowel obstruction due to internal hernias occurs at a rate of 2% to 3% and continues to be a problem in laparoscopic bariatric surgery. It is mainly due to technical error—failure to adequately close potential hernia defects. Although few data exist on the rate of intestinal obstruction in malabsorptive operations, it can be extrapolated from the laparoscopic gastric bypass literature. Stenosis of the small bowel typically occurs at either the distal anastomosis at a rate of 0.73% or at the mesenteric window through which the Roux limb traverses in the retrocolic path (0.4–0.9%) (23,24). The majority of adhesive small bowel obstructions resolve with conservative management. In contrast, obstruction from internal hernia is a surgical emergency, needing reduction of herniated small bowel, resection of nonviable bowel, possible revision of the anastomosis, and repair of the defect. For this reason, aggressive operative management of patients presenting with mechanical small bowel obstruction is recommended.

Incorrect bowel limb anastomosis (Roux-en-O) is not often reported in the literature, but unfortunately still occurs. The incorrect limb is anastomosed to the gastric pouch/duodenum, causing a prolonged, complete obstruction that is diagnosed notoriously late. All proximal radiology is normal.

Obstruction of the alimentary limb or common channel presents as small bowel obstruction, with the typical symptoms of nausea, vomiting, and obstipation. In contrast, obstruction of the biliopancreatic limb is more elusive. It may cause abdominal fullness and bloating, and pain from visceral distention or from pancreatitis. Laboratory values may show hyperamylasemia or elevation in hepatic enzymes. One must always be aware of obstructions involving the biliopancreatic limb, leading to duodenal distention with bile and pancreatic enzymes, and eventually blow-out of the duodenal stump.

Bertolotto et al. (27) found that of 15 BPD patients with small bowel obstruction, 67% had obstruction of the biliopancreatic limb. They found that plain abdominal films were useless, but that abdominal ultrasound and abdominal computed tomography (CT) scan (oral and IV contrast) revealed abnormal nonspecific findings, typically dilated or thick-walled small bowel (particularly the duodenum), or pelvic ascites. Even in the face of negative radiologic findings, if a high clinical suspicion for intestinal obstruction is present, surgical exploration is indicated. Laparoscopy can be both diagnostic and therapeutic.

Intestinal Bacterial Overgrowth

No blind limb exists in either BPD or BPD-DS. However, deleterious intestinal bacterial overgrowth occurs occasionally after these malabsorptive operations. The incidence is not certain, but the effect of antibiotics on many postoperative gastrointestinal symptoms provides some evidence for bacterial overgrowth. Metronidazole in particular is effective in treating abdominal distention, pseudo-obstruction, nocturnal diarrhea, proctitis, and acute arthralgia (28). Evidence exists that the short length of intestine (29), protein malnutrition (30), absence of bile and pancreatic secretions (31), and presence of undigested food in the colon (32) may all contribute to creating a milieu for bacterial overgrowth. One study has shown a 27% incidence of bacterial overgrowth that was successfully treated with antibiotics (1). A protein-deficient diet with an excess of simple carbohydrates may increase an individual's risk of bacterial overgrowth, and if chronic, may require surgical revision. Lengthening of the alimentary limb by incorporating a portion of the biliopancreatic limb will increase carbohydrate absorption. This decreases the quantity of unabsorbed carbohydrates entering the colon, one location where bacteria may proliferate (33).

Nutritional Deficiencies

Careful patient selection and education, and long-term follow-up are the cornerstones to successful maintenance of weight loss. Compliance plays a significant role in the success and avoidance of malnutrition after malabsorptive procedures. There are no certain variables that predict compliance, which is critical but not in the surgeon's control. The patient's failure to comply with dietary guidelines, nutritional supplementation, and office visits has been shown to be the most common reason for weight loss failure and for malnutrition (34). The patient must be instructed about changes in eating habits, nutritional supplements that must be taken postoperatively, and the importance of long-term follow-up appointments and laboratory evaluation. Preoperative literature and instruction, combined with postoperative reinforcement, should be instituted with the assistance of the team nutritionist. Screening must be done to identify patients who are unlikely to comply. Patients must have a grasp of these issues. Mental retardation and substance abuse are relative contraindications. Psychosis can interfere in adaptation to new behavioral and lifestyle changes. This may lead to surgical reversal, or occasionally, suicide.

Protein Malnutrition

Protein malnutrition may be mild or severe, and the literature has often failed to distinguish this difference. Typically, hypoalbuminemia refers to mild malnutrition that requires dietary supplementation or a short course of TPN. Severe protein malnutrition refers to the need for prolonged hospitalization for TPN, the recurrent need for TPN, or malnutrition recalcitrant to TPN that eventually requires surgical revision. The incidence of severe protein malnutrition ranges from 2% to 7% for both BPD (2,4,7,33) and BPD-DS (4,10,12,13). It is caused by either insufficient absorption or insufficient intake of protein.

The classic BPD with a 150- to 250-mL gastric pouch, 200-cm alimentary (Roux), and a 50-cm common channel results in approximately 57% absorption of ingested protein (3). The absorptive capacity of the alimentary and common channel depends on (1) number of villi per square centimeter, (2) transit time, and (3) the total intestinal length from the proximal anastomosis to the ileocecal valve. Any event that interferes with postoperative villous hypertrophy, increases transit time (e.g., gastroenteritis, bacterial overgrowth, high lumen osmolality), or decreases the length of the functional alimentary or common channel (e.g., fistula, inflammatory bowel disease) will put the patient at risk for severe protein malnutrition. Increased number of bowel movements or severe diarrhea may be precedents to protein malnutrition. The offending etiology should be corrected with the appropriate medications, and the patient hydrated. Oral pancreatic enzymes (Pancrease) can be prescribed to facilitate protein absorption. Surgical revision may be necessary in individuals whose absorptive intestines do not adapt to *short gut syndrome* with villous hypertrophy. Elongation must be performed along the biliopancreatic limb, to increase the length of Roux plus common channel to 400 cm.

Poor patient compliance with protein intake is the leading cause of hypoalbuminemia. This is reflected by Scopinaro et al.'s (3) observation that southern Italians who eat less protein and more carbohydrates in their diet have a higher incidence of protein malnutrition than northern Italians. In addition, up to 20% of patients have low albumin levels 6 months after BPD-DS, but this decreases to less than 10% at 9 years (28). This reflects the initial restriction due to gastric resection, anastomotic edema, and delayed gastric emptying. Protein malnutrition is commonly seen in patients who have unsuspected psychiatric illness that leads them into a complete derangement of normal life (7).

The recommended dietary protein intake should be a minimum of 90 g/day, and patients must be counseled thoroughly. The patient must be able to eat this amount of protein, reflecting the need for a moderate-sized (150–300 mL) gastric pouch. This explains why distal RYGBP has been reported as having a 16% mortality from protein malnutrition (35). Other authors, however, have not observed this as a problem (36).

Protein malnutrition must not be underestimated. Two series had late deaths due to protein malnutrition (3,12). Complete intestinal restoration may be necessary in patients who are psychologically intolerant to the operation, or in disease states that worsen with malnutrition: liver cirrhosis, nephrotic syndrome, malignancy, or psychosis.

Anemia

Postoperative anemia is typically microcytic, and is almost always due to iron malabsorption and rarely from folate or vitamin B_{12} deficiency. Iron is absorbed primarily in the duodenum, which is excluded after surgery. Iron deficiency is an expected outcome, and empiric postoperative supplementation is required. Up to 6% of patients, usually menstruating women, have serious anemia that requires parenteral iron or blood transfusion (28). The addition of several centimeters of duodenum in the DS for iron absorption has never been studied and is variable depending on how much proximal duodenum is actually maintained. In fact, Dolan et al. (10) found no difference in iron-deficiency anemia between BPD and BPD-DS patients (12.8% vs. 36.1%) (10).

Metabolic Bone Disease

Hypocalcemia is a well-recognized complication of malabsorptive operations. Marceau et al. (4) observed a 20% incidence of hypocalcemia, with 2% of patients suffering bone fractures per year. BPD patients appear to absorb 26% of ingested calcium (3). Malabsorption of vitamin D interferes with the intestinal absorption of calcium, leading to secondary hyperparathyroidism. Secondary hyperparathyroidism and osteomalacia has been reported previously after biliopancreatic diversion but the long-term sequelae are not known. Elevated parathyroid hormone (PTH) exceeding 100 mg/L associated with a rise in alkaline phosphatase coincides with bone demineralization. Despite prescribing patients oral calcium supplementation of 2 g/day and monthly intramuscular (IM) injections of 400,000 IU vitamin D (in addition to greater supplementation when needed), Scopinaro et al. (33) found that almost one third of their 252 patients had histomorphologic signs of bone demineralization on transiliac bone biopsy. Although it appeared to improve over time, 11% still had bone demineralization at 10 years, and 6% complained of bone pain. They also found that bone demineralization was worse in older and heavier patients. Four patients required surgical reversal to restore the duodenum into the absorptive limb for increased calcium absorption. Marceau et al. similarly found complaints of bone pain in 41% of BPD patients and 29% of DS patients. Murr et al. (8) found metabolic bone disease to affect 18% of their patients.

Slater et al. (37) found that 85% of 376 patients were hypocalcemic 1 year after surgery, and 52% remained hypocalcemic after 4 years. Over half the patients had elevated PTH up to 4 years, with 27% having PTH >100 mg/L. This is similar to the findings of Marceau et al. (4). However, only 4% had evidence of metabolic bone disease by year 4.

Fat-Soluble Vitamin Deficiency

Initial weight loss is attributable to moderate gastric restriction. However, weight loss durability is thought to be due to the malabsorption created by the diversion of pancreatic enzymes and bile from the alimentary tract and food bypassing the jejunum and proximal ileum. The last 50 to 100 cm of distal ileum, the common channel, is where food is exposed to bile and pancreatic enzymes. This results in absorption of only 28% of ingested fat (3). The fat-soluble vitamins (vitamins A, D, E, and K) have various levels of importance and are recognized in the literature only in situations in which metabolic sequelae are evident. This is reflected by the 37 cases of night blindness (2.8%) in 1344 BPD patients as observed by Scopinaro et al. (33), and by occasional case reports (38–40). Only one study has looked at the actual incidence of fat-soluble vitamin deficiencies in patients after malabsorptive operations. A combined study between Wesley Medical Center (Brisbane, Australia) and New York University School of Medicine (New York, NY) looked at 376 patients who had undergone malabsorptive operations within comprehensive bariatric programs (37). The study showed that despite aggressive nutritional counseling and empiric supplementation, the incidence of vitamin A deficiency increased with time such that 70% of patients were affected by the fourth postoperative year. Vitamin D was also found to be deficient in 57% at 1 year and in 63% by 4 years. Vitamin K deficiency was seen in 14% 1 year after surgery, but gradually increased to 42% by 4 years. Vitamin E deficiency was very low, affecting only 4% at 4 years. Although the benefits of zinc are not clearly defined, it was found to be abnormally low in over 50% of patients from year 1 to 4.

Conclusion

Laparoscopic malabsorption procedures offer effective weight loss. The relative value of reduced obesity-related comorbidity should be weighed against the significant long-term consequences of malabsorption. Due to the increased technical complexity of the procedures, the surgeon must have advanced laparoscopic skills to successfully perform them. With such a relatively high incidence of nutritional complications, the surgery must be performed within a comprehensive bariatric program that will offer lifelong patient follow-up.

References

1. Michielson D, Hendrickx L, van Hee R. Complications of biliopancreatic diversion surgery as proposed by Scopinaro in the treatment of morbid obesity. Obes Surg 1996;6: 416–420.
2. Nanni G, Balduzzi GF, Capoluongo R, et al. Biliopancreatic diversion: clinical experience. Obes Surg 1997;7:26–29.
3. Scopinaro N, Adami GF, Marinari GM, et al. Biliopancreatic diversion. World J. Surg 1998;22:936–946.
4. Marceau P, Hould FS, Simard S, et al. Biliopancreatic diversion with duodenal switch. World J.Surg 1998;22:947–954.
5. Noya G, Cossu ML, Coppola M, et al. Biliopancreatic diversion for treatment of morbid obesity: experience in 50 cases. Obes Surg 1998;8:61–66.
6. Rabkin RA. Distal gastric bypass/duodenal switch procedure, Roux-en Y gastric bypass and biliopancreatic diversion in a community practice. Obes Surg 1998;8:53–59.
7. Totte E, Hendrickx L, van Hee R. Biliopancreatic diversion for treatment of morbid obesity: experience in 180 consecutive cases. Obes Surg 1999;9:161–165.
8. Murr MM, Balsiger BM, Kennedy FP, et al. Malabsorptive procedures for severe obesity: comparison of pancreaticobiliary bypass and very very long limb Roux-en Y gastric bypass. J Gastrointest Surg 1999;3:607–612.
9. Bajardi G, Ricevuto G, Mastrandrea G, et al. Surgical treatment of morbid obesity with biliopancreatic diversion and gastric banding: report on an 8-year experience involving 235 cases. Ann Chir 2000;125:155–162.
10. Dolan K, Hatzifotis M, Newbury L, et al. A clinical and nutritional comparison of biliopancreatic diversion with and without duodenal switch. Ann Surg 2004;240(1):51–56.
11. Hess DS, Hess DW. Biliopancreatic diversion with a duodenal switch. Obes.Surg 1998;8:267–282.
12. Baltasar A, Bou R, Bengochea M, et al. Duodenal switch: an effective therapy for morbid obesity—intermediate results. Obes Surg 2001;11:54–58.
13. Anthone G. Malabsorptive Procedures. Boston: American Society for Bariatric Surgery, Essentials Course, June 2003.
14. Paiva D, Bernardes L, Suretti L. Laparoscopic biliopancreatic diversion for the treatment of morbid obesity: initial experience. Obes Surg 2002;12:358–361.
15. Scopinaro N, Marinari GM, Camerini G. Laparoscopic standard biliopancreatic diversion: technique and preliminary results. Obes Surg 2002;12:362–365.
16. Ren CJ, Patterson E, Gagner M. Early results of laparoscopic biliopancreatic diversion with duodenal switch for morbid obesity: a case series of 40 consecutive patients. Obes Surg 2000;10:514–523.
17. Baltasar A, Bou R, Miro J, et al. Laparoscopic biliopancreatic diversion with duodenal switch: technique and initial experience. Obes Surg 2002;12:245–248.
18. Rabkin RA, Rabkin JM, Metcalf B, et al. Laparoscopic technique for performing duodenal switch with gastric reduction. Obes Surg 2003;13:263–268.
19. Prem KA, Mensheha NM, McKelvey JL. Operative treatment of adenocarcinoma of the endometrium in obese women. Am J Obstet Gynecol 1965;92:16–22.
20. Fernandez AZ, DeMaria EJ, Tichansky DS, et al. Experience with over 3000 open and laparoscopic bariatric procedures: multivariate analysis of factors related to mortality and leak. Surg Endosc 2004;18(2):193–197.
21. Dolan K, Fielding G. Biliopancreatic diversion following failure of laparoscopic adjustable gastric banding. Surg Endosc 2004;18:45–47.
22. Wu EC, Barba CA. Current practices in the prophylaxis of venous thromboembolism in bariatric surgery. Obes Surg 2000;10:7–13.
23. Higa KD, Boone KB, Ho T, Davies OG. Laparoscopic Roux-en-Y gastric bypass for morbid obesity: technique and preliminary results of our first 400 patients. Arch Surg 2000;135:1029–1034.
24. Schauer PR, Ikramuddin S, Gourash WF, Ramanathan R, Luketich J. Outcomes after laparoscopic Roux-en-Y gastric bypass for morbid obesity. Ann Surg 2000;232:515–529.
25. Pelligrini CA, Patti MG, Lewin M, et al. Alkaline reflux gastritis and the effect of biliary diversion on gastric emptying of solid food. Am J Surg 1985;150:166.
26. Bell RH. Neoplasms of the exocrine pancreas. In: Bell RH, Rikkers LF, Mulholland MW, eds. Digestive Tract Surgery: A Text and Atlas, 1st ed. Philadelphia: Lippincott-Raven, 1996:867.
27. Bertolotto M, Gianetta E, Rollandi GA, et al. Imaging of patients with pancreaticobiliary diversion for obesity: postoperative anatomy and findings in small bowel obstruction. Br J Radiol 1996;69:708–716.
28. Marceau P, Hould FS, Lebel S, et al. Malabsorptive obesity surgery. Surg Clin North Am 2001;81:1113–1127.
29. Vanderhoof JA, Young RJ, Murray N, et al. Treatment strategies for small bowel bacterial overgrowth in short bowel syndrome. J Pediatr Gastroenterol Nutr 1998;27: 155–160.
30. Li M, Specian RE, Berg RD, et al. Effects of protein malnutrition and endotoxin on the intestinal mucosal barrier to

the translocation of indigenous flora in mice. J Parenter Enteral Nutr 1989;13:572–578.

31. Slocum MM, Sittig KM, Specian RD, et al. Absence of intestinal bile promotes bacterial translocation. Am Surg 1992;58:305–310.

32. Sedman PC, Macfie J, Sagar P, et al. The prevalence of gut translocation in humans. Gastroenterology 1994;107:643–649.

33. Scopinaro N, Adami GF, Marinari GM, et al. Biliopancreatic diversion: two decades of experience. In: Deitel M, Cowan G, eds. Update: Surgery for the Morbidly Obese Patient: The Field of Extreme Obesity Including Laparoscopy and Allied Care. Toronto: FD-Communications, 2000:227–258.

34. Brolin RE, Leung M. Survey of vitamin and mineral supplementation after gastric bypass and biliopancreatic diversion for morbid obesity. Obes Surg 1999;9(2):150–154.

35. Fox SR, Fox KS, Oh KH. The gastric bypass for failed bariatric surgical procedures. Obes Surg 1996;6:145–150.

36. Skroubis G, Sakellaropoulos G, Pouggouras K, et al. Comparison of nutritional deficiencies after Roux-en-Y gastric bypass and after biliopancreatic diversion with Roux-en-Y gastric bypass. Obes Surg 2002;12:551–558.

37. Slater G, Ren CJ, Siegel N, et al. Serum fat-soluble vitamin deficiency and abnormal calcium metabolism after malabsorptive bariatric surgery. J Gastrointest Surg 2004;8:48–55.

38. Smets RM, Waeben M. Unusual combination of night blindness and optic neuropathy after biliopancreatic bypass. Bull Soc Belge Ophtalmol 1999;271:93–96.

39. Huerta S, Rogers LM, Li Z, et al. Vitamin A deficiency in a newborn resulting from maternal hypovitaminosis A after biliopancreatic diversion for the treatment of morbid obesity. Am J Clin Nutr 2002;76(2):426–429.

40. Hatzifotis M, Dolan K, Newbury L, Fielding GA. Symptomatic vitamin A deficiency following biliopancreatic diversion. Obes Surg 2003;13(4):655–657.

22.6
Laparoscopic Malabsorption Procedures: Controversies

George A. Fielding

Since Scopinaro published his landmark paper on biliopancreatic bypass for obesity in 1979, this operation, now more commonly known as biliopancreatic diversion (BPD), has been surrounded by controversy (1). It carries perceptions of being more dangerous to perform than other procedures and of having more severe metabolic sequelae. Many surgeons have thought that it should be reserved as a revisional procedure or used to advantage only in the super-obese. But surgeons who perform the operation point to its proven track record in maintaining weight loss, which they cite as the most cogent reason to use BPD as a primary bariatric operation. This dichotomy may be best summed up in a communication by Scopinaro in response to an algorithm for selecting bariatric procedures written by Buchwald (2). Buchwald described the BPD as being popular in Italy. Scopinaro (3) replied, "The BPD was conceived in Italy and is popular everywhere."

There are elements of truth in both arguments—for and against. I will explore these controversies, as raised by the following questions:

- Should the BPD be a primary operation?
- Should the BPD be used only for the super-obese?
- When should the BPD be used as a revisional procedure?
- Is there a benefit in performing the duodenal switch rather than primary BPD?
- What is the place for BPD in Prader-Willi syndrome and in obese children?
- How does BPD affect pregnancy?

Should the Biliopancreatic Diversion Be a Primary Operation?

Does It Work?

The BPD is a very effective weight loss tool. Scopinaro et al.'s (4) data attest to the long-term maintenance of early weight loss. They have shown a mean permanent reduction of 75% of excess weight in 2241 patients during a 20-year period. The initial weight loss is rapid, probably due to restriction, and is maintained purely by malabsorption. It is maintained indefinitely, Scopinaro believes, because of the existence of a threshold absorption for fat and starch, which is compounded by increased resting energy expenditure. The BPD does not rely on restriction for maintenance of weight loss, as does the laparoscopic adjustable gastric band or Roux-en-Y gastric bypass (RYGBP).

The appeal of the BPD is not so much the magnitude of the weight loss but rather its maintenance. The bariatric surgery field is currently enamored with percentages and degrees of difference of excess weight loss, such as the distinctions among 55%, 65%, and 75%. There is little difference in actual weight lost by a 300-lb woman with a body mass index (BMI) of 48 who achieves 65% excess weight loss (EWL) versus 55% EWL. It represents about 16 lb, or $1^1/_2$ dress sizes. That difference has no further impact on the reduction of comorbidity, which will already have been reduced by this time. The actual numbers mean little if they are not maintained. The BPD has the greatest weight loss, maintained for the longest time.

Not all these patients lose a lot of weight (Table 22.6-1). Strangely enough, given the magnitude of the malabsorption with BPD, there is a substantial cohort of patients who fail to lose a large amount of weight with the BPD. Thirteen percent of Marceau et al.'s (5) patients lost less than 50% EWL. Marceau et al. found that only 41% BPD and 61% biliopancreatic diversion with duodenal switch (BPD-DS) had resolution of hunger after the surgery. Sanchez-Cabezudo and Larrad (6) reviewed 75 patients with 5-year follow-up after BPD and found nine (12%) had an EWL of less than 50% with a mean EWL of 36.9%. Patients who failed were statistically more likely to have lack of satiety and to be unmarried or unemployed. However, despite only achieving 36.9% EWL, most of these patients had at least an improvement in all preoperative comorbidities. In a series of BPD as revision for failed Lap-Band, 21% had failed ongoing

TABLE 22.6-1. Incidence of excess weight loss (EWL) <50%

First author (reference)	Common channel	Percent
Marceau (5)	100	13
Sanchez-Cabezudo (6)	100	12
Anthone (8) BMI ≥50	100	27
Anthone (8) BMI <50	100	18
Fielding (42) (revisions)	50	21

BMI, body mass index.

weight loss despite, in some cases, having a revision to only a 30-cm common channel (7). Anthone et al. (8), in a series of 701 BPD-DSs, found 18% of patients at 5 years had failed to maintain 50% EWL. In the group with a starting BMI >50, 27% had failed to maintain 50% EWL. In this group the BMI fell from 52 to 32 at 5 years. Once again there was a precipitous fall to 32 at 1 year, which was maintained at 5 years.

Is It a Safe Operation?

Until the recent advent of the laparoscopic adjustable gastric band, all bariatric surgery involved bowel surgery and bowel anastomoses of some kind. These carry an inherent risk of leak, sepsis, and death. In the hands of surgeons who are experienced in dealing with this difficult group of patients, the incidence of leak, sepsis, and death is relatively small. It is extremely small when one considers these patients' comorbidities; operative mortality ranges, in most large series, from 0.5% to 1.5%, compared to national averages for mortality from gastrectomy, pancreatectomy, and esophagectomy, which range from 8% to 10% in the United States, the United Kingdom, and other European countries (9,10).

Bariatric surgery is experiencing explosive growth. Over 100,000 patients have had a Lap-Band. There have been similar numbers of RYGBPs in the U.S. The 100,000 Lap-Band procedures have resulted in 34 procedure-related deaths (11). Several groups have published series of over 1000 cases without a death (12,13). Far fewer patients have had BPDs or BPD-DSs. As a way of interpreting the differences in risk, 100,000 RYGBPs or BPDs, which have a mortality of 0.5% to 1.5% in the best hands, would generate 500 to 1500 deaths, compared to the 34

in the Lap-Bands. In the super- and massively obese, the risk differential is even greater.

Operative Technique

There is no evidence that BPD per se is more dangerous an operation than a bypass when performed openly. Sarr et al. (14) compared 11 BPDs and 26 very, very long limb gastric bypasses in super-obese patients, and found no difference in morbidity or mortality.

Laparoscopic procedures may have different results. The key technical difference between the laparoscopic BPD and the laparoscopic RYGBP is that the Roux limb is distally based. Even though the gastric anastomosis is 14 to 15 cm more distal than in the RYGBP, the alimentary limb is fixed much more distally and to the right. Mobilization of the cecum and deeper division and thinning of the mesentery help bring the alimentary limb to the stomach. However, it can sometimes be very difficult to achieve a BPD anastomosis without tension by laparoscopic means.

Early results are promising for laparoscopic standard BPD (Table 22.6-2), as there has been no mortality in the first three small series. Paiva et al. (15) had a mean operating time of 210 minutes (range, 130 to 480) in 40 cases, and a mean BMI of 43 (range, 36 to 65) without conversion to an open procedure. Scopinaro et al. (16) converted five of 26 patients to an open procedure, with a mean BMI of 43 (range, 36 to 56). Fielding's group had a mean operating time of 181 minutes (range, 92 to 315) in 30 cases, with a mean BMI of 46 (range 30 to 67) with no conversions. Baltasar et al.'s (18) operating times ranged from 195 to 270 minutes in their first 16 cases, with a BMI of 43 to 56 for laparoscopic BPD-DS.

Super-obesity adds another degree of difficulty. The mesentery is thick and heavy, and the bowel is difficult to move in the cephalad direction, which can lead to longer operating times with an increased risk of deep vein thrombosis (DVT) and rhabdomyolysis. It also takes longer to perform the anastomoses under tension. There is solid evidence that laparoscopic BPD-DS is relatively dangerous in patients with a BMI over 60. Ren et al. (19), publishing Gagner's experience, showed the degree of difficulty added by super-obesity to laparoscopic BPD-DS, with a mean operating time of 210 minutes (range, 110 to 360) in 40 patients with one conversion, one

TABLE 22.6-2. Laparoscopic biliopancreatic diversion (BPD) and biliopancreatic diversion with duodenal switch (BPD-DS)

First author (reference)	Operation	n	BMI	Conversion to open procedure	Mean OR time (range)
Ren (19)	BPD-DS	40	60	2.5	210 (110–360)
Baltasar (18)	BPD-DS	26	45	0	(195–270)
Dolan (17)	BPD-DS	30	46	0	181 (92–315)
Paiva (15)	BPD	40	43	0	210 (130–480)
Scopinaro (16)	BPD	26	43	20.0	—
Dolan (17)	BPD	14	45	0	169 (140–239)

operative death, and one further in-hospital death, with a mean BMI of 60 (range, 42 to 85). However, laparoscopic Roux-en-Y is also more dangerous in this group of patients. Oliak et al. (20) had twice the rate of complications and 5% mortality, compared to 0.4%, in patients with a BMI >60. Fernandez et al. (21), reviewing Sugerman's extensive experience of over 3000 RYGBPs, found the leak and mortality rate was highest in male patients with a high BMI, which is similar to findings in laparoscopic BPD-DSs.

Laparoscopic BPD or BPD-DS is a long, complex, tiring, and challenging procedure. Surgeons must have a high degree of laparoscopic skill, particularly in manipulating the bowel and suturing. The benefits accrued, primarily in reduced wound complications and earlier return to normal activity, must be considered along with the disadvantages of a longer operating time with attendant complications.

Is It Safe in the Long Term?

The BPD seems to keep working in the long term, but at what cost? The debate is centered largely on anemia and protein malnutrition. Anemia is a fixed risk in this group of patients, particularly in menstruating women, and all patients should be prescribed iron supplementation (22). If iron levels remain low, patients need parenteral supplementation with either intramuscular or intravenous iron infusion. The protein malnutrition is dramatic. These patients become very cachectic and require intravenous feeding prior to limb lengthening or reversal of the BPD. However, the actual incidence is low and probably overstated by opponents of BPD (Table 22.6-3). Scopinaro et al. (4) reported this in 6% of patients that have a 50-cm common channel. Clare (23) reported 3.2%, Hess and Hess (24) 2.2%, and Marceau et al. (5) 0.9% per year with a 100-cm common channel. Anthone et al. (8) reported 5.5% with a 100-cm common channel at 5 years.

All authors stress the need for lifelong follow-up to assess nutritional status, and that lifelong maintenance of supplementation is mandatory.

The reality is that follow-up for these patients is often mediocre at best. Most large series report between 50% and 70% follow-up after 5 years (25,26). Scopinaro (27) would have us believe that this relatively low follow-up

rate is because all patients with a BPD are happy and thin. This may well be true. However, the concern is that they may be too thin and severely malnourished, and have vitamin deficiencies. This concern for long-term malnutrition has probably limited the broad adoption of BPD in the field of bariatric surgery.

We have previously shown only 80% compliance with supplementation in our patients despite maximum preoperative education and ongoing encouragement to take vitamins postoperatively (28). Furthermore, we recently documented vitamin levels in 4-year follow-up in a series of BPDs and found alarming levels of vitamin insufficiency, at 40% for vitamin A, D, and K, and for zinc and calcium (29). These deficiencies deteriorated further over time, and occurred despite intensive preoperative counseling and postoperative follow-up. Brolin et al. (30) had previously reported similar findings with distal Roux-en-Y bypass. They also carefully reviewed the estimates of bariatric surgeons about the degree of vitamin insufficiency in these patients (31). Alarmingly, most surgeons thought it was only 4% to 5%, rather than the roughly 40% that we have shown across the board for all the vitamins, zinc, and calcium. This is possibly an insurmountable problem, given the vagaries of human nature. Surgeons must have strategies in place to follow up and measure nutrient levels in these patients.

Should the Biliopancreatic Diversion Be Used Only for the Super-Obese?

There is a broadly held perception that the BPD is the procedure of choice for massive obesity. The landmark paper by Ren, Patterson, and Gagner (19) reported the high morbidity and mortality entailed in performing a BPD in patients with a BMI over 60. Gagner's group (32) and Anthone et al. (33) have suggested performing a sleeve gastrectomy alone, as an initial procedure, in these very big patients. This allows initial good weight loss by restriction alone. Once this restrictive loss stops, the patient can then return for a laparoscopic duodenal switch to allow ongoing weight loss by malabsorption. I have performed nine of these two-stage procedures; the second stage procedures with duodenal anastomoses have been very straightforward as laparoscopic techniques, with the weight loss resulting in great shrinkage of the liver, omentum, and mesentery, and making the bowel much more mobile. These developments, however, are predicated upon the belief that the BPD is the only satisfactory operation for super-obese patients. Advocates of the Lap-Band (34,35) and the RYGBP (36–38) for super-obesity would disagree, and they question the need for two procedures when, in their hands, one procedure has been shown to be very satisfactory in the majority of cases.

TABLE 22.6-3. Revision for malnutrition

First author (reference)	Common channel (cm)	Revision (%)
Clare (23)	100	3.2
Hess (24)	100	2.2
Marceau (5)	100	0.9
Anthone (8)	100	5.7
Scopinaro (4)	50	2.7
Dolan (17)	50	5.1

The advent of the Lap-Band has broadened the vision of bariatric surgery, showing that minimally invasive procedures have a place in the management of these patients. Gagner's group (39) is certainly no fan of the Lap-Band. However, they recently reported on five patients with mean BMI of 52 (range, 40 to 64) who had laparoscopic banding combined with duodenal switch, without gastrectomy, and showed satisfactory weight loss at 12 months (40). Yashkov et al. (41) previously described the same principle, adding a duodenal switch to a failed vertical banded gastroplasty (VBG).

I have a series of patients in whom this combination has been used to salvage a failed Lap-Band by adding the duodenal switch alone (seven patients) or to salvage a failed BPD by adding a Lap-Band to control hunger (seven patients). Eleven of 14 procedures were performed laparoscopically and three by open techniques. Standard BPD or BPD-DS has previously been used as revision for a failed band, but, like Gagner, I feel there is great benefit to be gained by eliminating gastric resection altogether (42). As he has said, "Even a sleeve gastrectomy carries morbidity with leak and stenosis" (40). I feel this combination therapy has real merit in revisional cases.

Stucki et al. (4) stated that the BPD is the only weight reduction method with no significant direct correlation between the initial and the final body weight. It has certainly been shown to be equally beneficial in the obese and super-obese. We have shown this in a series comparing BPD in the obese and the super-obese (43). In a group of 68 patients undergoing primary BPD between 1998 and 2002, 44 were morbidly obese, with a mean BMI of 42 (range, 33 to 49.9) and 24 were super-obese, with a mean BMI of 57 (range, 51 to 84). At 3 years the mean BMI fell to 27.5 in the obese group and 37 in the super-obese group. The %EWL was greater in the morbidly obese group compared to the super-obese group.

Perhaps more importantly, there was no significant difference in the incidence of vitamin, mineral, or protein deficiency in patients who are only morbidly obese. Further evidence for the safety of BPD in lower BMI patients exists in a series of 79 BPDs performed as revision for a failed Lap-Band (42). Two years after the procedure, the mean BMI of 37 in this group of 79 patients at the time of BPD had fallen to 29 and stabilized at that point.

We have seen no evidence that BPD in lower BMI patients has caused an increased incidence of malnutrition-based complications. In contrast, Sugerman et al. (44) concluded that the incidence of complications after BPD was too great to justify its use as a primary operation for treatment of patients with super-obesity. This has been an area of great controversy. Fobi's group (45) discussed revision of the standard Roux-en-Y to a distal Roux-en-Y, leaving a small gastric pouch rather than a BPD. The maintenance of adequate gastric size to allow adequate intake of a good protein meal is essential to the safe performance of BPD. Fox et al. (46) showed very worrying levels of malnutrition after revising a failed VBG to a BPD.

Biliopancreatic Diversion as Revision

The BPD is seen by some as an effective revisional procedure. There is, however, a caveat to this view: a malabsorptive operation superimposed on a tiny gastric pouch is a recipe for serious trouble. Scopinaro has warned of this, and, as previously mentioned, others who have revised an RYGBP to a distal RYGBP would agree with him. Furthermore, in a group of primary operations in massively obese individuals, Sarr et al. (14) reported that one patient died of liver failure and two became ill with metabolic bone disease in a group of 11 BPD patients at 8 years, compared to none in a group of 26 very, very long limb gastric bypasses (VVLGBs). In contrast, Brolin et al. (47) and Skroubis et al. (48) take a different view. They have not found increased nutritional complications with a distal RYGBP. Even though the BPD group lost more weight, the VVLGB group had equal resolution of its comorbidities. This is one of the main issues for the RYGBP—how to revise a failure.

This issue is most certainly not the case with the Lap-Band. One of the great advantages of the band is its ease of removal. Despite what Gagner and others have said about the difficulties of laparoscopic removal of a Lap-Band, it is a very straightforward procedure (22). This leaves virtually the whole stomach untouched and available for use in a BPD if desired. There is no doubt that if one's preference is for a sleeve gastrectomy, then the very apex of the sleeve can involve some of the fibrous tissue. The answer surely is to use a different procedure in that setting. As discussed, that can either be a standard BPD, well away from the area of the band, or simply a loosening of the band and performing a duodenal switch. With a normal adequate volume stomach, the BPD is an ideal revisional procedure. There is no evidence that it is dangerous to perform a BPD in this setting. I have performed 79 such procedures after a Lap-Band, 59 of which were completed laparoscopically with minimal morbidity (42). A further 20 had an open procedure, following previous VBG, and then a band. These cases had higher morbidity but no mortality. I no longer band previous VBG. Lemmens (49) has had a similar experience with 37 BPDs, as revision for 20 failed VBG and 17 bands, in a series of 1620 BPDs. There were no deaths, three leaks, three cases of malnutrition needing common channel lengthening, and five patients who did not lose weight

In time there will be two camps in bariatric surgery: those who believe that the Roux-en-Y is the answer to everything, and those who see a combination of a band as a primary procedure due to its inherent great safety, followed by some version of a BPD if the band fails. In my experience in 7 years with over 1600 bands, the incidence of band removal is 5.5%.

Biliopancreatic Diversion Versus Biliopancreatic Diversion with Duodenal Switch

Much has been made of the supposed benefits of the duodenal switch variant of the BPD over the standard BPD. Marceau et al. (5) and Hess (24) presented strong arguments in favor of the use of this procedure in an attempt to reduce protein malnutrition and iron deficiency anemia. Ren's group (19) first published Gagner's experience with the laparoscopic variant of this operation.

More recently Anthone et al. (8) presented the large experience from the University of Southern California (Los Angeles, CA). As with all American surgeons who have published on the duodenal switch, a 100-cm common channel was used in distinction to the European, Scopinaro-based, 50-cm channel. It was thought that this would improve malnutrition in these patients. This excellent series of 701 patients outlines all the dilemmas of the argument for performing DS versus BPD. It also illustrates some of the realities of BPD as a primary operation:

1. This procedure is major bowel surgery. There is a 1.4% mortality (10 of 701 patients died). Twenty-one further patients had significant nonfatal complications. All the usual culprits are present: pulmonary embolus, pneumonia, rhabdomyolysis, duodenal stump leak, gastric leak and anastomotic leaks, bleeding, and splenectomy.

2. There is a different outcome in patients with a BMI <50 and patients with a BMI ≥50. In the first group there is a 70% EWL at 5 years, with a BMI of 28. In the second group there is a 63% EWL at 5 years and a BMI of 36. In fact, in this group the BMI stabilized at 36 at 12 months and did not change over the next 4 years. Overall at 5 years for the total group there is an EWL of 65%, and the BMI remained at 31 for 1 to 5 years. In this large series, the BPD-DS did not provide any particular advantage in the super-obese.

The duodenal switch has been advocated primarily as a way of reducing anemia and protein malnutrition. The evidence in these 701 cases is that this is not the case. Forty-eight percent of patients were anemic with a duodenal switch with a 100-cm common channel. The results for serum albumin in these patients reflect, as already mentioned, that the actual incidence of protein malnutrition is low, at about 2%. Despite the use of a duodenal switch, revisional surgery to lengthen the common channel was necessary in 40 patients (5.7%) due to overt malnutrition in 34, persistent diarrhea in four, and chronic pain in two.

We have found similar results in Brisbane, after comparing 73 patients with standard BPD and 61 patients with duodenal switch, both groups with a 50-cm common channel (17). We found no evidence of any improvement in weight loss or lessening of gastrointestinal or nutritional side effects of BPD by the use of the duodenal switch at a median follow-up of 28 months. The EWL at 36 months was 72% and the mean BMI was 31.5 in both groups. There was no difference in meal size, intake of fats, nausea or vomiting, diarrhea, or nutritional parameters. Eighty percent confirmed compliance with vitamin supplementation. In the group as a whole 18% of patients were low in albumin, 32% were anemic, 25% were hypocalcemic, and nearly 50% had low vitamin A, D, and K. Seven patients required shortening of the common channel due to insufficient weight loss following BPD compared with eight patients following BPD-DS (9.6% and 13.1%). Four patients required lengthening of their common channel due to excessive weight loss with BPD compared to three patients with BPD-DS. There was once again no difference between BPD and BPD-DS.

There are significant technical issues with the BPD-DS. The one possible benefit, as pointed out by Anthone, is that the anastomosis, when done as an open procedure, is probably a lot easier, as the anastomosis is almost completely without tension. However, this advantage is counterbalanced by the difficulty of achieving a good sleeve gastrectomy in the open approach toward the top of the stomach, as evidenced by Anthone et al.'s incidence of splenectomy. In the laparoscopic approach, mobilization and division of the duodenum, while preserving its blood supply and dissecting the duodenum off the pancreas in obese patients, can be challenging. The anastomosis can also be difficult, performed at the end of what can be a long, tiring procedure. Furthermore, a heavy, fat-laden colon can make visualizing the duodenum difficult.

The anastomosis has been performed by transoral end-to-end anastomosis (EEA), side-to-side gastrointestinal anastomosis (GIA), laparoscopic hand sewn, and laparoscopic-assisted, using a small incision to perform the anastomosis (50). The last option has real merit. I have occasionally used a small subcostal incision, which provides good visualization, has minimal morbidity, and virtually never herniates. Jones (51) has been recommending this approach for years.

The BPD-DS has prompted rapidly increasing interest in the United States. This interest has been, to a significant extent, Internet driven, based on a perception of the sanctity of the pylorus. There is little evidence to suggest that BPD-DS confers any functional advantage over a standard BPD. I no longer perform BPD-DS with sleeve gastrectomy, having found the laparoscopic standard BPD to be a much more straightforward procedure, with exactly the same functional outcome as BPD-DS.

What Is the Place for Biliopancreatic Diversion in Prader-Willi Syndrome and in Obese Children?

There is little data on bariatric surgery for children. Until recently the procedure of choice in the U.S. has been RYGBP. Brolin's group (52), Sugerman et al. (53), and Endres and Wittgrove (54) have all shown good results with RYGBP. We have recently reported a series of Lap-Bands in this group with comparable results (55). Sugerman et al. describe doing three distal gastric bypasses in their series, one of which was revised for malnutrition. I have found only one published report of BPDs in children: Breaux (56) reported four BPDs in a group of 22 children aged 8 to 18 with very severe obesity, many of whom also had severe sleep apnea. The patients did well from a weight loss point of view, but three of the four BPDs developed protein deficiency, and all four patients developed either vitamin A and D deficiency or folate deficiency. There were also two late deaths at 15 months and 3.5 years.

It is difficult to see any place for BPD, in any of its forms, for children or adolescents. Compliance is always an issue in any form of bariatric surgery with children, and certainly compliance with multiple levels of supplementation would be extremely difficult in this group.

Another area of conflict in children is in the use of BPD in Prader-Willi syndrome. Advocates for BPD in these patients include Antal and Levin (57) and Scopinaro's group (58). Even though there was weight regain in Scopinaro's group at 10 years, the EWL was maintained at 40%, an excellent result for this difficult group of patients.

Grugni et al. (59) presented a case report with complete weight regain at 3 years combined with anemia, hyperproteinemia, and diarrhea. The lack of compliance in voluntary food restriction suggests that restrictive procedures have no part to play in this group of patients, and there is no definitive answer regarding the correct approach.

Pregnancy

Contraception is a major issue after BPD. Fertility increases after BPD, as it does after all weight loss procedures. Oral contraception may be variable due to very little absorption. Gerrits et al. (60) from Belgium reported that two of nine patients on oral contraception after BPD became pregnant. Most practitioners counsel against patients becoming pregnant during the first year after BPD due to the rapid weight loss and almost certain associated anemia and folate deficiency, with predisposition to spinal cord abnormalities. Scopinaro's group (61) found that 21% of 239 pregnant patients required parenteral nutritional support during their pregnancy and 27.8% of the infants were small for gestational age. Patients must be counseled preoperatively about the increased risk of pregnancy and about the variability of contraception.

References

1. Scopinaro N, Gianette E, Civalleri D. Biliopancreatic bypass for obesity: II. Initial experiences in man. Br J Surg 1979; 66:618–620.
2. Buchwald H. A bariatric surgery algorithm. Obes Surg 2002;12(6):733–746.
3. Scopinaro N. Comments to presidential address: gastric bypass and biliopancreatic diversion operations. Obes Surg 2002;12:881–883.
4. Scopinaro N, Adami GF, Marinari GM, et al. Biliopancreatic diversion. World J Surg 1998;22(9):936–946.
5. Marceau P, Hould F-S, Simard S, et al. Biliopancreatic diversion with duodenal switch. World J Surg 1998;22:947–954.
6. Sanchez-Cabezudo DC, Larrad JA. Analysis of weight loss with the biliopancreatic diversion of Larrad: absolute failures or relative successes? Obes Surg 2002;12(2):253.
7. Slater GH, Duncombe J, Fielding GA. Poor weight loss after revised bilio-pancreatic diversion for laparoscopic gastric band failure: an analysis of 18 cases. Surg Obes Relat Dis 2005;1:573–579.
8. Anthone GA, Lord RNV, DeMeester TR, et al. The Duodenal Switch Operation for the Treatment of Morbid Obesity: A 10-Year Experience. Presented at American Society for Bariatric Surgery (ASBS) Essentials in Bariatric Surgery, Course, Boston, MA: 2003.
9. Goodney PP, Siewers AE, Stukel TA, et al. Is Surgery getting safer? National trends in operative mortality. J Am Coll Surg 2002;195(2):219–227.
10. Grossmann EM, Longo WE, Virgo KS. Morbidity and mortality of gastrectomy for cancer in Department of Veterans Affairs Medical Centers. Surgery 2002;131(5):484–490.
11. O'Brien PE, Dixon JB. Weight loss and early and late complications—the international experience. Am J Surg 2002;184(6B):42S–45S.
12. Angrisani L, Alkilani M, Basso N, et al. Laparoscopic Italian experience with the Lap Band. Obes Surg 2001;11(3):307–310.
13. Weiner R, Blanco-Eugert R, Weiner S, et al. Outcome after laparoscopic adjustable gastric banding—8 years' experience. Obes Surg 2003;13(3):427–434.
14. Sarr MG, Felty CL, Hilmer DM, et al. Technical and practical considerations involved in operations on patients weighing more than 270 kg. Arch Surg 1995;130(1):L102–105.

15. Paiva D, Bernardes L, Suretti L. Laparoscopic biliopancreatic diversion: technique and initial results. Obes Surg 2002; 12(3):358–361.

16. Scopinaro N, Marinari GM, Camerini G. Laparoscopic standard biliopancreatic diversion: technique and preliminary results. Obes Surg 2002;12(3):362–365.

17. Dolan K, Hatzifotis M, Newbury L, Lowe N, Fielding G. A clinical and nutritional comparison of biliopancreatic diversion with and without duodenal switch. Ann Surg 2004;240: 51–56.

18. Baltasar A, Bou R, Miro J, et al. Laparoscopic biliopancreatic diversion with duodenal switch: technique and initial experience. Obes Surg 2002;12:245–248.

19. Ren C, Patterson E, Gagner M. Early results of laparoscopic bilio-pancreatic diversion with duodenal switch. Obes Surg 2000;10:514–523.

20. Oliak D, Ballantyne GH, Davies RJ. Short-term results of laparoscopic gastric bypass in patients with BMI ≥60. Obes Surg 2002;12:643–647.

21. Fernandez AZ, DeMaria EJ, Tichansky DS, et al. Experience with over 3000 open and laparoscopic bariatric procedures: multivariate analysis of factors related to mortality and leak. Surg Endosc 2003;17(suppl).

22. Stucki A, Grob JP, Chapuis G, et al. Biliopancreatic bypass and disorders of iron absorption. Schweiz Med Wochenschr 1991;121(50):1894–1896.

23. Clare MW. An analysis of 37 reversals on 504 biliopancreatic surgeries over 12 years. Obes Surg 1993;3:169–173.

24. Hess DW, Hess DS. Biliopancreatic diversion with a duodenal switch. Obes Surg 1998;8:267–282.

25. Jones KB. Quo Vadis? Obes Surg 2002;12:617–622.

26. Brolin RE, Gorman RC, Milgrim LM, et al. Multivitamin prophylaxis in prevention of post-gastric bypass vitamin and mineral deficiencies. Int J Obes 1991;15:661–668.

27. Scopinaro N. Comments to presidential address: gastric bypass and biliopancreatic diversion operations. Obes Surg 2002;12:881–884.

28. Newbury L, Dolan K, Hatzifotis M, et al. Calcium, vitamin D, alkaline phosphatase and parathyroid hormone following pancreatico-biliary diversion. Obes Surg 2003;13: 893–895.

29. Slater GH, Ren CJ, Siegel N, et al. Serum fat-soluble vitamin deficiency and abnormal calcium metabolism after malabsorptive bariatric surgery. J Gastrointest Surg 2004; 8:48–55.

30. Brolin RE, Gorman JH, Gorman RC, et al. Prophylactic iron supplementation after Roux-en-Y gastric bypass: a prospective, double-blind, randomized study. Arch Surg 1998;133:740–744.

31. Brolin RE, Leung M. Survey of vitamin and mineral supplementation after gastric bypass and biliopancreatic diversion for morbid obesity. Obes Surg 1999;9(2):150–154.

32. Chu CA, Gagner M, Quinn T, et al. Two-stage laparoscopic biliopancreatic diversion with duodenal switch: an alternative approach to super-super morbid obesity. Surg Endosc 2002;16:S187–S231.

33. Anthone G, Lord R, Almogy G, et al. Gastrectomy alone as surgical treatment for morbid and super-morbid obesity. Obes Surg 2003;13:209–210.

34. Dixon JB, O'Brien P. Selecting the optimal patient for lapband placement. Am J Surg 2002;184:175–205.

35. Fielding GA. Laparoscopic adjustable gastric banding for massive super obesity BMI >60. Surg Endosc 2003;17:1541–1545.

36. Gibbs K, White N, Vaimakis S, et al. Laparoscopic gastric bypass in the "massive superobese." Obes Surg 2003;13: 221–222.

37. Schauer PR, Ikramuddin S, Gourash W, et al. Outcomes after laparoscopic Roux-en-Y gastric bypass for morbid obesity. Ann Surg 2000;232:515–529.

38. DeMaria EJ, Sugerman HJ, Kellum JM, et al. Results of 281 consecutive total laparoscopic Roux-en-Y gastric bypasses to treat morbid obesity. Ann Surg 2002;235:640–647.

39. De Csepel J, Quinn T, Pomp A, Gagner M. Conversion to a laparoscopic biliopancreatic diversion with a duodenal switch for a failed laparoscopic adjustable silicone gastric banding. J Laparoendosc Adv Surg Tech A 2002;12(4):237–240.

40. Gagner M, Steffen R, Biertho L, et al. Laparoscopic adjustable gastric banding with duodenal switch for morbid obesity: technique and preliminary results. Obes Surg 2003;13:444–449.

41. Yashkov YI, Oppel TA, Shishlo LA, et al. Improvement of weight loss and metabolic effects of vertical banded gastroplasty by an added duodenal switch procedure. Obes Surg 2001;11:635–639.

42. Dolan K, Fielding G. Bilio pancreatic diversion following failure of laparoscopic adjustable gastric banding. Surg Endosc 2004;18:60–63.

43. Dolan K, Hatzifotis M, Newbury L, Fielding G. A comparison of laparoscopic adjustable gastric banding and biliopancreatic diversion in superobesity. Obes Surg 2004;14: 165–169.

44. Sugerman HJ, Kellum JM, Engle K, et al. Randomized trial of proximal and distal gastric bypass in the super-obese: early results [abstract]. Presented at the 4th International Symposium on Obesity Surgery, London, UK, August 24, 1989.

45. Fobi M, Lee H, Igwe D, et al. Revision of failed gastric bypass to distal Roux-en-Y gastric bypass: a review of 65 cases. Obes Surg 2001;11:190–195.

46. Fox SR, Fox KS, Oh KH. The gastric bypass for failed bariatric surgical procedures. Obes Surg 1996;6:145–150.

47. Brolin RE, Kenler HA, Gorman JH, et al. Long-limb gastric bypass in the superobese. A prospective randomized study. Ann Surg 1992;21:387–395.

48. Skroubis G, Sakellaropoulos G, Pouggouras K, et al. Comparison of nutritional deficiencies after Roux-en-Y gastric bypass and after biliopancreatic diversion with Roux-en-Y gastric bypass. Obes Surg 2002;12:551–558.

49. Lemmens L. Biliopancreatic diversion as a redo operation for failed restrictive gastric surgery. Obes Surg 2002;12: 479.

50. Rabkin RA, Rabkin JM, Metcalf B, et al. Laparoscopic technique for performing duodenal switch with gastric reduction. Obes Surg 2003;13:263–268.

51. Jones KB. The superiority of the left subcostal incision compared to mid-line incisions in surgery for morbid obesity. Obes Surg 1993;3:201–205.
52. Strauss RS, Bradley LJ, Brolin RE. Gastric bypass surgery in adolescents with morbid obesity. J Pediatr 2000;138:499–504.
53. Sugerman HJ, Sugerman EL, DeMaria EJ, et al. Bariatric surgery for severely obese adolescents. J Gastrointest Surg 2003;7:102–108.
54. Endres JE, Wittgrove AC. Laparoscopic Roux-en-Y gastric bypass in adolescents. Obes Surg 2003;13:206.
55. Dolan K, Creighton L, Hopkins G, et al. Laparoscopic gastric banding for morbidly obese adolescents. Obes Surg 2003;13:101–104.
56. Breaux CW. Obesity surgery in children. Obes Surg 1995;5: 279–284.
57. Antal S, Levin H. Biliopancreatic diversion in Prader-Willi syndrome associated with obesity. Obes Surg 1996;6:58–62.
58. Marinari GM, Camerini G, Novelli GB, et al. Outcome of biliopancreatic diversion in subjects with Prader-Willi syndrome. Obes Surg 2001;11:491–495.
59. Grugni G, Guzzaloni G, Morabito F. Failure of biliopancreatic diversion in Prader-Willi syndrome. Obes Surg 2000; 10:179–181.
60. Gerrits EG, Ceulemans R, van Hee R, et al. Contraceptive treatment after biliopancreatic diversion needs consensus. Obes Surg 2003;13:378–382.
61. Friedman D, Cuneo S, Valenzano M, et al. Pregnancies in an 18-year follow-up after biliopancreatic diversion. Obes Surg 1995;5:308–313.

23
Hand-Assisted Laparoscopic Bariatric Surgery

Dean J. Mikami and W. Scott Melvin

Surgery for the treatment of morbid obesity provides long-term relief for weight-related diseases. It is currently recognized as a safe and effective treatment for patients with a body mass index (BMI) greater than or equal to 35. The advancement of laparoscopic and video instrumentation and technology has allowed the application of minimally invasive surgical techniques to bariatric surgery. Currently, laparoscopic approaches provide a recognized advantage to surgery for obesity, and specifically the laparoscopic Roux-en-Y gastric bypass has been demonstrated to provide optimal outcomes in selected patients. However, laparoscopic bariatric surgery remains challenging. These challenges include difficulty in access, retraction, tissue manipulation, and identifying anatomic landmarks. These challenges make laparoscopic bariatric surgery difficult to learn and difficult for surgeons who lack an experienced assistant. Hand-assisted laparoscopic surgery (HALS) is an effective technique, applicable on a wide variety of advanced laparoscopic procedures (1). It provides the benefits of precise tissue manipulation, tactile feedback, blunt tissue dissection, and retraction, and it can be a valuable tool for the transition into and completion of minimally invasive bariatric surgery.

Hand-assisted laparoscopic surgery requires specialized instrumentation that allows access to the abdominal cavity by the surgeon's hand, while maintaining a pressure-tight seal to maintain pneumoperitoneum. Additional advantages are realized if other instruments or hands can be exchanged easily without losing pressure and with no pressure loss.

Hand-assisted laparoscopic surgery and minimally invasive approaches for bariatric surgery can be individualized for the unique situation of each surgeon, patient, and institution. Hand-assisted laparoscopic surgery is an effective and beneficial technique when applied selectively in bariatric surgery. We would select HALS in several situations, including surgeons early in the learning curve, a surgeon operating alone without a skilled assistant, in a difficult patient, and as a salvage technique prior to conversion to an open surgery.

During the development and application of a totally laparoscopic technique in bariatric surgery, we chose HALS as an enabling technique to facilitate laparoscopic bariatric surgery. The technique as described here enables the completion of a Roux-en-Y gastric bypass using single-surgeon techniques and incorporating many of the techniques used by the experienced open bariatric surgeon. Exposure of the proximal stomach, identification and blunt dissection in the lesser sac, and identification of the ligament of Treitz and the proximal jejunum are aided by HALS. Bowel approximation and manipulation of the stapling devices by the sensation of tactile feedback and subsequent manipulation of the operating surgeon's hands allows for a more efficient operation. Even correct placement of a nasogastric tube is aided by HALS. Initially, our program sought to reproduce our generally good results, including low mortality and leak rates, which were seen with open surgery. Our goal by adding HALS was to reduce our wound-related complications and speed recovery.

The additional value of HALS was seen by the application of minimally invasive surgical techniques to a patient population that included the super-obese. In our first series, the average BMI of patients treated was over 55 (2). Initial experience was also gained with a surgeon performing gastric bypass with only resident staff or fellowship-level trainees with little experience in bariatric surgery. The skills and experience gained in HALS bariatric surgery was subsequently applied to totally laparoscopic bariatric surgical techniques and continues to be refined with practice. As experience has been gained, HALS is now rarely the first approach for most patients requiring bariatric surgery.

The HALS technique is selected in several other situations. These include reoperative surgery or for super-obese patients in whom HALS may provide an advantage for surgeons early in their experience with these difficult cases.

Numerous hand-assisted abdominal procedures have been reported in the literature. A review by Kurian et al. (3) demonstrated more than 100 cases managed by the use of the hand-assisted technique. Hand-assisted laparoscopic surgery allows for direct manipulation of tissues by a surgeon's hand. In situations in which visibility is sometimes limited due to patient body habitus or difficult exposure, the sense of palpation and the direct manipulation of the tissues are greatly increased by HALS.

As a bridge to a total laparoscopic approach, hand-assisted Roux-en-Y gastric bypass can be as effective as open surgery in terms of weight loss and has been shown to have a lower complication rate (4). Hand-assisted laparoscopy allows surgeons to use their nondominant hand to manipulate and retract tissue, which is much easier than in traditional laparoscopic surgery. In the total laparoscopic techniques, both the surgeon and the assistant need to be well trained in advanced laparoscopic procedures. The HALS approach can serve as a stepping stone from the open to the total laparoscopic approach. The hand-assisted approach has been shown to be associated with shorter operative times when compared with a total laparoscopic approach in surgeons learning to perform gastric bypass surgery (2).

Equipment

There are multiple hand-assisted devices available in the United States. Those that are approved by the Food and Drug Administration include the Pneumo Sleeve (Dexterity, Atlanta, GA), the HandPort (Smith and Nephew, Andover, MA), the Intromit (MedTech, Dublin, Ireland), the Gel Port (Applied Medical, Rancho Santa Margarita, CA), and the Lapdisk (Johnson & Johnson, Cincinnati, OH). The different devices vary in their application and setup. The basic theory behind hand ports is to prevent the loss of pneumoperitoneum and to aid in hand exchange. In a study by Stielman (5), different kinds of hand ports were randomized and prospectively compared in a series of 133 porcine nephrectomies. In the study, the Intromit was rated the best in terms of instructions, overall design, and overall satisfaction. It had a failure rate of 15%, which was defined as a leak around the port site. The HandPort was rated as the easiest to set up, but it had the highest rate of failure at 27%. The Pneumo Sleeve, which was the first device available in the United States, had the lowest incidence of failure at 13%. The study concluded that all three devices were effective but each had their specific advantages and disadvantages.

Methods: Operative Technique for Hand-Assisted Roux-en-Y Gastric Bypass

The protocol and technique we use are comparable with those of many centers across the United States. Patients are administered 2 g of cefazolin and 5000 units of subcutaneous heparin approximately 30 minutes before the start of the operation. For patients with penicillin allergies, 900 mg of clindamycin is substituted. All patients wear intermittent lower leg venous compression devices during the entire procedure as well as postoperatively.

Patients are placed in the supine position. After induction of general anesthesia, a Foley catheter is placed. A 1-cm supraumbilical incision is made. A Veress needle is used in the standard fashion to obtain pneumoperitoneum. Next, a 10-mm trocar is placed in the supraumbilical position. Additional trocars are then placed under direct vision (Fig. 23-1). A 15-mm trocar is placed in the right upper quadrant near the midclavicular line. We first complete an exploration of the abdomen to be sure there is no abnormal pathology. The hand-assist device is then applied to the distended abdomen over the supraumbilical port (Fig. 23-2).

The greater omentum and transverse colon are then reflected cephalad to expose the ligament of Treitz. The small bowel is then traced back about 30 cm from the ligament of Treitz to a redundant portion of bowel that would easily reach up to the gastroesophageal (GE) junction. A 60 mm linear stapling device with a 2.5 mm staple load is then used to transect the bowel at this point. A 2.0-mm/45-mm load is then used to further transect the mesentery. A Penrose drain is sutured to the distal stapled end to allow

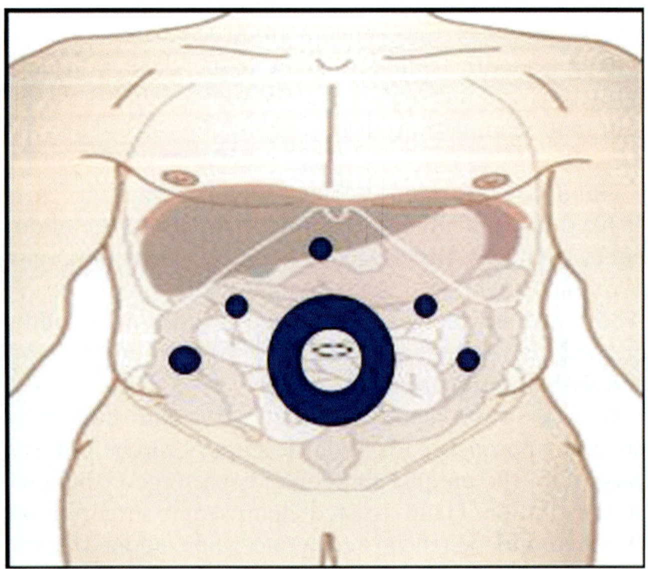

FIGURE 23-1. Diagram demonstrating port placement for the hand-assisted laparoscopic gastric bypass.

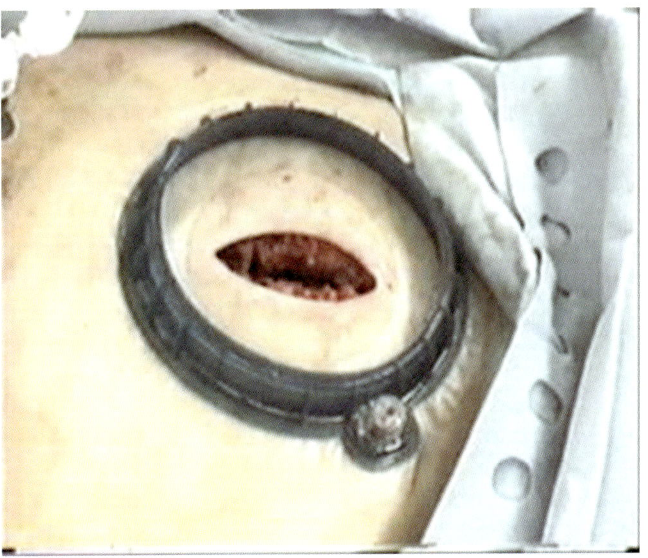

FIGURE 23-2. Pneumo Sleeve device on the patient abdomen.

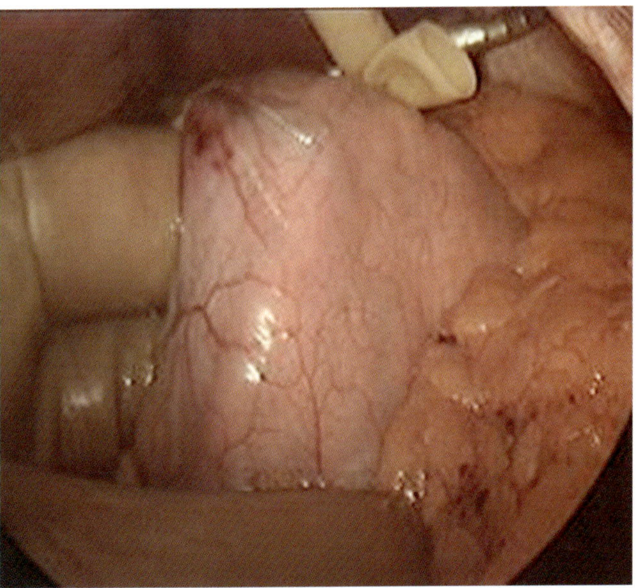

FIGURE 23-3. The surgeon's nondominant hand is inserted through the hand port. With blunt dissection, a window is created posterior to the stomach to allow for the creation of the gastric pouch.

for easy identification. The small bowel is then measured 150 cm distally. Bowel continuity is reestablished with a stapled side-to-side jejunojejunostomy using 2.5-mm/60-mm staple loads. The mesenteric defect is oversewn, and stay sutures are placed to avoid torsion of the anastomosis. Intracorporeal suturing is facilitated with standard sutures and a laparoscopic needle holder. The knots are tied intracorporeally with the inserted nondominant hand. The Roux limb is then traced back to the Penrose drain to make sure that it has not twisted.

Once the small bowel anastomosis is completed, the greater omentum is then divided up to the transverse colon to make room for an antecolic/antegastric Roux limb. Alternatively, a retrocolic passage of the limb can be facilitated with the nondominant hand elevating the transverse colon and palpating a thin portion in the mesocolon. A window is then created and the jejunal limb passed through the mesocolon to the lesser sac for positioning of the gastrojejunostomy. The liver retractor is then inserted and the liver is then retracted to expose the esophageal hiatus. The orogastric tube is removed at this point. Attention is then turned to the gastroesophageal junction, and this area is then dissected under direct visualization (Fig. 23-3).

Next, a point is selected on the anterior lesser curvature of the stomach just distal to the fat pad overlying the GE junction. This is the area from which the anvil is to exit. Just distal to this selected point, a window is created with blunt finger dissection posterior to the stomach from the lesser curvature to the greater curvature. This is done to preserve the neurovascular supply to the distal stomach. We prefer to create the gastrojejunostomy using a circular 25-mm stapler placed through the 15-mm right upper quadrant port. The anvil is then placed into the proximal stomach through a distal gastrostomy made

before creation of the pouch, or more commonly, when using the hand-assisted technique, by making a small gastrostomy and placing a purse-string suture with a laparoscopic needle driver and tied with the inserted hand.

The stomach pouch is created with multiple fires from a reticulating 3.5-mm/45-mm linear stapling device. Multiple firings are then performed in a curvilinear fashion up to the angle of His to completely transect the stomach and create a 30-mL gastric pouch (Fig. 23-4). The

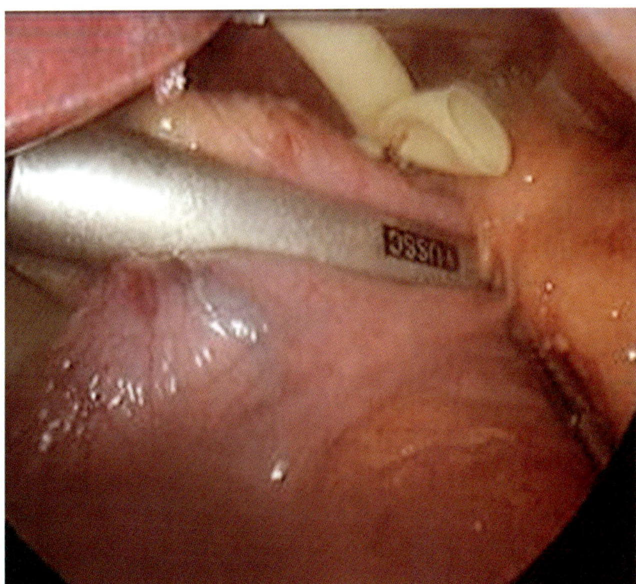

FIGURE 23-4. The creation of the gastric pouch using the linear 45-mm U.S. Surgical (Norwalk, CT) stapling device is demonstrated.

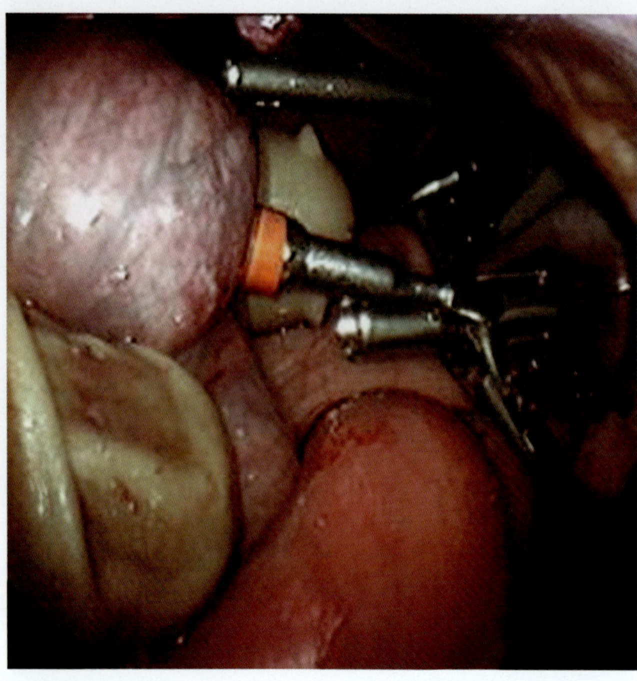

FIGURE 23-5. A 25-mm U.S. Surgical end-to-end anastomosis (EEA) stapler is used to create an end-to-side anastomosis with the jejunum and the gastric pouch.

surgeon's nondominant hand is used to guide the stapler into place.

Finally, the Roux limb is brought up to the anvil. The mesentery is further taken down with the ultrasonic shears. The staple line on the Roux-en-Y limb is also opened with the ultrasonic shears. The 25-mm end-to-end

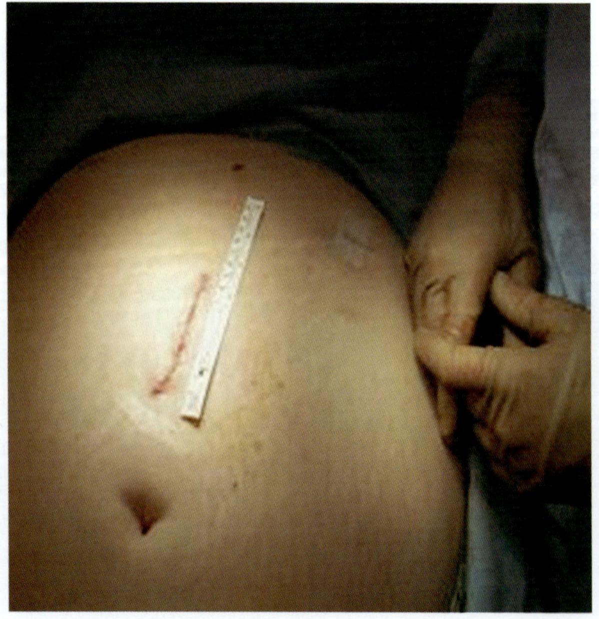

FIGURE 23-6. The final appearance of the hand port site. The length of the incision is 7 cm.

anastomosis (EEA) stapler is then inserted into the lumen of the Roux limb (Fig. 23-5). The remaining enterotomy of the Roux limb is then closed with a firing of a 2.5-mm/60-mm stapling device. A stitch is placed laterally on each side of the anastomosis to remove tension from and reinforce the staple line. The hand port is then removed and the incisions are closed appropriately. The incision used for the hand port is generally 6 to 8 cm in size (Fig. 23-6).

Discussion

At the Ohio State Medical Center we conducted a study comparing patients undergoing Roux-en-Y gastric bypass for morbid obesity. There were 40 hand-assisted cases compared with 80 open cases (4). The overall rate of wound infections is similar; however, fewer patients required reoperations in the first month in the hand-assisted Roux-en-Y gastric bypass group. After a learning curve of 10 cases, the operation times in the open and the hand-assisted groups were similar. Weight loss in the early postoperative period appears to be excellent in both groups, and almost all patients reported being satisfied with the outcome of their operations. Hand-assisted Roux-en-Y gastric bypass surgery may be associated with lower cost when postoperative complications are factored in. We concluded that the hand-assisted approach was associated with shorter operative times, improved tactile sensation, and reduced wound complications.

When first learning the technique of Roux-en-Y gastric bypass, tactile feedback to ensure anastomotic integrity is important. The hand-assisted device allows the surgeon to have more control over the operation and provides the ability to both visualize and feel the operation. Hand-assisted laparoscopy also allows intracorporeal suturing and knot tying, which can be a difficult skill to master laparoscopically. Naitoh et al. (6) demonstrated that hand-assisted laparoscopic digestive surgery provides improved safety for patients undergoing surgery for malignancy or obesity. In the study, the average length of incision for the hand port was 7.8 cm.

With the rapid advancement of laparoscopic instrumentation, totally laparoscopic Roux-en-Y gastric bypasses are performed routinely. We are currently offering gastric bypass completely laparoscopically as the first treatment option. With the aid of the hand port, the transition from open to total laparoscopic Roux-en-Y gastric bypass surgery is easier (7). The key for some surgeons is to do this procedure open at first, learn the skills needed to complete the operation safely, and then proceed laparoscopically with or without the assistance of the hand port.

Once the laparoscopic Roux-en-Y gastric bypass is mastered, the hand-assisted technique is still a valuable skill to have. This technique can be used if the surgeon thinks that there may be a need to convert to an open operation. Many times, just having one hand to retract or control bleeding is enough to complete he operation without opening.

Conclusion

Hand-assisted bariatric surgery has been proven to be safe and effective. It has been associated with reduced operative times, aids in retracting, and provides tactile feedback when compared with the total laparoscopic approach. Intracorporal suturing can be done quickly and easily, which is important if rapid control of hemorrhage is needed. As the field of laparoscopy advances, many new techniques have been developed. These new techniques allow surgeons to perform more complicated cases. Still, all surgeons performing advanced laparoscopy should be able to perform hand-assisted laparoscopic surgery. It is a valuable tool to aid in the transition from open to total laparoscopic surgery.

References

1. Westling A. Laparoscopic vs. open Roux-en-Y gastric bypass: a prospective, randomized trial. Obes Surg 2001;11(3):284–292.
2. Gould JC, Needleman BJ, Ellison EC, Muscarella P, Schneider C, Melvin WS. Evolution of minimally invasive bariatric surgery. Surgery 2002;132(4):565–571; discussion 571–572.
3. Kurian MS, Patterson E, Andrei VE, Edye MB. Hand-assisted laparoscopic surgery: an emerging technique. Surg Endosc 2001;15:1277–1281.
4. Needleman BJ, Damore LJ, Ellison EC, Cook CH, Dominguez E, Melvin WS. Hand-assisted laparoscopic Roux-en-Y gastric bypass: a safe alternative in minimally invasive bariatric surgery. SAGES Scientific Session, March 2000.
5. Stielman M. Prospective comparison of hand-assisted laparoscopic devices. Urology 2002;59(5):668–672.
6. Naitoh T, Gagner M, Garcia-Ruiz A, Heniford BT, Ise H, Matsuno S. Hand-assisted laparoscopic digestive surgery provides safety and tactile sensation for malignancy or obesity. Surg Endosc 1999;13:157–160.
7. McGrath V, Needleman BJ, Melvin WS. Evolution of the laparoscopic gastric bypass. J Laparoendosc Adv Surg Tech A 2003;13(4):221–227.

24
Risk–Benefit Analysis of Laparoscopic Bariatric Procedures

Stacy A. Brethauer and Philip R. Schauer

Bariatric surgery has evolved significantly over the last decade. The laparoscopic approach to bariatric surgery and the growing body of knowledge regarding the benefits of surgical weight loss has increased patient demand for these procedures. Surgeons are rapidly gaining interest in these challenging minimally invasive procedures as well. As we gain more experience with each of these procedures, though, it has not become clear which bariatric procedure is best suited for a specific patient. Currently, there are no clear data available to match a patient's characteristics (fat distribution, eating behavior, comorbidities, psychosocial factors) with a specific procedure. The decision is made primarily based on the procedures offered by the surgeon and the patient's willingness to accept a given level of risk and invasiveness (1).

In 1987, Sugerman proposed that sweet-eaters should undergo gastric bypass rather than a restrictive procedure. Maladaptive eating behavior (high calorie liquids and sweets) can certainly lead to failure after restrictive procedures, and this was demonstrated with the high long-term failure rate of the vertical banded gastroplasty (VBG). Dixon and O'Brien (2), though, analyzed 440 laparoscopic adjustable gastric banding (LAGB) patients and found no association between sweet-eating preoperatively and postoperative weight loss. They recommend that sweet-eating behavior not be used in the decision to proceed with surgery or in the selection of the operation to be performed. Negative predictors of postoperative weight loss in this LAGB study included increasing age, increasing body mass index (BMI) (>50), insulin resistance, poor physical activity, high pain scores, and poor general health. The authors are careful to point out, though, that the overall benefits of surgery, even in patients with these negative predictors who lost less weight, were great and these patients should still be offered surgery. Lindroos et al. (3) compared restrictive procedures (VBG and gastric banding) to Roux-en-Y gastric bypass (RYGBP) and found that the patient who consumed the most sweets lost more weight

at 2 years than patients who consumed fewer sweets preoperatively.

Psychological evaluation is a preoperative requirement for most bariatric programs and payers. This evaluation can identify patients who are at high risk for psychological reasons, particularly those with ongoing substance abuse, who are likely to be noncompliant with follow-up. For the most part, though, psychological evaluation prior to bariatric surgery does not accurately predict success or failure of the operation.

Ultimately, the type of bariatric procedure performed is determined by the patient who is well informed regarding the risks and benefits of each procedure offered. Undoubtedly, the surgeon's experience and preference affect the decision as well. Additionally, patients most often seek out surgeons who perform specific procedures based on their own research and referrals or recommendations from other physicians or patients. Each bariatric procedure has its merits and unique set of risks and complications that must be thoroughly discussed prior to embarking on this life-changing surgery. If performed by an experienced surgeon in the appropriate setting, each procedure can have impressive results in terms of weight loss and resolution of comorbidities with acceptable risks. As with most surgical procedures, careful patient selection can significantly affect outcomes. Proper patient selection in bariatric surgery goes beyond choosing appropriate candidates for surgical weight loss and should involve thorough discussions regarding the pros and cons for each type of procedure. This chapter highlights some of the important differences in laparoscopic RYGBP, LAGB, and laparoscopic biliopancreatic diversion with duodenal switch (BPD-DS) that should be considered when selecting patients for a bariatric procedure. Laparoscopic sleeve gastrectomy (LSG) has been used as the first stage procedure for high-risk patients prior to laparoscopic Roux-en-Y gastric bypass (LRYGBP) or biliopancreatic diversion (BPD). More recently, though, it has been used successfully as a primary procedure at some centers. There are currently limited data on LSG, which is discussed in Chapter 19.2.

Risks

Conversion Rate

The laparoscopic technique is used exclusively with the laparoscopic adjustable gastric band, and this procedure has a low rate of conversion to an open procedure (0–3.1%) (4–14). The lack of gastrointestinal anastomoses, the lower complexity of this procedure, and careful patient selection account for this lower conversion rate. Conversion rates to an open procedure ranges from 0% to 8% for LRYGBP (6,15–25) and from 0% to 26% for laparoscopic BPD or DS (26–29). In a review of 3464 cases, Podnos et al. (21) reported conversion to laparotomy in the LRYGBP of 2.2%. The most common reason for conversion was hepatomegaly (48%). The average conversion rate for the 467 patients in all of the laparoscopic BPD-DS series was 6%, though one study reported a 26% conversion rate that occurred early in the author's laparoscopic experience with the procedure (30). As more laparoscopic experience is gained with BPD-DS, it will likely achieve a conversion rate similar to that of RYGBP (less than 5% in experienced hands). The possibility that the laparoscopic procedure may be converted to open should not be a major factor in deciding which procedure to perform, but bariatric surgeons should know their own conversion rates for the procedures they perform and convey them to their patients preoperatively.

Early Postoperative Complications

There is a wide range of early postoperative complication rates in the literature for all three procedures. Major and minor complications occur after LRYGBP up to 30% of the time. In Podnos et al.'s (21) review of 3464 patients (10 studies), the most common perioperative complication after LRYGBP was wound infection (2.9%), followed by anastomotic leak (2%) and gastrointestinal hemorrhage (1.9%). Schauer et al. (22) reported early minor complications in 27% of patients and these included wound infection or erythema (5.1%), atelectasis (4.4%), urinary tract infection (2.5%), and asymptomatic or contained anastomotic leaks (2.5%). In this series of 275 patients, early major complications occurred in nine patients (3.3%). Early postoperative complications occur less frequently after LAGB, primarily because there are no gastrointestinal anastomoses. O'Brien et al. (9) reported an early postoperative complication rate of only 1.2% in 648 patients undergoing LAGB, and these were primarily infections at the reservoir site. Overall, the laparoscopic BPD series are primarily initial feasibil-

ity studies by highly experienced surgeons. The data are limited, but demonstrate acceptable rates of major early complications such as anastomotic leaks, wound infections, and thromboembolic events. In the largest series by Rabkin et al. (27) (duodenal switch, primarily hand-assisted) the overall perioperative complication rate was 10%. Higher postoperative complication rates were associated with BMI ≥ 65 in Ren's series. Patients with a BMI less than 65 had an 8.3% complication rate and patients with a BMI > 65 had a postoperative complication rate of 38%. Conversion rates and mortality were also higher for patients in the higher BMI group.

Bleeding complications occur more frequently with BPD-DS, primarily from longer staple lines in the gastric remnant. Among studies that reported this complication, the bleeding rate ranged from 5% to 10%. Ren reported four staple-line hemorrhages in 40 patients undergoing laparoscopic BPD-DS. One study showed improvement in bleeding rates with the use of absorbable buttress material on these staple lines (31). Postoperative bleeding occurs less than 5% of the time after LRYGBP and is rare after LAGB. In a review of the world's literature including 8504 patients, postoperative bleeding, including gastrointestinal bleeding, was reported in four patients (0.05%) after LAGB. In a review of 3464 LRYGBP patients, the postoperative gastrointestinal bleeding rate was 1.93%.

Anastomotic leaks after LRYGBP or BPD-DS can have devastating consequences. Anastomotic leak is a fatal complication up to 30% of the time and can have an insidious or delayed presentation. Anastomotic leak rates for LRYGBP and laparoscopic BPD-DS are comparable and occur less than 5% of the time. Leak rates decrease with surgeon experience as demonstrated by Wittgrove and Clark's (24) experience. Gastric perforation occurs 0.5% to 0.8% of the time after LAGB.

Wound infections are relatively uncommon in laparoscopic procedures and occur less frequently than in open bariatric procedures (18). The high infection rate shown in Table 24-1 for the laparoscopic BPD group reflects 3 of 18 patients (16.7%) who had wound infections in one series (32). Unlike many wound infections after open surgery, laparoscopic port-site infections are easily managed with local wound care and contribute little to overall postoperative morbidity when they do occur. Port site infection rates are generally low after LRYGBP and LAGB and occur <9% of the time in case series. In Chapman's (74) review of the LAGB literature, wound infections occurred in 0.28% of patients and Podnos et al.'s (21) review of LRYGBP series reported a wound infection rate of 2.98%. The lower wound infection rate with LAGB is explained by the fact that the gastrointestinal tract is not opened during the procedure, a factor that contributes to many of the advantages associated with LAGB.

TABLE 24.1. Risk–benefit analysis of laparoscopic bariatric procedures

	Laparoscopic RYGBP	LAGB	Laparoscopic BPD, BPD-DS*
Risks			
Conversion to open procedure	0–8%[6,15–19,21–25,58]	0–3.1%[5–12,14,63–65]	0–26%[26–29]
Early postoperative complications	4.2–30%[6,22,66,67]	0.8–12%[5–9,14,65,68–71]	2.6–22.5%[26–28]
Major and minor			
Bleeding	0.4–4%[6,15–19,21–25,58]	0.1%[5,6]	5–10%[26,28,32]
Leak	0–4.4%[6,15–19,21–25,58,72,73]	0.5–0.8%[5,74]	2.5–3.2%[26–28]
Wound infection	0–8.7%[15–19,21–25,58]	0.1–8.8%[5,7–11,14,63–65]	2.5–18.7%[26,28,29,32]
DVT	0–1.3%[15,16,18,19,22,24,58]	0.01–0.2%[9,74,75]	0.5–2.5%[27,28]
PE	0–1.1%[15,16,18,19,21–24,58,72]	0.1%[5,74]	0.9%[27]
Late complications	8.1–47%[6,22,66,67,76]	6–26%[5–8,14,65,68,69]	1.5–7.6%[27,29]
Major and minor			(no long-term f/u)
Anastomotic stricture	2–16%[6,15–19,21–25,33,58]	N/A	1.7–7.6%[27,29]
Marginal ulcer	0.7%–5.1%[15–17,19,22,58]	N/A	1.6%[77] (DS)
Bowel obstruction	1.1–10.5%[15–17,19,22,58,67,72]	0[74]	1.5%[27]**
Reoperation rate	9.8–13.8%[18,22,67]	4–19%[5,8–12,63,75,78]	0–12.5%[26,27,32,79]
Band-related complications			
Prolapse	N/A	2–25%[6–12,14,63,64,71,75,78,80]	N/A
Erosion	N/A	0–3%[5,7–12,14,63,64,74,75]	N/A
Gastric outlet obstruction/pouch dilation	N/A	0.2–14%[5,8,63,74,75,80]	N/A
Tube or port malfunction	N/A	0.4–7%[5,6,8–11,63,74,80]	N/A
Band intolerance	N/A	0.4–3.1%[6,75]	N/A
Nutritional deficiencies			
Iron	6–52%[81]	NR	23–44%[81]
Vitamin B_{12}	3–37%[81]	NR	22%[81]
Fat-soluble vitamins	10–51% (distal RYGBP)[81]	NR	5–69%[81]
Calcium	10% (distal RYGBP)[81]	NR	25–48%[81]
Protein malnutrition	0–13% (distal RYGBP)[81]	NR	3–18%[81]
Mortality rate	0–2%[15–19,21,22,24,58,72]	0–0.7%[5–10,12,34,63,64,74,78,80,82]	0–2.5%[26–28]
Benefits			
Excess weight loss	68–80% 12–60 months follow-up[15–19,22,24,58]	44–68%[9,34,74,80,83,84]	65–91.5%[26–29]
EWL for BMI >50	51–69%[6,35,36]	47–49%[36,37]	77%[36]
Hospital stay (mean)	2–4 days[15–19,22,24,58]	1–2 days[34,39,80]	4[27,28]
Durability	49–75% EWL at 10–14 years (open series)[85,86]	57% EWL at 6 years[9]	No long-term laparoscopic data 77% at 18 years (open series)[38]
Resolution of comorbidities			
Diabetes	82–98%[15,22,24]	54–64%[9,83]	100%[28]
Hypertension	36–92%[15,22,24]	55%[9]	80%[28]
Hyperlipidemia	63%[22]	74%[9]	55%[28]
GERD	72–98%[15,22,24]	76–89%[9,83]	NR
Sleep apnea	74–98%[22,24]	94%[9,83]	70%[28]
DJD	41–76%[15,22]	NR	NR
Urinary incontinence	44–88%[15,22]	NR	NR
Other factors			
Patient compliance	High priority for patient selection	High priority for band adjustments. Follow-up associated with EWL[87]	High priority in patient selection due to potential nutritional deficiencies
	Vitamin, protein intake postoperatively	More frequent postop visits required	Vitamin, protein intake postoperatively
Pregnancy	Limited data showing pregnancy safe after RYGBP[42,43]	Limited data showing safe pregnancy with band in place[12,40]	Limited data suggest improved birth outcomes after weight loss[40,41]
Adolescents	Safe, effective in carefully selected patients[47,50,51]	Safe, effective in carefully selected patients[52]	No data
Elderly	Overall, higher mortality rates for patients over 65[56] Safe, effective in carefully selected patients[57–59]	Safe, effective in carefully selected patients[61]	Trend toward higher complication rates for age >55 in open series[62]
Reversibility	Yes, restore gastric continuity	Yes, low difficulty to remove band laparoscopically	Yes, can reverse malabsorption but not partial gastrectomy
Surgeon learning curve	Steep 75–100 cases[88]	Moderate 50–75 cases	Very steep 150 cases
Operating time (minutes)	75–260 (mean 130)[15,17–19,22,25,58,89]	55–70[9,34,80]	210–240[26–29,32]

* Five studies, 347 patients, short-term follow-up (6–24 months).

** Hand-assisted.

LRYGBP, laparoscopic Roux-en-Y gastric bypass; LAGB, laparoscopic adjustable gastric banding; BPD, biliopancreatic diversion; DS, duodenal switch; NR, not reported; DJD, degenerative joint disease; GERD, gastroesophageal reflux disease; EWL, excess weight loss; BMI, body mass index.

Fortunately, *deep venous thrombosis* (DVT) and *pulmonary embolism* (PE) are rare complications in all series. Pulmonary embolism is the major cause of postoperative mortality after bariatric surgery. There are two laparoscopic BPD-DS series that reported DVT rates ranging from 0.5% (27) to 2.5% (one DVT in 40 patients) (28). In LRYGBP series with over 100 patients, DVTs occur 0% to 0.3% of the time and the PE rate is 0.3% to 1.1% (15,16,20,22). O'Brien (71) reported a 0.15% DVT rate in over 700 LAGB patients and the PE rate after LAGB is equally low (<0.2%). The low rate of DVT/PE after LAGB may be explained by patient selection (lower BMI) and shorter operative times with this procedure compared to LRYGBP and BPD-DS. These reported rates occurred in patients who received a variety of prophylactic regimens and were clinically significant events (not detected in asymptomatic patients as part of a surveillance protocol).

Late Complications

The LAGB has a lower rate of early postoperative complications, primarily because there are no anastomoses or staple lines to potentially leak or bleed. Late complications (>30 days postoperative for most series) do occur with all three procedures and are procedure-specific. The LAGB patients avoid late anastomotic and nutritional complications, but band, tubing, and port complications requiring reoperation can occur several months to years after band placement. There is no long-term data (>10 years) available for any laparoscopic bariatric procedure. Ultimately, the long-term effects of placing a silicone band around the gastric cardia are unknown. Late erosion and esophageal dilation have been concerns but, with 6 years of follow-up, these have not become major clinical problems with the adjustable band. Some of the late complications associated with open RYGBP and BPD-DS would be expected in the laparoscopically treated patients as well (bowel obstruction, anastomotic strictures, nutritional deficiencies), but late complications such as incisional hernia have been significantly reduced with the laparoscopic approach.

The way in which late complications are reported varies among series, and there is no uniformity regarding the classification of major and minor complications. Schauer et al. (22) reported an overall late complication range of 47% after LRYGBP. This included major and minor complications such as anastomotic stricture or ulcer, gastrogastric fistula, DVT, hernia, anemia, and hypokalemia as well as side effects such as prolonged nausea or vomiting and symptomatic cholelithiasis.

Anastomotic strictures after LRYGBP are typically seen 2% to 11% of the time in larger series, but the use of the circular end-to-end anastomosis (EEA) stapler for the gastrojejunostomy (especially the 21-mm size) has resulted in higher stricture rates up to 26% (33). Stricture rates for laparoscopic BPD-DS range from 1.7% to 7.6%, an acceptable range for this complication that can be easily treated endoscopically in most cases. There are no data available for marginal ulcer rates in laparoscopic BPD-DS, though open series report the occurrence of this complication 3% to 10% of the time. Bowel obstructions can occur at the transverse mesocolon for a retrocolic Roux limb, through Peterson's space, or through a defect in the mesenteries at the enteroenterostomy. This can occur up to 10% of the time with RYGBP. There are limited data for the laparoscopic BPD-DS that showed a 1.5% incidence of postoperative bowel obstruction in Rabkin's hand-assisted series of 345 patients.

Reoperation rates are fairly consistent among the different procedures, with a higher rate in the LAGB due to band slippage or port problems, particularly early in several authors' experiences. The LAGB has its unique set of delayed complication that include band slippage, prolapse of the stomach through the band, erosion of the band into the stomach, gastric outlet obstruction at the level of the band, and tube or port malfunction or infection. Occasionally, patients simply cannot tolerate the gastric restriction provided by the band and request removal (3.1%) (6).

Overall, LAGB has the lower rates of early and late postoperative complications. The incidence of band-specific complications (prolapse, tube or port problems), though, is similar to procedure-specific problems seen with LRYGBP (leak, stricture, bowel obstruction). The LRYGBP has acceptable rates of complications in the postoperative period that falls between LAGB and BPD-DS. To date, there are very few data regarding late complication rates for laparoscopic BPD-DS. If open BPD-DS complication rates are used as a surrogate, a higher price is paid in terms of complications after BPD-DS in return for the excellent and durable weight loss this procedure provides.

Nutritional deficiencies can occur following any procedure that bypasses a segment of the bowel. Restrictive procedures such as LAGB are not typically associated with any micronutrient deficiencies. Malabsorptive procedures such as BPD-DS and distal RYGBP have the highest rates of nutritional problems that can include protein-calorie malnutrition. Vitamin and mineral deficiencies can usually be prevented or easily treated with adequate supplementation. Patients undergoing these procedures must understand the lifelong commitment to supplementation and have the financial means to be compliant. The inability or unwillingness of patients to take lifelong supplementation should preclude them from undergoing a bypass procedure.

Mortality Rate

In Buchwald's (90) meta-analysis, 30-day perioperative mortality was 1.1% for BPD (all open), 0.5% for RYGBP (open and laparoscopic), and 0.1% for restrictive procedures (including LAGB). The range of mortality rates from large laparoscopic bariatric series are shown in Table 24.1. Laparoscopic BPD has the highest mortality rate among the laparoscopic procedures. Even though numbers are smaller in these series, which gives a 2.5% mortality rate for one death in the series of 40 patients, it is generally accepted, and supported by meta-analysis, that BPD has a higher mortality rate than the other two procedures. This may be explained, in part, by patient selection. Patients undergoing BPD-DS generally have higher BMIs than patients undergoing LRYGBP or LAGB, and increasing BMI is a predictor of perioperative morbidity and mortality.

Benefits

Excess Weight Loss

The BPD and BPD-DS provide the most excess weight loss (EWL) and have proven to be durable when performed as an open procedure. Weight loss for LRYGBP is excellent and falls between the EWL for LAGB and for BPD. Weight loss after LAGB is more gradual than with the bypass procedures, and patients must be informed about this preoperatively. Many LAGB studies report weight loss that is less than the EWL typically seen after LRYGBP. Several studies, though, have reported an EWL of 57% to 64% at 4 to 6 years after LAGB, and this weight loss is comparable to that seen with LRYGBP (9,34). Patient who choose to undergo LAGB over LRYGBP are typically more risk-averse and willing to accept less weight loss because the risk of having a major life-threatening complication is lower for the LAGB.

The EWL for super-obese patients (BMI > 50) is generally less after LAGB and LRYGBP (6,35–37). The EWL for super-obese patients undergoing BPD-DS is excellent in open series and is reported at 77% in one laparoscopic series of super-obese patients (36). Scopinaro et al.'s (38) open BPD series found no difference in EWL for patients who had initial excess weight of 120% compared to those who had an initial excess weight less than 120%.

Durability

There are currently insufficient data to compare long-term results among procedures. The longest reported follow-up after LRYGBP is 5 years with >75% EWL in the majority of patients (24). Pories's (85) open series of RYGBP reported 49% EWL at 15 years, and it is rea-sonable to expect the laparoscopic result to achieve at least that same level of effectiveness. The longest follow-up reported for the LAGB is O'Brien and Dixon's (9) 6-year results. They report 57% EWL at 6 years, which is comparable to that achieved by LRYGBP. In the U.S. Ponce et al. (34) reported 64% EWL 4 years after LAGB (>85% follow-up). There is no long-term follow-up available for the laparoscopic BPD-DS. Open series of BPD report 77% EWL at 18 years (38), and this procedure and the duodenal switch are considered the most durable bariatric procedures.

Resolution of Comorbidities

There are several large series documenting the improvement or resolution of various comorbidities after LRYGBP and LAGB. There is only one small series of laparoscopic BPD-DS that evaluated reduction of comorbidities, and this demonstrated excellent results similar to open series of BPD (28). The LRYGBP is more effective in eliminating diabetes than is the LAGB, which may be due to more rapid weight loss or, more likely, alteration in the entero-insular axis and gut hormones after RYGBP that rapidly improves glucose metabolism (prior to weight loss). Because of this difference, the presence of insulin resistance or diabetes influences many bariatric surgeons to perform a LRYGBP rather than a LAGB for these patients.

Hospital Stay

One of the major benefits of laparoscopy is a shorter hospital stay. In bariatric surgery, hospitalization is typically 1 day less for a laparoscopic procedure compared to its open counterpart. Most LRYGBP patients are discharged in 2 or 3 days. Laparoscopic BPD-DS patients have a longer hospital stay than the other two procedures, but this may reflect a higher risk patient population undergoing this procedure. Currently, LAGB has the shortest hospital stay among laparoscopic bariatric procedures, and some centers perform LAGB as a same-day surgery in selected patients (39).

Other Factors

Pregnancy

Pregnancy outcomes have been evaluated after gastric bypass, gastric banding, and biliopancreatic diversion. Most patients undergoing bariatric surgery are women of childbearing age, and contraception during the period of rapid weight loss should be emphasized. Pregnancies do occur during this period, though, as well as during the later weight-stable period, and fertility can significantly improve after surgically induced weight loss.

Laparoscopic adjustable gastric banding is unique in that it can be actively managed during the pregnancy based on maternal weight gain. The safety of the LAGB in pregnancy has been demonstrated in several small studies. Birth weight, pregnancy-induced hypertension, and gestational diabetes rates in LAGB patients were lower than in pre-band pregnancies and matched controls and were comparable to community norms (40).

Weight loss after BPD provides benefits in terms of normalizing gestational weight changes, normalizing infant birth weight, and reducing rates of fetal macrosomia. Children of mothers who conceived after BPD have normal growth patterns (41). Because protein and calorie absorption may not be adequate to sustain a pregnancy, up to 20% of women require parenteral nutrition during pregnancy following BPD. Therefore, delaying pregnancy until weight loss stabilizes is recommended.

After gastric bypass, patients becoming pregnant have fewer pregnancy-related complications than obese patients who delivered prior to gastric bypass. There was less gestational diabetes (42), hypertension, and large-for-gestational-age infants in post–gastric bypass surgery pregnancies (43). Nutritional status should be closely monitored, with specific attention to iron, calcium, folate, and vitamin B_{12} supplementation.

Adolescent Bariatric Surgery

Obesity in the pediatric and adolescent population has increased significantly over the last two decades, and the prevalence has nearly doubled in the last 10 years (44). Obesity in adolescence is associated with the same comorbidities seen in the adult population and the incidence of hypertension, hypercholesterolemia, type 2 diabetes, sleep apnea, pseudotumor cerebri, polycystic ovarian syndrome, nonalcoholic fatty liver disease, and musculoskeletal problems is higher in obese adolescents than normal-weight adolescents. The metabolic syndrome is present in 30% of overweight and 50% of severely obese adolescents (45,46). Childhood and adolescent obesity is also associated with a myriad of severe psychological and social problems and poor health-related quality of life (47–49).[47–49]

Small series support the safety and efficacy of RYGBP (47,50,51) and LAGB (52) in carefully selected adolescents. The selection criteria for these patients are strict, and the BMI criteria are generally higher than for adults (≥40 with severe obesity-related comorbidity or ≥50 with less severe comorbidities) (53). To be considered for surgery, these patients must have achieved skeletal maturity (13 to 14 years in girls, 15 to 16 years in boys) and failed at least 6 months of a medically supervised weight loss program. Psychologic evaluations in this group of patients is important to determine emotional maturity, motivation, and family support, and to identify any psychological or social contraindications to performing the surgery (54).

Short-term results with open and laparoscopic RYGBP have been favorable in this group, with 62% to 87% EWL and resolution of comorbidities in nearly all patients 1 to 2 years after surgery (47,50). Long-term results of studies with large numbers of adolescents undergoing laparoscopic bariatric surgery are not yet available.

The laparoscopic adjustable gastric band is currently not approved for use in adolescents in the United States, but success with this procedure has been demonstrated elsewhere for this age group. Dolan et al. (52) reported 59% EWL 24 months after surgery in 17 patients. There were only two band-related complications in this series. The LAGB is an attractive option for the adolescent population due to its reversibility, but long-term follow-up data are limited.

Biliopancreatic diversion is the most effective bariatric procedure in terms of weight loss and durability, but the higher morbidity and mortality associated with the procedure and the high incidence of nutritional deficiencies make this operation much less attractive in the adolescent population.

Bariatric Surgery in the Elderly

As with the adolescent age group, there was insufficient evidence in 1991 for the National Institutes of Health (NIH) consensus conference to make recommendations about bariatric surgery for patients older than 60 years. Currently, 33% of the U.S. population 60 years or older are obese, and 3.9% are severely obese (BMI ≥ 40). These patients frequently have multiple comorbidities and are generally higher risk operative candidates due to long-standing cardiovascular and pulmonary disease. Age over 55 has been shown to be an independent predictor of mortality after bariatric surgery (55). Flum et al. (56) reported higher all-cause perioperative mortality rates in Medicare patients over 65 years of age. Mortality rates for patients aged 65 years or older were 4.8% at 30 days and 6.9% at 90 days compared to 1.7% and 2.3%, respectively, for patients younger than 65. Nevertheless, carefully selected patients in this age group can benefit greatly from surgical weight loss. More important than the chronological age, patients' physiologic age, comorbidity severity, and functional status determine how they will tolerate, and benefit from, bariatric surgery. Recent evidence supporting bariatric surgery in older patients consists of case series of open and laparoscopic RYGBP (57–59), laparoscopic gastric banding (60,61), and biliopancreatic diversion (62). In a series by Papasavas et al. (58), patients over age 59 had excellent EWL at 2 years (67%) and over 70% had resolution of diabetes, hypertension, and sleep apnea at 1 year. Only three patients (4%) required rehabilitation postoperatively. Other reports have also confirmed the safety of gastric bypass in older patients, but have demonstrated less weight loss and less complete resolution of comorbidities in the older patient groups (57,59).

Gastric banding has been evaluated in patients over 50 years of age with EWL of 68% at 1 year. Complications requiring reoperation occurred in 10% of patients, and 97% had improvement in their obesity-related comorbidities (61). A study comparing long-term weight loss and complication rates between older and younger patients who underwent biliopancreatic diversion demonstrated similar weight loss at 5 years, but a trend toward higher rates of protein malnutrition, anastomotic ulcer, and need for reversal in patients over 55 years (62).

Reversibility

All three operations are potentially reversible. Certainly, the LAGB can simply be removed to restore the normal anatomy. This is an attractive feature for many patients who may be tentative about having their gastrointestinal anatomy significantly altered. Additionally, it may prove to be the most beneficial option for the adolescent population in which psychosocial factors can change rapidly. Gastric bypass can be reversed by re-creating gastric continuity and removing or reanastomosing the Roux limb to maintain bowel length. This restores normal alimentary flow through the duodenum. The BPD-DS can be reversed physiologically by creating a proximal enteroenterostomy to effectively eliminate the effects of the short common channel. Obviously, the gastric anatomy is permanently altered by the hemigastrectomy or sleeve gastrectomy.

Surgeon Learning Curve

Based on current reports in the literature, the BPD-DS is the most complex laparoscopic bariatric procedure to perform. Even in experienced hands, the procedure is associated with a higher rate of complications and longer operative time. This procedure has not been widely adapted by community surgeons as the LRYGBP has, and the data regarding the learning curve are limited. Based on small published series, it is safe to say that the learning curve for laparoscopic BPD-DS is very steep. More research has been conducted on the learning curve for LRYGBP, which is discussed in Chapter 7. In general the learning curve for LRYGBP is 75 to 100 cases. At this point in a surgeon's experience, operative times and complication rates should equal national standards.

Patient Compliance

A motivated, compliant patient is required for the success of any bariatric procedure. In reality, though, there is a wide spectrum of adherence to the postoperative plan among the bariatric surgery population. In addition, many patients travel considerable distances to undergo surgery and frequent follow-up visits with the primary surgeon are not practical or financially realistic. Nevertheless, efforts should be made during the preoperative evaluation to determine the likelihood of patient compliance.

For malabsorptive procedures, compliance is critical to follow nutritional parameters and reinforce patient adherence to supplementation. Patients who are lost to follow-up after BPD or DS risk developing severe protein or micronutrient deficiencies. Follow-up is important after LRYGBP as well, since many of these patients may develop iron deficiency anemia or B_{12} deficiency. Compliance with protein intake and nutritional supplements should be emphasized at each follow-up appointment. Patient adherence to the follow-up schedule after LAGB has been shown to impact weight loss. This procedure is unique from the others in that it requires adjustments that directly impact the success of the operation. In a study by Shen et al. (87), patient follow-up and weight loss were compared in the first year after surgery for 186 LAGB and 115 RYGBP patients. Overall EWL was 42% for LAGB patients who returned six or fewer times in the first year compared to 50% EWL for patients who returned more than six times ($p = .005$). Overall EWL for RYGBP at 1 year was 66% and was not affected by the number of patient follow-up visits.

Conclusion

There are currently no randomized prospective data to guide our decision regarding which laparoscopic procedure should be offered to a specific patient. The decision is primarily based on surgeon experience and the patient's expectations. Patients who are more risk-averse tend to choose the LAGB, and those who desire greater weight loss and can accept a potentially higher complication rate choose RYGBP or BPD. Currently, LRYGBP is the most commonly performed bariatric procedure in the world. This is largely due to its good safety profile and excellent long-term weight loss and comorbidity reduction. Laparoscopic adjustable gastric banding, though, is growing in popularity due to its low morbidity and mortality rates and encouraging medium-term results. Laparoscopic malabsorptive procedures are currently performed at specialized centers and, because of their technical complexity and potential for nutritional deficiencies, are unlikely to gain wide acceptance in the United States.

References

1. Ren CJ, Cabrera I, Rajaram K, Fielding GA. Factors influencing patient choice for bariatric operation. Obes Surg 2005;15(2):202–206.
2. Dixon JB, O'Brien PE. Selecting the optimal patient for LAP-BAND placement. Am J Surg 2002;184(6B):17S20S.
3. Lindroos AK, Lissner L, Sjostrom L. Weight change in relation to intake of sugar and sweet foods before and after weight reducing gastric surgery. Int J Obes Relat Metab Disord 1996;20(7):634–643.
4. Angrisani L, Alkilani M, Basso N, et al. Laparoscopic Italian experience with the Lap-Band. Obes Surg 2001;11(3):307–310.
5. Belachew M, Belva PH, Desaive C. Long-term results of laparoscopic adjustable gastric banding for the treatment of morbid obesity. Obes Surg 2002;12(4):564–568.
6. Biertho L, Steffen R, Ricklin T, et al. Laparoscopic gastric bypass versus laparoscopic adjustable gastric banding: a comparative study of 1,200 cases. J Am Coll Surg 2003;197(4):536–544; discussion 544–545.
7. Cadiere GB, Himpens J, Hainaux B, et al. Laparoscopic adjustable gastric banding. Semin Laparosc Surg 2002;9(2):105–114.
8. Dargent J. Laparoscopic adjustable gastric banding: lessons from the first 500 patients in a single institution. Obes Surg 1999;9(5):446–452.
9. O'Brien PE, Dixon JB, Brown W, et al. The laparoscopic adjustable gastric band (Lap-Band): a prospective study of medium-term effects on weight, health and quality of life. Obes Surg 2002;12(5):652–660.
10. Ren CJ, Horgan S, Ponce J. US experience with the LAP-BAND system. Am J Surg 2002;184(6B):46S–50S.
11. Rubenstein RB. Laparoscopic adjustable gastric banding at a U.S. center with up to 3–year follow-up. Obes Surg 2002;12(3):380–384.
12. Weiner R, Blanco-Engert R, Weiner S, et al. Outcome after laparoscopic adjustable gastric banding—8 years experience. Obes Surg 2003;13(3):427–434.
13. DeMaria EJ, Sugerman HJ, Meador JG, et al. High failure rate after laparoscopic adjustable silicone gastric banding for treatment of morbid obesity. Ann Surg 2001;233(6):809–818.
14. Fielding GA, Rhodes M, Nathanson LK. Laparoscopic gastric banding for morbid obesity. Surgical outcome in 335 cases. Surg Endosc 1999;13(6):550–554.
15. DeMaria EJ, Sugerman HJ, Kellum JM, et al. Results of 281 consecutive total laparoscopic Roux-en-Y gastric bypasses to treat morbid obesity. Ann Surg 2002;235(5):640–645; discussion 645–647.
16. Higa KD, Boone KB, Ho T. Complications of the laparoscopic Roux-en-Y gastric bypass: 1,040 patients–what have we learned? Obes Surg 2000;10(6):509–513.
17. Lujan JA, Frutos MD, Hernandez Q, et al. Laparoscopic versus open gastric bypass in the treatment of morbid obesity: a randomized prospective study. Ann Surg 2004;239(4):433–437.
18. Nguyen NT, Goldman C, Rosenquist CJ, et al. Laparoscopic versus open gastric bypass: a randomized study of outcomes, quality of life, and costs. Ann Surg 2001;234(3):279–289; discussion 289–291.
19. Nguyen NT, Ho HS, Palmer LS, Wolfe BM. A comparison study of laparoscopic versus open gastric bypass for morbid obesity. J Am Coll Surg 2000;191(2):149–155; discussion 155–157.
20. Papasavas PK, Hayetian FD, Caushaj PF, et al. Outcome analysis of laparoscopic Roux-en-Y gastric bypass for morbid obesity. The first 116 cases. Surg Endosc 2002;16(12):1653–1657.
21. Podnos YD, Jimenez JC, Wilson SE, et al. Complications after laparoscopic gastric bypass: a review of 3464 cases. Arch Surg 2003;138(9):957–961.
22. Schauer PR, Ikramuddin S, Gourash W, et al. Outcomes after laparoscopic Roux-en-Y gastric bypass for morbid obesity. 2000;232(4):515–529.
23. Westling A, Gustavsson S. Laparoscopic vs open Roux-en-Y gastric bypass: a prospective, randomized trial. Obes Surg 2001;11(3):284–292.
24. Wittgrove AC, Clark GW. Laparoscopic gastric bypass, Roux-en-Y- 500 patients: technique and results, with 3–60 month follow-up. Obes Surg 2000;10(3):233–239.
25. de la Torre RA, Scott JS. Laparoscopic Roux-en-Y gastric bypass: a totally intra-abdominal approach–technique and preliminary report. Obes Surg 1999;9(5):492–498.
26. Paiva D, Bernardes L, Suretti L. Laparoscopic biliopancreatic diversion: technique and initial results. Obes Surg 2002;12(3):358–361.
27. Rabkin RA, Rabkin JM, Metcalf B, et al. Laparoscopic technique for performing duodenal switch with gastric reduction. Obes Surg 2003;13(2):263–268.
28. Ren CJ, Patterson E, Gagner M. Early results of laparoscopic biliopancreatic diversion with duodenal switch: a case series of 40 consecutive patients. Obes Surg 2000;10(6):514–523; discussion 524.
29. Scopinaro N, Marinari GM, Camerini G. Laparoscopic standard biliopancreatic diversion: technique and preliminary results. Obes Surg 2002;12(2):241–244.
30. Gagner M, Steffen R, Biertho L, Horber F. Laparoscopic adjustable gastric banding with duodenal switch for morbid obesity: technique and preliminary results. Obes Surg 2003;13(3):444–449.
31. Consten EC, Gagner M, Pomp A, Inabnet WB. Decreased bleeding after laparoscopic sleeve gastrectomy with or without duodenal switch for morbid obesity using a stapled buttressed absorbable polymer membrane. Obes Surg 2004;14(10):1360–1366.
32. Baltasar A, Bou R, Miro J, et al. Laparoscopic biliopancreatic diversion with duodenal switch: technique and initial experience. Obes Surg 2002;12(2):245–248.
33. Nguyen NT, Stevens CM, Wolfe BM. Incidence and outcome of anastomotic stricture after laparoscopic gastric bypass. J Gastrointest Surg 2003;7(8):997–1003; discussion 1003.
34. Ponce J, Paynter S, Fromm R. Laparoscopic adjustable gastric banding: 1,014 consecutive cases. J Am Coll Surg 2005;201(4):529–535.
35. Farkas DT, Vemulapalli P, Haider A, et al. Laparoscopic Roux-en-Y gastric bypass is safe and effective in patients with a BMI > or = 60. Obes Surg 2005;15(4):486–493.

36. Parikh MS, Shen R, Weiner M, et al. Laparoscopic bariatric surgery in super-obese patients (BMI > 50) is safe and effective: a review of 332 patients. Obes Surg 2005;15(6):858–863.

37. Dolan K, Hatzifotis M, Newbury L, Fielding G. A comparison of laparoscopic adjustable gastric banding and biliopancreatic diversion in superobesity. Obes Surg 2004; 14(2):165–169.

38. Scopinaro N, Gianetta E, Adami GF, et al. Biliopancreatic diversion for obesity at eighteen years. Surgery 1996;119(3): 261–268.

39. Kormanova K, Fried M, Hainer V, Kunesova M. Is laparoscopic adjustable gastric banding a day surgery procedure? Obes Surg 2004;14(9):1237–1240.

40. Dixon JB, Dixon ME, O'Brien P E. Birth outcomes in obese women after laparoscopic adjustable gastric banding. Obstet Gynecol 2005;106(5):965–972.

41. Marceau P, Kaufman D, Biron S, et al. Outcome of pregnancies after biliopancreatic diversion. Obes Surg 2004; 14(3):318–324.

42. Wittgrove AC, Jester L, Wittgrove P, Clark GW. Pregnancy following gastric bypass for morbid obesity. Obes Surg 1998;8(4):461–464; discussion 465–466.

43. Richards DS, Miller DK, Goodman GN. Pregnancy after gastric bypass for morbid obesity. J Reprod Med 1987; 32(3):172–176.

44. Kimm SY, Barton BA, Obarzanek E, et al. Obesity development during adolescence in a biracial cohort: the NHLBI Growth and Health Study. Pediatrics 2002;110(5):e54.

45. Cook S, Weitzman M, Auinger P, et al. Prevalence of a metabolic syndrome phenotype in adolescents: findings from the third National Health and Nutrition Examination Survey, 1988–1994. Arch Pediatr Adolesc Med 2003;157(8):821–827.

46. Weiss R, Dziura J, Burgert TS, et al. Obesity and the metabolic syndrome in children and adolescents. N Engl J Med 2004;350(23):2362–2374.

47. Strauss RS, Bradley LJ, Brolin RE. Gastric bypass surgery in adolescents with morbid obesity. J Pediatr 2001;138(4): 499–504.

48. Falkner NH, Neumark-Sztainer D, Story M, et al. Social, educational, and psychological correlates of weight status in adolescents. Obes Res 2001;9(1):32–42.

49. Schwimmer JB, Burwinkle TM, Varni JW. Health-related quality of life of severely obese children and adolescents. Jama 2003;289(14):1813–1819.

50. Stanford A, Glascock JM, Eid GM, et al. Laparoscopic Roux-en-Y gastric bypass in morbidly obese adolescents. J Pediatr Surg 2003;38(3):430–433.

51. Sugerman HJ, Sugerman EL, DeMaria EJ, et al. Bariatric surgery for severely obese adolescents. J Gastrointest Surg 2003;7(1):102–107; discussion 107–108.

52. Dolan K, Creighton L, Hopkins G, Fielding G. Laparoscopic gastric banding in morbidly obese adolescents. Obes Surg 2003;13(1):101–104.

53. Inge TH, Garcia V, Daniels S, et al. A multidisciplinary approach to the adolescent bariatric surgical patient. J Pediatr Surg 2004;39(3):442–447; discussion 446–447.

54. Inge TH, Zeller M, Garcia VF, Daniels SR. Surgical approach to adolescent obesity. Adolesc Med Clin 2004; 15(3):429–453.

55. Livingston EH, Huerta S, Arthur D, et al. Male gender is a predictor of morbidity and age a predictor of mortality for patients undergoing gastric bypass surgery. Ann Surg 2002;236(5):576–582.

56. Flum DR, Salem L, Elrod JA, et al. Early mortality among Medicare beneficiaries undergoing bariatric surgical procedures. AMA 2005;294(15):1903–1908.

57. St Peter SD, Craft RO, Tiede JL, Swain JM. Impact of advanced age on weight loss and health benefits after laparoscopic gastric bypass. Arch Surg 2005;140(2):165–168.

58. Papasavas PK, Gagne DJ, Kelly J, Caushaj PF. Laparoscopic Roux-En-Y gastric bypass is a safe and effective operation for the treatment of morbid obesity in patients older than 55 years. Obes Surg 2004;14(8):1056–1061.

59. Sugerman HJ, DeMaria EJ, Kellum JM, et al. Effects of bariatric surgery in older patients. Ann Surg 2004;240(2): 243–247.

60. Abu-Abeid S, Keidar A, Szold A. Resolution of chronic medical conditions after laparoscopic adjustable silicone gastric banding for the treatment of morbid obesity in the elderly. Surg Endosc 2001;15(2):132–134.

61. Weiss HG, Nehoda H, Labeck B, et al. Pregnancies after adjustable gastric banding. Obes Surg 2001;11(3):303–306.

62. Cossu ML, Fais E, Meloni GB, et al. Impact of age on long-term complications after biliopancreatic diversion. Obes Surg 2004;14(9):1182–1186.

63. Angrisani L, Furbetta F, Doldi SB, et al. Lap Band adjustable gastric banding system: the Italian experience with 1863 patients operated on 6 years. Surg Endosc 2003; 17(3):409–412.

64. DeMaria EJ. Laparoscopic adjustable silicone gastric banding. Surg Clin North Am 2001;81(5):1129–1144, vii.

65. Weiner R, Gutberlet H, Bockhorn H. Preparation of extremely obese patients for laparoscopic gastric banding by gastric-balloon therapy. Obes Surg 1999;9(3):261–264.

66. Fobi MA, Lee H. The surgical technique of the Fobi-Pouch operation for obesity (the transected silastic vertical gastric bypass). Obes Surg 1998;8(3):283–288.

67. Higa KD, Boone KB, Ho T, Davies OG. Laparoscopic Roux-en-Y gastric bypass for morbid obesity: technique and preliminary results of our first 400 patients. Arch Surg 2000;135(9):1029–1033;discussion 1033–1034.

68. Chelala E, Cadiere GB, Favretti F, et al. Conversions and complications in 185 laparoscopic adjustable silicone gastric banding cases. Surg Endosc 1997;11(3):268–271.

69. Belachew M, Legrand M, Vincent V, et al. Laparoscopic adjustable gastric banding. World J Surg 1998;22(9):955–963.

70. Hauri P, Steffen R, Ricklin T, et al. Treatment of morbid obesity with the Swedish adjustable gastric band (SAGB): complication rate during a 12–month follow-up period. Surgery 2000;127(5):484–488.

71. O'Brien PE, Dixon JB. Weight loss and early and late complications—the international experience. Am J Surg 2002;184(6B):42S–45S.

72. Fernandez AZ, Jr., Demaria EJ, Tichansky DS, et al. Multivariate analysis of risk factors for death following gastric bypass for treatment of morbid obesity. Ann Surg 2004; 239(5):698–702; discussion 702–703.

73. Fernandez AZ, Jr., DeMaria EJ, Tichansky DS, et al. Experience with over 3,000 open and laparoscopic bariatric

procedures: multivariate analysis of factors related to leak and resultant mortality. Surg Endosc 2004;18(2):193–197.

74. Chapman AE, Kiroff G, Game P, et al. Laparoscopic adjustable gastric banding in the treatment of obesity: a systematic literature review. Surgery 2004;135(3):326–351.

75. Vertruyen M. Experience with Lap-band System up to 7 years. Obes Surg 2002;12(4):569–572.

76. Christou NV, Sampalis JS, Liberman M, et al. Surgery decreases long-term mortality, morbidity, and health care use in morbidly obese patients. Ann Surg 2004;240(3):416–423; discussion 423–424.

77. Weiner RA, Blanco-Engert R, Weiner S, et al. Laparoscopic biliopancreatic diversion with duodenal switch: three different duodeno-ileal anastomotic techniques and initial experience. Obes Surg 2004;14(3):334–340.

78. Favretti F, Cadiere GB, Segato G, et al. Laparoscopic banding: selection and technique in 830 patients. Obes Surg 2002;12(3):385–390.

79. Gagner M, Matteotti R. Laparoscopic biliopancreatic diversion with duodenal switch. Surg Clin North Am 2005; 85(1):141–149, x–xi.

80. Watkins BM, Montgomery KF, Ahroni JH. Laparoscopic adjustable gastric banding: early experience in 400 consecutive patients in the USA. Obes Surg 2005;15(1):82–87.

81. Bloomberg RD, Fleishman A, Nalle JE, et al. Nutritional deficiencies following bariatric surgery: what have we learned? Obes Surg 2005;15(2):145–154.

82. DeMaria EJ, Jamal MK. Laparoscopic adjustable gastric banding: evolving clinical experience. Surg Clin North Am 2005;85(4):773–787, vii.

83. O'Brien PE, Dixon JB. Lap-band: outcomes and results. J Laparoendosc Adv Surg Tech A 2003;13(4):265–270.

84. O'Brien PE, Brown WA, Smith A, et al. Prospective study of a laparoscopically placed, adjustable gastric band in the treatment of morbid obesity. Br J Surg 1999;86(1):113–118.

85. Pories WJ, Swanson MS, MacDonald KG, et al. Who would have thought it? An operation proves to be the most effective therapy for adult-onset diabetes mellitus. Ann Surg 1995;222(3):339–350; discussion 350–352.

86. White S, Brooks E, Jurikova L, Stubbs RS. Long-term outcomes after gastric bypass. Obes Surg 2005;15(2):155–163.

87. Shen R, Dugay G, Rajaram K, et al. Impact of patient follow-up on weight loss after bariatric surgery. Obes Surg 2004;14(4):514–519.

88. Schauer P, Ikramuddin S, Hamad G, Gourash W. The learning curve for laparoscopic Roux-en-Y gastric bypass is 100 cases. Surg Endosc 2003;17(2):212–215.

89. Dresel A, Kuhn JA, McCarty TM. Laparoscopic Roux-en-Y gastric bypass in morbidly obese and super morbidly obese patients. Am J Surg 2004;187(2):230–232; discussion 232.

90. Buchwald H, Avidor Y, Braunwald E, et al. Bariatric surgery: a systematic review and meta-analysis. JAMA 2004;292(14):1724–1737.

25.1
Alternative Minimally Invasive Options: Gastric Pacing

Scott Shikora

It is estimated that 66% of all adult Americans are overweight or obese (1). Furthermore, 4.8% are extremely (morbidly) obese, which is defined as a body mass index (BMI) greater than or equal to 40. Calculations suggest that the number of extremely obese adults in the United States has reached a staggering 14 to 16 million people. These individuals suffer from a wide range of comorbidities and make up the second largest group of preventable deaths after smoking (>300,000 yearly) (2). The cost of treating the obese is staggering, at approximately $70 billion yearly (3). The impact of obesity is also not limited to the United States but is spreading worldwide. Globally, the prevalence of overweight/obesity was recently estimated at 1.7 billion people (4). This accounts for over 2.5 million deaths per year (5). Not far behind obesity in adults is the growing epidemic of overweight adolescents. Currently, surgery is rarely offered to these patients for fear of operative complications and long-term noncompliance.

Bariatric surgery is now a widely accepted treatment for severe obesity. Numerous studies have demonstrated dramatic improvement in the obesity-associated comorbidities from the weight loss achieved with all of these procedures (6–8). However, currently fewer than 1% of those who meet standard criteria for eligibility for surgical therapy will have bariatric surgery in a given calendar year. While many potential candidates are denied surgery secondary to lack of medical insurance coverage, the lack of knowledge about the efficacy of these treatments, or other disqualifications, a great number will avoid surgery because of fear of the potential operative complications and long-term consequences of the current operative procedures.

Implantable gastric stimulation for weight loss is an exciting new concept for the treatment of obesity. It is unique in that it involves the least invasive surgery and does not alter the gastrointestinal tract anatomy. Since its inception in the mid-1990s, international investigations have demonstrated it to be the safest of all bariatric procedures in terms of both operative complications and long-term consequences. In addition, advances in this technology have led to improving efficacy. This chapter reviews the theory and current experience with gastric implantable stimulation for weight loss.

Gastric Electrophysiology and Motility

Motility is one of the most critical physiological functions of the human gut. Without coordinated motility, digestion and absorption of dietary nutrients could not take place. To accomplish its functions effectively, the gut needs to generate contractions that are coordinated. This produces the transit of luminal contents (peristalsis) to a position where the nutrients can be maximally absorbed. In addition, hypermotility must be avoided, which would negatively impact nutrient absorption by decreasing nutrient exposure to the mucosa. In a similar fashion, the stomach requires coordinated gastric contractions for normal emptying.

Gastric contractions are regulated by the myoelectrical activity of the stomach. Normal gastric myoelectrical activity consists of two components: slow waves and spike potentials (9). The slow wave is omnipresent and occurs at regular intervals whether or not the stomach contracts. It originates in the proximal stomach and propagates distally toward the pylorus (Fig. 25.1-1). The gastric slow wave determines the maximum frequency, propagation velocity, and propagation direction of gastric contractions. The normal frequency of the gastric slow wave is about 3 cycles per minute (cpm) in humans and 5 cpm in dogs. When a spike potential (similar to an action potential) is superimposed on the gastric slow wave, a strong lumen-occluding contraction occurs.

Gastric dysrhythmias represent aberrations from the normal gastric myoelectrical activity. Similar to cardiac dysrhythmias, they include abnormally rapid contraction (tachygastria) and abnormally slow contraction

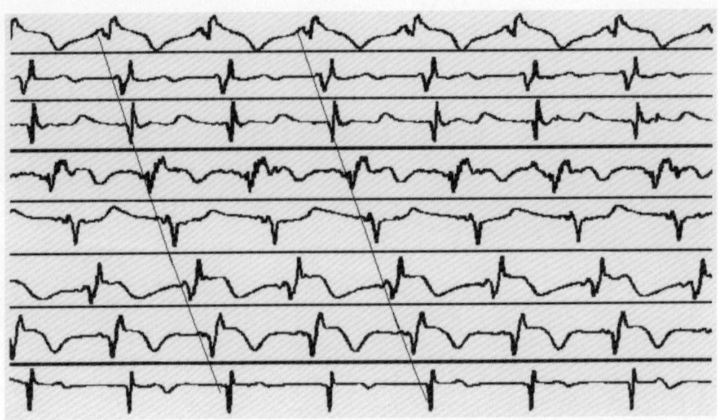

FIGURE 25.1-1. Normal gastric slow waves. Gastric slow waves recorded from electrodes implanted on the serosal surface of the stomach along the greater curvature in a healthy dog (1.5–min recording). The top tracing was obtained from a pair of electrodes 16 cm above the pylorus and the bottom one was from the electrodes 2 cm above the pylorus. (Courtesy of Jiande Chen, Ph.D.)

(bradygastria). For example (Fig. 25.1-2), there can be an ectopic pacemaker in the distal stomach in addition to the normal pacemaker in the proximal stomach. The ectopic pacemaker generates slow waves with a higher frequency than normal (tachygastria), and with a retrograde propagation toward the proximal stomach. These abnormal waves may interfere with the normal slow wave propagation and possibly disrupt normal gastric contractions.

Recently, the prevalence and origin of various gastric dysrhythmias was investigated (10). It was found that the majority of bradygastrias (80.5% ± 9.4%) originated in the proximal stomach ($p < .04$, vs. other locations) and propagated all the way to the distal antrum, that is,

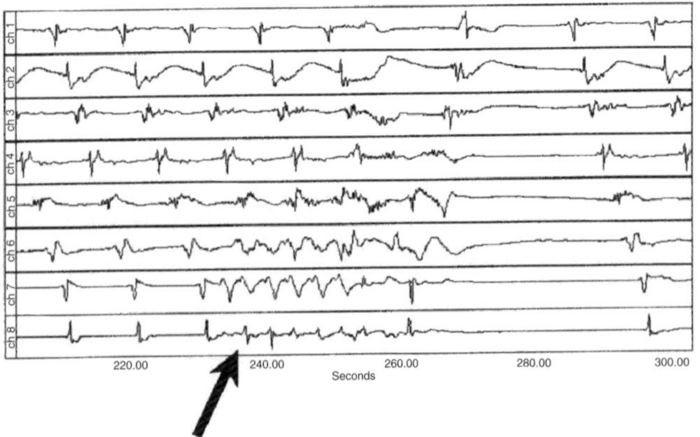

FIGURE 25.1-2. Tachygastria. Gastric slow waves recorded from electrodes implanted on the serosal surface of the stomach along the greater curvature showing the ectopic tachygastrial activity in the distal stomach (arrow). The top tracing was obtained from a pair of electrodes 16 cm above the pylorus and the bottom one was from the electrodes 2 cm above the pylorus. (Courtesy of Jiande Chen, Ph.D.)

bradygastria is attributed to a decrease in the frequency of the normal pacemaker. In contrast, tachygastria mainly originated in the distal antrum (80.6% ± 8.8%) ($p < .04$, vs. other locations) and propagated partially or all the way to the proximal stomach. During tachygastria, the normal pacemaker in the proximal stomach may still be present. That is, it is not uncommon for the proximal stomach to be dominated with normal slow waves, and the distal stomach to be dominated with tachygastria. Overall, the prevalence of dysrhythmia was highest in the distal antrum and lowest in the proximal part of the stomach.

The patterns of gastric motility are different in the fed and the fasting states (11). In the fed state, the human stomach contracts at its maximum frequency of 3 cpm. The contraction originates in the proximal stomach and propagates distally toward the pylorus. In healthy humans, 50% or more of the ingested food is usually emptied from the stomach by 2 hours after the meal and over 95% or more has been emptied by 4 hours after the meal (12). When the stomach is emptied, the pattern of gastric motility changes. The gastric motility pattern in the fasting state undergoes a cycle of periodic fluctuation divided into three phases: phase I (no contractions, 40–60 minutes), phase II (intermittent contractions, 20–40 minutes), and phase III (regular rhythmic contractions, 2–10 minutes).

Gastric emptying plays an important role in regulating food intake. Several studies have shown that gastric distention acts as a satiety signal to inhibit food intake (13). In addition, rapid gastric emptying is closely related to overeating and obesity. This is especially true for animals with lesions in the hypothalamic region of the brain (14). In a study of 77 human subjects composed of 46 obese and 31 age-, sex-, and race-matched nonobese individuals, obese subjects were found to have a more rapid gastric emptying rate than nonobese subjects (15). Obese men were found to empty much more rapidly than their nonobese counterparts. It was concluded that the rate of solid gastric emptying in the obese subjects is abnormally rapid. The significance and cause of this change in gastric emptying remains to be definitively established. However, from work performed at the University of Chicago in 1913, Carlson (16) proposed that a relationship existed between the gastrointestinal tract and the hypothalamus that regulated dietary intake. It has more recently been shown that several peptides, including cholecystokinin (CCK) and corticotropin-releasing factor (CRF), suppress feeding and decrease gastric transit. Peripherally administered CCK-8 was found to decrease the rate of gastric emptying and food intake in various species (17). CRF, when injected, has also been shown to decrease food intake and the rate of gastric emptying (18). More recently, it was shown that in ob/ob mice (a genetic model of obesity), the rate of gastric emptying was accelerated compared with that in lean mice

(19). Urocortin, a 40 amino acid peptide member of the CRF family, dose-dependently and potently decreased food intake and body weight gain as well as the rate of gastric emptying, in ob/ob mice. This suggests that rapid gastric emptying may contribute to hyperphagia and obesity in ob/ob mice and opens new possibilities for the treatment of obesity.

Gastric Stimulation and Pacing

Gastric stimulation involves the application of an electrical current to the stomach to alter its function. The utility of gastric pacing may be realized only if artificially generated electrical current could entrain normal gastric pacesetter potentials. This, in fact, has been demonstrated in canines (20) and in humans (21). How this affects gastric function is still to be determined.

Electrical stimulation of the stomach can be directed from proximal to distal (antegrade pacing) or from distal to proximal (retrograde pacing). While it would be attractive to assume that antegrade stimulation could improve normal gastric emptying, and retrograde stimulation would be used to retard or adversely impact normal gastric emptying, in human subjects these relationships have not been conclusively proven.

However, a number of papers have been published on gastrointestinal electrical stimulation for the treatment of gastrointestinal motility disorders in both dogs and humans. These disorders are characterized by poor contractility and delayed emptying (in contrast to obesity), and the aim of electrical stimulation in this setting is to normalize the underlying electrical rhythm and improve these parameters. In general, this is done by antegrade or forward gastric (or intestinal) stimulation.

Previous work on antegrade gastrointestinal stimulation has been focused on its effects on (1) gastric myoelectrical activity, (2) gastric motility, (3) gastric emptying, and (4) gastrointestinal symptoms (22–29). These studies have shown that entrainment of gastric slow waves is possible using an artificial pacemaker. The studies have indicated that such entrainment is dependent on certain critical parameters, including the width and frequency of the stimulation pulse (22). Furthermore, antegrade intestinal electrical stimulation can entrain intestinal slow waves using either serosal electrodes or intraluminal ring electrodes (25,28). McCallum et al. (26) demonstrated in patients suffering from gastroparesis that antegrade gastric pacing could entrain gastric slow waves in all nine patients. They paced the greater curvature of the stomach at frequencies approximately 10% higher than the slow wave frequencies measured. In two patients, it converted tachygastria to normal slow waves. In fact, electrical pacing significantly improved gastric emptying and symptoms in these patients. In a case

report, Familoni et al. (30) also were able to improve gastric emptying and symptoms in a patient with severe diabetic gastroparesis by pacing the stomach at a high frequency (12 cpm). In contrast, Hocking (31) was unable to treat postgastrectomy gastric dysrhythmias with pacing in a patient who underwent vagotomy and gastrojejunostomy for an obstructing duodenal ulcer.

Retrograde pacing may be of benefit for patients with abnormally rapid gastric emptying such as those patients with dumping syndrome and the morbidly obese (23). The principle of retrograde gastric electrical stimulation is the opposite of what has been described for patients with impaired gastric emptying. Retrograde gastric electrical stimulation employs retrograde pacing (Fig. 25.1-3). As previously stated, the original working concept was that retrograde pacing might retard the propulsive activity of the stomach and slow gastric emptying. This could be useful in the treatment of obesity, where it is postulated that a delay in gastric emptying would lead to early satiety and decreased food intake. Again, delayed gastric emptying as a mechanism of action for electrical stimulation has not been proven in humans.

To accomplish retrograde gastric electrical stimulation, an artificial pacemaker is connected to the distal stomach along the lesser curvature, resulting in electrical waves propagating from the distal to the proximal stomach. These waves conflict with the normal and physiologic electrical waves that propagate from the proximal to the distal stomach. Consequently, gastric dysrhythmia is induced and the regular propagation of gastric electrical waves is impaired. The severity of impairment is determined by the strength of the electrical stimulation.

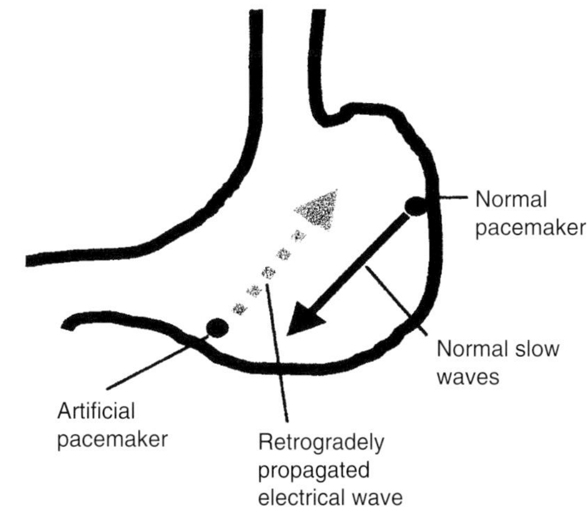

FIGURE 25.1-3. Retrograde gastric electrical stimulation. Electrical stimulation from an ectopic gastric pacemaker located in the distal stomach may delay gastric emptying. (Courtesy of Jiande Chen, Ph.D.)

Implantable Gastric Stimulation for Weight Loss

Whether delayed gastric emptying can be accomplished by electrical gastric stimulation or not, this modality has been shown to be safe and effective for the treatment of severe obesity. The concept was first developed by an Italian surgeon, Valerio Cigaina, in the late 1980s. At that time, he hypothesized that exogenous electrical impulses could be used to dysregulate normal gastric electromotor activity in obese patients, resulting in weight loss. Although the mechanism of action is still not elucidated, gastric stimulation has been shown to achieve meaningful weight loss. A more current theory that also has been supported by animal study is the effect of electrical stimulation on fundic relaxation. This relaxation is seen with normal postprandial gastric distention and may result in satiety (32).

Studies investigating the potential for gastric electrical stimulation to induce weight loss were first reported by Cigaina et al. (33) in 1996 in a porcine model. The results showed that retrograde gastric electrical stimulation was both safe and effective in moderating weight gain in growing swine. Animals were divided into three groups, two of which had electrodes implanted into the muscle layer of the distal antrum. Control animals received sham surgery. Implanted swine experienced either 3 or 8 months of electrical antral stimulation at 5 or 100 Hz, respectively. All animals were fed *ad libitum*. As expected, immature swine in the control group increased feeding and progressively gained weight. Over the first 12 weeks of the study, there were no differences in animal feed intake or weight between the groups (both control and stimulated groups increased intake and weight). However, after 13 weeks, animals subjected to high-frequency stimulation decreased their feed intake relative to the control group and then their weight. After 8 months, the swine stimulated at 100 Hz weighed 10.5% less than the control animals. The overall feed intake in the group stimulated at 100 Hz was 12.8% lower than in the control group. However, animals in the group stimulated at the lower frequency (5 Hz) for only 3 months demonstrated dramatically less change from the control group.

Gastric peristalsis has also been studied in the swine model. Peristalsis was noted to be altered with electrical stimulation. In a study with swine, those stimulated at 40 Hz were noted to have decreased peristalsis (34). However, the exact mechanism of action was not elucidated and gastric emptying not evaluated.

As a consequence of the animal study results, the initial human studies began in 1995 (35). Four women with a BMI of 40 or greater were implanted and followed for up to 40 months. Via laparoscopy, patients had platinum electrodes implanted intramuscularly on the anterior gastric wall, adjacent to the lesser curve and proximal to the pes anserinus. The system was bipolar in design so that two electrodes, one an anode and one a cathode, were inserted into the gastric muscle layer. A prototype electrical stimulator was implanted in a subcutaneous pocket of the anterior abdominal wall. All four patients were permitted food and drink *ad libitum*. At 40 months after implantation, one patient had lost 32 kg, and a second had lost 62 kg. In the other two patients, malfunctions in their stimulator system were discovered. One patient was found to have a fracture of the lead, which compromised its effectiveness. At 40 months after implantation, the patient had lost only 2 BMI units. Similarly, in a second patient there was also an apparent fracture of the lead, and that patient did not lose weight. In both of these patients, lead fracture led to unipolar pacing (only one electrode was presumed to be functional) versus the intended bipolar stimulation. The two subjects who had no lead problems and received bipolar pacing had much better results. Therefore, it was concluded that bipolar electrical stimulation was necessary. In addition, chronic gastric electrical stimulation was considered safe as no side effects were reported.

In 1998, a second study was initiated in human subjects to investigate the safety and efficacy of a first-generation, dedicated, gastric stimulator, the Prelude implantable gastric system (36). All enrolled patients had a BMI of more than 40, a history of unsuccessful weight loss, and an absence of serious cardiac, respiratory, or psychiatric problems. Ten patients underwent a minimally invasive surgical procedure to implant the system. Stimulation was initiated 30 days after implantation. After implant, all subjects were permitted food and drink *ad libitum* during three regular meals, but told not to eat between meals. Only sweet and alcoholic beverages were discouraged. Patients were followed at approximately monthly intervals. The stimulator was interrogated using transcutaneous radiofrequency telemetry, which linked the implanted device to a computerized programmer. Data collated included stimulation parameters, lead impedance, and residual battery capacity.

This study demonstrated both safety and efficacy. There were no deaths or other significant medical problems during the study, no complications related to the procedure, and no long-term complications. Specifically, there were no lead fractures or failures of the electrical components of the system. After receiving 51 months of stimulation, the mean weight loss of all 10 patients was 23% of excess weight and appears to be well maintained (Fig. 25.1-4). Not surprising, battery depletion led to weight regain and device replacement with a new battery resulted in renewed weight loss.

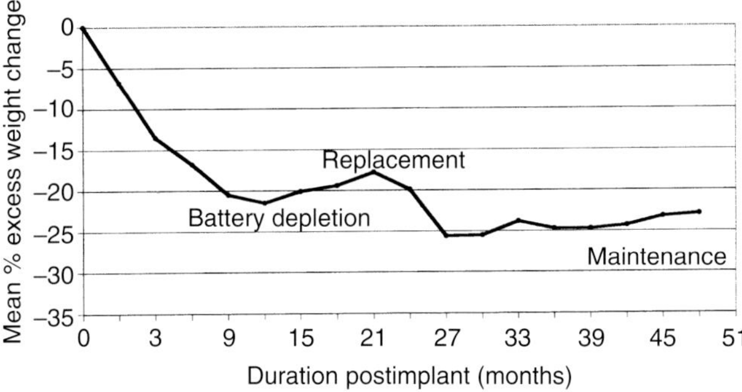

FIGURE 25.1-4. Long-term results from the preliminary pilot study of Cigaina et al. (36). Ten patients were followed for over 51 months. The patients achieved a mean of 23% excess weight loss. Also note that patients gained weight when there was battery depletion and lost weight once the devices were replaced.

Current International Experience with Implantable Gastric Stimulation for Weight Loss

The Implantable Gastric Stimulation (IGS), a pacemaker-like device (Transcend, Transneuronix, Mt. Arlington, NJ), includes a battery-operated pulse generator and a bipolar lead. The generator is similar to a heart pacemaker and about the size of a pocket watch. It is implanted under the skin in the left upper quadrant (Fig. 25.1-5). The system lead is laparoscopically inserted into the seromuscular layer of the anterior stomach wall. In most cases, the operation was performed in less than 1 hour. Most patients were discharged on the same day as the procedure or the next day. The programmer is a standard computer connected to a programming wand. The programmer communicates via the computer and wand with the implanted IGS using transcutaneous radiofrequency telemetry. The IGS can be quickly and easily interrogated or programmed in the clinic or office setting. Presently, over 800 patients have been enrolled worldwide in research trials and had the IGS system implanted. There have been no deaths or major complications.

European Multicenter Study

After the pioneering work of Cigaina et al., a multicenter trial was initiated in Europe. Fifty patients were implanted at seven clinical centers (in Italy, France, Germany, Sweden, Greece, Austria, and Belgium). While study design varied somewhat at each of the clinical centers, most were open-label. There were no significant complications in any of the patients. Mean weight loss has surpassed 40% of excess after a 2-year follow-up (Fig. 25.1-6).

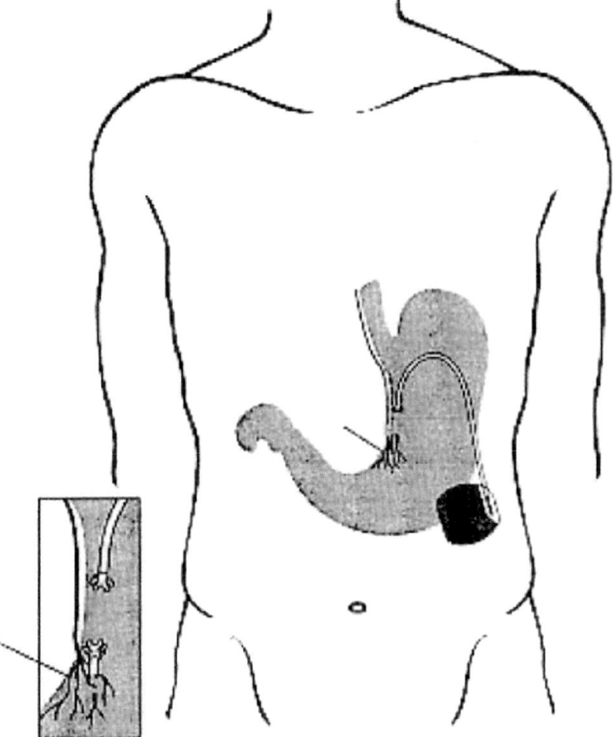

FIGURE 25.1-5. The Implantable Gastric Stimulation (IGS) system. Implantable gastric stimulator with the bipolar lead is inserted in the muscular layer along the lesser curvature. The lead is placed close to the pes anserinus.

Laparoscopic Obesity Stimulation Survey (LOSS)

A second multicenter investigation has been undertaken in Europe. This effort initially enrolled 60 patients at eight participating sites. As with the previous study, there have been no significant complications. After a 10-month period of follow-up, a mean excess weight loss of over 20% has been achieved (Fig. 25.1-7). Average excess weight loss was sustained at 25% in 91 patients two years after implantation (37).

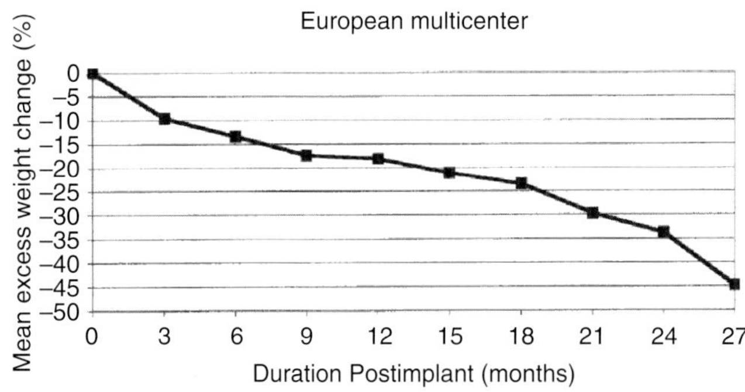

FIGURE 25.1-6. European multicenter study. Fifty patients at seven clinical sites were enrolled. Weight loss achieved was 40% of excess with a mean follow-up of 27 months.

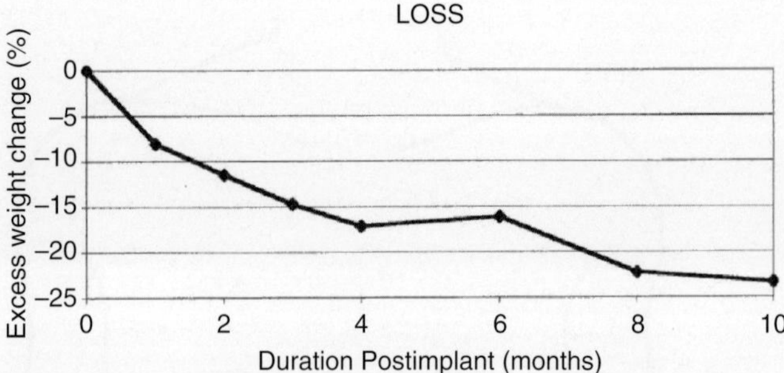

FIGURE 25.1-7. Laparoscopic Obesity Stimulation Survey (LOSS). Interim results from this multicenter European trial involving 60 patients at eight clinical centers. At a mean of 10 months of follow-up, patients lost over 20% of their excess weight and this was sustained two years after implantation.

U.S. O-01 Trial

In the United States, the first research investigation was a multicenter, randomized, controlled, double-blinded trial that was developed to evaluate both the safety and efficacy of the IGS system; 103 patients were enrolled. The IGS lead was laparoscopically placed in 100 of the patients (three patients had it placed via a small midline incision to assess the practicality of also placing the device by traditional surgery). One month after implant, patients were randomized to device activation or having the devices remain in the *off* mode. After 7 months, the off group was activated. Device settings were universal for all patients. Patients were clinically evaluated monthly for 24 months and carefully monitored for complications and for weight loss. No dietary or behavioral counseling was provided.

No deaths or complications from implantation occurred. Although none of the patients has experienced any untoward effects from this procedure, 17 of the first 41 leads were discovered to be dislodged from the stomach wall (38). This complication led to an alteration in technique to ensure better lead security. However, lead dislodgment almost certainly affected weight loss results. In addition, the lack of dietary and behavioral counseling, and the inclusion of patients with binge-eating disorders, may have also affected the weight loss results. Interestingly, during the first 6 months, many patients admitted to having deliberately overeaten or experimented with their diets to discern whether their devices were activated. Despite these drawbacks, after 1 year of stimulation, 20% of the patients lost greater than 5% of their total body weight and the mean total weight loss was 11%.

U.S. Dual-Lead Implantable Gastric Electrical Stimulator Trial

In hopes of building on the lessons learned from the European and U.S. O-01 trials, a pilot study was designed for the United States to see if the results could be improved. This open label pilot trial, the Dual-Lead Implantable Gastric Electrical Simulation Trial (DIGEST), enrolled 30 patients at two clinical sites. This trial is unique for several reasons. First, binge eaters are excluded, as they performed poorly in earlier trials. Second, behavioral support and dietary counseling are included. Third, the system includes two leads (four electrodes) that can be programmed separately or together. Finally, the device is programmed individually for each patient. A clinical breakthrough was discovered early in this investigation. It was found that by programming high electrical outputs, most patients immediately developed symptoms of bloating, nausea, retching, or abdominal pain. This finding may be similar to the *capture* of cardiac rhythm during heart pacing. The output is then reduced slightly, below the symptom threshold. Patients who experience symptoms have dramatic reductions in appetite and most have achieved weight loss. Overall, there was a 15% excess weight loss at 38 weeks (Fig. 25.1-8) and 23% excess weight loss at 16 months. However, at our site, we have achieved a mean excess weight loss of 30.4% at a mean follow-up of 9.5 months (8–14); 80% of our patients have lost weight and 60% of patients have lost more than 10% of their excess weight (14.7–104% of excess weight loss). The dramatic differences between the results from the two investigative sites may reflect differences in patient selection and administrative resources and suggests the importance of proper patient selection and support.

Need for Careful Patient Selection

Thus far, the worldwide experience with the IGS system has proven that like all other surgical procedures for weight loss, no procedure is effective for all patients. This has recently been validated when a simple screening tool (BaroScreen™) was developed and retrospectively

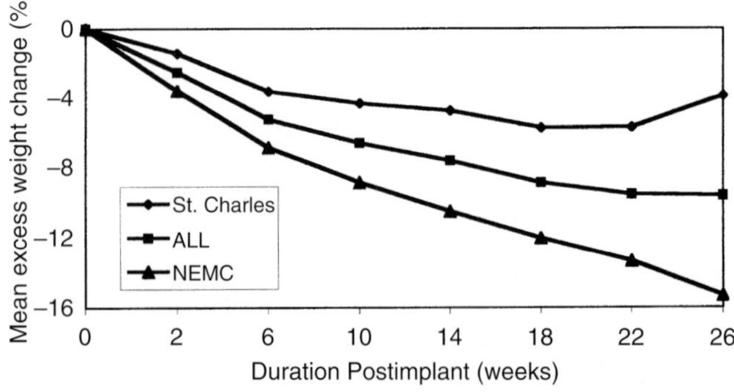

FIGURE 25.1-8. Dual-Lead Implantable Gastric Electrical Stimulation Trial (DIGEST). Preliminary results for the 30 enrolled patients at two clinical centers (New England Medical Center and St. Charles Hospital). Results varied at the two sites that may reflect differences in patient selection.

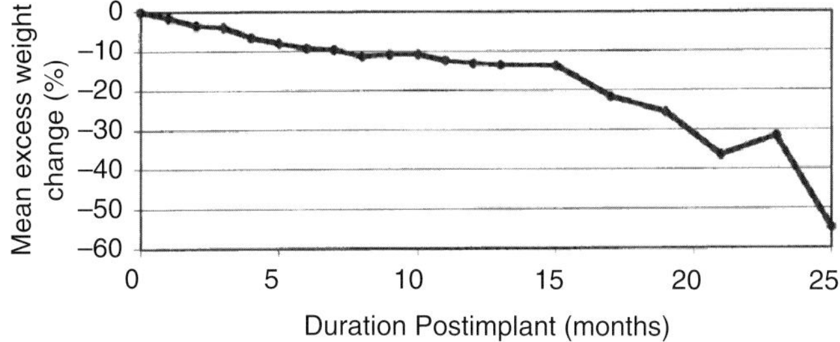

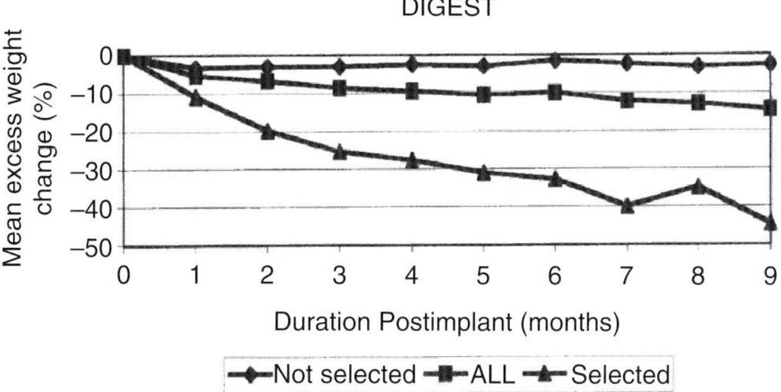

FIGURE 25.1-9. U.S. trial results with enhanced patient screening. A patient screening tool was used to predict responders and nonresponders. These graphs depict the weight loss results for both U.S. trials when only responders were included. Dramatically improved weight loss was seen. U.S. Trial O-01 is on the top and DIGEST is on the bottom.

applied to approximately 252 IGS patients internationally. The screening tool is based on demographics and responses to questionnaire items, and it appeared to accurately predict both responders, and nonresponders. Motivational factors seem to be most important. Applying this strategy retrospectively demonstrated that those patients who screened favorably for these motivational factors performed significantly better than those who screened unfavorably. For both U.S. trials, its implementation would have eliminated approximately 75% of the participants. However, those who scored favorably had dramatic results (Fig. 25.1-9). Further prospective analysis is necessary to confirm these preliminary findings.

Superficially, screening out 75% of potential patients seems to be a concern for the future of this technology. However, it should be remembered that 25% of the tens of millions of potential patients who might benefit from this procedure is still a significant number of patients who may benefit from treatment with gastric stimulation.

Future Considerations for Implantable Gastric Stimulation

While the IGS system is an exciting new approach for the treatment of severe obesity, there are still questions that need to be answered. Further animal and human research

is needed to better clarify its mechanism of action, patient selection, and proper application.

While delayed gastric emptying was initially entertained as a potential mechanism of action, this has not been demonstrated in a limited human investigation. Other etiologies are also being considered, such as the influence of gastric electrical stimulation on the secretion of gastrointestinal hormones and on nerve function. In a preliminary study on 11 patients, Cigaina and Hirshberg (39) found that IGS pacing resulted in meal-related responses of cholecystokinin and somatostatin, and basal levels of glucagon-like peptide-1 and leptin were significantly decreased as compared with controls. Further studies of gastrointestinal (GI) hormones such as ghrelin are underway.

Appropriate patient selection also needs to be better defined. Development of a simple patient screening tool (BaroScreen™) to segregate responders from nonresponders is a significant first step. As with electrical stimulation for other conditions such as epilepsy and urinary incontinence, avoiding implantation in those patients not likely to respond would dramatically improve results. In addition, determining the best subgroups of obese patients for this technology is also important. Obesity is a very heterogeneous condition. For instance, this device may prove very effective for patients with a BMI of 35 to 45, but less so for patients with a BMI of greater than 60. It may be most effective for patients with a BMI of 30 to 40. Approximately 50 million American adults have a BMI in this range, and they are generally not considered for surgery and are poorly served by medical weight loss strategies. The IGS may be attractive for the adolescent obese or could be used as a weight maintenance strategy for patients who have lost weight by nonoperative means.

Further work also needs to be performed to refine the most appropriate stimulation parameters for the device as well as the optimal location for the leads in the stomach wall. Are two leads better than one, or should multiple leads be considered? Lastly, additional applications for the IGS can also be entertained. For example, the IGS may be considered for other gastrointestinal conditions such as severe gastrointestinal reflux. Preliminary work out of Germany found that the IGS improved both lower esophageal pressures and lowered DeMeester scores in five patients with severe reflux (40).

Conclusion

Significant obesity has become a worldwide health concern that is growing in prevalence at alarming proportions. While surgery currently offers the only therapeutic option that consistently achieves meaningful and sustained weight loss, the majority of eligible surgical candidates will choose not to undergo surgery for fear of surgical complications or long-term sequelae. Implantable gastric stimulation is a new and unique surgical modality that offers safe and effective weight loss. Worldwide results have demonstrated that it is the safest of all the surgical procedures and is currently achieving near-comparable results.

While there is still much to be learned about this technology, it is clear that the IGS is introducing a paradigm shift in the surgical management of severe obesity and is close to joining the other procedures as a reliable option.

References

1. Ogden CL, Carroll MD, Curtin LR, McDowell MA, Tabak CJ, Flegal KM. Prevalence of overweight and obesity in the United States, 1999–2004. JAMA 2006;295(13):1549–1555.
2. Mokdad AH, Ford ES, Bowman BA, et al. Prevalence of obesity, diabetes, and obesity-related health risk factors, 2001. JAMA 2003;289:76–79.
3. Colditz GA. Economic costs of obesity and inactivity. Med Sports 1999;31:S663–S667.
4. Deitel M. Overweight and obesity worldwide now estimated at 1.7 billion people. Obes Surg 2003;13:329–330.
5. World Health Report 2002. www.iotf.org.
6. Schauer P, Ikramuddin S, Gourash W, et al. Outcomes after laparoscopic Roux-en-Y gastric bypass for morbid obesity. Ann Surg 2000;232:515–529.
7. Pories WJ, Swanson MS, MacDonald KG, et al. Who would have thought it? An operation proves to be the most effective therapy for adult-onset diabetes mellitus. Ann Surg 1995;222:339–352.
8. Dixon JB. O'Brien P. Health outcomes of severely obese type 2 diabetic subjects 1 year after laparoscopic adjustable silicone gastric banding. Diab Care 2002;25:358–363.
9. Chen JDZ, McCallum RW, ed. Electrogastrography: Principles and Applications. New York: Raven, 1995.
10. Qian LW, Pasricha PJ, Chen JDZ. Origins and patterns of spontaneous and drug-induced canine gastric myoelectrical dysrhythmia. Dig Dis Sci 2003;48;508–515.
11. Hasler WL. The physiology of gastric motility and gastric emptying. In: Yamada T, Alpers DH, Owyang C, Powell DW, Silverstein FE, eds. Textbook of Gastroenterology, 2nd ed. Philadelphia: Lippincott Williams & Wilkins, 1995:181–206.
12. Tougas G, Eaker EY, Abell TL, et al. Assessment of gastric emptying using a low fat meal: establishment of international control values. Am J Gastroenterology 2000;95:1456–1462.
13. Phillips RJ, Powley TL. Gastric volume rather than nutrient content inhibits food intake. Am J Physiol 1996;271:R766–R779.
14. Duggan JP, Booth DA. Obesity, overeating, and rapid gastric emptying in rats with ventromedial hypothalamic lesions. Science 1986;231:609–611.
15. Wright RA, Krinsky S, Fleeman C, et al. Gastric emptying and obesity. Gastroenterology 1983;84:747–751.
16. Carlson AJ. The Control of Hunger in Health and Disease (Psychic Secretion in Man). Chicago: University of Chicago Press, 1916.
17. Moran TH, McHugh PR. Cholecystokinin suppresses food intake by inhibiting gastric emptying. Am J Physiol 1982;242:R491–R497.
18. Sheldon RJ, Qi JA, Porreca F, et al. Gastrointestinal motor effects of corticotropic-releasing factor in mice. Regul Pept 1990;28:137–151.
19. Asakawa A, Inui A, Ueno N, et al. Urocortin reduces food intake and gastric emptying in lean and ob/ob obese mice. Gastroenterology 1999;116:1287–1292.
20. Kelly KA. Differential responses of the canine gastric corpus and antrum to electrical stimulation. Am J Physiol 1974;226:230–234.
21. Miedema BW, Sarr MG, Kelly KA. Pacing the human stomach. Surgery 1992;111:143–150.
22. Lin ZY, McCallum RW, Schirmer BD, et al. Effects of pacing parameters in the entrainment of gastric slow waves in patients with gastroparesis. Am J Physiol (Gastrointes Liver Physiol) 1998;37:G186–G191.
23. Eagon JC, Kelly KA. Effects of gastric pacing on canine gastric motility and emptying. Am J Physiol 1993;265:G767–G774.
24. Hocking MP, Vogel SB, Sninsky CA. Human gastric myoelectrical activity and gastric emptying following gastric surgery and with pacing. Gastroenterology 1992;103:1811–1816.
25. Lin XM, Peters LJ, Hayes J, et al. Entrainment of segmental small intestinal slow waves with electrical stimulation in dogs. Dig Dis Sci 2000;45:652–656.
26. McCallum RW, Chen JDZ, Lin ZY, et al. Gastric pacing improves emptying and symptoms in patients with gastroparesis. Gastroenterology 1998;114:456–461.
27. Qian LW, Lin XM, Chen JDZ. Normalization of atropine-induced postprandial dysrhythmias with gastric pacing. Am J Physiol (Gastrointest Liver Physiol 39) 1999;276:G387–G392.
28. Abo M, Liang J, Qian LW, et al. Normalization of distention-induced intestinal dysrhythmia with intestinal pacing in dogs. Dig Dis Sci 2000;45:129–135.
29. Bellahsene BE, Lind CD, Schlimer BD, et al. Acceleration of gastric emptying with electrical stimulation in canine model of gastroparesis. Am J Physiol 1992;262:G826–G834.
30. Familoni BO, Abell TL, Voeller G, et al. Electrical stimulation at a frequency higher than usual rate in human stomach. Dig Dis Sci 1997;42:885–891.
31. Hocking MP. Postoperative gastroparesis and tachygastria-response to electrical stimulation and erythromycin. Surgery 1993;114:538–542.
32. Xing JH, Brody F, Brodsky J, et al. Gastric electrical stimulation at proximal stomach induces gastric relaxation in dogs. Neurogastroenterol Motil 2003;15:15–23.
33. Cigaina V, Saggioro A, Rigo V, et al. Long-term effects of gastric pacing to reduce feed intake in swine. Obes Surg 1996;6:250–253.
34. Cigaina V. Gastric peristalsis control by mono situ electrical stimulation: a preliminary study. Obes Surg 1996;6:247–249.
35. Cigaina V, Rigo V, Greenstein RJ. Gastric myo-electrical pacing as therapy for morbid obesity: Preliminary results. Obes Surg 1999;9:333.

36. Cigaina V. Gastric pacing as therapy for morbid obesity: Preliminary results. Obes Surg 2002;12:12S–16S.

37. Miller K, Hoeller E, Aigner F. The implantable gastric stimulator for obesity: an update of the European Experience in the LOSS (Laparoscopic Obesity Stimulation Survey) Study. Treat Endocrinol 2006;5(1):53–58.

38. Shikora SA, Knox TA, Bailen L, et al. Successful use of endoscopic ultrasound (EU) to verify lead placement for the implantable gastric stimulator (IGS™). Obes Surg 2001;11:403.

39. Cigaina V, Hirshberg A. Gastric pacing for morbid obesity: Plasma levels of gastrointestinal peptides and leptin. Obes Res 2003;11:1456–1462.

40. Knippig C, Wolff S, Weigt H, et al. Gastric pacing has a positive effect on gastrointestinal reflux disease. Obes Surg 2002;12:473.

25.2

The BioEnterics Intragastric Balloon for the Nonsurgical Treatment of Obesity and Morbid Obesity

Franco Favretti, Maurizio De Luca, Gianni Segato, Luca Busetto, Enzo Bortolozzi, Alessandro Magon, and Tommaso Maccari

The development of nonsurgical treatments for morbid obesity has garnered widespread and renewed interest in the last few years. Behind these new approaches is an increased sensibility regarding the quality-of-life issue, which requires careful evaluation of the risk–benefit ratio for each intervention and for each patient, as well as a renewed respect for anatomy and function.

Intragastric balloons have been used since the early 1980s for the temporary, nonsurgical treatment of obesity and morbid obesity. In the early 1990s a new intragastric balloon was developed to optimize safety and effectiveness. The new device, the BioEnterics Intragastric Balloon (BIB; Inamed Health, Santa Barbara, CA) is a spherical, saline-filled durable device with a fill range of 400 to 700 mL.

Between January 1999 and April 2003, at the Padua Center (Padua, Italy), we treated 225 patients with the BIB. In conducting this study our aim was to determine the most appropriate indications and contraindications for BIB treatment. Additionally, we wanted to establish the best methods for balloon positioning and removal and the best approach to follow-up, drug and dietary support, and management of complications.

Historical Background

In the treatment of obesity, the intragastric balloon acts as an artificial bezoar that floats freely in the stomach. It supports weight loss by inducing a feeling of satiety that enables patients to reduce their food intake and eventually to adopt new dietary habits.

Over the years, several types of balloons have been marketed, balloons of varying sizes and shapes, made of various materials and employing different filling systems. Initially enthusiastic about this new technology, the medical community soon saw that the device could not live up to expectations in terms of safety and efficacy, and critical reports began to appear in the literature.

The two earliest balloons were the Garren-Edwards Bubble (made and sold in the United States, 1984) and the Ballobes (produced in Denmark). The Garren-Edwards, air-filled with a maximum fill volume of 220 mL, had a recommended placement of 3 months, was shaped like a tin can with sharp edges, and was made of plastic elastomer. The Ballobes, also air-filled, had a maximum fill volume of 500 mL, a sharp-edged ovoidal shape, and allowed a maximum placement of 4 months.

Both of these devices were found to produce high rates of complications, usually caused by the sharp edges. These complications included decubitus ulcers (3–7%) (1–3) and spontaneous balloon deflation (5–11%) (1–3). Several cases of bowel obstruction were also reported (1–3). Additionally, they failed the efficacy test by not producing adequate weight loss in patients due to their low maximum fill volume and the fact that they were air-filled. Nevertheless, these balloons were sold to physicians with little or no obesity surgery treatment experience. All of these problems led to the intragastric balloon falling out of favor and to its eventual demise.

Then, a scientific conference was held in Tarpon Springs, Florida, in 1987 that brought together 75 international experts from the fields of gastroenterology, surgery, obesity, nutrition, and behavior medicine. The purpose was to study the intragastric balloon and come to a consensus for the future development and use of this technology and treatment option. The conference recommended that the intragastric balloon have the following attributes:

- It should be effective at promoting weight loss.
- It should be filled with liquid (not air).
- It should be capable of adjustment to various sizes.
- It should have a smooth surface and low potential for causing ulcers and obstructions.

- It should contain a radiopaque marker that allows proper follow-up of the device if it deflates.
- It should be constructed of durable materials that do not leak.

Today, a better intragastric balloon is available. Based on the principles laid out at the Tarpon Springs Conference, Inamed Health developed the BIB. It is made of high-quality silicone. It is durable and elastic and has a smooth surface, without external seams or protuberances to irritate the gastric mucosa and lead to erosions and ulcers (Fig. 25.2-1). It can be filled with up to 700 mL of saline solution (larger size for greater weight loss) plus 10 mL of methylene blue (to individuate blue urine in case of balloon deflation) and can be left in place for up to 6 months. The inflated BIB is spherical in shape; the deflated balloon is encased in a smooth silicone sheath (which opens as the balloon inflates) for easier esophageal insertion (Fig. 25.2-2). The radiopaque markers allow the operator to radiographically visualize the orientation of the balloon and identify the position of the self-sealing valve.

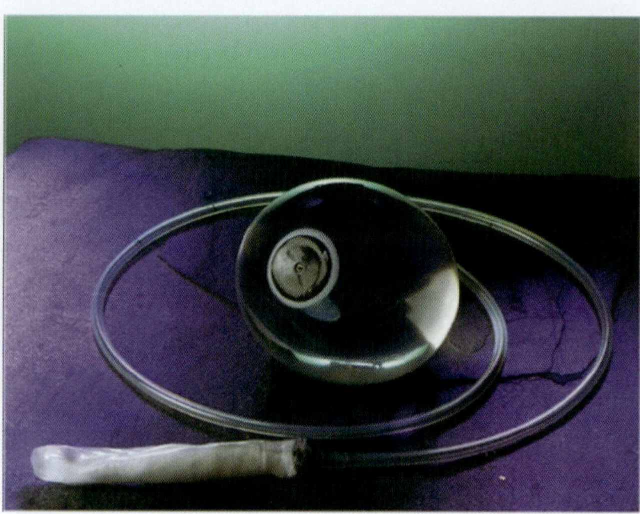

FIGURE 25.2-2. Intragastric balloon ex vivo demonstrating the inflated balloon (center) and the deflated balloon within a thin silicone sheath prior to placement. (Courtesy of Inamed Health, Santa Barbara, CA.)

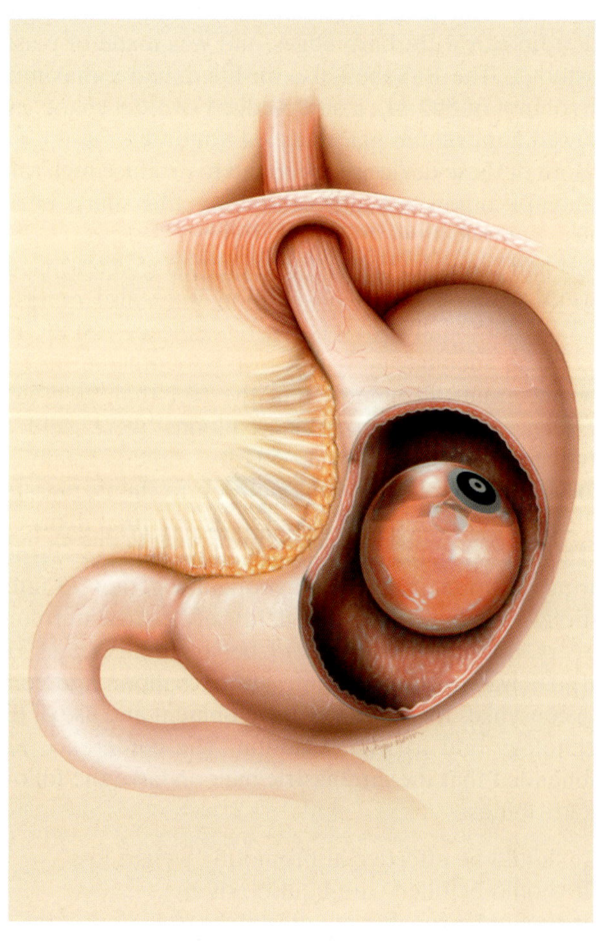

FIGURE 25.2-1. Bioenterics Intragastric Balloon (Inamed Health, Santa Barbara, CA) in place within the lumen of the stomach.

Indications

The indications for using the intragastric balloon are as follows (4,5):

- Preparation and selection in view of further surgery (Lap-Band; Inamed Health, Santa Barbara, CA) of super-obese patients with very high operative risk
- BIB test for evaluation and selection of patients for restrictive procedure (Lap-Band in our series)
- BMI ≥ 35 with resistance to clinical treatment and refusal or present contraindication to surgical treatment
- BMI < 35 with comorbidities and resistance to clinical treatment
- Reduction of anesthetic risk (general surgery, orthopedic surgery, cardiovascular surgery, etc.)

Contraindications

The absolute and relative contraindications to the intragastric balloon are as follows (4–8):

Absolute

- Severe and active esophagitis
- Active gastric or duodenal ulceration
- Inflammatory bowel disease
- Cancers
- Active and gastrointestinal bleeding
- Alcoholism or drug addiction

Relative

- Large hiatal hernia (>5 cm)
- Prior gastric or intestinal surgery
- Patients receiving anticoagulants or other gastric irritants
- Psychiatric disorders

BioEnterics Intragastric Balloon Positioning/Removal

Sedation and Anesthesia

For sedation and anesthesia during the BIB positioning and removal (5,6,9), diazepam, 10 mg, plus Dosine n-butyl bromure, 30 mg, and propofol are used. The presence of an anesthesiologist is necessary (without endotracheal intubation).

Placement

The procedure begins with examination of the stomach using the endoscope (diagnostic endoscopy). If no abnormalities are observed, the physician proceeds with placement of the BIB through the mouth and down the esophagus into the stomach under endoscopic guidance (previous lubrication of the BIB with Xylocaine gel). Once the BIB is inside the stomach, it is immediately filled with sterile saline (700 mL) and 10 mL of methylene blue through a small filling tube (catheter) attached to the balloon. Once the balloon is filled, the operator removes the catheter by gently pulling on the external end. The BIB has a self-sealing valve and at this point it is floating freely in the stomach. A check of the valve is performed and the endoscope is removed.

Postplacement Pharmaceutical Therapy

The following postplacement pharmaceutical therapy is recommended:

- Liquid IV (glucose and electrolytes), 2500-3000 cc/day for 1 to 2 days
- Metoclopramide IV 60 mg/day for 1 to 2 days
- Metoclopramide IM 40 mg/day for 2 to 3 days
- Proton pump inhibitor (PPI) 40 mg/day for 2 days
- Proton pump inhibitor (PPI) po 20 mg/day for 15 days while balloon is in place
  - —Proton pump inhibitor (PPI) po 40 mg/day in symptomatic patients
  - —In case of epigastric pain: Scopalamine butylbromide (Buscopan) 1 fL IM, and eventually Ketorolac tromethamine 1 fL 30 mg IM
  - —In case of vomiting, metoclopramide, 40 mg IM

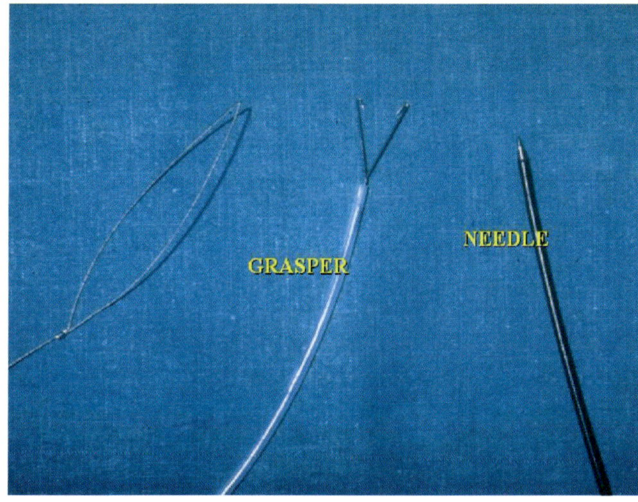

FIGURE 25.2-3. Endoscopic devices used for puncture and removal of the intragastric balloon (Aprime, Brussels, Belgium; Scandimed, Glastrup, Denmark; Olympus, Hamburg, Germany).

Removal

The BIB currently can be kept in place for 6 months. Before removal, the patient must be kept on a liquid diet for 3 days. The BIB is normally removed in the same way it was placed, via the esophagus and the mouth under endoscopic guidance. Using the endoscope, the operator introduces the BIB removal device (needle, Aprime, Brussels, Belgium) to puncture and deflate the balloon. Using a foreign body grasper (Aprime; Scandimed, Glastrup, Denmark; Olympus, Hamburg, Germany) the balloon is then removed (Fig. 25.2-3).

Our BioEnterics Intragastric Balloon Experience

From January 1999 to April 2003 a group of 225 obese or morbidly obese patients underwent BIB treatment in our institution (Table 25.2-1).

TABLE 25.2-1. Patient features in the total series of 225 patients

	n	Male	Female
All patients	225	108	117
BMI	52.6 ± 4.8	53.7 ± 4.9	49.2 ± 4.7
Sequential treatment (BIB + Lap-Band)	41	23	18
BMI	58.6 ± 5.8	57.7 ± 5.9	59.9 ± 5.6
BIB test	16	6	10
BMI	51.3 ± 7.9	52.1 ± 4.7	50.8 ± 6.6
Low BMI with resistance to clinical treatment	65	7	58
BMI	34.6 ± 2.8	34.9 ± 1.9	34.6 ± 1.6
Patients with comorbidities	51	26	25
BMI	46.0 ± 7.6	47.9 ± 6.9	45.6 ± 6.8

BIB, BioEnterics Intragastric Balloon; BMI, body mass index.

TABLE 25.2-2. Results: all groups by indication

BIB Indication	No. of Patients	Weight (kg)	BMI	%EWL
Total	225	129.1 ± 27.4	45.9 ± 6.2	22.1 ± 18.5
BIB Test	16	119.7 ± 19.3	44.9 ± 7.0	21.3 ± 13.4
With low BMI	65	79.2 ± 12.7	29.8 ± 3.6	30.2 ± 11.9
With comorbidities	51	112.9 ± 17.8	40.5 ± 8.2	17.8 ± 16.4
Previous failed Lap-Band surgery	3 (1 patient ended BIB treatment)	114.3 ± 13.8	42.2 ± 7.1	9.7 ± 7.4

%EWL, percent of excess weight loss.

Indications for BioEnterics Intragastric Balloon Treatment: Total Series of 225 Patients

Ninety patients were initially scheduled for Lap-Band surgery; 68 of them underwent presurgical balloon treatment. However, two patients suffered fatal pulmonary emboli and six patients had the BIB removed before the scheduled date; thus 60 patients completed presurgical BIB treatment. Since then, eight have refused an operation and 11 patients are still awaiting Lap-Band procedures. Forty-one patients have completed the sequential treatment (BIB + Lap-Band).

Sixteen patients (BMI ≈ 51) were scheduled for the BIB test only (evaluation of patient compliance and suitability for a future restrictive surgical procedure) (Lap-Band). Sixty-five patients with low BMI (<35) and resistance to clinical treatment were scheduled for BIB only. Fifty-one patients (BMI ≈ 46) with comorbidities were scheduled for BIB only. Three patients with previously unsuccessful Lap-Band surgery were scheduled for BIB.

Results

At the conclusion of balloon treatment in this series of 225 patients, the mean weight was 129.1 ± 27.4 kg, BMI was 45.9 ± 6.2, and percent of excess weight loss (%EWL) was 22.1 ± 18.5. Results of all patient groups are shown in Table 25.2-2. Results of the 41 patients who underwent BIB treatment prior to Lap-Band surgery (BIB + Lap-Band) are shown 2 years post–Lap-Band.

Our follow-up consists of surgical and nutritional assessment in weeks 1, 4, 12, and 24 after placement; abdominal ultrasound to evaluate the size and position of the BIB; contrast or endoscopic study of the stomach in symptomatic patients; and checking of urine and stool color by patients themselves.

Complications: Total Series of 225 Patients

Complications in the total series of 225 patients included 10 cases (4.4%) of leakage and deflation of the BIB; four cases (1.8%) of BIB elimination by stool; no small bowel obstruction (0%); five cases of BIB intolerance (2.2%);

12 cases (5.3%) of vomiting more than 2 weeks; one case (0.4%) of Mallory-Weiss syndrome; one case (0.4%) of pressure ulcer; two cases (0.8%) of gastric bleeding; and two cases (0.8%) of fatal pulmonary embolism.

Discussion

In our experience, the most appropriate clinical indications for BIB treatment are (1) preparation for and selection to further surgery (Lap-Band) of super-obese patients with very high operative risk, and (2) BIB test for evaluation and selection of patients for restrictive procedure (Lap-Band in our series) (5).

The Brazilian multicenter study (July 2001) of 219 cases revealed that in the group of 24 super-obese patients (BMI > 50) with a mean weight loss (WL) of 39 kg and mean %EWL of 31.7, all patients who were American Society of Anesthesiologists (ASA) IV before BIB treatment became ASA II after treatment (6).

Reducing anesthetic risk and perioperative complications with preoperative weight loss is considered very important in our clinical practice and is one of the main reasons our group has approached this so-called sequential treatment in selected patients (BIB + Lap-Band). Our series of 41 sequential treatment patients showed that the %EWL of BIB + Lap-Band at 2 years after Lap-Band was 35.3 ± 16.2 (Table 25.2-3); %EWL after BIB and before the operation was 23.1 ± 11.5. In terms of weight loss, mean weight at BIB positioning was 172.3 ± 27.4 kg, at Lap-Band surgery was 148.5 ± 22.9 kg, and at 2 years postoperatively was 131.8 ± 21.9 kg. In our experience and from an anesthesia point of view, this treatment has proven to be very effective.

Doldi et al.'s (10) comparison of BIB + diet vs. diet alone showed that BIB + diet could produce better weight loss in a shorter time than BIB alone; diet alone

TABLE 25.2-3. Results: sequential treatment (BIB + Lap-Band)

Time	No. of Patients	Weight (kg)	BMI	%EWL
BIB	41	172.3 ± 27.4	58.6 ± 5.8	—
Lap-Band	41	148.5 ± 22.9	50.7 ± 5.8	23.1 ± 11.5
6 months	30	139.7 ± 21.1	47.1 ± 5.6	31.3 ± 12.8
1 year	26	134.5 ± 24.0	46.3 ± 6.9	34.8 ± 16.5
2 years	12	131.8 ± 21.9	46.6 ± 7.9	35.3 ± 16.2

at 12 months produced weight loss similar to BIB + diet at 6 months. A more recent study of 349 BIB patients by Doldi and colleagues helped to further define the optimal indications for BIB. These patients had BIB placed for 4 months in conjunction with a 1000 kcal/day diet. At the end of the treatment period, the mean reduction in BMI was 4.8. The conclusions from this study were that BIB is best suited for morbidly or super-obese patients in preparation for bariatric operations, and for patients with a BMI of 35 to 40 with severe comorbidity prior to bariatric surgery. Patients with a BMI of <35 had a BIB placed as part of a multidisciplinary approach to weight loss to control chronic comorbidities (11). A large retrospective study of 2515 patients who underwent BIB and a 1000 kcal/day diet for 6 months reported an overall complication rate of 2.8% with five gastric perforations (0.2%), four of whom had undergone prior gastric surgery. Additional complications included 19 gastric obstructions (0.76%) requiring balloon removal, nine balloon ruptures (0.36%), 32 cases of esophagitis (1.27%), and five gastric ulcers (0.2%). Preoperative comorbidities improved in 44.8% of patients and resolved in 44.3% of patients. After 6 months of treatment, this study reported a mean BMI decrease of 9.3 and EWL of 33.9% ± 18% (12).

In a randomized, controlled, crossover study in 32 patients with an average BMI of 43.7, Genco et al. (13) reported a decrease in BMI of 5.5 in the first 3 months of BIB in 16 patients randomized to receive the balloon and diet. At 3 months, the balloon was removed and there was an additional decrease of one BMI point in this group for the last 3 months of the study. The second group of patients underwent a sham procedure initially and lost only 0.5 BMI points with the 1000 kcal/day diet. After receiving the BIB at the 3-month crossover, this group achieved weight loss similar to the first group (BMI decrease of 4.3). This study showed that BIB can be a useful adjunct to diet for preoperative weight loss prior to bariatric surgery (13).

The indication of BIB placement in patients with BMI < 35 and resistance to clinical treatment has shown the best results in our series. The weight at BIB placement was 91.6 ± 9.7 kg while at BIB removal was 79.2 ± 12.7 kg and %EWL was 30.2 ± 11.9. It will be important to evaluate the results in terms of weight loss maintenance at least at 24 months.

The BMI in the group of patients who underwent BIB placement for comorbidity reduction (51 patients) averaged 46 at BIB placement and 40.5 at BIB removal (Table 25.2-4). Sixty-three percent of patients with hypertension were able to reduce medication and 26% were able to eliminate drugs completely after BIB use. In the subset of patients with type 2 diabetes, 47% were able to reduce medication and 26% eliminated it completely. Fifty-seven percent of sleep apnea patients discontinued continuous positive airway pressure (CPAP).

TABLE 25.2-4. Results: BIB for comorbidities

Comorbidities Pre-BIB	BIB removal—results	
	Drug reduction	Drug elimination
Type 2 diabetes—19 patients	9 (47%)	5 (26%)
Hypertension—27 patients	17 (63%)	7 (26%)
Post-heart attack—2 patients	2 (100%)	—
Sleep apnea (CPAP)—14 patients	4 (29%)	8 (57%)
Arthrosis—26 patients	9 (35%)	4 (15%)
Depression—9 patients	3 (33%)	—
Posttraumatic spinal cord injury—2 patients	—	—

In three subjects we registered a failure of the Lap-Band in terms of weight loss (from 129.4 ± 15.9 kg to 124.2 ± 13.1 kg in a mean time of 26 months). When this occurs we usually advise patients to undergo a malabsorptive procedure involving a duodenal switch with gastric preservation (Bandinaro, Chapter 20.5). However, in these three selected patients, with strict multidisciplinary support (surgical, dietary, and psychological), we tried a more conservative and less permanent approach (BIB) to produce the weight loss yet avoid the malabsorptive elements. One patient ended the treatment prematurely due to cardiac arrhythmia and the other two patients are currently in treatment. While we do not consider these three patients with failed Lap-Bands to have any statistical relevance, we are encouraged by the results so far: mean weight at 4 months post-BIB positioning is 114.3 ± 13.8 kg with a %EWL of 9.7 ± 7.4. And though the results in this group of patients were not significant, we do believe that in these cases the BIB could be a good conservative alternative prior to submitting patients to an additional (malabsorptive) surgical procedure.

In the last 75 patients of our series BIB inflation has been more or less maximum (about 700 mL), so almost all patients of this series presented with epigastric pain and some episodes of vomiting for 1 to 2 days. Because of this early discomfort, it is rare for us after placement of the BIB to be able to discharge the patient the same day or the next day as we do at BIB removal. Even so, the results, in terms of %EWL, have been better in this group of patients.

The five cases of BIB intolerance for which the patients required endoscopic removal of the BIB all occurred in the group of patients with BMI < 35 whose need and motivation for adequate results could probably not be compared with those of super-obese patients in preoperative preparation. One case of pressure ulcer of the antrum was discovered at the time of BIB removal. The patient continued the therapy with PPI and endoscopic control. One month after BIB removal the ulcer was healed.

Conclusion

We have used the BIB as a temporary nonsurgical treatment for obesity and morbid obesity and found that it succeeds in inducing >20% EWL with minimal complication risk. The most appropriate indications in our series are (1) preparation and selection for further surgery (Lap-Band) of super-obese patients with very high operative risk; and (2) BIB test to select patients for restrictive surgery (Lap-Band). While the best results were achieved in the group of patients with BMI < 35, good results were observed in patients with high BMI and comorbidities as well.

References

1. Garren L. Garren Gastric bubble. Bariatr Surg 1985;3: 14–15.
2. Mathus Vliegen EMH, Tytgat GNJ, Veldhuizen-Offermans EAML. Intragastric balloon in the treatment of super-morbid obesity. Double blind, sham controlled, crossover evaluation of 500 milliliter balloon. Gastroenterology 1990;99:362–369.
3. Siardi C, Vita PM, Granelli P, De Roberto F, Doldi SB, Montorsi W. Il trattamento dell'obesità con palloncino gastrico. Minerva Dietol Gastroenterol 1990;36(1):13–17.
4. Nieben OG, Harboe H. Intragastric balloon as an artificial bezoar for treatment for obesity. Lancet 1990;1:189–199.
5. Bortolozzi L, Maccari T, De Luca M, Segato G, Busetto L, Favretti F. BioEnterics Intragastric Balloon (BIB). The University of Padua Obesity Center series. The Intragastric Balloon. Endoscopic gastroplasty for the treatment of obesity. Caminho Editorial, San Paolo, Brazil, 2002.
6. Sallet JA. The Intragastric Balloon. Endoscopic gastroplasty for the treatment of obesity. Caminho Editorial, Sao Paolo, Brazil, 2002.
7. Tottè E, Hendrickx L, Pauwels M, Van Hee R. Weight reduction by means of intragastric device: experience with the BioEnterics Intragastric Balloon. Obes Surg 2001; 11(4):519–523.
8. Weiner R, Gutberlet H, Bockhom H. Pre-surgical treatment of extremely obese patients with the intragastric balloon. Obes Surg 1998;8:367–368.
9. Walhen CH, Bastens B, Herve J, et al. The BioEnterics Intragastric Balloon (BIB): How to use it. Obes Surg 2001;11(4):524–527.
10. Doldi SB, Micheletto G, Di Prisco F, et al. Intragastric Balloon in obese patients. Obes Surg 2000;7:361–366.
11. Doldi SB, Micheletto G, Perrini MN, Rapetti R. Intragastric balloon: another option for treatment of obesity and morbid obesity. Hepatogastroenterology 2004;51(55):294–297.
12. Genco A, Bruni T, Doldi SB, et al. BioEnterics Intragastric Balloon: the Italian experience with 2,515 patients. Obes Surg 2005;15(8):1161–1164.
13. Genco A, Cipriano M, Bacci V, et al. BioEnterics(R) Intragastric Balloon (BIB(R)): a short-term, double-blind, randomised, controlled, crossover study on weight reduction in morbidly obese patients. Int J Obes (Lond) 2006;30:129–133.

25.3
The Emerging Field of Endoluminal and Transgastric Bariatric Surgery

Philip R. Schauer, Bipan Chand, and Stacy A. Brethauer

Gastrointestinal endoluminal technology is emerging as the next major revolution in minimally invasive surgery. A similar trend is already well underway in vascular surgery with the widespread endoluminal vascular therapy. The endoluminal approach to bariatric surgery will have numerous advantages. These techniques will potentially be performed as outpatient procedures without the need for skin incisions or general anesthesia and they may reduce the risk, discomfort, and cost of bariatric procedures. Innovative devices have been developed and Food and Drug Administration (FDA) approved for the treatment of gastroesophageal reflux disease (GERD), and they may be adapted as, or lead to, new devices that can be used for weight loss procedures. This chapter reviews endoluminal technologies currently in development, preliminary clinical and preclinical data describing their use in bariatric applications, and the future of endoluminal bariatric surgery.

By combining the high success rates of weight loss achieved with current surgical procedures (1) with the low complications and benefits of natural orifice access surgery, these approaches may represent a potentially safer, simpler, and less costly option than current minimally invasive procedures. The annual rate of bariatric procedures increased fivefold between 1998 and 2002 (2), and the demand will certainly continue to rise over the next several decades. The continued pressure to provide ambulatory surgery, though, remains, and endoluminal and transgastric therapy has the potential to significantly change the way obesity is treated.

The emerging field has recently been referred to as natural orifice transluminal endoscopic surgery (NOTES) (3). The Natural Orifice Surgery Consortium for Assessment and Research (NOSCAR) is a newly organized group of surgeons and gastrointestinal endoscopists devoted to establishing guidelines for development and clinical use of this technology (3).

The potential applications for endoscopic bariatric surgery include procedures for preoperative weight loss, revisional procedures for stoma and gastric pouch enlargement, and stand-alone or primary weight loss procedures.

Endoluminal Surgery: Proof of Principle

The first major indication in endoluminal surgery to be tackled widely by medical device companies was the treatment of GERD. The invention of the endoscopic "sewing machine" by Swain led to the development of several endoluminal suturing devices, beginning with the EndoCinch™ Suturing System (Davol, Cranston, RI) (Fig. 25.3-1) (4,5). Other suturing devices ensued, including the Endoscopic Suturing Device® (ESD; Wilson Cook Medical, Winston-Salem, NC) (Fig. 25.3-2) and the Plicator™ (NDO Surgical, Mansfield, MA) (Fig. 25.3-3). Both the EndoCinch and the Plicator are FDA approved for GERD. These suturing devices have enabled the endoluminal creation of a mechanical barrier to reflux at the esophagogastric junction that attempts to mimic Nissen fundoplication. Other technologies now FDA approved for GERD include the Stretta® device (Curon Medical, Sunnyvale, CA), which uses radiofrequency energy (RFE) to ablate tissues, and an implantable copolymer, Enteryx® (Boston Scientific, Natick, MA). Several other devices are in various stages of clinical development for GERD.

The long-term outcomes with endoluminal devices, together with initial data from recently published sham-controlled trials, indicate that the endoluminal treatment of GERD is relatively efficacious and durable, but this approach remains controversial (5–7).

Successful studies of endoluminal GERD therapies provide proof of principle for endoluminal bariatric surgery. Numerous established device companies, as well

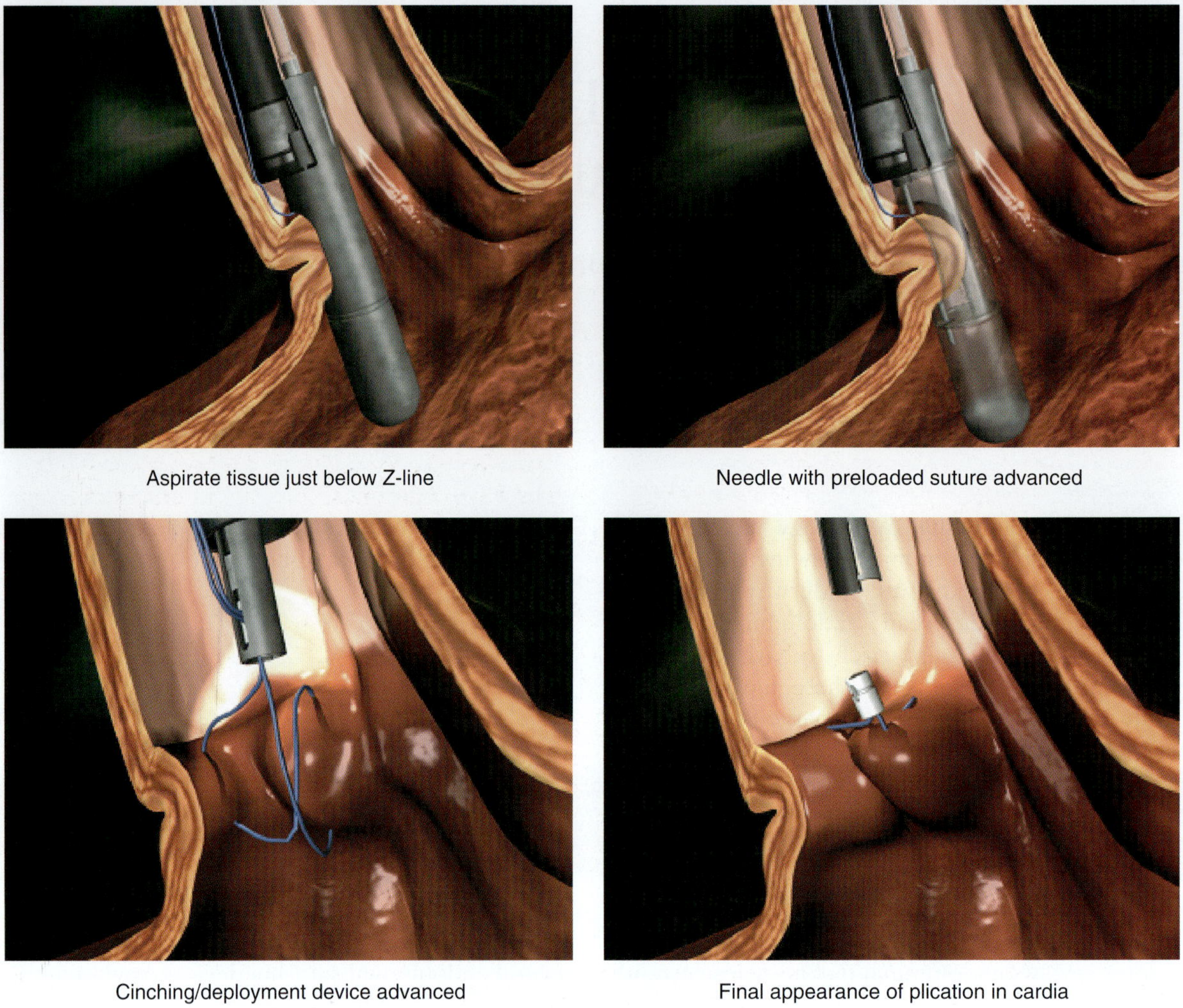

Aspirate tissue just below Z-line

Needle with preloaded suture advanced

Cinching/deployment device advanced

Final appearance of plication in cardia

FIGURE 25.3-1. *EndoCinch.* (Courtesy of Davol Inc., Cranston, RI.)

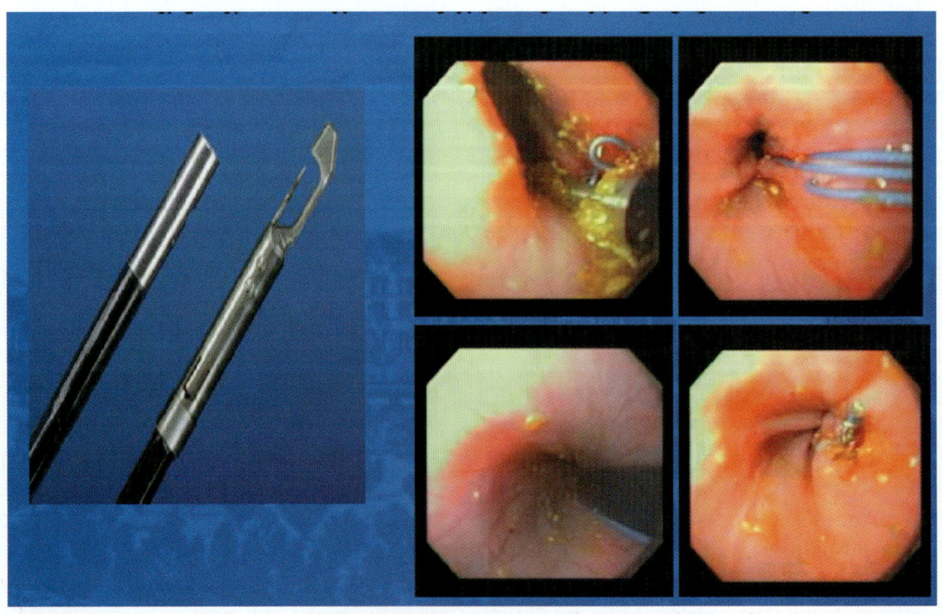

FIGURE 25.3-2. Wilson Cook Endoscopic Suturing Device. (Courtesy of Wilson Cook Medical, Winston-Salem, NC.)

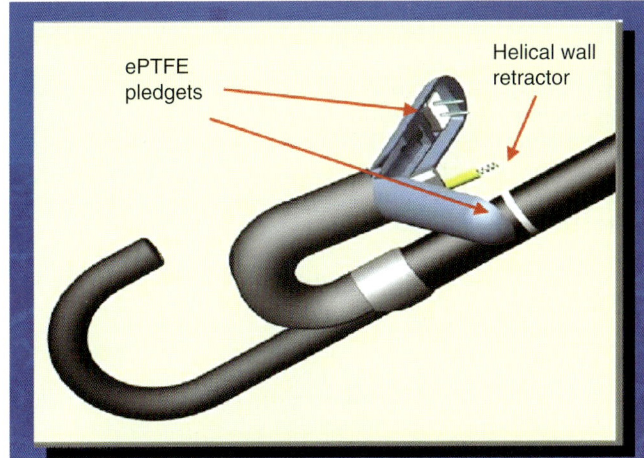

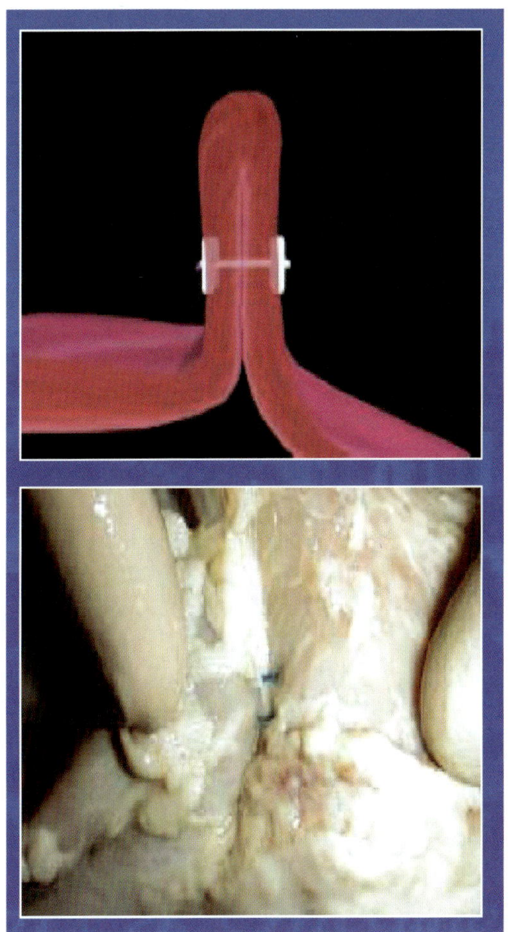

FIGURE 25.3-3. (A) NDO Plicator. ePTFE, expanded polyte-trafluoroethylene. (B) Full-thickness plication of gastric wall. (Courtesy of NDO Surgical, Inc., Mansfield, MA.)

as start-up ventures, are currently investigating endoluminal approaches to treat obesity (Table 25.3-1).

Suturing and Stapling Devices

As mentioned above, several suturing platforms were developed based on Swain's "sewing machine" for the treatment of GERD, including the above-mentioned EndoCinch, ESD, and Plicator. Many of these devices, which include partial- and full-thickness plication technologies, may be adapted for use in bariatric procedures. In addition, endoluminal suturing techniques are being developed with the goal of simulating a gastric sleeve (Fig. 25.3-4). The utility of these devices in bariatric surgery is being explored in both preclinical and clinical studies, including revisional surgeries and potential primary weight loss procedures.

One of the major obstacles to overcome with endoscopic suturing is durability. Mucosa to mucosa apposition in the stomach may not provide a durable partition unless tissue bridging can be induced or division of the tissue can be accomplished. Endoscopic stapling devices, then, have enormous potential in endoluminal bariatric surgery. The SurgASSIST® flexible endoscopy stapler (Power Medical Interventions, New Hope, PA) is currently available, but this circular endoluminal stapler currently has limited applications. Ultimately, an endoluminal linear cutting stapler that can safely create a divided partition may offer a durable endoluminal solution. This type of procedure, though, would certainly entail the risk of staple line leakage, which could potentially increase the risk-benefit ratio for this type of procedure. There are many engineering obstacles to overcome before a device such as this would be available for use. Other techniques such as endoluminal clamping or a nondivided staple line are concepts that are being developed (Fig. 25.3-5).

Intragastric Prostheses

The intragastric balloon (BioEnterics Intragastric Balloon, BIB, Inamed Health, Santa Barbara, CA) is the only device currently available in this category. In clinical studies, it has been used to induce preoperative weight loss to decrease anesthetic risk and technical challenges in super-obese patients undergoing bariatric surgery (8). New prosthetic devices are under development for bariatric applications. The types of devices being considered include a prosthetic gastric partitioning, other space-occupying devices (Fig. 25.3-6), and endoluminal tubes or stents (Fig. 25.3-7) that would exclude food from the body of the stomach or the absorptive surface of the small bowel.

Mucosal Ablation

Devices that cause tissue ablation include injection (sclerotherapy) and RFE (e.g., the above-mentioned Stretta device). These have been used in the treatment of GERD and patients who regain weight after Roux-en-Y gastric bypass (RYGBP). These technologies are being adapted for use in natural orifice bariatric surgery in both preclinical and clinical investigations. Spaulding (9) provided

TABLE 25.3-1. Available and emerging endoluminal technologies

Technology class	Company	Trade name	Mechanism of action and clinical applications
Endoluminal suturing and stapling	Davol, Inc., a subsidiary of C.R. Bard, Inc. (Cranston, RI)	EndoCinch Suturing System*	Partial-thickness plication for GERD
	Wilson Cook Medical (Winston-Salem, NC)	Endoscopic Suturing Device	Partial-thickness plication for GERD
	NDO Surgical, Inc. (Mansfield, MA)	Plicator*	Full-thickness plication for GERD
	Syntheon (Miami, FL)	Antireflux Device	Full-thickness plication for GERD
	Olympus (Tokyo, Japan)	Eagle Claw	Intragastric suturing apparatus for obesity
	USGI Medical (San Clemente, CA)		Intragastric suturing apparatus for obesity
	Power Medical Interventions, Inc. (New Hope, PA)	SurgASSIST	Intraluminal flexible circular stapler
Injection or prosthesis	Boston Scientific Corp. (Natick, MA)	Enteryx**	Biocompatible copolymer bulking agent for GERD
	Wilson Cook Medical (Winston-Salem, NC)		Space-occupying bezoar-like plastic ribbon for obesity
	GI Dynamics (Newton, MA)		Disk with nitinol clips to create gastric pouch for obesity
	GI Dynamics (Newton, MA)		Tube/stent for placement in duodenum for malabsorption for obesity
	BaroSense (Menlo Park, CA)		Cup valve used to create gastric pouch for obesity
	Cook Surgical (Bloomington, IN)	Surgisis	Prolene mesh used in gastric partitioning for obesity
	Allergan (Irvine, CA), formerly Inamed Corp. (Santa Barbara, CA)	BioEnterics Intragastric Balloon	Endoluminal balloon for obesity
	Satiety (Palo Alto, CA)		Fastening element for gastric restriction for obesity
	Polymorfix (Emeryville, CA)		Acid-sensitive capsule releases polymer in stomach to curb hunger for obesity
Electrical stimulation	IntraPace (Menlo Park, CA)		Intragastric electrodes to slow gastric emptying for obesity
	Enteromedics		Vagal nerve downregulation to slow gastric emptying, slow digestion, and curb hunger for obesity
Ablation	Curon Medical (Sunnyvale, CA)	Stretta*	RFE delivery to distal esophagus or rectum, used for GERD
	Silhouette Medical (Mountain View, CA)		RFE ablation of gastric antrum for obesity
Other technologies	USGI Medical (San Clemente, CA)	Shape Locking Endoscopic Overtube	Overtube can be locked into different positions for multiple endoscopic uses
	Barosense (Menlo Park, CA)	Articulating endoscope	Articulating endoscope for new techniques for multiple endoscopic uses

GERD, gastroesophageal reflux disease; RFE, radiofrequency energy.
* FDA cleared for use in United States
** FDA cleared for use in United States, but not currently available for clinical use.
Source: U.S. Patent Office, available at http://www.uspto.gov/patft/index.html. European Patent Office, available at www.european-patent-office.org.

data on a series of 20 patients with dilated gastrojejunal stomas after gastric bypass and following sclerotherapy; 75% of the patients lost weight after the procedure. Treatment using RFE, which causes localized tissue ablation through the generation of heat within targeted tissues, may have an application in bariatrics. The Silhouette™ Medical ablation system (Silhouette Medical, Mountain View, CA) used RFE ablation to target the antrum or pylorus to impair gastric emptying (10).

Electrical Stimulation

There has been much enthusiasm regarding electrical stimulation and devices that innervate the stomach for bariatric applications, the most widely known being the Transcend® system (Medtronic, Minneapolis, MN). These devices may be implanted through open or laparoscopic means, but new ventures are generating interest with electrical stimulation systems that are deployed endoluminally (Fig. 25.3-8). IntraPace (Menlo Park, CA) is in

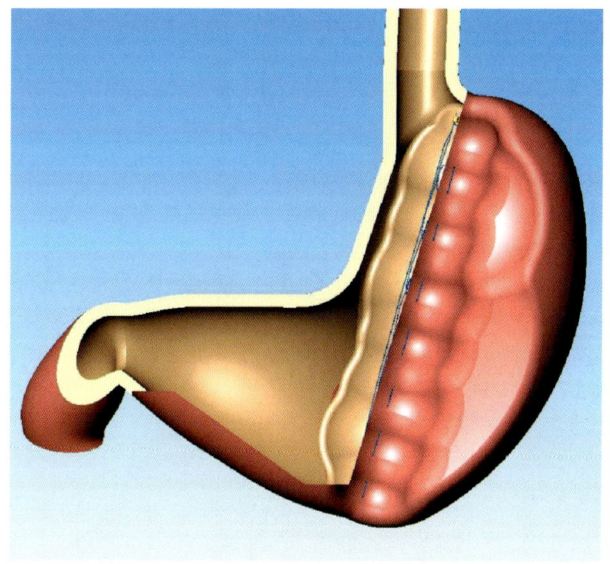

FIGURE 25.3-4. Endoluminal suturing. (Courtesy of Davol Inc., Cranston, RI.)

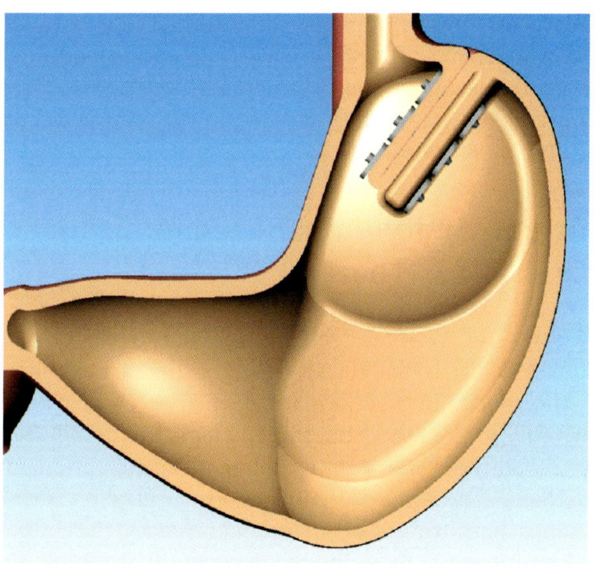

FIGURE 25.3-5. Clamping/stapling. (Courtesy of Davol Inc., Cranston, RI.)

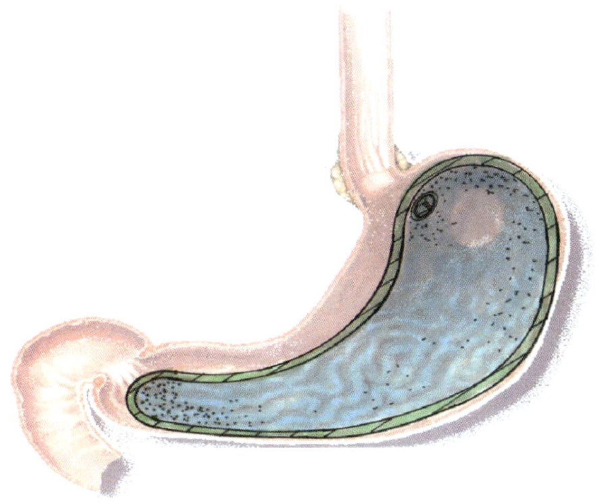

FIGURE 25.3-6. Endoscopically placed space-occupying balloon. (Courtesy of Davol Inc., Cranston, RI.)

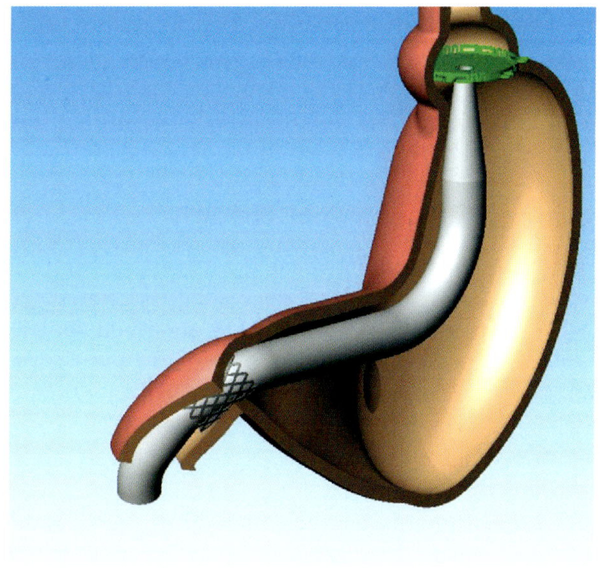

FIGURE 25.3-7. Outlet restriction. (Courtesy of Davol Inc., Cranston, RI.)

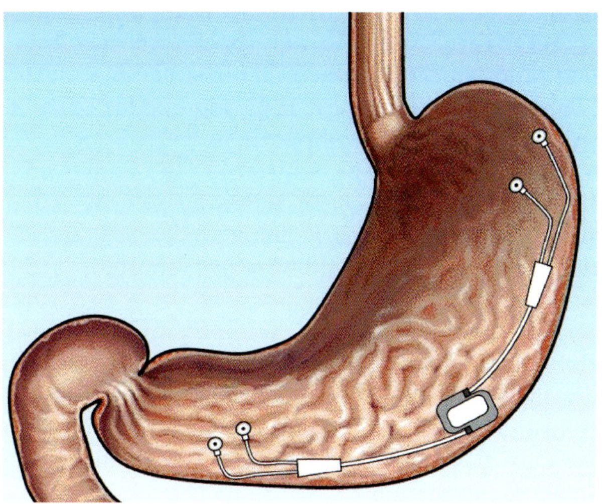

FIGURE 25.3-8. Endoscopically placed electrical gastric stimulation. (Courtesy of Davol Inc., Cranston, RI.)

the process of developing an endoscopically delivered gastric pacemaker for obesity. The addition of endoluminal gastric pacing further augments the expanding possibilities of natural orifice surgery in its efforts to treat obesity.

Current Endoluminal Modalities for Weight-Loss Therapy

As new and existing technologies are developed for endoluminal bariatric surgery, the question arises regarding the specific indications for each type of procedure. Currently in the literature, three categories of endoluminal modalities undergoing clinical investigation are described: presurgical weight loss, postsurgical revision of previous bariatric procedures, and primary procedures. The presurgical modality represents procedures that induce short-term weight reductions in patients with super-obesity to reduce anesthetic risk and surgical complications. Postsurgical repairs are performed to reduce a dilated gastrojejunal anastomosis, treat stenoses, or repair suture or staple lines. Primary procedures performed endoluminally may eventually become a mainstream part of bariatric surgery, but major obstacles regarding feasibility and durability will need to be overcome.

Presurgical Endoluminal Therapy

Several surgeons have advocated a two-stage approach to bariatric surgery to reduce obesity-related risk (11–13). Regan and colleagues (11) described the two-stage operation, which consists of a sleeve gastrectomy (first stage) to be followed by a RYGBP or duodenal switch (second stage). The rationale is that the first-stage operation, sleeve gastrectomy, is comparatively simple (requiring no anastomosis), less operative time (1 to 2 hours), and results in a predictable 40- to 50-kg weight loss. Such weight loss reduces operative risk for the second-stage procedure, which presumably results in more weight loss and greater durability. Other multistage operations utilize the BIB as the first-stage procedure in patients with super-obesity. The limited data available suggest that the presurgical use of an intragastric balloon can reduce presurgical weight and perioperative risk, as well as operative and inpatient recovery time (14,15).

Postsurgical Revision Procedures

Multiple endoluminal technologies have been used to address complications of bariatric surgeries. Experience with endoscopic suturing devices, intragastric balloons, ablation therapy, fibrin glues, and other techniques have been reported in the literature. Late complications following a bariatric surgical procedures such as RYGBP and gastroplasty procedures can include staple line dis-

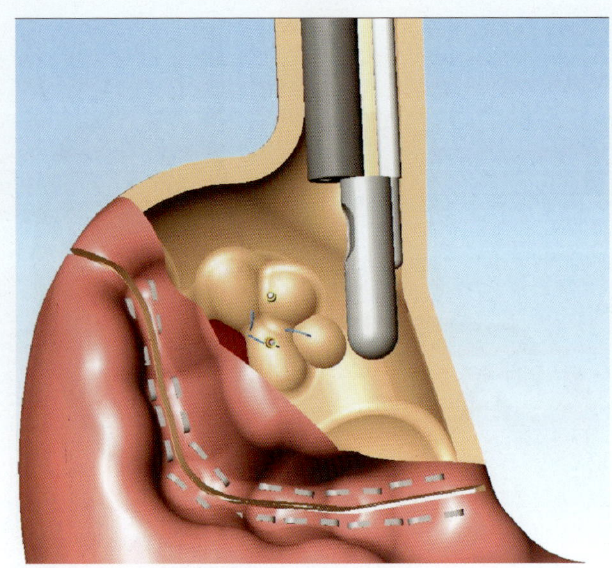

FIGURE 25.3-9. Anastomotic outlet reduction with suturing device. (Courtesy of Davol Inc., Cranston, RI.)

ruption, dilation of the gastric pouch or stoma, stomal stenosis, anastomotic stricture, and gastrogastric fistula (16). Multiple endoluminal technologies are being used to address these complications, including the use of suturing devices, ablation therapy, fibrin glues, and other technologies.

One of the more exciting endoluminal revisional treatments reported has been the endoluminal suturing platforms. Reports of experience with both the EndoCinch and the ESD have been published recently. In one study reported by Thompson (17), eight patients who had undergone RYGBP but had dilated gastrojejunal anastomoses and significant weight regain (an average of 24 kg from the lowest weight) were treated with the EndoCinch (Fig. 25.3-9). Plications were placed at the rim of the anastomosis to reduce the diameter of the anastomosis. After the revision procedure, six of eight patients experienced weight loss (average 10 kg) at 4 months. Four patients reported significant improvements in satiety. Three reported only brief improvements in satiety, and underwent a second anastomotic reduction. Of these 3 patients, one lost 19 kg and one lost 20 kg at 5 months. No significant complications were reported. The second study, reported by Schweitzer (18), employed the ESD to address weight regain following RYGBP. All four patients in this study reported improved satiety and early weight loss. Long-term data were not reported.

The preliminary data reported in these two studies demonstrate the feasibility and potential efficacy of endoluminal suturing as a means to address weight regain following RYGBP. While the long-term outcomes of plications in bariatric surgery are not known, current long-term data from the treatment of GERD suggest that benefits are durable for 1 to 2 years (5).

Other endoluminal techniques used in postsurgical repair include sclerotherapy and the use of fibrin glues. In two studies, endoscopic sclerotherapy was used to treat complications of RYGBP and vertical banded gastroplasty (VBG), and in one study, weight loss was achieved (9,19). The successful use of fibrin glue has also been reported in a limited study of patients following VBG. Papavramidis et al. (20) described the use of fibrin sealant to treat gastrocutaneous fistula in two patients with VBG and one patient with biliopancreatic diversion. After one or more endoscopic applications, treatment was successful in all three patients.

Primary Endoluminal Weight Loss Therapies

The use of endoluminal techniques as stand-alone treatments for obesity is in its infancy. Nevertheless, it is an active and rapidly evolving field. The intragastric balloon has been used in patients with varying degrees of obesity to induce weight loss independent of intended bariatric surgery (21). Endoluminal suturing techniques are also under development, with the goal of replicating surgical gastric restriction through endoscopic means. The expected end points for such procedures are yet to be determined. Most certainly, the safety profile will be expected to exceed that of current laparoscopic procedures. Weight loss and durability, though, are more difficult to predict. The ultimate measure of success for any bariatric procedure will be the resolution or improvement of obesity-related comorbid conditions that accompanies weight loss. The endoluminal procedures of the future will need to demonstrate these effects to gain acceptance. Patients and referring physicians may be fearful of bariatric surgery, which may explain why only 1% of patients who meet the National Institutes of Health (NIH) criteria for bariatric surgery undergo these procedures (22). A safe and effective endoluminal procedure will go a long way toward alleviating these fears and should increase referrals for weight loss procedures.

Intragastric Balloon as Primary Weight Loss Therapy

The only long-term data with the BIB come from a study by Mathus-Vliegen and Tytgat (23). This single-center study randomized 43 patients to one of two groups: 3-month balloon treatment ($n = 20$) or 3-month sham treatment ($n = 23$). After this initial treatment period, sham-treated patients received balloon treatment. All patients treated with the BIB had the balloon exchanged for a new balloon every 3 months for 1 year (or 9 months in patients initially in the sham group). After 1 year of treatment, patients were further evaluated during a 1-year balloon-free follow-up period. A significant sham treatment effect was demonstrated in this study, as sham and balloon-treatment groups lost similar amounts of weight after the 3-month sham-controlled period [11.2 kg (9%) control group vs. 12.9 kg (10.4%) balloon group; p = NS]. Nevertheless, over 70% of patients lost ≥15% body weight after 12 months of treatment, and nearly half lost ≥20% body weight. Although patients did regain weight during the 1-year balloon-free follow-up period, overall weight remained 12.7 kg (9.9%) below body weight at study entry. The results of this study suggest that some proportion of weight loss with the intragastric balloon is durable up to 24 months.

Endoscopic Gastroplasty Concepts

Endoluminal suturing to create gastric restriction is currently being investigated. To date, all but one study of this approach have been preclinical. Of these preclinical studies, two studies evaluated a technique called the butterfly endoluminal gastroplasty procedure (24,25). This endoluminal technique involves the creation of a small gastric pouch with a restrictive outlet that can be adjusted endoscopically at a later date. The first study compared the simulated effect of food intake on four different groups (25). Twelve porcine stomachs were divided into control, VBG, adjustable gastric band, and butterfly groups. The authors noted that pressure and flow characteristics of simulated food intake with the butterfly procedure correlated well with VBG and adjustable gastric banding (AGB). Yield pressure and flow rate were not different between treatment groups, but were significantly different from controls in all three restrictive groups ($p < .001$). The second study compared different methods of tightening the restrictive outlet in a porcine model (24). Two methods (tubular lengthening and pleating) were shown to produce effective tightening of the outlet, indicating the feasibility of this approach. Comparison of the butterfly technique to established gastroplasty techniques suggests that the butterfly procedure may restrict pressure and flow in a similar manner.

The only clinical study of endoluminal suturing for weight loss reported to date was undertaken by Fogel et al. (26). The investigators enrolled 10 voluntary overweight patients with body mass index (BMI) ranging from 28 to 43, and performed an endoscopic gastric plication along the lesser curvature using the EndoCinch. Plications were placed successfully in all 10 patients. Time required for the procedure ranged from 60 to 90 minutes. There were no immediate complications. All patients lost weight, with total weight loss ranging from 15 to 49 kg at 9 months postprocedure. A repeat procedure was performed in one patient following rupture of the plication 9 months after the first procedure. These preliminary data suggest that this endoluminal suturing technique is feasible, safe, and effective in producing short-term weight loss in overweight individuals.

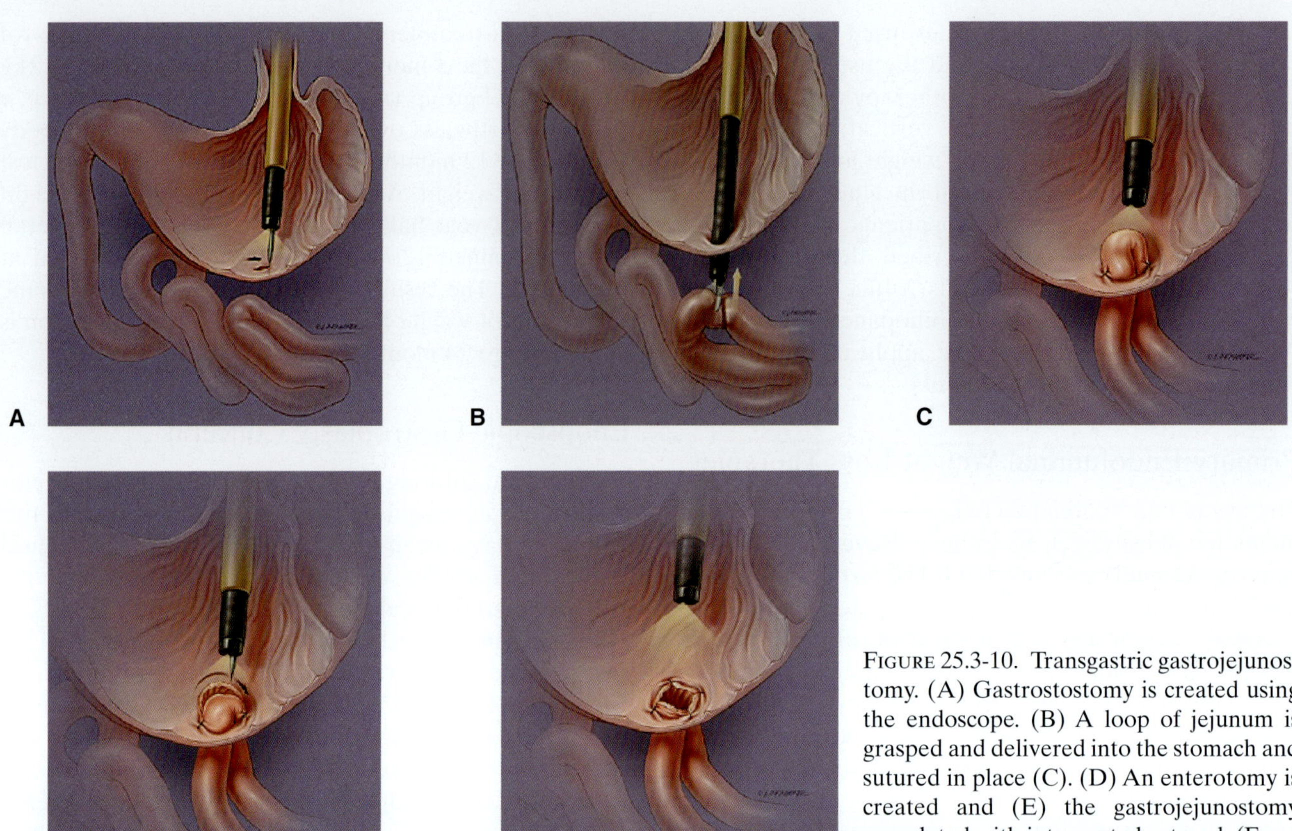

FIGURE 25.3-10. Transgastric gastrojejunostomy. (A) Gastrostostomy is created using the endoscope. (B) A loop of jejunum is grasped and delivered into the stomach and sutured in place (C). (D) An enterotomy is created and (E) the gastrojejunostomy completed with interrupted sutured. (From Kantsevoy et al. (27), with permission.)

Emerging Transluminal Technologies

The excitement surrounding transluminal approaches has prompted investigators to begin developing procedures and tools to operate beyond the gastric lumen. Such approaches are being adapted for use in weight-loss procedures. While the developments are still in their infancy, a handful of animal studies have been reported. Two independent studies have developed methodologies to perform gastrojejunal anastomoses or bypasses using natural orifice surgery (27,28). Kantsevoy et al. (27) reported a procedure in which a flexible endoscope enters the peritoneal cavity through the stomach wall, grasps a small bowel-loop, retracts the loop into the gastric lumen, and creates a gastrojejunostomy (Fig. 25.3-10). Park et al. (28) describe a novel intestinal anastomotic device, deployable with a flexible endoscope, that allows the joining of two bowel lumens.

Continued development has also focused on new tools and instrumentation to meet the unique demands of transluminal surgery. Swanstrom et al. (29) developed a new access device specifically designed for transgastric procedures (Fig. 25.3-11). The new device facilitates multi-instrument access, tissue retraction, improved maneuverability, platform stability, and some limited tri-angulation of instruments in the operative field. This device has been used successfully to explore the peritoneal cavity and perform transgastric cholecystectomy in the porcine model. After the intraperitoneal procedure is completed, the gastrotomy is closed with a suturing device that is placed through one of the device's working channels. While this device represents the greatest advancement in transgastric surgery to date, there are many technical refinements that will need to occur before it is ready for human use.

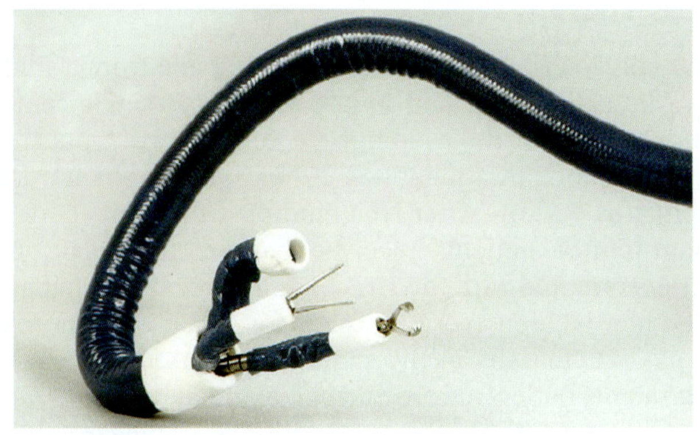

FIGURE 25.3-11. Novel access device for transgastric surgery. (From Swanstrom et al. (29), with permission.)

The Role of Endoluminal Surgery in Bariatric Practice

Questions abound regarding the relative efficacy, durability, and safety of these procedures, as well as their place within general and bariatric surgery. Skeptics will point to the low morbidity rates associated with current laparoscopic techniques and the ability to complete a laparoscopic procedure without violating the gastrointestinal tract. Current and future clinical trials are essential to address these concerns, guide treatment choices, and drive advances in this technology. The first indications likely to emerge are in presurgical weight loss and postsurgical repair applications, where preliminary data indicate the safety and relative effectiveness of endoluminal techniques. The NOTES community has proactively determined the path that this field will follow. A careful, stepwise approach for each endoluminal application will be necessary to achieve safe applications in humans. Prospective, randomized trials will need to be conducted after appropriate preclinical and clinical work is complete.

The application of endoluminal techniques in bariatric practice is promising. Such procedures have the potential to reduce or eliminate many risks associated with current surgeries, and to create a new outpatient obesity therapy (Table 25.3-2). Endoluminal surgery may also bring costs

TABLE 25.3-2. Comparison of bariatric surgery and endoluminal technologies

Approach	Type	Procedure	Application	Weight loss	Durability	Risks/complications
Laparoscopic	*Restrictive*	Lap-band	Morbidly obese	50% excess weight on average (31)	Stable over long-term follow-up (31)	Perioperative: — Infection — Bleeding Postoperative: — Band slippage — Gastric pouch dilation — Gastric erosion — Acid reflux — Obstruction — Noncompliance
	Malabsorptive	Biliopancreatic diversion	Morbidly obese	Over 75% excess weight (32)	Average 70% excess weight loss after 15 years (32)	Perioperative — Infection — Bleeding Postoperative — Malnutrition — Anemia — Bone demineralization — Gastric ulcer — Dumping syndrome
	Combination	Roux-en-Y gastric bypass	Morbidly obese	Up to 50% to 75% excess weight (33,34)	Stable over long-term follow-up (33,34)	Perioperative: — Infection — Bleeding Postoperative: — Leakage — Staple-line disruption — Stricture — Fistulae — Weight regain
	Electrical stimulation	Implanted gastric stimulator	Morbidly obese	Variable; over 20% excess weight in some patients (35)	Up to 19% at 14 months (35)	Gastric perforation, lead dislodgment
Endoluminal	*Space-occupying*	Intragastric balloon	Presurgical, staging	Up to 26% excess weight (14,36,15)	Regained upon balloon removal (14,36,15)	Vomiting, reflux, hypokalemia, renal dysfunction, intestinal blockage
			Primary	Up to 38% excess weight (8,22)	Approx. 10% total weight loss at 1 year (8,22)	Vomiting, reflux, hypokalemia, renal dysfunction, intestinal blockage
	Suturing	Endoluminal suturing	Repair	10 kg average (17)	Up to 4 months follow-up (17)	None reported
			Primary	15–49 kg at 9 months (26)	1 in 10 suture rupture at 9 months (26)	No intraprocedure complications; no late complications reported

of intervention within reach for many more patients, and may be appropriate for patients with less severe obesity.

The question of who will conduct these endoluminal bariatric procedures is another important issue. Currently, endoluminal procedures for GERD are performed mostly by gastroenterologists, but the growing number of surgeons involved in this discipline is encouraging (30). Endoluminal surgery represents a combination of disciplines that will include surgical skills and highly specific flexible endoscopy skills. Furthermore, each individual device is technically challenging to operate and requires extensive training and experience to be effective. The future, however, may demand the development of novel training programs to address the specific demands of bariatric endotherapy. It will be imperative for the fields of gastroenterology and surgery to work together within a multidisciplinary culture and structure to ensure safe adoption of these new techniques.

Acknowledgments. Bard is a registered trademark and EndoCinch is a trademark of C. R. Bard, Inc. or an affiliate. Plicator is a trademark of NDO Surgical, Inc. SurgASSIST is a registered trademark of Gerald Dorros, M.D. BioEnterics is a registered trademark of BioEnterics Corporation. Silhouette is a trademark of Silhouette Medical, Inc. Transcend is a registered trademark of Medtronic Transneuronix, Inc. Eagle Claw is a trademark of Olympus America, Inc. Enteryx is a registered trademark of Boston Scientific Scimed, Inc. Surgisis is a registered trademark of Cook Biotech, Inc.

References

1. Buchwald H, Avidor Y, Braunwald E, et al. Bariatric surgery: a systematic review and meta-analysis. JAMA 2004;292:1724–1737.
2. Nguyen NT, Root J, Zainabadi K, et al. Accelerated growth of bariatric surgery with the introduction of minimally invasive surgery. Arch Surg 2005;140:1198–1202.
3. Hawes R. ASGE/SAGES Working Group on Natural Orifice Translumenal Endoscopic Surgery. Gastrointest Endosc 2006;63:199–203.
4. Kadirkamanathan SS, Evans DF, Gong F, Yazaki E, Scott M, Swain CP. Antireflux operations at flexible endoscopy using endoluminal stitching techniques: an experimental study. Gastrointest Endosc 1996;44:133–143.
5. Chen YK, Raijmann I, Ben-Menachem T, et al. Long-term outcomes of endoluminal gastroplication: a U.S. multicenter trial. Gastrointest Endosc 2005;61:659–667.
6. Corley DA, Katz P, Wo JM, et al. Improvement of gastroesophageal reflux symptoms after radiofrequency energy: a randomized, sham-controlled trial. Gastroenterology 2003;125:668–676.
7. Deviere J, Costamagna G, Neuhaus H, et al. Nonresorbable copolymer implantation for gastroesophageal reflux disease: a randomized sham-controlled multicenter trial. Gastroenterology 2005;128:532–540.
8. Doldi SB, Micheletto G, Perrini MN, Rapetti R. Intragastric balloon: another option for treatment of obesity and morbid obesity. Hepatogastroenterology 2004;51:294–297.
9. Spaulding L. Treatment of dilated gastrojejunostomy with sclerotherapy. Obes Surg 2003;13:254–257.
10. European Patent Office. www.european-patent-office.org. Accessed October 2005.
11. Regan JP, Inabnet WB, Gagner M, Pomp A. Early experience with two-stage laparoscopic Roux-en-Y gastric bypass as an alternative in the super-super obese patient. Obes Surg 2003;13:861–864.
12. Cottam D, Mattar S, Sharma S, et al. Sleeve gastrectomy as an initial weight loss procedure for high risk patients with morbid obesity. Surg Endosc 2006;20:859–863.
13. Almogy G, Crookes PF, Anthone GJ. Longitudinal gastrectomy as a treatment for the high-risk super-obese patient. Obes Surg 2004;14:492–497.
14. Sallet JA, Marchesini JC, Ribeiro MR, Pizani CE, Kamoto K, Sallet PC. Utilization of the intragastric balloon (BIB) in pre-operative preparation for super obese patients with high surgical risk. Presented at the 21st Annual Meeting of American Society for Bariatric Surgery, 2004:P69.
15. Busetto L, Segato G, De Luca M, et al. Preoperative weight loss by intragastric balloon in super-obese patients treated with laparoscopic gastric banding: a case-control study. Obes Surg 2004;14:671–676.
16. Livingston EH. Complications of bariatric surgery. Surg Clin North Am 2005;85:853–868, vii.
17. Thompson CC. Per-oral endoscopic reduction of dilated gastrojejunal anastomosis following Roux-en-Y gastric bypass: a possible new option for patients with weight regain. SOARD 2005;1:223.
18. Schweitzer M. Endoscopic intraluminal suture plication of the gastric pouch and stoma in postoperative Roux-en-Y gastric bypass patients. J Laparoendosc Adv Surg Tech A 2004;14:223–226.
19. Catalano MJ, George S, Thomas M, Geenen JE, Chua T. Weight gain following bariatric surgery secondary to staple line disruption and stomal dilation: endotherapy using sodium morrhuate to induce stomal stenosis prevents need for surgical revision. Gastrointest Endosc 2004;59:P149.
20. Papavramidis ST, Eleftheriadis EE, Papavramidis TS, Kotzampassi KE, Gamvros OG. Endoscopic management of gastrocutaneous fistula after bariatric surgery by using a fibrin sealant. Gastrointest Endosc 2004;59:296–300.
21. Roman S, Napoleon B, Mion F, et al. Intragastric balloon for "non-morbid" obesity: a retrospective evaluation of tolerance and efficacy. Obes Surg 2004;14:539–544.
22. U.S. surgical procedure volumes. MedTech Insight 2005;7:136.
23. Mathus-Vliegen EM, Tytgat GN. Intragastric balloon for treatment-resistant obesity: safety, tolerance, and efficacy of 1-year balloon treatment followed by a 1-year balloon-free follow-up. Gastrointest Endosc 2005;61:19–27.
24. Kelleher B, Stone C, Burns M, Gaskill H. The butterfly procedure for endoluminal treatment of obesity. Gastrointest Endosc 2003;57:AB186
25. Swain CP, Park P-O, Savides T, Kelleher B, Stone C, Burns M. In vivo evaluation of the butterfly endoluminal gastro-

plasty procedure for obesity. Gastrointest Endosc 2003; 57:AB83.

26. Fogel R, De La Fuente R, Bonilla Y. Endoscopic vertical gastroplasty: a novel technique for treatment of obesity: a preliminary report Gastrointest Endosc 2005;61:AB106.

27. Kantsevoy S, Jagannath S, Niiyama H, et al. Endoscopic gastrojejunostomy with survival in a porcine model. Gastrointest Endosc 2005;62:287–292.

28. Park A, Adrales G, McKinlay R, Knapp C. A novel anastomotic device in a porcine model. Am Surg 2004;70:767–773.

29. Swanstrom L, Kozarek R, Pasricha P, et al. Development of a new access device for transgastric surgery Surg 2005;9: 1129–1137.

30. MacFadyen BV Jr, Cuschieri A. Endoluminal surgery. Surg Endosc 2005;19:1–3.

31. O'Brien PE, Brown WA, Smith A, McMurrick PJ, Stephens M. Prospective study of a laparoscopically placed, adjustable gastric band in the treatment of morbid obesity. Br J Surg 1999;86(1):113–118.

32. Scopinaro N, Gianetta E, Adami GF, Friedman D, Traverso E, Marinari GM, Cuneo S, Vitale B, Ballari F, Colombini M, Baschieri G, Bachi V. Biliopancreatic diversion for obesity at eighteen years. Surgery 1996;119(3):261–268.

33. Wittgrove AC, Clark GW. Laparoscopic gastric bypass, Roux-en-Y-500 patients: technique and results, with 3-60 month follow-up. Obes Surg 2000;10(3):233–239.

34. Schauer PR, Ikramuddin S, Gourash W, Ramanathan R, Luketich J. Outcomes after laparoscopic Roux-en-Y gastric bypass for morbid obesity. Ann Surg 2000;232(4):515–529.

35. Shikora SA, Storch K, Investigational team, 2004 ABS Consensus Conference. Implantable gastric stimulation for the treatment of severe obesity: the American experience. Surg Obes Relat Dis 2005;1(3):334–342.

36. Weiner R, Gutberlet H, Bockhorn H. Preparation of extremely obese patients for laparoscopic gastric banding by gastric-balloon therapy. Obes Surg 1999;9:261–264.

26
Venous Thrombosis and Pulmonary Embolism

Gianluca Bonanomi, Giselle Hamad, and Franklin A. Bontempo

Risk of Deep Venous Thrombosis and Pulmonary Embolism in Obese Patients

Morbid obesity is a major risk factor for the development of deep venous thrombosis (DVT) and pulmonary embolism (PE). Thromboembolic complications are the most common cause of death in bariatric surgery and contribute significantly to postoperative morbidity (1). A study of risk factors for venous thromboembolism in hospitalized patients demonstrated an association with age over 40 years, obesity, and major surgery (2). The increased risk in the morbidly obese is attributable to a sedentary lifestyle, increased abdominal pressure, and the excessive weight resting on the inferior vena cava drainage. Additional risk factors include prior history of DVT or PE, immobility, pregnancy, oral contraceptive use, smoking, hypercoagulable states, malignancy, and trauma (Table 26-1). Although they are usually diagnosed as postoperative complications, DVT and PE may also occur in nonhospitalized patients. Studies of risk factors for thromboembolism in the general population have demonstrated an association with obesity, suggesting that morbid obesity is an independent risk factor for DVT and PE (3,4).

Coagulation Abnormalities in Obesity

Thrombosis is a complex process resulting from the balance between the procoagulant clotting cascades, the anticoagulant fibrinolytic mechanisms, and the physiologic anticoagulant proteins. The procoagulant forces are represented by the intrinsic and extrinsic coagulation pathways, while the major anticoagulant forces are the plasminogen-based fibrinolytic mechanism along with the natural clot inhibitors antithrombin III, protein C, and protein S. Any congenital or acquired disorder of clotting may alter this balance and lead to thrombosis. Obesity is associated with a number of coagulation abnormalities. Elevated plasma concentration of fibrino-gen, von Willebrand factor, tissue-type plasminogen activator (t-PA), factor VII, and plasminogen activator inhibitor-1 (PAI-1) have been found in obese patients. Moreover, platelet aggregation appears to be augmented and leptin has been implicated as a promoter of platelet aggregation. The obesity-associated metabolic syndrome might be responsible for the coagulation disorders and the increased thrombotic risk (5).

Interestingly, weight loss may lead to normalization of several coagulation parameters. The deficiency of antithrombin III (AT-III) found in obese patients may be reversed with weight loss (6). Likewise, significant reductions in fibrinogen, t-PA, PAI-1, and factor VII have been correlated with the amount of weight loss (7,8). Therefore, the medical or surgical treatment of morbid obesity may reverse some of the coagulation abnormalities and subsequently reduce the associated thromboembolic and cardiovascular risk. Obese patients who have a history of prior DVT or PE should be screened for congenital or acquired hypercoagulable states in order to identify patients who are at higher risk of postoperative thromboembolic events, and who could benefit from close surveillance and possibly anticoagulation therapy. Testing recommendations for the diagnosis of hypercoagulable states should include screening for the lupus anticoagulants (LACs), the AT-III, protein C and protein S deficiencies, the activated protein C (APC) resistance to identify factor V Leiden mutations, and the prothrombin gene variant. Common coagulation abnormalities observed in obese patients and predisposing to DVT and PE are listed in Table 26-2.

Intraoperative Factors Contributing to Deep Venous Thrombosis

Patients with morbid obesity undergoing surgery are at risk for development of DVT and PE. Thromboembolic events continue to be the most common cause of death

TABLE 26-1. Risk factors for deep venous thrombosis and pulmonary embolism

Age over 40 years
History of thromboembolism
Obesity
Smoking
Pregnancy
Oral contraceptive use
Malignancy
Trauma
Major surgery
Immobilization
Hypercoagulable states

in bariatric surgery. In a survey of members of the American Society for Bariatric Surgery the self-reported incidence of DVT and PE was 2.63% and 0.95%, respectively (9). Forty-eight percent of bariatric surgeons reported at least one death from PE in their practice. The development of DVT has been ascribed to the Virchow's triad of stasis, endothelial damage, and hypercoagulability. Laparoscopic bariatric surgery has its own intraoperative factors that may contribute to the development of DVT. Factors contributing to venous stasis during laparoscopy include reverse Trendelenburg positioning and pneumoperitoneum causing an impaired venous return from compression of the iliac veins and inferior vena cava. A reduction in femoral venous flow that was reversed with the use of sequential pneumatic compression devices has been demonstrated during laparoscopic cholecystectomy (10). Moreover, a number of studies demonstrate a hypercoagulable state associated with laparoscopy in both animals and humans (11–13). However, the factors that contribute to DVT during laparoscopy may be offset by a lower degree of operative injury, early mobilization, and reduced postoperative acute-phase response (14).

TABLE 26-2. Coagulation abnormalities associated with morbid obesity

Elevated fibrinogen levels
Elevated factor VII
Elevated von Willebrand factor
Elevated tissue-type plasminogen activator (t-PA)
Elevated plasminogen activator inhibitor-1 (PAI-1)
Antithrombin III deficiency
Protein C deficiency
Protein S deficiency
Lupus anticoagulants
Factor V Leiden mutation
Prothrombin gene variant
Dysfibrinogens
Increased platelet aggregation

The Importance of Prophylaxis

Deep venous thrombosis and PE occur in approximately 20% to 30% of patients undergoing general surgery without any prophylaxis. Perioperative prophylaxis may reduce the incidence of DVT and PE by 70% and 50%, respectively (15). The rationale for prophylaxis of DVT is based on the high prevalence of venous thromboembolism among obese patients, the clinically silent nature of the disease, and the associated morbidity, mortality, and costs. Clinical diagnosis of DVT is often unreliable and may expose the patient to the risk of PE. Therefore, primary prevention of venous thromboembolism and its associated morbidity and mortality has been suggested. Traditional pharmacologic agents for prophylaxis and treatment of thromboembolism include unfractionated heparin (UFH), low molecular weight heparins (LMWHs), and warfarin (16,17). Other prophylactic measures include graduated compression stockings, intermittent pneumatic compression, and early mobilization. In a small subgroup of patients at high risk for thromboembolism and in whom anticoagulants are contraindicated, the preoperative insertion of a vena caval filter may be considered (18).

The most widely used prophylactic agent for DVT is UFH. An initial subcutaneous dose of 5000 units is typically given preoperatively and continued postoperatively every 8 or 12 hours until the patient is fully ambulatory. Many reports have demonstrated the beneficial prophylactic effect of UFH in general surgery patients (19,20).

Low molecular weight heparins have a lower degree of plasma protein binding, an improved subcutaneous bioavailability, a dose-independent clearance, and longer half-life than UFH. The efficacy of these agents for prevention and treatment of DVT and PE is well established (21,22). The LMWHs allow once-a-day injection as opposed to UFH, which requires two or three doses per day.

There is no consensus in the literature regarding the best approach to prevent this problem in the morbidly obese population. It is unclear whether the same dosage regimens may be safely applied. Because of the increased body mass, obese patients may be undertreated with standard non–weight-based prophylactic doses. Conversely, the use of a treatment dosage regimen based on actual body weight may conceivably lead to excessive anticoagulation and bleeding. Obesity is associated with physiologic changes in drug pharmacokinetics (23). However, uncertainty remains on whether pharmacologic prophylaxis dosage should be based on body weight, renal function, or both in obese patients. The volume of distribution of heparin approximates blood volume, and the blood content of adipose tissue is relatively low. Therefore, the use of total weight in heparin dosage calculations might lead to excessive heparin concentrations in obese patients. Assays for direct measurement of LMWHs levels are not commercially available. As a result, most pharmacokinetic studies of LMWHs have used surrogate biologic markers such as the anti–factor Xa and AT-III activities. Several authors have demonstrated variability in the correlation between anti-Xa activity, the body weight, and the incidence of thrombosis and hemorrhagic events, raising concerns about the consistency of anticoagulation achieved with LMWHs in the morbidly obese patient (24,25).

According to a survey among members of the American Society for Bariatric Surgery, routine prophylaxis for venous thromboembolism in bariatric patients is adopted by 95% of surgeons, and the most frequently used combination is low-dose UFH or LMWHs associated with intermittent pneumatic compression (9).

Definitive data on thromboembolic prophylaxis in this high-risk and growing population are needed. The only way to determine the best prophylaxis would be a multicenter prospective randomized trial in which all the different strategies are considered and screening of all patients is performed.

Diagnosis

The clinical diagnosis of DVT is often misleading and unreliable. Clinical findings associated with DVT include lower extremity edema, erythema and warmth, fever, calf pain and tenderness, pain induced by calf dorsiflexion (Homans' sign), and a palpable venous cord. Duplex imaging is the standard noninvasive examination for the detection of DVT and has supplanted contrast venography. Unlike impedance plethysmography and portable Doppler, duplex imaging enables the visualization of the thrombus and the evaluation of its anatomic level and extent. Duplex scanning has been shown to be an accurate investigation when compared to ascending contrast venography (26). However, the accuracy of duplex scanning may be impaired by the body habitus of obese patients.

Pulmonary embolism is a devastating potential consequence of DVT. However, fewer than 30% of patients diagnosed with PE present with clinical signs of lower extremity DVT. Clinical manifestations of PE include dyspnea, chest pain, tachycardia, tachypnea, hypotension, fever, and hemoptysis. The mortality rate associated with PE is 30%, but if the condition is recognized and treated promptly the mortality decreases to 2.5%. Pulmonary embolism must be differentiated from another potentially life-threatening complication of bariatric surgery represented by anastomotic leaks. Anastomotic leaks may also present with tachycardia, chest pain, fever, and respiratory distress. Therefore, awareness, early recognition, and differential diagnosis between PE and anasto-

motic leaks are key elements in the postoperative management of bariatric surgery patients. Whether an evaluation for either PE or anastomotic leak will be instituted first should be dictated by the clinical presentation. A chest computed tomography (CT) scan or a ventilation/perfusion (V/Q) scan should be obtained promptly if the clinical picture strongly suggests the occurrence of PE. An upper gastrointestinal (UGI) study or surgical exploration should be undertaken if an anastomotic leak is suspected.

Spiral CT scan of the chest is currently the diagnostic modality of choice for the diagnosis of PE (27). Spiral CT scan has been shown to have higher sensitivity, specificity, and positive and negative predictive value for the detection of PE as compared to V/Q scan (28). Special equipment should be available to accommodate morbidly obese patients. This investigation involves intravenous injection of contrast dye and therefore is contraindicated in patients with advanced renal failure or dye allergy.

Ventilation/perfusion scanning is the most commonly used imaging modality when PE is suspected. However, the accuracy of this investigation is low, and up to 70% of scans are reported as indeterminate. The Prospective Investigation of Pulmonary Embolism Diagnosis (PIOPED) study found that 88% of patients with high probability V/Q scans had PE, as did 12% of those with low probability scans (29). Therefore, V/Q scan should be interpreted in conjunction with the clinician's suspicion, and further confirmatory testing is often required to establish the diagnosis of PE.

Pulmonary angiography is considered the gold standard for the diagnosis of PE. It should be ordered when the V/Q or the CT scan are suspicious but indeterminate. However, the recent advances in spiral CT technology have increasingly replaced the adoption of this invasive imaging technique for the diagnosis of PE.

The D-dimer blood test is able to detect fibrin proteolysis and intravascular thrombus formation. Pulmonary embolism and DVT are associated with high levels of D-dimer. Although not diagnostic, this test has a high negative predictive value and therefore is useful in excluding the diagnosis of PE.

Magnetic resonance imaging is a promising noninvasive diagnostic tool that needs further evaluation and has not been introduced yet in the routine workup for the diagnosis of PE.

Therapy

The standard treatment of acute DVT and PE is heparin followed by sodium warfarin therapy. Heparin prevents the extension of existing thrombus as well as the formation of new thrombus and enables the physiologic fibrinolytic system to work more effectively. Heparin is administered intravenously, consisting of an initial bolus of 1000 units followed by a continuous drip of 10 to 15 units/kg/hour to maintain the partial thromboplastin time at a level 1.5 to 2 times the control value. Complications of heparin treatment include heparin-induced thrombocytopenia and hemorrhage. Oral warfarin is usually started 24 hours after initiation of heparin therapy when the patient's condition is stable. Heparin is continued for 1 week or until warfarin has reached its therapeutic window. Generally treatment with warfarin is continued for 3 to 6 months. The prothrombin time is maintained at 1.5 to 2 times the normal value. Treatment with oral warfarin may be problematic in obese patients who have undergone bariatric surgery and whose oral intake and vitamin absorption is reduced. Patients may develop a vitamin K deficiency, and therefore their prothrombin time should be monitored frequently after treatment with warfarin has been initiated.

Acute DVT and PE may be managed with LMWHs. In several studies, LMWHs have been proved to be safe and equal or superior in efficacy when compared with UFH or warfarin (30). Similar complications to UFH treatment occur but less frequently. Moreover, LMWHs have the advantage of an improved bioavailability, predictable anticoagulation that makes monitoring of anticoagulation unnecessary, and potential use in the outpatient setting. Data evaluating the safety of using weight-based dosing of LMWHs in obese patients are limited (31). Usually a body mass weight-based dosage of LMWHs has been adopted, not exceeding the maximum daily dose suggested by manufacturers.

Conclusion

Obesity has been shown to be an independent risk factor for the development of thromboembolism. Deep venous thrombosis and PE are a major cause of morbidity and mortality in patients undergoing bariatric surgery. Prevention of thromboembolism in the perioperative period is critical, but there is no consensus as to the ideal method for prophylaxis in the morbidly obese patient. Differential diagnosis and early recognition of DVT and PE may be difficult in the postoperative management of bariatric patients.

References

1. Eriksson S, Backman L, Ljungstrom KG. The incidence of clinical postoperative thrombosis after gastric surgery for obesity during 16 years. Obes Surg 1997;7:332–335.
2. Anderson FA, Wheeler B, Goldberg RJ, Hosmer DW, Forcier A. The prevalence of risk factors for venous thromboembolism among hospital patients. Arch Intern Med 1992; 152:1660–1664.
3. Goldhaber SZ, Savage DD, Garrison RJ, et al. Risk factors for pulmonary embolism. The Framingham study. Am J Med 1983;74:1023–1028.
4. Hansson PO, Eriksson H, Welin L, Svardsudd K, Wilhemsen L. Smoking and abdominal obesity. Risk factors for venous thromboembolism among middle-aged men. Arch Intern Med 1999;159:1886–1890.
5. Bosello O, Zamboni M. Visceral obesity and metabolic syndrome. Obes Rev 2000;1:47–56.
6. Batist G, Bothe A, Bern M, Bistrian BR, Blackburn GL. Low antithrombin III in morbid obesity: return to normal with weight reduction. JPEN 1983;7:447–449.
7. Folsom AR, Qamhieh HT, Wing RR, et al. Impact of weight loss on plasminogen activator inhibitor (PAI-1), factor VII, and other hemostatic factors in moderately overweight adults. Arterioscler Thromb 1993;13:162–169.
8. Primrose JN, Davies JA, Prentice CRM, Hughes R, Johnston D. Reduction in factor VII, fibrinogen and plasminogen activator inhibitor-1 activity after surgical treatment of morbid obesity. Thromb Haemost 1992;68:396–399.
9. Wu EC, Barba Ca. Current practices in the prophylaxis of venous thromboembolism in bariatric surgery. Obes Surg 2000;10:7–13.
10. Schwenk W, Bohm B, Fugener A, Muller JM. Intermittent pneumatic sequential compression (ISC) of the lower extremities prevents venous stasis during laparoscopic cholecystectomy. A prospective randomized study. Surg Endosc 1998;12:7–11.
11. Caprini JA, Arcelus JI, Laubach M, Size G, Hoffman KN, Coats RW, Blattner S. Postoperative hypercoagulability and deep vein thrombosis after laparoscopic cholecystectomy. Surg Endosc 1995;9:304–309.
12. Nguyen NT, Luketich JD, Shurin MR, et al. Coagulation modifications after laparoscopic and open cholecystectomy in a swine model. Surg Endosc 1998;12:973–978.
13. Lindberg F, Rasmussen I, Siegbahn A, Bergqvist Dl. Coagulation activation after laparoscopic cholecystectomy in spite of thromboembolism prophylaxis. Surg Endosc 2000; 14:858–861.
14. Nguyen NT, Goldman CD, Ho HS, Gosselin RC, Singh A, Wolfe BM. Systemic stress response after laparoscopic and open gastric bypass. J Am Coll Surg 2002;194:557–566.
15. Clagett G, Reisch J. Prevention of venous thromboembolism in general surgical patients. Results of meta-analysis. Ann Surg 1988;208:227–240.
16. Hirsh J, Warkentin TE, Shaughnessy SG, et al. Heparin and low-molecular weight heparin. Chest 2001;119:64S-94S.
17. Geerts WH, Heit JA, Clagett GP, et al. Prevention of venous thromboembolism. Chest 2001;119:132S–175S.
18. Sugerman HJ, Sugerman EL, Wolfe L, Kellum JM, Schweitzer MA, DeMaria EJ. Risks and benefits of gastric bypass in morbidly obese patients with severe venous stasis disease. Ann Surg. 2001;234:41–46.
19. National Institutes of Health. Consensus conference on prevention of venous thrombosis and pulmonary embolism. JAMA 1986;256:744–748.
20. Prevention of fatal postoperative pulmonary embolism by low doses of heparin: an international multicentre study. Lancet 1975;2:45–51.

21. Kakkar VV, Cohen AT, Edmonson RA, et al. Low molecular weight heparin versus standard heparin for prevention of venous thromboembolism after major abdominal surgery. Lancet 1993;341:256–259.

22. Palmer AJ, Schramm W, Kirchof B. Low molecular weight heparin and unfractionated heparin for prevention of thromboembolism in general surgery: a meta-analysis of randomized clinical trials. Haemostasis 1997;27:65–74.

23. Cleymol G. Effects of obesity on pharmacokinetics: implications for drug therapy. Clin Pharmacol 2000;39:215–231.

24. Levine MN, Planes A, Hirsh J, Goodyear M, Vochelle N, Gent M. The relationship between anti-factor Xa level and clinical outcome in patients receiving enoxaparin low molecular weight heparin to prevent deep vein thrombosis after hip replacement. Thromb Haemost 1989;62:940–944.

25. Kovacs MJ, Weir K, MacKinnon K, Keeney M, Brien WF, Cruickhank MK. Body weight does not predict for anti-Xa levels after fixed dose prophylaxis with enoxaparin after orthopedic surgery. Thromb Res 1998;91:137–142.

26. Vogel P, Laing PC, Jeffrey RB. Deep venous thrombosis of the lower extremity: ultrasound evaluation. Radiology 1987;163:747–751.

27. Tapson VF. Pulmonary embolism—new diagnostic approaches. N Engl J Med 1997;336:1449–1451.

28. Blachere H, Latrabe V, Montaudon M. Pulmonary embolism revealed on helical CT angiography: comparison with ventilation-perfusion radionuclide lung scanning. Am J Roentgenol 2000:174:1041–1047.

29. The PIOPED Investigators. Value of the ventilation/perfusion scan in acute pulmonary embolism. Results of the prospective investigation of pulmonary embolism diagnosis (PIOPED). JAMA 1990;263:2753–2759.

30. Quader MA, Stump LS, Sumpio BE. Low molecular weight heparins: current use and indications. J Am Coll Surg 1998;187:641–658.

31. Wilson SJ, Wilbur K, Burton E, Anderson DR. Effect of patient weight on the anticoagulant response to adjusted therapeutic dosage of low molecular weight heparin for the treatment of venous thromboembolism. Haemostasis 2001;31:42–48.

27
Role of Flexible Endoscopy in the Practice of Bariatric Surgery

Bruce R. Schirmer

Bariatric surgery underwent an explosion in terms of patient demand, the number of procedures performed, and the number of surgeons performing it from the years 1998 to 2003. Since then, the insurance industry has successfully limited the growth of this field with blanket denials for coverage, adopting policies that require expensive riders for bariatric coverage, and otherwise limiting expenditures for bariatric surgery with the undocumented excuse that the rise in volume has led to increased complications. This has served to halt the beneficial spread of the only known successful treatment for the comorbid medical problems caused by severe obesity.

Much of the reason for the rapid expansion of the field of bariatric surgery around the turn of the 21st century was the availability of a laparoscopic approach for performing all the major bariatric operations. Other factors contributed as well, including increased patient awareness resulting from increased media coverage, use of the Internet by patients for obtaining information and information exchange, and the increased interest in performing minimally invasive bariatric surgery among young surgeons completing their training. Thus, bariatric surgery has become much more mainstream in the United States. Clearly this is a positive transformation in the care of the severely obese patient population.

Since many of the bariatric surgeons who are now performing minimally invasive bariatric surgery are relatively new to the field, it is important that they learn all the aspects of bariatric surgical practice, which will enhance their patients' long-term outcomes. In this regard, it is therefore important that the bariatric surgeon give strong consideration to being adept at flexible upper endoscopy as an important tool in the management of patients pre-, intra-, and postoperatively who are undergoing bariatric surgical procedures of all types. This discussion centers on the reasons for acquiring this skill set as well as the methods and applications of flexible upper endoscopy in the current practice of bariatric surgery.

Preoperative Assessment

There has been ample documentation in the surgical literature about the potential advantages of performing routine flexible upper endoscopy in patients planning to undergo Roux-en-Y gastric bypass (RYGBP). While the data are largely published about this particular operation, there is certainly adequate reason to expect that some of the strongest indications for preoperative screening of bariatric surgery patients, such as those with a significant history of gastroesophageal reflux disease (GERD) to rule out Barrett's esophagitis, are applicable to all bariatric operations, and not just RYGBP.

At the University of Virginia, from 1986 to near the end of 2001, a total of 596 patients undergoing RYGBP as well as an additional 71 patients undergoing vertical banded gastroplasty (VBG) had a preoperative screening flexible upper endoscopy examination prior to surgery. While the vast majority of patients did have normal anatomy on this screening examination, there was a small but significant percentage of patients (31, or 4.6% of the total) for whom their operation was altered by pathologic findings at the time of flexible endoscopy. The most common pathologic findings that altered surgery were severe gastritis, duodenal ulcer, and duodenitis. For the majority of these patients, a distal gastrostomy was added to RYGBP, but in two instances a VBG was performed instead. Other less common causes for alteration of operation included gastric polyps, large hiatal hernia, and Barrett's esophagitis with dysplasia.

Between 1997 and 2001 at the University of Virginia, the preoperative endoscopy has included routine prepyloric biopsy for testing for *Helicobacter pylori*. The incidence of *H. pylori* was over 30% for patients tested. In the untested patients prior to that date, the incidence of marginal ulcer postoperatively was 24 of 354 patients (6.8%). Since 1997, patients who have undergone preoperative screening for *H. pylori* and subsequent treatment if positive have had a cumulative marginal ulcer rate of

2.6%. This is a significantly (p <.05) lower rate of marginal ulcer than was seen prior to testing and treating for *H. pylori* (1). Ramaswamy et al. (2) found that the preoperative incidence of *H. pylori* infection in their patients undergoing bariatric surgery was 24%. Postoperative foregut symptoms were significant in 48% of the *H. pylori*–positive group, and in only 19% of the *H. pylori*–negative group, a significant difference.

Based on these data, we now recommend routine testing for *H. pylori* prior to bariatric surgery. If the patient undergoes a flexible upper gastrointestinal endoscopy prior to surgery, then prepyloric biopsies are obtained for histologic analysis for *H. pylori*. If no endoscopy is performed, a serum test to determine exposure is obtained. While a positive serum test does not necessarily confer active presence of the bacteria, it warrants treatment in the previously untreated patient. We have not subjected patients treated for *H. pylori* to posttreatment breath testing to determine efficacy of treatment. This is because we question the cost-effectiveness of such an additional step in view of the relatively low incidence (usually in the 10% range) of ineffective medical therapy and the minimal likely effect that would have on marginal ulcer rates in the overall bariatric population. However, such a decision is not a data-driven one.

Other investigators have reported the advantages of performing preoperative flexible upper endoscopy prior to bariatric surgery. Sharaf et al. (3) evaluated 195 patients by upper endoscopy prior to bariatric surgery, and found one or more lesions of the upper gastrointestinal tract in 89.7% of cases. Of these, 61.5% were felt to be clinically important. The most common findings were hiatal hernia (40%), gastritis (29%), esophagitis (9%), gastric ulcer (3.6%), Barrett's esophagus (3%), and esophageal ulcer (3%). Verset et al. (4) reported an incidence of 37% gastroduodenal lesions and 31% esophagitis in a group of 159 patients undergoing routine flexible upper endoscopy prior to VBG. Most of these gastroduodenal lesions were asymptomatic, and the esophagitis was almost always associated with a hiatal hernia or incompetent lower esophageal sphincter. A high incidence of esophagitis in severely obese patients is not surprising and is well documented in other studies as well (5).

Preoperative assessment of patients undergoing VBG was reported by Papavramidis et al. (6). They found a 16.6% incidence of hiatal hernia, a 13.3% incidence of esophagitis, a 30% incidence of gastritis, and a 6.6% incidence of duodenitis.

Preoperative endoscopy is also an essential component of the evaluation of a patient who has experienced failure of a previous bariatric operation. Often such patients present for consideration for reoperation due to poor weight loss or other more acute symptoms. For example, GERD is reported as a complaint of between 15% and 18% of patients who underwent previous VBG (4,6). Assessment of the size of a previously created gastric pouch, the integrity of a previously placed gastric staple line, the size and location of previously created anastomoses, and the presence of any upper gastrointestinal pathology as a result of the previous operation is essential for the surgeon to determine if reoperative surgery is possible, appropriate, and indicated. It also allows for the appropriate treatment of anatomic problems and ongoing pathology with the reoperation. The best outcomes for reoperative surgery can only be achieved if such appropriate evaluation and planning are part of the preoperative plan.

Intraoperative Endoscopy

Based on the operative technique used, flexible endoscopy may become an integral part of bariatric, particularly laparoscopic bariatric surgery. Wittgrove and Clark (7) have described a technique of performing the gastrojejunostomy of their laparoscopic RYGBP using an endoscopically guided placement of the anvil of the end-to-end anastomosis (EEA) stapler. Schauer et al. (8) described the use of flexible upper endoscopy to inspect the staple line of all gastrojejunostomies during laparoscopic RYGBP, as well as to perform a leak test using air under pressure. Gagner et al. (9) described the use of intraoperative endoscopy for passage of the EEA stapler using a nasogastric tube during the performance of RYGBP as well. Champion et al. (10) used intraoperative endoscopy during 825 bariatric operations, most of them RYGBPs, and found a 4.1% incidence of intraoperative error in the creation of the pouch or anastomosis. Of these 34 errors found, most of them leaks, only one persisted as a postoperative problem after repair was performed. Thus flexible endoscopy has become an integral part of the performance of RYGBP in these experts' hands. Many bariatric surgeons now routinely use intraoperative flexible upper endoscopy as a standard part of their operative procedure, most commonly for RYGBP but for other operations as well.

Revisional bariatric surgery often relies on intraoperative upper endoscopy to confirm the size and borders of previously created proximal gastric pouches, as well as to confirm the appropriate location for performing an anastomosis to such proximal gastric pouches. Upper endoscopy is also then used to confirm the integrity and patency of anastomoses created when revising a previous bariatric operation.

Intraoperative endoscopy is also a valuable tool, in an academic setting, for the training of the future gastrointestinal and bariatric surgeon. Recently the American Board of Surgery required defined numbers of upper and lower flexible endoscopic procedures.

There is also good documentation in the literature of the efficacy and safety of resident-performed intraoperative endoscopy (11).

Postoperative Endoscopy

Flexible endoscopy in the surgeon's hands becomes most valuable in the postoperative period. Patients who have undergone previous bariatric operations may present with a variety of symptoms suggestive of postoperative upper gastrointestinal pathology. Flexible endoscopy allows the surgeon to assess the anatomy and pathology. Only the surgeon who has performed the previous operation has the unique first-hand knowledge of what was done and created at the time of surgery. Postoperative endoscopy provides the next surgeon feedback on the anatomic construction of the operation in addition to facilitating the determination of existing pathology. It permits immediate assessment as to the best treatment strategy for the existing pathology, which may often occur during the endoscopic setting. Despite the expertise of medical gastroenterologists in flexible endoscopy, often their lack of familiarity with the anatomy of the bariatric operation performed leads to misinterpretation of the findings on upper endoscopy.

Obstruction

Postoperative symptoms of obstruction, pain, bleeding, and reflux are the most common indications for which flexible upper endoscopy is performed after bariatric surgery. Obstructive symptoms may or may not coincide with a true anatomic stricture of the gastrojejunostomy after RYGBP, or gastric outflow after a VBG. Upper endoscopy is less often used in diagnosing problems of food intolerance and reflux after laparoscopic adjustable gastric banding (LAGB), where band prolapse is responsible for most such symptoms and an upper GI series is diagnostic. For RYGBP, a pattern of progressive dysphagia for solid and then for liquid food, most frequently starting 3 to 8 weeks postoperatively, is highly suggestive of proximal anastomotic stenosis. While an upper GI series usually provides definitive evidence for the presence of a stricture of the anastomosis, flexible upper endoscopy can provide even more certain assessment of the anastomotic size as well as allow the performance of a simultaneous balloon dilatation of the stricture.

For RYGBP, our proximal anastomotic stenosis rate has ranged from a high of 14% with the use of a 21-mm EEA stapler and oversewing the staple line with nonabsorbable suture, to a recent low rate of under 2% with a linear stapled anastomosis reinforced only anteriorly with absorbable suture during laparoscopic RYGBP. Peak incidence of symptoms occurs in the 4- to 6-week postoperative range. An initial flexible upper endoscopy confirms the stenosis and allows balloon dilatation to be done at that setting. The typical dilatation is performed under direct endoscopic vision using an inflatable 18- to 20-French (F) balloon passed through the anastomosis for performance of balloon dilatation. The anastomotic opening can be dilated up to virtually the size of the flexible therapeutic endoscope using this approach. Often the anastomotic opening is 3mm or smaller in diameter, when first visualized endoscopically.

The endoscopist must be certain that if a balloon dilatation is to be performed, the relatively rigid end of the balloon is not passed blindly through the anastomotic opening and then forced against resistance. The end-to-side configuration of many RYGBP gastrojejunal anastomoses presents a potentially hazardous anatomic configuration for dilatation. The endoscopist must only pass the end of the dilating balloon just past the anastomotic stricture on the first dilation. Once the anastomotic opening is enlarged enough to see across it further, the balloon can be positioned in a more advantageous position to allow maximal balloon size and pressure to be exerted on the anastomosis with subsequent balloon insufflation. Once the flexible endoscope itself can be passed through the anastomotic opening, the dilatation is essentially completed. However, a final dilatation may be performed by passing the balloon into the visible lumen of the jejunum beyond the anastomosis, and then withdrawing the scope to position the balloon directly across the anastomosis for one final insufflation and dilatation.

Symptoms of anastomotic obstruction may be verbalized by the patient, only to find a normal-sized anastomosis on endoscopy. In our first 560 patients undergoing RYGBP, there were 72 patients with symptoms suggestive of anastomotic stricture postoperatively. Of these, 54 (75%) had that problem (defined as an anastomotic opening too small to allow passage of the flexible diagnostic endoscope). However, 25% did not. These 18 patients underwent 28 flexible upper endoscopies for false-positive symptoms suggestive of anastomotic stricture. The 54 patients who did have anastomotic stenosis underwent 80 dilatations to successfully treat their anastomotic stenosis (1).

While initial flexible upper endoscopy facilitates simultaneous diagnosis and treatment of stenosis, the limitation of the dilatation is that the maximum size balloon that will fit down the channel of a therapeutic endoscope is 20F. Therefore, when we encounter a patient with a tight stenosis who returns with recurrent symptoms after one endoscopic dilatation, we often refer the patient to the radiology department for a fluoroscopic balloon dilatation with a 30F to 36F balloon, which is routinely used for the procedure, providing a larger stretch of the tight area. The technique employed by the radiologist is to provide topical anesthetic to the hypopharynx, followed by passage of an orogastric guidewire, which is passed through the anastomosis under fluoroscopic guidance. The dilating balloon is passed over this guidewire. The safety and efficacy of both fluoroscopic and endoscopic balloon dilatation is excellent. Of all the patients with stenosis after RYGBP in our series, only four patients, all with postoperative marginal ulcer, failed to be adequately treated with serial balloon dilatations for postoperative anastomotic stenosis and required reoperation. All other patients were treated with three dilatations or fewer.

Go et al. (12) also reported a 6.8% stenosis rate after laparoscopic RYGBP, with a mean time to presentation of 7.7 weeks. The average number of balloon dilatations required to treat the stenosis in their series was 2.1, with 29% requiring three or more dilatations. Final treatment was similarly effective in the vast majority of patients, as in our experience. Goitein et al. (13) reviewed their incidence of postoperative gastrojejunal stenosis following laparoscopic RYGBP and found an incidence of 5.1%. Most (90%) of these patients were amenable to endoscopic balloon dilatation. Mean time to presentation was 32 days, and most patients in this series required more than two dilatations. However, all who underwent dilatation were symptom-free at 21-month follow-up.

Schwartz et al. (14) described their experience treating stenosis of the gastrojejunostomy following RYGBP. Their technique in performing the anastomosis, however, involved suturing of a piece of fascia lata around the anastomosis at the time of surgery. Though the incidence of stenosis in the series was low (3.3%), perhaps the operative technique accounted for the fact that in their experience stenosis presented significantly later (almost half after 3 months postoperative), was unable to be successfully dilated in 25% of cases, and 12.5% of the patients experienced perforation with dilatation.

Stenosis following VBG is usually a result of progressive stricturing and scarring of the outflow tract of the proximal stomach through the fixed band. The band can create a rim of hypertrophic scar that may progressively thicken with time. In our experience, 17% of patients after VBG required treatment for gastric outlet obstruction (15). Balloon dilatation, done either endoscopically or fluoroscopically or both, was needed for these patients. In over half of these cases, serial dilatations proved ineffective in producing adequate relief of obstruction, and reoperation was required. Papavramidis et al. (6) reported a 13.3% incidence of stenosis after VBG, comparable to our experience. Others have reported similar but slightly lower rates: Wayman et al. (16) found 8% of their patients after VBG developed stomal stenosis, with all but one responding to balloon dilatation.

The other postoperative symptoms that elicit the use of flexible endoscopy for diagnostic and therapeutic purposes include bleeding and abdominal pain. At our institution, these symptoms were the indications for another 74 patients from the initial series report undergoing 99 additional flexible upper endoscopic procedures (1). Of the two symptoms, the more common indication for these procedures was abdominal pain, suggestive of marginal ulcer. Often such diagnostic evaluations were negative for marginal ulcer (over 60% of cases). Actual life-threatening bleeding following RYGBP has been rare in our series, and in only one patient in that reported group was active bleeding seen during endoscopy. When bleeding is encountered early in the postoperative period, it most often is a result of staple line bleeding at the anastomosis. Standard endoscopic injection technique using epinephrine is the treatment of choice for the problem. The surgeon endoscopist must be careful about manipulating the bowel around a fresh anastomosis, but endoscopy is not contraindicated at any time postoperatively due to concerns of anastomotic disruption. Rather, if performed with expertise, it can avoid reoperation for the patient.

Overall, patients undergoing bariatric surgery at our institution had an over 20% incidence of having a flexible upper endoscopy performed by their surgeon during the time of their postoperative follow-up. This figure also emphasizes the significant frequency for which upper endoscopy may play a helpful diagnostic and therapeutic role in caring for the patient who has undergone bariatric surgery.

It should also be noted that the attitude of our patients, when faced with a postoperative need for flexible upper endoscopy, is almost uniformly relaxed and relieved, due to their experience and familiarity with the procedure from preoperative screening and the knowledge that reoperation is unlikely to be needed.

Conclusion

Flexible upper endoscopy may be a helpful screening tool for detecting preoperative upper gastrointestinal pathology in patients undergoing bariatric surgery. In our experience with routine use, it changed the operative procedure in 4.6% of cases. Others have reported a higher incidence on routine screening. Selective application would likely result in an even higher percentage.

Preoperative screening for and treatment of *H. pylori*, when added as a routine step in upper endoscopy, has significantly decreased our marginal ulcer rate following RYGBP from 6.8% to 2.6%. Biopsy for *H. pylori* should be strongly considered when performing preoperative screening endoscopy.

Several high-volume centers of bariatric surgery in the U.S. routinely use intraoperative flexible endoscopy as part of their performance of laparoscopic RYGBP.

Postoperative anastomotic stenosis after RYGBP occurs in from 2% to 15% of patients after RYGBP. This condition is amenable to endoscopic diagnosis and simultaneous balloon dilatation. Endoscopic balloon dilatation, used either alone or in combination with fluoroscopic balloon dilatation, is highly successful in treating anastomotic stenosis after RYGBP.

Over 20% of patients undergoing RYGBP have, in our experience, returned with signs and symptoms for which flexible upper endoscopy were indicated. The surgeon who performed the operation is the most knowledgeable in interpreting postoperative findings at the time of flexible upper endoscopy. Bariatric surgeons should strongly consider incorporating the practice of flexible upper endoscopy into their overall treatment program for their patients.

References

1. Schirmer B, Erenoglu C, Miller A. Flexible endoscopy in the management of patients undergoing Roux-en-Y gastric bypass. Obes Surg 2002;12:634–638.
2. Ramaswamy A, Lin E, Ramshaw BJ, Smith CD. Early effects of Helicobacter pylori infection in patients undergoing bariatric surgery. Arch Surg 2004;139:1094–1096.
3. Sharaf RN, Weinshel EH, Bini EJ, Rosenberg J, Sherman A, Ren CJ. Endoscopy plays an important preoperative role in bariatric surgery. Obes Surg 2004;14:1367–1372.
4. Verset D, Houben J-J, Gay F, Elcheroth J, Bourgeois V, Van Gossum A. The place of upper gastrointestinal tract endoscopy before and after vertical banded gastroplasty for morbid obesity. Dig Dis Sci 1997;42:2333–2337.
5. Hagen J, Deitel M, Khanna RK, Ilves R. Gastroesophageal reflux in the massively obese. Int Surg 1987;72:1–3.
6. Papavramidis ST, Theorcharidis AJ, Zaraboukas TG, et al. Upper gastrointestinal endoscopic and histologic findings before and after vertical banded gastroplasty. Surgical Endoscopy 1996;10:825–830.
7. Wittgrove AC, Clark GW. Laparoscopic gastric bypass: a five-year prospective study of 500 patients followed from 3 to 60 months. Obes Surg 1999;9:123–143.
8. Schauer PR, Ikramuddin S, Gourash W, Ramanathan R, Luketich J. Outcomes after laparoscopic Roux-en-Y gastric bypass for morbid obesity. Ann Surg 2000;232:515–529.
9. Gagner M, Garcia-Ruiz A, Arca MJ, Heniford TB. Laparoscopic isolated gastric bypass for morbid obesity. Surg Endosc 1999;S19:S6.
10. Champion JK, Hunt T, DeLisle N. Role of routine intraoperative endoscopy in laparoscopic bariatric surgery. Surg Endosc 2002;16:1663–1665.
11. Mittendorf EA, Brandt CP. Utility of intraoperative endoscopy: implications for surgical education. Surg Endosc 2002;16:703–706.
12. Go MR, Muscarella P, Needleman BJ, et al. Endoscopic management of stomal stenosis after Roux-en-Y gastric bypass. Surg Endosc 2004;18:56–59.
13. Goitein D, Papasavas PK, Gagne D, et al. Gastrojejunal strictures following laparoscopic Roux-en-Y gastric bypass for morbid obesity. Surg Endosc 2005;19:628–632.
14. Schwartz ML, Drew RL, Roiger RW, Ketover SR, Chazin-Caldie M. Stenosis of the gastroenterostomy after laparoscopic gastric bypass. Obes Surg 2004;484–491.
15. Vance PL, de Lange EE, Shaffer HA Jr, Schirmer B. Gastric outlet obstruction following surgery for morbid obesity: efficacy of fluoroscopically guided balloon dilatation. Radiology 2002;222:70–72.
16. Wayman CS, Nord JH, Combs WM, Rosemurgy AS. The role of endoscopy after vertical banded gastroplasty. Gastrointest Endosc 1992;38:44–46.

28
Bariatric Surgery in Adolescents

Timothy D. Kane, Victor F. Garcia, and Thomas H. Inge

Paralleling the epidemic of adult obesity are increasing trends in the prevalence and incidence of childhood obesity. Nearly two-thirds of adults in the United States are overweight and one-third obese (1), and 17% of children and adolescents are overweight or obese (2). The immediate and long-term health consequences of childhood obesity as well as the psychosocial and economic effects increasingly are cited as compelling arguments to perform bariatric surgery on adolescents to achieve aggressive weight loss. To provide a framework for considering and performing adolescent bariatric surgery, this chapter discusses the basic concepts of pediatric obesity, including definitions, risk factors, and consequences of obesity unique to adolescents. Additionally, we review the available evidence for the efficacy of bariatric procedures in the adolescent population and provide the reader with a suggested guideline and pathway for the application of bariatric surgery among adolescents.

Definition of Pediatric Obesity

The body mass index (BMI) is a relatively simple means to define overweight adults who have attained full growth. Adults with a BMI > 25 are considered overweight, whereas those with BMI ≥ 30 are considered obese. But in children and adolescents, we expect physiologic increases in adiposity, height, and weight during growth, and thus we cannot simply use a single BMI value to make accurate predictions about adiposity. Instead, for the vast majority of children and adolescents, growth charts are used to assign cutoffs for obesity that are age, race, and sex specific (3). In this context, some authors have defined pediatric obesity as BMI greater than the 95th percentile for age and sex. Overweight, or *at risk* for overweight, has been defined as a BMI > 85th percentile (4,5). It is important to first recognize that these percentile definitions of obesity and overweight become unreliable at the extreme categories of obesity. In essence, for the very severe categories of obesity, which might prompt consideration for

bariatric surgery in adolescence, there are currently no strong, reliable population-based data by which one can calculate percentile boundaries. This is because children and adolescents with BMI values in the >40 range are very poorly represented in the National Health and Nutrition Examination Survey (NHANES)—the data set that provides the weight and height information used to create the commonly used pediatric growth charts. For example, there are solid epidemiologic data to determine that a 20-year-old man with a BMI of 40 has a BMI for age at the 98.5th percentile. While it may be possible in the future to consider applying this 98.5th percentile (or perhaps a 99th percentile) definition of morbid obesity to younger age groups, the scientific basis for this has not yet been established. Alternatively, for the present time, most authors use BMI > 40 as a conservative threshold for defining morbid obesity in children and adolescents, which is congruent with the World Health Organization's definition for adults.

Adopting a BMI threshold as a general guideline for considering adolescent bariatric surgery is done with the understanding that an obese adolescent with an advanced, severe, and incontrovertibly weight-related comorbidity also should be considered for weight loss surgery without the strictest regard for the level of the BMI. To state this differently, there are some, albeit few, obese individuals for whom bariatric surgery may be required to relieve an urgent, life-threatening health problem, and thus they should not be required to meet an arbitrary BMI threshold to gain access to services.

Risk Factors for Adolescent Obesity

When considering bariatric surgery for adolescents, it may be useful to identify those patients who are at highest risk of persistent obesity and its sequelae. Indeed, recent insights into the developmental origins of obesity may inform the clinical evaluation of the adolescent candidate for bariatric surgery (6). The risk of a child carrying obesity into adulthood is influenced by genetic, biologic, psychological, cultural, and environmental factors (7). There are critical phases in the development of adolescent obesity in the period between preconception and adolescence (8,9). In neonates, lower birth weight has been linked to higher BMI in childhood and adulthood (10–14). The phenomenon of *adiposity rebound* also significantly affects the risk of chronic obesity (7). Adiposity rebound is defined as the age at which the physiologic low point of BMI occurs, typically around age 6 years. Patients who are at highest risk of chronic obesity can demonstrate adiposity rebound as early as age 3 or 4 years. Childhood obesity risks are also higher for offspring of mothers with diabetes mellitus (15). Extended duration of breast-feeding in the postnatal period reduces the risk of adolescent overweight (16,17). Conversely, longer duration of bottle feeding, maternal smoking during pregnancy, and low social status are risk factors for childhood overweight and adiposity. In fact, early bottle feeding accelerates the age of obesity rebound, which predicts obesity in later life (18).

Due in part to the rapid hormonal changes, puberty also is a critical period for the development of both insulin resistance (19) and obesity (20). Earlier menarche is seen in obese children, suggesting that the obese experience an earlier onset of physiologic maturation compared with children of normal weight (21).

Obesity in family members is an additional and important risk factor for adolescent obesity. The risk for persistence of childhood obesity into adulthood is elevated threefold if one parent and 10-fold if both parents are obese (22,23). The risk of obesity persisting into adulthood is far higher among obese adolescents than among overweight younger children (24). Finally, there is a preexisting racial-ethnic disparity in the risk of obesity (5), with lower socioeconomic groups being especially vulnerable because of poor diet and limited opportunity for physical activity (25).

In summary, important risk factors for childhood and adolescent obesity are (1) low birth weight, (2) bottle feeding, (3) earlier adiposity rebound, (4) a diabetic mother, and (5) parental obesity. Knowledge of these important risk factors for adolescent obesity and its persistence into adulthood gives some insight into the phenotypes of those individuals who may be least likely to succeed with nonsurgical management of obesity, and by inference, those who may benefit most from early application of surgical therapy.

Consequences of Obesity Unique to Adolescents

Obesity in adolescents is associated with many of the immediate and long-term consequences seen in adults. Important complications of obesity in adults include increased risk of cardiovascular disease (especially hypertension), dyslipidemia, diabetes mellitus, gallbladder disease, increased prevalences and mortality ratios of selected types of cancer, lower socioeconomic status, and psychosocial impairment (26). The magnitude of the adverse health consequences of obesity in adults is underscored by multiple studies that demonstrate an increased incidence of morbidity, mortality, and in particular early death in obese adults (27–29). These factors elevate the level of concern about the significance of medical consequences of obesity among adolescents.

The incidence of premature disease in obese adolescents is increased, and a wide range of organ systems is affected (30,31). Risk factors for atherosclerosis and coronary artery disease coexist in obese adolescents with hyperlipidemia and are also more common in this group (32,33). Almost 60% of obese children in the Bogalusa Heart Study had one risk factor for cardiovascular disease, with 20% having two or more risk factors (34).

Glucose intolerance is a frequent consequence of adult obesity as manifested by non–insulin-dependent diabetes mellitus (NIDDM). Derangements in carbohydrate metabolism, primarily insulin resistance, are clearly associated with childhood obesity (19). In 1996, a group from Cincinnati Children's Hospital reported a 10-fold increased incidence of type 2 diabetes in adolescents (35). Among new adolescent diagnoses of diabetes, type 2 diabetes accounted for one third. From 19% to 27% of severely obese adults (36,37), and 17% to 25% of obese children and adolescents (38,39), have impaired glucose tolerance, while the prevalence of type 2 diabetes is 24% to 27% for adults and only 4% to 6% in obese youth. Therefore, both insulin resistance and impaired glucose tolerance are highly prevalent among obese adults and children. Insulin resistance may also represent the fundamental defect underlying development of the cardiometabolic syndrome—a disorder with severe consequences, including premature mortality (40). Given the current increases in childhood diabetes and obesity prevalence, epidemiologists at the Centers for Disease Control (CDC) have recently made a sobering prediction: type 2 diabetes is expected to develop in 33% to 50% of all Americans born in the year 2000 (41).

Other health problems associated with pediatric obesity include reduced sleep efficiency and frank obstructive sleep apnea. Sleep deprivation and excessive daytime sleepiness are more common in obese children, and poor school performance has been associated with disordered sleep patterns in these children (42,43). Some data also demonstrate that correction of obstructive sleep apnea problems improves school performance. Of particular concern is the fact that children with obstructive sleep apnea also exhibit early cardiac abnormalities such as left ventricular hypertrophy and abnormal ventricular dimensions (44) not ameliorated by modest weight loss (45).

Skeletal disorders related to obesity demonstrate the toll that excessive weight takes over time on developing bone and cartilaginous structures. In Blount's disease, characterized by the abnormal bowing of the tibia (tibia vara) and resultant overgrowth of the medial aspect of the proximal tibial metaphysis in children, over two thirds of affected children are obese (46). Slipped capital femoral epiphysis stems from the effects of increased body weight on the cartilaginous growth plate of the hip. Up to 50% of children with slipped capital femoral epiphysis are overweight, and recurrence after surgical correction is likely if weight loss is not achieved (47).

Hypertension, which is less frequently found in children overall, occurs at a ninefold increased risk in the obese (48). Pseudotumor cerebri is a rare childhood disorder associated with increased intracranial pressure. Although pseudotumor presents with headaches and pulsatile tinnitus, it can progress to papilledema and require optic nerve fenestration for palliation. As many as 50% of children with this disorder are obese; however, the relationship between obesity and symptom onset is unclear (49).

A consequence of the epidemic of adolescent obesity is the increasing incidence of polycystic ovarian syndrome (PCOS) and hyperandrogenism related to insulin resistance and hyperinsulinism, which affect ovarian function (50). Obesity is present in approximately 50% of adolescents with PCOS; thus sustained weight loss can ameliorate the clinical manifestations of acne and hirsutism, as well as favorably impact insulin resistance (50).

Nonalcoholic fatty liver disease and steatohepatitis occur more frequently in obese children and adolescents (51). The most serious consequence of liver injury associated with obesity is fibrosis and accelerated cirrhosis, which can lead to end-stage liver disease. Finally, the risks of certain cancers, in particular gynecologic malignancies, have been associated with obesity in adolescents (52–54).

Psychosocial and quality of life issues are among the most prevalent in obese adolescents. The patterns of discrimination against obese children are established early in life and become ingrained in a culture in which thinness is admired (16,55). Although young children do not exhibit negative self-esteem or low self-image (56), adolescents develop a negative self-concept that may persist into adulthood (57). Moreover, obese individuals report that their weight has a negative impact on several aspects of their daily lives including physical function, self-esteem, sexual function, and employment (58).

Wang and Dietz (59) determined that over the past two decades (1979–1999), the cost of health care for children between 6 and 17 years of age with obesity-related diagnoses had more than tripled from $35 million to $127 million. They attributed increased incidences of diabetes, complications from gallbladder disease, and obstructive sleep apnea as responsible for the overall increase.

Bariatric Surgery in Adolescents

The rationale for performing bariatric procedures on adolescents is to prevent or alter the pattern of adverse health consequences that potentially impact obesity-related early mortality, which has been shown to exist in obese adults. The undeniable health benefits of bariatric surgery seen in adults will most likely be realized in the adolescent population as well. Thus, the use of bariatric surgery for carefully selected adolescents with severe obesity and comorbidities, who are unable to achieve a healthy weight with conventional measures, seems reasonable.

Guidelines and recommendations for offering bariatric surgery to adolescents have been proposed by the authors in conjunction with a group of pediatric obesity specialists and surgeons (58). Inclusion and exclusion criteria should be considered for adolescent patients seeking bariatric surgery (Table 28-1).

An alternative approach to these conservative indications is to offer bariatric surgery to adolescents earlier in

TABLE 28-1. Indications and contraindications for bariatric surgery in adolescence

Indications
Patient has failed at least 6 months of organized, medically supervised weight loss attempts; and
Patient has attained physiologic maturity (unless comorbidity is extreme); and
Patient is severely obese (BMI > 40) with obesity related comorbidities or have BMI >50; and
Patient exhibits commitment to comprehensive medical and psychological evaluation both before and after surgery; and
Patient agrees to avoid pregnancy for at least 1 year postoperatively; and
Patient is capable of adhering to and complying with postoperative nutritional guidelines; and
Patient signs informed consent form for surgical management; and
Patient demonstrates decisional capacity; and
Patient has a supportive family environment

Contraindications
Patient has been a substance abuser within the preceding year; or
Patient has a psychiatric diagnosis that would impair ability to adhere to postoperative dietary or medication regimen (e.g., psychosis); or
Patient has medical causes of obesity (endocrine, hypothalamic, or pituitary); or
Patient (or parent) is unable or unwilling to fully comprehend the surgical procedure and its medical consequences; or
Patient is unable or refuses to participate in lifelong medical surveillance

the course of their disease. Offering bariatric surgery only to those adolescents who have severe comorbidities or severe obesity may result in higher complication rates and potentially less weight loss for these patients. Offering the procedure to patients with lower BMIs at an earlier point in the disease process, however, may decrease their operative risk and optimize results. This concept of selecting patients based on risk factors analysis rather than BMI has not yet been widely accepted, but may be applicable to obese adults as well as adolescents. Further data are required, however, before this concept can be implemented and the use of arbitrary BMI cutoffs to select patients abandoned.

The American Society of Bariatric Surgery (ASBS) does not support a strict BMI cutoff of 40 for morbidly obese adolescents to qualify for bariatric surgery. Such a cutoff may prevent access to surgery for adolescents with lower BMIs and severe comorbidities who are in need of surgical intervention. Additionally, the ASBS has questioned the need to include established comorbidities as an indication for bariatric surgery in the adolescent group. Given the natural history of obesity, morbidly obese children will almost certainly develop severe comorbidities as they progress to adulthood. The ASBS has emphasized the need to prevent comorbidities by offering surgery earlier rather than waiting for them to develop in this patient population. In summary, the ASBS supports using the same criteria for bariatric surgery in the adolescent as those set forth by the 1991 National Institutes of Health (NIH) Consensus Conference for morbidly obese adults (60).

Adolescent bariatric surgery should be available as an integral part of comprehensive pediatric weight management programs. Expertise in a number of disciplines should be represented in such comprehensive programs to ensure optimal outcomes. These specialties include adolescent medicine, psychology, nutrition, and exercise physiology. Other specialists may be required, depending on individuals' needs. These include pediatric experts in endocrinology, pulmonology, gastroenterology, cardiology, and orthopedics.

Unique Features of Adolescents Relevant to Bariatric Surgery

Since adolescence represents an extensive period of substantial growth and maturation, both physically and emotionally, special attention to developmental issues in adolescents is critical when considering bariatric procedures that will have marked impact on future growth and development. For adolescents who have attained the vast majority (>95%) of linear growth, there is clearly little reason to believe that growth would be impaired by a bariatric procedure (61). Based on peak height velocity measurements in normal weight girls (8 to 9 cm/year) and boys (9 to 10 cm/year), girls should achieve >95% linear growth by 13 years of age and boys by 15 years of age (62). The onset of menarche is also a marker for physiologic maturity in girls, and growth is generally completed within 2 years after menarche. Bone age can also be assessed by plain radiography of the hand and wrist if there is uncertainty about status of physiologic maturation. Nomograms are used by radiologists to accurately predict the percentile of adult stature that a child has attained.

The importance of a dedicated pediatric psychologist and continued postprocedural follow-up cannot be overstated. As a corollary to physiologic growth, adolescents are also rapidly maturing psychologically. As chronologic age does not accurately correlate with maturity of thought, adolescents present along a continuum relative to their ability to understand health and disease and the implications of treatment decisions. Historically, adolescents with chronic illnesses have demonstrated poor compliance with medical treatment regimens and clinical follow-up (63,64). Rand and Macgregor (65) reported that less than one in five adolescent gastric bypass patients were completely compliant with postoperative dietary multivitamin and nutrient supplementations. Conversely, studies have suggested that in this age group, adherence to medication and dietary regimens can be improved with family-based behavioral therapy (66–68). For instance, adolescents with cystic fibrosis, asthma, or type 1 diabetes have demonstrated significantly enhanced regimen adherence with defined behavioral interventions. Thus, there is scientifically rigorous evidence from other chronic disease models that would suggest that ongoing behavioral therapy offers the best chance at long-term success with compliance with postoperative regimens after bariatric procedures in adolescence.

Clinical Pathway for the Management of the Adolescent Undergoing Bariatric Surgery

Gastric bypass surgery reduces the intake and decreases the absorption of food items rich in essential fatty acids, vitamins, and other specific nutrients, the long-term results of which are unknown and are of legitimate concern. This is particularly relevant given the fact that a majority of adolescents seeking bariatric surgery are girls who are or soon will be considering planning families of their own. Undernutrition of the mother during fetal development may well result in adverse health consequences or subsequent obesity in the offspring, as suggested by the Dutch famine cohort (11). Therefore, success of adolescent bariatric surgery should be examined along the life course, not only in terms of sustained weight loss but also in terms of normal progression through adolescence and adulthood, and eventually in terms of uncomplicated reproduction and normal offspring.

Adolescents should be considered a high-risk population, and thus bariatric operations should be performed only in specialized regional programs and centers that provide comprehensive and extended preoperative and postoperative medical surveillance. The potential benefits of regionalizing complex surgical procedures have been recognized for at least two decades (69–72). Recent data suggests that nearly 3000 adolescents have undergone bariatric surgery over the past decade, representing <1% of the adult bariatric volume. In addition, a threefold increase in adolescent bariatric surgical volume was seen between 2000 and 2003 (Dr. R. Burd, personal communication, May 2006). These findings suggest that centers offering adolescent bariatric surgery should be dedicated to the collection of quality outcome data. The long-term sequelae of adolescent bariatric surgery are currently unclear; thus, clinical pathways should have the goal not only of achieving significant and sustained weight loss and comorbidity resolution, but also of identifying potential adverse effects of bariatric procedures and risk factors for late weight regain, and contributing to determining which operations are the most effective.

There is good reason to have a heightened concern for development of postoperative hypovitaminosis syndromes after gastric bypass surgery in adolescents (65). Obesity is a risk factor for preoperative micronutrient malnutrition (73), and this could be compounded postoperatively, since gastric bypass patients are at risk for noncompliance with supplementation regimens (65). Indeed, adolescents have developed symptomatic beriberi requiring a period of parenteral supplementation for resolution, despite receiving adequate multivitamin supplementation (74).

Postoperative vitamin and mineral supplementation should mimic best practice used for adult bariatric patients; unfortunately, there are no evidence-based guidelines for micronutrient management after bariatric surgery. However, many agree that at a minimum, patients should be prescribed two pediatric chewable multivitamins, in addition to a calcium supplement, and an iron supplement for menstruating females. Strong consideration should also be given to additional supplementation of B complex vitamins beyond what is contained in multivitamin preparations, to augment thiamine supplementation (74). However, the risk of noncompliance with supplements in the younger age group also provides the rationale for simplification of the regimen and for more extensive postoperative surveillance. When there is any question of compliance with supplement intake, it is reassuring to document the adequacy of intake by measuring levels (e.g., folate, vitamins A, B_1, B_6, and B_{12}).

Body composition assessment should also be considered for adolescents undergoing rapid weight loss. This can be performed with either bioelectrical impedance (for patients weighing in excess of 300 pounds) or dual energy x-ray absorptiometry analysis (DEXA, for patients weighing less than 300 pounds) preoperatively and at regular intervals postoperatively. DEXA measures the rate and relative amounts of fat and lean body mass loss, and a dedicated lumbar spine study provides a quantitative assessment of bone mineral density. Bone density measurements can be reassuring, given the fact that bone mineral accretion continues to occur throughout the first three decades of life and is not complete until the mid-20s. Evidence suggesting that even as little as a two standard deviation change in bone mineral content of the adolescent can significantly increase the risk of osteoporosis and bone fractures in later life underscores the importance of meticulous and extended monitoring of nutrient, vitamin, and mineral absorption (75,76). Body composition analysis is also used to modify dietary plans intended to preserve lean body mass during weight loss.

Outcomes of Bariatric Surgery in Adolescents

Bariatric surgery in adolescents has not been evaluated or compared with nonoperative approaches in a prospective manner. However, the limited experience accrued in several small series suggests that gastric bypass and adjustable gastric banding can be performed safely and effectively in adolescents (65,77–81).

Whereas most of the published accounts have reported results of the open Roux-en-Y gastric bypass technique, laparoscopic gastric bypass has been used successfully in adolescents with few complications (82,83). Stanford et al. (83) reported an excess weight loss over 80% in three of four patients who were followed >20 months following laparoscopic gastric bypass surgery. Excess weight loss following gastric bypass has been satisfactory in most series, with Strauss et al. (78) reporting nine of 10 patients who lost over 59% of their initial excess weight, and similarly, Sugerman et al. (79) reported a 56% excess weight loss in 20 patients >10 years after gastric bypass surgery was performed in their adolescence (ages 12 to 17 years) (78,79).

There has been an ongoing debate over whether gastric bypass (open or laparoscopic) versus the laparoscopically placed adjustable gastric band should be the preferred procedure for weight loss in severely obese adolescents. Despite consideration of the Roux-en-Y gastric bypass as the gold standard for the achievement of sustained weight loss (36), adjustable gastric banding has been used with success in the obese adolescent population. The appeal of adjustable gastric banding for adolescents lies in the reversibility, low incidence of morbidity and mortality, and potential avoidance of severe nutritional risks associated with malabsorptive procedures (84). Dolan et al. (81) reported on 17 adolescents (ages 12 to 19 years) who underwent laparoscopic adjustable gastric banding for obesity (mean preoperative BMI = 44.7) with an average of 2 years follow-up, who had achieved 59.3% excess weight loss, and the majority (76.5%) lost at least 50% of their excess weight (postoperative BMI = 30.2). Many patients in this study experienced marked improvement in obesity-related comorbidities. Other authors have observed similar results in adolescents following adjustable gastric banding (85). Long-term follow-up is necessary to determine whether the elimination of comorbidities and maintenance of weight loss are sustained, and whether complications related to the gastric banding approach are acceptable. In the United States, Food and Drug Administration (FDA) approval of this device in June 2001 was confined to the adult population. An FDA panel meeting in November 2005 was dedicated to the design of trials for weight loss devices in pediatric morbidly obese patients. However, as of yet there have been no weight loss devices approved for use in children or adolescents.

There has been no reported procedure-related mortality in adolescents undergoing gastric bypass. Early complications have included pulmonary embolism, wound infection, stomal stenoses, and marginal ulcers. Late complications have included small bowel obstructions, incisional hernias, symptomatic cholelithiasis, protein calorie and micronutrient deficiencies, and late weight regain (10–15% incidence) (77–80). The predictability of such complications parallels those of adult series and therefore necessitates lifelong follow-up. In 2001, the first children's hospital-based comprehensive weight management program including bariatric surgery was developed at Cincinnati Children's Hospital Medical Center. Institutional consensus was achieved for a multidisciplinary team early in the process (86). Modification of a number of processes was also needed to accommodate care delivery to morbidly obese adolescents, most notably, assessment of weight limits for diagnostic equipment used in the radiology department (87).

Over 70 adolescents have undergone laparoscopic Roux-en-Y gastric bypass at Cincinnati Children's Hospital. The average age of adolescent patients was 17 years. While all patients have had comorbidities of obesity, more than half have suffered from obstructive sleep apnea (88). The youngest patient was a 14-year-old girl with type 2 diabetes mellitus. Most adolescents have demonstrated some features of metabolic syndrome (89). Eighty-three percent have evidence of fatty liver disease, with a quarter of patients demonstrating steatosis alone, one third with some inflammation and steatosis, and 20% formally demonstrated nonalcoholic steatohepatitis (90).

Most patients have demonstrated markedly impaired quality of life, worse on average than patients who suffer from pediatric cancer (91).

The mean preoperative weight in our patients is 361 pounds (164 kg), and the BMI ranged from 44 to 85, with a mean of 57. After 1 year, the mean weight was 222 pounds (101 kg) and BMI ranged from 26 to 58 with a mean of 35. This represents a 39% reduction in BMI over the year. The excess weight loss is 63%. By comparison, BMI in a comparable cohort ($n = 12$) enrolled for 1 year in our nonsurgical pediatric weight management program fell 2.6% from 47.2 to 46 (p = NS). Postoperative polysomnography (6 months) showed a dramatic reduction in the severity of obstructive sleep apnea (OSA) in all patients, with complete resolution of OSA in 90% (87); similarly, type 2 diabetes resolved at 1 year after surgical weight loss in all six patients with this diagnosis. Metabolic outcomes have shown that insulin resistance and hypertriglyceridemia resolve after adolescent gastric bypass as well (89). Patient and parental satisfaction have been very good overall. A support group is considered useful for allowing a frank exchange of information among families who are considering surgery and those who have had bariatric surgery, although overall participation has been less than ideal.

Conclusion

Surgical approaches may be reasonable for clinically severely obese adolescents who have obesity-related comorbidities and have been unsuccessful in achieving sustained weight loss following organized attempts. Suggested indications and contraindications for operative intervention should not be inflexibly applied to every patient but rather should be considered guidelines for performing bariatric surgery in adolescents. Individuals should be considered based on the degree of obesity, the severity of comorbid conditions, their physical and emotional maturity level, and the stability of family support. The benefits of a multidisciplinary approach in adolescent weight management and bariatric surgery cannot be overemphasized. Families and patients alike must participate fully in all aspects of preoperative decision making, and must fully understand the potential complications before bariatric interventions are made. Families and patients must understand that bariatric surgery is a valuable weight loss tool, as opposed to a *cure* for obesity, to promote continued compliance with lifestyle and dietary changes postoperatively. Adolescent bariatric surgery should be conducted only in institutions capable of managing adolescents with complications of severe obesity and where detailed clinical data collection and outcome studies can be done. Finally, highly trained and skilled bariatric surgeons must have an integral role within the multidisciplinary team to guarantee safe and appropriate application of bariatric surgical procedures in adolescents.

References

1. Flegal KM, Carroll MD, Ogden CL, Johnson CL. Prevalence and trends in obesity among US adults, 1999–2000. JAMA 2002;288:1723–1727.
2. Ogden CL, et al. Prevalence of overweight and obesity in the United States, 1999–2004. JAMA 2006;295(13):1549–1555.
3. Himes JH, Dietz WH. Guidelines for overweight in adolescent preventive services: recommendations from an expert committee. The Expert Committee on Clinical Guidelines for Overweight in Adolescent Preventive Services. Am J Clin Nutr 1994;59:309–316.
4. Yanovski JA. Pediatric obesity. Rev Endocr Metab Disord 2001;2(4):371–383.
5. Strauss RS, Pollack HA. Epidemic increase in childhood overweight, 1986–1998. JAMA 2001;286:2845–2848.
6. Oken E, Gillman MW. Fetal origins of obesity. Obes Res 2003;11(4):496–506.
7. Cameron N, Demerath EW. Critical periods in human growth and their relationship to diseases of aging. Am J Phys Anthropol 2002;suppl 35:159–184.
8. Michels KB. Early life predictors of chronic disease. J Womens Health (Larchmt) 2003;12(2):157–161.
9. Wahlqvist ML. Chronic disease prevention: a life-cycle approach which takes account of the environmental impact and opportunities of food, nutrition and public health policies—the rationale for an eco-nutritional disease nomenclature. Asia Pac J Clin Nutr 2002;11(suppl 9):S759–762.
10. Bavdekar A, Yanik CS, Fall CH, et al. Insulin resistance syndrome in 8-year-old Indian children: small at birth, big at 8 years, or both? Diabetes 1999;48(12):2422–2429.
11. Ravelli AC, van Der Meulen S, Osmond C, et al. Obesity at the age of 50 y in men and women exposed to famine prenatally. Am J Clin Nutr 1999;70(5):811–816.
12. Parsons TJ, Powers C, Logan S, et al. Childhood predictors of adult obesity: a systematic review. Int J Obes Relat Metab Disord 1999;23(suppl 8):S1–107.
13. Sorensen HT, Sabroe S, Rothman KJ, et al. Relation between weight and length at birth and body mass index in young adulthood: cohort study. BMJ 1997;315(7116):1137.
14. Byberg L, McKeigue PM, Zethelius B, et al. Birth weight and the insulin resistance syndrome: association of low birth weight with truncal obesity and raised plasminogen activator inhibitor-1 but not with abdominal obesity or plasma lipid disturbances. Diabetologia 2000;43(1):54–60.
15. Silverman BL, Rizzo TA, Cho NH, et al. Long-term effects of the intrauterine environment. The Northwestern University Diabetes in Pregnancy Center. Diabetes Care 1998; 21(suppl 2):B142–149.
16. Gillman MW. Breast-feeding and obesity. J Pediatr 2002; 141(6):749–757.
17. Gillman MW, Rifas-Shiman SL, Camargo CA Jr, et al. Risk of overweight among adolescents who were breastfed as infants. JAMA 2001;285(19):2461–2467.
18. Bergmann KE, Bergmann RL, Von Kries R, et al. Early determinants of childhood overweight and adiposity in a birth cohort study: role of breast-feeding. Int J Obes Relat Metab Disord 2003;27(2):162–172.
19. Caprio S. Insulin resistance in childhood obesity. J Pediatr Endocrinol Metab 2002;15(suppl 1):487–492.
20. Heald FP, Khan MA. Teenage obesity. Pediatr Clin North Am 1973;20(4):807–817.
21. Wattigney WA, Srinivasan SR, Chen W, et al. Secular trend of earlier onset of menarche with increasing obesity in black and white girls: the Bogalusa Heart Study. Ethn Dis 1999; 9(2):181–189.
22. Whitaker RC, Wright JP, Peper MS, et al. Predicting obesity in young adulthood from childhood and parental obesity. N Engl J Med 1997;337(13):869–873.
23. Pi-Sunyer FX. The obesity epidemic: pathophysiology and consequences of obesity. Obes Res 2002;10(suppl 2):97S–104S.
24. Whitaker RC. Understanding the complex journey to obesity in early adulthood. Ann Intern Med 2002;136(12): 923–925.
25. Gordon-Larsen P, Adair LS, Popkin BM. Ethnic differences in physical activity and inactivity patterns and overweight status. Obes Res 2002;10(3):141–149.
26. Health implications of obesity. National Institutes of Health Consensus Development Conference Statement. Ann Intern Med 1985;103(pt 2):1073.
27. Peeters A, Barendregt JJ, Willekens F, et al. Obesity in adulthood and its consequences for life expectancy: a lifetable analysis. Ann Intern Med 2003;138:24–32.
28. Raman RP. Obesity and health risks. J Am Coll Nutr 2002; 21:134S–139S.
29. Sonne-Holm S, Sorensen TI, Christensen U. Risk of early death in extremely overweight young men. Br Med J (Clin Res Ed) 1983;287:795–797.
30. Must A, Jacques PF, Dallal GE, et al. Long-term morbidity and mortality of overweight adolescents: a follow-up of the Harvard Growth Study of 1922–1935. N Engl J Med 1992; 327:1350–1355.
31. Dietz WH. Health consequences of obesity in youth: childhood predictors of adult disease. Pediatrics 1998;101;(3 pt 2): 518–525.
32. Daniels SR. Cardiovascular disease risk factors and atherosclerosis in children and adolescents. Curr Atheroscler Rep 2001;3:479–485.
33. Freedman DS, Srinivasan SR, Harsha DW, et al. Relation of body fat patterning to lipid and lipoprotein concentrations in children and adolescents: the Bogalusa Heart Study. Am J Clin Nutr 1989;50:930–939.
34. Freedman DS, Khan LK, Dietz WH, et al. Relationship of childhood obesity to coronary heart disease risk factors in adulthood: the Bogalusa Heart Study. Pediatrics 2001;108: 712–718.
35. Pinhas-Hamiel O, Dolan LM, Daniels SR, et al. Increased incidence of non-insulin dependent diabetes mellitus among adolescents. J Pediatr 1996;128:608–615.
36. Pories WJ, Swanson MS, MacDonald KG, et al. Who would have thought it? An operation proves to be the most effective therapy for adult-onset diabetes mellitus. Ann Surg 1995;222(3):339–350.

37. Cowan GS Jr, Buffington CK. Significant changes in blood pressure, glucose, and lipids with gastric bypass surgery. World J Surg 1998;22(9):987–992.

38. Sinha R, Fisch G, Teague B, et al. Prevalence of impaired glucose tolerance among children and adolescents with marked obesity. N Engl J Med 2002;346(11):802–810.

39. Paulsen EP, Richenderfer L, Ginsberg-Fellner F. Plasma glucose, free fatty acids, and immunoreactive insulin in sixty-six obese children. Studies in reference to a family history of diabetes mellitus. Diabetes 1968;17(5):261–269.

40. Steinberger J, Daniels SR. Obesity, insulin resistance, diabetes, and cardiovascular risk in children: an American Heart Association scientific statement from the Atherosclerosis, Hypertension, and Obesity in the Young Committee (Council on Cardiovascular Disease in the Young) and the Diabetes Committee (Council on Nutrition, Physical Activity, and Metabolism). Circulation 2003;107(10):1448–1453).

41. Narayan K, Boyle J, Thompson T, Sorensen S. Lifetime risk for diabetes mellitus in the United States. Diabetes 2003; suppl 1:A225(abstract 967–P).

42. Gozal D, Wang M, Pope DW. Objective sleepiness measures in pediatric obstructive sleep apnea. Pediatrics 2001;108:693–697.

43. Gozal D. Sleep-disordered breathing and school performance in children. Pediatrics 1998;102:616–620.

44. Amin RS, Kimball TR, Bean JA, et al. Left ventricular hypertrophy and abnormal ventricular geometry in children and adolescents with obstructive sleep apnea. Am J Respir Crit Care Med 2002;165:1395–1399.

45. Witt SA, Glascock BJ, Khoury P, Kimball, TR, Daniels SR. Does obesity and weight reduction affect cardiac geometry and function in normotensive children? Presented at the 74th Scientific Sessions of the American Heart Association, Anaheim, CA, November 13, 2001.

46. Dietz WH, Gross WL, Kirkpatrick JA. Blount disease (tibia vara): another skeletal disorder associated with childhood obesity. J Pediatr 1982;101:735–737.

47. Kelsey JL, Acheson RM, Keggi KJ. The body build of patients with slipped capital femoral epiphysis. Am J Dis Child 1972;124:276–281.

48. Rosner B, Prineas R, Daniels SR, et al. Blood pressure difference between blacks and whites in relation to body size and among US children and adolescents. Am J Epidemiol 2000;151:1007–1019.

49. Weisberg LA, Chutorian AM. Pseudotumor cerebri of childhood. Am J Dis Child 1977;131:1243–1248.

50. Gordon CM. Menstrual disorders in adolescents. Excess androgens and polycystic ovarian syndrome. Pediatr Clin North Am 1999;46(3);519–543.

51. Xanthakos S, Miles L, Bucuvalas J, Daniels S, Garcia V, Inge T. Histologic spectrum of NASH in morbidly obese adolescents differs from adults. Clin Gastroenterol Hepatol 2006;4(2):226–232.

52. Bergstrom A, Pisani P, Tenet V, et al. Overweight as an avoidable cause of cancer in Europe. Int J Cancer 2001;91:421–430.

53. Wolk A, Gridley G, Svensson M, et al. A prospective study of obesity and cancer risk (Sweden). Cancer Causes Control 2001;12:13–21.

54. Lubin F, Chetrit A, Freedman LS, et al. Body mass index at age 18 years and during adult life and ovarian cancer risk. Am J Epidemiol 2003;157:113–120.

55. Richardson SA, Goodman N, Hastorf AH, et al. Cultural uniformity in reaction to physical disabilities. Am Soc Rev 1961;26:241–247.

56. Kaplan KM, Wadden TA. Childhood obesity and self-esteem. J Pediatr 1986;109:367–370.

57. Stunkard A, Burt V. Obesity and the body image II. Age at onset of disturbances in the body image. Am J Psychiatry 1967;123:1443–1447.

58. Kolotkin RL, Crosby RD, Williams GR, et al. The relationship between health-related quality of life and weight loss. Obes Res 2001;9:564–567.

59. Wang G, Dietz WH. Economic burden of obesity in youths aged 6 to 17 years: 1979–1999. Pediatrics 2002;109(6):E81.

60. Wittgrove AC, Buchwald H, Sugerman H, Pories W. Surgery for severely obese adolescents: further insight from the American Society for Bariatric Surgery. Pediatrics 2004; 114(1):253–254.

61. Inge TH, et al. Bariatric surgery for overweight adolescents? Concerns and recommendations. Pediatrics 2004; 114:217–223.

62. Tanner JM, Davies PS. Clinical longitudinal standards for height and weight velocity for North American children. J Pediatr 1985;107:317–329.

63. Borowitz D, Wegman T, Harris M. Preventive care for patients with chronic illness. Multivitamin use in patients with cystic fibrosis. Clin Pediatr (Phila) 1994;33:720–725.

64. Phipps S, De Cuir-Whalley S. Adherence issues in pediatric bone marrow transplantation. J Pediatr Psychol 1990;15:459–475.

65. Rand CS, Macgregor AM. Adolescents having obesity surgery: a 6-year follow-up. South Med J 1994;87:1208–1213.

66. Wysocki T, Harris MA, Greco P, et al. Randomized, controlled trial of behavioral therapy for families of adolescents with insulin-dependent diabetes mellitus. J Pediatr Psychol 2000;25:23–33.

67. Lemanek KL, Kamps J, Chung NB. Empirically supported treatments in pediatric psychology: regimen adherence. J Pediatr Psychol 2001;26:253–275.

68. Fielding D, Duff A. Compliance with treatment protocols: interventions for children with chronic illness. Arch Dis Child 1999;80 196–200.

69. Norton EC, Garfinkel SA, McQuay LJ, et al. The effect of hospital volume on the in-hospital complication rate in knee replacement patients. Health Serv Res 1998;33(5 pt 1):1191–1210.

70. Flood AB, Scott WR, Ewy W. Does practice make perfect? Part II: the relation between volume and outcomes and other hospital characteristics. Med Care 1984;22(2):115–125.

71. Gordon TA, Bowman HM, Tielsch JM, et al. Statewide regionalization of pancreaticoduodenectomy and its effect on in-hospital mortality. Ann Surg 1998;228(1):71–78.

72. Hamilton SM, Letourneau S, Pekeles E, et al. The impact of regionalization on a surgery program in the Canadian health care system. Arch Surg 1997;132(6):605–609; discussion 609–611.

73. Harnroongroj T, Jintaridhi P, Vudhivai N, et al. B vitamins, vitamin C and hematological measurements in overweight and obese Thais in Bangkok. J Med Assoc Thai 2002; 85(1):17–25.

74. Towbin A, Inge TH, Garcia VF, et al. Beriberi after gastric bypass surgery in adolescence. J Pediatr 2004;145(2): 263–267.

75. Nguyen TV, Maynard LM, Towne B, et al. Sex differences in bone mass acquisition during growth: the Fels Longitudinal Study. J Clin Densitom 2001;4(2):147–157.

76. Whiting SJ. Obesity is not protective for bones in childhood and adolescence. Nutr Rev 2002;60(1):27–30.

77. Breaux CW. Obesity surgery in children. Obes Surg 1995;5: 279–284.

78. Strauss RS, Bradley LJ, Brolin RE. Gastric bypass in adolescents with morbid obesity. J Pediatr 2001;138:499–504.

79. Sugerman HJ, Sugerman EL, DeMaria EJ, Kellum JM, Kennedy C, Mowery Y. Bariatric surgery for severely obese adolescents. J Gastrointestinal Surg 2003;7:102–108.

80. Lawson L, Harmon C, Chen M, et al. One year outcomes of Roux en Y gastric bypass in adolescents: a multicenter report from the Pediatric Bariatric Study Group. J Pediatr Surg 2006 41(1):137–143; discussion 137–143.

81. Dolan K, Creighton L, Hopkins G, Fielding G. Laparoscopic gastric banding in morbidly obese adolescents. Obes Surg 2003;13:101–105.

82. Garica VF, Langford L, Inge T. Application of laparoscopy for bariatric surgery in adolescents. Cur Opinion in Pediatrics 2003;15:248–255.

83. Stanford A, Glascock JM, Eid GM, et al. Laparoscopic Roux-en Y gastric bypass in morbidly obese adolescents. J Pediatr Surg 2003;38(3):430–433.

84. O'Brien PE, Dixon JB. Laparoscopic adjustable gastric banding in the treatment of morbid obesity. Arch Surg 2003;138:376–382.

85. Angrisani L, Favretti F, Furbetta F, et al. Obese teenagers treated by Lap-Band System: the Italian experience. Surgery 2005;138:877–881.

86. Inge TH, Garcia VF, Daniels SR, et al. A multidisciplinary approach to the adolescent bariatric surgical patient. J Pediatr Surg 2004;39:442–447

87. Inge TH, Donnelly LF, Vierra M, Cohen A, Daniels SR, Garcia VF. Managing bariatric patients in a children's hospital: radiologic considerations and limitations. J Pediatr Surg 2005;40:609–617.

88. Kalra M, Inge T, Garcia V, et al. Obstructive sleep apnea in morbidly obese adolescents: effect of bariatric surgical intervention. Obes Res 2005;13:1175–1179.

89. Lawson L, Harmon C, Chen M, et al. One year outcomes of Roux-en-Y gastric bypass in adolescents: a multicenter report from the Pediatric Bariatric Study Group. J Pediatr Surg 2006;41(1):137–143; discussion 137–143.

90. Xanthakos S, Miles L, Bucuvalas J, Daniels S, Garcia V, Inge T. Histologic spectrum of NASH in morbidly obese adolescents differs from adults. Clin Gastroenterol Hepatol 2006;4(2):226–232.

91. Zeller MH, Roehrig HR, Modi AC, Daniels SR, Inge TH. Adolescents seeking bariatric surgery: an examination of health-related quality of life and depressive symptoms. Pediatrics 2006;117(4):1155–1161.

29
Bariatric Surgery in the Elderly

Julie Kim, Scott Shikora, and Michael Tarnoff

Advances in health care enable people to live longer and healthier lives than ever before. The average life span is now well into the 70s. This is a dramatic increase since Roman times, when the average life span was only 25 to 30 years. In 1990, more than 30 million people were above the age of 65 in the United States. This figure is estimated to nearly double to 58.9 million, comprising nearly 20% of the population, by the year 2025 (1). Individuals above the age of 65 currently undergo more surgical procedures than any other age group, the incidence of which is only expected to increase over the next several decades (2). This raises many potential areas of concern for all surgeons, including bariatric surgeons.

Before discussing bariatric surgery in the elderly, however, one must first define "elderly," as there is no standard criterion and little consensus in the surgical literature. Publications use different age definitions, ranging from 50 to above 80 (3–5). For our discussion purposes, elderly will be defined as individuals of ages 60 or older, based on the federal age classifications that are currently in place.

Assessing the effect of age on operative risk is also difficult. Age is relative to the time in question, which is why there are no absolute standards; for example, a study from the 1950s regarding age and operative risk may not be as relevant today as it once had been. The wide heterogeneity of operations in question also adds bias. There are unfortunately few studies specifically addressing bariatric surgery in the elderly. Bariatric surgery in the elderly may entail a risk profile that is inherently different from that for cataract, cancer, or cardiac surgery. Most analyses of perioperative care in the elderly have been extrapolated from the literature on younger patients, making them prone to error. Finally, the advancement of minimally invasive techniques adds another parameter that may affect operative risk.

Approximately 20% of obese Americans are elderly. As this percentage continues to rise it will become increasingly important that standard guidelines are created to help facilitate the process of patient selection and perioperative care for this group of bariatric patients. Until sufficient evidence is obtained from prospective randomized trials, the decision to operate on the elderly will be left to the discretion of each individual bariatric surgeon or practice. We have performed bariatric procedures in our practice on patients into their seventh decade of life without any significant increase in morbidity or mortality.

How Does Obesity Impact the Elderly?

Most research on obesity is derived from young and middle-aged patients. There are limited data regarding the prognostic importance of overweight and obesity in the elderly. Surprisingly, overweight and mild obesity do not seem to be associated with any significant increase in cardiovascular mortality in individuals 65 years of age or older, as compared with younger cohorts. The data, in fact, suggest that individuals 65 and older may require a higher optimum body mass index (BMI) than the ideal weight currently defined in federal guidelines for all individuals as a BMI between 18.7 and 24.9 (6). Several studies have shown that the excess mortality associated with obesity actually declines with age (7). Therefore, until age-specific recommendations are made, elderly patients who are being considered for weight reduction surgery should meet strict National Institutes of Health (NIH) weight criteria. There are also few data involving medical weight loss in the elderly. Most studies on supervised diets or medications have been performed in younger patients. Thus, it is probably prudent that elderly patients have attempted a serious effort at documented medical weight loss before undergoing surgical treatment.

Patient Selection and Preoperative Assessment of Surgical Risk in the Elderly

Due to the lack of any uniform consensus, the onus of patient selection falls on the bariatric surgeon.

Chronologic age alone is a poor predictor of outcome. After establishing fulfillment of the general NIH criteria for weight reduction surgery, emphasis should be placed on the evaluation of the functional status of the individual (8). The impact of age on surgical risk arises from a decrease in vital organ function. This is attributable to the normal aging process in conjunction with any preexisting disease, resulting in a decreased ability to respond optimally to operative stress (1). Age in and of itself, however, is not the risk. Patients should be stratified into a high- or low-risk category based on the number of associated diseases. The literature suggests that the preoperative condition of the patient is more important than intraoperative events in predicting adverse outcomes after surgery. A dramatic increase in perioperative deaths has been seen in elderly patients with multisystem disease. Premorbid conditions that may increase perioperative risk include congestive heart failure and coronary artery disease (9). The goal of any bariatric operation should be to improve the quality of postoperative life, or at minimum, not impair it. Therefore, preoperative optimization of the elderly patient's overall condition, without undue delay in surgery, is advocated.

There are several normal age-related physiologic changes that may or may not have any overt clinical findings. These age-related changes result in altered end-organ function, most importantly cardiac, pulmonary, and renal function. Cardiac output can be decreased from a blunted response to catecholamines, which can lead to increased ectopy that may not be seen in the resting state. Hypertrophy of the left ventricular mass can add to any underlying diastolic dysfunction already present. It may be prudent in elderly patients to evaluate the functional cardiac status under stressed conditions (using a treadmill stress test or a Persantine thallium scan), even in the presence of a normal electrocardiogram. A transthoracic echocardiogram should also be considered in any patient with history of congestive heart failure (CHF).

The changes in the respiratory system include decreased chest wall compliance, decreased lung volumes, and decreased strength of the respiratory musculature, resulting in an overall decline of pulmonary function. Elderly patients, therefore, may be more susceptible to postoperative respiratory complications. Pulmonary function tests are not normally required in the workup of a routine bariatric candidate but may be informative, particularly if there is a question regarding pulmonary reserve in a patient with baseline chronic lung disease (previous episodes of pneumonia, long smoking history, pulmonary embolus, asthma) or obesity hypoventilation syndrome.

Normal renal changes include decreased renal blood flow with resultant decreased glomerular filtration rate and decreased creatinine clearance. Patients who present with marginal renal function should have close attention to their perioperative fluid status. Gentle hydration without large volume shifts is generally better tolerated. Any potentially nephrotoxic drugs should be discontinued prior to surgery (1).

One postoperative complication that is relatively unique to the elderly population is delirium. Delirium is defined as a "clinical syndrome in which there is an acute disruption of attention and cognition" (10). Delirium has been associated most commonly with cardiac and orthopedic procedures, but has been reported in all types of surgery. When delirium occurs postoperatively, it has been associated with increased morbidity and mortality (11). Preoperative risk factors include age, history of or current alcohol abuse, history of depression, dementia, and the presence of any metabolic derangements (11). Screening for these risk factors and correction preoperatively as necessary should be attempted.

Immobility is a problem associated with morbid obesity that can become aggravated in elderly patients. The incidence of degenerative joint disease increases with age, and many obese elderly patients may be denied corrective joint repair due to their excess weight. Their immobility, however, may limit their ability to lose weight through more conservative measures such as diet and exercise, leaving surgery as one of the few options for effective treatment. Immobility can also result in wound care issues, with the formation of decubitus ulcers. Elderly bariatric patients requiring long-term intensive care are at high risk for the development of such ulcers. For the uncomplicated postoperative patient, early ambulation is essential, which in the elderly may require assistance from physiotherapists or the nursing staff.

Outcomes of Bariatric Surgery in the Elderly

There are several studies in the literature that suggest an increased risk of mortality in the elderly after surgery. Most of these studies, however, have small sample size, include patients in their eighth and ninth decades of life, as well as those undergoing cancer operations, cardiac procedures, or semi-emergent operations (12–15). It is on the basis of such a wide range of operations that much of our outcomes data on the elderly has been gathered. Studies showing poor outcome may have created a bias that until recently prevented many elderly patients from undergoing necessary procedures. Although we are still gaining insight on the safest way to manage elderly patients, certain trends have been established. Emergency surgery is associated with higher morbidity and mortality in all age groups, but particularly in the elderly. Elderly patients often present with more advanced disease, forcing surgical therapy once complications have already occurred. Elderly patients are less likely to tolerate complications, if they occur; therefore, prevention is essential (9).

There are unfortunately few studies specifically addressing outcomes of bariatric surgery in the elderly, most being limited to retrospective reviews or nonrandomized prospective studies. Some studies combine a mixture of procedures, ranging from open procedures such as vertical banded gastroplasty, Roux-en-Y gastric bypass, and biliopancreatic diversion to laparoscopic gastric banding and laparoscopic Roux-en-Y gastric bypass, limiting their applicability.

Until recently, many bariatric centers refused surgery to patients over 50. In 1977, Printen et al. (3) reported a greater than twofold increase in mortality in patients older than 50 of 8.0%, compared with 2.8% in those younger than 50 undergoing gastric bypass procedures. This, however, was an evaluation of only 36 patients during a time when the overall mortality for gastric bypass was significantly higher than what is seen today. In contrast, MacGregor and Rand (4) in 1993 did not find a statistical difference in mortality (1.1% vs. 0.6%) in those patients aged 50 or older as compared with younger patients undergoing a variety of obesity operations. Similar findings were shown by Murr et al. (5) in 1995. A later study by Livingston et al. (16) suggested that increasing age was not associated with increased morbidity after gastric bypass. However, if a complication were to occur in this population, the incidence of mortality associated with an adverse event was threefold in older patients.

These data reinforce the concept that elderly patients may have less physiologic reserve than younger patients to overcome an adverse event. With a better understanding of bariatric medicine and refinements in minimally invasive techniques, the overall mortality and complication rates have fallen dramatically. Laparoscopic gastric bypass seems to result in less operative stress, earlier postoperative recovery, and reduced postoperative pain without a concomitant increase in morbidity or mortality (17,18). It has been suggested by Gonzalez et al. (19) that the laparoscopic gastric bypass resulted in fewer intensive care unit admissions and shorter length of hospital stay than the open technique in patients 50 years or older. Laparoscopic gastric banding has also been shown to be safe in the elderly and may prove to be another viable option for the older patient (20,21). Several other studies of nonbariatric laparoscopic procedures have shown them to be safe and effective in the elderly, including laparoscopic cholecystectomies, laparoscopic Nissen fundoplications, and laparoscopic colectomies (22–25).

An argument against performing bariatric surgery on the elderly is that it may offer limited benefits with respect to prolongation of life and provision of quality-of-life years than in the younger severely obese population. At a time when approximately 1% of individuals eligible to undergo bariatric surgery with its expected benefits are actually receiving surgical treatment, one would pose an argument in favor of continuing to target these procedures to younger patients or to elderly patients who by physiologic assessment are low risk for surgery.

Conclusion

Performing bariatric surgery in the elderly remains a controversial issue for which there are currently no standard guidelines to follow. The elderly comprise the fastest growing segment of the population in the United States. The proportion of elderly patients who will be candidates for weight reduction surgery is likely to increase over the next several decades. It is therefore an area of serious concern to all bariatric surgeons. As our understanding of geriatric physiology and our ability to identify risk factors increase, we will be better able to select the low-risk elderly patient. Careful preoperative screening is advocated in elderly patients in hopes of optimizing functional status and improving outcome. Chronologic age will probably prove to be less clinically significant than previously thought. Minimally invasive surgery techniques have revolutionized the field of bariatric surgery. As more surgeons become skilled in minimally invasive surgery techniques, the likelihood of performing safe and effective bariatric procedures in the elderly seems more promising.

References

1. Beliveau MM, Multach M. Perioperative care for the elderly patient. Med Clin North Am 2003;87:273–289.
2. Ergina P, Gold S, Meakin J. Perioperative care of the elderly patient. World J Surg 1993;17:192–198.
3. Printen KJ, Mason EE. Gastric bypass for morbid obesity in patients more than fifty years of age. Surg Gynecol Obstet 1977;144:192–194.
4. MacGregor AMC, Rand CS. Gastric surgery in morbid obesity. Outcome in patients aged 55 and older. Arch Surg 1993;128:1153–1157.
5. Murr MM, Siadati MR, Sarr MG. Results of bariatric surgery for morbid obesity in patients older than 50 years. Obes Surg 1995;5:399–402.
6. Heiat A, Vaccarino V, Krunholz HM. An evidence-based assessment of federal guidelines for overweight and obesity as they apply to elderly persons. Arch Intern Med 2001;161: 1194–1203.
7. Bender R, Jockel KH, Trautner C, et al. Effect of age on excess mortality in obesity. JAMA 1999;281:1498–1504.
8. Gastrointestinal surgery for severe obesity. National Institutes of Health Consensus Development Conference Statement. Am J Cli Nutr 1992;55:615s–619s.
9. Liu L, Leung JM. Predicting adverse postoperative outcomes in patients aged 80 years or older. J Am Geritr Soc 2000;48:405–412.

10. Marcantonio ER, Goldman L, Mangione CM, et al. A clinical prediction rule for delirium after elective non-cardiac surgery. JAMA 1994;271:134–139.
11. Marcantonio ER, Goldman L, Ovar EJ, et al. The association of intraoperative factors with the development of postoperative delirium. Am J Med 1998;105:380–384.
12. Bender J, Magnunsun T, Zenilman M et al. Outcome following colon surgery in the octogenarian. Am Surg 1996;62:276–279.
13. Keating J III. Major surgery in nursing home patients: procedures, morbidity and mortality in the frailest of the frail elderly. J Am Geriatr Soc 1992;40:8–11.
14. Adkins RJ, Scott HJ. Surgical procedures in patients aged 90 years and older. South Med J 1984;77:1357–1364.
15. Osaki T, Shirakusa T, Kodate M, et al. Surgical treatment of lung cancer in the octogenarian. Ann Thorac Surg 1994;57:188–193.
16. Livingston EH, Huerta S, Arthur D, et al. Male gender is a predictor of morbidity and age a predictor of mortality in patients undergoing gastric bypass surgery. Ann Surg 2002;236:576–582.
17. Ngyuyen NT. Systemic response after laparoscopic and open gastric bypass. J Am Coll Surg 2002;194:557–566.
18. Schauer PR, Ikramuddin S, Gourash WF, et al. Outcomes after laparoscopic Roux-en-Y gastric bypass for morbid obesity. Ann Surg 2000;232:515–529.
19. Gonzalez R, Lin E, Mattar SG, et al. Gastric bypass for morbid obesity in patients 50 years or older: laparoscopic technique safer? Am Surg 2003;69:547–553.
20. Nehoda H, Hourmont K, Sauper T, et al. Laparoscopic gastric banding in older patients. Arch Surg 2001;136:1171–1176.
21. Abu-Abeid S, Keider A, Szoid A. Resolution of chronic medical conditions after laparoscopic adjustable silicone gastric banding for the treatment of morbid obesity in the elderly. Surg Endsc 2001;15:132–134.
22. Trus TL, Laycock WS, Wo JM, et al. Laparoscopic antireflux surgery in the elderly. Am J Gastroenterol 1998;93:351–353.
23. Bammer T, Hinder RA, Klaus A, et al. Safety and long-term outcome of laparoscopic antireflux surgery in patients in their eighties and older. Surg Endosc 2002;16:40–42.
24. Law WL, Chu KW, Tung PH. Laparoscopic colorectal resection: a safe option for elderly patients. J Am Coll Surg 2002;195:768–773.
25. Bingener J, Richards ML, Schwesinger WH. Laparoscopic cholecystectomy for elderly patients: gold standard for golden years? Arch Surg 2003;138:535–536.

30
The High-Risk Bariatric Patient

Vicki March and Kim M. Pierce

With the increased incidence of obesity, there has been a concomitant rise in the number of patients referred for surgical weight loss, as well as the number of surgeons and centers offering bariatric surgery. Although surgery offers the greatest odds for durable weight loss for many of the most obese individuals, the incidence of perioperative mortality with these procedures has been reported to be as high as 1.5%, and morbidity exceeds 10% in most series.

As with all surgery, determining the size of the risk is critical, not only to guide the physician in the management of this special group of patients, but also to help these surgical candidates make informed decisions about their own care.

Well-established guidelines regarding preoperative risk stratification have led to improved surgical outcomes. These standards remain useful in the appraisal of the obese patient. Therefore, the current American College of Cardiology Foundation and the American Heart Association recommendations, along with the American Society of Anesthesia class, should be incorporated into the preoperative evaluation.

In addition, there is evidence that obesity itself is a surgical risk factor. Both the predictors of morbidity and mortality after bariatric surgery and the complications of the surgery may be unique to the morbidly obese population, that is, those with a body mass index (BMI) greater than 40. Ironically, it seems that the very population for whom bariatric surgery is indicated and beneficial may be at increased risk for having the surgery because of excessive weight.

Based on the available evidence about postoperative outcomes, this chapter characterizes the high-risk bariatric surgical patient and recommends strategies for preoperative risk reduction in the clinically severely obese patient.

Identifying the High-Risk Patient

Who is the high-risk bariatric patient? The definition is still evolving and is based on limited evidence. Only a few studies have attempted to define predictors of outcomes in morbidly obese patients for either bariatric or non-bariatric surgery. Despite a rapid increase in the number of bariatric procedures in the United States in the last 5 years and a growing body of bariatric literature, accurate preoperative risk stratification remains elusive. Risk stratification for morbidly obese patients not only provides valuable preoperative information for surgeons and patients but also provides a tool for accurate comparison of outcome data among centers (1).

Early mortality in the bariatric patient has been linked both to preoperative patient characteristics and to perioperative complications (2). Adverse events most common to bariatric surgical patients include pulmonary embolism, pneumonia, anastomotic leaks, marginal ulcers, wound dehiscence, and small bowel obstruction. The complications most predictive of early postoperative mortality (within 30 days of surgery) include pulmonary embolism and intestinal leak. Lastly, the greater the BMI preoperatively, the more likely that a patient will sustain these poor outcomes.

Known operative risks factors and recommendations that apply to the general population also should be applied to bariatric patients, including conditions that are considered contraindications to surgery. Guidelines specific to this unique population have not yet been established. The identification of the high-risk bariatric patient provides the necessary step in the development such guidelines.

Probability analysis has been used to help determine the relative contribution of individual risk factors to a patient's overall outcome after bariatric surgery (Table 30-1). Livingston and Ko (3) performed such an analysis for 1067 patients who underwent Roux-en-Y gastric bypass (RYGBP) and found an overall complication rate of 5.8%. The average patient, a 42-year-old woman who weighed 334 pounds, had a complication rate of 3.9%. On the other hand, a 62-year-old diabetic, hypertensive male smoker with sleep apnea who weighed 646 pounds and was undergoing revisional surgery had a predicted complication rate of 33.7%. These two examples emphasize

TABLE 30-1. Sensitivity analysis of preoperative risk factors predictive of adverse events

Risk factor: $C_o{}^a$	Age 1.43E^{-2}	Sex 0.48	Weight 2.08E^{-3}	Smoke 0.16	HTN 0.16	OA$^-$ 9.71E^{-2}	DM 0.31	SA 0.33	CPAP −0.27	Redo 0.55	Risk (%)
Avg. patient	42.3	F	334	N	N	N	N	N	N	N	3.9
+CPAP	42.3	F	334	N	N	N	N	N	**Y**	N	3.0
+OA	42.3	F	334	N	N	**Y**	N	N	N	N	3.5
+1 SD weight	42.3	F	**399**	N	N	N	N	N	N	N	4.4
+2 SD weight	42.3	F	**464**	N	N	N	N	N	N	N	5.0
+1 SD age	**52.1**	F	334	N	N	N	N	N	N	N	4.4
+2 SD age	**61.6**	F	334	N	N	N	N	N	N	N	5.0
+HTN	42.3	F	334	N	**Y**	N	N	N	N	N	4.5
+Smoke	42.3	F	334	**Y**	N	N	N	N	N	N	4.5
+DM	42.3	F	334	N	N	N	**Y**	N	N	N	5.2
+SA	42.3	F	334	N	N	N	N	**Y**	N	N	5.3
+Male	42.3	**M**	334	N	N	N	N	N	N	N	6.1
+Redo	42.3	F	334	N	N	N	N	N	N	**Y**	6.5
Male + factors	42.3	**M**	334	**Y**	**Y**	N	**Y**	**Y**	N	**Y**	22.7
Redo/large female	42.3	F	**464**	N	N	N	N	N	N	**Y**	8.4
Redo/large male	42.3	**M**	**464**	N	N	N	N	N	N	**Y**	12.9
Old/large + factors	61.6	**M**	**464**	**Y**	**Y**	N	**Y**	**Y**	N	**Y**	33.7

Note: The first column summarizes addition of individual or combinations of risk factors for the purposes of sensitivity analysis. The first row of numbers represents the regression equation coefficients. The last column represents the predicted risk of major complications when individual risk factors were entered into the regression equation. Risk factors denoted in boldface are those that were changed in reference to the average patient during the sensitivity analysis.
[a] Coefficient for the logistic regression equation. The intercept value (C_O) = −4.52. HTN, hypertension; OA, osteoarthritis; DM, diabetes mellitus; SA, sleep apnea; CPAP, continuous positive airway pressure.
Source: Livingston and Ko (3), with permission.

the importance of risk stratification for individual bariatric surgery patients as well as for bariatric outcomes analysis.

The operative risk of the bariatric surgical candidate may be divided into several categories: patient characteristics; medical conditions (including comorbidities) of the obese patient; and surgical factors in bariatric surgery.

Patient Characteristics

Age and Gender

As obese patients age, their risk of developing complications and other poor surgical outcomes increase. Age greater than 50 years is identified as a risk factor for postoperative complications (4). A threefold risk of mortality has been noted for patients older than 55 years in a multivariate analysis that evaluates causes of mortality associated with gastric bypass surgery (2). In a review of over 16,000 Medicare patients who underwent bariatric surgery from 1997 to 2002, Flum and colleagues (5) found higher mortality rates for patients aged 65 years or older compared with younger patients (4.8% vs. 1.7% at 30 days, 6.9% vs. 2.3% at 90 days, and 11.1% vs. 3.9% at 1 year; $p < .001$).

An increased risk of morbidity and mortality in the obese patient is also associated with male gender. Although males are usually heavier than females, male gender has been found to be an independent risk factor.

Although gender and age cannot be modified, patients in these more vulnerable groups can be educated about their increased risk prior to surgery.

Body Mass Index

A BMI greater than 50 is an independent risk factor for increased morbidity and mortality (2). It is postulated that this increased risk is due to both an increase in comorbidities and the technical difficulty of the surgery as BMI increases. Initial retrospective studies have demonstrated that preoperative weight loss of about 5% can result in technically easier operations with decreased blood loss (6) as well as shorter operative time and greater postoperative weight loss (7) compared to patients who did not lose weight prior to surgery. If presurgical weight loss is found to be beneficial in larger prospective studies, further analysis should consider the percentage of weight loss necessary to confer a risk reduction.

Sedentary Lifestyle

Most severely obese patients are deconditioned, and it has been shown that a sedentary lifestyle increases morbidity and mortality. A patient's activity history should be included in the preoperative evaluation along with an assessment of cardiovascular fitness. A clinically appropriate exercise prescription should be considered, such as walking daily for 5 to 10 minutes. Improved cardiopulmonary conditioning preoperatively may favorably affect surgical outcomes.

Tobacco

Smoking is a modifiable patient characteristic that may adversely influence outcome. While smoking is not specific to obesity, it can exacerbate the hypercoagulable state in an obese person, increase the odds of postoperative atelectasis and pneumonia, and aggravate asthma, obesity hypoventilation syndrome, and obstructive sleep apnea. Additionally, smoking has been implicated as a risk factor for marginal ulceration after gastric bypass. Therefore, patients should be counseled on smoking cessation prior to bariatric surgery.

Medical Conditions Including Comorbidities

As with all surgeries, preoperative risk stratification is dependent on determining cardiopulmonary status. However, when evaluating a patient for bariatric surgery, cardiopulmonary risk reduction is only one of several goals.

Algorithms and scoring systems have proven useful for stratifying risk and optimizing control of illnesses before, during, and after surgery. With stabilization of many chronic illnesses, operative risk can be reduced to acceptable levels.

Patients seeking bariatric surgery frequently present with comorbidities (see Table 2-1 in Chapter 2)—medical conditions that are exacerbated by, or the consequence of, obesity. These comorbidities may adversely affect outcomes. Since preventive screening is done less often in obese patients than in the normal weight population, it is often the presurgical visit where these conditions are diagnosed or found to be undertreated (8). Comorbidities that confer increased operative risk include cardiovascular disease (hypertension, congestive heart failure, cardiomyopathy, unstable angina, myocardial infarction or revascularization within 12 months, and stroke), pulmonary disease [obstructive and central sleep apnea, asthma, chronic obstructive pulmonary disease (COPD), and restrictive lung disease], hypercoagulable states (inherited, acquired, or trauma- or medication-induced), pregnancy, diabetes, renal insufficiency, liver disease [nonalcoholic steatohepatitis (NASH), and hepatic insufficiency], vasculitis, and immunodeficiencies.

Hypertension

In a multivariate analysis that examined the risk factors for mortality following bariatric surgery, hypertension was an independent risk factor (2). Hypertension was defined as a sitting blood pressure of ≥150 mm Hg systolic, or ≥90 mm Hg diastolic, or the use of antihypertensive medications.

Hypercoagulability

Postoperative pulmonary embolism has been found to be an independent risk factor for perioperative mortality in a study of 2000 bariatric patients (2). Patients undergoing bariatric surgery are at increased risk of thromboembolic events because of their obesity, the abdominal surgery, the high probability of venous stasis disease, and postoperative immobility. Other factors that contribute to the hypercoagulable condition include endothelial dysfunction secondary to the obesity itself, smoking, and erythrocytosis from either smoking or the obesity hypoventilation syndrome, and the existence of underlying hypercoagulable disorders such as hyperhomocystinemia. Preoperative patients should be carefully screened for a personal or family history of thromboembolic disorders, such as deep venous thrombosis (DVT), pulmonary embolism, or stroke. Aggressive DVT prophylaxis in the perioperative period is essential to minimize risk.

Diabetes Mellitus

Uncontrolled diabetes mellitus, either type 1 or 2, increases the risk of postoperative infection and poor wound healing. Careful screening and management of diabetes in the bariatric patient is required and is addressed in more detail in Chapter 33.

Obstructive Sleep Apnea

While often undiagnosed preoperatively, both obstructive sleep apnea and obesity hypoventilation syndrome impart significant perioperative risk. In addition to the increased prevalence of pulmonary hypertension, cardiovascular risk, and life-threatening arrhythmias seen in patients with obstructive sleep apnea, difficulty with extubation and CO_2 narcosis with an increased sensitivity to narcotics are common complications seen postoperatively in these patients. Preoperative questionnaires and sleep studies are recommended with continuous positive airway pressure (CPAP) treatment prior to and during hospitalization.

Surgical Factors

In a number of series, predictors of perioperative and post-operative death have been identified (2). It has been shown that the procedure performed influences outcome, and restrictive procedures have a lower mortality rate than gastric bypass or malabsorptive procedures (9). In a pooled analysis of 3464 laparoscopic and 2771 open gastric bypasses, there was a higher mortality rate in the open series (0.87 vs. 0.23, $p = .001$) (10). In three randomized controlled trials comparing open to laparoscopic RYGBP, however, mortality rates between the open and laparoscopic techniques were not significantly different (11–13). These studies, though, were not adequately powered to detect this relatively small difference. Patient characteristics often influence the type of surgical procedure performed. Patients with higher BMIs (higher risk patients) often undergo more invasive procedures such as RYGBP or a biliopancreatic diversion to achieve greater weight loss than they could reasonably expect with a restrictive operation. In patients with BMI greater than 65, one-stage bariatric procedures have been associated with a 38% major complication rate and 6.25% mortality rate, much higher than in most series of patients undergoing bariatric surgery (14). The risk-benefit analysis for these super-obese patients should be different from those for patients with lower BMIs, but they should not automatically be dismissed as being "too sick" for bariatric surgery. Careful planning and optimization of their medical conditions preoperatively can lead to successful outcomes in these patients with acceptable risk.

The fatty infiltration and increased liver size found in NASH has not been satisfactorily addressed in terms of mitigating preoperative risk. However, the size of the liver has implications regarding the technical aspects of the surgery. Both visualization of and access to the surgical site may be greatly diminished, thus leading to a higher conversion rate from laparoscopic procedures to open procedures, or an increased number of staged procedures and prolonged operating room time.

Surgeon volume has repeatedly been shown to impact outcomes in bariatric surgery. When assessing the patient's risk, surgeons should consider their own bariatric experience before taking on high-risk patients. For all patients undergoing bariatric surgery, mortality is significantly lower in high-volume hospitals and with high-volume surgeons (2,15).

Conclusion

If comorbid conditions and risk factors are identified, they may be modified preoperatively to reduce surgical risk. An interdisciplinary medical and surgical preoperative evaluation, which includes an extensive history, physical examination, and diagnostic studies to identify and assess existing comorbidities, is critical to modify a patient's surgical risk. Appropriate clinical management of the patient's comorbidities should occur prior to

surgery. The management of many of these medical conditions are discussed in further detail elsewhere in this book.

It is clear that the most severely obese patients who are at the highest risk of peri- and postoperative complications are also at extremely high risk of premature death because of their excessive weight. Therefore, the risk-benefit ratio of bariatric surgery must be carefully assessed on a case-by-case basis. In addition, while preparation for surgery has been established for many disease states, the standard of care for the preoperative evaluation and management of the bariatric surgical candidate is in evolution. While much that is already known about preoperative risk assessment should be applied to the bariatric patient, the rapid advances of bariatric surgery, as well as the increasing population of severely obese patients, have not been accompanied by clearly defined preoperative recommendations. As outcomes data accumulate and are analyzed from multiple institutions now performing bariatric surgery, more comprehensive recommendations can be formulated. These recommendations will provide guidance not only for bariatric surgery but also for all surgical procedures in the obese population.

References

1. Jamal MK, DeMaria EJ, Johnson JM, et al. Impact of major co-morbidities on mortality and complications after gastric bypass. Surg Obes Relat Dis 2005;1:511–516.
2. Fernandez AZ Jr, Demaria EJ, Tichansky DS, et al. Multivariate analysis of risk factors for death following gastric bypass for treatment of morbid obesity. Ann Surg 2004; 239(5):698–702; discussion 702–703.
3. Livingston EH, Ko CY. Assessing the relative contribution of individual risk factors on surgical outcome for gastric bypass surgery: a baseline probability analysis. J Surg Res 2002;105(1):48–52.
4. Nguyen NT, Rivers R, Wolfe BM. Factors associated with operative outcomes in laparoscopic gastric bypass. J Am Coll Surg 2003;197(4):548–555; discussion 555–557.
5. Flum DR, Salem L, Elrod JA, et al. Early mortality among Medicare beneficiaries undergoing bariatric surgical procedures. JAMA 2005;294(15):1903–1908.
6. Liu RC, Sabnis AA, Forsyth C, Chand B. The effects of acute preoperative weight loss on laparoscopic Roux-en-Y gastric bypass. Obes Surg 2005;15(10):1396–1402.
7. Alvarado R, Alami RS, Hsu G, et al. The impact of preoperative weight loss in patients undergoing laparoscopic Roux-en-Y gastric bypass. Obes Surg 2005;15(9):1282–1286.
8. Residori L, Garcia-Lorda P, Flancbaum L, et al. Prevalence of co-morbidities in obese patients before bariatric surgery: effect of race. Obes Surg 2003;13(3):333–340.
9. Buchwald H, Avidor Y, Braunwald E, et al. Bariatric surgery: a systematic review and meta-analysis. JAMA 2004;292(14):1724–1737.

10. Podnos YD, Jimenez JC, Wilson SE, et al. Complications after laparoscopic gastric bypass: a review of 3464 cases. Arch Surg 2003;138(9):957–961.

11. Lujan JA, Frutos MD, Hernandez Q, et al. Laparoscopic versus open gastric bypass in the treatment of morbid obesity: a randomized prospective study. Ann Surg 2004; 239(4):433–437.

12. Nguyen NT, Goldman C, Rosenquist CJ, et al. Laparoscopic versus open gastric bypass: a randomized study of outcomes, quality of life, and costs. Ann Surg 2001;234(3): 279–289; discussion 289–291.

13. Westling A, Gustavsson S. Laparoscopic vs open Roux-en-Y gastric bypass: a prospective, randomized trial. Obes Surg 2001;11(3):284–292.

14. Regan JP, Inabnet WB, Gagner M, Pomp A. Early experience with two-stage laparoscopic Roux-en-Y gastric bypass as an alternative in the super-super obese patient. Obes Surg 2003;13(6):861–864.

15. Schauer P, Ikramuddin S, Hamad G, Gourash W. The learning curve for laparoscopic Roux-en-Y gastric bypass is 100 cases. Surg Endosc 2003;17(2):212–215.

31
Gastroesophageal Reflux Disease in the Bariatric Surgery Patient

Paul A. Thodiyil, Samer G. Mattar, and Philip R. Schauer

The increasing incidence of esophageal and gastric cardia adenocarcinoma has been paralleled by the rising prevalence of obesity in the United States population. Risk factors for esophageal adenocarcinoma are high body mass index (BMI) (1–4), gastroesophageal reflux symptoms (5,6), hiatal hernia, and esophagitis (7).

Higher BMI is associated with a number of factors that predispose to gastroesophageal reflux and complicate its therapy. Furthermore, weight loss surgery substantially alters the surgical anatomy of the foregut so as to make conventional antireflux fundoplication procedures unusable. For example, a gastric pouch or a sleeve gastrectomy precludes creation of a gastric pressure transmitting fundal wrap.

Definition and Presentation

Gastroesophageal reflux disease is a condition characterized by pathologic acidification of the esophagus. This may be symptomatic or asymptomatic and erosive or nonerosive. Typical reflux symptoms include heartburn, regurgitation, chest pain, and dysphagia, while atypical symptoms include hoarseness, wheezing or asthma, cough, and sinus discharge. Nonerosive reflux disease (NERD) affects about 5% of patients, and they are a more challenging group to treat in terms of symptom resolution.

Epidemiology and Risk Factors

The prevalence of morbid obesity in the United States has increased at epidemic proportions (8), with about 66% of adults overweight and an additional 32% obese (BMI > 30) (9). Obesity carries the significant risk of the development of multiple diseases. Gastroesophageal reflux disease (GERD) is a common comorbidity that symptomatically affects about 58% of morbidly obese

individuals and is proven objectively in 21% (10). The Bristol Helicobacter project (11), a cross-sectional population-based study of 10,537 subjects aged 20 to 59 years, showed that a BMI > 30 confers an adjusted odds ratio of 1.8 of experiencing at least weekly symptoms of reflux (11), while the Olmsted County cross-sectional population-based study of 1524 subjects aged 25 to 76 years showed that a BMI > 30 conferred an adjusted odds ratio of 2.8 of experiencing reflux symptoms (12). In study of 65 patients with BMI > 35, heartburn and regurgitation were found respectively in 79% and 66%, with erosive esophagitis (49%), short columnar epithelium (18%), and Barrett's metaplasia in 9% (13). This study, however, did not show any significant association between the degree of obesity and esophageal lesions. However, others have shown a significant association between degree of obesity and the frequency of endoscopic esophagitis [odds ratio (OR), 1.8; 95% confidence interval (CI), 1.4–2.1) (14). Others have shown greater severity of GERD in those with higher BMI, accompanied by higher pH scores in the more obese, but with no differences in lower esophageal sphincter (LES) length or pressure (15). Notably, LES pressure and abdominal length were significantly higher in subjects with a BMI over 50 compared to those with a BMI between 35 and 39.9, but with no differences in 24-hour pH monitoring between these two groups (13). These observations would be consistent with the known contribution of raised intraabdominal pressure in the etiology of GERD in the obese subject (15).

Obesity is a significant independent risk factor for hiatal hernia and is significantly associated with esophagitis, attributable in part to the higher incidence of hiatal hernia in this population (14). Excessive body weight significantly increases the probability of a hiatal hernia with increasing BMI ($p < .01$).

There are, however, a number of studies suggesting a lack of association between morbid obesity and GERD (16–18). While heartburn and acid regurgitation is reported respectively in 37% and 28% in subjects with

BMI > 35, neither weight, BMI, nor the waist-hip ratio were significantly correlated with any of the reflux variables in a 24-hour pH study when compared to an age- and sex-matched control (16). This lack of association is said to be limited to morbidly obese males, unlike females where estrogenization is thought to increase risk of GERD (17).

Pathophysiology of Gastroesophageal Reflux Disease in Morbid Obesity

Raised intraabdominal pressures coupled with an increased frequency of hiatal hernias appears to contribute to the problem of GERD in the morbidly obese.

Increased Intraabdominal Pressure

Obesity disrupts the barrier to gastroesophageal reflux in subjects with a structurally intact lower esophageal sphincter mechanism (15). The principal mechanism for this appears to be a rise in intraabdominal pressure (Fig. 31-1). In-vitro studies have confirmed the crucial importance of LES length and pressure in maintaining antireflux competency in the face of intraabdominal pressure, with higher pressures placing higher demands on the LES in terms of length and pressures in maintaining competency (Fig. 31-2) (19). This is confirmed by an in-vivo study demonstrating the higher gastroesophageal pressure gradient in the obese subject (20). Several studies have confirmed raised intraabdominal pressure in the morbidly obese, and have further shown its significant association with some of the comorbidities of obesity, including GERD (21–23). Urinary bladder pressure, a reliable indicator of intraabdominal pressure, is higher in the obese than the nonobese (18 ± 0.7 vs. 7 ± 1.6 cm H_2O, $p < .001$) and also rises with BMI (22) (Fig. 31-3) with a strong correlation (24). Intraabdominal pressure falls fol-

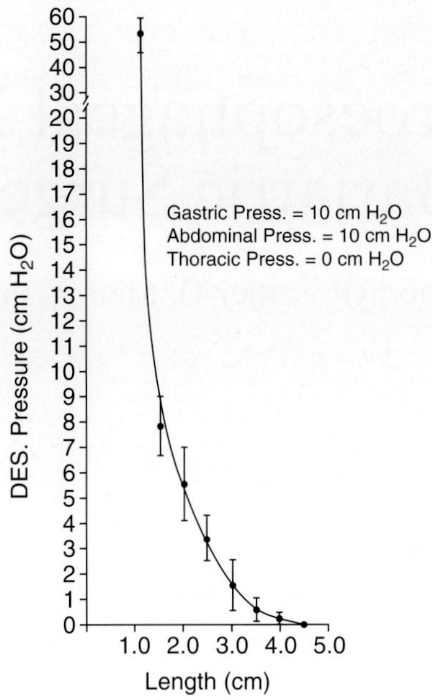

FIGURE 31-2. Relationship between LES pressure and length to competency of the intraabdominal esophagus.

lowing weight loss surgery and is of relevance to therapy (Fig. 31-4).

Hiatal Hernia

Lower esophageal sphincter disruption by hiatal hernias occurs in as many as 13% of subjects with twice the ideal body weight (25). However, a more recent study by the same group showed that the prevalence of hiatal hernia in patients with BMI > 35 (22% of 201 patients) is similar to that of a group of asymptomatic volunteers (27% of 56) (26). The relevance of this observation is not clear and remains to be validated in a cross-sectional population-based study. The presence of a hiatal hernia has pre-

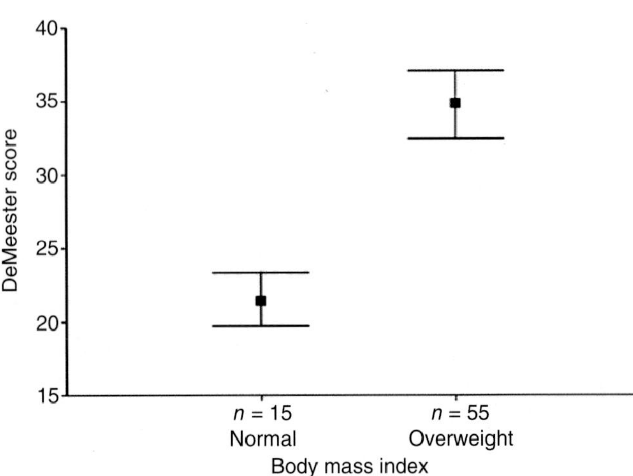

FIGURE 31-1. Elevated body mass disrupts the reflux barrier in subjects with an intact lower esophageal sphincter (LES).

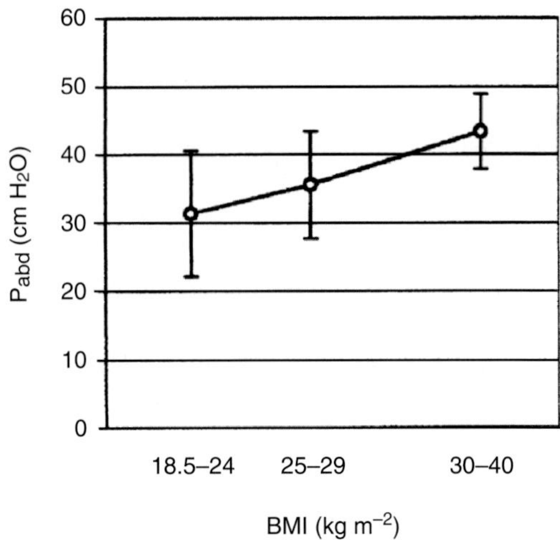

FIGURE 31-3. Abdominal pressure in BMI groups ($r = 0.52$, $p < .01$).

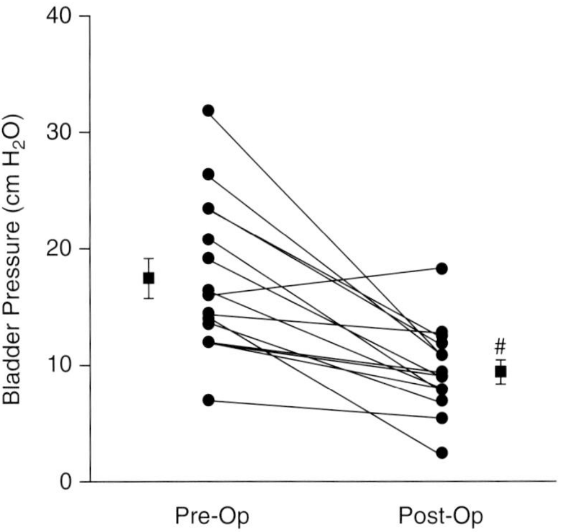

FIGURE 31-4. Urinary bladder pressure before and 1 year after weight loss surgery. *$p < .001$.

viously been shown to be the strongest predictor of esophagitis (27–29).

Esophageal Transit Time

Esophageal body pump function, as measured by peak velocity, is also adversely affected by raised afterload created by elevated intraabdominal pressures in the obese. Radionuclide esophageal transit study shows significantly elevated transit time in obese patients with gastroesophageal reflux compared to lean subjects with or without reflux with LES manometry showing prolonged transit was related to elevated gastroesophageal pressure gradient (Fig. 31-5), with the latter caused by increased intraabdominal pressure (30). Prolonged transit time

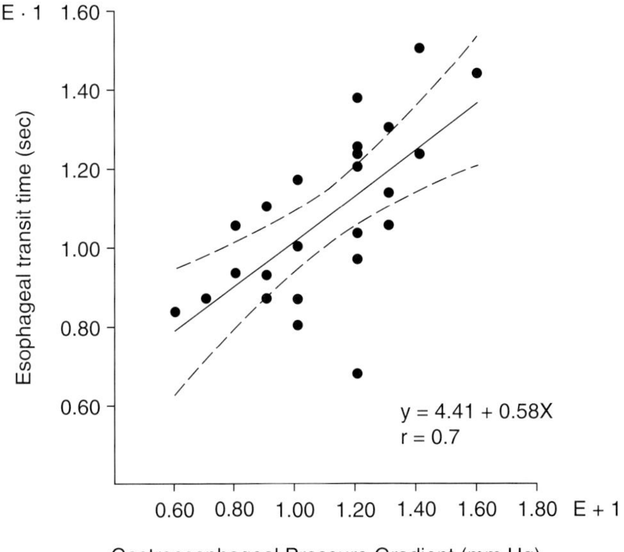

FIGURE 31-5. Effect of esophageal pressure gradient on esophageal transit time.

means delayed esophageal clearance of acid and consequent injury to the mucosa.

Clinical Presentation

Heartburn and regurgitation are present in over 70% of obese subjects with twice the ideal body weight [25], with nocturnal aspiration or globus in 4%. About 55% of morbidly obese patients have some GERD symptoms. Among those with chronic GERD, symptoms included heartburn (87%), water brash (18%), wheezing (40%), laryngitis (17%), and aspiration (14%) (31).

Hiatal hernias (13%) and low LES pressures (50%) were found in one series of 55 morbidly obese patients (25). In patients with BMI >50 and without hiatal hernias, LES pressure and intraabdominal lengths are significantly higher than normal controls (13).

Diagnosis

Diagnosis of GERD is made on the basis of history and physical examination supplemented by upper gastrointestinal endoscopy and selective use of esophageal manometry and 24-hour ambulatory pH study (32). A composite score (DeMeester score) of more than 14.8 or a percentage time pH below 4 and greater than 4% confirms pathologic esophageal acidification.

Esophageal impedance studies are useful in determining acid exposure and clearance times (33–35) and are particularly useful in the 60% of patients with non–acid reflux who are not detected with pH monitoring. Multiple biopsies from the gastroesophageal junction and cardia are valuable in assessing mucosal injury including Barrett's metaplasia. In considering surgical treatment of GERD, it is essential to establish the presence or absence of dysplasia, as in such cases an antireflux procedure may have to be supplemented with resection or close endoscopic surveillance (36). A 24-hour pH study is also strongly recommended, as a normal study should prompt a search for an alternative diagnosis (36,37). A video esophagogram is helpful in identifying an irreducible hiatal hernia. An irreducible hiatal hernia larger than 5 cm suggests esophageal shortening and serves as a warning sign of a high likelihood of failure of the antireflux procedure. Such a situation would call for extensive esophageal mobilization through a thoracic access, supplemented if necessary with a Collis gastroplasty and creation of a transthoracic Nissen or Belsey fundoplication (38).

Treatment Options

Standard surgical treatment for GERD consists of hiatal reconstruction and fundoplication. In the general population, a Nissen fundoplication carries a 93% actuarial success rate at 96 months (39). Obesity adversely affects long-term outcomes after Nissen fundoplication, with recurrent GERD in 31% of 224 patients at a mean 37-month follow-up (40), compared to 4.5% in the nonobese group. Furthermore, a fundoplication addresses only one of the several comorbidities present.

The pathophysiology of GERD in the morbidly obese suggests that therapy for GERD in this group should include the following elements:

1. Improve esophageal transit by reducing gastroesophageal pressure gradient. This is most effectively achieved by reducing weight.
2. Repair structural defects of the LES caused by hiatal hernias.

Weight loss of 5% to 10% can be achieved with dietary and lifestyle strategies. Weight loss surgery, whether gastric bypass, adjustable gastric banding, or biliopancreatic diversion, is the only proven treatment modality that causes a significant weight loss of more than 50% excess body weight that is sustained in 65% of patients for over 10 years (10,41–43).

Gastric bypass effectively reduces GERD symptoms, with data at 1 year showing complete relief of GERD symptoms, accompanied by a significant decreases in urinary bladder pressure (17 ± 2 to $10 \pm 1\,cm\,H_2O$), weight (140 ± 8 to $87 \pm 6\,kg$, $69\% \pm 4\%$ excess weight loss), and BMI (52 ± 3 to 33 ± 2) (44). Laparoscopic Roux-en-Y gastric bypass (RYGBP) results in a significant decrease in heartburn (from 87% to 22%, $p < .001$), water brash (from 18% to 7%, $p < .05$), wheezing (from 40% to 5%, $p < .001$), laryngitis (from 17% to 7%, $p < .05$), and aspiration (from 14% to 2%, $p < .01$) (31), and is accompanied by improvement in physical and mental function as recorded by the Short Form (SF-36) and patient satisfaction in 97%. The postoperative use of acid suppressants also decreases significantly for proton pump inhibitors (from 44% to 9%, $p < .001$) and H2 blockers (from 60% to 10%, $p < .01$) (31).

There are very few studies reporting on the management of hiatal hernias in association with RYGBP. The addition of an anterior crural repair with a posterior gastropexy to the RYGBP has been shown in one study to improve the Visick class from a preoperative class IV to a postoperative class I or II in 94% of 121 patients (45). Here, anterior crural repair and a gastropexy with interrupted silk or braided nylon sutures to anchor the gastroesophageal junction below the diaphragm was combined with an RYGBP (45).

This impressive improvement in symptoms is not seen in the subgroup of morbidly obese patients with GERD symptoms who have acid reflux proven by 24-hour pH monitoring. In patients with pH-proven GERD undergoing RYGBP, 42% remained symptomatic and on antisecretory medication at 13 months after RYGBP despite an average weight loss equivalent to 18.6 BMI units. Only 41% of the 19 patients in this study achieved normalization of DeMeester scores. Gastric pouch mucosa was Congo red positive in 84% of patients with biopsies confirming the presence of parietal cells in 89% of patients. Gastric pouch length did not influence GERD symptoms, pH scores, or the presence of parietal cells (46). Surprisingly, the well-recognized correlation between reflux symptoms and DeMeester score was absent in this postoperative group, with no relation between postoperative GERD symptoms and postoperative DeMeester scores (46).

Laparoscopic gastric banding is also effective in treating GERD in the morbidly obese, including atypical manifestations such as asthma where significant improvement in asthma scores occurs in all patients (47). It corrects the pH abnormality and LES resting pressure (48). At 6 months postoperatively, there is a significant impairment of LES relaxation (from 16% to 42%) and deterioration of esophageal transport (in preoperatively 23% to 47% postoperatively) with dilatation of the esophagus in 28% (12 of 43) of patients. Although increased outflow resistance is caused by the band, the band did not cause dysphagia or necessitate a reoperation (48). Outcomes in centers performing fewer gastric bands are poor (49), with pouch dilatation associated with increased esophageal acid exposure (50).

There is little data on the effect of malabsorptive procedures such as biliopancreatic diversion (BPD) on acid reflux in the morbidly obese (51). Both BPD alone or with a duodenal switch effectively diverts bile (52) and may exert a beneficial effect on GERD through its effect on weight loss.

Prognosis

Roux-en-Y gastric bypass and adjustable gastric banding are effective treatment options for treatment of gastroesophageal reflux symptoms in morbidly obese patients. However, GERD outcomes are less satisfactory in the subgroup of patients with pH-proven acid reflux. These patients continue to suffer GERD symptoms despite weight loss surgery and constitute a difficult group to treat. About 2% have persistent reflux symptoms after gastric banding (48). The value of malabsorptive procedures in morbidly obese patients with GERD remains unproven.

References

1. Chow WH, et al. Body mass index and risk of adenocarcinomas of the esophagus and gastric cardia. J Natl Cancer Inst 1998;90:150–155.
2. Lagergren J, Bergstrom R, Adami HO, Nyren O. Association between body mass and adenocarcinoma of the esophagus and gastric cardia. Ann Intern Med 2000;130:883–890.

3. Wu AH, Wan P, Bernstein L. A multiethnic population-based study of smoking, alcohol and body size and risk of adenocarcinomas of the stomach and esophagus (United States). Cancer Causes Control 2001;12:721–732.

4. Vaughan TL, Davis S, Kristal A, Thomas DB. Obesity, alcohol, and tobacco as risk factors for cancers of the esophagus and gastric cardia: adenocarcinoma versus squamous cell carcinoma. Cancer Epidemiol Biomarkers Prev 1995;4:85–92.

5. Lagergren J, Bergstrom R, Lindgren A, Nyren O. Symptomatic gastroesophageal reflux as a risk factor for esophageal adenocarcinoma. N Engl J Med 1999;340:825–831.

6. Shaheen N, Ransohoff DF. Gastroesophageal reflux, Barrett esophagus, and esophageal cancer: scientific review. JAMA 2002;287:1972–1981.

7. Chow WH, et al. The relation of gastroesophageal reflux disease and its treatment to adenocarcinomas of the esophagus and gastric cardia. JAMA 1995;274:474–477.

8. Kuczmarski RJ, Flegal KM, Campbell SM, Johnson CL. Increasing prevalence of overweight among US adults. The National Health and Nutrition Examination Surveys, 1960 to 1991. JAMA 1994;272:205–211.

9. Ogden CL, Carroll MD, Curtin LR, McDowell MA, Tabak CJ, Flegal KM. Prevalence of overweight and obesity in the United States, 1999–2004. JAMA 2006;295(13)1549–1555.

10. Schauer PR, Ikramuddin S, Gourash W, Ramanathan R, Luketich J. Outcomes after laparoscopic Roux-en-Y gastric bypass for morbid obesity. Ann Surg 2000;232:515–529.

11. Murray L, et al. Relationship between body mass and gastro-oesophageal reflux symptoms: The Bristol Helicobacter Project. Int J Epidemiol 2003;32:645–650.

12. Locke GR 3rd, Talley NJ, Fett SL, Zinsmeister AR, Melton LJ 3rd. Risk factors associated with symptoms of gastroesophageal reflux. Am J Med 1999;106:642–649.

13. Csendes A, Burdiles P, Rojas J, Burgos A, Henriquez A. [Pathological gastroesophageal reflux in patients with severe, morbid and hyper obesity]. Rev Med Chil 2001;129:1038–1043.

14. Wilson LJ, Ma W, Hirschowitz BI. Association of obesity with hiatal hernia and esophagitis. Am J Gastroenterol 1999;94:2840–2844.

15. Wajed SA, Streets CG, Bremner CG, DeMeester TR. Elevated body mass disrupts the barrier to gastroesophageal reflux. Arch Surg 2001;136:1014–1018; discussion 1018–1019.

16. Lundell L, Ruth M, Sandberg N, Bove-Nielsen M. Does massive obesity promote abnormal gastroesophageal reflux? Dig Dis Sci 1995;40:1632–1635.

17. Nilsson M, Lundegardh G, Carling L, Ye W, Lagergren J. Body mass and reflux oesophagitis: an oestrogen-dependent association? Scand J Gastroenterol 2002;37:626–630.

18. Lagergren J, Bergstrom R, Nyren O. No relation between body mass and gastro-oesophageal reflux symptoms in a Swedish population based study. Gut 2000;47:26–29.

19. DeMeester TR, Wernly JA, Bryant GH, Little AG, Skinner DB. Clinical and in vitro analysis of determinants of gastroesophageal competence. A study of the principles of antireflux surgery. Am J Surg 1979;137:39–46.

20. Mercer CD, Wren SF, DaCosta LR, Beck IT. Lower esophageal sphincter pressure and gastroesophageal pressure gradients in excessively obese patients. J Med 1987;18:135–146.

21. Sugerman H, Windsor A, Bessos M, Wolfe L. Intra-abdominal pressure, sagittal abdominal diameter and obesity comorbidity. J Intern Med 1997;241:71–79.

22. McIntosh S, et al. Relationship of abdominal pressure and body mass index in men with LUTS. Neurourol Urodyn 2003;22:602–605.

23. Sanchez NC, et al. What is normal intra-abdominal pressure? Am Surg 2001;67:243–248.

24. Noblett KL, Jensen JK, Ostergard DR. The relationship of body mass index to intra-abdominal pressure as measured by multichannel cystometry. Int Urogynecol J Pelvic Floor Dysfunct 1997;8:323–326.

25. Hagen J, Deitel M, Khanna RK, Ilves R. Gastroesophageal reflux in the massively obese. Int Surg 1987;72:1–3.

26. Hamoui N, Hagen JA, Tamhankar AP, Anthone G, Crookes P. In: Digestive Diseases Week. New Orleans, 2004.

27. Jones MP, et al. Hiatal hernia size is the dominant determinant of esophagitis presence and severity in gastroesophageal reflux disease. Am J Gastroenterol 2001;96:1711–1717.

28. Fein M, et al. Role of the lower esophageal sphincter and hiatal hernia in the pathogenesis of gastroesophageal reflux disease. J Gastrointest Surg 1999;3:405–410.

29. Kahrilas PJ, Lin S, Chen J, Manka M. The effect of hiatus hernia on gastro-oesophageal junction pressure. Gut 1999;44:476–482.

30. Mercer CD, Rue C, Hanelin L, Hill LD. Effect of obesity on esophageal transit. Am J Surg 1985;149:177–181.

31. Frezza EE, et al. Symptomatic improvement in gastroesophageal reflux disease (GERD) following laparoscopic Roux-en-Y gastric bypass. Surg Endosc 2002;16:1027–1031.

32. American Gastroenterological Association. Medical position statement: guidelines on the use of esophageal pH recording. Gastroenterology 1996;110:1981.

33. Kahrilas PJ. Will impedance testing rewrite the book on GERD? Gastroenterology 2001;120:1862–1864.

34. Balaji NS, Blom D, DeMeester TR, Peters JH. Redefining gastroesophageal reflux (GER). Surg Endosc 2003;17:1380–1385.

35. Sifrim D, Castell D, Dent J, Kahrilas PJ. Gastro-oesophageal reflux monitoring: review and consensus report on detection and definitions of acid, non-acid, and gas reflux. Gut 2004;53:1024–1031.

36. Guidelines for surgical treatment of gastroesophageal reflux disease (GERD). Society of American Gastrointestinal Endoscopic Surgeons (SAGES). Surg Endosc 1998;12:186–188.

37. Klingman RR, Stein HJ, DeMeester TR. The current management of gastroesophageal reflux. Adv Surg 1991;24:259–291.

38. Kauer WK, et al. A tailored approach to antireflux surgery. J Thorac Cardiovasc Surg 1995;110:141–146; discussion 146–147.

39. Bremner RM, et al. The effect of symptoms and nonspecific motility abnormalities on outcomes of surgical therapy for gastroesophageal reflux disease. J Thorac Cardiovasc Surg 1994;107:1244–1249; discussion 1249–1250.

40. Perez AR, Moncure AC, Rattner DW. Obesity adversely affects the outcome of antireflux operations. Surg Endosc 2001;15:986–989.

41. MacLean LD, Rhode BM, Sampalis J, Forse RA. Results of the surgical treatment of obesity. Am J Surg 1993;165:155–160; discussion 160–162.

42. Hall JC, et al. Gastric surgery for morbid obesity. The Adelaide Study. Ann Surg 1990;211:419–427.

43. Mason EE, Printen KJ, Blommers TJ, Scott DH. Gastric bypass for obesity after ten years experience. Int J Obes 1978;2:197–206.

44. Sugerman H, et al. Effects of surgically induced weight loss on urinary bladder pressure, sagittal abdominal diameter and obesity co-morbidity. Int J Obes Relat Metab Disord 1998;22:230–235.

45. Smith SC, Edwards CB, Goodman GN. Symptomatic and clinical improvement in morbidly obese patients with gastroesophageal reflux disease following Roux-en-Y gastric bypass. Obes Surg 1997;7:479–484.

46. Schauer P-R, et al. Objective evidence of persistent acid reflux after Roux-en-Y gastric bypass for morbid obesity. Digestive Disease Week Abstracts and Itinerary Planner 2003, abstract No. 2003.

47. Dixon JB, Chapman L, O'Brien P. Marked improvement in asthma after Lap-Band surgery for morbid obesity. Obes Surg 1999;9:385–389.

48. Weiss HG, et al. Treatment of morbid obesity with laparoscopic adjustable gastric banding affects esophageal motility. Am J Surg 2000;180:479–482.

49. DeMaria EJ, et al. High failure rate after laparoscopic adjustable silicone gastric banding for treatment of morbid obesity. Ann Surg 2001;233:809–818.

50. Iovino P, et al. Abnormal esophageal acid exposure is common in morbidly obese patients and improves after a successful Lap-band system implantation. Surg Endosc 2002;16:1631–1635.

51. Scopinaro N, et al. Biliopancreatic diversion. World J Surg 1998;22:936–946.

52. Welch NT, et al. Effect of duodenal switch procedure on gastric acid production, intragastric pH, gastric emptying, and gastrointestinal hormones. Am J Surg 1992;163:37–44; discussion 44–45.

32
Gallbladder Disease in the Bariatric Surgery Patient

Carol A. McCloskey and Giselle Hamad

Obesity, a major nutrition-related health problem in the United States, is a well-known risk factor for the development of cholesterol gallstones. The reported incidence of biliary tract disease in the morbidly obese varies from 28% to 45.2% (1–3), three to four times greater than in the general population (4).

Cholesterol gallstones occur when bile becomes supersaturated, which occurs when there is a relative excess of cholesterol or an insufficiency of bile salts (5). Analysis of gallbladder bile in morbidly obese patients has demonstrated increased biliary cholesterol saturation, secondary to increased cholesterol excretion from the liver, while the secretion rate of bile salt remains unchanged (1). There is a linear correlation between body weight and cholesterol secretion into bile (6). This supersaturation of bile with cholesterol is a major predisposition to cholesterol stone formation, and the presence of stones enhances the propensity to gallbladder inflammation. Therefore, acute and chronic cholecystitis are much more common in obese persons (4). Even in the absence of stones, ultrasonographically normal gallbladders removed from obese patients were noted to have a high proportion of mucosal abnormalities (7). The most frequent abnormality was cholesterolosis (37%), followed by chronic cholecystitis with cholesterolosis (18%). In a study by Amaral and Thompson (8), 46% of patients had cholesterolosis. The frequency of gallstones in patients with cholesterolosis was 18.2%. The frequency of cholesterolosis in patients with gallstones was 50%. While some studies have suggested that cholesterolosis is a precursor to the development of cholelithiasis or cholecystitis (9), the link remains unclear and the indications for removal of a gallbladder with cholesterolosis remain debatable.

Other identified risk factors for the development of cholesterol gallstones include rapid weight loss, dietary, genetic and ethnic influences, ileal disease, and increased alcohol use (10). Weight loss is associated with a reduction in the bile salt pool. However, cholesterol secretion is reduced to a lesser degree than bile salt secretion, pos-

sibly due to increased mobilization of adipose tissue. This results in a bile composition that favors cholesterolosis and stone formation (6,11). Gallbladder contractility is also decreased, possibly secondary to diminished sensitivity to cholecystokinin. Impaired emptying of the gallbladder also predisposes these patients to gallstone formation (12).

Therefore, morbidly obese patients who undergo surgery for weight reduction are at additional risk for gallstone formation (Table 32-1). Shiffman et al. (13) observed that 49% of patients developed sludge or stones after gastric bypass, 95% of which developed within 6 months after surgery. Wattchow et al. (3) reported a 33% incidence during 4 to 27 months of follow-up, and found that patients with gallstones had greater early weight loss than those who did not form stones. In a study by Amaral and Thompson (8), cholecystectomy was required in 28.7% of patients within 3 years of Roux-en-Y gastric bypass (RYGBP). The indications for postoperative cholecystectomy in these patients were acute cholecystitis, gallstone pancreatitis, and choledocholithiasis. However, a study by O'Brien and Dixon (14) has demonstrated that the incidence of cholecystectomy after laparoscopic adjustable gastric banding surgery was not different from the expected rate for the nonsurgical obese population. They suggest that other mechanisms, such as the malabsorption associated with gastric bypass, may play a role in stone formation. The increased risk of gallbladder disease in morbidly obese patients who undergo procedures for surgical weight loss has appropriately raised the issue of performing routine prophylactic cholecystectomy regardless of the presence of cholelithiasis or symptoms. In contemplating simultaneous cholecystectomy with gastric bypass, there are multiple factors to be considered. These include increased operative time, technical difficulties secondary to hepatomegaly or anomalous biliary/arterial anatomy, and possible increased perioperative morbidity of an additional procedure. In addition, some argue that certain patients will never go

TABLE 32-1. The incidence of postoperative biliary disease following gastric bypass surgery

Author	Postoperative incidence of biliary disease (%)	Period of follow-up (months)
Knecht et al. (2)	13.8	6–24
Amaral et al. (8)	28.7	36
Wattchow et al. (3)	33.0	4–27
Schmidt et al. (15)	40	6
Schiffman et al. (13)	5.0	24

on to develop gallstones, or may develop gallstones that are not symptomatic, and therefore should not be subjected to an unnecessary procedure. Conversely, those in favor of simultaneous cholecystectomy cite the risk of morbidity from subsequent gallbladder disease as well as the additional expense of a second surgery if not performed simultaneously.

Combined gastric bypass and prophylactic cholecystectomy have been advocated for open bariatric procedures by several studies. Schmidt et al. (15) performed a retrospective study to evaluate the preoperative and postoperative incidence of cholelithiasis in 218 patients who underwent open RYGBP. Thirty percent of patients had clinically detectable gallbladder disease before or at the time of surgery. The authors found that 40% went on to develop cholelithiasis and/or required cholecystectomy by 24 months postoperatively, leading to their recommendation of prophylactic cholecystectomy at the time of bariatric surgery. Likewise, a study by Amaral and Thompson (8) reported that cholecystectomy was required in 28.7% of patients who underwent open RYGBP within 3 years following surgery, and they therefore recommended routine cholecystectomy at the time of surgery. Fobi et al. (16) reviewed the records of their patients who underwent prophylactic cholecystectomy (regardless of preoperative ultrasound results) at the time of transected Silastic ring vertical RYGBP; 23% had prior cholecystectomy, 20% had gallstones at the time of surgery, and 324 of 429 patients with negative preoperative ultrasound had pathologic evidence of disease. Therefore, only 14% of patients had no evidence of gallbladder pathology at the time of surgery. The authors concluded that the incidence of gallbladder disease despite negative preoperative findings is high enough to warrant routine cholecystectomy at the time of weight loss surgery.

In light of the potential risks of a combined procedure, many surgeons have adopted a selective approach, attempting to identify those patients at highest risk for subsequent biliary disease. However, the criteria for a selective approach vary widely among surgeons. Some surgeons who perform a selective approach base their decision on the presence of gallstones diagnosed by preoperative abdominal ultrasound. Others select the patients based solely on the presence of symptoms, or intraoperative evidence of disease, such as palpable stones, cholesterolosis, chronic inflammation, or even intraoperative ultrasound. Sugerman et al. (17) reported performing simultaneous cholecystectomy only if stones or sludge was noted by intraoperative ultrasound. Jones (18) based his approach from 1983 to 1986 on cholelithiasis and cholesterolosis, with a 13% second operation for biliary disease postoperatively. From 1986 to 1993, he added a strong family history of biliary disease and clinical evidence of chronic cholecystitis at the time of surgery to the criteria, and his reoperation rate for biliary disease during the second time period decreased to 9%. This demonstrates the importance of careful selection criteria for the identification and treatment of those with the highest risk for postoperative biliary disease.

Hamad et al. (19) were the first to report outcomes for selective laparoscopic cholecystectomy during laparoscopic gastric bypass (LGBP). All patients who had gallstones on routine preoperative ultrasound examination underwent simultaneous cholecystectomy at the time of LGBP. Simultaneous cholecystectomy was safe and feasible because it neither affected conversion rates to laparotomy nor increased the incidence of biliary-related complications. However, it did significantly increase operating time and hospital stay.

An important issue in adopting a selective approach is the reliability of the diagnosis of cholelithiasis in morbidly obese patients. Amaral and Thompson (8) reported that only 14.9% percent of patients who had normal preoperative ultrasound examinations had normal gallbladders on gross and microscopic pathologic examination following gastric exclusion surgery. The sensitivity of ultrasonographic examination of the gallbladder in detecting gallstones in this study was only 63%, compared with the previously reported sensitivity of 92% in the general population (20,21). The high false-negative rate was attributed to the poor quality of ultrasonograms obtained through a large adipose mass. Seinage et al. (22) found that preoperative ultrasonography or cholescintigraphy was inaccurate at reliably predicting the patients who would benefit from cholecystectomy. They also concluded that intraoperative findings other than palpable gallstones were unreliable.

In contrast, Oria (23) addressed the issue of false-negative sonographic findings in morbid obesity. He retrospectively compared radiology results, surgical findings, and pathology reports in 5257 patients and found discrepancy in only 1.1% of cases. He therefore concluded that ultrasound results are accurate in the setting of experienced sonographers or radiologists, stating that false-negative results are commonly caused by soft stones, microlithiasis, polypoid cholesterolosis, or hydrops, and that nonvisualization is usually due to technical problems, not the patient's size.

An alternative to cholecystectomy at the time of bariatric surgery for patients without gallstones is the utilization of bile salt therapy (ursodiol) to prevent gallstone formation during the phase of rapid postoperative weight loss. In a multicenter, placebo-controlled, randomized clinical trial, 233 patients without gallstones by intraoperative ultrasound were begun on ursodiol within 10 days of RYGBP, and treated for 6 months. The authors found that gallstone formation was significantly decreased from 32% to 2% in patients receiving 600 mg and 6% in patients receiving 1200 mg compared with placebo controls (17). In this study, the recommended length of treatment was 6 months to correspond with the period of most rapid weight loss, but the optimal length of treatment is not conclusive. There is a lack of information on long-term usage of ursodiol, although few adverse drug reactions have been reported. A second study found that ursodiol therapy was not efficacious; however, this was attributed to a poor compliance rate of 28% (24).

Given the increase in the prevalence and severity of obesity, the increased use of bariatric surgery for weight reduction, as well as the conversion from an open to laparoscopic approach, the concept of routine cholecystectomy in patients undergoing bariatric surgery remains an ongoing controversy. Overall, analysis of the bariatric literature is hampered by the fact that various procedures done both open and laparoscopically are difficult to compare. In addition, the patient populations vary in sex, age, and initial body mass index.

To assess the current standard of practice, Mason and Renquist (25) collected data from participants in the 28th report of the International Bariatric Surgery Registry as well as from members of the American Society for Bariatric Surgery. Overall, they reported an increase in concurrent cholecystectomy during the last 15 years. When extensive bypass procedures were performed (distal RYGBP or biliopancreatic diversion with a duodenal switch) all patients were reported to have undergone cholecystectomy. However, only 30% of surgeons performing RYGBP remove normal appearing gallbladders, while a majority have adopted a selective approach. Ursodiol is used to prevent gallstone formation in one third of patients when a normal-appearing gallbladder is left in place. However, both prophylactic cholecystectomy and selective cholecystectomy continue to fall within the current standard of care as dictated by current practice.

In conclusion, the prevalence of morbid obesity in developed countries continues to steadily increase, and weight reduction surgery is now sought with increased frequency in those patients who fail nonsurgical management. Obesity as well as rapid weight loss places this population at significantly increased risk for biliary disease. There is ongoing debate over routine versus selective cholecystectomy. Both approaches are acceptable, and the decision often depends on the type of surgery performed, careful selection criteria, and reliable diagnostic tools. Further studies on preventive therapies with drugs such as ursodiol may also provide a useful adjunct to the selective approach. It is hoped that the increased number of surgeries now performed for morbid obesity will provide additional insight into this continuing controversy. In the meantime, it is essential for each bariatric surgeon to develop a protocol for the diagnosis and management of gallstones in this patient population as part of the routine assessment and plan.

References

1. Mabee TM, Meyer P, DenBesten L, et al. The mechanism of increased gallstone formation in obese human subjects. Surgery 1976;79(4):460–468.
2. Knecht BH. Experience with gastric bypass for massive obesity. Am Surg 1978;44(8):496–504.
3. Wattchow DA, Hall JC, Whiting MJ, et al. Prevalence and treatment of gallstones after gastric bypass surgery for morbid obesity. Br Med J (Clin Res Ed) 1983;286(6367):763.
4. Friedman GD, Kannel WB, Dawber TR. The epidemiology of gallbladder disease: observations in the Framingham Study. J Chronic Dis 1966;19(3):273–292.
5. Carey MC, Small DM. The physical chemistry of cholesterol solubility in bile. Relationship to gallstone formation and dissolution in man. J Clin Invest 1978;61(4):998–1026.
6. Bennion LJ, Grundy SM. Effects of obesity and caloric intake on biliary lipid metabolism in man. J Clin Invest 1975;56(4):996–1011.
7. Csendes A, Burdiles P, Smok, et al. Histologic findings of gallbladder mucosa in 87 patients with morbid obesity without gallstones compared to 87 control subjects. J Gastrointest Surg 2003;7(4):547–551.
8. Amaral JF, Thompson WR. Gallbladder disease in the morbidly obese. Am J Surg 1985;149(4):551–557.
9. Acalovschi M, Dumitrascu D, Grigorescu M, et al. Pathogenetic interrelations between cholesterolosis and cholesterol gallstone disease. Med Interne 1983;21(3):175–179.
10. Scragg RK, McMichael AJ, Baghurst PA. Diet, alcohol, and relative weight in gall stone disease: a case-control study. Br Med J (Clin Res Ed) 1984;288(6424):1113–1119.
11. Schlierf G, Schellenberg B, Stiehl A, et al. Biliary cholesterol saturation and weight reduction—effects of fasting and low calorie diet. Digestion 1981;21(1):44–49.
12. Liddle RA, Goldstein RB, Saxton J. Gallstone formation during weight-reduction dieting. Arch Intern Med 1989;149(8):1750–1753.
13. Shiffman ML, Sugerman HJ, Kellum JM, et al. Gallstone formation after rapid weight loss: a prospective study in patients undergoing gastric bypass surgery for treatment of morbid obesity. Am J Gastroenterol 1991;86:1000–1005.
14. O'Brien PE, Dixon JB. A rational approach to cholelithiasis in bariatric surgery. Arch Surg 2003;138:908–912.
15. Schmidt JH, Hocking MP, Rout WR, et al. The case for prophylactic cholecystectomy concomitant with gastric restriction for morbid obesity. Am Surg 1988;54(5):269–272.

16. Fobi M, Lee H, Igwe D, Felahy B, et al. Prophylactic chole-cystectomy with gastric bypass operation: incidence of gall-bladder disease. Obes Surg 2002;12(3):350–353.
17. Sugerman HJ, Brewer WH, Shiffman ML, et al. A multi-center, placebo-controlled, randomized, double-blind, pro-spective trial of prophylactic ursodiol for the prevention of gallstone formation following gastric-bypass-induced rapid weight loss. Am J Surg 1995;169(1):91–96.
18. Jones KB, Jr. Simultaneous cholecystectomy: to be or not to be. Obes Surg 1995;5(1):52–54.
19. Hamad GG, Ikramuddin S, Gourash WF, et al. Elective cholecystectomy during laparoscopic Roux-en-Y gastric bypass: is it worth the wait? Obes Surg 2003;13:76–81.
20. Cooperberg PL, Burhenne HJ. Real-time ultrasonography. Diagnostic technique of choice in calculous gallbladder disease. N Engl J Med 1980;302(23):1277–1279.
21. Lee JK, Melson GL, Koehler RE, et al. Cholecystosonog-raphy: accuracy, pitfalls and unusual findings. Am J Surg 1980;139(2):223–228.
22. Seinige UL, Sataloff DM, Lieber CP, et al. Gallbladder disease in the morbidly obese patient. Obes Surg 1991;1(1):51–56.
23. Oria HE. Pitfalls in the diagnosis of gallbladder disease in clinically severe obesity. Obes Surg 1998;8(4):444–451.
24. Wudel LJ Jr, Wright JK, Debelak JP, et al. Prevention of gallstone formation in morbidly obese patients undergoing rapid weight loss: results of a randomized controlled pilot study. J Surg Res 2002;102(1):50–56.
25. Mason EE, Renquist KE. Gallbladder management in obesity surgery. Obes Surg 2002;12(2):222–229.

33
Diabetes in the Bariatric Surgery Patient

Panduranga Yenumula, Carolina Gomes Goncalves,
Stacy A. Brethauer, Sangeeta Kashyap, and Philip R. Schauer

Incidence

According to the recently updated National Diabetes Statistics Fact Sheet, an estimated 18.2 million people, or approximately 6.3% of the United States population, have diabetes. Of those, 13 million are diagnosed with overt diabetes and 5.2 million are undiagnosed. Each year, approximately 1.3 million persons aged 20 years or older are diagnosed with the disease.

Obesity and type 2 diabetes mellitus (T2DM) are two of the most common chronic, debilitating diseases of Western society, and both have experienced an alarming growth in the last few decades. Indeed, the close association of the two metabolic disorders has led to the coined term "diabesity." Thirty-four percent of the U.S. adult population is overweight [body mass index (BMI) 25 to 29.9], and another 32% is obese (BMI > 30) (1). The prevalence of obesity has increased by more than 75% since 1980 (2). In the U.S. there are 800,000 new cases of diabetes per year (almost all are type 2), and almost 8% of the adult population and 19% of the population older than the age of 65 years have diabetes (3). The understanding that obesity is a central feature and an etiologic factor in the pathophysiologic development of T2DM is well established (4). There is no medical cure for T2DM, and despite treatment with antidiabetic medication, the natural course of the disease is characterized by progression to microvascular and macrovascular complications, which include neuropathy, nephropathy, erectile dysfunction, retinopathy, and accelerated atherosclerotic cardiovascular disease (5). Type 2 diabetes mellitus in the U.S. is the most common cause of blindness, renal failure, and amputation, and up to 70% of diabetic patients die of cardiovascular disease (5,6). The cost of treating diabetes and its complications in the U.S. is estimated to be $100 billion per year (7).

Diagnosis

The diagnosis of diabetes mellitus is based on three criteria: (1) a fasting plasma glucose equal to or greater than 126 mg/dL, (2) a random plasma glucose equal to or greater than 200 mg/dL together with classic symptoms of diabetes mellitus (polyuria, polydipsia, unexplained weight loss), or (3) a 2-hour plasma glucose of 200 mg/dL or greater following a 75-g glucose load. A random elevation must be repeated with a separate test on a different day, if possible, to confirm the diagnosis (8,9).

Those individuals whose blood glucose is intermediate between normal and diabetic range have impaired fasting glucose (IFG), which is a fasting plasma glucose ≥100 mg/dL but <126 mg/dL, and impaired glucose tolerance (IGT), which is a 2-hour plasma glucose of ≥140 mg/dL but <200 mg/dL. Both IFG and IGT are not specific clinical entities but represent risk factors for the future development of diabetes and cardiovascular disease (8,9). However, both IFG and IGT individuals are characterized by the presence of insulin resistance and the predisposition to an increased risk for atherosclerotic cardiovascular disease.

Type 1 Diabetes Mellitus

Type 1 diabetes is caused by loss of insulin secretion caused by progressive destruction of the pancreatic β cells (10). It is again divided into two types. Type 1A is an autoimmune disease characterized by cellular antibodies that may form against islet cells (islet cell antibodies, ICAs), insulin (insulin autoantibodies antibodies, IAAs), and glutamic acid decarboxylase$_{65}$ (GAD$_{65}$). These antibodies gradually destroy endogenous insulin production until the patient becomes metabolically unstable. Type 1B is an idiopathic, nonautoimmune disease state with loss of β-cell function (11). Type 1 patients demonstrate hyperglycemia and weight loss, and are prone to ketoacidosis. This acute metabolic syndrome requires prompt treatment with exogenous insulin and fluid resuscitation. The mortality rate increases if the acidotic state is not promptly reversed. Following stabilization, continuous exogenous insulin therapy is required to replace the endogenous insulin deficit.

Insulin deficiency is the primary metabolic defect in type 1 diabetes; however, several studies suggest that a majority of patients with diabetes of long duration are characterized by varying degrees of insulin resistance (12–18). Insulin resistance is strongly related to abdominal fat. In type 1 diabetes, the administration of exogenous insulin can produce relative systemic hyperinsulinemia, which may contribute to abdominal fat deposition. It has been shown that insulin increases the activity of 11β-hydroxysteroid dehydrogenase, which enhances the differentiation of adipose stromal cells to adipocytes from omental fat, but not subcutaneous fat, and this constant exposure of glucocorticoid in the omental adipose tissue can promote abdominal obesity (19,20).

Type 2 Diabetes Mellitus

Type 2 diabetes is a complex metabolic disorder that results from coexisting defects at multiple organ sites that progress over many years. Comprehension of these complexities allows a better use of the currently available therapeutic modalities by clinicians. The Third Report of the National Cholesterol Education Program Expert Panel on Detection, Evaluation, and Treatment of High Blood Cholesterol in Adults (ATP III) defined a cluster of closely associated metabolic abnormalities, or the metabolic syndrome, as an individual meeting three or more of the following criteria:

1. Abdominal obesity: waist circumference >102 cm in men and >88 cm in women
2. Hypertriglyceridemia: >150 mg/dL
3. Low high-density lipoprotein (HDL) cholesterol: <40 mg/dL in men and <50 mg/dL in women
4. High blood pressure: >130/85 mm Hg
5. High fasting glucose: >110 mg/dL

Insulin resistance is believed to be an underlying feature of metabolic syndrome. Recent studies demonstrate that dietary modifications and enhanced physical activity, including the use of metformin, may delay or prevent the transition from impaired glucose tolerance to type 2 diabetes mellitus (21).

Type 2 diabetes is a complex, chronic metabolic disease that results from defects in both insulin secretion and insulin action. The hallmarks of type 2 diabetes are fasting and postprandial hyperglycemia. This hyperglycemia results from complex interplay between insulin resistance and relatively decreased pancreatic insulin secretion. An elevated rate of basal hepatic glucose production in the presence of hyperinsulinemia is the primary cause of fasting hyperglycemia; after a meal, impaired suppression of hepatic glucose production by insulin and decreased insulin-mediated glucose uptake by muscle contribute almost equally to postprandial hyperglycemia. In patients with type 2 diabetes and established fasting hyperglycemia, the rate of basal hepatic glucose production is excessive, despite two- to fourfold increased plasma insulin concentrations. These findings provide evidence for hepatic resistance to insulin, and these data are substantiated by an impaired ability of insulin to suppress hepatic glucose production.

Insulin resistance is also demonstrated in the muscles where higher concentrations of insulin are required to allow glucose to enter the cells. The presence of insulin resistance predicts the development of type 2 diabetes and can be detected in normal first-degree relatives of patients with diabetes. Insulin resistance results in compensatory hyperinsulinemia to maintain normal glucose tolerance in obese individuals. However, with progressive impairment in insulin secretion there is deterioration of blood glucose levels leading to overt diabetes.

The risk for development of type 2 diabetes is positively correlated with BMI, and this disease is 20 times more likely to develop in persons with BMI 35.0 or greater (22). Therefore, a modest weight loss of 10% in overweight and obese persons results in significant health benefits by reducing various comorbid conditions such as glucose intolerance, non–insulin-dependent diabetes mellitus, hypertension, and dyslipidemia (23,24). Diet and exercise therapy have been the fundamental cornerstones for the initial treatment of T2DM and have been shown to reduce the incidence of T2DM by 58% (25).

Medical Versus Surgical Management of the Obese T2DM Patient

Given the complexity of the pathophysiology of type 2 diabetes, medical therapy is targeted in a multimodal fashion to ameliorate the metabolic derangements that result in T2DM. Therefore, the best medical strategy should be based on effective reduction of weight coupled with drug therapy targeting insulin resistance (metformin, thiazoledinediones) and restoration of B-cell function with thiazoledinediones and stimulation of incretin hormones (exenatide). In obese diabetic patients microvascular disease is principally related to the presence of hyperglycemia; consequently, tight glycemic control is fundamental. The aims for glycemic control include preprandial glucose of 90 to 130 mg/dL, bedtime glucose of 110 to 150 mg/dL, and hemoglobin A_{1c} (HbA$_{1c}$) of less than 7% (9). Figure 33-1 delineates the standard

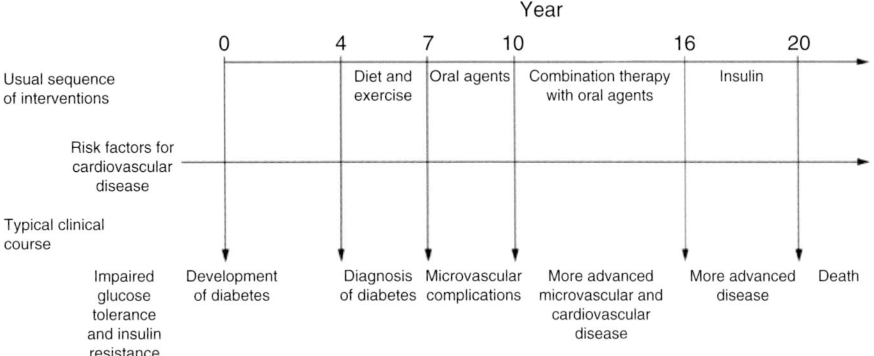

FIGURE 33-1. The typical clinical course of type 2 diabetes, including the progression of glycemia and the development of complications, and the usual sequence of interventions. [Nathan (5), with permission. Copyright 2004 Massachusetts Medical Society. All rights reserved.]

of care management of type 2 diabetes, featuring a stepwise increase in pharmacotherapy from oral agents to insulin as the disease progresses from microvascular complications to end-organ failure. The 2006 American Diabetes Association's (ADA) position on bariatric surgery for the treatment of T2DM is that "gastric bypass or gastroplasty may be appropriate and may allow significant improvement in glycemic control with reduction or discontinuation of medication." This is the first time that bariatric surgery has received recognition in the ADA guidelines as a treatment option for DM. Despite ample evidence of the therapeutic benefit of bariatric surgery in treating T2DM, there still remains a curious reluctance from medical specialists to recommend bariatric surgery for their severely obese type 2 diabetic patients (26).

Two randomized studies (United Kingdom Prospective Diabetes Study, UKPDS, and Diabetes Control and Complications Trial, DCCT) (27,28) demonstrated that tight glycemic control with medication decreased the risk of microvascular complications associated with diabetes. These studies reported that for every drop of 1% in HbA_{1c} there was a relative risk reduction of 25% to 45%. However, in some patients, the insulin dose to achieve glycemic control ($HbA_{1c} \leq 7\%$) was as high as 100 units per day. Furthermore, in community settings where more than 95% of T2DM patients are treated, HbA_{1c} levels vary from 8.5% to 9%, demonstrating that tight control with medication is difficult to accomplish (27).

Physical activity improves insulin sensitivity, independent of weight loss, and thus plays an important role in the achievement of glycemic control in the obese diabetic patient (29). Diet and exercise usually needs supplementation with oral pharmacotherapy to maintain glycemic control. Oral agents address two of the main defects in T2DM, insulin resistance and β-cell dysfunction (30). Because of the progressive β-cell dysfunction in T2DM, eventually the insulin secretory capacity is not enough to overcome the insulin resistance, and a state of relative insulin resistance develops. Therefore, when other therapeutic measures fail, insulin therapy becomes necessary (31).

Weight control is a key component of diabetes management. However, despite good success in the short term, most obese patients are unable to achieve long-term weight control with conventional treatment even with the addition of pharmacologic therapy (32).

Table 33-1 summarizes the results of studies using non-surgical weight loss approaches in patients with obesity but not morbid obesity (BMI generally <35) (33–40). Only two studies promoted sustained weight loss (beyond 1 year) (34,36), and the other studies demonstrated modest weight loss (3 to 5 kg or 2 to 3 BMI units). Despite the improvement in blood glucose, the mean HbA_{1c} remained above 7% in most series. Shi et al. (40) demonstrated a mean HbA_{1c} lower than 7%; however, the patients studied were newly diagnosed T2DM and had lower mean HbA_{1c} starting levels (7.3%).

In the severely obese patient (BMI > 40), diet, behavior modification, and drug therapy are often unsuccessful in the long term. The recidivism rate for diet therapy is close to 100% at 5 years (41,42). Furthermore, sibutramine and orlistat have limited weight reduction, and are not acceptable treatment for severely obese patients who need to lose a larger amount of weight and maintain the weight loss (43).

Bariatric surgery has proven to promote significant and long-lasting weight loss, glycemic control, and resolution of obesity-related comorbidities in the severely obese patients. Within 2 years of gastric bypass, nearly two thirds of excess body weight is lost and most of this weight loss is maintained for up to 14 years (44). Schauer et al. (45) have demonstrated successful glycemic control and restoration of HbA_{1c} levels after laparoscopic Roux-en-Y gastric bypass (LRYGBP), with morbidity and mortality of 13.6% and 0.5%, respectively.

TABLE 33-1. Outcomes of medical weight loss on type 2 diabetes mellitus

Study	n	Time	Rx	T2DM severity	Pre-Rx Wt or BMI	Post-Rx Wt or BMI	Pre-Rx HbA$_{1c}$	Post-Rx HbA$_{1c}$	Pre-FPG	Post-FPG	Post-Rx Anti-DM change
Uusitupa (33)	86	1 yr	Controlled meal diet plan	DC-T2DM	91 kg	86 kg	8.4%	6.6%	7.6 mmol/L	6.2 mmol/L	N/A
Agurs-Collins et al. (38)	64	6 mo	Fen-Phen† and diet counseling	OA or I-T2DM	93 kg	90 kg	11%	9.9%	N/A	N/A	N/A
Pan et al. (34)	577	6 yr	Diet and exercise counseling	IFG	29 BMI	27 BMI	N/A	N/A	5.9 mmol/L	7.6 mmol/L	OA added to patients with T2DM
Redmon et al. (35)	44	1 yr	Diet and exercise counseling	OA or I-T2DM	37 BMI	33.6 BMI	8.3%	7.6%	175 mg/dL	137 mg/dL	Reduced OA usage
Metz et al. (37)	119	1 yr	VLCD or VLCD and exercise	DC or OA-T2DM	33 BMI	32 BMI	8.7%	8.5%	10.7 mmol/L	9.96 mmol/L	N/A
Paisey et al. (36)	45	5 yr	Diet and exercise counseling	OA or I-T2DM	36 BMI	33 BMI	N/A	N/A	13* mmol/L	14* mmol/L	N/A
Halpern et al. (39)	280	6 mo	Orlistat and diet or placebo and diet	DC or OA-T2DM	89.5 kg / 89.7 kg	84.8 kg / 86.7 kg	8.4% / 8.5%	7.8% / 8.3%	11.05 mmol/L / 11.50 mmol/L	10.05 mmol/L / 11.49 mmol/L	N/A
Shi et al. (40)	249	6 mo	Orlistat and diet or placebo and diet	DC-T2DM	78.7 kg / 79.4 kg	73.3 kg / 77 kg	7.3% / 7.3%	6.8% / 6.4%	8.0 mmol/L / 8.1 mmol/L	6.7 mmol/L / 7.6 mmol/L	N/A

* Not a fasting plasma glucose 2 hours postprandially.
† FenPhen, fenfluramine and phentermine used with diet to induce weight loss.
Fasting plasma glucose: 125 mg/dL or 7.0 mmol/L is considered indicative of T2DM.
Anti-DM, antidiabetic medications; DC, diet controlled; I, insulin; N/A, not available; OA oral agent; Rx, treatment; VLCD, very low calorie diet.
Source: Modified from Schauer et al. (45), with permission from Lippincott Williams & Wilkins.

Antidiabetic Effect of Bariatric Surgery

At present, bariatric surgery is the only therapeutic modality proven to produce long-term weight loss and reduce associated comorbidity in morbidly obese patients (46). One of the dramatic effects of various types of bariatric surgery, including Roux-en-Y gastric bypass (RYGBP), biliopancreatic diversion/duodenal switch, and gastric band, is the amelioration or resolution of type 2 diabetes mellitus, which is traditionally regarded as a progressive, unrelenting disease.

In five published studies examining a total of 3685 people undergoing RYGBP, diabetic patients experienced complete remission of their disease at rates ranging from 82% to 98%, with most studies demonstrating resolution in approximately 83% of cases (44,45,47–50).

In a study published by Schauer et al., (45) 1160 morbidly obese patients underwent LRYGBP, and 240 (21%) preoperatively were known to have IFG or T2DM. Follow-up information was obtained in 191 of 240 patients (80%). Following gastric bypass surgery, fasting plasma glucose and glycosylated hemoglobin concentrations returned to normal levels (83%) or markedly improved (17%) in all patients. A significant reduction in the use of oral antidiabetic agents (80%) and insulin (79%) followed surgical treatment. Patients with the shortest duration (<5 years), the mildest form of T2DM (diet controlled), and the greatest weight loss after surgery were most likely to achieve complete resolution of T2DM. Therefore, it was concluded that LRYGBP resulted in significant weight loss (60% of excess body weight loss) and resolution (83%) of T2DM. Furthermore, early surgical intervention in morbidly obese patients with T2DM (duration ≤5 years) results in a higher resolution rate (95%) compared to patients with T2DM for 6 to 10 years (75%) or more than 10 years (54%) ($p < .001$).

The reversal of impaired glucose tolerance without frank T2DM was nearly universal. Patients whose DM remitted were able to discontinue all diabetic medications and manifest normal fasting glucose and glycosylated hemoglobin levels. In a longitudinal study of obese people with impaired glucose tolerance followed for approximately 5.5 years, bariatric surgery lowered the rate of progression to T2DM by more than 30-fold (51).

Recent studies demonstrated significant improvement in T2DM after major types of bariatric operations, including vertical banded gastroplasty, laparoscopic adjustable silicone gastric banding (LAGB), RYGBP, and biliopancreatic diversion (Table 33-2) (45,47,48,50,52–58). Direct comparison of these studies is problematic because they are quite variable in terms of the distribution of severity of T2DM within the study population (e.g., % IFG vs. diet-controlled T2DM vs. oral agent T2DM vs. insulin T2DM) and methodology of evaluating improvement by biochemical or clinical assessment.

Buchwald et al. (58), in a meta-analysis (Table 33-2), summarized the effects on diabetes mellitus of all types of obesity surgery. When defined as the ability to discontinue all diabetes-related medications and maintain blood glucose levels within the normal range, strong evidence for improvement in type 2 diabetes and impaired glucose tolerance was found across all the surgery types. Within studies reporting resolution of diabetes, 1417 (76.8% [meta-analytic mean, 76.8%; 95% confidence interval (CI), 70.7–82.9%]) of 1846 patients experienced complete resolution. Within studies reporting both resolution and improvement or only improvement of diabetes, 414 (85.4% [meta-analytic mean, 86.0%; 95% CI, 78.4–93.7%]) of 485 patients experienced resolution or improvement of diabetes.

There was a difference in diabetes outcomes analyzed according to the four categories of operative procedures. With respect to diabetes resolution, there was a gradation of effect from 98.9% (95% CI, 96.8–100%) for biliopancreatic diversion or duodenal switch to 83.7% (95% CI, 77.3–90.1%) for gastric bypass to 71.6% (95% CI, 55.1–88.2%) for gastroplasty, and to 47.9% (95% CI, 29.1–66.7%) for gastric banding. The percentage of patients with diabetes resolved or improved showed different results; this variation from the trend solely for diabetes resolved may be due to the far greater number of patients assessed for this variable ($n = 1846$) compared with the number assessed for the combined variable ($n = 485$) in the total population (58).

Torquati et al. (50), in a recent study, also showed significant resolution of T2DM (74% of patients) and interestingly demonstrated that peripheral fat distribution (smaller waist circumference) and absence of insulin treatment were independent and significant predictors of complete resolution of T2DM.

There are several mechanisms to explain the beneficial effect of bariatric surgery on amelioration of T2DM. Weight loss from surgery is associated with dramatic improvements in insulin sensitivity, and this may lessen the burden on the pancreas to restore insulin secretion. Weight loss is also associated with improvement in glucose ("glucotoxicity") and lipid levels (e.g., free fatty acids, adipokines), which can also restore B-cell function and improve insulin resistance. Indeed, patients who have lost substantial weight after surgery display increased levels of an adipocyte-derived hormone known as adiponectin (which increases muscle insulin sensitivity) and muscle insulin-receptor concentration, as well as reductions in intramyocellular lipids and fatty acyl-coenzyme A (molecules that are known to cause insulin resistance from "lipotoxicity") (59–61). As predicted, insulin sensitivity, measured by minimal modeling, is increased approximately four- to fivefold after RYGBP-induced weight loss (59,61). The beneficial effects of RYGBP on diabetes mellitus (DM), however, cannot be accounted for by weight loss alone. Perhaps the most

TABLE 33-2. Effects of surgical weight loss on type 2 diabetes mellitus

Study	Procedure	n	Weight (BMI, kg, or %IBW)	% pts with T2DM	T2DM severity (IFG, T2DM, DC, OA, IU)	F/U (years)	%EWL T2DM pts All pts	Preop vs. postop FPG	Preop vs. postop HbA$_{1c}$	Resolved, improved, or unchanged
Pasquali.et al. (52)	VBG	52	46	N/A	N/A	15 mo	T2DM = N/A All = 46 kg lost	6.4 vs. 5.5 mmol/L	N/A	N/A
SOS Study (53) (1999, 2000)	70% VBG 24% RYGBP 6% RYGBP	1029	42	19%	N/A	2	RYGB = 33% EWL VBG = 23% EWL GB = 21% EWL	N/A	N/A	R = 46% I/U = N/A
Dixon and O'Brien (54)	LAGB	500	48	11%	67 IFG 51 DC 4 IU	1	T2DM = 38% All = 47%	6.2 mmol/L	7.8 vs. 6.2	R = 64% I = 26% U = 10%
Pontiroli et al. (55)	LAGB	143	45	47% IFG 19% T2DM	47 IGF 19 T2DM	3	T2DM = N/A All = BMI 45 to 37	6.2 vs. 5.4 mmol/L	6.3 vs. 5.3	R = 80% I/U = N/A
Pories et al. (44)	RYGBP	608	134 kg	27%	165 IFG 165 DC/OA	10	T2DM = N/A All = 54% @ 10 yr	117 mg/dL	12.3 vs. 6.6	R = 89% I = 7% U = 4%
Schauer et al. (45)	LRYGBP	1160	50.4	20%	14 IFG 32 DC 93 OA 52 IU	4	T2DM = 60% All = N/A	180 vs. 98 mg/dL	8.2 vs. 5.6	R = 83% I = 17%
Wittgrove and Clark (48)	LRYGBP	500	N/A	17%	50 IFG 46 DC 30 OA 9 IU	5	T2DM = 72% All = 82%	N/A	N/A	R = 98% I = 2%
Sugerman et al. (47)	LRYGBP RYGBP	1025	51	15%	40 DC 114 OA/I	1–10	T2DM = N/A All = 66%	N/A	N/A	R = 86%
Marceau et al. (56)	BPD/DS	465	47	15%	72 T2DM	4	T2DM = N/A BPD = 61% DS = 73%	N/A	N/A	R = 96% I = 2.5% U = 1.5%
Scopinaro et al. (57)	BPD	2241	117% IBW	8%	275 IFG 137 OA 39 IU	1–21	T2DM = N/A All = 75%	NL postop	N/A	R = 100%
Buchwald et al. (58)	VBG LABG BPD/DS RYGB	22094	47	N/A	N/A	N/A	T2DM = 57.25% RYGB = 61% VBG = 68% GB = 47.5% BPD/DS = 70.1%	N/A	N/A	R = 77% I = 86%
Torquati et al. (50)	LRYGBP	117		100%	117 T2DM	1	RYGB = 69% EWL	NA	7.7 vs. 6.0	R = 74% I = 26%

BPD, biliopancreatic diversion; DC, diet controlled; DS, BPD with duodenal switch; I, improved; IU, insulin user; LAGB, laparoscopic adjustable gastric banding; LRYGBP, laparoscopic Roux-en-Y gastric bypass; OA, oral agents; R, resolved; RYGBP, open Roux-en-Y gastric bypass; U, unchanged; VBG, vertical banded gastroplasty; %EWL, percent excess weight loss; N/A, not available; %IBW, percent of ideal body weight; PTS, patients; NL, normal.
Source: Modified from Schauer et al. (45), with permission from Lippincott Williams & Wilkins.

impressive observation is that previously diabetic patients typically discontinue all of their DM medications at the time of discharge from the hospital after RYGBP (~1 week), long before major weight loss has occurred (62).

Other mechanisms for rapid recovery from diabetes include negative caloric balance. Patients consume very little food in the immediate postoperative period, so their pancreatic β cells are not challenged. Alleviation of DM with starvation is well described. By the time they begin to eat reasonably normally at home, they are losing weight and in a state of negative energy balance, a condition that improves glucose tolerance. Eventually, amelioration of DM can be accounted for by the well-known effect of weight loss to increase insulin sensitivity, thereby decreasing glucotoxicity and lipotoxicity and improving β-cell function.

Another important mechanism that may act in concert with weight loss is favorable alterations in gut hormone release, which improve insulin secretion or action. Ghrelin ("hunger hormone"), which decreases after the RYGBP, exerts several diabetogenic effects. Exogenous injections of ghrelin in humans increase levels of growth hormone (GH), cortisol, and epinephrine, three of the four classical counterregulatory hormones (63). Ghrelin administration also suppresses insulin levels in humans, even in the face of ghrelin-induced hyperglycemia (64). Finally, ghrelin directly antagonizes insulin-mediated intracellular signaling events pertaining to glucose metabolism in cultured hepatocytes (65). Thus, at least at pharmacologic doses, ghrelin hinders insulin secretion and action, and chronic administration of ghrelin receptor agonists impairs glucose tolerance in human (66). If these effects are physiologic and ghrelin acts as an anti-incretin to limit peripheral glucose utilization in the fasting and preprandial state, then suppression of ghrelin levels could enhance glucose disposal. Decreased ghrelin levels also account for the preservation of weight loss in the bariatric population. Many forms of medical weight loss including cancer cachexia are characterized by increased ghrelin levels, which can stimulate weight gain.

An important mediator of the antidiabetic effects of RYGBP is glucagon-like peptide-1 (GLP-1). Glucose-dependent insulinotropic peptide (GIP) and GLP-1 are the classic incretins that stimulate insulin secretion in response to enteral nutrients. Furthermore, GLP-1 exerts proliferative and antiapoptotic effects on pancreatic β cells (67). It may also improve insulin sensitivity, at least indirectly (68). Accordingly, methods to enhance GLP-1 signaling show great promise for the treatment of T2DM (63). Moreover, GLP-1 inhibits gastric emptying and can decrease food intake (69). GLP-1 is secreted primarily by the hindgut after food ingestion, and part of this response results from direct contact between enteral nutrients and the intestinal L cells that produce GLP-1. After RYGBP,

ingested nutrients reach the hindgut more readily, bypassing part of the foregut. The larger postprandial bolus of nutrients in the hindgut should increase GLP-1 levels after RYGBP. Several studies of jejunoileal bypass (JIB), which also expedites nutrient delivery to the hindgut, show increased GLP-1 levels after surgery, both within the first year and as late as 20 years postoperatively (70–72). Biliopancreatic diversion creates a similar shortcut to the ileum; this operation also increases hormone secretion from L cells and is at least as effective as RYGBP at ameliorating T2DM (73). A recent study evaluated the gut hormonal responses after RYGBP. At 1, 3, and 6 months after operation, progressively increasing GLP-1 responses were observed (74). Le Roux et al. (75) also demonstrated increased postprandial plasma GLP-1 in patients following RYGBP.

The secretion of other hindgut hormones, if similarly enhanced after RYGBP, could also contribute to the effects of this procedure on glucose homeostasis and energy balance. Recently, peptide YY_{3-36} (PYY) was shown to decrease food intake in humans and body weight in rodents (76,77); PYY is primarily a hindgut hormone, and its levels, especially postprandial, increase after RYGBP (74,75), an effect that might contribute to weight loss. Fasting and postprandial PYY levels do increase after other surgeries that expedite nutrient delivery to the hindgut, including extensive small bowel resection (78) 9 months and 20 years postoperatively (70,72).

Role of the Foregut and Hindgut in the Effects of Gastric Bypass on Diabetes Resolution

Although all bariatric operations promote weight loss and improve glucose homeostasis, gastric bypass and biliopancreatic diversion (BPD) are the fastest and most effective procedures for both end points (45,79,80). Both operations cause durable remissions of DM in more than 80% of cases, typically within a few days after surgery (46,79,80,81). Because these two procedures exclude the intestinal foregut from digestive continuity, whereas other bariatric operations do not, it has been hypothesized that bypass of this hormonally active region is an important determinant of the effects of bariatric surgery (79). As mentioned above, suppression or constraint of ghrelin secretion from the bypassed foregut is one mechanism to explain some of the effects of RYGBP on weight loss and glucose homeostasis. To integrate ghrelin data into the foregut hypothesis, one would predict that standard BPD, which leaves the ghrelin-rich gastric fundus in digestive continuity, would not significantly impair ghrelin secretion, whereas the duodenal switch, in which most ghrelin-producing tissue is either resected or bypassed, would suppress ghrelin levels.

Using Goto-Kakizaki rats, a spontaneous, nonobese model of T2DM, Rubino and Marescaux (82) provided additional data supporting the foregut hypothesis and isolated the effects of RYGBP that are related to exclusion of the duodenum and proximal jejunum from those related to gastric restriction and bypass. The most interesting finding in this study was that gastrojejunal bypass (GJB) rats showed significant improvement in glucose tolerance compared with sham-operated controls, despite equivalent body weights in the two groups. The GJB resulted in better glycemic control than did either rosiglitazone therapy or substantial weight loss from food restriction. The implication of these findings is that bypass of the intestinal foregut and the early arrival of a meal in the terminal ileum (e.g., as accomplished by RYGBP and BPD) can ameliorate T2DM independently of weight loss, through mechanisms that remain unclear. The authors hypothesize that there are alterations in gut hormones, but candidate molecules are not obvious. The incretin hormone glucose-dependent insulinotropic peptide (GIP), produced primarily by the foregut, is stimulated by ingested nutrients and promotes insulin secretion. Bypass of the foregut theoretically should decrease GIP levels, and there is little consensus on the actual effect of intestinal bypass operations on this hormone; various reports claim decreased postoperative levels (83,84).

An alternative mechanism, called the hindgut hypothesis, claims that the expedited delivery of ingested nutrients to the hindgut promotes weight loss by accentuating the ileal brake. In this phenomenon, the presence of nutrients in the ileum suppresses gastrointestinal motility, gastric emptying, small intestinal transit, and, thus, food intake. Neural mechanisms are implicated in this response, as well as hormones, including PYY, GLP-1, neurotensin, and enteroglucagon—all of which are increased in response to meals or at baseline after JIB (70–73,85,86); PYY and GLP-1 have also demonstrated increased levels after RYGBP (74,75). Enteroglucagon, a marker of secretion from the intestinal L cells that produce GLP-1, is also increased after RYGBP and BPD (81–87). As detailed previously, enhanced GLP-1 secretion from facilitated delivery of nutrients to the hindgut could plausibly account for some of the antidiabetic effects of RYGBP, JIB, and BPD. In support of the hindgut hypothesis are intriguing rodent experiments in which a portion of the ileum was resected and inserted into the mid-duodenum (88). Without creating any restrictive or malabsorptive physiology, such ileal interpositions caused major weight loss, possibly by placing the hormone-rich ileum in close contact with ingested nutrients and enhancing the ileal brake. Consistent with this mechanism, ileal interposition increases levels of PYY, GLP-1, and enteroglucagon, and it delays gastric motility and emptying (88–90).

The various mechanisms mediating weight loss and improved glucose tolerance after bariatric surgery may be summarized as following: (1) gastric restriction, causing early satiety, small meal size; (2) bypass of the foregut, impairing ghrelin secretion via unknown mechanisms, and causing mild malabsorption in the case of long-limb variations only; and (3) increased rate of delivery of nutrients to the hindgut, enhancing the ileal brake, and stimulating the release of PYY and GLP-1, which may decrease food intake and increase insulin secretion via the incretin effect. Dumping symptoms accompanying ingestion of concentrated carbohydrates may contribute in some people. In addition to the above hypotheses, there can be numerous gut hormones that have yet to be examined in the resolution of diabetes. Clearly, this is an arena rich with opportunities for research that should ultimately elucidate all of the mechanisms underlying the dramatic effects of bariatric operations. The National Institutes of Health (NIH) has recently sponsored a six-center program, the Longitudinal Assessment of Bariatric Surgery (LABS), to address some of these questions over the next 5 years or longer. It is hoped that insights from this and other studies will facilitate the development of new medications that can achieve at least some of the beneficial effects of bariatric surgery, without the surgery.

References

1. Ogden CL, Carroll MD, Curtin LR, McDowell MA, Tabak CJ, Flegal KM. Prevalence of overweight and obesity in the United States, 1999–2004. JAMA 2006;295(13):1549–1555.
2. Flegal K, Carroll M, Kuczmarski R, et al. Overweight and obesity in the United States: prevalence and trends, 1960–1994. Int J Obes Relat Metab Dis 1998;22:39–47.
3. Harris M, Flegal K, Cowie C, et al. Prevalence of diabetes, impaired fasting glucose, and impaired glucose tolerance in U.S. adults. Diabetes Care 1998;21:518–524.
4. National Task Force on the Prevention and Treatment of Obesity. Over-weight, obesity, and health risk. Arch Intern Med 2000;160:898–904.
5. Nathan D. Initial management of glycemia in type 2 diabetes mellitus. N Engl J Med 2002;347:1342–1349.
6. Panzram G. Mortality and survival in type 2 (non-insulin-dependent) diabetes mellitus. Diabetologia 1998;30:123–131.
7. Rubin R, Altman W, Mendelson D. Health care expenditures for people with diabetes mellitus, 1992. J Clin Endocrinol Metab 1994;78:809A–809F.
8. American Diabetes Association. Report of the expert committee on the diagnosis and classification of diabetes mellitus. Diabetes Care 2002;25(suppl 1):S5–S20.
9. American Diabetes Association. Diagnosis and classification of diabetes mellitus. Diabetes Care 2006;29(suppl 1):S43–S48.
10. Atkinson MA, Maclaren NK. The pathogenesis of insulin-dependent diabetes mellitus. N Engl J Med 1994;331:1428–1436.
11. Imagawa A, Hanafusa T, Miyagawa J, et al. A novel subtype of type 1 diabetes mellitus characterized by a rapid onset

and an absence of diabetes-related antibodies. N Engl J Med 2000;342:301–307.

12. Lager I, Lonnroth P, von Schenck H, Smith U. Reversal of insulin resistance in type I diabetes after treatment with continuous subcutaneous insulin infusion. Br Med J (Clin Res Ed) 1983;287:1661–1664.

13. DeFronzo RA, Hendler R, Simonson D. Insulin resistance is a prominent feature of insulin-dependent diabetes. Diabetes 1982;31:795–801.

14. Yki-Jarvinen H, Koivisto VA. Natural course of insulin resistance in type I diabetes. N Engl J Med 1986;315:224–230.

15. DeFronzo RA, Simonson D, Ferrannini E. Hepatic and peripheral insulin resistance: a common feature of type 2 (non-insulin-dependent) and type 1 (insulin-dependent) diabetes mellitus. Diabetologia 1982;23:313–319.

16. Samaras K, Nguyen TV, Jenkins AB, et al. Clustering of insulin resistance, total and central abdominal fat: same genes or same environment? Twin Res 1999;2:218–225.

17. Carey DG, Jenkins AB, Campbell LV, Freund J, Chisholm DJ. Abdominal fat and insulin resistance in normal and overweight women: direct measurements reveal a strong relationship in subjects at both low and high risk of NIDDM. Diabetes 1996;45:633–638.

18. Kabadi UM, Vora A, Kabadi M. Hyperinsulinemia and central adiposity: influence of chronic insulin therapy in type 1 diabetes. Diabetes Care 2000;23:1024–1025.

19. Bujalska IJ, Kumar S, Stewart PM. Does central obesity reflect "Cushing's disease of the omentum"? Lancet 1997;349:1210–1213.

20. Pernet A, Trimble ER, Kuntschen F, et al. Insulin resistance in Type 1 (insulin-dependent) diabetes: dependence on plasma insulin concentration. Diabetologia 1984;26:255–260.

21. Shahady E. Exercise as medication: how to motivate your patients. Consultant 2000;40:2174–2178.

22. Levey AS, Adler S, Caggiula AW, et al. Effects of dietary protein restriction on the progression of advanced renal disease in the Modification of Diet in Renal Disease Study. Am J Kidney Dis 1996;27:652–663.

23. Koivisto VA, DeFronzo RA. Physical training and insulin sensitivity. Diabetes Metab Rev 1986;1:445–481.

24. DeFronzo RA, Ferrannini E, Sato Y, et al. Synergistic interaction between exercise and insulin on peripheral glucose uptake. J Clin Invest 1981;68:1468–1474.

25. Tuomilehto J, Lindstrom J, Eriksson JG, et al. Finnish Diabetes Prevention Study Group. Prevention of type 2 diabetes mellitus by changes in lifestyle among subjects with impaired glucose tolerance. N Engl J Med 2001;344:1343–1350.

26. Dixon JB, Pories WJ, O'Brien PE, Schauer PR, Zimmet P. Surgery as an effective early intervention for diabesity: Why the reluctance? Diabetes Care 2005;28:472–474.

27. Intensive blood glucose control with sulphonylureas or insulin compared with conventional treatment and risk of complications in patients with type 2 diabetes (UKPDS 33). Lancet 1998;352:837–853.

28. The relationship of glycemic exposure (HbA sub1c) to the risk of development and progression of retinopathy in the diabetes control and complications trial. Diabetes 1995;44:968–983.

29. Helmrich SP, Ragland DR, Leung RW, Paffenbarger RS Jr. Physical activity and reduced occurrence of non-insulin-dependent diabetes mellitus. N Engl J Med 1991;325(3):147–152.

30. Inzucchi SE. Oral antihyperglycemic therapy for type 2 diabetes. JAMA 2002;287:360–372.

31. American Diabetes Association. The pharmacologic treatment of hyperglycemia in NIDDM. Diabetes Care 1995;18:1510–1518.

32. Halford JC. Clinical pharmacotherapy for obesity: current drugs and those in advanced development. Curr Drug Targets 2004;5:637–646.

33. Uusitupa MIJ. Early lifestyle intervention in patients with non-insulin dependent diabetes mellitus and impaired glucose tolerance. Ann Med 1996;28:445–449.

34. Pan X, Li G, Hu Y, et al. Effects of diet and exercise in preventing NIDDM in people with impaired glucose tolerance: the Da Qing IGT and Diabetes Study. Diabetes Care 1997;20:537–544.

35. Redmon J, Raatz S, Kwong C, et al. Pharmacologic induction of weight loss to treat type 2 diabetes. Diabetes Care 1999;22:896–903.

36. Paisey R, Frost J, Harvey A, et al. Five year results of a prospective very low calorie diet or conventional weight loss programme in type 2 diabetes. J Hum Nutr Dietet 2002;15:121–127.

37. Metz J, Stern JS, Kris-Etherton P, et al. A randomized trial of improved weight loss with a prepared meal plan in overweight and obese patients: impact on cardiovascular risk reduction. Arch Intern Med 2000;160:2150–2158.

38. Agurs-Collins T, Kumanyika S, Ten Have T, et al. A randomized controlled trial of weight reduction and exercise for diabetes management in older African American subjects. Diabetes Care 1997;20:1503–1511.

39. Halpern A, Mancini MC, Suplicy H, et al. Latin-American trial of orlistat for weight loss and improvement in glycaemic profile in obese diabetic patients. Diabetes, Obesity and Metaboism, 2003;5:180–188.

40. Shi YF, Pan CY, Hill J, Gao Y. Orlistat in the treatment of overweight or obese Chinese patients with newly diagnosed type 2 diabetes. Diabet Med 2005;22:1737–1743.

41. Johnson D, Drenick EJ. Therapeutic fasting in morbid obesity. Arch Intern Med 1977;137:1381–1382.

42. Andersen T, Backer OG, Stokholm KH, et al. Randomized trial of diet and gastroplasty compared with diet alone in morbid obesity. N Engl J Med 1984;310:352–356.

43. NIH Technology Assessment Conference Panel. Methods for voluntary weight loss and control. Ann Intern Med 1992;116:942–949.

44. Pories WJ, Swanson MS, MacDonald KG, et al. Who would have thought it? An operation proves to be the most effective therapy for adult-onset diabetes mellitus. Ann Surg 1995;222:339–352.

45. Schauer PR, Burguera B, Ikramuddin S, et al. Effect of laparoscopic Roux-en Y gastric bypass on type 2 diabetes mellitus. Ann Surg 2003;238:467–484; discussion 484–485.

46. Crookes PF. Surgical treatment of morbid obesity. Annu Rev Med 2006;57:243–264.

47. Sugerman HJ, Wolfe LG, Sica DA, Clore JN. Diabetes and hypertension in severe obesity and effects of gastric bypass-induced weight loss. Ann Surg 2003;237:751–756; discussion 757–758.

48. Wittgrove AC, Clark GW. Laparoscopic gastric bypass, Roux-en-Y—500 patients: technique and results, with 3–60 month follow-up. Obes Surg 2000;10:233–239.

49. Schauer PR, Ikramuddin S, Gourash W, et al. Outcomes after laparoscopic Roux-en-Y gastric bypass for morbid obesity. Ann Surg 2000;232:515–529.

50. Torquati A, Lutfi R, Abumrad N, Richards WO. Is Roux-en-Y gastric bypass surgery the most effective treatment for type 2 diabetes mellitus in morbidly obese patients? J Gastrointest Surg 2005;9:1112–1116.

51. Long SD, O'Brien K, MacDonald KG Jr, et al. Weight loss in severely obese subjects prevents the progression of impaired glucose tolerance to type II diabetes. A longitudinal interventional study. Diabetes Care 1994;17:372–375.

52. Pasquali R, Vicennati V, Scopinaro N, et al. Achievement of near-normal body weight as the prerequisite to normalize sex hormone-binding globulin concentrations in massively obese men. Int J Obes 1997;21:1–5.

53. Sjostrom C, Lissner L, Wedel H, et al. Reduction in incidence of diabetes, hypertension and lipid disturbances after intentional weight loss induced by bariatric surgery: the SOS Intervention Study. Obes Res 1999;7:477–484.

54. Dixon JB, O'Brien PE. Health outcomes of severely obese type 2 diabetic subjects 1 year after laparoscopic adjustable gastric banding. Diabetes Care 2002;25:358–363.

55. Pontiroli A Pizzocri P, Librenti M, et al. Laparoscopic adjustable gastric banding for the treatment of morbid (grade 3) obesity and its metabolic complications: a three year study. J Clin Endocrinol Metab 2002;87:3555–3561.

56. Marceau P Hould FS, Simard S, et al. Biliopancreatic diversion with duodenal switch. World J Surg 1998;22:947–954.

57. Scopinaro N, Gianetta E, Adani GF, et al. Biliopancreatic diversion for obesity at eighteen years. Surgery 1996;119:261–268.

58. Buchwald H, Avidor Y, Braunwald E, et al. Bariatric surgery: a systematic review and meta-analysis. JAMA 2004;292:1724–1737.

59. Pender C, Goldfine ID, Tanner CJ, et al. Muscle insulin receptor concentrations in obese patients post bariatric surgery: relationship to hyperinsulinemia. Int J Obes Relat Metab Disord 2004;28:363–369.

60. Gray RE, Tanner CJ, Pories WJ, MacDonald KG, Houmard JA. Effect of weight loss on muscle lipid content in morbidly obese subjects. Am J Physiol Endocrinol Metab 2003; 284:E726–E732.

61. Houmard JA, Tanner CJ, Yu C, et al. Effect of weight loss on insulin sensitivity and intramuscular long-chain fatty acyl-CoAs in morbidly obese subjects. Diabetes 2002;51: 2959–2963.

62. Pories WJ. Diabetes: the evolution of a new paradigm. Ann Surg 2004;239:12–13.

63. Cummings DE, Shannon MH. Roles for ghrelin in the regulation of appetite and body weight. Arch Surg 2003;138: 389–396.

64. Broglio F, Arvat E, Benso A, et al. Ghrelin, a natural GH secretagogue produced by the stomach, induces hyperglycemia and reduces insulin secretion in humans. J Clin Endocrinol Metab 2001;86:5083–5086.

65. Murata M, Okimura Y, Iida K, et al. Ghrelin modulates the downstream molecules of insulin signaling in hepatoma cells. J Biol Chem 2002;277:5667–5674.

66. Svensson J, Lonn L, Jansson JO, et al. Two-month treatment of obese subjects with the oral growth hormone (GH) secretagogue MK-677 increases GH secretion, fat-free mass, and energy expenditure. J Clin Endocrinol Metab 1998;83: 362–369.

67. Drucker DJ. Glucagon-like peptide-1 and the islet β-cell: augmentation of cell proliferation and inhibition of apoptosis. Endocrinology 2003;144:5145–5148.

68. Zander M, Madsbad S, Madsen JL, Holst JJ. Effect of 6-week course of glucagon-like peptide 1 on glycemic control, insulin sensitivity, and β-cell function in type 2 diabetes: a parallel-group study. Lancet 2002;359:824–830.

69. Drucker DJ. Enhancing incretin action for the treatment of type 2 diabetes. Diabetes Care 2003;26:2929–2940.

70. Naslund E, Gryback P, Backman L, et al. Distal small bowel hormones: correlation with fasting antroduodenal motility and gastric emptying. Dig Dis Sci 1998;43:945–952.

71. Naslund E, Backman L, Holst JJ, Theodorsson E, Hellstrom PM. Importance of small bowel peptides for the improved glucose metabolism 20 years after jejunoileal bypass for obesity. Obes Surg 1998;8:253–260.

72. Naslund E, Gryback P, Hellstrom PM, et al. Gastrointestinal hormones and gastric emptying 20 years after jejunoileal bypass for massive obesity. Int J Obes Relat Metab Disord 1997;21:387–392.

73. Sarson DL, Scopinaro N, Bloom SR. Gut hormone changes after jejunoileal (JIB) or biliopancreatic (BPB) bypass surgery for morbid obesity. Int J Obes 1981;5:471–480.

74. Borg CM, le Roux CW, Ghatei MA, Bloom SR, Patel AG, Aylwin SJ. Progressive rise in gut hormone levels after Roux-en-Y gastric bypass suggests gut adaptation and explains altered satiety. Br J Surg 2006;93:210–215.

75. Le Roux CW, Aylwin SJ, Batterham RL, et al. Gut hormone profiles following bariatric surgery favor an anorectic state, facilitate weight loss, and improve metabolic parameters. Ann Surg 2006;243:108–114.

76. Batterham RL, Cohen MA, Ellis SM, et al. Inhibition of food intake in obese subjects by peptide YY3–36. N Engl J Med 2003;349:941–948.

77. Batterham RL, Cowley MA, Small CJ, et al. Gut hormone PYY(3–36) physiologically inhibits food intake. Nature 2002;418:650–654.

78. Andrews NJ, Irving MH. Human gut hormone profiles in patients with short bowel syndrome. Dig Dis Sci 1992;37: 729–732.

79. Greenway SE, Greenway FL, Klein S. Effects of obesity surgery on non-insulin-dependent diabetes mellitus. Arch Surg 2002;137:1109–1117.

80. Rubino F, Gagner M. Potential of surgery for curing type 2 diabetes mellitus. Ann Surg 2002;236:554–559.

81. Scopinaro N, Adami GF, Marinari GM, et al. Biliopancreatic diversion. World J Surg 1998;22:936–946.

82. Rubino F, Marescaux J. Effect of duodenal-jejunal exclusion in a nonobese animal model of type 2 diabetes: a new perspective for an old disease. Ann Surg 2004;239:1–11.

83. Clements RH, Gonzalez QH, Long CI, Wittert G, Laws HL. Hormonal changes after Roux-en Y gastric bypass for morbid obesity and the control of type-II diabetes mellitus. Am Surg 2004;70:1–4.

84. Rubino F, Gagner M, Gentileschi P, et al. The early effect of the Roux-en-Y gastric bypass on hormones involved in body weight regulation and glucose metabolism. Ann Surg 2004;240:236–242.

85. Kellum JM, Kuemmerle JF, O'Dorisio TM, et al. Gastrointestinal hormone responses to meals before and after gastric bypass and vertical banded gastroplasty. Ann Surg 1990;211:763–770.

86. Sorensen TI, Lauritsen KB, Holst JJ, Stadil F, Andersen B. Gut and pancreatic hormones after jejunoileal bypass with 3:1 or 1:3 jejunoileal ratio. Digestion 1983;26:137–145.

87. Meryn S, Stein D, Straus EW. Pancreatic polypeptide, pancreatic glucagon, and enteroglucagon in morbid obesity and following gastric bypass operation. Int J Obes 1986;10:37–42.

88. Koopmans HS, Ferri GL, Sarson DL, Polak JM, Bloom SR. The effects of ileal transposition and jejunoileal bypass on food intake and GI hormone levels in rats. Physiol Behav 1984;33:601–609.

89. Ueno T, Shibata C, Naito H, et al. Ileojejunal transposition delays gastric emptying and decreases fecal water content in dogs with total colectomy. Dis Colon Rectum 2002; 45:109–116.

90. Ohtani N, Sasaki I, Naito H, Shibata C, Tsuchiya T, Matsuno S. Effect of ileojejunal transposition of gastrointestinal motility, gastric emptying, and small intestinal transit in dogs. J Gastrointest Surg 1999;3:516–523.

34
Cardiovascular Disease and Hypertension in the Bariatric Surgery Patient

Daniel Edmundowicz

Obesity increases an individual's risk for cardiovascular disease by causing a variety of cardiac structural changes, hemodynamic alterations, and metabolic dyscrasias that lead to both myocardial and endothelial dysfunction. Obesity is associated with an increase in both total blood volume and cardiac output due to the increased metabolic demands of excessive fat accumulation. This increased workload leads to an increased left ventricular mass and hypertrophy, which predispose to a clinically significant imbalance between perfusion and metabolic demand known as the syndrome of obesity cardiomyopathy (1).

Obesity cardiomyopathy (OC) occurs most frequently in patients with a body mass index (BMI) of 40 or more (or greater than 75% ideal body weight). Over 10% of individuals meeting these criteria, typically for longer than 10 years, are likely to develop OC. The predominant causes of death in this syndrome are progressive congestive heart failure and sudden cardiac death (2).

Hemodynamically, Alexander et al. (3) demonstrated that the increased cardiac output in OC is a result of an increased left ventricular (LV) stroke volume rather than increased heart rate alone. Further, De Divitiis et al. (4) demonstrated that oxygen demand, cardiac output, LV stroke volume, right ventricular (RV) end diastolic pressure, mean pulmonary artery pressure, and mean pulmonary capillary wedge pressure all exceeded the normal range in obese individuals. These factors may potentially lead to LV dilatation, increased LV wall stress, compensatory LV hypertrophy, and LV diastolic dysfunction. Finally, LV systolic dysfunction may occur if inadequate hypertrophy results in sustained LV wall stress.

Clinically, exertional dyspnea, orthopnea, paroxysmal nocturnal dyspnea, and edema are typical of early OC frequently occurring in the setting of normal left ventricular systolic function. Concomitant sleep apnea/hypoventilation syndrome, occurring in at least 10% of such patients, may exacerbate symptoms of right heart failure. Even in the absence of such sleep-disordered breathing, however, symptoms of OC may be accompanied by abnormal heart gallops, pulmonary rales, edema, and ascites.

Importantly, the relation between obesity and coronary artery disease (CAD) has been under considerable debate. The relationship is less clear when the measure of adiposity is expressed with a classic anthropometric variable such as weight and BMI, which may be inadequate surrogates for adiposity itself. For example, Gillum et al. (5) and Hodgson et al. (6) found that the increased risk for CAD present in abdominal adiposity is indirectly mediated by the presence of the other classical risk factors. The Nurses' Health Study, during an 8-year observation of 121,700 females, demonstrated that obesity is a determinant of CAD. After controlling for cigarette smoking, which is essential to assess the true effect of obesity, even mild-to-moderate overweight increased the risk of CHD (7).

Finally, the Munster Heart Study (PROCAM), in which 16,288 men aged 40.6 ± 11.3 years and 7328 women aged 36.0 ± 12.3 years were enrolled between 1979 and 1991 (8). In this study the BMI-associated increase in congestive heart disease (CHD) death was accounted for by traditional CAD risk factors.

The association between obesity and CHD becomes more robust when the distribution of body fat is considered. In a study of African-American women, Clark et al. (9) found the strongest predictor of CAD to be a waist to hip ratio (WHR) of greater than 0.85. Gaudet et al. (10) also found isolated abdominal obesity to be a powerful predictor of CHD in men in a group of patients with raised low-density lipoprotein (LDL) cholesterol levels due to familial hypercholesterolemia.

Hypertension

There is strong evidence that severe obesity is frequently accompanied by arterial hypertension. Because the adverse effects of obesity and hypertension on cardiac work are additive, the latter remains one of the major components of OC. The combination of obesity and hypertension increases the risk of developing congestive heart failure, and studies have clearly shown the greatest heart weight in obese, hypertensive patients (11).

Hypertension, particularly in obese individuals, is the final manifestation of a complex series of hemodynamic and metabolic alterations. Many of the latter appear to be closely linked to the presence of insulin resistance. As previously mentioned, Alexander's early work established the presence of an increased cardiac output in the setting of obesity, most likely related to the increased metabolic demand of excessive fat accumulation. Despite an early compensatory decrease in systemic vascular resistance to accommodate the increased output, the effect is not sustained. This unexpectedly normal peripheral resistance is potentially mediated by enhanced adrenergic tone, altered endothelial function, activation of renin-angiotensin systems, and increased levels of neuropeptide Y (NPY), which has been shown to be a potent vasoconstrictor (12). In most, but not all, obese individuals, these neurohumoral and hemodynamic alterations, as well as blood pressure levels, significantly improved after weight loss.

Sodium excess is known to be an initial factor in the development of hypertension in both obese and lean individuals. Increased sympathetic activity, perhaps exacerbated by insulin resistance in the obese individual, leads to the release of renin and, subsequently, angiotensin. Angiotensin I is converted to angiotensin II, which stimulates the secretion of aldosterone, a mineralocorticoid responsible for a portion of renal retention of sodium and water. Defective renal excretion of sodium and transport of sodium across cell membranes provide the predisposition for sodium excess and lead to an increase in overall effective circulating blood volume completing the cycle of higher preload, increased cardiac output and resultant systemic hypertension.

As has been alluded to so far, hypertension and atherosclerotic vascular disease in the obese individual are closely linked to the concomitant metabolic dyscrasias. The cluster of metabolic disorders associated with hypertension, atherosclerosis, and resultant increased risk for clinically evident CAD in obesity have been well described (13). Mounting clinical and experimental data have demonstrated that central obesity, dyslipidemia, hypertension, and insulin resistance make up a particular clinical profile predicting the development of type 2 diabetes and cardiovascular disease (14–17). The clustering of these variables clearly occurs simultaneously to a greater degree than would be expected by chance alone (18,19), and their expression has been referred to as the metabolic syndrome (20,21). While not all obese patients exhibit the metabolic syndrome, the cardiovascular implications, both in terms of concurrent risks of bariatric surgery and issues of postoperative management, should be considered.

Adipose tissue is no longer seen as just an inert storage for excess fat deposition. In fact, it is now evident that it is an important source of cytokines (22), and that adiposity in itself contributes to a proinflammatory milieu (23). Therefore, fat is both a dynamic endocrine organ and a highly active metabolic tissue that produces and secretes inflammatory factors collectively called adipocytokines or adipokines and including tumor necrosis factor-α (TNF-α), leptin, plasminogen activator inhibitor-1 (PAI-1), interleukin-6 (IL-6), resistin, and angiotensinogen (22). The levels of these serum adipokines are elevated in humans and animals with excess adiposity (23–26). More importantly, visceral fat that was previously noted to be worse in terms of clinical outcomes than subcutaneous fat has been found to be more active in the production of several of these adipokines than the subcutaneous adipose tissue (27–30).

Importantly, reduction in fat mass correlates well with decrease in the serum levels of many of these adipokines (31–35), implying that approaches designed to promote fat loss should be useful in attenuating these proinflammatory factors associated with obesity.

New evidence also supports an association between some of these adipokines and insulin metabolism. In particular, TNF-α is known to inhibit the tyrosine kinase phosphorylation of the insulin receptor, resulting in defects in insulin signaling and ultimately leading to insulin resistance and impaired glucose transport (36), crucial steps in the development of this syndrome and in the development of the cardiovascular comorbidities such as hypertension. In addition, these adipokines have also been shown to enhance the attachment and migration of monocytes into the vessel wall and their conversion into macrophages that are recognized key elements in the development of vascular atherosclerosis (37). Specifically, TNF-α activates the transcription factor nuclear factor (NF)-κB, which facilitates the expression of adhesion molecules of intracellular adhesion molecule-1 and vascular cell adhesion molecule-1 (38–41), which enhance monocyte adhesion to the vessel wall (30–34); production of monocyte chemoattractant protein-1 and macrophage colony-stimulating factor (M-CSF) (42–44); and activation of a proinflammatory macrophage state, resulting in increased macrophage expression of inducible nitric oxide synthase, interleukins, and superoxide dismutase (45–48). T lymphocytes are also activated and are responsible for enhancing macrophage atherosclerotic activity (49).

Additionally, leptin is a plasma protein secreted by adipocytes and involved in the control of body weight (50). Plasma concentrations of leptin are increased in human obesity and are positively correlated with body fat mass (51). More recently, in addition to long-term regulation of the body weight, a role for leptin has been suggested in atherosclerosis (52). In this large prospective study, leptin was noted to be a novel risk factor for coronary artery disease. It was later noted that leptin-dependent prothrombotic properties and a platelet proaggregatory effect were responsible for this risk factor association (53). In addition, leptin has been shown to enhance cellular immune responses (54) as well as to raise blood pressure (55,56). Leptin has also been reported to stimulate cholesterol accumulation by the macrophage, particularly in the presence of high glucose (57).

Finally, cardiovascular risk in the obese individual is perpetuated by the presence of hyperinsulinemia, which is invariably found in insulin resistance, and stimulates PAI-1 release from fat and other tissues (58). In fact, the simple consumption of a high-calorie, high-carbohydrate meal stimulates insulin release, and this is enough to increase plasma PAI-1 levels, whereas fasting or administration of metformin or insulin sensitizers are associated with decreased circulating insulin and PAI-1 levels (59,60). Whether PAI-1 is related to diabetes beyond inflammation or insulin resistance, perhaps through genetics, adrenal steroids, or other factors, remains to be investigated. Nevertheless, plasma PAI-1 appears to be a useful predictor of diabetes, and therapeutic approaches that lower circulating PAI-1 levels may be associated with prevention of diabetes (61).

Although insulin resistance is generally accepted as the primary underlying abnormality preceding and contributing to most of the observed metabolic derangements seen in the metabolic syndrome, truncal obesity appears to be a key element in this sequence of events. It has been proposed that insulin resistance and the metabolic syndrome occur as a result of lipotoxicity in various organs (62). Furthermore, there is also emerging evidence that suggests that adipocytes are very active and secrete or influence actions of a variety of cytokines, including adiponectin, leptin, tissue factor, angiotensinogen, lipoprotein lipase, IL-6, PAI-1, and many others, not only causing vascular damage but also perpetuating this damage by altering both the oxidative stress balance and by the proinflammatory actions (62).

Cardiovascular disease is a good example of a disease process whose phenotypic profile is quite diverse. As described above, several cardiovascular risk factors tend to cluster, and this clustering of metabolic risk factors has been referred to as the insulin resistance syndrome (63–65). More importantly, a crucial association among obesity, metabolic syndrome, and adverse cardiovascular clinical outcomes has raised important questions about the underlying pathophysiologic processes.

Preoperative Assessment of the Obese Patient

The initial evaluation of any patient prior to surgery requires a detailed history and physical examination, which can often indicate the potential for serious cardiovascular risk. The history and physical exam establish the pretest probability of significant cardiovascular disease and provide important information for subsequent interpretation of cardiac tests.

Symptoms and Signs

Symptoms related to underlying cardiovascular disease or obesity cardiomyopathy are similar in obese and nonobese patients. Chest pain syndromes should be ascertained and carefully elicited in obese patients given the clustering of coronary artery disease risk factors seen in this population.

Dyspnea is defined as an abnormal uncomfortable awareness of breathing. Exertional dyspnea has often been described as an "anginal equivalent," as it is often the primary complaint in myocardial ischemia. In the obese patient, however, it may occur with diastolic or systolic dysfunction as elevated intracardiac pressures and pulmonary congestion persist. Dyspnea can also manifest as a deconditioned response to exercise or activity, making it difficult to separate from the possibility of underlying cardiomyopathy or coronary artery disease.

As remodeling of the left ventricle progresses, symptoms other than angina and dyspnea are seen. Orthopnea, paroxysmal nocturnal dyspnea, lower extremity swelling, and weight gain are frequently experienced. In obesity, these symptoms are commonly seen with diastolic dysfunction alone, and they do not necessarily herald the presence of systolic dysfunction. These symptoms may also be due to sleep apnea and the obesity-hypoventilation syndrome, as increased chronic arterial hypertension inevitably leads to right heart failure.

Palpitations with or without light-headedness and dizziness may occur in the setting of atrial or ventricular arrhythmias. The incidence of syncope in obese patients is no greater than that in the general population but, if present, must be evaluated cautiously.

The clinical exam should be focused on detecting signs of underlying cardiomyopathy. Heart gallops, such as an S3 or S4, suggest that LV remodeling has already occurred. In addition to gallop rhythms, pulmonary crackles suggest underlying volume overload or increased ventricular filling pressures. Jugular venous distention, hepatojugular reflex, and lower extremity swelling are seen in right heart failure, which may be due to either left ventricular dysfunction or sleep apnea/obesity-hypoventilation syndrome. Hepatomegaly and ascites are often present but are more difficult to appreciate with large body mass and central obesity.

Electrocardiogram (ECG)

The ECG is a mainstay in the preoperative evaluation for cardiovascular risk. It can detect past myocardial infarction and current myocardial ischemia, perhaps helping to further identify patients at higher than average risk prior to surgery. The ECG in obesity has been long studied (3,4), and it is abundantly clear that obesity alters the resting ECG. With increasing body mass index and soft tissue between the heart and the anterior surface of the chest wall, low QRS voltage is seen in the precordial leads (17). Leftward deviation of the P-wave, QRS, and T-wave axis is seen in obese patients as compared to normals (18), possibly due to the presence of left ventricular hypertrophy (LVH) and horizontal displacement of the heart due to abdominal adiposity. T-wave abnormalities are also seen in the obese (16). T-wave flattening is far more common than T-wave inversions, and these changes are frequently seen in the inferior, lateral, and inferolateral leads (17). These abnormalities are not specific for ischemia but rather are felt to be due to the horizontal position of the heart in obese individuals. Left atrial abnormality is another ECG finding seen in obesity. Its presence was best predicted with a p-terminal force in lead V_1 greater than 0.04 ms (17),

Left ventricular hypertrophy is known to be present in obese patients given the presence of increased LV mass and chronic effects of systemic hypertension. The Cornell voltage criteria for LVH (the sum of the R-wave amplitude in lead aVL plus the S wave amplitude in lead V_3) has been shown to yield a higher sensitivity as compared to other voltage criteria for LVH, especially when obesity is taken into account (19). This has been validated when compared to echocardiographic data (20). However, the accuracy of the ECG in diagnosing LVH remains poor and should not be used alone.

Substantial weight reduction produces a variety of favorable cardiac hemodynamics and structural alterations in morbid obesity (21,66). These structural alterations have been shown to reverse many of the ECG alterations associated with morbid obesity in a population of patients who underwent gastric bypass surgery (67).

References

1. Benotti PN, Bistrain B, Benotti JR, Blackburn G, Forse RA. Heart disease and hypertension in severe obesity: the benefits of weight reduction. Am J Clin Nutr 1992;55:586S–590S.
2. Alpert MA. Obesity cardiomyopathy: pathophysiology and evolution of the clinical syndrome. Am J Med Sci 2001;321(4):225–236.
3. Alexander JK, Dennis EW, Smith WG, et al. Blood volume, cardiac output and distribution of systemic blood flow in extreme obesity. Cardiovasc Res Center Bull 1961;1:39–44.
4. DeDivitiis O, Fazio S, Pettitto M, et al. Obesity and cardiac function. Circulation 1981;64:477–482.
5. Gillum RF, Mussolino ME, Madans JH. Body fat distribution and hypertension incidence in women and men. The NHANES I Epidemiologic Follow-up Study. Int J Obes Relat Metab Disord 1998;22:127–134.
6. Hodgson JM, Wahlqvist ML, Balazs ND, Boxall JA. Coronary atherosclerosis in relation to body fatness and its distribution. Int J Obes Relat Metab Disord 1994;18:41–46.
7. Manson JE, Colditz GA, Stampfer MJ, et al. A prospective study of obesity and risk of coronary heart disease in women (see comments). N Engl J Med 1990;322:882–889.
8. Schulte H, Cullen P, Assmann G. Obesity, mortality and cardiovascular disease in the Munster Heart Study (PROCAM). Atherosclerosis 1999;144:199–209.
9. Clark LT, Karve MM, Rones KT, et al. Obesity: distribution of body fat and coronary heart disease in black women. Am J Cardiol 1994;73:895–896.
10. Gaudet D, Vohl MC, Perron P, et al. Relationships of abdominal obesity and hyperinsulinemia to angiographically assessed coronary artery disease in men with known mutations in the LDL receptor gene. Circulation 1998;97:871–877.
11. Benotti PN, Bistrian B, Benotti JR, et al. Heart disease and hypertension in severe obesity: the benefits of weight reduction. Am J Clin Nutr 1992;55:586S.
12. Clarke J, Benjamin N, Larkin S, et al. Interaction of neuropeptide Y and the sympathetic nervous system in vascular control in man. Circulation 1991;83:774–777.
13. Reaven GM. Role of insulin resistance in human disease. Diabetes 1988;37:1595–1607.
14. Kannel WB, McGee DL. Diabetes and cardiovascular disease: the Framingham Study. JAMA 1979;241:2035–2038.
15. Haffner SM, Stern MP, Hazuda HP, Mitchell BD, Patterson JK. Cardiovascular risk factors in confirmed prediabetic individuals: does the clock for coronary heart disease start ticking before the onset of diabetes? JAMA 1990;263:2893–2898.
16. Despres J-P, Lamarche B, Mauriege P, et al. Hyperinsulinemia as an independent risk factor for ischemic heart disease. N Engl J Med 1996;334:952–957.
17. Wilson PW, McGee DL, Kannel WB. Obesity, very low density lipoproteins, and glucose intolerance over fourteen years: the Framingham Study. Am J Epidemiol 1981;114:697–704.
18. Schmidt MI, Watson RL, Duncan BB, et al. Clustering of dyslipidemia, hyperuricemia, diabetes, and hypertension and its association with fasting insulin and central and overall obesity in a general population. Metabolism 1996;45:699–706.
19. Wilson PWF, Kannel WB, Silbershatz H, D'Agostino RB. Clustering of metabolic factors and coronary heart disease. Arch Intern Med 1999;159:1104–1109.
20. Meigs JB, D'Agostino RB, Wilson PWF, Cupples LA, Nathan DM, Singer DE. Risk variable clustering in the insulin resistance syndrome: the Framingham Offspring Study. Diabetes 1997;46:1594–1600.
21. Meigs JB. Invited commentary: insulin resistance syndrome? Syndrome X? Multiple metabolic syndrome? A syndrome at all? Factor analysis reveals patterns in the fabric of correlated metabolic risk factors. Am J Epidemiol 2000;152:908–911.
22. Ahima RS, Flier JS. Adipose tissue as an endocrine organ. Trends Endocrinol Metab 2000;11:327–332.

23. Yudkin JS, Stehouwer CD, Emeis JJ, Coppack SW. C-reactive protein in healthy subjects: associations with obesity, insulin resistance, and endothelial dysfunction: a potential role for cytokines originating from adipose tissue? Arterioscler Thromb Vasc Biol 1999;19:972–978.

24. Samad F, Loskutoff DJ. Tissue distribution and regulation of plasminogen activator inhibitor-1 in obese mice. Mol Med 1996;2:568–582.

25. Samad F, Yamamoto K, Pandey M, Loskutoff DJ. Elevated expression of transforming growth factor-β in adipose tissue from obese mice. Mol Med 1997;3:37–48.

26. Zhang B, Graziano MP, Doebber TW, et al. Down-regulation of the expression of the obese gene by an antidiabetic thiazolidinedione in Zucker diabetic fatty rats and db/db mice. J Biol Chem 1996;271:9455–9459.

27. Dusserre E, Moulin P, Vidal H. Differences in mRNA expression of the proteins secreted by the adipocytes in human subcutaneous and visceral adipose tissues. Biochim Biophys Acta 2000;1500:88–96.

28. Fried SK, Bunkin DA, Greenberg AS. Omental and subcutaneous adipose tissues of obese subjects release interleukin-6: depot difference and regulation by glucocorticoid. J Clin Endocrinol Metab 1998;83:847–850.

29. Eriksson P, Van Harmelen V, Hoffstedt J, et al. Regional variation in plasminogen activator inhibitor-1 expression in adipose tissue from obese individuals. Thromb Haemost 2000;83:545–548.

30. Giacchetti G, Faloia E, Mariniello B, et al. Overexpression of the renin-angiotensin system in human visceral adipose tissue in normal and overweight subjects. Am J Hypertens 2002;15:381–388.

31. Dandona P, Weinstock R, Thusu K, Abdel-Rahman E, Aljada A, Wadden T. Tumor necrosis factor-α in sera of obese patients: fall with weight loss. J Clin Endocrinol Metab 1998;83:2907–2910.

32. Ziccardi P, Nappo F, Giugliano G, et al. Reduction of inflammatory cytokine concentrations and improvement of endothelial functions in obese women after weight loss over one year. Circulation 2002;105:804–809.

33. Primrose JN, Davies JA, Prentice CR, Hughes R, Johnston D. Reduction in factor VII, fibrinogen and plasminogen activator inhibitor-1 activity after surgical treatment of morbid obesity. Thromb Haemost 1992;68:396–399.

34. Folsom AR, Qamhieh HT, Wing RR, et al. Impact of weight loss on plasminogen activator inhibitor (PAI-1), factor VII, and other hemostatic factors in moderately overweight adults. Arterioscler Thromb 1993;13:162–169.

35. Itoh K, Imai K, Masuda T, et al. Relationship between changes in serum leptin levels and blood pressure after weight loss. Hypertens Res 2002;25:881–886.

36. Feinstein R, Kanety H, Papa MZ, Lunenfeld B, Karasik A. Tumor necrosis factor-α suppresses insulin-induced tyrosine phosphorylation of insulin receptor and its substrates. J Biol Chem 1993;268:26055–26058.

37. Libby P. Changing concepts of atherogenesis. J Intern Med 2000;247:349–358.

38. Landry DB, Couper LL, Bryant SR, Lindner V. Activation of the NF-κB and IκB system in smooth muscle cells after rat arterial injury. Induction of vascular cell adhesion molecule-1 and monocyte chemoattractant protein-1. Am J Pathol 1997;151:1085–1095.

39. Iademarco MF, McQuillan JJ, Dean DC. Vascular cell adhesion molecule 1: contrasting transcriptional control mechanisms in muscle and endothelium. Proc Natl Acad Sci USA 1993;90:3943–3947.

40. Eck SL, Perkins ND, Carr DP, Nabel GJ. Inhibition of phorbol ester-induced cellular adhesion by competitive binding of NF-κB in vivo. Mol Cell Biol 1993;13:6530–6536.

41. Clesham GJ, Adam PJ, Proudfoot D, Flynn PD, Efstathiou S, Weissberg PL. High adenoviral loads stimulate NFκB-dependent gene expression in human vascular smooth muscle cells. Gene Ther 1998;5:174–180.

42. Martin T, Cardarelli PM, Parry GC, Felts KA, Cobb RR. Cytokine induction of monocyte chemoattractant protein-1 gene expression in human endothelial cells depends on the cooperative action of NF-κB and AP-1. Eur J Immunol 1997;27:1091–1097.

43. Peng HB, Rajavashisth TB, Libby P, Liao JK. Nitric oxide inhibits macrophage-colony stimulating factor gene transcription in vascular endothelial cells. J Biol Chem 1995;270:17050–17055.

44. Rajavashisth TB, Yamada H, Mishra NK. Transcriptional activation of the macrophage-colony stimulating factor gene by minimally modified LDL. Involvement of nuclear factor-κB. Arterioscler Thromb Vasc Biol 1995;15:1591–1598.

45. Xie QW, Kashiwabara Y, Nathan C. Role of transcription factor NF-κB/Rel in induction of nitric oxide synthase. J Biol Chem 1994;269:4705–4708.

46. Goto M, Katayama KI, Shirakawa F, Tanaka I. Involvement of NF-κB p50/p65 heterodimer in activation of the human pro-interleukin-1β gene at two subregions of the upstream enhancer element. Cytokine 1999;11:16–28.

47. Kawashima T, Murata K, Akira S, et al. STAT5 induces macrophage differentiation of M1 leukemia cells through activation of IL-6 production mediated by NF-κB p65. J Immunol 2001;167:3652–3660.

48. Kelly KA, Hill MR, Youkhana K, Wanker F, Gimble JM. Dimethyl sulfoxide modulates NF-κB and cytokine activation in lipopolysaccharide-treated murine macrophages. Infect Immun 1994;62:3122–3128.

49. Frostegard J, Ulfgren AK, Nyberg P, et al. Cytokine expression in advanced human atherosclerotic plaques: dominance of pro-inflammatory (Th1) and macrophage-stimulating cytokines. Atherosclerosis 1999;145:33–43.

50. Mantzoros CS. The role of leptin in human obesity and disease: a review of current evidence. Ann Intern Med 1999;130:671–680.

51. Considine RV, Sinha MK, Heiman ML, et al. Serum immunoreactive-leptin concentrations in normal-weight and obese human. N Engl J Med 1996;334:292–295.

52. Wallace AM, McMahon AD, Packard CJ, et al. Plasma leptin and the risk of cardiovascular disease in West of Scotland Coronary Prevention Study (WOSCOPS). Circulation 2001;104:3052–3056.

53. Konstantinides S, Schafer K, Koschnick S, Loskutoff DJ. Leptin-dependent platelet aggregation and arterial thrombosis suggests a mechanism for atherothrombotic disease in obesity. J Clin Invest 2001;108:1533–1540.

54. Lord GM, Matarese G, Howard JK, Baker RJ, Bloom SR, Lechler RI. Leptin modulates the T-cell immune response and reverses starvation-induced immunosuppression. Nature 1998;394:897–901.

55. Shek EW, Brands MW, Hall JE. Chronic leptin infusion increases arterial pressure. Hypertension 1998;31:409–414.

56. Correia ML, Morgan DA, Sivitz WI, Mark AL, Haynes WG. Leptin acts in the central nervous system to produce dose-dependent changes in arterial pressure. Hypertension 2001; 37:936–942.

57. O'Rourke L, Gronning LM, Yeaman SJ, Shepherd PR. Glucose-dependent regulation of cholesterol ester metabolism in macrophages by insulin and leptin. J Biol Chem 2002;277:42557–42562.

58. Samad F, Loskutoff DJ. Tissue distribution and regulation of plasminogen activator inhibitor-1 in obese mice. Mol Med 1996;2:568–582.

59. Loskutoff DJ, Samad F. The adipocyte and hemostatic balance in obesity: studies of PAI-1. Arterioscler Thromb Vasc Biol 1998;18:1–6.

60. Chu NV, Kong APS, Kimm DD, et al. Differential effects of metformin and troglitazone on cardiovascular risk factors in patients with type 2 diabetes. Diabetes Care 2002; 25:542–549.

61. Lyon CJ, Hsueh WA. Effect of plasminogen activator inhibitor-1 in diabetes mellitus and cardiovascular disease. Am J Med 2003;115:62–68.

62. Unger RH. Lipotoxic diseases. Annu Rev Med 2002;53: 319–336.

63. Reaven GM. Banting lecture 1988: Role of insulin resistance in human disease. Diabetes 1988;37:1595–1607.

64. Haffner SM. Epidemiology of hypertension and insulin resistance syndrome. J Hypertens Suppl 1997;15:S25–30.

65. Lopez-Candales A. Metabolic syndrome X: a comprehensive review of the pathophysiology and recommended therapy. J Med 2001;32:283–300.

66. Deedwania PC. The deadly quartet revisited. Am J Med 1998;105(1A):1S–3S.

67. Alberti KG, Zimmet PZ. Definition, diagnosis and classification of diabetes mellitus and its complications. Part 1: Diagnosis and Classification of Diabetes Mellitus, provisional report of a WHO consultation. Diabet Med 1998;15:539–553.

35
Sleep Apnea in the Bariatric Surgery Patient

Rachel J. Givelber and Mark H. Sanders

Obstructive sleep apnea hypopnea (OSAH) is a chronic medical condition characterized by repetitive episodes of breathing disturbance, characterized by upper airway obstruction, occurring during sleep. It is extremely common in patients undergoing bariatric surgery and may impact perioperative complications. It is also one of the medical comorbidities of obesity that may be cured after the weight loss resulting from bariatric surgery. This chapter reviews the pathophysiology and clinical aspects of OSAH, emphasizing the relationship with obesity, bariatric preoperative workup and management, and the perioperative implications of OSAH.

Pathophysiology and Epidemiology

Obstructive sleep apnea hypopnea is characterized by repetitive episodes of obstructive apnea (complete upper airway closure with consequent cessation of airflow; Fig. 35-1) or hypopnea (partial closure of the upper airway with reduction but not cessation of airflow) during sleep. Conventional definitions require apneas and hypopneas to be at least 10 seconds in duration, and both apneas and hypopneas may be associated with similar physiologic disturbance. Conventional estimates of disease severity rely on the number of respiratory events per hour of sleep (1) (Apnea + Hypopnea Index, AHI; Table 35-1) as well as patient symptoms. Obstructive sleep apnea hypopnea patients may not have any clinically evident pulmonary compromise during wakefulness. Upper airway (or pharyngeal) size is determined by the balance between outward-directed or dilating forces that promote luminal patency and inward-directed forces that predispose to collapse. During sleep several factors contribute to airway narrowing. With sleep onset, there is a physiologic reduction in neural activation of the upper airway dilator muscles; moreover, the tonic activity of these muscles (including the genioglossus, geniohyoid, and tensor palatini) decreases more than the neural drive

to the respiratory pump muscles. The negative intrathoracic and intra-airway pressure that is generated during inspiration is transmitted to the less stable pharynx, which, as a consequence of sleep-associated instability, is narrowed. Thus, there is a normal, sleep-related increase in upper airway resistance that is generally without adverse clinical impact. However, in the setting of an abnormal decrement in pharyngeal dilator muscle activity during sleep, or an upper airway that is anatomically susceptible to collapse, there is clinically significant limitation or cessation of airflow with consequent oxyhemoglobin desaturation and sleep disruption.

A small pharyngeal cross-sectional area is a risk factor for OSAH. Obesity, particularly central obesity and increased neck circumference, are well recognized predispositions for OSAH, possibly due to airway narrowing by excess adipose tissue in the lateral fat pads of the pharynx and thickening of the muscles compromising the lateral pharyngeal walls. In addition, craniofacial abnormalities, such as retrognathia and micrognathia, reduce upper airway size and predispose to OSAH. These features do not compromise airflow during wakefulness, when there is a compensatory increase in upper airway dilator muscle activation, but do become significant during the physiologic reduction in upper airway dilator tone and loss of neural compensation that is normally associated with sleep.

The immediate physiologic consequences of apneas and hypopneas include oxyhemoglobin desaturation as well as arousal from sleep. The rate and degree of desaturation is dependent on the baseline oxyhemoglobin saturation as well as the duration of the apnea or hypopnea. In the morbidly obese patient, oxygen saturation may be diminished even during wakefulness, because excess weight on the chest and abdomen decreases the resting volume of the lungs and may be associated with small airway closure and ventilation/perfusion inequality. In addition, the oxygen storage capacity of the lungs may be diminished by virtue of the reduced lung volume, and this

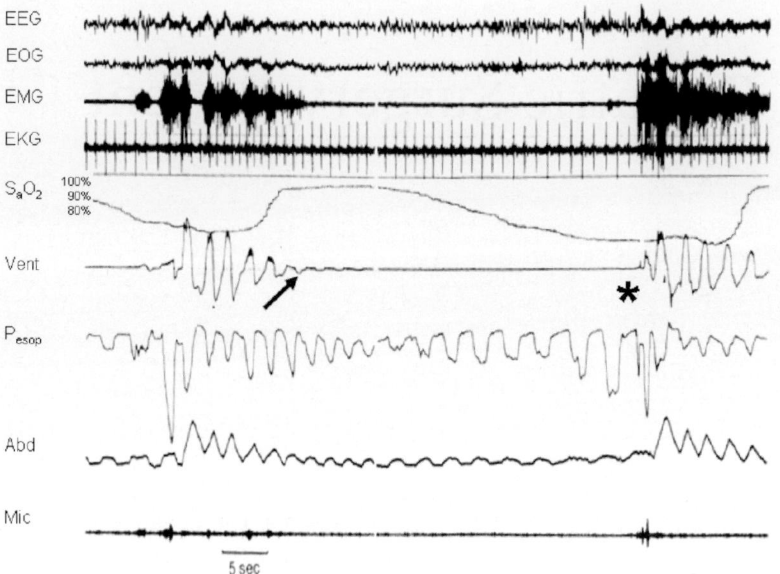

FIGURE 35-1. Obstructive apnea in a patient with severe obstructive sleep apnea hypopnea (OSAH). At the arrow, airflow stops while respiratory effort recorded by negative swings in esophageal pressure and abdominal movement continues, indicating the airway is occluded. Resumption of airflow (at the asterisk) is accompanied by increased chin muscle tone, heart rate and EEG frequency indicating arousal from sleep. EEG, electroencephalogram, C$_4$–A$_1$; EOG, electro-oculogram; EMG, electromyogram; EKG, electrocardiogram; S$_a$O$_2$, oxygen saturation; Vent, minute ventilation in liters/minute; P$_{esop}$, esophageal pressure; Abd, abdominal movement; Mic, microphone recording snoring. (Adapted from Kryger MH, Roth T, Dement WC. Principles and Practices of Sleep Medicine, 3rd ed. Philadelphia: WB Saunders, 2000.)

also may accentuate the rate and depth of desaturation in conjunction with sleep-disordered breathing events such as apneas and hypopneas. An important subset of obese patients exhibits alveolar hypoventilation even during wakefulness (defined by an elevated arterial carbon dioxide tension, PaCO$_2$ >45 mm Hg), further reducing daytime oxygen saturation and consequent worsening of sleep-related desaturation. Assuming a recumbent position accentuates the abnormalities in oxygenation. A lower baseline saturation places the patient closer to the steep portion of the oxyhemoglobin dissociation curve where even small decrements in arterial oxygen tension (PaO$_2$) result in relatively greater desaturation. Termination of an apnea or hypopnea is usually associated with arousal from sleep, and repetitive events lead to sleep fragmentation. During the obstructive breathing event, heart rate often falls and blood pressure may rise, fall, or remain unchanged. However, as the obstruction is relieved, there is a surge in sympathetic nervous system activity with consequent relative hypertension and tachycardia.

Obstructive sleep apnea hypopnea is common in the general population. Samples drawn from the community estimate that at least one in five adults aged 20 to 80 has mild sleep apnea, defined as five or more episodes of

breathing disturbance per hour of sleep, and one in 15 adults has 15 or more of these episodes (2). The prevalence of sleep apnea increases from young adulthood to approximately age 65, and then levels off (3). Men are more commonly affected than women, although after menopause the prevalence among women rises to a level that approximates that in males. Obstructive sleep apnea hypopnea affects all racial groups, with the rate in African Americans slightly higher than in Caucasians.

In the general population, OSAH is highly associated with obesity, with the risk increasing threefold for each standard deviation increase in body mass index (BMI), neck circumference, or waist-to-hip ratio (4). Paradoxically, in the severely obese patients likely to undergo bariatric surgery, this strong relation is lost, perhaps because the prevalence of OSAH is so high in this group. In series of bariatric patients that did not screen all patients for OSAH, one quarter to one third of the subjects were known to have OSAH at the time of surgery (5–7), but this probably underestimates the prevalence in this population. In a series of 170 consecutive patients undergoing bariatric surgery, sleep data were available in 96%, and the overall prevalence of OSAH was 77% (8), confirming the findings of smaller studies (9,10). In the general population and among bariatric surgery patients, at any given level of obesity men have more severe OSAH than women. Thus although greater numbers of women undergo bariatric surgery than men, the women on average have less severe OSAH (8).

Some patients with OSAH also have daytime hypercapnia and chronic respiratory acidosis, known as the obesity hypoventilation syndrome. Often these patients will have concomitant chronic obstructive pulmonary disease (COPD). Patients with resting hypercapnia tend to be more obese, and have worse nocturnal oxygenation

TABLE 35-1. Severity of obstructive sleep apnea hypopnea (OSAH)

Severity	Apnea + Hypopnea Index
Mild	5–15 events/hour
Moderate	16–30 events/hour
Severe	More than 30 events/hour

Source: Data from American Academy of Sleep Medicine Task Force (1).

and greater pulmonary hypertension (11,12). The risk for perioperative pulmonary and cardiac complications for subjects with obesity hypoventilation syndrome is believed to be worse than for OSAH alone, although prospective clinical data are lacking.

Clinical Features

Patients with OSAH may have nocturnal or diurnal complaints, or both or neither (Table 35-2). Snoring with resuscitative snorting and witnessed apneas may be reported by bed partners or roommates of patients. Patients often complain of nonrestorative sleep, excessive daytime sleepiness, and less commonly of awakening with a sensation of choking or gasping (13). They may also acknowledge nocturia (14), frequent awakenings for uncertain reason, and morning headaches (15). Family members may note changes in mood or increased irritability, and the prevalence of depression is increased (16). However, epidemiologic studies indicate that most subjects with OSAH are asymptomatic and have never sought medical care (4,17).

Many of the prototypical symptoms of OSAH are non-specific. For example, sleepiness is pervasive in modern society (18). Further confounding risk assessment for a diagnosis of sleep apnea, sleepiness and unrefreshing sleep are common complaints in obese patients even in the absence of OSAH (19). This has been attributed to an association between high levels of inflammatory cytokines, including interleukin-6 (IL-6) and tumor necrosis factor-α (TNF-α), which have been shown in animal models to be somnogenic (20). In a series of 313 patients undergoing laparoscopic gastric band placement, 52% of men and 26% of women reported witnessed apneas, and only 25% rated their sleep quality as good (21). Thus, while daytime sleepiness is neither specific nor sensitive for OSAH in the bariatric surgery population, additional diagnostic investigation is usually warranted in this high-risk group.

TABLE 35-2. Common symptoms of OSAH

Symptom	Prevalence (%) (28)
Events during sleep	
Snoring ≥3 nights/wk	>50
Loud snoring	>50
Breathing pauses ≥1 night/wk	7–25
Leg kicks ≥1 night/wk	13
Symptoms during wakefulness	
Nonrestorative sleep ≥1 time/wk	>33
Dozing while watching television ≥1 night/wk	30–50
Difficulty maintaining sleep	10–25
Waking with a headache	5–15

Although the prevalence of sleep-related mortality attributable to OSAH is not known, it is increasingly evident that this disorder is associated with significantly adverse health consequences. Obstructive sleep apnea hypopnea is an independent risk factor for hypertension (22), and is associated with cardiovascular disease, congestive heart failure, stroke, diabetes mellitus, and the metabolic syndrome (23–25). Patients with sleep apnea are at increased risk of motor vehicle accidents (26).

Diagnosis

Use of Clinical Measures to Predict Obstructive Sleep Apnea Hypopnea

While OSAH is often suspected based on clinical symptoms, these symptoms alone are poorly predictive of the presence or severity of disease. Women with OSAH are less likely to report habitual snoring, and more likely to complain of daytime fatigue than men (27,28). Several studies have identified witnessed apneas as predictive, but this historical information is lacking in subjects without regular bed partners. The Epworth Sleepiness Scale is an eight-item self-administered questionnaire that asks patients to rate the chance that they would doze in everyday situations such as reading a book or after lunch (29). While it is commonly used in sleep clinics to screen for sleep apnea, Epworth Sleepiness Scale Score is a poor predictor of individual risk, particularly in the bariatric population (10,30). The Multivariable Apnea Risk Index, which combines questionnaire and demographic information, has been validated in patients presenting to sleep clinics, but not in patients undergoing bariatric surgery (31).

Several groups have attempted to create prediction models for OSAH based on symptoms and physical examination. All models include measures of obesity, either body mass index (BMI) or neck circumference, as well as report of habitual snoring and witnessed apnea. In general, the positive predictive power of these models have not been assessed by investigators other than those who created them, so their use in practice has been limited. Furthermore, to the extent that these models have been validated, it has been in general sleep clinic populations, and they have not been validated in the bariatric population.

Dixon and colleagues (30) identified predictors of OSAH in 99 subjects undergoing bariatric surgery. Their sample included only subjects with symptoms of OSAH, so virtually all were habitual snorers. Demographic factors, clinical symptoms, measures of obesity, and biochemical measures were each assessed for the ability to predict AHI. In multivariate analyses, *B*MI ≥45, *a*ge ≥38 years, observed *s*leep apnea, *h*emoglobin A$_{1c}$ ≥6%, fasting plasma *i*nsulin $\geq$28 μmol/L, and *m*ale sex (BASH 'IM) were independent predictors of an AHI $\geq$15. These independent predictors were equally weighted in this model (which is easy to remember, as the acronym BASH 'IM is often the response of a male subject's bed partner to his sleep apnea), yielding a scale from 0 to 6. In their population, a BASH 'IM score of $\geq$3 had a sensitivity of 89% and specificity of 81% for AHI $\geq$15. Obstructive sleep apnea hypopnea (defined as an AHI >15) was diagnosed in none of the 31 subjects with a BASH 'IM score of 0 or 1 and in only four of 24 subjects with a score of 2. Thus, this model is potentially very useful in identifying subjects at low risk of OSAH who do not need further workup. Potential limitations of the model include the need to measure fasting insulin and hemoglobin A_{1c} levels and the lack of information on subjects who were not suspected of OSAH, and so did not undergo polysomnography. This is problematic given the poor predictive value of symptoms for diagnosing OSAH in a severely obese population. The model has not yet been validated in another population or at another center.

Objective Testing for Obstructive Sleep Apnea Hypopnea

The gold standard for diagnosing OSAH is a polysomnogram (PSG) in a sleep laboratory with a trained technician in attendance to ensure optimal data collection. A polysomnogram measures electroencephalography, eye movements, and muscle tone to identify and stage sleep, oxygen saturation by transcutaneous oximetry, heart rate, and measures of respiratory effort and airflow. Polysomnography has several limitations. Patients may perceive the testing as inconvenient or time consuming. Demand for PSG exceeds the supply of sleep laboratory slots in many areas, so testing may be delayed. It requires both skilled personnel and sophisticated equipment, and hence is relatively expensive. However, only a PSG can accurately assess the presence of sleep and gauge sleep continuity.

Because of the inherent barriers to laboratory PSG, researchers have attempted to design portable monitors that can be used in the patient's home to rule in or rule out OSAH. The technology ranges from devices that record only oximetry and heart rate to full PSG done in the home, but more commonly used are biomonitors that assess four or more cardiopulmonary signals (for example, thoracoabdominal movement to reflect breathing effort, airflow, oxygen saturation, and heart rate). Unfortunately, no unattended technology has been studied with enough rigor to recommend clinical use (32), and their utility has not been proven in the bariatric population. In general, portable monitors underestimate OSAH severity because the denominator for the AHI is time in bed rather than sleep time, and displaced sensors cannot be replaced, so missing data are more common than in the sleep laboratory. In addition, respiratory events that result in minimal oxygen desaturation may be missed. Paradoxically, manual scoring of portable monitors may overestimate AHI (33). In the event that OSAH is strongly suspected based on an unattended portable sleep study, a laboratory PSG is still required to initiate therapy with positive airway pressure (see below).

No prospective trials clearly indicate which patients require preoperative evaluation for OSAH as part of their workup prior to bariatric surgery. Our practice is to perform PSG in patients with subjective sleep complaints including nonrefreshing sleep and excessive daytime sleepiness, or subjects who have been told by bed partners that they have breathing pauses during sleep. In addition, subjects with cardiac comorbidity, particularly congestive heart failure, are at markedly increased risk of OSAH; therefore, these subjects also undergo mandatory PSG. Finally, subjects with coexistent pulmonary disease, low oxygen saturation during wakefulness, or daytime hypercapnia are likely to have profound nocturnal desaturation and should undergo laboratory PSG. In our practice, portable monitoring is reserved for triage of subjects who cannot be accommodated promptly in the sleep laboratory.

Treatment of Obstructive Sleep Apnea Hypopnea

Effective treatment of OSAH must provide upper airway patency and adequate oxyhemoglobin saturation during sleep, as well as restore good sleep continuity. The most common and rapidly acting treatment to achieve these goals is with positive airway pressure (continuous positive airway pressure, CPAP) or bilevel positive airway pressure (BiPAP). Each of these devices deliver pressurized airflow through a nasal or full-face mask interface into the upper airway (Fig. 35-2). The increased intraluminal pressure splints the upper airway open and prevents collapse. Continuous positive airway pressure is a mode of positive airway pressure therapy in which the same level of pressure is applied continuously throughout the ventilatory cycle. Bilevel positive airway pressure has the capability to provide pressure levels that alternate between a higher pressure during inspiration and a relatively lower pressure during exhalation, based on the observation that higher pressures are required to maintain upper airway patency during inspiration in sleep compared to expiration (34). Both modalities permit patients to initiate inspiration and expiration and thereby largely determine their own breathing pattern. In patients with OSAH, CPAP is preferred initially over BiPAP based on data demonstrating better compliance with CPAP (35) and the higher costs associated with

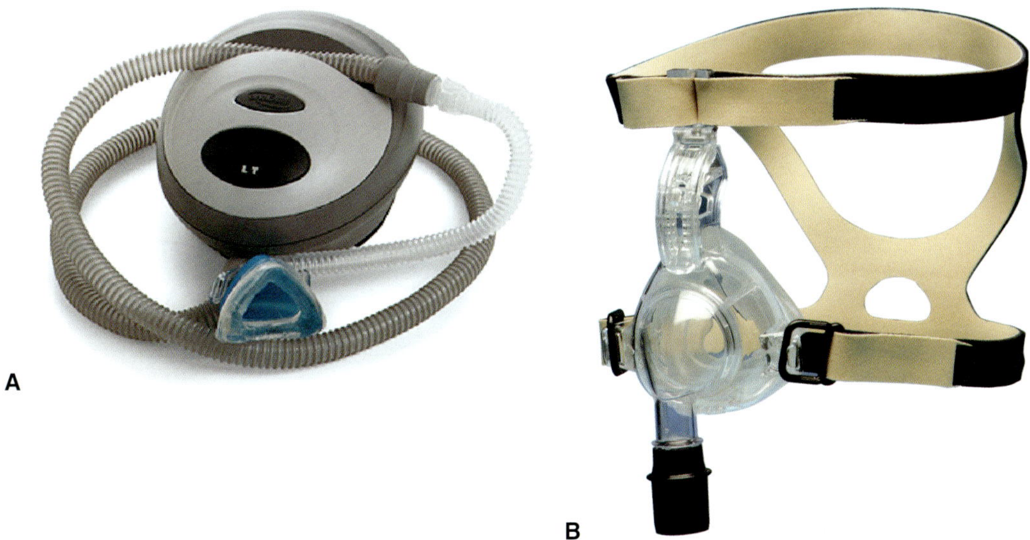

FIGURE 35-2. Continuous positive airway pressure (CPAP) device (A) with face mask (B). (Courtesy of Invacare, Elyria, OH.)

bilevel therapy. However, BiPAP is effective at lower mean airway pressure and may be more comfortable than conventional CPAP (36). In our center, BiPAP is the preferred treatment in patients with concomitant hypoventilation and in those intolerant of CPAP due to nasal discomfort or mouth leaks, difficulty exhaling against an expiratory pressure, or chest discomfort arising from breathing at elevated lung volumes.

Therapeutic positive pressure levels are usually determined during a PSG, conducted in a sleep laboratory during which a technician titrates the CPAP or BiPAP settings to eliminate apneas, hypopneas, oxyhemoglobin desaturation, and sleep fragmentation. Autotitrating CPAP units are also commercially available, but there are no data addressing their efficacy in a bariatric surgery population. These devices incorporate proprietary algorithms designed to "recognize" impending apneas and hypopneas and increase the delivered pressure accordingly. When no further apneas or hypopneas detected over an ensuing time interval, the pressure gradually decreases until events again are again "recognized," precipitating an increase in pressure delivery. These devices are not currently mainstream therapy for OSAH, and their use is not recommended in excessively obese patients, those with obesity hypoventilation syndrome or lung or cardiac disease, and others in whom its safety and efficacy have not been validated (37). Moreover, in our experience, bariatric patients, like most OSAH patients, may have difficulty accommodating to CPAP or BiPAP therapy and benefit from an initial laboratory titration. Positive airway pressure is safe and effective. It is often, but not always, embraced by patients. Poorly fitting masks, nasal dryness or stuffiness, and claustrophobia may interfere with willingness to use positive pressure

therapy. Simple interventions and well-trained sleep technicians can significantly improve compliance with CPAP (38).

Upper airway patency may also be maintained with the use of an oral appliance, fitted by a dentist with experience in this modality in the treatment of OSAH patients. There are a wide variety of oral appliance designs that are intended to stabilize the upper airway during sleep by advancing the mandible to increase the size of the retrolingual airway (Fig. 35-3). Periodontal disease and inadequate dentition to support retention of these appliances are contraindications. Temporomandibular joint disease is also an absolute or relative contraindication (such determinations are usually best made by an appropriately trained and experienced dental practitioner). Although oral appliance therapy is well tolerated and often preferred by patients to CPAP, it is less effective than CPAP, particularly in patients with more pronounced oxygen desaturation (39,40). Use in the United States is limited by lack of insurance coverage. In addition, fitting and advancing the oral appliance often takes several weeks to months, which may not be desirable in a patient planning bariatric surgery. Use of these devices has not been validated in a bariatric population, and lower BMI is a predictor of successful oral appliance therapy (41), suggesting bariatric patients would be suboptimal candidates for their use.

Several surgical procedures are used to treat OSAH. Uvulopalatopharyngoplasty is effective in about 50% of cases, and may be less efficacious in patients with morbid obesity who are more likely to have retrolingual than retropalatal airway obstruction (42–44). Some centers have reported that maxillomandibular osteotomy and advancement procedures cure OSAH in 75% to 90% of

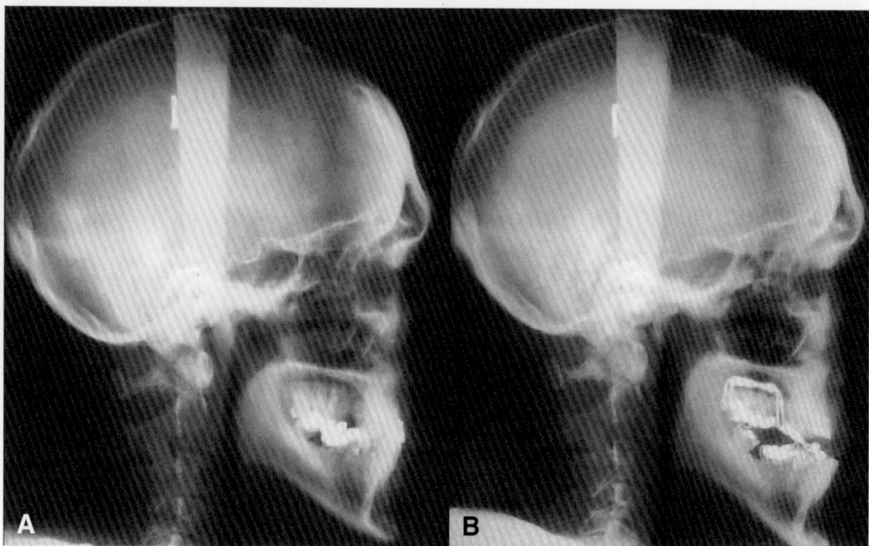

FIGURE 35-3. Lateral cephalogram in a patient with sleep apnea without (A) and with (B) a mandibular repositioning appliance in place. The mandibular reposition appliance advances the mandible forward increasing the size of the retrolingual airway. (Courtesy of Dr. Kathleen Ferguson, University of Western Ontario.)

selected patients, but these individuals were not excessively obese (45,46). Enthusiasm for surgical intervention in morbidly obese patients is diminished by their increased anesthesia and perioperative risks, especially without a high likelihood of successful outcome. Tracheostomy effectively bypasses the site of obstruction in OSAH and so is highly effective. As may be expected, it is not well accepted by patients. However, it is indicated in patients with life-threatening OSAH, especially those who have failed positive pressure therapy. Furthermore, tracheostomy may be the safest therapeutic option for patients with severe OSAH in whom positive pressure therapy has been unsuccessful, patients with obesity-hypoventilation, and patients with severe cardiopulmonary disorders, who are to undergo bariatric surgery.

The decision to treat OSAH is based on a compilation of symptoms and pathophysiologic derangements. Patients with excessive daytime sleepiness, bothersome nocturnal awakenings (especially those associated with sensations of choking, gasping, or smothering), or other symptoms warrant a therapeutic trial, even if the AHI is only moderately increased (AHI >5 but 10 or less). The benefit of treating patients without sleepiness is less clear (47). Bariatric patients often have severe oxygen desaturation that is likely to be even worse in the postoperative period, particularly after receiving narcotics and muscle relaxants. The impact of treating sleep apnea of any severity prior to bariatric surgery has not been investigated prospectively. It is intuitively appealing to consider that effective preoperative treatment will reduce preoperative night hypoxemia and cardiovascular stress as well as decrease upper airway edema with consequently easier and safer airway and peri- and postoperative management. These considerations, as well as the clinical experience that demonstrates that accommodation of some patients to CPAP or BiPAP requires an acclimatization period, suggest that it is prudent to treat these conditions before surgery. In addition, preoperative assessment of therapeutic requirements provides guidelines for postoperative CPAP or BiPAP pressure requirements. The possibility exists for higher pressure requirements in the postoperative period mandating careful monitoring of treatment adequacy (see below).

Effect of Obstructive Sleep Apnea Hypopnea on Outcomes After Bariatric Surgery

Pulmonary and Cardiac Complications

Patients undergoing bariatric surgery have numerous risk factors for pulmonary complications even in the absence of OSAH. Abdominal surgery, particularly upper abdominal surgery, causes reversible impairment in pulmonary function that persists at least 48 hours (48). Early and late postoperative hypoxemia has been observed in otherwise healthy patients undergoing abdominal surgery (49). However, patients with OSAH are at even greater risk. The American Academy of Sleep Medicine has published a short questionnaire to help identify OSAH in patients in whom the disorder has not been investigated (50) (Table 35-3).

Anesthetic agents and narcotics adversely affect upper airway tone, worsening upper airway obstruction, and leading to hypoxic and hypercapnic respiratory failure. Therefore, premedication with opiates or sedatives when the patient is unsupervised prior to intubation should be avoided, and nonopioid analgesia is preferred postoperatively, to the extent possible (51). In addition, patients with OSAH may have a difficult airway, since excess pharyngeal tissue increases the odds of sleep-related upper

TABLE 35-3. Questionnaire for exploring OSAH symptoms

People tell me that I snore.	Y	N
I wake up at night with a feeling of shortness of breath or choking.	Y	N
People tell me that I gasp, choke, or snort while I am sleeping.	Y	N
People tell me that I stop breathing while I am sleeping.	Y	N
I awake feeling almost as tired as, or more tired than, when I went to bed.	Y	N
I often awake with a headache.	Y	N
I often have difficulty breathing through my nose.	Y	N
I fight sleepiness during the day.	Y	N
I fall asleep when I relax before or after dinner.	Y	N
Friends, colleagues, or family comment on my sleepiness.	Y	N

Source: Meoli et al. (50), with permission.

airway obstruction. Intubation and extubation, periods when the potential for loss of airway control is present, are critical times in the management of patients with known or suspected OSAH. Patients should demonstrate return of purposeful movement and recovery from neuromuscular blockade by maneuvers such as sustained head lift for a minimum of 5 seconds before the endotracheal tube is removed. The timing and dose of intraoperative analgesia and sedation must be carefully titrated to achieve pain control without excessive sedation or upper airway compromise.

Unexpected and unexplained postoperative deaths in the first week most commonly occur at night (52), and hypoxemia has been proposed as the most likely mediator of these deaths (53). On the first postoperative night rapid eye movement (REM) sleep decreases significantly, with a rebound in the percentage of REM sleep on postoperative nights 2 and 3. Rapid eye movement sleep is the most vulnerable sleep period for OSAH because neural input to respiratory muscles is maximally inhibited; thus the observed nocturnal hypoxemia may be exacerbated by REM rebound (54).

Most reports of perioperative complications in patients with OSAH concern upper airway surgery to alleviate OSAH; however, complications related to OSAH may occur in any type of surgery. For example, CPAP in the postoperative period in patients with known OSAH undergoing CABG is associated with better outcomes (55). The effect of undiagnosed OSAH on postoperative complications and length of stay was investigated retrospectively in 101 matched pairs of patients with and without sleep apnea, undergoing hip or knee replacement (56). In this study, the incidence of orthopedic complications was the same in both groups; however, the patients with OSAH had 24% incidence of serious complications, defined as an acute cardiac event, unplanned intensive care unit transfer, or need for urgent respiratory support, compared with only 9% of the matched controls. Hospital stay was on average 1.7 days longer for the subjects

with OSAH. Patients treated for OSAH with CPAP did not experience this high rate of cardiac or pulmonary decompensation, albeit in a nonrandomized study. Thus, although no randomized controlled trial evidence proves that therapy for OSAH prevents respiratory complications after bariatric surgery, theoretical considerations and the preponderance of data support its use.

Obstructive sleep apnea hypopnea is associated with cardiac arrhythmias, including atrial fibrillation and supraventricular and ventricular tachycardia, but severe sinus bradycardia and atrioventricular block are reported most commonly (57). The severity of rhythm disturbance correlates with the severity of OSAH and nocturnal desaturation (58). Electrophysiologic studies are usually normal, suggesting that excess vagal tone, generally in the setting of oxyhemoglobin desaturation, is responsible for the bradyarrhythmias (59). Effective treatment for OSAH abolishes these sleep-related arrhythmias without specific cardiac therapy (59–62). The experience in the postoperative period is similar to the findings in patients with OSAH who are not undergoing surgery. Episodes of asymptomatic heart block occurring during sleep postoperatively following weight loss surgery have been reported in three subjects with proven or suspected sleep apnea (63). No subject required pacing, and no syncope was reported even in the absence of therapy for OSAH.

Both OSAH (the Sleep Heart Health Study, SHHS) and obesity are associated with congestive heart failure. Subjects with coexisting structural heart disease and OSAH are likely at increased risk of cardiac complications. Guidelines for intensive care unit or step-down unit of telemetry monitoring vary among institutions. Our practice is to recommend increased monitoring for patients with severe OSAH that has not been adequately treated preoperatively or with OSAH and cardiac disease, as well as for patients with respiratory compromise in the early postoperative period. While the site of monitoring for these higher risk patients (intensive care unit versus step-down unit versus telemetry floor) depends on the patient's acuity and the hospital resources, minimum requirements include continuous pulse oximetry and cardiac monitoring for arrhythmia.

Anastomotic Complications

Two large series of consecutive patients have identified OSAH as a risk factor for postoperative complications, mainly related to the anastomosis. Perugini and colleagues (5) reported a series of 188 patients, 22% with OSAH who underwent laparoscopic Roux-en-Y gastric bypass (RYGBP). Subjects with sleep apnea had three times the odds [95% confidence interval (CI), 1.3–7.1] of suffering a complication that required an invasive therapeutic intervention compared with subjects without OSAH in a multivariate analysis. The only factor more significant than OSAH was the surgeon's experience. The majority of complications reported related to stenosis at the gastrojejunal anastomosis, but a variety of other complications including hemorrhage, hernia, leak or fistula formation, and mortality were also included. The numbers were too small to permit analysis of association between particular complication and OSAH or other comorbidity. The impact of positive pressure therapy for OSAH was not discussed.

Outcomes and risk factors for complications were reported in 3073 patients treated with either open or laparoscopic bariatric procedures at Virginia Commonwealth University (64). In this sample, 23.4% of patients without OSAH developed an anastomotic leak while the rate for patients with OSAH was significantly higher at 34.3% ($p = .0037$). In a multivariate analysis, OSAH was no longer a significant risk factor for leak in the whole sample, while it remained an independent risk in those patients who underwent an open gastric bypass procedure. Again, the influence of treatment for OSAH with CPAP was not addressed. In contrast, Livingston and colleagues (65) did not associate CPAP with increased risk for complications, including increased rate of anastomotic leak, in patients with OSAH.

None of these series identified OSAH as a risk factor for mortality. Severe OSAH was associated with increased hospital costs in one study, likely because of an association with postoperative complications, prolonged ventilatory support, and intensive care unit admission (66).

Positive airway pressure therapy, in which pressurized air is applied to the upper airway via a nasal or oronasal mask, can transmit positive pressure to the gastrointestinal tract. Gastric distention may occur when CPAP is used to treat acute respiratory failure, although the distention tends to be mild and rarely limits therapy. Of note, CPAP may reduce gastroesophageal reflux by virtue of mildly increasing intraesophageal pressure (67) (e.g., mid-esophageal pressure increasing from −3.5 cm to −0.9 cm while on 8 cm of nasal CPAP). Concern has been raised that postoperative positive airway pressure could lead to anastomotic breakdown in the setting of a bowel anastomosis, particularly one that is associated with bypassing the potentially protective area of the pylorus. These problems were not observed in the largest prospective case series to examine the effect of perioperative CPAP therapy, in which there was no difference in the risk of anastomotic leak or pulmonary complications between the 159 subjects treated with CPAP or the 908 subjects not treated with CPAP undergoing RYGBP (68). However, recently two cases of postoperative bowel dilation and anastomotic leak were reported in patients with a history of sleep apnea treated with BiPAP (69). It is uncertain whether these reported cases represent a risk of BiPAP that is greater than the risk of CPAP, or whether

these complications were unrelated to the BiPAP, as the case reports indicated neither the total number of patients who underwent gastric surgery nor the total number of patients with postoperative bowel dilation. Both patients were experienced users of BiPAP, so difficulty accommodating to the machine is unlikely to explain the complications. No studies have examined the relative risk of anastomotic or other complications in patients with OSAH treated with CPAP versus untreated OSAH patients.

Effect of Bariatric Surgery on Severity of Obstructive Sleep Apnea Hypopnea

Weight loss associated with successful bariatric surgery is often also associated with improvement or even cure of OSAH, although the studies to date are limited by incomplete follow-up and lack of confirmatory polysomnography. In the prelaparoscopic era, respiratory insufficiency was initially considered a contraindication to bariatric surgery; however, early case reports and series suggested that surgically induced weight loss was effective therapy for sleep apnea and obesity hypoventilation syndrome in these patients (70–73). Studies that assessed pre– and post–weight loss arterial blood gases during wakefulness or polysomnography measures reported improvement, but not necessarily normalization. Several investigators have noted that patients generally feel their sleep is improved even if OSAH persists (74,75), thus highlighting the need for objective follow-up assessment of sleep and breathing (e.g., PSG), rather than reliance on improved symptoms as a reflection of improved OSAH. One series reported initial improvement in OSAH 4.5 months after weight reduction surgery, followed by recurrence an average of 7.5 years after surgery without intervening weight gain (76).

More recent studies of larger series of patients have noted improvements in snoring, sleep apnea, and daytime sleepiness, although the ability to draw conclusions is limited by the self-report rather than by the objective nature of the data (77,78). Dixon and colleagues (21) reported marked 1-year improvements in self-reported habitual snoring, witnessed apnea, morning headaches, Epworth Sleepiness Score, and sleep quality. This sample included 313 subjects, but only 39% returned for follow-up with a mean weight loss of $31.2 \pm 13.0\,kg$ or $48\% \pm 16\%$ of excess weight loss. Only 10 subjects used CPAP therapy for OSAH preoperatively, and only three required positive pressure therapy after 1 year.

Polysomnographic outcomes of bariatric surgery have been reported in three series of patients. Scheuller et al. (79) reported a series of 15 patients who underwent biliopancreatic bypass or gastroplasty and had polysomnograms preoperatively and at least 1 year after surgery. These patients lost an average 54.7 kg. The average number of sleep-disordered breathing events per hour of sleep fell from 97 to 11 and nocturnal oxygen saturation improved significantly. However, four of the 15 patients still had an AHI >20 despite an average weight loss of 35 kg, but none elected to have treatment for OSAH. Eight subjects had required tracheostomy before weight loss surgery for prolonged apneas and desaturation, and all were decannulated postoperatively. Rasheid and colleagues (80) reported that BMI decreased from 54 ± 1 to 38 ± 1 and the Epworth Sleepiness Scale decreased from 12 ± 0.1 to 6 ± 1 in 100 patients a median of 6 months after gastric bypass. Before surgery, 58 subjects were treated with positive airway pressure therapy, but only 11 returned for a postoperative polysomnogram. In this selected group, AHI fell from 56 ± 13 to 23 ± 7, and oxygen saturation and sleep efficiency improved significantly. Regression analysis did not show correlation between percent of excess weight loss and postoperative AHI in the small sample. In the most recent publication, eight of 34 subjects with OSAH returned for a follow-up sleep study an average of 28 ± 8 months after gastric bypass (81). In this group, the mean reduction in BMI was 13.4 ± 7.8. AHI improved by at least 50% in all subjects except one, but three subjects still had enough sleep apnea to require CPAP therapy.

The data strongly suggests that significant weight loss occurring after bariatric surgery leads to an improvement in symptoms of sleepiness and sleep apnea such as habitual snoring and nonrefreshing sleep. The data on objective improvement in OSAH is less clear, but the preponderance of evidence suggests most subjects improve. Unfortunately, some patients who lose weight still have significant, though perhaps improved, OSAH, and predictors of patients who are less likely to improve their sleep apnea are not yet known. Patients who do not lose weight are unlikely to improve. The substantial loss to follow-up in the studies with objective outcomes allows for considerable bias in the estimate of how much sleep apnea will improve. Patients with the best outcomes who are feeling well may not want to bother returning for follow-up. Alternatively, patients with poorer outcomes may feel discouraged and thus be less likely to comply with follow-up visits.

Conclusion

Obstructive sleep apnea hypopnea is likely to affect between one quarter and three quarters of all patients who undergo bariatric surgery, and the disorder should influence workup and management. The optimal strategy for selecting patients to screen for OSAH has not been determined; however, patients with higher BMI or witnessed apnea are at particularly high risk, and patients with concomitant cardiac or pulmonary disease may have

more severe oxygen desaturation and physiologic derangement. Confirmation of clinical prediction rules like the BASH 'IM acronym will be helpful in identifying patients at low risk of OSAH who do not need further testing. The perioperative period is a time of particular risk for patients with OSAH, particularly unsuspected OSAH. Anesthesiologists participating in the care of bariatric patients should be judicious in the use of sedatives and analgesics and vigilant for signs of airway compromise before and after surgery. Further studies utilizing objective outcomes with longer-term follow-up are necessary to confirm the lasting impact of bariatric surgery on improvement of OSAH, and to identify subsets of patients likely to have good or poor response. Finally, the degree to which CPAP use can mitigate any adverse associations of OSAH with complications following bariatric surgery warrants further study.

References

1. Sleep-related breathing disorders in adults: recommendations for syndrome definition and measurement techniques in clinical research. The Report of an American Academy of Sleep Medicine Task Force. Sleep 1999;22:667–689.
2. Young T, Peppard PE, Gottlieb DJ. Epidemiology of obstructive sleep apnea: a population health perspective. Am J Respir Crit Care Med 2002;165:1217–1239.
3. Young T, Shahar E, Nieto FJ, et al. Predictors of sleep-disordered breathing in community-dwelling adults: The Sleep Heart Health Study. Arch Intern Med 2002;162:893–900.
4. Young T, Palta M, Dempsey J, Skatrud J, Weber S, Badr S. The occurrence of sleep-disordered breathing among middle-aged adults. N Engl J Med 1993;328:1230–1235.
5. Perugini RA, Mason R, Czerniach DR, et al. Predictors of complication and suboptimal weight loss after laparoscopic Roux-en-Y gastric bypass: a series of 188 patients. Arch Surg 2003;138:541–545; discussion 545–546.
6. Fernandez AZ Jr, Demaria EJ, Tichansky DS, et al. Multivariate analysis of risk factors for death following gastric bypass for treatment of morbid obesity. Ann Surg 2004; 239:698–702; discussion 702–703.
7. Schauer PR, Ikramuddin S, Gourash W, Ramanathan R, Luketich J. Outcomes after laparoscopic Roux-en-Y gastric bypass for morbid obesity. Ann Surg 2000;232:515–529.
8. O'Keeffe T, Patterson EJ. Evidence supporting routine polysomnography before bariatric surgery. Obes Surg 2004; 14:23–26.
9. Frey WC, Pilcher J. Obstructive sleep-related breathing disorders in patients evaluated for bariatric surgery. Obes Surg 2003;13:676–683.
10. Serafini FM, MacDowell Anderson W, Rosemurgy AS, Strait T, Murr MM. Clinical predictors of sleep apnea in patients undergoing bariatric surgery. Obes Surg 2001;11: 28–31.
11. Akashiba T, Kawahara S, Kosaka N, et al. Determinants of chronic hypercapnia in Japanese men with obstructive sleep apnea syndrome. Chest 2002;121:415–421.

12. Kessler R, Chaouat A, Schinkewitch P, et al. The obesity-hypoventilation syndrome revisited: a prospective study of 34 consecutive cases. Chest 2001;120:369–376.

13. Kimoff RJ, Cosio MG, McGregor M. Clinical features and treatment of obstructive sleep apnea. Can Med Assoc J 1991;144:689–695.

14. Pressman MR, Figueroa WG, Kendrick-Mohamed J, Greenspon LW, Peterson DD. Nocturia. A rarely recognized symptom of sleep apnea and other occult sleep disorders. Arch Intern Med 1996;156:545–550.

15. Loh NK, Dinner DS, Foldvary N, Skobieranda F, Yew WW. Do patients with obstructive sleep apnea wake up with headaches? Arch Intern Med 1999;159:1765–1768.

16. Ohayon MM. The effects of breathing-related sleep disorders on mood disturbances in the general population. J Clin Psychiatry 2003;64:1195–200; quiz, 1274–1276.

17. Gottlieb DJ, Whitney CW, Bonekat WH, et al. Relation of sleepiness to respiratory disturbance index: the Sleep Heart Health Study. Am J Respir Crit Care Med 1999;159: 502–507.

18. Foley D, Ancoli-Israel S, Britz P, Walsh J. Sleep disturbances and chronic disease in older adults: results of the 2003 National Sleep Foundation Sleep in America Survey. J Psychosom Res 2004;56:497–502.

19. Vgontzas AN, Bixler EO, Tan T-L, Kantner D, Martin LF, Kales A. Obesity without sleep apnea is associated with daytime sleepiness. Arch Intern Med 1998;158:1333–1337.

20. Vgontzas AN, Papanicolaou DA, Bixler EO, et al. Sleep apnea and daytime sleepiness and fatigue: relation to visceral obesity, insulin resistance, and hypercytokinemia. J Clin Endocrinol Metab 2000;85:1151–1158.

21. Dixon JB, Schachter LM, O'Brien PE. Sleep disturbance and obesity: changes following surgically induced weight loss. Arch Intern Med 2001;161:102–106.

22. Peppard PE, Young T, Palta M, Skatrud J. Prospective study of the association between sleep-disordered breathing and hypertension. N Engl J Med 2000;342:1378–1384.

23. Shahar E, Whitney CW, Redline S, et al. Sleep-disordered breathing and cardiovascular disease: cross-sectional results of the Sleep Heart Health Study. Am J Respir Crit Care Med 2001;163:19–25.

24. Resnick HE, Redline S, Shahar E, et al. Diabetes and sleep disturbances: findings from the Sleep Heart Health Study. Diabetes Care 2003;26:702–709.

25. Punjabi NM, Sorkin JD, Katzel LI, Goldberg AP, Schwartz AR, Smith PL. Sleep-disordered breathing and insulin resistance in middle-aged and overweight men. Am J Respir Crit Care Med 2002;165:677–682.

26. Teran-Santos J, Jimenez-Gomez A, Cordero-Guevara J. The association between sleep apnea and the risk of traffic accidents. Cooperative Group Burgos-Santander. N Engl J Med 1999;340:847–851.

27. Chervin RD. Sleepiness, fatigue, tiredness, and lack of energy in obstructive sleep apnea. Chest 2000;118:372–379.

28. Young T, Hutton R, Finn L, Badr S, Palta M. The gender bias in sleep apnea diagnosis. Are women missed because they have different symptoms? Arch Intern Med 1996; 156:2445–2451.

29. Johns MW. A new method for measuring daytime sleepiness: the Epworth Sleepiness Scale. Sleep 1991;14:540–545.

30. Dixon JB, O'Brien PE. Predicting sleep apnea and excessive day sleepiness in the severely obese: indicators for polysomnography. Chest 2003;123:1134–1141.

31. Maislin G, Pack AI, Kribbs NB, et al. A survey screen for prediction of apnea. Sleep 1995;18:158–166.

32. Chesson AL Jr, Berry RB, Pack A. Practice parameters for the use of portable monitoring devices in the investigation of suspected obstructive sleep apnea in adults. Sleep 2003; 26:907–913.

33. Baltzan MA, Verschelden P, Al-Jahdali H, Olha AE, Kimoff RJ. Accuracy of oximetry with thermistor (OxiFlow) for diagnosis of obstructive sleep apnea and hypopnea. Sleep 2000;23:61–69.

34. Schwab RJ, Gefter WB, Hoffman EA, Gupta KB, Pack AI. Dynamic upper airway imaging during awake respiration in normal subjects and patients with sleep disordered breathing. Am Rev Respir Dis 1993;148:1385–1400.

35. Reeves-Hoche MK, Hudgel DW, Meck R, Witteman R, Ross A, Zwillich CW. Continuous versus bilevel positive airway pressure for obstructive sleep apnea. Am J Respir Crit Care Med 1995;151:443–449.

36. Sanders MH, Kern N. Obstructive sleep apnea treated by independently adjusted inspiratory and expiratory positive airway pressures via nasal mask. Physiologic and clinical implications. Chest 1990;98:317–324.

37. Littner M, Hirshkowitz M, Davila D, et al. Practice parameters for the use of auto-titrating continuous positive airway pressure devices for titrating pressures and treating adult patients with obstructive sleep apnea syndrome. An American Academy of Sleep Medicine report. Sleep 2002;25:143–147.

38. Chervin RD, Theut S, Bassetti C, Aldrich MS. Compliance with nasal CPAP can be improved by simple interventions. Sleep 1997;20:284–289.

39. Ferguson KA, Ono T, Lowe AA, Keenan SP, Fleetham JA. A randomized crossover study of an oral appliance vs nasal-continuous positive airway pressure in the treatment of mild-moderate obstructive sleep apnea. Chest 1996;109: 1269–1275.

40. Ferguson KA, Ono T, Lowe AA, al-Majed S, Love LL, Fleetham JA. A short-term controlled trial of an adjustable oral appliance for the treatment of mild to moderate obstructive sleep apnoea. Thorax 1997;52:362–368.

41. Liu Y, Lowe AA, Fleetham JA, Park YC. Cephalometric and physiologic predictors of the efficacy of an adjustable oral appliance for treating obstructive sleep apnea. Am J Orthod Dentofacial Orthop 2001;120:639–647.

42. Larsson LH, Carlsson-Nordlander B, Svanborg E. Four-year follow-up after uvulopalatopharyngoplasty in 50 unselected patients with obstructive sleep apnea syndrome. Laryngoscope 1994;104:1362–1368.

43. Sher AE, Schechtman KB, Piccirillo JF. The efficacy of surgical modifications of the upper airway in adults with obstructive sleep apnea syndrome. Sleep 1996;19:156–177.

44. Walker-Engstrom ML, Tegelberg A, Wilhelmsson B, Ringqvist I. 4-year follow-up of treatment with dental appliance or uvulopalatopharyngoplasty in patients with obstructive sleep apnea: a randomized study. Chest 2002; 121:739–746.

45. Riley RW, Powell NB, Li KK, Troell RJ, Guilleminault C. Surgery and obstructive sleep apnea: long-term clinical outcomes. Otolaryngol Head Neck Surg 2000;122:415–421.

46. Hochban W, Conradt R, Brandenburg U, Heitmann J, Peter JH. Surgical maxillofacial treatment of obstructive sleep apnea. Plast Reconstr Surg 1997;99:619–626; discussion 627–628.

47. Barbe F, Mayoralas LR, Duran J, et al. Treatment with continuous positive airway pressure is not effective in patients with sleep apnea but no daytime sleepiness: a randomized, controlled trial. Ann Intern Med 2001;134:1015–1023.

48. Meyers JR, Lembeck L, O'Kane H, Baue AE. Changes in functional residual capacity of the lung after operation. Arch Surg 1975;110:576–583.

49. Siler JN, Rosenberg H, Mull TD, Kaplan JA, Bardin H, Marshall BE. Hypoxemia after upper abdominal surgery: comparison of venous admixture and ventilation-perfusion inequality components, using a digital computer. Ann Surg 1974;179:149–155.

50. Meoli AL, Rosen CL, Kristo D, et al. Upper airway management of the adult patient with obstructive sleep apnea in the perioperative period—avoiding complications. Sleep 2003;26:1060–1065.

51. Boushra NN. Anaesthetic management of patients with sleep apnoea syndrome. Can J Anaesth 1996;43:599–616.

52. Rosenberg J, Pedersen MH, Ramsing T, Kehlet H. Circadian variation in unexpected postoperative death. Br J Surg 1992;79:1300–1302.

53. Rosenberg-Adamsen S, Kehlet H, Dodds C, Rosenberg J. Postoperative sleep disturbances: mechanisms and clinical implications. Br J Anaesth 1996;76:552–559.

54. Rosenberg J, Wildschiodtz G, Pedersen MH, von Jessen F, Kehlet H. Late postoperative nocturnal episodic hypoxaemia and associated sleep pattern. Br J Anaesth 1994; 72:145–150.

55. Rennotte M, Baele P, Aubert G, Rodenstein D. Nasal continuous positive airway pressure in the perioperative management of patients with obstructive sleep apnea submitted to surgery. Chest 1995;107:367–374.

56. Gupta RM, Parvizi J, Hanssen AD, Gay PC. Postoperative complications in patients with obstructive sleep apnea syndrome undergoing hip or knee replacement: a case-control study. Mayo Clin Proc 2001;76:897–905.

57. Guilleminault C, Connolly SJ, Winkle RA. Cardiac arrhythmia and conduction disturbances during sleep in 400 patients with sleep apnea syndrome. Am J Cardiol 1983;52: 490–494.

58. Roche F, Xuong AN, Court-Fortune I, et al. Relationship among the severity of sleep apnea syndrome, cardiac arrhythmias, and autonomic imbalance. Pacing Clin Electrophysiol 2003;26:669–677.

59. Grimm W, Koehler U, Fus E, et al. Outcome of patients with sleep apnea-associated severe bradyarrhythmias after continuous positive airway pressure therapy. Am J Cardiol 2000;86:688–692.

60. Becker HF, Koehler U, Stammnitz A, Peter JH. Heart block in patients with sleep apnoea. Thorax 1998;53:29S–32.

61. Harbison J, O'Reilly P, McNicholas WT. Cardiac rhythm disturbances in the obstructive sleep apnea syndrome: effects of nasal continuous positive airway pressure therapy. Chest 2000;118:591–595.

62. Fichter J, Bauer D, Arampatzis S, Fries R, Heisel A, Sybrecht GW. Sleep-related breathing disorders are associated with ventricular arrhythmias in patients with an implantable cardioverter-defibrillator. Chest 2002;122:558–561.

63. Block M, Jacobson LB, Rabkin RA. Heart block in patients after bariatric surgery accompanying sleep apnea. Obes Surg 2001;11:627–630.

64. Fernandez AZ Jr, DeMaria EJ, Tichansky DS, et al. Experience with over 3,000 open and laparoscopic bariatric procedures: multivariate analysis of factors related to leak and resultant mortality. Surg Endosc 2004;18:193–197. Epub 2003 Dec 29.

65. Livingston EH, Huerta S, Arthur D, Lee S, De Shields S, Heber D. Male gender is a predictor of morbidity and age a predictor of mortality for patients undergoing gastric bypass surgery. Ann Surg 2002;236:576–582.

66. Cooney RN, Haluck RS, Ku J, et al. Analysis of cost outliers after gastric bypass surgery: what can we learn? Obes Surg 2003;13:29–36.

67. Fournier MR, Kerr PD, Shoenut JP, Yaffe CS. Effect of nasal continuous positive airway pressure on esophageal function. J Otolaryngol 1999;28:142–144.

68. Huerta S, DeShields S, Shpiner R, et al. Safety and efficacy of postoperative continuous positive airway pressure to prevent pulmonary complications after Roux-en-Y gastric bypass. J Gastrointest Surg 2002;6:354–358.

69. Vasquez TL, Hoddinott K. A potential complication of bilevel positive airway pressure after gastric bypass surgery. Obes Surg 2004;14:282–284.

70. Victor DW Jr, Sarmiento CF, Yanta M, Halverson JD. Obstructive sleep apnea in the morbidly obese. An indication for gastric bypass. Arch Surg 1984;119:970–972.

71. Sugerman HJ, Fairman RP, Lindeman AK, Mathers JA, Greenfield LJ. Gastroplasty for respiratory insufficiency of obesity. Ann Surg 1981;193:677–685.

72. Hamazoe R, Furumoto T, Kaibara N, Inoue Y. Vertical banded gastroplasty for sleep apnea syndrome associated with morbid obesity. Obes Surg 1992;2:271–274.

73. Boone KA, Cullen JJ, Mason EE, Scott DH, Doherty C, Maher JW. Impact of vertical banded gastroplasty on respiratory insufficiency of severe obesity. Obes Surg 1996;6: 454–458.

74. Sugerman HJ, Fairman RP, Sood RK, Engle K, Wolfe L, Kellum JM. Long-term effects of gastric surgery for treating respiratory insufficiency of obesity. Am J Clin Nutr 1992;55:597S–601S.

75. Charuzi I, Lavie P, Peiser J, Peled R. Bariatric surgery in morbidly obese sleep-apnea patients: short- and long-term follow-up. Am J Clin Nutr 1992;55:594S–596S.

76. Pillar G, Peled R, Lavie P. Recurrence of sleep apnea without concomitant weight increase 7.5 years after weight reduction surgery. Chest 1994;106:1702–1704.

77. Dhabuwala A, Cannan RJ, Stubbs RS. Improvement in co-morbidities following weight loss from gastric bypass surgery. Obes Surg 2000;10:428–435.

78. Frigg A, Peterli R, Peters T, Ackermann C, Tondelli P. Reduction in co-morbidities 4 years after laparoscopic adjustable gastric banding. Obes Surg 2004;14:216–223.

79. Scheuller M, Weider D. Bariatric surgery for treatment of sleep apnea syndrome in 15 morbidly obese patients: long-term results. Otolaryngol Head Neck Surg 2001;125:299–302.

80. Rasheid S, Banasiak M, Gallagher SF, et al. Gastric bypass is an effective treatment for obstructive sleep apnea in patients with clinically significant obesity. Obes Surg 2003; 13:58–61.

81. Guardiano SA, Scott JA, Ware JC, Schechner SA. The long-term results of gastric bypass on indexes of sleep apnea. Chest 2003;124:1615–1619.

36
Ventral Hernias in the Bariatric Patient

Paul A. Thodiyil and George M. Eid

Ventral hernia, a collective term for incisional, umbilical, and other anterior abdominal wall hernias, are common occurrences in the morbidly obese population. The correct management of these hernias in the morbidly obese has an important bearing on the overall outcome of the surgical management of this group of patients. Morbidly obese patients who have concurrent ventral hernias pose a therapeutic dilemma for two reasons: their weight predisposes them to a high recurrence rate, and the field contamination that invariably accompanies opening bowel in the operative field precludes the use of prosthetic meshes. In addition, new incisional hernias have been common long-term complications of open bariatric surgical procedures.

Epidemiology and Risk Factors

Incisional hernias complicate 3% to 13% of laparotomies in the general surgical population (1) and as many as 20% of morbidly obese patients undergoing an open gastric bypass (2). They are more common in the older population, mean age 51 (3), with a male-to-female ratio of 1.6:1. Umbilical hernias are also relatively common, and most likely occur in the fifth and sixth decades of life (3,4). Still, many hernias remain undetected until patients undergo another procedure; Nassar et al. (5) report a 12% incidence of umbilical or paraumbilical defects in patients undergoing laparoscopic cholecystectomy.

Etiology

Morbid obesity is a major risk factor for incisional hernias, with about 20% of patients undergoing open gastric bypass developing an incisional hernia. It has been considered to be five times more potent as a risk factor compared to chronic steroid use (2). Within the morbidly obese population undergoing gastric bypass surgery, previous incisional hernia, severe wound infection, type 2 diabetes, sleep apnea, and obesity hypoventilation are independently associated with increased risk. On the other hand, preoperative weight, gender, and age do not appear to be associated with increased risk of incisional hernia formation (2).

Primary hernias, like umbilical hernias, tend to be an acquired defect in over 90% of adults (6). About 8% of these are recurrent, with omental incarceration in 30%. The average size of the hernia defect in this population is $25.4\,\mathrm{cm}^2$ with multiple defects in 5% (7).

Clinical Presentation

While most patients with a ventral hernia present with a bulge on the abdominal wall, this may not be the case in a morbidly obese patient where the diagnosis presents a challenge (8). Morbidly obese patients may present for the first time with abdominal pain, nausea, or small bowel obstruction. It should be noted that due to patient body habitus, it is difficult to feel the hernia defect due to a thick abdominal wall, and a computed tomography (CT) scan of the abdomen may be warranted (9). As a matter of fact, in about 10% of morbidly obese patients, the diagnosis is first made intraoperatively.

Treatment

The challenge of managing ventral hernias in the morbidly obese patient arises from the dangers of deferring surgical repair and the risk of mesh infection where repair is undertaken concurrently with gastric bypass. In the authors' experience, 36% of patients whose hernia repair was deferred at the time of gastric bypass develop small bowel obstruction due to incarceration in the postoperative period. The time interval for this complication is an average of 63 days (range 10–150 days) from the gastric bypass. The risk of infecting a prosthetic mesh by contamination with enteric contents is also well documented.

There have been considerable advances in the surgical repair of abdominal wall hernias, from the open primary repair to the laparoscopic approach using prosthetic meshes. Primary open repair is attended by high recurrence rates (49%) (10–12), in large part due to the considerable tension in the repair line with subsequent ischemic failure of the wound as well as high risk of wound infection. The development of the concept of tension-free repair has had a major impact with reduced recurrence (8% to 17%) with the use of prosthetic materials (13,14).

However, the use of mesh in open repair is associated with increased wound complications and infections (15,16). Prefascial polypropylene mesh repair is complicated by minor wound infection (12%), major wound infection (5%), seroma (5%), hematoma (3%), and chronic pain (6%), with a 4% incidence of recurrent hernia at 20 months (2).

Further advances in the tension-free concept have come from the understanding of the mechanics of intraabdominal pressure. By placing the mesh posterior to the deep fascia, a rise in intraabdominal pressure has the effect of further bolstering the repair. This underlies the principle of the open Rives-Stoppa technique, which has been taken a step further by deploying it through a transperitoneal laparoscopic approach (11,15) using an inlay prosthetic mesh, with a resultant reduction in recurrence rates to 0% to 5% (17–19). In addition to allowing a wide overlay of the defect, the laparoscopic view may identify otherwise unrecognized multiple fascial defects.

The technique we use to place the mesh during the closing stages of the laparoscopic gastric bypass (LGB) is based on the modified Rives-Stoppa technique. This involves reduction of the hernia, and under laparoscopic vision, outlining the hernia defect on anterior abdominal wall skin using a marker pen. A further outline adds an extra 3-cm overlay margin. A rehydrated mesh of biomaterial mesh is placed and then tailored to size using the outline on the abdominal wall. Nonabsorbable sutures are placed onto the corners of the mesh, which is then rolled up and introduced into the abdomen through a trocar. Using a Carter-Thomason device, the mesh is anchored into the desired position using the previously placed sutures. The mesh is further anchored with several titanium helical tacks placed circumferentially at about 1-cm intervals. Through several small stab incisions, the mesh is secured in place using nonabsorbable sutures at 3-cm intervals along its circumference, placed with the Carter-Thomason device.

The laparoscopic approach with mesh has many advantages over the open technique, especially in a reduced incidence of wound complications (17,20,21). However, the laparoscopic approach is complicated by seroma formation (16,22–24) occurring in 21% to 32% of patients. The seroma typically is an accumulation of serous fluid in the potential space between the mesh and the anterior abdominal wall. The natural history of seromas, in a prospective study using ultrasound (25), showed peak volumes in 100% of patients on day 7, with 80% resolving by day 90. The majority of these resolve spontaneously or with repeated aspiration and only 0.2% of patients require reexploration at 6 weeks (26).

The considerations for umbilical hernia repair are slightly different from the incisional hernia, as the former tends to be a smaller defect with a healthier muscle and fascial layer. Open umbilical herniorrhaphy using suture technique has been widely used over the last century. Despite attempts to vary suturing techniques, primary repair of umbilical hernias yielded unfavorable results with recurrence rates of 10% to 20% (27,28). These rates have been markedly reduced to 1% with the use of mesh to achieve a tension-free repair (27). However, the use of synthetic mesh for repair of umbilical hernias may not be appropriate when combined with another procedure that violates a biliary or enteric lumen, because of the potential risk of contamination and chronic wound infection.

Laparoscopic transfascial suture repair of these defects, an approach that allows wider fascial closure, may offer an attractive alternative in these cases. In the course of the primary operation, if incarcerated omentum was encountered, blunt dissection was performed to reduce it. A 2-mm stab incision is performed over the umbilicus to allow for the insertion of the tip of the Carter-Thomason device (29). Using the device, and under direct vision, a nonabsorbable suture is introduced into the abdominal cavity on one side of the defect and retrieved back on the other side of the defect after once more passing the Carter-Thomason device, as shown in Figure 36-1. At least three sutures are placed across the fascial defect and left untied (Fig. 36-2). After all sutures are placed, the pneumoperitoneum pressure is released and the sutures are then tied. The suture knots are buried under the skin and the incision is closed with a subcutaneous suture.

For the patient undergoing an LGB who is incidentally found to have one or more ventral hernias, every available option is suboptimal. Primary repair invites well-known failure rates (22% to 49%) (7,10), while use of synthetic materials in the contaminated field risks a graft infection with subsequent failure. Deferring repair until significant weight loss has been shown to be dangerous, with 36% of patients developing small bowel obstruction within a 6-month period (7). The use of absorbable mesh (e.g., Vicryl mesh) is associated with recurrence rates of 75% (30) and may not be a viable option.

The advent of newer biomaterial mesh may make ventral hernia repair in this group more successful. They provide a collagen framework containing several growth factors (31) that encourages native tissue in-growth into the collagen matrix that is gradually and completely reab-

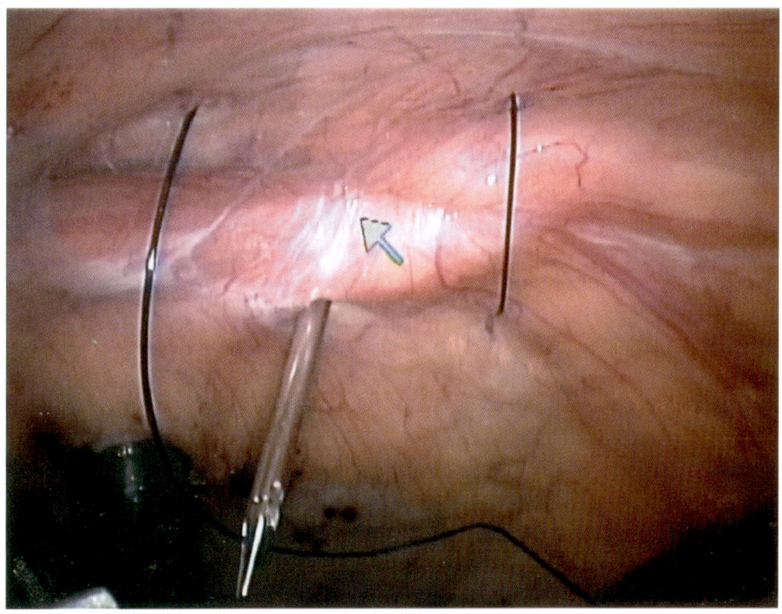

Figure 36-1. A Carter-Thomason device is used to introduce and then retrieve a nonabsorbable suture into the abdominal cavity on either side of the defect (arrow).

sorbed (30). Its potential to act as a focus of infection is minimal, making it more suitable for use in contaminated fields.

In the largest study of ventral hernia management in patients undergoing LGB (7), the lowest recurrence rate (0/12 at 13 months) was obtained with biomaterial mesh compared to a primary repair. Seroma formation is common, with most resolving without specific intervention. About 8% (1/12) develop wound cellulites that resolve with antibiotics. With adequate preoperative and postoperative patient counseling and perseverance, a satisfactory outcome is achieved. Two patients developed persistent focal wound pain that responded to one or two local infiltrations with bupivacaine.

In this study, umbilical hernias that were smaller than 3 to 4 cm in diameter were closed primarily with transfixion transabdominal suture using a technique similar to that used for closure of 12-mm trocar sites. Unfortunately, recurrence rate with this method was 22%. However, in defects smaller than 2 cm, there were no recurrences (0/8) at 36 months' follow-up (3). This suggests that for defects larger than 2 cm, a Rives-Stoppa type of tension-free repair with a biomaterial graft would be a preferred option.

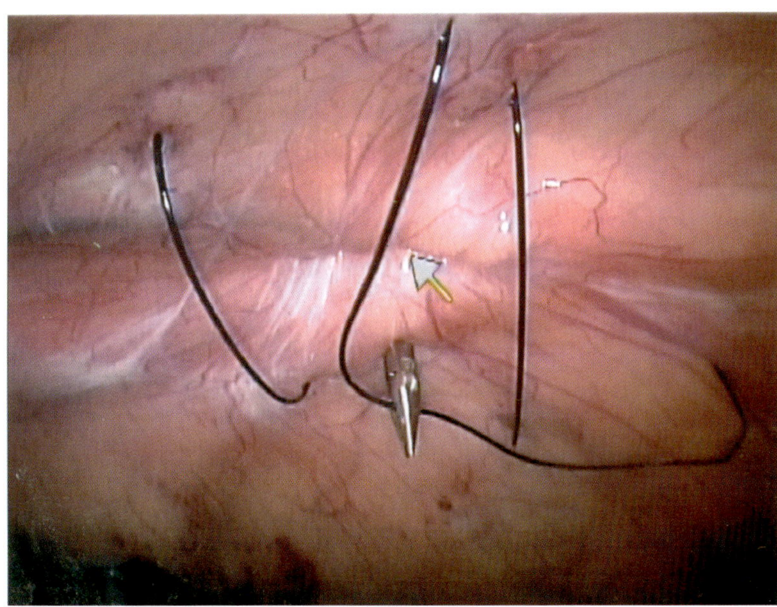

Figure 36-2. At least three sutures are placed across the fascial defect (arrow) but only tied after release of the pneumoperitoneum.

Clinical Pearls

Hernias still present a therapeutic challenge in the morbidly obese. It is important to make the morbidly obese patient aware of the potential intraoperative discovery of incidental hernias and the high risk of recurrence associated with their repair. It is also essential to repair all incisional hernias in the morbidly obese population undergoing bariatric surgery, especially in the presence of omental incarceration (7), because of the high risk of strangulating bowel obstruction in the postoperative period.

Reinforcing all defects with biomaterial mesh has been suggested in an attempt to reduce recurrence. If the defects are small (<2 cm diameter), these could be repaired using the Carter-Thomson suture device with figure-of-8 stitches. If large (≥2 cm diameter), the use of biomaterial mesh can be a viable option for a repair concurrent with the gastric bypass (3). However, for defects larger than 5 cm in diameter, the authors suggest a formal hernia repair using a dual layer [expanded polytetrafluoroethylene (PTFE) polypropylene] mesh as previously described (32) at least 3 months prior to a gastric bypass. With the PTFE side facing the peritoneal cavity, adhesions are minimal at reexploration.

References

1. Mudge M, Hughes LE. Incisional hernia: a 10 year prospective study of incidence and attitudes. Br J Surg 1985;72:70–71.
2. Sugerman HJ, et al. Greater risk of incisional hernia with morbidly obese than steroid-dependent patients and low recurrence with prefascial polypropylene mesh. Am J Surg 1996;171:80–84.
3. Eid GM, et al. Laparoscopic repair of umbilical hernias in conjunction with other laparoscopic procedures. JSLS 2006;10:63–65.
4. Harmel RP. Umbilical hernia. In: Nyhus LM, Condon RE. eds. Hernia. Philadelphia: Lippincott, 1989;347–352.
5. Nassar AH, Ashkar KA, Rashed AA, Abdulmoneum MG. Laparoscopic cholecystectomy and the umbilicus. Br J Surg 1997;84:630–633.
6. Morgan WW, White JJ, Stumbaugh S, Haller JA Jr. Prophylactic umbilical hernia repair in childhood to prevent adult incarceration. Surg Clin North Am 1970;50:839–845.
7. Eid GM, et al. Repair of ventral hernias in morbidly obese patients undergoing laparoscopic gastric bypass should not be deferred. Surg Endosc 2004;18:207–210.
8. Ianora AA, Midiri M, Vinci R, Rotondo A, Angelelli G. Abdominal wall hernias: imaging with spiral CT. Eur Radiol 2000;10:914–919.
9. Rubio PA, Del Castillo H, Alvarez BA. Ventral hernia in a massively obese patient: diagnosis by computerized tomography. South Med J 1988;81:1307–1308.
10. Anthony T, et al. Factors affecting recurrence following incisional herniorrhaphy. World J Surg 2000;24:95–100; discussion 101.
11. van der Linden FT, van Vroonhoven TJ. Long-term results after surgical correction of incisional hernia. Neth J Surg 1988;40:127–129.
12. Hesselink VJ, Luijendijk RW, de Wilt JH, Heide R, Jeekel J. An evaluation of risk factors in incisional hernia recurrence. Surg Gynecol Obstet 1993;176:228–234.
13. Liakakos T, Karanikas I, Panagiotidis H, Dendrinos S. Use of Marlex mesh in the repair of recurrent incisional hernia. Br J Surg 1994;81:248–249.
14. Rios A, et al. Factors that affect recurrence after incisional herniorrhaphy with prosthetic material. Eur J Surg 2001;167:855–859.
15. Stoppa RE. The treatment of complicated groin and incisional hernias. World J Surg 1989;13:545–554.
16. White TJ, Santos MC, Thompson JS. Factors affecting wound complications in repair of ventral hernias. Am Surg 1998;64:276–280.
17. Ramshaw BJ, et al. Comparison of laparoscopic and open ventral herniorrhaphy. Am Surg 1999;65:827–831; discussion 831–832.
18. Birgisson G, Park AE, Mastrangelo MJ Jr, Witzke DB, Chu UB. Obesity and laparoscopic repair of ventral hernias. Surg Endosc 2001;15:1419–1422.
19. Costanza MJ, Heniford BT, Arca MJ, Mayes JT, Gagner M. Laparoscopic repair of recurrent ventral hernias. Am Surg 1998;64:1121–1125; discussion 1126–1127.
20. Park A, Birch DW, Lovrics P. Laparoscopic and open incisional hernia repair: a comparison study. Surgery 1998;124:816–821; discussion 821–822.
21. Holzman MD, Purut CM, Reintgen K, Eubanks S, Pappas TN. Laparoscopic ventral and incisional hernioplasty. Surg Endosc 1997;11:32–35.
22. Chowbey PK, et al. Laparoscopic ventral hernia repair. J Laparoendosc Adv Surg Tech A 2000;10:79–84.
23. Temudom T, Siadati M, Sarr MG. Repair of complex giant or recurrent ventral hernias by using tension-free intraparietal prosthetic mesh (Stoppa technique): lessons learned from our initial experience (fifty patients). Surgery 1996;120:738–743; discussion 743–744.
24. Leber GE, Garb JL, Alexander AI, Reed WP. Long-term complications associated with prosthetic repair of incisional hernias. Arch Surg 1998;133:378–382.
25. Susmallian S, Gewurtz G, Ezri T, Charuzi I. Seroma after laparoscopic repair of hernia with PTFE patch: is it really a complication? Hernia 2001;5:139–141.
26. Schwab JR, et al. After 10 years and 1903 inguinal hernias, what is the outcome for the laparoscopic repair? Surg Endosc 2002;16:1201–1206.
27. Arroyo A, et al. Randomized clinical trial comparing suture and mesh repair of umbilical hernia in adults. Br J Surg 2001;88:1321–1323.
28. Celdran A, Bazire P, Garcia-Urena MA, Marijuan JL. H-hernioplasty: a tension-free repair for umbilical hernia. Br J Surg 1995;82:371–372.
29. Carter JE. A new technique of fascial closure for laparoscopic incisions. J Laparoendosc Surg 1994;4:143–148.

30. Dayton MT, Buchele BA, Shirazi SS, Hunt LB. Use of an absorbable mesh to repair contaminated abdominal-wall defects. Arch Surg 1986;121:954–960.

31. Voytik-Harbin SL, Brightman AO, Kraine MR, Waisner B, Badylak SF. Identification of extractable growth factors from small intestinal submucosa. J Cell Biochem 1997;67: 478–491.

32. Eid GM, et al. Medium-term follow-up confirms the safety and durability of laparoscopic ventral hernia repair with PTFE. Surgery 2003;134:599–603; discussion 603–604.

37
Plastic Surgery Following Weight Loss

Dennis Hurwitz

Minimally invasive gastrointestinal bypass surgery for morbid obesity is being successfully applied at the University of Pittsburgh Bariatric Center (1). With over 1000 patients treated last year, the demand for body contouring has skyrocketed. Following massive weight loss, these patients develop disheartening changes in body contour with repulsive hanging skin and bizarre rolls of skin and fat. In the course of achieving extraordinary weight loss and alleviation of comorbidities, successful bariatric surgery creates these problems that diminish patients' quality of life. Our Bariatric Center clinical staff anticipates these issues and encourages completion of rehabilitation through skilled body contouring surgery.

Over the past decade, many plastic surgeons agree that skin redundancy of the trunk and thigh is best treated by a circumferential abdominoplasty and a lower body lift (2–8). However, results vary, and there is no consensus on technique. There are few reports that include body contouring surgery after massive weight loss, and none after minimally invasive surgery. Hence, I explored a variety of approaches, procedures, and positioning. An innovative technique evolved. Consistent patterns of deformity were discovered, necessitating individualization of procedures. These are extensive and complex operations over large portions of the body, running from 6 to 12 hours under general anesthesia, with significant risks.

By diligent assessment of outcomes and feedback from numerous presentations at scientific meetings, treatment for body contouring has been developed that can be tailored to the deformities and desires of the patient. A complete medical evaluation and comprehensive consideration of the total body deformity is essential. The plan is based on the application of basic plastic surgical principles that incorporate artistry, efficiency, and tight closures, with minimal trauma to tissues (Table 37-1).

This chapter presents the patient profile, operative planning, and a summary of the operative technique, as well as selected cases. The principles of treatment are detailed, followed by an evaluation of the surgical outcomes. From March 2000 to July 2003, the author has performed 208 procedures on 54 patients after massive weight loss. These include abdominoplasty ($n = 48$), lower body lift ($n = 44$), upper body lift ($n = 15$), medial thighplasty ($n = 34$), vertical medial thighplasty ($n = 7$), brachioplasty ($n = 17$), mastopexy/breast reduction ($n = 19$), facelift ($n = 8$), gynecomastia corrections ($n = 8$), and other cosmetic procedures ($n = 8$). None of the patients had a body mass index (BMI) over 35. Due to the high rate of complications, we have not treated patients with severe obesity (9).

Patient Profile

Obesity is a stigmatizing disorder, especially among women, which may explain why women predominate in seeking treatment (2). The increased demand is due to word of mouth comments on the improved results and lower morbidity, supported by reports in scientific journals, the Internet, and the media (10). Eighty-four percent of the patients in this series seeking body contouring after weight loss are women.

Most patients report that the laparoscopic bypass operation was brief, followed by easily controlled pain. Through five or six small incisions their peritoneal cavity has been inflated to expose intestines for rerouting over what has routinely become a 2- to 3-hour session. They are discharged within days to return to work within a week. Those who are converted to open procedures due to technical considerations tend to have a slightly more prolonged postoperative course. Delayed wound healing and incisional hernia are common in the open group.

With small gastric pouches and a moderately long Roux-en-Y jejunal bypass [the length varies directly with the degree of obesity (11)], the patients shed pounds rapidly due to limited intake, reduced absorption, and

TABLE 37-1. Plastic surgical principles

1. Analyze deformity and patient.
2. Be efficient in design and execution.
3. Excise excess as much as possible transversely.
4. Position incisions favorably, and respect scars.
5. Focus on the ultimate contour and tissue tension.
6. Preserve healthy dermis and subcutaneous fascia.
7. Remove fat from flaps gently and effectively.
8. Make closure tight and secure.
9. Minimize swelling, infection, phlebitis, and seroma.
10. Analyze your experience.

early satiety. Many experience mild gastrointestinal dumping after minimal sugar or fat intake. Most become uninterested in food, which may be a hormonally mediated change. All are encouraged to maintain a small caloric multiple-meal diet and an active exercise program, in anticipation of increased gastrointestinal capacity over time. In general, patients lose weight because of reduced food intake and increased physical activity and not intestinal malabsorption. Many become champions of bariatric surgery and encourage others in their organized support group meetings. Most have been introduced to the results of plastic surgery at these group meetings and individually through the bariatric nurse coordinators, who have personal experience. A referral program called Life after Bypass has been instituted at the University of Pittsburgh. Patients receive automatic appointments and an informative brochure about body contouring surgery, shortly after their bypass. Patients find their way to the Hurwitz Center for Plastic Surgery through Internet searches, word of mouth referrals, and national television programs featuring the total body lift (the author's signature procedure).

After a steady weight loss to about 70% of their excess weight over 18 months, most regain about 20% over the next few years (12). Therefore, if a patient's weight loss has plateaued, waiting beyond 18 months before initiating body contouring surgery is counterproductive. Commonly, over the next year patients gain much of the weight removed during body contouring surgery. On the other hand, in some patients unanticipated further weight loss occurs, from 20 to 60 pounds, because of partial gastrointestinal mechanical obstruction. This causes subclinical malnutrition reflected in low serum prealbumin fraction and additional skin laxity. The nutritional deficiency may prolong what would otherwise be minor wound healing problems. Additional weight loss results in new skin laxity, which will detract from what could have been an optimal outcome.

The patients who struggle with their layers of hanging skin and fat and have the courage to do something about it present to plastic surgeons, When obese, their massive size presented an unappealing but recognizable shape. Hanging skin distorts the body shape and patient age and appearance, and it flaps around during vigorous activity. Skin beneath folds becomes moist, malodorous, and inflamed. Clothes fit poorly. Embarrassment of their hanging pannus, mons pubis, and inner thighs thwarts sexual intimacy. While many comprehend that plastic surgery is an anticipated part of their rehabilitation, they still may resent and even regret the bypass operation. The plastic surgeon's empathy is important, especially when asking the patient to accept the new risks and self-pay costs of body contouring surgery. If the patient has limited financial means, we offer national cosmetic surgery finance plans at reasonable rates for those with good credit.

With the ease of convalescence, effective weight loss, improved exercise habits, and encouragement from others who have gone before them, patients are accepting of the arduous body contouring procedures yet ahead. The opportune time to perform body contouring is when the patient has completed the catabolism and has reduced comorbidities. These include sleep apnea, hypertension, gastroesophageal reflux disease (GERD), cardiomyopathy, diabetes, leg edema, osteoarthritis, and mental depression. Because of their diseases and prolonged postoperative negative nitrogen balance (starvation), we avoid panniculectomy coincidental to the intestinal bypass. Moreover, the panniculectomy scar may preclude optimal subsequent surgical planning for definitive contour correction.

We find most patients understand the goals and limitations and the need for multiple stages and possible revisions. We impress upon them that optimal contour improvement entails a very tight closure with risk of suture line dehiscence. If that complication is unacceptable, then less pull will be made. While the scars are generally thin, they may be thickened and uneven. After revealing the common and serious risks of their operations, we offer a detailed consent form for each procedure. We have established a Web site (www.usabodycontouring.com) that patients may visit before the first office appointment. They learn about the surgery, see results of operations on a variety of patients, and are cautioned about the risks. There is a detailed intake form, which is instructive to the patient and gathers important information for the surgeon. The Hurwitz Center for Plastic Surgery sends each patient who seeks a consultation a complimentary copy of a consumer-friendly book, *Total Body Lift: Reshaping the Breasts, Chest, Arms, Thighs, Hips, Back, Waist, Abdomen, and Knees After Weight Loss, Aging, and Pregnancies*, published by MDPublish, New York, New York, 2005. We attempt to exclude candidates suffering from chronic medical and psychiatric illnesses and those with unrealistic expectations.

Digital imaging is used during the second visit several weeks before the scheduled surgery. The patient's preoperative photographs are displayed. Electronic pens allow for drawing anticipated incision lines, indicating the direction of tissue tensions and final scar placement on multiple views of their images. Their new silhouette can be drawn, but no promises are made. Technique and outcomes vary according to the patient's basic body habitus. Oversized people, endomorphs, cannot be transformed into ectomorphs. During office follow-up, impatient and disappointed patients, as well as pleased patients, are graphically reminded of the extent of their original deformity by having a monitor with all possible images available within view of the examination room.

The surgeon considers the body shape (endomorph, mesomorph, or ectomorph), extent of deformity, size, sex, patient priorities, lifestyle, and tolerance for risk. Before embarking on such lengthy procedures, the surgeon and the support team and hospital should have experience working together on less extensive procedures. Three days of hospital care are essential. The larger the patient and the longer the procedure, the more likely are complications.

The Deformity

The massive weight loss patient is a deflated shape based on familial and gender specific fat deposition and skin to fascia adherences. The most susceptible regions are the anterior neck, upper arms, breasts, lower back, flanks, abdomen, mons pubis, and thighs. In men there is a tendency to accumulate fat around the flanks, intraabdominally, and the breasts. In women the fullness lies in the subcutaneous fat of the abdomen, hips, and thighs. Patterns of deformity are emerging that seem to be affected by the magnitude of initial BMI and change in BMI.

Redundant skin hangs over regions of fibrous adherence to deep fascia (Fig. 37-1). The skin of the trunk is densely adherent along the inframammary fold, down the upper midline to the linea alba, and in the groin. Adherence is variably dense across the rectus abdominis transverse tendinous inscriptions (more so in the male), and along one or two transverse levels across the anterolateral ribs, flanks, and back. Skin flaps undermined beyond adherences will re-adhere after the operation and have less tension on the skin, which explains why the epigastrium usually maintains an unwanted roll after an abdominoplasty.

Both anteriorly and posteriorly, there is medial to lateral staggered sweep of redundant tissue. Thigh skin is adherent below the anterior superior iliac spine, along the midlateral and midmedial regions and to a lesser extent along the entire posterior thigh. By the time the weight loss plateaus, the amount of fat within this redundant skin varies considerably. With massive weight loss, there are extensive layered folds or wrinkling. The skin is like an oversized suit and in no dimension, vertical or horizontal, is there normal skin turgor. Unlike posttraumatic or congenital deformity surgery, there is no displaced normal tissue to relocate. All the skin is disordered and is treated accordingly.

Etiology of Skin Laxity

The etiology of skin laxity after rapid weight loss is inadequately understood. The subdermal to aponeurosis fibroelastic spans, overflowing with adipocytes in the obese, has fractured elastin fibers on microscopic study. The damaged elastin and collagen allow for no skin retraction after weight loss. With rapid weight loss, there is no way to prevent sagging of the abdominal skin, skin of the breasts and buttocks, and the inner portions of the arms and thighs. It is important to repair the abdomen with the best quality of skin, usually from the upper portions. Unfortunately, in massive and rapid weight loss patients there is usually no quality skin. The problem is compounded in individuals over 55, who lose considerable skin elasticity without weight loss. Until we are able to reverse this complex disorder of subcutaneous disease, we are forced to excise the widest possible areas of skin and then close the skin flaps as tightly as possible.

Three factors contribute to postoperative skin laxity. First is the diseased skin collagen and elastin. Second, the farther the skin is from the line of closure, the less effective the pull. I refer to this as the law of skin laxity. Otherwise stated, skin laxity is corrected closest to the line of closure and is progressively increased farther away. Third, the adherence of the skin to underlying fascia prevents tightening beyond the adherence. Surgical disruption of these customary and unique adherences mobilizes the flaps, but since perforating blood supply usually occurs there, flap vitality may be compromised.

As yet there are no proven means to improve skin and subcutaneous tissue elasticity. Currently, I am investigating the applicability of Endermologie (LPG, Miami, FL), a computer modulated differential vigorous massage and suction machine, to treat these patients. LPG claims that significant skin laxity can be reduced with about 20 twice weekly treatment sessions. We have initiated treatments to improve our surgical results and substantiate this claim. We are convinced that if expertly performed, Endermologie hastens resolution of postoperative

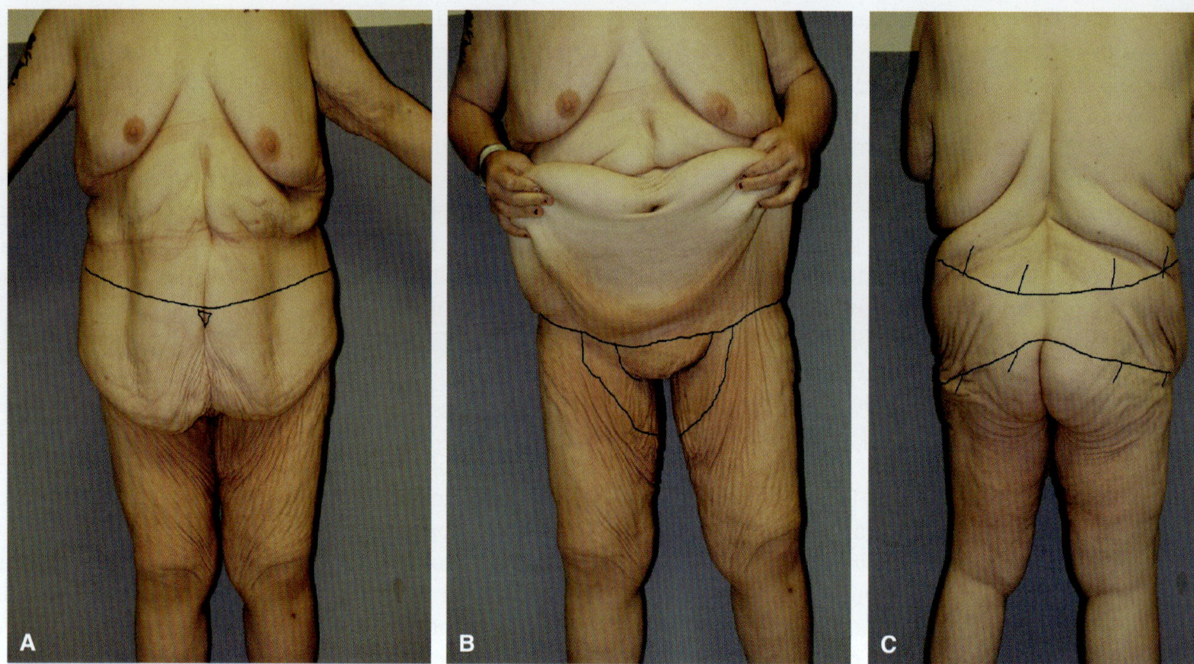

Figure 37-1. Massive weight loss deformity varies according to the original fat distribution and pattern of skin adherence. (A) This 33-year-old, 203-pound woman lost 300 pounds 2 years after Roux-en-Y gastrointestinal bypass. She has a large hanging pannus and considerable skin laxity in the mid-torso, hips, and medial thighs. The redundant skin and fat torso rolls cascade from midline to lateral. There is an anterior midline adherence along the linea alba and umbilicus, which is somewhat accentuated in the epigastrium by her vertical surgical scar. There are paramedian vertical folds reflective of the semilunary lines along the lateral rectus margins extend from the costal margins to the end of the hanging pannus. Beginning with the inframammary folds there is an asymmetrical stair-step array of transverse skin adherences. Immediately superior to the costal margin the skin is broadly adherent, more on the left than the right side. Inferiorly, two transverse lines reflecting the tendinous inscriptions cross from lateral rectus border to the midline in the epigastrium and at the umbilicus. (B) On lifting the pannus, one sees the broad adherence along the iliac crests, to across the suprapubic region, and diverting along each labial-thigh junction. There is a progressive laterally flowing of rippled skin from upper medial thigh to the suprapatella region. (C) Back folds begin inferior to the scapula. The left back has two oblique lines of back fascial adherence, while the right has a series of three. The last rolls overlap the pelvic rim. The firmly adherent central buttock fullness buttock is framed laterally and inferiorly by numerous thin folds of lax skin. The posterior and lower lateral thigh skin below the lateral trochanter is broadly adherent to the fascia lata. The markings for a circumferential abdominoplasty, lower body lift, and medial thighplasty are drawn. Surgical lines for the first stage have been drawn while the patient reclines, pulls her pannus out of the way and stands. The vertical lines ensure proper alignment for closure. The markings begin with the patient reclined and pulling up on her pannus. A 14-cm transverse line is centered about 8 cm above the labial commissure. With firm oblique upward pull on the pannis to the opposite costal margin, the incision line is continued across each groin and over the anterior superior iliac crests. The inferior incision continues across the hip with the patient in lateral decubitus and abducting the thigh. With all excisable skin drawn cephalad, the transverse line extends posteriorly to end immediately superior to the intergluteal fold. When the patient is standing, as seen here, the line dips inferiorly to the extent there is lateral thigh skin laxity. The anterior superior incision is along the umbilicus and is planned by pulling down the superior flap to the bikini line, because unraveling upper redundancy will be limited by costal margin skin adherences. The medial thighplasty has an inner line along the labial thigh groove extending to border the lateral mons pubis. The outer line is an estimate of skin removal, aided by the patient raising her leg while in the supine position. The posterior extension of the medial thighplasty overlies the ischial tuberosities and ends along the inferior gluteal folds.

swelling and induration. It softens most hypertrophic scars, and reduces scar-related neuralgia. It is Food and Drug Administration (FDA) approved to temporarily improve cellulite. We find that minor contour deformities are smoothed by these treatments. There is experimental evidence in pigs that subcutaneous organized collagen can be produced by these treatments over a short period of time (13). Clinical studies have failed to show a reliable improvement for contour deformity, but promising results for cellulite and as a helpful adjunct to ultrasonic and traditional liposuction (14–17). The introduction of advanced electronic technology into the Keymodule (LPG One, Inc., Miami, FL) is promising to deliver on improved results sooner. Over the first 6 months of 2006 we have successfully applied Thermage®, (Thermage, Inc., Hayward, CA), a radiofrequency energy source, to correct minor postoperative skin laxity.

Panniculectomy

Many patients request plastic surgery referral from the bariatric nurses for a panniculectomy. They know that most insurance companies will reimburse when overhanging pannus is symptomatic. Our bariatric nurses explain that panniculectomy is inadequate to treat their myriad skin redundancy problems. A panniculectomy is simply the removal of hanging panniculus by a long anterior transverse excision of skin and fat between the umbilicus and pubis. There is no undermining of the superior flap or alteration or reconstruction of the umbilicus. It is often complemented with liposuction of surrounding, nonundermined bulging skin. It satisfies the medical indications by correcting the inflammatory sequelae of an overhanging pannus. It is indicated in unusual patients who have most of their deformity between the umbilicus and pubis.

Operative Planning and Care

Operative planning and sequencing is based on the deformity and patient priorities. The majority are prepared for removal of excess tissue of the lower torso and thighs through a circumferential abdominoplasty and lower body lift. Unwanted redundancy distal to the mid-thighs requires long vertical medial excision of skin. Most patients accept this long scar, which usually heals favorably and is concealed by the thighs, in exchange for the distasteful skin redundancy. Many want the mid-back rolls and sagging breasts also corrected, which is usually performed many months later.

Upper and Total Body Lift

An upper body lift treats epigastric skin, and mid-back folds and flattened, distorted breasts. Similarly, upper body lifts treat ptotic gynecomastia in continuity with back rolls. In women the upper body lift focuses on establishing a higher and firm inframammary fold. In men the fold should be obliterated. Abdomens that have defined mid-level skin adherence resulting in a two-tiered pannus (Fig. 37-1) will not have adequate correction of the epigastrium without an upper body lift. Due to abdominal flap blood supply concerns and the magnitude of the operation, the total body lift is usually staged with the lower preceding the upper. In three men who were concerned with difficult gynecomastia, and in several female patients who wanted as much accomplished as possible in a single operative session, we have performed a single-stage total body lift lasting 8 to 12 hours. The single-staged procedure should be limited to the most experienced operative teams, including a second experienced plastic surgeon, a physician assistant, and talented residents in plastic surgery training for multiple concurrent procedures.

Each of the body contouring procedures takes 2 to 3 hours. Unless medically contraindicated, cosmetic procedures were added to a medically necessary (insurance reimbursed) procedure. At Magee Women's Hospital, which is part of the University of Pittsburgh Medical Center, facility and anesthesia-related costs and hospital convalescence costs are considerably reduced this way.

Experienced anesthesiologists will be prepared for the position change and protection of the face and weight-bearing surfaces. A foam rubber mask with a cut-out for the endotracheal tube has been our preferred approach (Gentle Touch™ 5″ headrest pillow by Orthopedic Systems Inc., Union City, CA). Intravenous fluids are scaled down in consideration of the use of tumescent subcutaneous injections. Intraoperative fluid and medical management are controlled by the anesthesia team. The need for colloid and blood replacement is discussed during the procedure. All patients are continuously monitored, which includes urine output. Larger patients predonate one to two units of blood for later transfusion. Hespan, colloids, and if necessary blood transfusions are given toward the end of the procedure.

Intermittent leg pressure pumps are activated and intravenous antibiotics are given before the induction of general anesthesia. Additional risk factors for thrombophlebitis, a history of phlebitis, thromboembolism, lower extremity swelling, or localized tenderness prompts the use of low-molecular-weight heparin.

Patients are hospitalized for about 3 days for fluids, electrolytes, and pain management. Also their movements are assisted to reduce excessive tension on tight suture lines.

In this series of patients, there have been no medical complications or thrombophlebitis. Minor wound dehiscence, requiring bedside suture line closure or allowed to heal secondarily, totaled eight incisions in the 52 patients. Minor skin necrosis occurred in 10 patients. Skin loss requiring debridement and grafting occurred in one cigarette smoking woman after an upper body lift. Multiple seroma aspiration was required in eight patients.

Summary of Operative Technique

Our basic operative technique has been reported elsewhere (18). In essence, a circumferential abdominoplasty with a lower body lift removes a wide swath of skin and fat along the bikini line (Figs. 37-1 to 37-5). The panniculectomy is a small portion of the procedure. This approach requires at least one turn of the patient. This

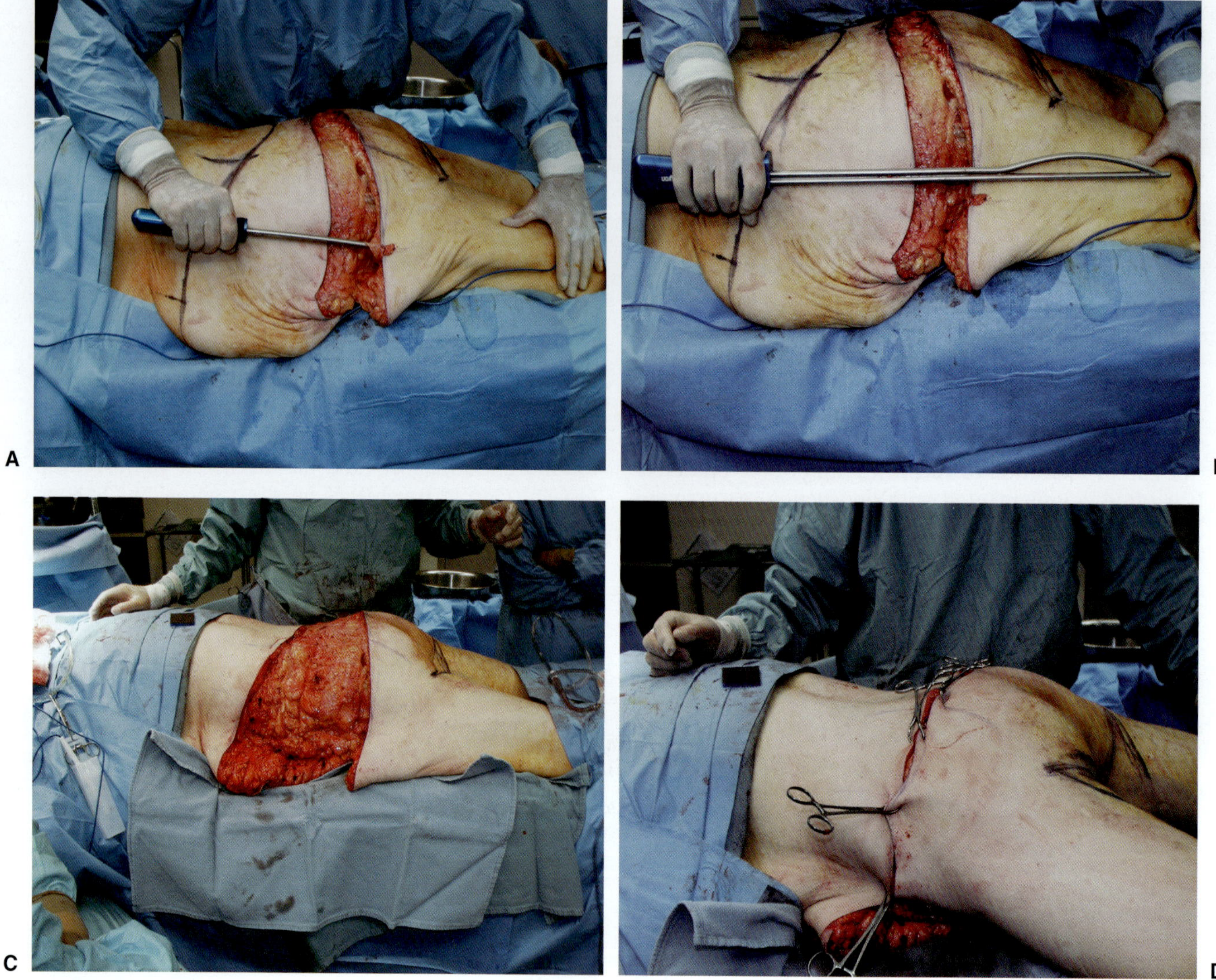

FIGURE 37-2. The operation was started with the patient in the prone position. A scalpel cut was made for the inferior incision. (A) After direct undermining to just beyond the lateral trochanter, a long blunt underminer designed by Dr. Ted Lockwood is used. (B) Pushing against the fascia lata, the surgeon repeatedly thrusts the underminer down the lateral, posterior, and anterior thigh. When skin mobilization is complete, the thigh flap is pulled up to the proposed superior incision. If appropriate, the superior transverse incision is made. (C) Then the intervening island of skin and fat is excised, leaving behind the appropriate amount of large globular fat along the flank. The wound is very large. (D) To avoid persistent thigh skin laxity, the incision should be closed as tightly as possible. Several maneuvers assist in obtaining a secure closure. The thigh is fully abducted onto a padded utility table placed next to the operating room table. The wound margins are approximated with towel clips. Closely placed large braided permanent sutures are used to approximate the subcutaneous fascial system as the clips are replaced. Before the patient is turned for the abdominoplasty, the lateral triangular shape extensions of the medial thighplasties are excised and closed.

procedure varies according to patterns of truncal skin adherence and the patient's BMI.

The full abdominoplasty features removal of all the redundant skin of the lower abdomen, central undermining to the xiphoid, and minimal lateral undermining of the superior flap. Large braided permanent sutures imbricate the central fascia from xiphoid to pubis. The operating table is flexed as the superior flap is approximated to the incision over the pubis and groins with high lateral oblique tension. That tension narrows the waist and raises the anterolateral thighs. The lower body lift, performed with the patient in the prone position, incorporates extensive undermining distally along the hips and thighs followed by a very tight subcutaneous fascial closure, aided by full abduction of the leg onto a utility table placed next the operating

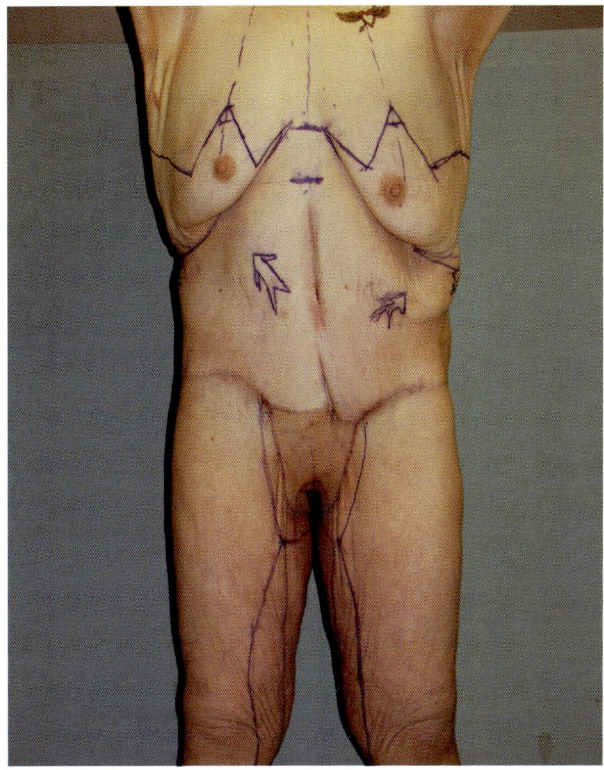 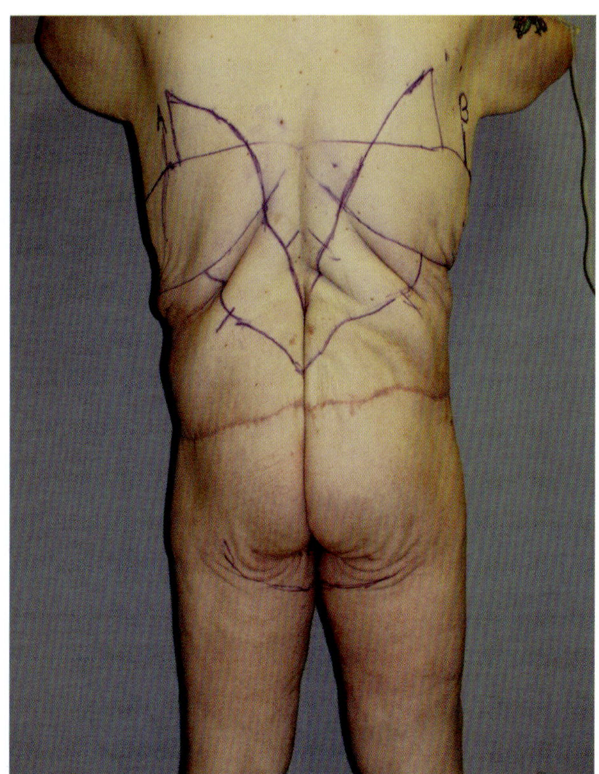

FIGURE 37-3. (A,B) The result 4 months after the first stage is seen as well as the surgical markings for the upper body lift, mastopexy, and vertical thighplasty. (A) The wide vertical resection of medial thigh skin was performed because of an inadequate correction from the high transverse medial thighplasty. A broad rim of skin is resected from the lower thorax to the infra-mammary fold. (B) The excision is continued around the back. Because of the severe skin redundancy a broad oblique excision of skin crosses the transverse band. The operation was begun with the patient in the prone position. After the reverse abdominoplasty is done, a Wise pattern mastopexy completed the upper body lift. Then the medial thighplasty was performed.

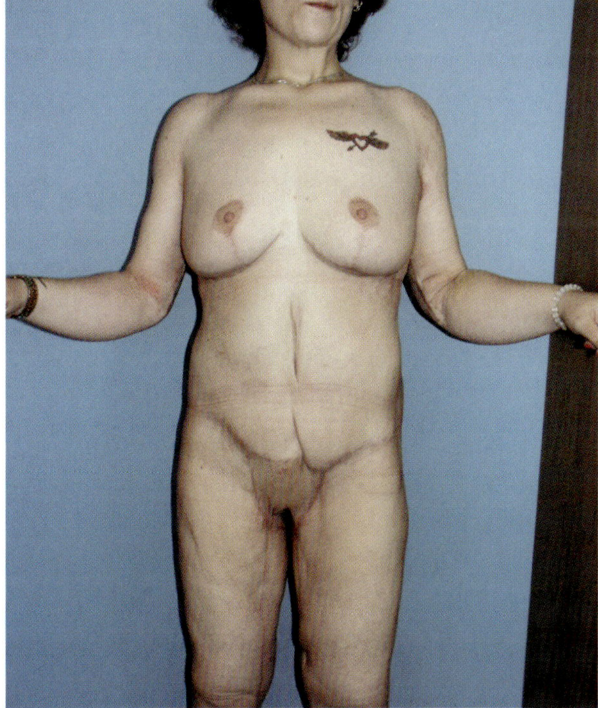 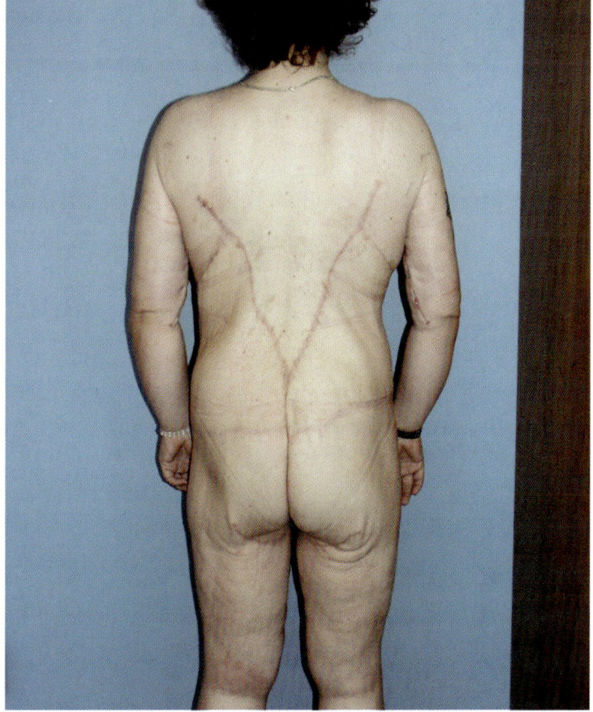

FIGURE 37-4. (A,B) The result 6 months later than in Figure 37-3 is seen, and immediately after bilateral brachioplasties. The patient had a staged total body lift. Prior to her body contouring surgery she weighed 210 pounds and now she weighs 170 pounds. (A) Her breasts are well shaped and symmetrical. All redundant skin is removed and a natural hip and waist contour is established. (B) The thighs have a natural tapered contour. Most of her extensive back scars can be covered by underwear.

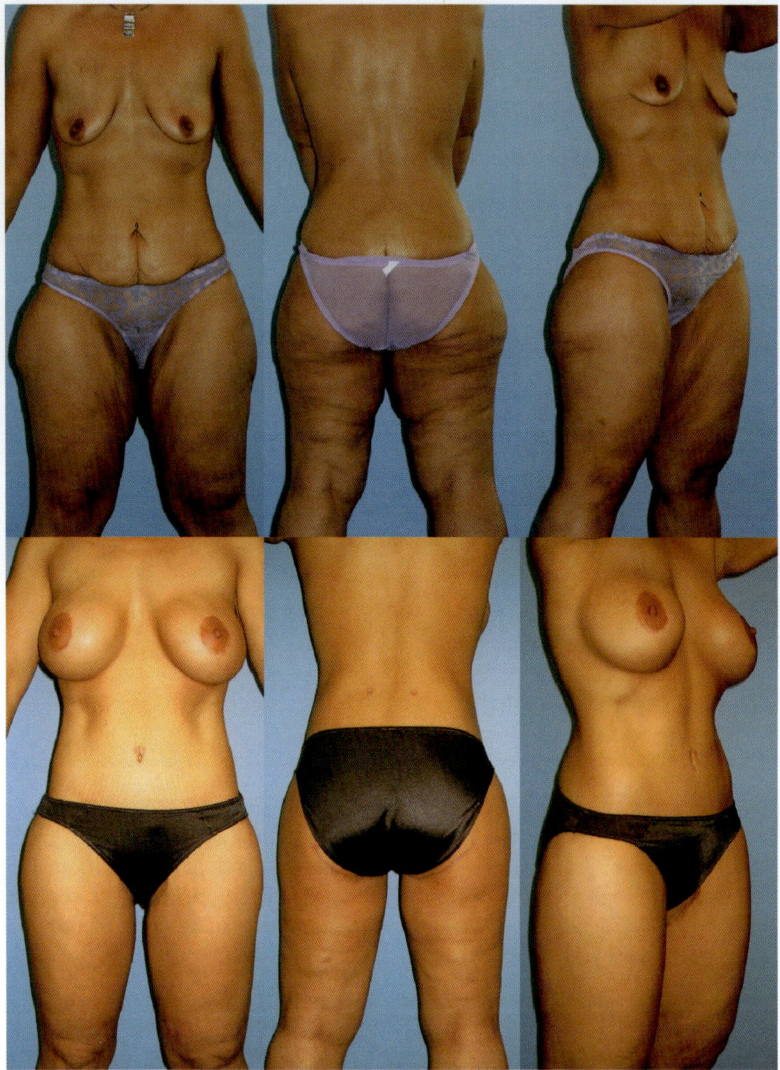

FIGURE 37-5. This is a composite before and after photograph of a 34-year-old female corporate executive. After losing 170 pounds, she weighed 160 pounds. A single-stage operation was done, consisting of a circumferential abdominoplasty, a lower body lift, medial thighplasties, and 450-mL silicone gel smooth round implant partial subpectoral breast augmentations beneath concentric ring mastopexies. Her scars lie within brief underpants and inconspicuously around the areolas. While the thighs are still large, they have excellent contour with no redundant and sagging skin. Her larger, symmetrical, shapely and soft breasts complement her full-sized hips and lateral thighs. Her sagging mons pubis has been raised and contoured with the lower central abdomen.

room table. Liposuction is liberally used except through the distal central flap. A medial thighplasty frequently accompanies the lower body lift in massive weight loss patients. Smaller patients may have additional coincidental major procedures, such as mastopexies and brachioplasties.

Proper preoperative marking of the incisions plans for the removal of excess skin and estimates the closure tension, which affects the contour for the surrounding tissues and final location of the scars. Long abdominal scars must be respected, to avoid a narrow segment of skin between the incision and scar. The surgeon can either include the scar in the incision or leave enough space between the incision and scar to ensure adequate blood supply to the intervening skin. Because of the physical difficulties of marking the hanging tissue while the patient is standing, many of the surgical lines are made with the patient reclined, and then reevaluated with the patient standing. Others have advocated a similar approach (4,6).

Principles of Treatment

These multiple operations are lengthy, envelop large portions of a big body, and require position changes and high-tension closure of undermined and thinned flaps. Accordingly, we have listed the relevant plastic surgery principles for successful results with a low complication rate. The precise technique varies according to the deformity and surgeon preferences, but the principles are inviolate (Table 37-1).

The first principle is to analyze the patient and the deformity, which has been discussed. We need to emphasize that the farther from the suture line, the less effective is the pull. Therefore, following a bikini line closure, residual laxity is seen in the epigastrium, midlateral trunk, and distal thighs. This laxity can be treated secondarily through a reverse abdominoplasty, which we have developed into the upper body lift and by direct excisions along the medial thighs. Excessive intraabdominal girth limits the effectiveness of tight skin closures. This may be reduced by a month of preoperative abdominal binding, several days of purging, and avoiding nitrous oxide anesthesia (gaseous distention) during abdominal wall plication.

Efficiency is the second principle. Inefficiency lengthens an already long operation, thereby increasing bleeding, medical and wound healing complications, surgeon fatigue, and costs. The surgeon should develop a consistent procedure so that the surgical assistants can anticipate the surgeon's needs. Unusual equipment or sutures should be requested ahead of time. With experience, preoperative assessment of the width of the resection becomes accurate (especially for the thinner patients), but does require nearly an hour of vigorous skin shoving while the patient lies, sits, and stands for the markings.

The most effective and efficient positioning and turning of the patient has not yet been determined. I believe that by operating with the patient in the prone and supine positions, including the recent modification of placing the leg in full abduction onto a nearby utility table, the best possible results have been achieved (19).

Prone followed by supine requires only one position change. The flap with the greatest movement is elevated first. The operation starts with the patient in the prone position, with the inferior incision of the lower body lift. Once suctioned and mobilized, the buttock and thigh flap is pulled superiorly and the intended superior incision line is confirmed and incised. The intervening low back and flank skin is removed as an island of skin and fat from side to side. Appropriate traction and countertraction permit rapid resection through a potentially bloody and difficult plane of dissection. Care is taken to leave behind the ideal amount of fat along the flanks. The central back closure is not tight; hence, it better tolerates the marked flexion needed for the abdominal closure later in the operation. Before the patient is turned, the posterior portion of the medial thighplasty is performed superficially along the inferior gluteal fold. Later the patient is turned and placed in the supine position onto a second operating room table and sterile sheets for the abdominoplasty. Experienced residents assist or perform portions of the procedure with both the attending and the residents suctioning fat or suturing simultaneously.

The third principle is to excise skin transversely. Skin redundancy is predominantly vertical, and crisscrossing with vertical excisions leaves compromised flap tips. Transverse scars are easily placed within underwear areas and are less likely to hypertrophy. Plan the trunk scar along the bikini line, which is easily covered, and represents the greatest circumference of the female torso (Fig. 37-5). When the relatively narrow waist level excess skin is advanced over the iliac crests, much of the transverse excess is taken in.

Inverted superior anterior midline V excision is reserved for removal of widened and depressed surgical scars. A posterior V-shaped excision is limited to the midline buttock flap, to help rotate in excessively redundant lateral thigh skin. A broad vertical segment of midline back skin is invariably adherent, and therefore it is only excised as the end of a transversely oriented ellipse. Further exceptions to the rule of transverse excisions are the correction of severe gynecomastia and mid-back rolls, where obliquely oriented ellipses have been used.

Proper incision planning, the fourth principle, as discussed previously, leaves level scars along the bikini line. Most incisions are made with the patient reclining, but checked standing. Mid- and upper abdominal transverse scars are included in the excision, to avoid possible skin necrosis, whenever possible.

The fifth principle is to focus on the contour and tension of the tissue left behind, much as in a breast reduction. When great closure tension is present, some late thinning of the subcutaneous tissues can be anticipated, particularly in the lateral buttock region. Nevertheless, the central buttock assumes a more spherical shape over time.

We follow the sixth principle, preservation of dermis and subcutaneous fascia, by preliminary infiltration along the anticipated incision of hundreds of milliliters of lactated Ringer's solution with 1 mg of epinephrine and 40 cc of 1% Xylocaine per liter. This preparation minimizes bleeding and limits the use of electrocautery. The incision is slightly beveled along the dermis and perpendicularly through the fat and subcutaneous fascia, as the flaps are retracted from each other. The use of a vasoconstrictor follows the second principle, efficiency, requiring interruption to coagulate bleeders only after considerable tissue is incised.

The seventh principle is gentle fat removal, which is possible by liposuction with prior infiltration of Xylocaine and epinephrine. A brief run with an ultrasound probe reduces the vigor of the liposuction cannula stokes. The smaller caliber, low-power multiringed VASER (Sound Surgical Technologies, Louisville, CO) ultrasound system has an advantage. Bleeding rarely occurs, and if it some blood is seen in the cannula, significant vessel damage is presumed and the liposuction is stopped. Flap edge direct resection of excess subscarpal fat does not diminish overlying skin blood supply.

The eighth principle dictates a high-tension skin flap closure. After massive weight loss the trunk skin flaps are relatively inelastic. The flap vessels are large, a remnant of the prior obesity, which appears to increase blood flow, permitting greater undermining and tension on the flaps than one would generally consider safe. Correction of the lateral thigh saddlebag deformity has been improved by fully abducting the leg onto a side utility table while closing with the patient in the prone position (Fig. 37-2) (19). Preliminary approximation with towel clips keeps the tension during closure of the wound minimal. Optimal abdominoplasty closure is achieved by flexing the trunk, approximating the wound edges with large towel clamps, and then closing with large subcutaneous tissue bites with closely placed No. 1 braided nylon. The reverse abdominoplasty, the central aspect of the upper body lift, is successful after establishing the new inframammary fold with high-tension advancement of the upper abdominal skin flap to the rib periosteum.

The ninth principle is that swelling, infection rate, phlebitis, and seroma are reduced by closing wounds as expeditiously as possible over long dwelling suction catheters. Elasticized garments with minimal pressure over the lower abdomen are comfortable and reassuring to the patient. Aside from some flap tacking sutures in the groins, we have not closed the dead space. Our occasional patient with multiple seroma aspirations has been a self-limiting annoyance.

The tenth principle is that analyzing the aesthetic results and the patient outcomes a year or more postoperative is very instructive. Persistent heavy tissues, particularly of the thighs, lower the transverse scars and depress the contours. Review of standard photography is the best gauge of our efforts. We have developed a deformity and outcome grading scale, which we have applied to our results (19,20).

The Surgical Challenge

The recent presentation of a large number of reasonably healthy, body-conscious weight-loss patients has offered me a rare surgical opportunity and challenge. Complex planning based on clinical experience and artistic skills, followed by a physically demanding and tedious procedure, is rewarded by incredible body transformations. The metamorphosis is greeted with patient elation and gratitude. This is plastic surgery that melds reconstructive and cosmetic procedures for eagerly anticipating patients. Effective, reliable, and reduced risk procedures are evolving so that future contributions are available to the legion of surgeons who want to commit their talents to this needy population (21–23).

References

1. Schauer PR, Ikramuddin S, Gourash W, Ramanathan R, Luketich J. Outcomes after laparoscopic Roux-en-Y gastric bypass for morbid obesity. Ann Surg 2000;4:515–529.
2. Lockwood TE. Lower body lift with superficial fascial system suspension. Plast Reconstr Surg 1993;92:1112–1122.
3. Lockwood TE. Lower body lift. Aesth Surg J 2001;21:355–360.
4. Hamra S. Circumferential body lift. Aesth Surg J 1999; 19(3):244–251.
5. Pascal JF, Le Louarn C. Remodeling body lift with high lateral tension. Aesth Plast Surg 2002;26:223–230.
6. Aly AS, Cram AE, Chao M, et al. Belt lipectomy for circumferential truncal excess: the University of Iowa experience. Plast Reconstr Surg 2003;111:398–413.
7. Van Geertruyden JP, Vandeweyer E, de Fontanie S, et al. Circumferential torsoplasty. Br J Plast Surg 1999;52:623–630.
8. Hunstad JP. Addressing difficult areas in body contouring with emphasis on combined tumescent and syringe techniques. Clin Plast Surg 1996;23:57–80.
9. Matory WE Jr, O'Sullivan J, Fudem G, et al. Abdominal surgery in patients with severe morbid obesity. Plast Reconstr Surg 1994;94:976–980.
10. Mitka M. Surgery for obesity, demand soars amid scientific, ethical questions. JAMA 2003;289(14):1761.
11. Schauer PR, Ikramuddin I. Laparoscopic surgery for morbid obesity. Surg Clin North Am 2001;81:1145–1151.
12. Buchwald H. Overview of bariatric surgery. J Am Coll Surg 2002;194:367–375.
13. Adcock D, Paulsen S, Davis S, Nanney L, Shack RB. Analysis of the cutaneous and systemic effects of Endermologie in the Porcine model. Aesth Surg J 1998;18:414–420.
14. Latrenta GS. Endermologie versus liposuction with external ultrasound assist. Aesth Surg J 1999;19:1110–1114.
15. Ersek RA, Mann GE II, Salisbury S, Salisbury AV. Noninvasive mechanical body contouring: a preliminary clinical outcome study. Aesth Plast Surg 1997;21:61–67.
16. Latrenta GS, Mick S. Endermologie after external ultrasonic assisted lipoplasty (EUAL) versus EUAL alone. Aesth Surg J 2001;21:128–136.
17. Dabb RW. A combined program of small-volume liposuction, Endermologie, and nutrition: a logical alternative. Aesth Surg J 1999;19:388–393.
18. Hurwitz DJ, Zewert TE. Body contouring after bariatric surgery. Oper Tech Plast Reconstr Surg 2002;8(2):77–85.
19. Hurwitz DJ, Rubin JP, Risen M, Sejjadian A, Serieka S. Correcting the saddlebag deformity in the massive weight loss patient. Plast Reconstr Surg 2004;114(5):1313–1325.
20. Song AY, Jean RD, Hurwitz DJ, Fernstrom MH, Scott JA, Rubin JP. A classification of contour deformities after massive weight loss: the Pittsburgh Rating Scale. Plast Reconstr Surg 2005;116(5):1535–1544.
21. Hurwitz DJ. Single stage total body lift after massive weight loss. Ann Plast Surg 2004;52(5):435–441.
22. Hurwitz DJ, Holland SW. The L brachioplasty: an innovative approach to correct excess tissue of the upper arm, axilla and lateral chest. Plast Reconstr Surg 2006;117(2):403–411.
23. Hurwitz DJ, Agha-Mohammadi S. Post bariatric surgery breast reshaping: the spiral flap. Ann Plast Surg 2006;56(5):481–486.

38
The Female Patient: Pregnancy and Gynecologic Issues in the Bariatric Surgery Patient

Giselle Hamad and George M. Eid

Polycystic Ovary Syndrome and Morbidly Obese Women

Polycystic ovary syndrome (PCOS) affects nearly 7% of reproductive age females (1). The syndrome was initially named Stein-Leventhal syndrome for the physicians who recognized in 1935 a clinical triad of hirsutism, amenorrhea, and obesity. Since then, the National Institutes of Health (NIH) has updated this definition to: "amenorrhea and hyperandrogenism, existing after the exclusion of all the secondary causes." The etiology of PCOS remains unclear, although there are a number of theories, including obesity as a prominent hypothesis. One theory suggests increased gonadotropin-releasing hormone (GnRH) pulsatility as the culprit, and another theory points to ovarian dysfunction and dysregulation of androgen synthesis (2). The role of genetics in PCOS is similarly uncertain.

Polycystic ovary syndrome is primarily a disorder of ovarian function, resulting in menstrual irregularities, infertility, and hyperandrogenism. Hyperandrogenism is manifested in a number of ways, including hirsutism and acne. In addition, PCOS is associated with metabolic abnormalities such as dyslipidemia and glucose intolerance (3). As a result of these endocrinopathies and metabolic aberrations, women with PCOS have an increased incidence of hypertension, diabetes mellitus, coronary artery disease, and endometrial cancer (4).

The role of obesity in PCOS is controversial. Whether it is a cause or manifestation of the disease remains unclear. Nonetheless, it is undoubtedly a significant component of the syndrome for many women. The reported incidence of obesity among women with PCOS ranges from 35% to 80%, depending on the population studied (3). Some investigators believe that obesity is the primary metabolic insult in women with PCOS. Others describe a subphenotype of obesity within PCOS (5). In the general population, obesity is fast becoming an epidemic in the United States. The prevalence of obesity among women is estimated at 33% to 49% (5), which represents approximately 35 million women or more. Obesity is associated with a number of well-known risks including cardiovascular disease, hypertension, diabetes mellitus, sleep apnea, osteoarthritis, dysfunctional uterine bleeding, and endometrial carcinoma. When compared to their nonobese PCOS counterparts or to obese women without PCOS, women with PCOS and obesity have an even higher risk of developing the comorbidities that overlap between the two conditions. In other words, the risks are additive (6).

As mentioned above, the etiology of PCOS is unknown. However, there is agreement regarding the manifestations of PCOS. In addition to the controversial role of obesity discussed above, two other common components of PCOS include hyperandrogenism and hyperinsulinemia. While there is agreement that each of these biochemical anomalies is frequently present in PCOS, which is the cause of the other remains controversial. As a result, there are treatments aimed at hyperinsulinemia, treatments that target hyperandrogenism, and treatments directed at obesity.

Insulin-sensitizing agents are one of the options aimed at hyperinsulinemia to treat PCOS. Advocates of their use believe that high insulin levels trigger the cascade of endocrinopathies that lead to anovulation and hyperandrogenism. Metformin has been shown to have an overall favorable effect on women with PCOS. It has proven effective in lowering serum insulin and glucose, decreasing hyperandrogenism, assisting in weight loss, and improving menstrual regularity. However, the reduction in serum androgens is often not enough to produce an improvement in clinical symptoms (7).

Hyperandrogenism is another target in the treatment of PCOS. One way to treat hyperandrogenism is to give antiandrogen medication. Proponents of antiandrogen therapy suggest that reducing serum androgen production not only restores normal ovulatory cycles but also treats insulin resistance. However, most studies of anti-androgen therapy point only to its treatment of hyperandrogenism and specifically hirsutism (8). Antiandrogens used to treat PCOS include cyproterone acetate, spironolactone, and flutamide.

Oral contraceptive pills are yet another treatment for PCOS that is aimed at reducing hyperandrogenism. They are useful in regulating menstrual cycles and improving hyperandrogenism, but generally cause no improvement in insulin resistance or obesity.

Currently, there is no ideal treatment for PCOS, as none of the treatments described can remedy all of the biochemical aberrations, signs, and symptoms of the disease. Rather, most treatments tend to target only one or a few components of PCOS. An exception to this tendency is weight loss, which commonly results in amelioration of most aspects of PCOS. The evidence supporting weight loss as an effective treatment for PCOS is abundant. Numerous studies report that weight loss improves many components of PCOS, including insulin resistance, menstrual dysfunction, and hyperandrogenism (9,10). Weight loss was also associated with a concomitant decrease in serum testosterone (11). In addition to these changes, weight loss has long been known to reduce the risk of cardiovascular disease, diabetes, and arthritis. It is well known that weight loss is difficult to achieve, particularly in the morbidly obese with PCOS (11). Current recommendations include nutritionist consultation, physician encouragement, hypocaloric diet, and initiation of an exercise program. Although weight loss is recommended as the first-line treatment for PCOS, patients are frequently unsuccessful in doing so with lifestyle modification alone (11).

Surgical weight loss has been proven to be an effective treatment of morbid obesity (12,13). The phenomenon of resumed menstruation after surgically induced weight loss has also been observed in patients who underwent the jejunoileal bypass operation (13). This procedure, while an effective form of weight loss, was associated with high rates of complications such as hepatic failure, renal stones, vitamin deficiencies, and other metabolic and hormonal problems, and thus has been condemned. More recent procedures such as the gastric band (adjustable silicone, Inamed, Santa Barbara, CA) (12,14) and the Roux-en-Y gastric bypass (13,15) have far fewer side effects. Additionally, these procedures can now be done laparoscopically, which dramatically reduces both morbidity and mortality (12,16).

Preliminary data from our institution showed a dramatic improvement of PCOS manifestations following gastric bypass. In this study of 24 women diagnosed with PCOS who underwent Roux-en-Y gastrojejunostomy at the University of Pittsburgh between 1997 and 2001, we looked at changes in menstrual cycles, hirsutism, infertility, and diabetes mellitus type 2 (17). Significant improvements were noted in each (Table 38-1). The mean weight was 306 lb with a corresponding mean body mass index (BMI) of 50. The mean follow-up was 27.5 months, and 81% of patients with menstrual irregularities developed normal menstrual cycles after an average of 3.4 months postoperatively. One third of the patients with hirsutism reported improvement or resolution, and one quarter of patients with infertility became pregnant 2 years postoperatively after losing 80% of their excess body weight. The 11 patients with type 2 diabetes no longer had the disease. While this retrospective study is evidence that gastric bypass can be an effective treatment for obese women with PCOS, it lacks the biochemical testing for diagnosis of PCOS. A prospective study is currently underway that, it is hoped, will provide more compelling evidence that gastric bypass leads to relief of many, if not all, of the signs, symptoms, and hormonal aberrations of PCOS.

TABLE 38-1. Patient characteristics pregastric bypass and postgastric bypass

	Preoperative	Postoperative	% change
Age (yr)	34 ± 9.7	N/A	N/A
Weight (lb)	306 ± 44	201 ± 30	—
BMI	50 ± 7.5	30 ± 4.5	—
HTN	9	2	77
DM	11	0	100
HbA_{1c} (%)	8.2	5.14	62*
GERD	12	0	100
Dyslipidemia	12	1	92
Hirsutism	23	5	79
Depression	10	0	100
Menstrual dysfunction	24	0	100
Medications per hypertensive	1.3 (9 patients on 12 medications)	0.67 (2 patients on 3 medications)	N/A
Diabetic medications	1.1 (11 patients on 12 medications)	0	100
Medications per patient	2.5	0.6	75

BMI, body mass index; HTN, hypertension; DM, diabetes mellitus; HbA_{1c}, hemoglobin A_{1c}; GERD, gastroesophageal reflux disease.
* Based on five patients who had preoperative HbA_{1c} levels and postoperative HbA_{1c} levels.
Source: From Eid et al. (17).

Pregnancy After Bariatric Surgery

A common question among women of reproductive age who are potential candidates for bariatric surgery concerns the safety and optimal timing of subsequent childbearing. Because preoperative menstrual irregularities frequently resolve following bariatric surgery, female patients of reproductive age are more fertile and therefore are at increased risk of becoming pregnant.

Obesity confers risks to the pregnancy, including preeclampsia, gestational diabetes, hypertension, macrosomia, postdatism, meconium staining, complications of labor, and cesarean delivery (18). However, rapid weight loss and the state of relative malnutrition following bariatric surgery may have deleterious effects on a fetus. Therefore, it is critical to discuss the importance of using birth control for up to 18 to 24 months following bariatric surgery. A urine pregnancy test should be performed preoperatively as well as on the day of surgery for women of reproductive age.

Pregnancy Following Gastric Bypass

The period of rapid weight loss following gastric bypass surgery is a vulnerable time period for a pregnancy. Printen and Scott (19) reported on 45 women having 54 pregnancies following gastric bypass, with 46 deliveries. Most delivered 24 months or less after gastric bypass. Twenty mothers gained weight while five lost weight. Eight spontaneous abortions occurred. Seven infants were premature at delivery and one was microcephalic. When the mothers of premature infants were analyzed, all but one were older than 30 years of age, and two had significant gynecologic histories that made previous pregnancies unsuccessful. Despite these premature births, however, the majority of infants were heavier at birth than their siblings who were delivered prior to gastric bypass. The authors advised that pregnancy should be avoided during the period of rapid weight loss.

Other authors have noted a lower rate of pregnancy-related complications because of the weight loss following gastric bypass surgery. Richards et al. (20) reported on 57 pregnancies in postoperative gastric bypass patients that were compared with morbidly obese controls. The gastric bypass group had a lower incidence of hypertension and large-for-gestational-age infants. No significant difference was found in complications of pregnancy. Wittgrove et al. (21) published a study of 41 women who reported their pregnancies out of 2000 bariatric surgery patients. A lower rate of pregnancy-related complications were noted, including gestational diabetes, macrosomia, and cesarean section, compared to the previous pregnancies while the patients were still morbidly obese.

Pregnancy Following Restrictive Procedures

A low rate of pregnancy-related complications has been noted among patients having purely restrictive procedures. In a study by Bilenka and colleagues (22), nine women who had previous undergone vertical banded gastroplasty (VBG) had 14 pregnancies. While seven of 18 pregnancies ended in miscarriage prior to VBG, only one of 14 pregnancies resulted in miscarriage from toxemia. Prior to VBG, five of six women had complications of pregnancy compared to three of nine women postoperatively.

An advantage of adjustable gastric banding is that the band may be deflated during pregnancy to decelerate weight loss or for hyperemesis. Martin and colleagues (23) studied 20 women with 23 pregnancies who had previously undergone adjustable gastric banding. Eighteen pregnancies were carried to term, with one ectopic pregnancy and four abortions (two elective and two spontaneous). Four out of the 18 full-term pregnancies were delivered by cesarean section. The mean birth weight was 3676 g. During pregnancy, five women lost 1.8 to 17.6 kg of body weight. Three women required band fluid removal because of nausea and vomiting. Two women without fluid in the bands experienced weight gain during pregnancy. In an Austrian study from Weiss et al. (24), seven unexpected pregnancies occurred in 215 morbidly obese women. Five were carried to term, while two women miscarried during the first trimester. All bands were decompressed for nausea and vomiting. In two patients, band-related complications required reoperation (one intragastric band migration and one balloon defect).

Dixon and colleagues (25) cite the adjustability of the gastric restriction of the Lap-Band (BioEnterics, Inamed Health, Santa Barbara, CA) as an ideal method to control the weight of pregnant bariatric patients (25). Of 1382 Lap-Band patients, 79 pregnancies were compared with the patients' previous pregnancies and with matched obese subjects and community outcomes data. Birth weights were comparable to the community birth weights. Gestational diabetes and pregnancy-induced hypertension were comparable to the community incidence and were more frequent compared to the obese cohort. Stillbirths, preterm deliveries, and abnormal birth weights were concordant with the community data.

Aggressive nutritional surveillance may be required if fetal abnormalities are noted in the prenatal period. A report of a 35-year-old Swedish gastric banding patient who became pregnant 15 months postoperatively was published by Granstrom and colleagues (26). She had lost 55 kg. During her third trimester, she suffered from severe emesis and lost an additional 6 kg. Oligohydramnios and fetal growth retardation of 38% was diagnosed by ultrasound. Normalization of the oligohydramnios and weight gain was achieved by enteral nutrition. A 2470-g infant was delivered by cesarean section.

Pregnancy Following Biliopancreatic Diversion

One study with 18-year follow-up has addressed pregnancy following biliopancreatic diversion (BPD) (27); 239 pregnancies occurred in 1136 women who had previously undergone BPD. Fourteen pregnancies were present at the time of publication. Seventy-three abortions occurred. Eighty-five percent delivered at term and 28% were small for gestational age. Total parenteral nutrition was required in 21%. Two birth malformations were observed and three fetal deaths occurred. Thirty-five women experienced improvement in fertility following surgically induced weight loss.

In another study of pregnancy in BPD patients, a survey of 783 women showed an improvement in fertility in 47% of patients who were unable to conceive preoperatively (28). Although fetal macrosomia improved after the BPD, the miscarriage rate remained elevated at 26%. The authors supported delaying pregnancy until weight stabilization.

Internal Hernia During Pregnancy

Internal herniation is a potentially catastrophic complication that may result in mortality for both mother and fetus (28–31). The gravid uterus displaces the intestines cephalad, and a closed-loop obstruction may occur, leading to infarction or perforation. In the pregnant bariatric patient presenting with abdominal pain, clinical manifestations and imaging studies may be vague and nondiagnostic. Therefore, in the patient with unexplained abdominal pain, exploratory laparotomy or diagnostic laparoscopy warrants consideration.

Nutritional Issues

Several essential micronutrients are malabsorbed in patients with gastric bypass. Therefore, compliance with vitamin and mineral supplementation is of utmost importance in pregnant patients following gastric bypass surgery.

Premenopausal women are already at risk of iron-deficiency anemia because of menstrual losses; following gastric bypass, these women are even more predisposed to iron deficiency. Gastric acid is required for release of iron and cobalamin from food. Iron is maximally absorbed in the duodenum, while cobalamin is absorbed in the termi-

nal ileum. Following gastric bypass, the parietal cells in the distal stomach are bypassed, thereby reducing gastric acidity and subsequent absorption of iron and cobalamin. Therefore, daily iron supplementation is mandatory in gastric bypass patients. Prenatal vitamins or multivitamin supplements containing additional iron are generally inadequate to meet the needs of the gastric bypass patient; a separate iron supplement is required.

Calcium is another divalent cation that is maximally absorbed in the duodenum. The anatomy of the gastric bypass therefore reduces the absorption of calcium. Metabolic bone disease has been reported in patients who have undergone bariatric surgery (32,33).

Neural Tube Defects

A common congenital malformation, neural tube defects (NTDs) are related to folate deficiency and obesity. The risk of neural tube defects is related to prepregnancy weight and BMI (34).

Several studies demonstrate the importance of vitamin supplementation and close surveillance in pregnant women following gastric bypass. Haddow and colleagues (35) reported on three women who delivered three NTD births from 2 to 7 years after gastric bypass. All three had vitamin B_{12} or folate deficiencies. None of the women was taking vitamin supplements at the beginning of the pregnancy, and one drank excessive amounts of alcohol, which may have affected folate metabolism. The latter had two miscarriages and the other two women had anencephalic fetuses.

In a study of discharge and birth registries in Sweden and Denmark, 77 infants born to mothers who had previous intestinal bypass had no NTDs (36). However, an increased proportion of low birthweight and growth retardation was found among the singleton infants compared to the total population of singleton births. Therefore, pregnant women who have had intestinal bypass or gastric bypass surgery should be observed closely for nutritional deficiencies.

In a study from the University of Iowa, three cases of NTDs were present in 110 pregnancies greater than 4 years after gastric bypass (37). Although all women had been advised to use vitamin supplementation, they failed to comply. The authors recommended pregnancy counseling for gastric bypass patients who are considering pregnancy because of an increased risk for NTDs.

Urinary Stress Incontinence in the Morbidly Obese

Urinary stress incontinence affects 15% of all women between the ages of 30 to 39 years and is significantly associated with elevated BMI (38). Epidemiologic data show prevalence of stress incontinence rising from 10% in patients with BMI <25 to 18% with BMI >40 (39) and is an independent risk factor for stress incontinence [odds ratio (OR), 4.2; 95% confidence interval (CI), 2.2–7.9].

This increased predisposition arises from an increase in intraabdominal pressure (40,41), while the bladder (detrusor muscles) itself remains stable (42). The intra-abdominal pressure raises intravesical pressure to a point higher than the maximum urethral closing pressure, precipitating incontinence (43).

Achieving weight loss appears to be an essential element in sustained improvement in stress incontinence. The effect of nonsurgical weight reduction (44) resulting in weight loss of ≥5% had a ≥50% reduction in incontinence frequency compared to only 25% of women with <5% weight loss ($p < .03$), demonstrating an association between weight reduction and improved urinary incontinence.

There are very few publications specifically addressing the effect of weight loss surgery on urinary stress incontinence. Deitel et al. (45) showed that surgical weight loss effectively reduces the incidence of stress incontinence. Among 138 women, a 50% or greater excess weight loss was associated with a decrease in incidence of urinary stress incontinence from 61.2% to 11.6% ($p < .001$).

The effectiveness of the tension-free vaginal tape in obese women (46) with genuine stress incontinence (GSI) had been demonstrated where almost 90% of the obese women with GSI were cured, while the remaining 10% noted a considerable improvement in their symptoms, with a significant improvement in quality of life in all groups ($p < .001$). Obesity is sometimes considered a relative contraindication to traditional surgical treatment with Burch colposuspension and slings or injectable agents (47), but others (48) have not found this to be the case.

Conclusion

Obesity and PCOS are closely related; surgically induced weight loss improves menstrual irregularities, hirsutism, and infertility. Postoperative bariatric patients are at increased risk of becoming pregnant. Bariatric surgeons should counsel patients about using birth control during the period of rapid weight loss. During pregnancy, compliance with vitamin supplementation is of utmost importance. Close surveillance should be instituted by an obstetrician with experience in high-risk pregnancies, if possible. Elevated BMI is a risk factor for urinary stress incontinence, which improves with surgically induced weight loss.

References

1. Franks S. Polycystic Ovary Syndrome. N Engl J Med 1995; 333:853–861.

2. Poretsky L. The insulin related ovarian regulatory system in health and disease. Endocr Rev 1999;20:535–582.

3. Patel SR, Korytkowski MT. Polycystic ovary syndrome: How best to establish the diagnosis. Women's Health in Primary Care 2000;3:55–67.

4. Rogerio CL. Importance of diagnosing the polycystic ovary syndrome. Ann Intern Med 2000;132:989–993.

5. Legro R. The genetics of obesity: Lessons for polycystic ovary syndrome. Ann NY Acad Sci 2000;900:193–202.

6. Hoeger K. Obesity and weight loss in polycystic ovary syndrome. Obstet Gynecol Clin North Am 2001;28:85–97.

7. Futterweit W. Polycystic ovary syndrome: clinical perspectives and management. Obstet Gynecol Surv 1999;54:403–413.

8. Diamanti-Kandarakis E, Zapatni E. Insulin sensitizers and antiandrogens in the treatment of polycystic ovary syndrome. Ann NY Acad Sci 2000;900:203–212.

9. Hollmann M, Runnebaum B, Gerhard I. Effects of weight loss on the hormonal profile in obese infertile women. Hum Reprod 1996;11:1884–1891.

10. Pasquali R, Antenucci D, Casimirri F, et al. Clinical and hormonal characteristics of obese amenorrheic hyperandrogenic women before and after weight loss. J Clin Endocrinol Metab 1989;68:173–179.

11. Kopelman PG, White N, Pilkington TRE, et al. The effect of weight loss on sex steroid secretion and binding in massively obese women. Clin Endocrinol 1981;15:113–116.

12. Dixon JB, Dixon ME, O'Brien PE. Birth outcomes in obese women after laparoscopic adjustable gastric banding. Obstet Gynecol 2005;106:965–972.

13. Schauer PR, Ikramuddin S. Laparoscopic surgery for morbid obesity. Surg Clin North Am 2001;81:1145–1179.

14. Favretti F, Cadiere GB, Segato G, et al. Laparoscopic banding: selection and technique in 830 Patients. Obes Surg 2002;12:385–390.

15. Pories WJ, Swanson MS, MacDonald KG, et al. Who would have thought it? An operation proves to be the most effective therapy for adult-onset diabetes mellitus. Ann Surg 1995;222:339–352.

16. O'Brien PE, Brown WA, Smith A, McMurrick PJ, Stephens M. Prospective study of a laparoscopically placed, adjustable gastric band in the treatment of morbid obesity. Br J Surg 1999;85:113–118.

17. Eid GM, Cottam DR, Velcu LM, et al. Effective treatment of polycystic ovarian syndrome with Roux-en-Y gastric bypass. Surg Obes Relat Dis 2005;1:77–80.

18. Johnson JWC, Longmate JA, Frentzen B. Excessive maternal weight and pregnancy outcome. Am J Obstet Gynecol 192;167:353–372.

19. Printen KJ, Scott D. Pregnancy following gastric bypass for the treatment of morbid obesity. Am Surg 1982;8:363–365.

20. Richards DS, Miller DK, Goodman GN. Pregnancy after gastric bypass for morbid obesity. J Reprod Med 1987;32: 172–176.

21. Wittgrove AC, Jester L, Wittgrove P, et al. Pregnancy following gastric bypass for morbid obesity. Obes Surg 1998;8:461–464; discussion 465–466.

22. Bilenka B, Ben-Shlomo I, Cozacov C, et al. Fertility, miscarriage, and pregnancy after vertical banded gastroplasty operation for morbid obesity. Acta Obstet Gynecol Scand 1995;74:42–44.

23. Martin LF, Finigan KM, Nolan TE. Pregnancy after adjustable gastric banding. Obstet Gynecol 2000;95(6 pt 1):927–930.

24. Weiss HG, Nehoda H, Labeck B, et al. Pregnancies after adjustable gastric banding. Obes Surg 2001;11(3):303–306.

25. Dixon JB, Dixon ME, O'Brien PE. Pregnancy after Lap-Band surgery: management of the band to achieve healthy weight outcomes. Obes Surg 2001;11:59–65.

26. Granstrom L, Granstrom L, Backman L. Fetal growth retardation after gastric banding. Acta Obstet Gynecol Scand 1990;69:533–536.

27. Friedman D, Cuneo S, Valenzano M, et al. Pregnancies in an 18–year follow-up after biliopancreatic diversion. Obes Surg 1995;5:308–313.

28. Marceau P, Kaufman D, Biron S, et al. Outcome of pregnancy after biliopancreatic diversion. Obes Surg 2004;14: 318–324.

29. Charles A, Domingo S, Goldfadden A, et al. Small bowel ischemia after Roux-en-Y gastric bypass complicated by pregnancy: a case report. Am Surg 2005;71:231–234.

30. Kakarla N, Dailey C, Marino T, et al. Pregnancy after gastric bypass surgery and internal hernia formation. Obstet Gynecol 2005;105:1195–1198.

31. Moore KA, Ouyang W, Whang EE. Maternal and fetal deaths after gastric bypass surgery for morbid obesity. N Engl J Med 2004;351:721–722.

32. Ott MT, Fanti P, Malluche H, et al. Biochemical evidence of metabolic bone disease in women following Roux-Y gastric bypass for morbid obesity. Obes Surg 1992;2; 341–348.

33. Goldner WS, O'Dorisio TM, Dillon JS, et al. Severe metabolic bone disease as a long-term complication of obesity surgery. Obes Surg 2002;12:685–692.

34. Werler MM, Louik C, Shapiro S, et al. Prepregnant weight in relation to risk of neural tube defects. JAMA 1996;275: 1089–1092.

35. Haddow JE, Hill LE, Kloza EM, et al. Neural tube defects after gastric bypass. Lancet 1986;1:1330.

36. Knudsen LB, Kallen B. Gastric bypass, pregnancy, and neural tube defects. Lancet 1986;2:227.

37. Martin L, Chavez GF, Adams MJ Jr, et al. Gastric bypass surgery as maternal risk factor for neural tube defects. Lancet 1988;1:640–641.

38. Mommsen S, Foldspang, A. Body mass index and adult female urinary incontinence. World J Urol 1994;12:319–322.

39. Hannestad YS, Rortveit G, Daltveit AK, Hunskaar S. Are smoking and other lifestyle factors associated with female urinary incontinence? The Norwegian EPINCONT Study. Bjog 2003;110:247–254.

40. Bai SW, Kang JY, Rha KH, et al. Relationship of urodynamic parameters and obesity in women with stress urinary incontinence. J Reprod Med 2002;47:559–563.

41. Noblett KL, Jensen, JK, Ostergard DR. The relationship of body mass index to intra-abdominal pressure as measured by multichannel cystometry. Int Urogynecol J Pelvic Floor Dysfunct 1997;8:323–326.

42. Dwyer PL, Lee ET, Hay DM. Obesity and urinary incontinence in women. Br J Obstet Gynaecol 1988;95:91–96.

43. Kolbl H, Riss P. Obesity and stress urinary incontinence: significance of indices of relative weight. Urol Int 1988;43: 7–10.

44. Subak LL, Johnson C, Whitcomb E, et al. Does weight loss improve incontinence in moderately obese women? Int Urogynecol J Pelvic Floor Dysfunct 2002;13:40–43.

45. Deitel M, Stone E, Kassam HA, et al. Gynecologic-obstetric changes after loss of massive excess weight following bariatric surgery. J Am Coll Nutr 1988;7:147–153.

46. Mukherjee K, Constantine G. Urinary stress incontinence in obese women: tension-free vaginal tape is the answer. BJU Int 2001;88:881–883.

47. Brieger G, Korda A. The effect of obesity on the outcome of successful surgery for genuine stress incontinence. Aust N Z J Obstet Gynaecol 1992;32:71–72.

48. Zivkovic F, Tamussino K, Pieber D. et al. Body mass index and outcome of incontinence surgery. Obstet Gynecol 1999; 93:753–756.

39
Medicolegal Issues: The Pitfalls and Pratfalls of the Bariatric Surgery Practice

Kathleen M. McCauley

With extraordinary gains in medical technology comes the increase in medical malpractice litigation. In no area of medicine has the increase in both been more evident than in the surgical management of obesity. The increase in litigation involving bariatric surgery has been attributed to several factors, including an increase in the number of bariatric procedures performed generally (1), inexperience of the operator (2), the inherent risk of these complicated surgical procedures, and the complex nature of the patient population. The consequences of this quantum leap include negative impacts on the cost of professional liability insurance (3,4), the physician credentialing process, and the regulation and discipline of licensed health care practitioners nationwide.

The American Society for Bariatric Surgery (ASBS) estimates that 140,600 bariatric procedures were performed in 2004. This estimate is eight times the number of procedures performed a decade ago (5). With the number of procedures performed annually on the rise and patient demand continuing to grow, this highly specialized area of practice will continue to thrive. However, with any growth spurt comes growing pains; among the most painful are the legal pitfalls and implications of obesity surgery.

Historical Perspective

There has been an explosion in the number of medical malpractice lawsuits filed in recent years, and general surgeons have experienced the effects of this boom in and out of the operating room. While medical negligence lawsuits have been recognized for over two centuries, the modern-day impact of this type of litigation in the United States has been simmering for decades. It has become manifest that we are now entering a period of crisis proportions, a period last observed in the mid-1980s (6).

The legal theory behind medical malpractice claims originates in English jurisprudence dating back to the 18th century; however, lawsuits alleging medical malpractice were filed sparingly in the United States until the middle of the 19th century (7). By 1850, medical malpractice litigation as we know it today was entrenched in the American legal landscape. Historians have attributed the precipitous increase in professional negligence actions in the United States to the cultural decline in fatalist philosophical thought and the marked increase in religious perfectionism, both concepts having grown out of the Christian revivals of the 1820s and 1830s (8). The increase in the number of suits filed in later decades of the 19th century has been attributed to the birth of what has been called "marketplace professionalism" (9). The concept of marketplace professionalism, unique to the United States during this stage in the country's development, illustrates the most dramatic American divergence from traditional European models of professional evolution (10). Historically, the learned professions of Western Europe were granted authority by the ruling class. In the United States, however, this sanction was not embraced by American society and became most evident in the 1830s when concepts of social status, economic class, monopoly, and elitism garnered great public criticism (11). The professions, including law and medicine, were thrust into the marketplace to fend for themselves in an environment of Darwinian competition. Consequently, the medical profession expanded to include those who were trained and untrained, alternative and traditional, with little quality control. At the same time, lawyers found themselves in an equally hostile culture of competition, and medical malpractice became an area of growth for the legal profession (12).

The result of this fight for professional survival was an unprecedented increase in the number of medical malpractice suits filed in the United States. Between 1840 and 1860, the number of lawsuits alleging medical negligence grew by 950% (13). Although medical malpractice litigation exploded onto the scene in the middle of the 19th century as a result of a cultural shift, the phenomenon has perpetuated in response to both scientific innovation and the call for professional regulation. Historically, with every new era of medical innovation or expansion came an increase in claims for negligence. Once the innovation became passé, the wave of litigation abated but it never fell back to zero (14).

Despite the recognition that medicine is not perfection and physicians are fallible, our culture demanded a standard by which mistakes could be measured. Accordingly, the mid-19th century saw the advent of various professional organizations, including the American Medical Association. As a result of this self-regulation, unqualified physicians were identified and driven from the profession. However, the impact on those who remained was the creation of uniform standards by which medical professionals would be judged. In the wake of these new licensing requirements and standards of care, the profession was exposed to more litigation as lawyers now judged physicians by the profession's own standards (15).

Finally, the introduction of professional liability insurance in the late 19th century proved to be both a champion and an enemy of the physician. Insurance virtually erased risk to the financial survival of the individual practitioner, but at the same time it guaranteed resources to the malpractice plaintiff (16). As a result, the introduction of insurance to the profession effectively guaranteed the survival of medical malpractice litigation into the 20th century and beyond (17). Today, medical malpractice litigation is pervasive. One economic study by the Joint Economic Committee of the U.S. Congress suggests that the current state of the medical malpractice litigation system has had a negative impact on the access to and the cost of professional liability insurance, the quality of health care, and the cost of and access to health care in this country (18). While the future of the current medical liability system in the United States is unknown, the prudent bariatric surgeon must be able to identify potential risks associated with litigation and how best to avoid it.

Medical Negligence Litigation and the Bariatric Surgeon

What is medical malpractice? How does a plaintiff prove medical malpractice? Why the surge in medical malpractice claims involving bariatric surgery? Why do people sue their physician? What is the impact of a medical malpractice lawsuit on the physician's career? What is the impact on the physician's job satisfaction and personal happiness? These are the questions that cause the medical profession angst, despair, and insomnia. For some, the topic inspires only ire and frustration.

The word *malpractice* has been defined as "any professional misconduct, unreasonable lack of skill or fidelity in the profession or fiduciary duties, evil practice or illegal or immoral conduct" (19). The term *medical malpractice* is derived from the Latin *mala praxis*—bad practice—and was first applied to the profession of medicine by Sir William Blackstone in 1768 (20). To prevail in a medical negligence suit, the plaintiff must prove by the greater weight of the evidence, all four elements of the cause of action. That is, to prove a prima facie case of medical negligence, the plaintiff must establish:

1. A duty to the patient;
2. A breach of that duty or standard of care;
3. A compensable injury; and
4. Proximate causation to the injury or damages (21,22)

Once the physician–patient relationship is established, the physician owes his patient the duty of due care. "Due care" is defined as the care required of a reasonably prudent physician in the same field of practice under the same or similar circumstances (23). In most cases, the duty of due care—or the standard of care—must be proved through expert testimony. Likewise, any alleged breach of the standard of care and proximate causation must be proved through the introduction of expert testimony. The plaintiff often uses documents such as medical records, medical literature, and demonstrative aids such as models, charts, medical chronologies, and diagrams at trial as well.

Physicians are sued for myriad reasons, from the sublime to the ridiculous. That said, most suits for malpractice allege the following:

- Failure to communicate or miscommunication
- Failure to diagnose
- Failure to treat
- Failure to document appropriately
- Failure to perform a procedure appropriately
- Failure to get appropriate consultations
- Inappropriate orders or delegation of duties
- Breach of confidentiality
- Failure to admit a patient to the hospital or premature discharge
- Failure to order appropriate diagnostic tests or studies
- Misinterpreted diagnostic tests or studies
- Bad outcomes and unreasonable expectations
- Complications and failure to timely address recognized complications
- Inadequate informed consent or no informed consent
- Failure to follow up or patient abandonment

However, patients and their families also sue because they are angry, offended, or grieving. As well, we know anecdotally that plaintiffs often use the litigation process to apportion blame, shift accountability, manage guilt or grief, and seek closure.

Bariatric surgeons see increasing claims of malpractice for similar reasons, although weight loss procedures and morbidly obese patients are unique in the medical litigation mise-en-scĕne. Cases against bariatric surgeons include many of those claims delineated above, but also may include the following allegations:

- Inexperience of the operator
- Inadequate facilities or equipment for the bariatric patient
- Failure to monitor or inadequate postoperative monitoring
- Failure to diagnose or to timely diagnose a lethal complication
- Inadequate preoperative workup or substandard patient selection
- Contraindications to surgery, including history of gallstones or cholecystitis
- Poor follow-up support after surgery
- Unrecognized or unaddressed psychiatric issues
- Misguided motivation for surgery

Today, the lion's share of litigation involving weight loss procedures concentrates on allegations of negligence during the postoperative period, immediate postoperative inpatient care, and follow-up once the patient is discharged to home (24). Regardless of the theory of liability against the bariatric surgeon, the claims are increasing as the numbers of procedures performed keep growing.

Informed Consent

Informed consent is a process, not a piece of paper. It is a common misconception that one proves informed consent with a signed "consent for treatment" form. To the contrary, the signed consent form is merely one piece of evidence that the attending physician completed the informed consent process. The doctrine of informed consent is based on the premise that people have a right to decide what happens to their own bodies and minds. It is based on the concept of autonomy—a concept firmly grounded in philosophy, not law. Autonomy—or self-determination—embraces the notion that people have the right to choose the course of their own medical treatment in accordance with their own values, mores, religious beliefs, and life goals. The principle is also grounded on the premise that no other person, institution, or other entity should be permitted to intervene to overrule an individual's wishes, whether or not those wishes are "right," as long as the decision does not negatively affect another individual (25). That choice, however, must be based on information regarding diagnosis, prognosis, risks and benefits of the procedure or course of therapy, as well as the consequences of refusing treatment.

The doctrine of informed consent is composed of two discrete components: permission and knowledge. A patient is entitled to give express permission for any touching by another and that permission is to be based on information that is deemed to be important by the patient's physician. That is, it is incumbent on the medical practitioner to impart all information necessary for the patient to make a well-reasoned, educated choice regarding treatment. Informed consent is of paramount importance when dealing with elective procedures, as consent is implied in the case of an emergency. As bariatric surgery is a high-risk elective procedure by its very nature, the informed consent process must be well planned and well executed.

Causes of action involving issues of informed consent fall into two categories: the tort of battery (no consent) or negligence (inadequate consent). Battery—or unauthorized touching—occurs when the physician fails to obtain informed consent or if the touching exceeds the scope of the informed consent. Negligent informed consent is consent that is based on inadequate information. In most jurisdictions, informed consent is based on the "reasonable" man standard; that is, consent is informed when it is based on the information that a reasonably prudent surgeon would convey to his patient during the informed consent process. Suits alleging negligent informed consent usually require expert testimony on the subject; cases alleging battery do not.

Generally, the informed consent process should include the following:

1. A discussion in laymen terms regarding the description of the surgical procedure to be performed;
2. A discussion of the significant risks and benefits of the procedure to be performed;
3. A discussion of the alternatives to the proposed surgical procedure;
4. A discussion of the consequences of the procedure being declined by the patient; and
5. Documentation of the informed consent process *and* the actual consent, including a signed consent form, a note in the Physicians Progress Notes, in the patient's clinic chart, and in the operative report.

It is important to be sensitive to false or unrealistic expectations in the patient population and to dispel any misconceptions about the procedures of anticipated outcome. It is reasonable to assume that any representation about obesity surgery made on a Web site, in promotional materials, or in informational pamphlets or videotapes will be relied upon by patients and their families. Surgeons should be wary of making promises and predictions.

Documentation

The most credible piece of evidence in litigation is medical record documentation. Accordingly, the medical record must be complete, concise, accurate, legible, timely, and authentic. While this may seem a daunting task, physicians may be asked to interpret or rely upon a medical record several years after the provided care and treatment to a patient. In the busy practice, particularly one in the academic milieu, it is of paramount importance to maintain an accurate and comprehensive medical record.

Why document in the medical record? Is the documentation strictly used to defend the surgeon who finds himself embroiled in litigation? No. The medical record memorializes care and treatment contemporaneously in an effort to promote continuity of care, accurate communication among the care team members, data for retrospective review and analysis, and to defend surgeons who find themselves embroiled in litigation.

Accurate and complete documentation may prove to be the most important tool in management of the bariatric patient. In this highly specialized practice of surgery, both the pre- and postsurgical phases of treatment require effective communication among various disciplines (i.e., medicine, surgery, nutrition, psychology, and occupational and physical therapy) and adequate data to provide comprehensive, timely, and safe treatment to this unique patient population. In general, effective inpatient documentation describes in an objective manner all noteworthy data regarding a patient's presentation, history and physical, recommendations for treatment, actual ongoing care and treatment, and follow-up. It is important to include the most current information available, which will ensure that the patient's chart will be the most reliable resource for ongoing patient care and the best evidence that appropriate and timely care was provided. As the medical record is the primary conduit for continuing care and communication among a patient's care providers, it should include all pertinent clinical information, including the physician's assessment and reaction to laboratory reports, radiology, and other studies. Surgeons often fail to include their rationale for clinical decisions, including data to support the differential diagnosis; however, this information is critical. Physicians should be sure to document a differential diagnosis when the facts permit a reasonable inference that something other than the primary diagnosis may be valid. It is far more difficult to allege that a surgeon failed to consider all of the options when faced with clinically pertinent data if it is documented in the medical record, especially in an area of medicine where potential complications are many, potentially lethal, and often occur quickly.

Regardless of the procedure, the operative note should be dictated expeditiously—ideally on the same day—and should include all findings and complications encountered and the related management of those findings. Operative notes dictated weeks or months after the procedure are a "red flag" in litigation, particularly in situations where complications were encountered by the surgical team. Despite the routine nature of some surgical procedures, the prudent surgeon should avoid using "boilerplate" language, rather endeavoring to personalize the operative note to the individual patient. Furthermore, all dictation should be reviewed, corrected, and signed promptly and include the results of the sponge and instrument counts. Likewise, postoperative orders should be legible and signed by the operating surgeon, and follow-up and discharge instructions should be signed by the patient or his or her responsible party.

In the bariatric clinic setting, it is important to document all preoperative patient encounters, referrals, and consultations. Preoperative screening should be comprehensive and noted in the patient's chart, as well as all relevant discussions with the patient and family and any consultants. All consultation reports should be contained in the record, as well as preoperative laboratory results, radiology, and other screening exams pertinent to the bariatric patient headed for surgery. When documenting the informed consent process, include the risks, benefits, and alternatives discussed, as well as whether additional information was provided to the patient and family (e.g., videotape, brochure, pamphlets, referral to support groups, or other forms of patient education). In most cases, the informed consent process for bariatric procedures is lengthy, candid, and may be included in the patient screening mechanism. That being said, it should be well documented to protect the care team from claims alleging inadequate consent after a bad outcome.

Postoperative follow-up is arguably the most important phase in caring for the bariatric patient. Accordingly, the surgeon or professional staff should document clearly all follow-up instructions, appointments, referrals, prescriptions and refills, and the plan of care going forward. As the medical record is used as a communication tool and for documentation of continuing care, it is critical that all telephone communications are entered in the chart, as well as missed, canceled, and rescheduled appointments. Above all, document and include all correspondence related to the physician's decision to terminate the physician–patient relationship or when the patient informs the physician that the physician's services are no longer necessary.

Do's of Effective Charting

- Do use precise, concise, specific language.
- Do use objective, factual statements.
- Do document a patient's verbatim statements.
- Do date and time each entry in the medical record.
- Do make sure the patient's name appears on the page before writing.
- Do draw diagonal lines through all blank space after an entry.

- Do document adverse reactions to medications or therapy.
- Do "red flag" all allergies.
- Do ensure that all procedure notes and chart entries are timely and accurate.
- Do be sure to read a medical record entry before co-signing.
- Do include time and specific action in all discharge instructions.
- Do include all pertinent communications with residents, attending physicians, nursing staff, and consults.
- Do include an addendum or late entry if necessary.
- Do include the words "addendum" or "late entry"; time and date the note.

Don'ts of Effective Charting

- Do not alter the medical record . . . ever. This is a criminal act.
- Do not obliterate errors or remove pages from the chart.
- Do not use personal abbreviations, initials, or ditto marks.
- Do not include derogatory or discriminatory remarks.
- Do not document conflicts with other physicians or nursing staff.
- Do not use subjective statements about prior treatment or poor outcomes.
- Do not include a late entry after an adverse event.
- Do not include non–patient care information.
- Do not perpetuate incorrect information.
- Do not write any finger-pointing or self-serving statements.
- Do not alter existing documentation or withhold portions of the chart once a claim has been made or after the record has been copied.
- Do not use phrases that imply a risk.
- Do not include incident reports, quality assurance information, or documents involving the legal process in the patient chart . . . ever.

While the patient chart is first and foremost a medical document, it is also a legal document. It is the best defense to any claim of medical malpractice and should reflect the attention to detail required of the prudent bariatric surgeon.

Confidentiality

Since the Clinton Administration, patient privacy and medical record confidentiality have garnered much public and political attention. Congress passed the Health Insurance Portability and Accountability Act (HIPAA), historically known as the Kassebaum-Kennedy Law, in 1996 (26). Its primary purpose was to improve continuity and portability in the delivery of health care while preserving the privacy of certain sensitive health information (27). Furthermore, it seeks to "combat waste, fraud and abuse in health insurance and health care delivery . . . [and] simplify the administration of health insurance" (28). In an effort to carry out these purposes in the age of technology, HIPAA targets three areas of the health care industry: (1) insurance portability, (2) fraud enforcement, and (3) administrative simplification (29). It is the administrative simplification section of HIPAA that concentrates on patient privacy and that is of most interest to health care professionals and their staff (30).

The privacy regulations (Privacy Rule) of HIPAA are designed to provide patients a process by which to maintain the confidential nature of certain protected health information (PHI). The final Privacy Rule was published in December 2000, to be effective in April 2001 (31). It applies to specific "covered" entities including health plans, health care clearinghouses, and health care providers who transmit health information in electronic form related to a transaction covered by the federal regulations (32). The final modifications to the Privacy Rule were published in August 2002 (33), and the previously specified entities were required to comply with the Privacy Rule by April 14, 2003 (34).

The Privacy Rule protects individually identifiable health information (the PHI) that is maintained or transmitted by a covered entity, whether oral or written (35). Individually identifiable health information includes even the most basic demographic information collected from an individual patient (36). It also includes any information created by or received by a health plan, a patient's employer, a health care clearinghouse, or health care provider that relates to past, present, or future physical or mental health condition of an individual (37). Further, the Privacy Rule relates to information regarding the past, present, or future payment for health care by the individual, if the information identifies the individual patient (38).

The Privacy Rule does not prohibit disclosure of PHI; rather, it requires that the information be disclosed only in accordance with the provisions of HIPAA (39). That is, when a covered entity discloses PHI or when it is requesting protected information from another covered entity, it must make reasonable efforts to limit the transmission of protected information to the minimum disclosure necessary to meet the requirements of the request (40). However, the Privacy Rule requirement does not apply to the release of PHI in the following scenarios:

1. Requests from or disclosure to a health care provider for the purpose of medical treatment;
2. Release of PHI to the patient himself;

3. Disclosure of PHI to the U.S. Department of Health and Human Services;
4. Disclosures or requests required by law; or
5. Release of or request for information in accordance with the Privacy Rule (41).

The Privacy Rule requires that a covered entity not disclose or use PHI without an authorization, unless the disclosure is contemplated by the regulations (42). For an authorization to be valid under HIPAA, it must include the following:

1. A description of the information to be disclosed;
2. Identification of the persons or class of persons authorized to use or disclose the PHI;
3. Identification of the persons or class of persons to whom disclosure will be made;
4. A description of the purpose of the use of disclosure;
5. An expiration date certain or precipitating event;
6. The individual's signature and date; and
7. A description of the authority of the signatory to act on behalf of the individual, if signed by a personal representative (43).

The authorization for disclosure under HIPAA must also include the following:

1. A statement that the individual may revoke authorization and instructions regarding how to do so;
2. A statement that medical treatment, payment, enrollment in a plan, or eligibility for benefits may not be predicated on obtaining the authorization from the individual if such a condition is prohibited by the Privacy Rule. To the degree it is not prohibited, the authorization must include a statement about the consequences of not authorizing use and/or disclosure; and
3. A statement about the likelihood that the recipient will disclose the PHI (44).

Patient authorization is *not* required for disclosure in accordance with public health activities; reporting victims of abuse, neglect, or domestic violence; health oversight activities; judicial and administrative proceedings; or law enforcement purposes (i.e., pursuant to court order or subpoena) (45).

As one would expect, patients are granted rights to their own PHI under HIPAA's Privacy Rule. Specifically, patients may request certain restrictions be placed on the disclosure of their PHI (46), the right to review and copy their PHI (47), the right to amend their PHI (48), the right to receive a copy of the HIPAA notice from the covered entity (49), and the right to receive an accounting of disclosures of PHI (50).

It is important to note that any provision of the HIPAA Privacy Rule that is contrary to individual state law pre-empts that provision of state law (51). That being said, federal law will not preempt state law if the state law is promulgated to prevent fraud and abuse related to payment for medical services; to ensure state regulation of the insurance industry and health care plans; to report on the delivery of health care and related costs; to serve a compelling need related to public health, safety, or welfare; or to regulate controlled substances (52). Furthermore, HIPAA will not preempt state law if the state law is more restrictive than the federal statute (53). It is extremely important for physicians to be aware of their state's confidentiality statutes that control when and how private health information may be disclosed.

With this recent attention to patient privacy, surgeons and their professional staff have become increasingly more sensitive to the requirements of HIPAA; however, the principles behind the law have been part and parcel of good medicine for centuries. The concept of patient privacy is based on the principles of fidelity and confidentiality; two ideals articulated in the Oath of Hippocrates and the Prayer of Maimonides. Accordingly, the ethics of HIPAA and the requirements to keep private that information imparted to the surgeon for purposes of treatment shall remain tantamount to the prudent practice of medicine.

Risk Management and Prevention

Physicians in modern American society cannot control whether or not they are sued; they can, however, control how they defend themselves. The best defense in litigation amounts to the best practices of the profession.

The Physician

While an excellent education is imperative to the practice of surgery, experience is the keystone to a successful bariatric surgery practice. Because obesity surgery has been in the media spotlight in recent years, dozens of surgeons have broadened their practices by adding weight loss procedures. By the surgical community's own admission, the procedures generate revenue and the practice area has proven to be lucrative. It has also provided hope and recovery to a large portion of the population for whom other weight-loss programs have proven to be a miserable failure. It saves lives. However, a fact that must not be ignored is that bariatric surgery is extraordinarily dangerous at the hand of the inexperienced or underexperienced surgeon. Obesity surgery was not included in the general surgery residency training as a matter of course until recent years and is not widely available even today. Accordingly, many surgeons learn the procedures in weekend classes and mini-fellowships. This training, while provided by the professional community's finest bariatric surgeons, is inadequate to arm the general practitioner with the skills and experience necessary to maintain a safe surgical weight loss practice.

The American Society of Bariatric Surgeons (ASBS) has prescribed guidelines for the credentialing of bariatric surgeons. While not a credentialing body itself, the ASBS in 2003 published guidelines for granting privileges in bariatric surgery (54). The guidelines are divided into five categories for various levels of experience and expertise: (1) surgeons who have established credentials to perform open bariatric procedures, (2) surgeons who have established credentials to perform open and laparoscopic procedures, (3) surgeons who can demonstrate 25 completed open and laparoscopic during the general surgery residency within the last 3 years, (4) surgeons trained in an approved fellowship and as a first assistant to an experienced bariatric surgeon, and (5) surgeons who do not meet the criterion of any category.

The guidelines contemplate four categories of hospital admitting privileges: (1) global bariatric surgery privileges, (2) provisional bariatric surgery privileges, (3) open bariatric surgery privileges, and (4) open and laparoscopic bariatric surgery privileges. Each level of credentials requires specific satisfaction of certain criteria. More importantly, these categories speak to the importance of experience when assessing the safety and ethics of performing these complicated procedures.

Global credentials require that the surgeon

(1) have surgery credentials at an accredited institution to perform gastrointestinal and biliary procedures;
(2) document that he or she is working within an integrated framework for the care and treatment of the morbidly obese patient with the appropriate ancillary services;
(3) document that there is a program to prevent, monitor, and manage the complications associated with bariatric procedures, and
(4) document that there is a program in place for follow-up of all patients for a period of at least 5 years.

Provisional credentials are conferred on surgeons with the understanding that they will go on to obtain global bariatric privileges. The provisional credential in bariatric surgery requires the surgeon to

(1) successfully complete bariatric surgery training of at least 2 days in a course that includes both didactic lecture and hands on cadaver work,
(2) document three proctored cases in which the assistant was a fully trained bariatric surgeon, or
(3) document completion of an approved preceptorship.

Open bariatric surgery credentials are conferred on the surgeon who meets the criteria of global credentials and documents

(1) three proctored cases in which the assistant was a fully trained bariatric surgeon, and
(2) successful outcomes for 10 open bariatric cases performed.

Laparoscopic bariatric credentials require that the surgeon meet the criteria for global privileges and

(1) have existing open bariatric credentials,
(2) have existing privileges to perform advanced laparoscopic surgery,
(3) document the completion of three proctored cases in which the assistant was a fully trained bariatric surgeon, and
(4) document outcomes in 15 laparoscopic bariatric cases performed as the primary surgeon with acceptable perioperative complication rates.

It is important for physicians to be aware of these recommendations even if the hospital at which they seek privileges has not adopted the ASBS guidelines, as the recommendations were crafted and endorsed by the leaders in bariatrics. In the current litigation climate where the experience of the operator increasingly has been called into question, expertise may be the best defense to such allegations at trial.

As discussed earlier in the chapter, the physician's best line of defense in litigation is documentation. The physician should be concise, clear, and complete, as malpractice litigation is often won or lost on the content and quality of the medical record. The documentation the physician creates today may be used years later in litigation; therefore, good record keeping should be an integral part of the bariatric surgeon's daily routine. Because meticulous medical records constitute the very best evidence at trial, this aspect of malpractice litigation remains in the exclusive control of the practitioner: Document, document, document . . . and document well.

Patients and their families sue for a variety of reasons, some that are within the control of the surgeon and some that are not. The most important human relationship in bariatric surgery exists between the patient and the surgeon, not between the surgeon and his or her attorney. Accordingly, surgeons should treat the physician–patient relationship with as much care as they treat the actual patient. This interpersonal relationship is becoming more important in the increasingly more hostile health care environment. Patients who are treated with compassion and respect are less likely to resolve their feelings or disagreements in court. Physicians must give the patient their time and their undivided attention.

While bad outcomes are not always preventable, it has been suggested that physicians who apologize for bad outcomes are less likely to be the subject of a malpractice claim. Because anger is often the driving force in a lawsuit, contrition and honesty have been shown to dispel anger long before litigation is ever contemplated (55). Good communication between physician and patient has been linked to a decrease in physician shopping, noncompliance, and malpractice claims as well (56). Not only have communication and honesty been shown to positively impact the physician–patient relationship, but the manner in which the information is communicated may dictate the likelihood of a lawsuit resulting from a bad outcome (57).

The Facility

With the unprecedented growth in obesity surgery programs nationwide, more and more hospitals are providing the surgical venue, but without the appropriate facilities and equipment for the bariatric patient population. The key to a successful and safe surgical weight-loss program is strategic planning for this unique population, adequate spending to retrofit or build the appropriate facilities, and appropriate staffing and staff education.

While bariatric procedures are elective, they are not cosmetic surgery. Because bariatric patients are often very ill and require complex care, hospitals and staff must be prepared and equipped to manage their preoperative, perioperative, and postoperative courses. Accordingly, facilities should be equipped with appropriately sized surgical instruments, blood pressure cuffs, endotracheal and nasogastric tubes, and adequate imaging equipment including computed tomography and magnetic resonance imaging. Further, surgical weight loss patients require specialty beds, chairs, and intensive care unit facilities.

Outpatient facilities should include large examination tables and enough chairs to accommodate patients and their families. It is important to be aware of the needs of this patient population and to respect their unique perspective. Every detail should be taken into consideration down to the magazines available in the waiting room.

In 2000, the American College of Surgeons published recommendations for facilities caring for the morbidly obese (58). These comprehensive guidelines provide facilities with recommendations for equipping and managing a safe and appropriate venue for weight-loss surgery and for the even more important follow-up period.

Staff education is as important as having the appropriate equipment. As the bariatric surgeon cannot be at the bedside 24 hours a day, well-trained staff must be the eyes and ears of the surgical team. Precious time is lost when postoperative complications manifest if the condition is not diagnosed and treated immediately. Accordingly, nursing staff must be attuned to the special needs of the bariatric population and must be quick to recognize and react to pertinent clinical information. The best solution is to have a devoted bariatric service and floor of the facility. When such a solution is unavailable, specialized training and education of hospital medical-surgical staff is the best defense to allegations of missed postoperative complications and negligent nursing care.

The Program

Bariatric surgeons treat the most complex patient population in the general surgery community—the morbidly obese. Bariatric surgical candidates often have multiple and varied comorbidities, which make the care and treatment of these special patients challenging. Patients who meet the criteria for weight-loss surgery present with myriad health problems, including asthma and sleep apnea, gout, heart disease, stroke, diabetes, gallbladder disease, hypertension, hypercholesterolemia, osteoarthritis, and a higher incidence of cancer. As a result, many of these patients have low reserves and a profoundly compromised ability to recover from the many complications associated with surgical weight-loss procedures. A comprehensive preoperative screening process, detailed informed consent discussions, and an appropriate and a well-supported long-term follow-up program are of paramount importance to the successful bariatric practice.

The safest and most successful bariatric surgery programs are built on an interdisciplinary approach to health care. This interdisciplinary approach contemplates the special needs of the morbidly obese and the health concerns with which they present. A successful program includes a comprehensive introduction to weight loss surgery, patient/family education, and sensitivity to the patients served.

The program should include a thorough preoperative workup and a well-documented informed consent process based on the interdisciplinary approach. Morbidly obese patients come with myriad diagnoses, which require attention and management throughout the patient's journey from surgery to follow-up. Therefore, preoperative and postoperative care should include consultations with various subspecialties of internal medicine (including cardiology, endocrinology, pulmonology, etc.), psychiatry, nutrition, and physical and occupational therapy. The program should include a process for choosing the appropriate weight-loss procedure for the individual patient, based on the patient's diagnoses, risk factors, and other needs. This decision should be well documented, including the thought process employed by the surgeon in formulating the patient's plan of care.

The prudent program should also include long-term follow-up with appropriate specialists, support staff, and a mechanism to ensure the continuity of care. Patients who are provided quality care and treatment in a friendly and respectful environment, by compassionate and patient practitioners, are likely to be happy and healthier. Likewise, a deliberate program designed to care for the morbidly obese protects the surgical professional from allegations involving poor planning, inadequate facilities, inappropriate equipment, and inadequately trained staff.

Conclusion

It is safe to expect that the bariatric surgical community will continue to grow as the demand for weight loss surgery continues to rise. As we move toward the future of bariatric medicine, it is important to recognize the risks of practicing in this exciting and rewarding field. With education, conscientious bariatric surgeons can avoid many of the legal pitfalls, despite the fact that it is impossible to insulate your practice from lawsuits. Nevertheless, prudent practices, complete medical record documentation, appropriate informed consent, and a healthy physician–patient relationship will provide the best defense for surgeons who find themselves exposed to the litigation process.

References and Notes

1. Mathias JM. Increase in bariatric surgery brings a surge in legal cases. OR Manager 2002;18(2).
2. Kowalczyk L. Gastric bypass risk is linked to inexperience. Boston Globe 2004, January 4.
3. Alt SJ. Market memo: liability insurance premiums on bariatric surgery soar. Health Care Strategic Manag 2004;22(1):1.
4. Rice B. How high now? Med Econ 2004;81:57–59.
5. Twiddy D. Associated Press 2004, August 26.
6. For a more extensive discussion about the current medical malpractice crisis in the United States, see Studdert DM, Mello MM, Brennan TA, Medical malpractice. N Engl J Med 2003;348(23):2281, corrected in N Engl J Med 2003; 349(10):1010; and Mello MM, Studdert DM, Brennan TA. The new medical malpractice crisis. N Engl J Med 2004; 350(3):283.
7. Mohr JC. American medical malpractice litigation in historical perspective, JAMA 2000;283(13):1731.
8. Ibid., p. 1732.
9. Ibid., citing Mohr JC. Doctors and the Law: Medical Jurisprudence in Nineteenth-Century America. New York: Oxford University Press, 1993.
10. Ibid.
11. Ibid.
12. Ibid.
13. Ibid.
14. Ibid., p. 1734.
15. Ibid.
16. Ibid., p. 1735.
17. Ibid.
18. Miller D. Liability for medical malpractice: issues and evidence. Joint Economic Committee, U.S. Congress, Vice Chair Jim Saxton (R-NJ), May 2003 (www.house.gov), accessed September 6, 2004.
19. Black's Law Dictionary, citing Mathews v. Walker, 34 Ohio App.2d 128, 296 N.E.ed 569, 571.
20. Mohr JC. American medical malpractice litigation in historical perspective. JAMA 2000;283(13):1731, citing Blackstone W. Commentaries on the Laws of England, vol 3. Oxford, England: Clarendon Press, 1768:122.
21. See, generally, Fiscina S, et al. Medical Liability. Eagan, MN: West Group, 2004:209. West Publishing, 1991.
22. It is important to note that the law of torts is customarily controlled by the individual states. Accordingly, medical negligence case law may vary from jurisdiction to jurisdiction, although it is based on the more general common law.
23. Pike v. Honsinger, 155 N.Y. 201, 49 N.E. 760 (1898).
24. Misreading Obesity Surgery Risk, www.rmf.harvard.edu, accessed August 7, 2004.
25. Furrow BR, et al. Bioethics: Health Care Law and Ethics, 3rd ed. St. Paul, MN.
26. Pub. L. No. 104–191, 110 Stat. 1936 (1996) (codified in portions of 29 U.S.C., 42 U.S.C., and 18 U.S.C.).
27. Ibid.
28. Ibid.
29. For a more comprehensive discussion of the administrative simplification process, see Perrow et al. The Health Insurance Portability and Accountability Act: An Overview of Administrative Simplification, XIV J. Civ. L. 231 (2002).
30. 42 U.S.C. § 1320d et seq (2002).
31. Standards for Privacy of Individually Identifiable Health Information. 65 Fed. Reg. 82462 (December 28, 2000).
32. Standards for Privacy of Individually Identifiable Health Information. 45 C.F.R. § 164.502 (2001).
33. Standards for Privacy of Individually Identifiable Health Information. 67 Fed. Reg. 53181 (August 14, 2002).
34. 42 U.S.C. § 1320d-3 (2002). Small health plans must have complied by April 14, 2004. Ibid.
35. 45 C.F.R. § 164.501 (2001).
36. Ibid.
37. Ibid.
38. Ibid.
39. 45 C.F.R. § 164.502 (2001).
40. Ibid.
41. 45 C.F.R. § 164.506.
42. 45 C.F.R. § 164.508 (2001).
43. 45 C.F.R. § 164.
44. Ibid.
45. 45 C.F. R. § 164.512 (2001).
46. 45 C.F.R. § 164.522 (2001).
47. 45 C.F.R. § 164.524 (2001).
48. 45 C.F.R. § 164.526 (2001).
49. 45 C.F.R § 164.520 (2001).
50. 45 C.F.R. § 164.528 (2001).
51. 42 U.S.C. § 1320d-7 (2002). "Contrary to state law" is defined as impossible to comport with both state and federal law or that the state law is a major obstacle to the implementation to the Privacy Rule. 45 C.F.R. § 160.203 (2001).
52. 45 C.F.R. § 160.203(a) (2001).
53. Ibid.
54. Guidelines for Granting Privileges in Bariatric Surgery, www.asbs.org/html/guidelines.html, accessed September 1, 2004.

55. Zimmerman R. Doctors' new tool to fight lawsuits: saying "I'm sorry." The Wall Street Journal 2004, May 18.
56. Levinson W, Roter DL, Mullooly JP, Dull VT, Frankel, RM. Physician-patient communication: the relationship with malpractice claims among primary care physicians and surgeons. JAMA 1997;277:553–559.
57. Ambady N, LaPlante D, Nguyen T, Rosenthal R, Chaumeton N, Levinson W. Surgeon's tone of voice: a clue to malpractice history. Surgery 2002;132:5–9.
58. Bariatric Surgery: American College of Surgeons Recommendations for Facilities Performing Bariatric Surgery. Bull Am Coll Surg 2000;85(9).

Index